THIRD EDITION

MODERN EPIDEMIOLOGY

Kenneth J. Rothman
Vice President, Epidemiology Research
RTI Health Solutions
Professor of Epidemiology and Medicine
Boston University
Boston, Massachusetts

Sander Greenland
Professor of Epidemiology and Statistics
University of California
Los Angeles, California

Timothy L. Lash
Associate Professor of Epidemiology and Medicine
Boston University
Boston, Massachusetts

Wolters Kluwer | Lippincott Williams & Wilkins
Health
New Delhi • Philadelphia • Baltimore • New York • London
Buenos Aires • Hong Kong • Sydney • Tokyo

Third Edition

530 Walnut Street
Philadelphia, PA 19106 USA
LWW.com

First Indian Reprint, 2009
Second Indian Reprint, 2010
Third Indian Reprint, 2010
Fourth Indian Reprint, 2011
Fifth Indian Reprint, 2013
Sixth Indian Reprint, 2014
Seventh Indian Reprint, 2015
Eighth Indian Reprint, 2016
Ninth Indian Reprint, 2017
Tenth Indian Reprint, 2019

Indian Reprint ISBN-13: 978-81-8473-112-5
Original ISBN: 978-0-7817-5564-1

Published by Wolters Kluwer (India) Pvt Ltd, New Delhi

Printed and bound at Sanat Printers

If you have difficulty buying LWW books, please write to us at:
marketing@wolterskluwerindia.co.in

Contents

Preface and Acknowledgments vii
Contributors ix

1 Introduction 1
Kenneth J. Rothman, Sander Greenland, and Timothy L. Lash

SECTION I
Basic Concepts

2 Causation and Causal Inference 5
Kenneth J. Rothman, Sander Greenland, Charles Poole, and Timothy L. Lash

3 Measures of Occurrence 32
Sander Greenland and Kenneth J. Rothman

4 Measures of Effect and Measures of Association 51
Sander Greenland, Kenneth J. Rothman, and Timothy L. Lash

5 Concepts of Interaction 71
Sander Greenland, Timothy L. Lash, and Kenneth J. Rothman

SECTION II
Study Design and Conduct

6 Types of Epidemiologic Studies 87
Kenneth J. Rothman, Sander Greenland, and Timothy L. Lash

7 Cohort Studies 100
Kenneth J. Rothman and Sander Greenland

8 Case-Control Studies 111
Kenneth J. Rothman, Sander Greenland, and Timothy L. Lash

9 Validity in Epidemiologic Studies 128
Kenneth J. Rothman, Sander Greenland, and Timothy L. Lash

10 Precision and Statistics in Epidemiologic Studies 148
Kenneth J. Rothman, Sander Greenland, and Timothy L. Lash

11 Design Strategies to Improve Study Accuracy 168
Kenneth J. Rothman, Sander Greenland, and Timothy L. Lash

12 Causal Diagrams 183
M. Maria Glymour and Sander Greenland

SECTION III
Data Analysis

13 Fundamentals of Epidemiologic Data Analysis 213
Sander Greenland and Kenneth J. Rothman

14 Introduction to Categorical Statistics 238
Sander Greenland and Kenneth J. Rothman

15 Introduction to Stratified Analysis 258
Sander Greenland and Kenneth J. Rothman

16 Applications of Stratified Analysis Methods 283
Sander Greenland

17 Analysis of Polytomous Exposures and Outcomes 303
Sander Greenland

18 Introduction to Bayesian Statistics 328
Sander Greenland

19 Bias Analysis 345
Sander Greenland and Timothy L. Lash

20 Introduction to Regression Models 381
Sander Greenland

21 Introduction to Regression Modeling 418
Sander Greenland

SECTION IV
Special Topics

22 Surveillance 459
James W. Buehler

23 Using Secondary Data 481
Jørn Olsen

24 Field Methods in Epidemiology 492
Patricia Hartge and Jack Cahill

25 Ecologic Studies 511
Hal Morgenstern

26 Social Epidemiology 532
Jay S. Kaufman

27 Infectious Disease Epidemiology 549
C. Robert Horsburgh, Jr., and Barbara E. Mahon

28 Genetic and Molecular Epidemiology 564
Muin J. Khoury, Robert Millikan, and Marta Gwinn

29 Nutritional Epidemiology 580
Walter C. Willett

30 Environmental Epidemiology 598
Irva Hertz-Picciotto

31 Methodologic Issues in Reproductive Epidemiology 620
Clarice R. Weinberg and Allen J. Wilcox

32 Clinical Epidemiology 641
Noel S. Weiss

33 Meta-Analysis 652
Sander Greenland and Keith O'Rourke

References 683

Index 733

Preface and Acknowledgments

This third edition of *Modern Epidemiology* arrives more than 20 years after the first edition, which was a much smaller single-authored volume that outlined the concepts and methods of a rapidly growing discipline. The second edition, published 12 years later, was a major transition, as the book grew along with the field. It saw the addition of a second author and an expansion of topics contributed by invited experts in a range of subdisciplines. Now, with the help of a third author, this new edition encompasses a comprehensive revision of the content and the introduction of new topics that 21st century epidemiologists will find essential.

This edition retains the basic organization of the second edition, with the book divided into four parts. Part I (Basic Concepts) now comprises five chapters rather than four, with the relocation of Chapter 5, "Concepts of Interaction," which was Chapter 18 in the second edition. The topic of interaction rightly belongs with Basic Concepts, although a reader aiming to accrue a working understanding of epidemiologic principles could defer reading it until after Part II, "Study Design and Conduct." We have added a new chapter on causal diagrams, which we debated putting into Part I, as it does involve basic issues in the conceptualization of relations between study variables. On the other hand, this material invokes concepts that seemed more closely linked to data analysis, and assumes knowledge of study design, so we have placed it at the beginning of Part III, "Data Analysis." Those with basic epidemiologic background could read Chapter 12 in tandem with Chapters 2 and 4 to get a thorough grounding in the concepts surrounding causal and non-causal relations among variables. Another important addition is a chapter in Part III titled, "Introduction to Bayesian Statistics," which we hope will stimulate epidemiologists to consider and apply Bayesian methods to epidemiologic settings. The former chapter on sensitivity analysis, now entitled "Bias Analysis," has been substantially revised and expanded to include probabilistic methods that have entered epidemiology from the fields of risk and policy analysis. The rigid application of frequentist statistical interpretations to data has plagued biomedical research (and many other sciences as well). We hope that the new chapters in Part III will assist in liberating epidemiologists from the shackles of frequentist statistics, and open them to more flexible, realistic, and deeper approaches to analysis and inference.

As before, Part IV comprises additional topics that are more specialized than those considered in the first three parts of the book. Although field methods still have wide application in epidemiologic research, there has been a surge in epidemiologic research based on existing data sources, such as registries and medical claims data. Thus, we have moved the chapter on field methods from Part II into Part IV, and we have added a chapter entitled, "Using Secondary Data." Another addition is a chapter on social epidemiology, and coverage on molecular epidemiology has been added to the chapter on genetic epidemiology. Many of these chapters may be of interest mainly to those who are focused on a particular area, such as reproductive epidemiology or infectious disease epidemiology, which have distinctive methodologic concerns, although the issues raised are well worth considering for any epidemiologist who wishes to master the field. Topics such as ecologic studies and meta-analysis retain a broad interest that cuts across subject matter subdisciplines. Screening had its own chapter in the second edition; its content has been incorporated into the revised chapter on clinical epidemiology.

The scope of epidemiology has become too great for a single text to cover it all in depth. In this book, we hope to acquaint those who wish to understand the concepts and methods of epidemiology with the issues that are central to the discipline, and to point the way to key references for further study. Although previous editions of the book have been used as a course text in many epidemiology teaching programs, it is not written as a text for a specific course, nor does it contain exercises or review questions as many course texts do. Some readers may find it most valuable as a reference or supplementary-reading book for use alongside shorter textbooks such as Kelsey et al. (1996), Szklo and Nieto (2000), Savitz (2001), Koepsell and Weiss (2003), or Checkoway et al. (2004). Nonetheless, there are subsets of chapters that could form the textbook material for epidemiologic methods courses. For example, a course in epidemiologic theory and methods could be based on Chapters 1 through 12, with a more abbreviated course based on Chapters 1 through 4 and 6 through 11. A short course on the foundations of epidemiologic theory could be based on Chapters 1 through 5 and Chapter 12. Presuming a background in basic epidemiology, an introduction to epidemiologic data analysis could use Chapters 9, 10, and 12 through 19, while a more advanced course detailing causal and regression analysis could be based on Chapters 2 through 5, 9, 10, and 12 through 21. Many of the other chapters would also fit into such suggested chapter collections, depending on the program and the curriculum.

Many topics are discussed in various sections of the text because they pertain to more than one aspect of the science. To facilitate access to all relevant sections of the book that relate to a given topic, we have indexed the text thoroughly. We thus recommend that the index be consulted by those wishing to read our complete discussion of specific topics.

We hope that this new edition provides a resource for teachers, students, and practitioners of epidemiology. We have attempted to be as accurate as possible, but we recognize that any work of this scope will contain mistakes and omissions. We are grateful to readers of earlier editions who have brought such items to our attention. We intend to continue our past practice of posting such corrections on an internet page, as well as incorporating such corrections into subsequent printings. Please consult <http://www.lww.com/ModernEpidemiology> to find the latest information on errata.

We are also grateful to many colleagues who have reviewed sections of the current text and provided useful feedback. Although we cannot mention everyone who helped in that regard, we give special thanks to Onyebuchi Arah, Matthew Fox, Jamie Gradus, Jennifer Hill, Katherine Hoggatt, Marshal Joffe, Ari Lipsky, James Robins, Federico Soldani, Henrik Toft Sørensen, Soe Soe Thwin and Tyler VanderWeele. An earlier version of Chapter 18 appeared in the *International Journal of Epidemiology* (2006;35:765–778), reproduced with permission of Oxford University Press. Finally, we thank Mary Anne Armstrong, Alan Dyer, Gary Friedman, Ulrik Gerdes, Paul Sorlie, and Katsuhiko Yano for providing unpublished information used in the examples of Chapter 33.

Kenneth J. Rothman
Sander Greenland
Timothy L. Lash

Contributors

James W. Buehler
Research Professor
Department of Epidemiology
Rollins School of Public Health
Emory University
Atlanta, Georgia

Jack Cahill
Vice President
Department of Health Studies Sector
Westat, Inc.
Rockville, Maryland

Sander Greenland
Professor of Epidemiology and Statistics
University of California
Los Angeles, California

M. Maria Glymour
Robert Wood Johnson Foundation Health and Society Scholar
Department of Epidemiology
Mailman School of Public Health
Columbia University
New York, New York
Department of Society, Human Development and Health
Harvard School of Public Health
Boston, Massachusetts

Marta Gwinn
Associate Director
Department of Epidemiology
National Office of Public Health Genomics
Centers for Disease Control and Prevention
Atlanta, Georgia

Patricia Hartge
Deputy Director
Department of Epidemiology and Biostatistics Program
Division of Cancer Epidemiology and Genetics
National Cancer Institute, National Institutes of Health
Rockville, Maryland

Irva Hertz-Picciotto
Professor
Department of Public Health
University of California, Davis
Davis, California

C. Robert Horsburgh, Jr.
Professor of Epidemiology, Biostatistics and Medicine
Department Epidemiology
Boston University School of Public Health
Boston, Massachusetts

Jay S. Kaufman
Associate Professor
Department of Epidemiology
University of North Carolina at Chapel Hill, School of Public Health
Chapel Hill, North Carolina

Muin J. Khoury
Director
National Office of Public Health Genomics
Centers for Disease Control and Prevention
Atlanta, Georgia

Timothy L. Lash
Associate Professor of Epidemiology and Medicine
Boston University
Boston, Massachusetts

Barbara E. Mahon
Assistant Professor
Department of Epidemiology and Pediatrics
Boston University
Novartis Vaccines and Diagnostics
Boston, Massachusetts

Robert C. Millikan
Professor
Department of Epidemiology
University of North Carolina at Chapel Hill, School of Public Health
Chapel Hill, North Carolina

Hal Morgenstern
Professor and Chair
Department of Epidemiology
University of Michigan School of Public Health
Ann Arbor, Michigan

Jørn Olsen
Professor and Chair
Department of Epidemiology
UCLA School of Public Health
Los Angeles, California

Keith O'Rourke
Visiting Assistant Professor
Department of Statistical Science
Duke University
Durham, North Carolina
Adjunct Professor
Department of Epidemiology and Community Medicine
University of Ottawa
Ottawa, Ontario
Canada

Charles Poole
Associate Professor
Department of Epidemiology
University of North Carolina at Chapel Hill, School of Public Health
Chapel Hill, North Carolina

Kenneth J. Rothman
Vice President, Epidemiology Research
RTI Health Solutions
Professor of Epidemiology and Medicine
Boston University
Boston, Massachusetts

Clarice R. Weinberg
National Institute of Environmental Health Sciences
Biostatistics Branch
Research Triangle Park, North Carolina

Noel S. Weiss
Professor
Department of Epidemiology
University of Washington
Seattle, Washington

Allen J. Wilcox
Senior Investigator
Epidemiology Branch
National Institute of Environmental Health Sciences/NIH
Durham, North Carolina

Walter C. Willett
Professor and Chair
Department of Nutrition
Harvard School of Public Health
Boston, Massachusetts

CHAPTER 1

Introduction

Kenneth J. Rothman, Sander Greenland, and Timothy L. Lash

Although some excellent epidemiologic investigations were conducted before the 20th century, a systematized body of principles by which to design and evaluate epidemiology studies began to form only in the second half of the 20th century. These principles evolved in conjunction with an explosion of epidemiologic research, and their evolution continues today.

Several large-scale epidemiologic studies initiated in the 1940s have had far-reaching influences on health. For example, the community-intervention trials of fluoride supplementation in water that were started during the 1940s have led to widespread primary prevention of dental caries (Ast, 1965). The Framingham Heart Study, initiated in 1949, is notable among several long-term follow-up studies of cardiovascular disease that have contributed importantly to understanding the causes of this enormous public health problem (Dawber et al., 1957; Kannel et al., 1961, 1970; McKee et al., 1971). This remarkable study continues to produce valuable findings more than 60 years after it was begun (Kannel and Abbott, 1984; Sytkowski et al., 1990; Fox et al., 2004; Elias et al., 2004; www.nhlbi.nih.gov/about/framingham). Knowledge from this and similar epidemiologic studies has helped stem the modern epidemic of cardiovascular mortality in the United States, which peaked in the mid-1960s (Stallones, 1980). The largest formal human experiment ever conducted was the Salk vaccine field trial in 1954, with several hundred thousand school children as subjects (Francis et al., 1957). This study provided the first practical basis for the prevention of paralytic poliomyelitis.

The same era saw the publication of many epidemiologic studies on the effects of tobacco use. These studies led eventually to the landmark report, *Smoking and Health,* issued by the Surgeon General (United States Department of Health, Education and Welfare, 1964), the first among many reports on the adverse effects of tobacco use on health issued by the Surgeon General (www.cdc.gov/Tobacco/sgr/index.htm). Since that first report, epidemiologic research has steadily attracted public attention. The news media, boosted by a rising tide of social concern about health and environmental issues, have vaulted many epidemiologic studies to prominence. Some of these studies were controversial. A few of the biggest attention-getters were studies related to

- Avian influenza
- Severe acute respiratory syndrome (SARS)
- Hormone replacement therapy and heart disease
- Carbohydrate intake and health
- Vaccination and autism
- Tampons and toxic-shock syndrome
- Bendectin and birth defects
- Passive smoking and health
- Acquired immune deficiency syndrome (AIDS)
- The effect of diethylstilbestrol (DES) on offspring

Disagreement about basic conceptual and methodologic points led in some instances to profound differences in the interpretation of data. In 1978, a controversy erupted about whether exogenous estrogens are carcinogenic to the endometrium: Several case-control studies had reported an extremely strong association, with up to a 15-fold increase in risk (Smith et al., 1975; Ziel and Finkle, 1975; Mack et al., 1976). One group argued that a selection bias accounted for most of the observed association (Horwitz and Feinstein, 1978), whereas others argued that the alternative design proposed by Horwitz and Feinstein introduced a downward selection bias far stronger than any upward bias it removed (Hutchison and Rothman, 1978; Jick et al., 1979; Greenland and Neutra, 1981). Such disagreements about fundamental concepts suggest that the methodologic foundations of the science had not yet been established, and that epidemiology remained young in conceptual terms.

The last third of the 20th century saw rapid growth in the understanding and synthesis of epidemiologic concepts. The main stimulus for this conceptual growth seems to have been practice and controversy. The explosion of epidemiologic activity accentuated the need to improve understanding of the theoretical underpinnings. For example, early studies on smoking and lung cancer (e.g., Wynder and Graham, 1950; Doll and Hill, 1952) were scientifically noteworthy not only for their substantive findings, but also because they demonstrated the efficacy and great efficiency of the case-control study. Controversies about proper case-control design led to recognition of the importance of relating such studies to an underlying source population (Sheehe, 1962; Miettinen, 1976a; Cole, 1979; see Chapter 8). Likewise, analysis of data from the Framingham Heart Study stimulated the development of the most popular modeling method in epidemiology today, multiple logistic regression (Cornfield, 1962; Truett et al., 1967; see Chapter 20).

Despite the surge of epidemiologic activity in the late 20th century, the evidence indicates that epidemiology remains in an early stage of development (Pearce and Merletti, 2006). In recent years epidemiologic concepts have continued to evolve rapidly, perhaps because the scope, activity, and influence of epidemiology continue to increase. This rise in epidemiologic activity and influence has been accompanied by growing pains, largely reflecting concern about the validity of the methods used in epidemiologic research and the reliability of the results. The disparity between the results of randomized (Writing Group for the Woman's Health Initiative Investigators, 2002) and nonrandomized (Stampfer and Colditz, 1991) studies of the association between hormone replacement therapy and cardiovascular disease provides one of the most recent and high-profile examples of hypotheses supposedly established by observational epidemiology and subsequently contradicted (Davey Smith, 2004; Prentice et al., 2005).

Epidemiology is often in the public eye, making it a magnet for criticism. The criticism has occasionally broadened to a distrust of the methods of epidemiology itself, going beyond skepticism of specific findings to general criticism of epidemiologic investigation (Taubes, 1995, 2007). These criticisms, though hard to accept, should nevertheless be welcomed by scientists. We all learn best from our mistakes, and there is much that epidemiologists can do to increase the reliability and utility of their findings. Providing readers the basis for achieving that goal is the aim of this textbook.

Section I

Basic Concepts

CHAPTER 2

Causation and Causal Inference

Kenneth J. Rothman, Sander Greenland, Charles Poole, and Timothy L. Lash

Causality 5
A Model of Sufficient Cause and Component Causes 6
The Need for a Specific Reference Condition 7
Application of the Sufficient-Cause Model to Epidemiology 8
Probability, Risk, and Causes 9
Strength of Effects 10
Interaction among Causes 13
Proportion of Disease due to Specific Causes 13
Induction Period 15
Scope of the Model 17
Other Models of Causation 18
Philosophy of Scientific Inference 18
Inductivism 18
Refutationism 20
Consensus and Naturalism 21
Bayesianism 22
Impossibility of Scientific Proof 24
Causal Inference in Epidemiology 25
Tests of Competing Epidemiologic Theories 25
Causal Criteria 26

CAUSALITY

A rudimentary understanding of cause and effect seems to be acquired by most people on their own much earlier than it could have been taught to them by someone else. Even before they can speak, many youngsters understand the relation between crying and the appearance of a parent or other adult, and the relation between that appearance and getting held, or fed. A little later, they will develop theories about what happens when a glass containing milk is dropped or turned over, and what happens when a switch on the wall is pushed from one of its resting positions to another. While theories such as these are being formulated, a more general causal theory is also being formed. The more general theory posits that some events or states of nature are causes of specific effects. Without a general theory of causation, there would be no skeleton on which to hang the substance of the many specific causal theories that one needs to survive.

Nonetheless, the concepts of causation that are established early in life are too primitive to serve well as the basis for scientific theories. This shortcoming may be especially true in the health and social sciences, in which typical causes are neither necessary nor sufficient to bring about effects of interest. Hence, as has long been recognized in epidemiology, there is a need to develop a more refined conceptual model that can serve as a starting point in discussions of causation. In particular, such a model should address problems of multifactorial causation, confounding, interdependence of effects, direct and indirect effects, levels of causation, and systems or webs of causation (MacMahon and Pugh, 1967; Susser, 1973). This chapter describes one starting point, the sufficient-component cause model (or sufficient-cause model), which has proven useful in elucidating certain concepts in individual mechanisms of causation. Chapter 4 introduces the widely used potential-outcome or counterfactual model of causation, which is useful for relating individual-level to population-level causation, whereas Chapter 12 introduces graphical causal models (causal diagrams), which are especially useful for modeling causal systems.

Except where specified otherwise (in particular, in Chapter 27, on infectious disease), throughout the book we will assume that disease refers to a nonrecurrent event, such as death or first occurrence of a disease, and that the outcome of each individual or unit of study (e.g., a group of persons) is not affected by the exposures and outcomes of other individuals or units. Although this assumption will greatly simplify our discussion and is reasonable in many applications, it does not apply to contagious phenomena, such as transmissible behaviors and diseases. Nonetheless, all the definitions and most of the points we make (especially regarding validity) apply more generally. It is also essential to understand simpler situations before tackling the complexities created by causal interdependence of individuals or units.

A MODEL OF SUFFICIENT CAUSE AND COMPONENT CAUSES

To begin, we need to define *cause*. One definition of the cause of a specific disease occurrence is an antecedent event, condition, or characteristic that was necessary for the occurrence of the disease at the moment it occurred, given that other conditions are fixed. In other words, a cause of a disease occurrence is an event, condition, or characteristic that preceded the disease onset and that, had the event, condition, or characteristic been different in a specified way, the disease either would not have occurred at all or would not have occurred until some later time. Under this definition, if someone walking along an icy path falls and breaks a hip, there may be a long list of causes. These causes might include the weather on the day of the incident, the fact that the path was not cleared for pedestrians, the choice of footgear for the victim, the lack of a handrail, and so forth. The constellation of causes required for this particular person to break her hip at this particular time can be depicted with the sufficient cause diagrammed in Figure 2–1. By *sufficient cause* we mean a complete causal mechanism, a minimal set of conditions and events that are sufficient for the outcome to occur. The circle in the figure comprises five segments, each of which represents a causal component that must be present or have occured in order for the person to break her hip at that instant. The first component, labeled A, represents poor weather. The second component, labeled B, represents an uncleared path for pedestrians. The third component, labeled C, represents a poor choice of footgear. The fourth component, labeled D, represents the lack of a handrail. The final component, labeled U, represents all of the other unspecified events, conditions, and characteristics that must be present or have occured at the instance of the fall that led to a broken hip. For etiologic effects such as the causation of disease, many and possibly all of the components of a sufficient cause may be unknown (Rothman, 1976a). We usually include one component cause, labeled U, to represent the set of unknown factors.

All of the component causes in the sufficient cause are required and must be present or have occured at the instance of the fall for the person to break a hip. None is superfluous, which means that blocking the contribution of any component cause prevents the sufficient cause from acting. For many people, early causal thinking persists in attempts to find single causes as explanations for observed phenomena. But experience and reasoning show that the causal mechanism for any effect must consist of a constellation of components that act in concert (Mill, 1862; Mackie, 1965). In disease etiology, a sufficient cause is a set of conditions sufficient to ensure that the outcome will occur. Therefore, completing a sufficient cause is tantamount to the onset of disease. Onset here may refer to the onset of the earliest stage of the disease process or to any transition from one well-defined and readily characterized stage to the next, such as the onset of signs or symptoms.

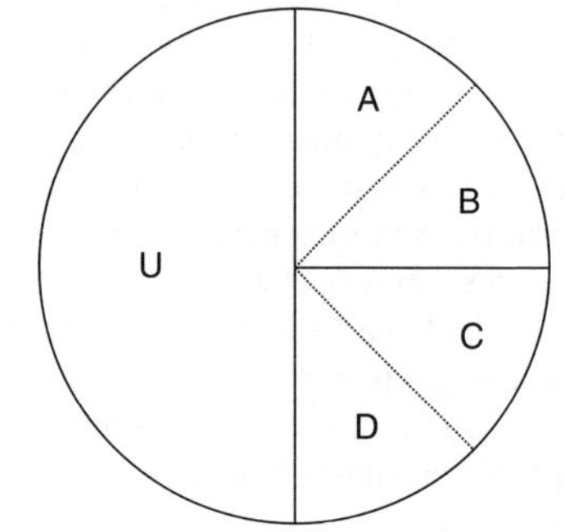

FIGURE 2–1 ● Depiction of the constellation of component causes that constitute a sufficient cause for hip fracture for a particular person at a particular time. In the diagram, A represents poor weather, B represents an uncleared path for pedestrians, C represents a poor choice of footgear, D represents the lack of a handrail, and U represents all of the other unspecified events, conditions, and characteristics that must be present or must have occured at the instance of the fall that led to a broken hip.

Consider again the role of the handrail in causing hip fracture. The absence of such a handrail may play a causal role in some sufficient causes but not in others, depending on circumstances such as the weather, the level of inebriation of the pedestrian, and countless other factors. Our definition links the lack of a handrail with this one broken hip and does not imply that the lack of this handrail by itself was sufficient for that hip fracture to occur. With this definition of cause, no specific event, condition, or characteristic is sufficient by itself to produce disease. The definition does not describe a complete causal mechanism, but only a component of it. To say that the absence of a handrail is a component cause of a broken hip does not, however, imply that every person walking down the path will break a hip. Nor does it imply that if a handrail is installed with properties sufficient to prevent that broken hip, that no one will break a hip on that same path. There may be other sufficient causes by which a person could suffer a hip fracture. Each such sufficient cause would be depicted by its own diagram similar to Figure 2–1. The first of these sufficient causes to be completed by simultaneous accumulation of all of its component causes will be the one that depicts the mechanism by which the hip fracture occurs for a particular person. If no sufficient cause is completed while a person passes along the path, then no hip fracture will occur over the course of that walk.

As noted above, a characteristic of the naive concept of causation is the assumption of a one-to-one correspondence between the observed cause and effect. Under this view, each cause is seen as "necessary" and "sufficient" in itself to produce the effect, particularly when the cause is an observable action or event that takes place near in time to the effect. Thus, the flick of a switch appears to be the singular cause that makes an electric light go on. There are less evident causes, however, that also operate to produce the effect: a working bulb in the light fixture, intact wiring from the switch to the bulb, and voltage to produce a current when the circuit is closed. To achieve the effect of turning on the light, each of these components is as important as moving the switch, because changing any of these components of the causal constellation will prevent the effect. The term *necessary cause* is therefore reserved for a particular type of component cause under the sufficient-cause model. If any of the component causes appears in every sufficient cause, then that component cause is called a "necessary" component cause. For the disease to occur, any and all necessary component causes must be present or must have occurred. For example, one could label a component cause with the requirement that one must have a hip to suffer a hip fracture. Every sufficient cause that leads to hip fracture must have that component cause present, because in order to fracture a hip, one must have a hip to fracture.

The concept of complementary component causes will be useful in applications to epidemiology that follow. For each component cause in a sufficient cause, the set of the other component causes in that sufficient cause comprises the complementary component causes. For example, in Figure 2–1, component cause A (poor weather) has as its complementary component causes the components labeled B, C, D, and U. Component cause B (an uncleared path for pedestrians) has as its complementary component causes the components labeled A, C, D, and U.

THE NEED FOR A SPECIFIC REFERENCE CONDITION

Component causes must be defined with respect to a clearly specified alternative or reference condition (often called a *referent*). Consider again the lack of a handrail along the path. To say that this condition is a component cause of the broken hip, we have to specify an alternative condition against which to contrast the cause. The mere presence of a handrail would not suffice. After all, the hip fracture might still have occurred in the presence of a handrail, if the handrail was too short or if it was old and made of rotten wood. We might need to specify the presence of a handrail sufficiently tall and sturdy to break the fall for the absence of that handrail to be a component cause of the broken hip.

To see the necessity of specifying the alternative event, condition, or characteristic as well as the causal one, consider an example of a man who took high doses of ibuprofen for several years and developed a gastric ulcer. Did the man's use of ibuprofen cause his ulcer? One might at first assume that the natural contrast would be with what would have happened had he taken nothing instead of ibuprofen. Given a strong reason to take the ibuprofen, however, that alternative may not make sense. If the specified alternative to taking ibuprofen is to take acetaminophen, a different drug that might have been indicated for his problem, and if he would not have developed the ulcer had he used acetaminophen, then we can say that using ibuprofen caused the ulcer. But ibuprofen did not cause his ulcer if the specified alternative is taking aspirin and, had he taken aspirin, he still would have developed the ulcer. The need to specify the alternative to a preventive is illustrated by a newspaper headline that read: "Rare Meat Cuts Colon Cancer Risk." Was this a story of an epidemiologic study comparing the colon cancer rate of a group of people who ate rare red meat with the rate in a group of vegetarians? No, the study compared persons who ate rare red meat with persons who ate highly cooked red meat. The same exposure, regular consumption of rare red meat, might have a preventive effect when contrasted against highly cooked red meat and a causative effect or no effect in contrast to a vegetarian diet. An event, condition, or characteristic is not a cause by itself as an intrinsic property it possesses in isolation, but as part of a causal contrast with an alternative event, condition, or characteristic (Lewis, 1973; Rubin, 1974; Greenland et al., 1999a; Maldonado and Greenland, 2002; see Chapter 4).

APPLICATION OF THE SUFFICIENT-CAUSE MODEL TO EPIDEMIOLOGY

The preceding introduction to concepts of sufficient causes and component causes provides the lexicon for application of the model to epidemiology. For example, tobacco smoking is a cause of lung cancer, but by itself it is not a sufficient cause, as demonstrated by the fact that most smokers do not get lung cancer. First, the term *smoking* is too imprecise to be useful beyond casual description. One must specify the type of smoke (e.g., cigarette, cigar, pipe, or environmental), whether it is filtered or unfiltered, the manner and frequency of inhalation, the age at initiation of smoking, and the duration of smoking. And, however smoking is defined, its alternative needs to be defined as well. Is it smoking nothing at all, smoking less, smoking something else? Equally important, even if smoking and its alternative are both defined explicitly, smoking will not cause cancer in everyone. So who is susceptible to this smoking effect? Or, to put it in other terms, what are the other components of the causal constellation that act with smoking to produce lung cancer in this contrast?

Figure 2–2 provides a schematic diagram of three sufficient causes that could be completed during the follow-up of an individual. The three conditions or events—A, B, and E—have been defined as binary variables, so they can only take on values of 0 or 1. With the coding of A used in the figure, its reference level, A = 0, is sometimes causative, but its index level, A = 1, is never causative. This situation arises because two sufficient causes contain a component cause labeled "A = 0," but no sufficient cause contains a component cause labeled "A = 1." An example of a condition or event of this sort might be A = 1 for taking a daily multivitamin supplement and A = 0 for taking no vitamin supplement. With the coding of B and E used in the example depicted by Figure 2–2, their index levels, B = 1 and E = 1, are sometimes causative, but their reference levels, B = 0 and C = 0, are never causative. For each variable, the index and reference levels may represent only two alternative states or events out of many possibilities. Thus, the coding of B might be B = 1 for smoking 20 cigarettes per day for 40 years and B = 0 for smoking 20 cigarettes per day for 20 years, followed by 20 years of not smoking. E might be coded E = 1 for living in an urban neighborhood with low average income and high income inequality, and E = 0 for living in an urban neighborhood with high average income and low income inequality.

A = 0, B = 1, and E = 1 are individual component causes of the sufficient causes in Figure 2–2. U_1, U_2, and U_3 represent sets of component causes. U_1, for example, is the set of all components other than A = 0 and B = 1 required to complete the first sufficient cause in Figure 2–2. If we decided not to specify B = 1, then B = 1 would become part of the set of components that are causally complementary to A = 0; in other words, B = 1 would then be absorbed into U_1.

Each of the three sufficient causes represented in Figure 2–2 is minimally sufficient to produce the disease in the individual. That is, only one of these mechanisms needs to be completed for

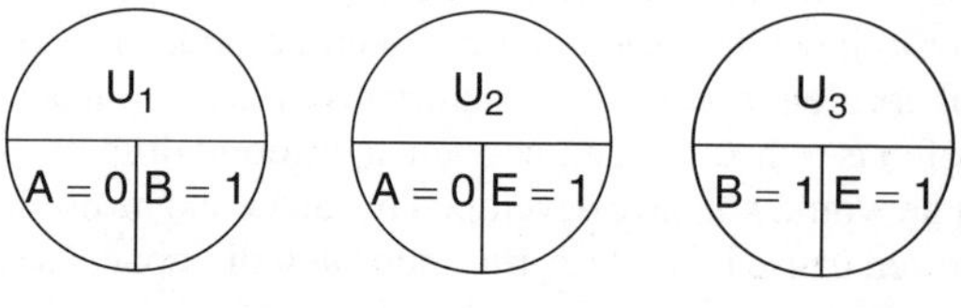

FIGURE 2–2 • Three classes of sufficient causes of a disease (sufficient causes I, II, and III from left to right).

disease to occur (sufficiency), and there is no superfluous component cause in any mechanism (minimality)—each component is a required part of that specific causal mechanism. A specific component cause may play a role in one, several, or all of the causal mechanisms. As noted earlier, a component cause that appears in all sufficient causes is called a *necessary* cause of the outcome. As an example, infection with HIV is a component of every sufficient cause of acquired immune deficiency syndrome (AIDS) and hence is a necessary cause of AIDS. It has been suggested that such causes be called "universally necessary," in recognition that every component of a sufficient cause is necessary for that sufficient cause (mechanism) to operate (Poole 2001a).

Figure 2–2 does not depict aspects of the causal process such as sequence or timing of action of the component causes, dose, or other complexities. These can be specified in the description of the contrast of index and reference conditions that defines each component cause. Thus, if the outcome is lung cancer and the factor B represents cigarette smoking, it might be defined more explicitly as smoking at least 20 cigarettes a day of unfiltered cigarettes for at least 40 years beginning at age 20 years or earlier (B = 1), or smoking 20 cigarettes a day of unfiltered cigarettes, beginning at age 20 years or earlier, and then smoking no cigarettes for the next 20 years (B = 0).

In specifying a component cause, the two sides of the causal contrast of which it is composed should be defined with an eye to realistic choices or options. If prescribing a placebo is not a realistic therapeutic option, a causal contrast between a new treatment and a placebo in a clinical trial may be questioned for its dubious relevance to medical practice. In a similar fashion, before saying that oral contraceptives increase the risk of death over 10 years (e.g., through myocardial infarction or stroke), we must consider the alternative to taking oral contraceptives. If it involves getting pregnant, then the risk of death attendant to childbirth might be greater than the risk from oral contraceptives, making oral contraceptives a preventive rather than a cause. If the alternative is an equally effective contraceptive without serious side effects, then oral contraceptives may be described as a cause of death.

To understand prevention in the sufficient-component cause framework, we posit that the alternative condition (in which a component cause is absent) prevents the outcome relative to the presence of the component cause. Thus, a preventive effect of a factor is represented by specifying its causative alternative as a component cause. An example is the presence of A = 0 as a component cause in the first two sufficient causes shown in Figure 2–2. Another example would be to define a variable, F (not depicted in Fig. 2–2), as "vaccination (F = 1) or no vaccination (F = 0)". Prevention of the disease by getting vaccinated (F = 1) would be expressed in the sufficient-component cause model as causation of the disease by not getting vaccinated (F = 0). This depiction is unproblematic because, once both sides of a causal contrast have been specified, causation and prevention are merely two sides of the same coin.

Sheps (1958) once asked, "Shall we count the living or the dead?" Death is an event, but survival is not. Hence, to use the sufficient-component cause model, we must count the dead. This model restriction can have substantive implications. For instance, some measures and formulas approximate others only when the outcome is rare. When survival is rare, death is common. In that case, use of the sufficient-component cause model to inform the analysis will prevent us from taking advantage of the rare-outcome approximations.

Similarly, etiologies of adverse health outcomes that are conditions or states, but not events, must be depicted under the sufficient-cause model by reversing the coding of the outcome. Consider spina bifida, which is the failure of the neural tube to close fully during gestation. There is no point in time at which spina bifida may be said to have occurred. It would be awkward to define the "incidence time" of spina bifida as the gestational age at which complete neural tube closure ordinarily occurs. The sufficient-component cause model would be better suited in this case to defining the event of complete closure (no spina bifida) as the outcome and to view conditions, events, and characteristics that prevent this beneficial event as the causes of the adverse condition of spina bifida.

PROBABILITY, RISK, AND CAUSES

In everyday language, "risk" is often used as a synonym for probability. It is also commonly used as a synonym for "hazard," as in, "Living near a nuclear power plant is a risk you should avoid." Unfortunately, in epidemiologic parlance, even in the scholarly literature, "risk" is frequently used for many distinct concepts: rate, rate ratio, risk ratio, incidence odds, prevalence, etc. The more specific, and therefore more useful, definition of *risk* is "probability of an event during a specified period of time."

The term *probability* has multiple meanings. One is that it is the relative frequency of an event. Another is that probability is the tendency, or propensity, of an entity to produce an event. A third meaning is that probability measures someone's degree of certainty that an event will occur. When one says "the probability of death in vehicular accidents when traveling >120 km/h is high," one means that the proportion of accidents that end with deaths is higher when they involve vehicles traveling >120 km/h than when they involve vehicles traveling at lower speeds (frequency usage), that high-speed accidents have a greater tendency than lower-speed accidents to result in deaths (propensity usage), or that the speaker is more certain that a death will occur in a high-speed accident than in a lower-speed accident (certainty usage).

The frequency usage of "probability" and "risk," unlike the propensity and certainty usages, admits no meaning to the notion of "risk" for an individual beyond the relative frequency of 100% if the event occurs and 0% if it does not. This restriction of individual risks to 0 or 1 can only be relaxed to allow values in between by reinterpreting such statements as the frequency with which the outcome would be seen upon random sampling from a very large population of individuals deemed to be "like" the individual in some way (e.g., of the same age, sex, and smoking history). If one accepts this interpretation, whether any actual sampling has been conducted or not, the notion of individual risk is replaced by the notion of the frequency of the event in question in the large population from which the individual was sampled. With this view of risk, a risk will change according to how we group individuals together to evaluate frequencies. Subjective judgment will inevitably enter into the picture in deciding which characteristics to use for grouping. For instance, should tomato consumption be taken into account in defining the class of men who are "like" a given man for purposes of determining his risk of a diagnosis of prostate cancer between his 60th and 70th birthdays? If so, which study or meta-analysis should be used to factor in this piece of information?

Unless we have found a set of conditions and events in which the disease does not occur at all, it is always a reasonable working hypothesis that, no matter how much is known about the etiology of a disease, some causal components remain unknown. We may be inclined to assign an equal risk to all individuals whose status for some components is known and identical. We may say, for example, that men who are heavy cigarette smokers have approximately a 10% lifetime risk of developing lung cancer. Some interpret this statement to mean that all men would be subject to a 10% probability of lung cancer if they were to become heavy smokers, as if the occurrence of lung cancer, aside from smoking, were purely a matter of chance. This view is untenable. A probability may be 10% conditional on one piece of information and higher or lower than 10% if we condition on other relevant information as well. For instance, men who are heavy cigarette smokers and who worked for many years in occupations with historically high levels of exposure to airborne asbestos fibers would be said to have a lifetime lung cancer risk appreciably higher than 10%.

Regardless of whether we interpret probability as relative frequency or degree of certainty, the assignment of equal risks merely reflects the particular grouping. In our ignorance, the best we can do in assessing risk is to classify people according to measured risk indicators and then assign the average risk observed within a class to persons within the class. As knowledge or specification of additional risk indicators expands, the risk estimates assigned to people will depart from average according to the presence or absence of other factors that predict the outcome.

STRENGTH OF EFFECTS

The causal model exemplified by Figure 2–2 can facilitate an understanding of some key concepts such as *strength of effect* and *interaction.* As an illustration of strength of effect, Table 2–1 displays the frequency of the eight possible patterns for exposure to A, B, and E in two hypothetical populations. Now the pie charts in Figure 2–2 depict classes of mechanisms. The first one, for instance, represents all sufficient causes that, no matter what other component causes they may contain, have in common the fact that they contain $A = 0$ and $B = 1$. The constituents of U_1 may, and ordinarily would, differ from individual to individual. For simplification, we shall suppose, rather unrealistically, that U_1, U_2, and U_3 are always present or have always occured for everyone and Figure 2–2 represents all the sufficient causes.

TABLE 2–1

Exposure Frequencies and Individual Risks in Two Hypothetical Populations According to the Possible Combinations of the Three Specified Component Causes in Fig. 2–1

Exposures					Frequency of Exposure Pattern	
A	B	E	Sufficient Cause Completed	Risk	Population 1	Population 2
1	1	1	III	1	900	100
1	1	0	None	0	900	100
1	0	1	None	0	100	900
1	0	0	None	0	100	900
0	1	1	I, II, or III	1	100	900
0	1	0	I	1	100	900
0	0	1	II	1	900	100
0	0	0	none	0	900	100

Under these assumptions, the response of each individual to the exposure pattern in a given row can be found in the response column. The response here is the risk of developing a disease over a specified time period that is the same for all individuals. For simplification, a deterministic model of risk is employed, such that individual risks can equal only the value 0 or 1, and no values in between. A stochastic model of individual risk would relax this restriction and allow individual risks to lie between 0 and 1.

The proportion getting disease, or incidence proportion, in any subpopulation in Table 2–1 can be found by summing the number of persons at each exposure pattern with an individual risk of 1 and dividing this total by the subpopulation size. For example, if exposure A is not considered (e.g., if it were not measured), the pattern of incidence proportions in population 1 would be those in Table 2–2.

As an example of how the proportions in Table 2–2 were calculated, let us review how the incidence proportion among persons in population 1 with $B = 1$ and $E = 0$ was calculated: There were 900 persons with $A = 1$, $B = 1$, and $E = 0$, none of whom became cases because there are no sufficient causes that can culminate in the occurrence of the disease over the study period in persons with this combination of exposure conditions. (There are two sufficient causes that contain $B = 1$ as a component cause, but one of them contains the component cause $A = 0$ and the other contains the component cause $E = 1$. The presence of $A = 1$ or $E = 0$ blocks these etiologic mechanisms.) There were 100 persons with $A = 0$, $B = 1$, and $E = 0$, all of whom became cases because they all had U_1, the set of causal complements for the class of sufficient causes containing $A = 0$ and

TABLE 2–2

Incidence Proportions (IP) for Combinations of Component Causes B and E in Hypothetical Population 1, Assuming That Component Cause A Is Unmeasured

	B = 1, E = 1	B = 1, E = 0	B = 0, E = 1	B = 0, E = 0
Cases	1,000	100	900	0
Total	1,000	1,000	1,000	1,000
IP	1.00	0.10	0.90	0.00

TABLE 2–3

Incidence Proportions (IP) for Combinations of Component Causes B and E in Hypothetical Population 2, Assuming That Component Cause A Is Unmeasured

	B = 1, E = 1	B = 1, E = 0	B = 0, E = 1	B = 0, E = 0
Cases	1,000	900	100	0
Total	1,000	1,000	1,000	1,000
IP	1.00	0.90	0.10	0.00

B = 1. Thus, among all 1,000 persons with B = 1 and E = 0, there were 100 cases, for an incidence proportion of 0.10.

If we were to measure strength of effect by the difference of the incidence proportions, it is evident from Table 2–2 that for population 1, E = 1 has a much stronger effect than B = 1, because E = 1 increases the incidence proportion by 0.9 (in both levels of B), whereas B = 1 increases the incidence proportion by only 0.1 (in both levels of E). Table 2–3 shows the analogous results for population 2. Although the members of this population have exactly the same causal mechanisms operating within them as do the members of population 1, the relative strengths of causative factors E = 1 and B = 1 are reversed, again using the incidence proportion difference as the measure of strength. B = 1 now has a much stronger effect on the incidence proportion than E = 1, despite the fact that A, B, and E have no association with one another in either population, and their index levels (A = 1, B = 1 and E = 1) and reference levels (A = 0, B = 0, and E = 0) are each present or have occured in exactly half of each population.

The overall difference of incidence proportions contrasting E = 1 with E = 0 is (1,900/2,000) − (100/2,000) = 0.9 in population 1 and (1,100/2,000) − (900/2,000) = 0.1 in population 2. The key difference between populations 1 and 2 is the difference in the prevalence of the conditions under which E = 1 acts to increase risk: that is, the presence of A = 0 or B = 1, but not both. (When A = 0 *and* B = 1, E = 1 completes all three sufficient causes in Figure 2–2; it thus does not increase anyone's risk, although it may well shorten the time to the outcome.) The prevalence of the condition, "A = 0 or B = 1 but not both" is 1,800/2,000 = 90% in both levels of E in population 1. In population 2, this prevalence is only 200/2,000 = 10% in both levels of E. This difference in the prevalence of the conditions sufficient for E = 1 to increase risk explains the difference in the strength of the effect of E = 1 as measured by the difference in incidence proportions.

As noted above, the set of all other component causes in all sufficient causes in which a causal factor participates is called the *causal complement* of the factor. Thus, A = 0, B = 1, U_2, and U_3 make up the causal complement of E = 1 in the above example. This example shows that the strength of a factor's effect on the occurrence of a disease in a population, measured as the absolute difference in incidence proportions, depends on the prevalence of its causal complement. This dependence has nothing to do with the etiologic mechanism of the component's action, because the component is an equal partner in each mechanism in which it appears. Nevertheless, a factor will appear to have a strong effect, as measured by the difference of proportions getting disease, if its causal complement is common. Conversely, a factor with a rare causal complement will appear to have a weak effect.

If strength of effect is measured by the ratio of proportions getting disease, as opposed to the difference, then strength depends on more than a factor's causal complement. In particular, it depends additionally on how common or rare the components are of sufficient causes in which the specified causal factor does *not* play a role. In this example, given the ubiquity of U_1, the effect of E = 1 measured in ratio terms depends on the prevalence of E = 1's causal complement and on the prevalence of the conjunction of A = 0 and B = 1. If many people have both A = 0 and B = 1, the "baseline" incidence proportion (i.e., the proportion of not-E or "unexposed" persons getting disease) will be high and the proportion getting disease due to E will be comparatively low. If few people have both A = 0 and B = 1, the baseline incidence proportion will be low and the proportion getting disease due to E = 1 will be comparatively high. Thus, strength of effect measured by the incidence proportion ratio depends on more conditions than does strength of effect measured by the incidence proportion difference.

Regardless of how strength of a causal factor's effect is measured, the public health significance of that effect does not imply a corresponding degree of etiologic significance. Each component cause in a given sufficient cause has the same etiologic significance. Given a specific causal mechanism, any of the component causes can have strong or weak effects using either the difference or ratio measure. The actual identities of the components of a sufficient cause are part of the mechanics of causation, whereas the strength of a factor's effect depends on the time-specific distribution of its causal complement (if strength is measured in absolute terms) plus the distribution of the components of all sufficient causes in which the factor does not play a role (if strength is measured in relative terms). Over a span of time, the strength of the effect of a given factor on disease occurrence may change because the prevalence of its causal complement in various mechanisms may also change, even if the causal mechanisms in which the factor and its cofactors act remain unchanged.

INTERACTION AMONG CAUSES

Two component causes acting in the same sufficient cause may be defined as *interacting causally* to produce disease. This definition leaves open many possible mechanisms for the interaction, including those in which two components interact in a direct physical fashion (e.g., two drugs that react to form a toxic by-product) and those in which one component (the *initiator* of the pair) alters a substrate so that the other component (the *promoter* of the pair) can act. Nonetheless, it excludes any situation in which one component E is merely a cause of another component F, with no effect of E on disease except through the component F it causes.

Acting in the same sufficient cause is not the same as one component cause acting to produce a second component cause, and then the second component going on to produce the disease (Robins and Greenland 1992, Kaufman et al., 2004). As an example of the distinction, if cigarette smoking (vs. never smoking) is a component cause of atherosclerosis, and atherosclerosis (vs. no atherosclerosis) causes myocardial infarction, both smoking and atherosclerosis would be component causes (cofactors) in certain sufficient causes of myocardial infarction. They would not necessarily appear in the same sufficient cause. Rather, for a sufficient cause involving atherosclerosis as a component cause, there would be another sufficient cause in which the atherosclerosis component cause was replaced by all the component causes that brought about the atherosclerosis, including smoking. Thus, a sequential causal relation between smoking and atherosclerosis would not be enough for them to interact synergistically in the etiology of myocardial infarction, in the sufficient-cause sense. Instead, the causal sequence means that smoking can act indirectly, through atherosclerosis, to bring about myocardial infarction.

Now suppose that, perhaps in addition to the above mechanism, smoking reduces clotting time and thus causes thrombi that block the coronary arteries if they are narrowed by atherosclerosis. This mechanism would be represented by a sufficient cause containing both smoking and atherosclerosis as components and thus would constitute a synergistic interaction between smoking and atherosclerosis in causing myocardial infarction. The presence of this sufficient cause would not, however, tell us whether smoking also contributed to the myocardial infarction by causing the atherosclerosis. Thus, the basic sufficient-cause model does not alert us to indirect effects (effects of some component causes mediated by other component causes in the model). Chapters 4 and 12 introduce potential-outcome and graphical models better suited to displaying indirect effects and more general sequential mechanisms, whereas Chapter 5 discusses in detail interaction as defined in the potential-outcome framework and its relation to interaction as defined in the sufficient-cause model.

PROPORTION OF DISEASE DUE TO SPECIFIC CAUSES

In Figure 2–2, assuming that the three sufficient causes in the diagram are the only ones operating, what fraction of disease is caused by E = 1? E = 1 is a component cause of disease in two of the sufficient-cause mechanisms, II and III, so all disease arising through either of these two mechanisms is attributable to E = 1. Note that in persons with the exposure pattern A = 0, B = 1, E = 1, all three sufficient causes would be completed. The first of the three mechanisms to be completed would be the one that actually produces a given case. If the first one completed is mechanism II or III, the case would be causally attributable to E = 1. If mechanism I is the first one to be completed, however, E = 1 would not be part of the sufficient cause producing that case. Without knowing the completion times of the three mechanisms, among persons with the exposure pattern A = 0, B = 1, E = 1 we cannot tell how many of the 100 cases in population 1 or the 900 cases in population 2 are etiologically attributable to E = 1.

Each of the cases that is etiologically attributable to E = 1 can also be attributed to the other component causes in the causal mechanisms in which E = 1 acts. Each component cause interacts with its complementary factors to produce disease, so each case of disease can be attributed to every component cause in the completed sufficient cause. Note, though, that the attributable fractions added across component causes of the same disease do not sum to 1, although there is a mistaken tendency to think that they do. To illustrate the mistake in this tendency, note that a necessary component cause appears in every completed sufficient cause of disease, and so by itself has an attributable fraction of 1, without counting the attributable fractions for other component causes. Because every case of disease can be attributed to every component cause in its causal mechanism, attributable fractions for different component causes will generally sum to more than 1, and there is no upper limit for this sum.

A recent debate regarding the proportion of risk factors for coronary heart disease attributable to particular component causes illustrates the type of errors in inference that can arise when the sum is thought to be restricted to 1. The debate centers around whether the proportion of coronary heart disease attributable to high blood cholesterol, high blood pressure, and cigarette smoking equals 75% or "only 50%" (Magnus and Beaglehole, 2001). If the former, then some have argued that the search for additional causes would be of limited utility (Beaglehole and Magnus, 2002), because only 25% of cases "remain to be explained." By assuming that the proportion explained by yet unknown component causes cannot exceed 25%, those who support this contention fail to recognize that cases caused by a sufficient cause that contains any subset of the three named causes might also contain unknown component causes. Cases stemming from sufficient causes with this overlapping set of component causes could be prevented by interventions targeting the three named causes, or by interventions targeting the yet unknown causes when they become known. The latter interventions could reduce the disease burden by much more than 25%.

As another example, in a cohort of cigarette smokers exposed to arsenic by working in a smelter, an estimated 75% of the lung cancer rate was attributable to their work environment and an estimated 65% was attributable to their smoking (Pinto et al., 1978; Hertz-Picciotto et al., 1992). There is no problem with such figures, which merely reflect the multifactorial etiology of disease. So, too, with coronary heart disease; if 75% of that disease is attributable to high blood cholesterol, high blood pressure, and cigarette smoking, 100% of it can still be attributable to other causes, known, suspected, and yet to be discovered. Some of these causes will participate in the same causal mechanisms as high blood cholesterol, high blood pressure, and cigarette smoking. Beaglehole and Magnus were correct in thinking that if the three specified component causes combine to explain 75% of cardiovascular disease (CVD) and we somehow eliminated them, there would be only 25% of CVD cases remaining. But until that 75% is eliminated, any newly discovered component could cause up to 100% of the CVD we currently have.

The notion that interventions targeting high blood cholesterol, high blood pressure, and cigarette smoking could eliminate 75% of coronary heart disease is unrealistic given currently available intervention strategies. Although progress can be made to reduce the effect of these risk factors, it is unlikely that any of them could be completely eradicated from any large population in the near term. Estimates of the public health effect of eliminating diseases themselves as causes of death (Murray et al., 2002) are even further removed from reality, because they fail to account for all the effects of interventions required to achieve the disease elimination, including unanticipated side effects (Greenland, 2002a, 2005a).

The debate about coronary heart disease attribution to component causes is reminiscent of an earlier debate regarding causes of cancer. In their widely cited work, *The Causes of Cancer*, Doll and Peto (1981, Table 20) created a table giving their estimates of the fraction of all cancers caused by various agents. The fractions summed to nearly 100%. Although the authors acknowledged that any case could be caused by more than one agent (which means that, given enough agents, the attributable fractions would sum to far more than 100%), they referred to this situation as a "difficulty" and an "anomaly" that they chose to ignore. Subsequently, one of the authors acknowledged that the attributable fraction could sum to greater than 100% (Peto, 1985). It is neither a difficulty nor an anomaly nor something we can safely ignore, but simply a consequence of the fact that no event has a single agent as the cause. The fraction of disease that can be attributed to known causes will grow without bound as more causes are discovered. Only the fraction of disease attributable to a single component cause cannot exceed 100%.

In a similar vein, much publicity attended the pronouncement in 1960 that as much as 90% of cancer is environmentally caused (Higginson, 1960). Here, "environment" was thought of as representing all nongenetic component causes, and thus included not only the physical environment, but also the social environment and all individual human behavior that is not genetically determined. Hence, environmental component causes must be present to some extent in every sufficient cause of a disease. Thus, Higginson's estimate of 90% was an underestimate.

One can also show that 100% of any disease is inherited, even when environmental factors are component causes. MacMahon (1968) cited the example given by Hogben (1933) of yellow shanks, a trait occurring in certain genetic strains of fowl fed on yellow corn. Both a particular set of genes and a yellow-corn diet are necessary to produce yellow shanks. A farmer with several strains of fowl who feeds them all only yellow corn would consider yellow shanks to be a genetic condition, because only one strain would get yellow shanks, despite all strains getting the same diet. A different farmer who owned only the strain liable to get yellow shanks but who fed some of the birds yellow corn and others white corn would consider yellow shanks to be an environmentally determined condition because it depends on diet. In humans, the mental retardation caused by phenylketonuria is considered by many to be purely genetic. This retardation can, however, be successfully prevented by dietary intervention, which demonstrates the presence of an environmental cause. In reality, yellow shanks, phenylketonuria, and other diseases and conditions are determined by an interaction of genes and environment. It makes no sense to allocate a portion of the causation to either genes or environment separately when both may act together in sufficient causes.

Nonetheless, many researchers have compared disease occurrence in identical and nonidentical twins to estimate the fraction of disease that is inherited. These twin-study and other heritability indices assess only the relative role of environmental and genetic causes of disease in a particular setting. For example, some genetic causes may be necessary components of every causal mechanism. If everyone in a population has an identical set of the genes that cause disease, however, their effect is not included in heritability indices, despite the fact that the genes are causes of the disease. The two farmers in the preceding example would offer very different values for the heritability of yellow shanks, despite the fact that the condition is always 100% dependent on having certain genes.

Every case of every disease has some environmental and some genetic component causes, and therefore every case can be attributed both to genes and to environment. No paradox exists as long as it is understood that the fractions of disease attributable to genes and to environment overlap with one another. Thus, debates over what proportion of all occurrences of a disease are genetic and what proportion are environmental, inasmuch as these debates assume that the shares must add up to 100%, are fallacious and distracting from more worthwhile pursuits.

On an even more general level, the question of whether a given disease does or does not have a "multifactorial etiology" can be answered once and for all in the affirmative. All diseases have multifactorial etiologies. It is therefore completely unremarkable for a given disease to have such an etiology, and no time or money should be spent on research trying to answer the question of whether a particular disease does or does not have a multifactorial etiology. They all do. The job of etiologic research is to identify components of those etiologies.

INDUCTION PERIOD

Pie-chart diagrams of sufficient causes and their components such as those in Figure 2–2 are not well suited to provide a model for conceptualizing the *induction period,* which may be defined as the period of time from causal action until disease initiation. There is no way to tell from a pie-chart diagram of a sufficient cause which components affect each other, which components must come before or after others, for which components the temporal order is irrelevant, etc. The crucial information on temporal ordering must come in a separate description of the interrelations among the components of a sufficient cause.

If, in sufficient cause I, the sequence of action of the specified component causes must be A = 0, B = 1 and we are studying the effect of A = 0, which (let us assume) acts at a narrowly defined point in time, we do not observe the occurrence of disease immediately after A = 0 occurs. Disease occurs only after the sequence is completed, so there will be a delay while B = 1 occurs (along with components of the set U_1 that are not present or that have not occured when A = 0 occurs). When B = 1 acts, if it is the last of all the component causes (including those in the set of unspecified conditions and events represented by U_1), disease occurs. The interval between the action of B = 1 and the disease occurrence is the induction time for the effect of B = 1 in sufficient cause I.

In the example given earlier of an equilibrium disorder leading to a later fall and hip injury, the induction time between the start of the equilibrium disorder and the later hip injury might be long, if the equilibrium disorder is caused by an old head injury, or short, if the disorder is caused by inebriation. In the latter case, it could even be instantaneous, if we define it as blood alcohol greater than a certain level. This latter possibility illustrates an important general point: Component causes that do not change with time, as opposed to events, all have induction times of zero.

Defining an induction period of interest is tantamount to specifying the characteristics of the component causes of interest. A clear example of a lengthy induction time is the cause–effect relation between exposure of a female fetus to diethylstilbestrol (DES) and the subsequent development of adenocarcinoma of the vagina. The cancer is usually diagnosed between ages 15 and 30 years. Because the causal exposure to DES occurs early in pregnancy, there is an induction time of about 15 to 30 years for the carcinogenic action of DES. During this time, other causes presumably are operating; some evidence suggests that hormonal action during adolescence may be part of the mechanism (Rothman, 1981).

It is incorrect to characterize a disease itself as having a lengthy or brief induction period. The induction time can be conceptualized only in relation to a specific component cause operating in a specific sufficient cause. Thus, we say that the induction time relating DES to clear-cell carcinoma of the vagina is 15 to 30 years, but we should not say that 15 to 30 years is the induction time for clear-cell carcinoma in general. Because each component cause in any causal mechanism can act at a time different from the other component causes, each can have its own induction time. For the component cause that acts last, the induction time equals zero. If another component cause of clear-cell carcinoma of the vagina that acts during adolescence were identified, it would have a much shorter induction time for its carcinogenic action than DES. Thus, induction time characterizes a specific cause–effect pair rather than just the effect.

In carcinogenesis, the terms *initiator* and *promotor* have been used to refer to some of the component causes of cancer that act early and late, respectively, in the causal mechanism. Cancer itself has often been characterized as a disease process with a long induction time. This characterization is a misconception, however, because any late-acting component in the causal process, such as a promotor, will have a short induction time. Indeed, by definition, the induction time will always be zero for at least one component cause, the last to act. The mistaken view that diseases, as opposed to cause–disease relationships, have long or short induction periods can have important implications for research. For instance, the view of adult cancers as "diseases of long latency" may induce some researchers to ignore evidence of etiologic effects occurring relatively late in the processes that culminate in clinically diagnosed cancers. At the other extreme, the routine disregard for exposures occurring in the first decade or two in studies of occupational carcinogenesis, as a major example, may well have inhibited the discovery of occupational causes with very long induction periods.

Disease, once initiated, will not necessarily be apparent. The time interval between irreversible disease occurrence and detection has been termed the *latent period* (Rothman, 1981), although others have used this term interchangeably with induction period. Still others use *latent period* to mean the total time between causal action and disease detection. We use *induction period* to describe the time from causal action to irreversible disease occurrence and *latent period* to mean the time from disease occurrence to disease detection. The latent period can sometimes be reduced by improved methods of disease detection. The induction period, on the other hand, cannot be reduced by early detection of disease, because disease occurrence marks the end of the induction period. Earlier detection of disease, however, may reduce the apparent induction period (the time between causal action and disease detection), because the time when disease is detected, as a practical matter, is usually used to mark the time of disease occurrence. Thus, diseases such as slow-growing cancers may appear to have long induction periods with respect to many causes because they have long latent periods. The latent period, unlike the induction period, is a characteristic of the disease and the detection effort applied to the person with the disease.

Although it is not possible to reduce the induction period proper by earlier detection of disease, it may be possible to observe intermediate stages of a causal mechanism. The increased interest in biomarkers such as DNA adducts is an example of attempting to focus on causes more proximal to the disease occurrence or on effects more proximal to cause occurrence. Such biomarkers may nonetheless reflect the effects of earlier-acting agents on the person.

Some agents may have a causal action by shortening the induction time of other agents. Suppose that exposure to factor $X = 1$ leads to epilepsy after an interval of 10 years, on average. It may be that exposure to a drug, $Z = 1$, would shorten this interval to 2 years. Is $Z = 1$ acting as a catalyst, or as a cause, of epilepsy? The answer is both: A catalyst is a cause. Without $Z = 1$, the occurrence of epilepsy comes 8 years later than it comes with $Z = 1$, so we can say that $Z = 1$ causes the onset of the early epilepsy. It is not sufficient to argue that the epilepsy would have occurred anyway. First, it would not have occurred at that time, and the time of occurrence is part of our definition of an event. Second, epilepsy will occur later only if the individual survives an additional 8 years, which is not certain. Not only does agent $Z = 1$ determine when the epilepsy occurs, it can also determine whether it occurs. Thus, we should call any agent that acts as a catalyst of a causal mechanism, speeding up an induction period for other agents, a cause in its own right. Similarly, any agent that postpones the onset of an event, drawing out the induction period for another agent, is a preventive. It should not be too surprising to equate postponement to prevention: We routinely use such an equation when we employ the euphemism that we "prevent" death, which actually can only be postponed. What we prevent is death at a given time, in favor of death at a later time.

SCOPE OF THE MODEL

The main utility of this model of sufficient causes and their components lies in its ability to provide a general but practical conceptual framework for causal problems. The attempt to make the proportion of disease attributable to various component causes add to 100% is an example of a fallacy that is exposed by the model (although MacMahon and others were able to invoke yellow shanks and phenylketonuria to expose that fallacy long before the sufficient-component cause model was formally described [MacMahon and Pugh, 1967, 1970]). The model makes it clear that, because of interactions, there is no upper limit to the sum of these proportions. As we shall see in Chapter 5, the epidemiologic evaluation of interactions themselves can be clarified, to some extent, with the help of the model.

Although the model appears to deal qualitatively with the action of component causes, it can be extended to account for dose dependence by postulating a set of sufficient causes, each of which contains as a component a different dose of the agent in question. Small doses might require a larger or rarer set of complementary causes to complete a sufficient cause than that required by large doses (Rothman, 1976a), in which case it is particularly important to specify both sides of the causal contrast. In this way, the model can account for the phenomenon of a shorter induction period accompanying larger doses of exposure, because a smaller set of complementary components would be needed to complete the sufficient cause.

Those who believe that chance must play a role in any complex mechanism might object to the intricacy of this seemingly deterministic model. A probabilistic (stochastic) model could be invoked to describe a dose–response relation, for example, without the need for a multitude of different causal mechanisms. The model would simply relate the dose of the exposure to the probability of the effect occurring. For those who believe that virtually all events contain some element of chance, deterministic causal models may seem to misrepresent the indeterminism of the real world. However, the deterministic model presented here can accommodate "chance"; one way might be to view chance, or at least some part of the variability that we call "chance," as the result of deterministic events that are beyond the current limits of knowledge or observability.

For example, the outcome of a flip of a coin is usually considered a chance event. In classical mechanics, however, the outcome can in theory be determined completely by the application of physical laws and a sufficient description of the starting conditions. To put it in terms more familiar to epidemiologists, consider the explanation for why an individual gets lung cancer. One hundred years ago, when little was known about the etiology of lung cancer; a scientist might have said that it was a matter of chance. Nowadays, we might say that the risk depends on how much the individual smokes, how much asbestos and radon the individual has been exposed to, and so on. Nonetheless, recognizing this dependence moves the line of ignorance; it does not eliminate it. One can still ask what determines whether an individual who has smoked a specific amount and has a specified amount of exposure to all the other known risk factors will get lung cancer. Some will get lung cancer and some will not, and if all known risk factors are already taken into account, what is left we might still describe as chance. True, we can explain much more of the variability in lung cancer occurrence nowadays than we formerly could by taking into account factors known to cause it, but at the limits of our knowledge, we still ascribe the remaining variability to what we call chance. In this view, chance is seen as a catchall term for our ignorance about causal explanations.

We have so far ignored more subtle considerations of sources of unpredictability in events, such as chaotic behavior (in which even the slightest uncertainty about initial conditions leads to vast uncertainty about outcomes) and quantum-mechanical uncertainty. In each of these situations, a random (stochastic) model component may be essential for any useful modeling effort. Such components can also be introduced in the above conceptual model by treating unmeasured component causes in the model as random events, so that the causal model based on components of sufficient causes can have random elements. An example is treatment assignment in randomized clinical trials (Poole 2001a).

OTHER MODELS OF CAUSATION

The sufficient-component cause model is only one of several models of causation that may be useful for gaining insight about epidemiologic concepts (Greenland and Brumback, 2002; Greenland, 2004a). It portrays qualitative causal mechanisms within members of a population, so its fundamental unit of analysis is the causal mechanism rather than a person. Many different sets of mechanisms can lead to the same pattern of disease within a population, so the sufficient-component cause model involves specification of details that are beyond the scope of epidemiologic data. Also, it does not incorporate elements reflecting population distributions of factors or causal sequences, which are crucial to understanding confounding and other biases.

Other models of causation, such as potential-outcome (counterfactual) models and graphical models, provide direct representations of epidemiologic concepts such as confounding and other biases, and can be applied at mechanistic, individual, or population levels of analysis. Potential-outcome models (Chapters 4 and 5) specify in detail what would happen to individuals or populations under alternative possible patterns of interventions or exposures, and also bring to the fore problems in operationally defining causes (Greenland, 2002a, 2005a; Hernán, 2005). Graphical models (Chapter 12) display broad qualitative assumptions about causal directions and independencies. Both types of model have close relationships to the structural-equations models that are popular in the social sciences (Pearl, 2000; Greenland and Brumback, 2002), and both can be subsumed under a general theory of longitudinal causality (Robins, 1997).

PHILOSOPHY OF SCIENTIFIC INFERENCE

Causal inference may be viewed as a special case of the more general process of scientific reasoning. The literature on this topic is too vast for us to review thoroughly, but we will provide a brief overview of certain points relevant to epidemiology, at the risk of some oversimplification.

INDUCTIVISM

Modern science began to emerge around the 16th and 17th centuries, when the knowledge demands of emerging technologies (such as artillery and transoceanic navigation) stimulated inquiry into the origins of knowledge. An early codification of the scientific method was Francis Bacon's *Novum Organum,* which, in 1620, presented an inductivist view of science. In this philosophy, scientific reasoning is said to depend on making generalizations, or inductions, from observations to general laws of nature; the observations are said to induce the formulation of a natural law in the mind of the scientist. Thus, an inductivist would have said that Jenner's observation of lack of smallpox among milkmaids induced in Jenner's mind the theory that cowpox (common among milkmaids) conferred immunity to smallpox. Inductivist philosophy reached a pinnacle of sorts in the canons of John Stuart Mill (1862), which evolved into inferential criteria that are still in use today.

Inductivist philosophy was a great step forward from the medieval scholasticism that preceded it, for at least it demanded that a scientist make careful observations of people and nature rather than appeal to faith, ancient texts, or authorities. Nonetheless, in the 18th century the Scottish philosopher David Hume described a disturbing deficiency in inductivism. An inductive argument carried no logical force; instead, such an argument represented nothing more than an *assumption* that certain events would in the future follow the same pattern as they had in the past. Thus, to argue that cowpox caused immunity to smallpox because no one got smallpox after having cowpox corresponded to an unjustified assumption that the pattern observed to date (no smallpox after cowpox) would continue into the future. Hume pointed out that, even for the most reasonable-sounding of such assumptions, there was no logical necessity behind the inductive argument.

Of central concern to Hume (1739) was the issue of causal inference and failure of induction to provide a foundation for it:

> Thus not only our reason fails us in the discovery of the ultimate connexion of causes and effects, but even after experience has inform'd us of their constant conjunction, 'tis impossible for us to satisfy ourselves by our reason, why we shou'd extend that experience beyond those particular instances, which have fallen under our observation. We suppose, but are never able to prove, that there must be a resemblance betwixt those objects, of which we have had experience, and those which lie beyond the reach of our discovery.

In other words, no number of repetitions of a particular sequence of events, such as the appearance of a light after flipping a switch, can prove a causal connection between the action of the switch and the turning on of the light. No matter how many times the light comes on after the switch has been pressed, the possibility of coincidental occurrence cannot be ruled out. Hume pointed out that observers cannot perceive causal connections, but only a series of events. Bertrand Russell (1945) illustrated this point with the example of two accurate clocks that perpetually chime on the hour, with one keeping time slightly ahead of the other. Although one invariably chimes before the other, there is no direct causal connection from one to the other. Thus, assigning a causal interpretation to the pattern of events cannot be a logical extension of our observations alone, because the events might be occurring together only because of a shared earlier cause, or because of some systematic error in the observations.

Causal inference based on mere association of events constitutes a logical fallacy known as *post hoc ergo propter hoc* (Latin for "after this therefore on account of this"). This fallacy is exemplified by the inference that the crowing of a rooster is necessary for the sun to rise because sunrise is always preceded by the crowing.

The *post hoc* fallacy is a special case of a more general logical fallacy known as the *fallacy of affirming the consequent*. This fallacy of confirmation takes the following general form: "We know that if H is true, B must be true; and we know that B is true; therefore H must be true." This fallacy is used routinely by scientists in interpreting data. It is used, for example, when one argues as follows: "If sewer service causes heart disease, then heart disease rates should be highest where sewer service is available; heart disease rates are indeed highest where sewer service is available; therefore, sewer service causes heart disease." Here, H is the hypothesis "sewer service causes heart disease" and B is the observation "heart disease rates are highest where sewer service is available." The argument is logically unsound, as demonstrated by the fact that we can imagine many ways in which the premises could be true but the conclusion false; for example, economic development could lead to both sewer service and elevated heart disease rates, without any effect of sewer service on heart disease. In this case, however, we also know that one of the premises is not true—specifically, the premise, "If H is true, B must be true." This particular form of the fallacy exemplifies the problem of *confounding*, which we will discuss in detail in later chapters.

Bertrand Russell (1945) satirized the fallacy this way:

> 'If p, then q; now q is true; therefore p is true.' E.g., 'If pigs have wings, then some winged animals are good to eat; now some winged animals are good to eat; therefore pigs have wings.' This form of inference is called 'scientific method.'

REFUTATIONISM

Russell was not alone in his lament of the illogicality of scientific reasoning as ordinarily practiced. Many philosophers and scientists from Hume's time forward attempted to set out a firm logical basis for scientific reasoning.

In the 1920s, most notable among these was the school of logical positivists, who sought a logic for science that could lead inevitably to correct scientific conclusions, in much the way rigorous logic can lead inevitably to correct conclusions in mathematics. Other philosophers and scientists, however, had started to suspect that scientific hypotheses can never be proven or established as true in any logical sense. For example, a number of philosophers noted that scientific statements can only be found to be consistent with observation, but cannot be proven or disproven in any "airtight" logical or mathematical sense (Duhem, 1906, transl. 1954; Popper 1934, transl. 1959; Quine, 1951). This fact is sometimes called the problem of *nonidentification* or *underdetermination* of theories by observations (Curd and Cover, 1998). In particular, available observations are always consistent with several hypotheses that themselves are mutually inconsistent, which explains why (as Hume noted) scientific theories cannot be logically proven. In particular, consistency between a hypothesis and observations is no proof of the hypothesis, because we can always invent alternative hypotheses that are just as consistent with the observations.

In contrast, a valid observation that is inconsistent with a hypothesis implies that the hypothesis as stated is false and so refutes the hypothesis. If you wring the rooster's neck before it crows and the sun still rises, you have disproved that the rooster's crowing is a necessary cause of sunrise. Or consider a hypothetical research program to learn the boiling point of water (Magee, 1985). A scientist who boils water in an open flask and repeatedly measures the boiling point at 100°C will never, no matter how many confirmatory repetitions are involved, prove that 100°C is always the boiling point. On the other hand, merely one attempt to boil the water in a closed flask or at high altitude will refute the proposition that water always boils at 100°C.

According to Popper, science advances by a process of elimination that he called "conjecture and refutation." Scientists form hypotheses based on intuition, conjecture, and previous experience. Good scientists use deductive logic to infer predictions from the hypothesis and then compare observations with the predictions. Hypotheses whose predictions agree with observations are confirmed (Popper used the term "corroborated") only in the sense that they can continue to be used as explanations of natural phenomena. At any time, however, they may be refuted by further observations and might be replaced by other hypotheses that are more consistent with the observations. This view of scientific inference is sometimes called *refutationism* or *falsificationism*. Refutationists consider induction to be a psychologic crutch: Repeated observations did not in fact induce the formulation of a natural law, but only the belief that such a law has been found. For a refutationist, only the psychologic comfort provided by induction explains why it still has advocates.

One way to rescue the concept of induction from the stigma of pure delusion is to resurrect it as a psychologic phenomenon, as Hume and Popper claimed it was, but one that plays a legitimate role in hypothesis formation. The philosophy of conjecture and refutation places no constraints on the origin of conjectures. Even delusions are permitted as hypotheses, and therefore inductively inspired hypotheses, however psychologic, are valid starting points for scientific evaluation. This concession does not admit a logical role for induction in confirming scientific hypotheses, but it allows the process of induction to play a part, along with imagination, in the scientific cycle of conjecture and refutation.

The philosophy of conjecture and refutation has profound implications for the methodology of science. The popular concept of a scientist doggedly assembling evidence to support a favorite thesis is objectionable from the standpoint of refutationist philosophy because it encourages scientists to consider their own pet theories as their intellectual property, to be confirmed, proven, and, when all the evidence is in, cast in stone and defended as natural law. Such attitudes hinder critical evaluation, interchange, and progress. The approach of conjecture and refutation, in contrast, encourages scientists to consider multiple hypotheses and to seek crucial tests that decide between competing hypotheses by falsifying one of them. Because falsification of one or more theories is the goal, there is incentive to depersonalize the theories. Criticism leveled at a theory need not be seen as criticism of the person who proposed it. It has been suggested that the reason why certain fields of science advance rapidly while others languish is that the rapidly advancing fields are propelled by scientists who are busy constructing and testing competing hypotheses; the other fields, in contrast, "are sick by comparison, because they have forgotten the necessity for alternative hypotheses and disproof" (Platt, 1964).

The refutationist model of science has a number of valuable lessons for research conduct, especially of the need to seek alternative explanations for observations, rather than focus on the chimera of seeking scientific "proof" for some favored theory. Nonetheless, it is vulnerable to criticisms that observations (or some would say their interpretations) are themselves laden with theory (sometimes called the *Duhem-Quine thesis*; Curd and Cover, 1998). Thus, observations can never provide the sort of definitive refutations that are the hallmark of popular accounts of refutationism. For example, there may be uncontrolled and even unimagined biases that have made our refutational observations invalid; to claim refutation is to assume as true the unprovable theory that no such bias exists. In other words, not only are theories underdetermined by observations, so are refutations, which are themselves theory-laden. The net result is that logical certainty about either the truth or falsity of an internally consistent theory is impossible (Quine, 1951).

CONSENSUS AND NATURALISM

Some 20th-century philosophers of science, most notably Thomas Kuhn (1962), emphasized the role of the scientific community in judging the validity of scientific theories. These critics of the conjecture-and-refutation model suggested that the refutation of a theory involves making a choice. Every observation is itself dependent on theories. For example, observing the moons of Jupiter through a telescope seems to us like a direct observation, but only because the theory of optics on which the telescope is based is so well accepted. When confronted with a refuting observation, a scientist faces the choice of rejecting either the validity of the theory being tested or the validity of the refuting observation, which itself must be premised on scientific theories that are not certain (Haack, 2003). Observations that are falsifying instances of theories may at times be treated as "anomalies," tolerated without falsifying the theory in the hope that the anomalies may eventually be explained. An epidemiologic example is the observation that shallow-inhaling smokers had higher lung cancer rates than deep-inhaling smokers. This anomaly was eventually explained when it was noted that lung tissue higher in the lung is more susceptible to smoking-associated lung tumors, and shallowly inhaled smoke tars tend to be deposited higher in the lung (Wald, 1985).

In other instances, anomalies may lead eventually to the overthrow of current scientific doctrine, just as Newtonian mechanics was displaced (remaining only as a first-order approximation) by relativity theory. Kuhn asserted that in every branch of science the prevailing scientific viewpoint, which he termed "normal science," occasionally undergoes major shifts that amount to scientific revolutions. These revolutions signal a decision of the scientific community to discard the scientific infrastructure rather than to falsify a new hypothesis that cannot be easily grafted onto it. Kuhn and others have argued that the consensus of the scientific community determines what is considered accepted and what is considered refuted.

Kuhn's critics characterized this description of science as one of an irrational process, "a matter for mob psychology" (Lakatos, 1970). Those who believe in a rational structure for science consider Kuhn's vision to be a regrettably real description of much of what passes for scientific activity, but not prescriptive for any good science. Although many modern philosophers reject rigid demarcations and formulations for science such as refutationism, they nonetheless maintain that science is founded on reason, albeit possibly informal common sense (Haack, 2003). Others go beyond Kuhn and maintain that attempts to impose a singular rational structure or methodology on science hobbles the imagination and is a prescription for the same sort of authoritarian repression of ideas that scientists have had to face throughout history (Feyerabend, 1975 and 1993).

The philosophic debate about Kuhn's description of science hinges on whether Kuhn meant to describe only what has happened historically in science or instead what ought to happen, an issue about which Kuhn (1970) has not been completely clear:

> Are Kuhn's [my] remarks about scientific development. . . to be read as descriptions or prescriptions? The answer, of course, is that they should be read in both ways at once. If I have a theory of how and why science works, it must necessarily have implications for the way in which scientists should behave if their enterprise is to flourish.

The idea that science is a sociologic process, whether considered descriptive or normative, is an interesting thesis, as is the idea that from observing how scientists work we can learn about how scientists ought to work. The latter idea has led to the development of *naturalistic* philosophy of science, or "science studies," which examines scientific developments for clues about what sort of methods scientists need and develop for successful discovery and invention (Callebaut, 1993; Giere, 1999).

Regardless of philosophical developments, we suspect that most epidemiologists (and most scientists) will continue to function as if the following classical view is correct: The ultimate goal of scientific inference is to capture some objective truths about the material world in which we live, and any theory of inference should ideally be evaluated by how well it leads us to these truths. This ideal is impossible to operationalize, however, for if we ever find any ultimate truths, we will have no way of knowing that for certain. Thus, those holding the view that scientific truth is not arbitrary nevertheless concede that our knowledge of these truths will always be tentative. For refutationists, this tentativeness has an asymmetric quality, but that asymmetry is less marked for others. We may believe that we know a theory is false because it consistently fails the tests we put it through, but our tests could be faulty, given that they involve imperfect reasoning and sense perception. Neither can we know that a theory is true, even if it passes every test we can devise, for it may fail a test that is as yet undevised.

Few, if any, would disagree that a theory of inference should be evaluated at least in part by how well it leads us to detect errors in our hypotheses and observations. There are, however, many other inferential activities besides evaluation of hypotheses, such as prediction or forecasting of events, and subsequent attempts to control events (which of course requires causal information). Statisticians rather than philosophers have more often confronted these problems in practice, so it should not be surprising that the major philosophies concerned with these problems emerged from statistics rather than philosophy.

BAYESIANISM

There is another philosophy of inference that, like most, holds an objective view of scientific truth and a view of knowledge as tentative or uncertain, but that focuses on evaluation of knowledge rather than truth. Like refutationism, the modern form of this philosophy evolved from the writings of 18th-century thinkers. The focal arguments first appeared in a pivotal essay by the Reverend Thomas Bayes (1764), and hence the philosophy is usually referred to as Bayesianism (Howson and Urbach, 1993), and it was the renowned French mathematician and scientist Pierre Simon de Laplace who first gave it an applied statistical format. Nonetheless, it did not reach a complete expression until after World War I, most notably in the writings of Ramsey (1931) and DeFinetti (1937); and, like refutationism, it did not begin to appear in epidemiology until the 1970s (e.g., Cornfield, 1976).

The central problem addressed by Bayesianism is the following: In classical logic, a deductive argument can provide no information about the truth or falsity of a scientific hypothesis unless you can be 100% certain about the truth of the premises of the argument. Consider the logical argument called *modus tollens:* "If H implies B, and B is false, then H must be false." This argument is logically valid, but the conclusion follows only on the assumptions that the premises "H implies B" and "B is false" are true statements. If these premises are statements about the physical world, we cannot possibly know them to be correct with 100% certainty, because all observations are subject to error. Furthermore, the claim that "H implies B" will often depend on its own chain of deductions, each with its own premises of which we cannot be certain.

For example, if H is "Television viewing causes homicides" and B is "Homicide rates are highest where televisions are most common," the first premise used in *modus tollens* to test the hypothesis that television viewing causes homicides will be: "If television viewing causes homicides, homicide rates are highest where televisions are most common." The validity of this premise is doubtful—after all, even if television does cause homicides, homicide rates may be low where televisions are common because of socioeconomic advantages in those areas.

Continuing to reason in this fashion, we could arrive at a more pessimistic state than even Hume imagined. Not only is induction without logical foundation, *deduction* has limited scientific utility because we cannot ensure the truth of all the premises, even if a logical argument is valid.

The Bayesian answer to this problem is partial in that it makes a severe demand on the scientist and puts a severe limitation on the results. It says roughly this: If you can assign a degree of certainty, or personal probability, to the premises of your valid argument, you may use any and all the rules of probability theory to derive a certainty for the conclusion, and this certainty will be a logically valid consequence of your original certainties. An inescapable fact is that your concluding certainty, or *posterior probability,* may depend heavily on what you used as initial certainties, or *prior probabilities.* If those initial certainties are not the same as those of a colleague, that colleague may very well assign a certainty to the conclusion different from the one you derived. With the accumulation of consistent evidence, however, the data can usually force even extremely disparate priors to converge into similar posterior probabilities.

Because the posterior probabilities emanating from a Bayesian inference depend on the person supplying the initial certainties and so may vary across individuals, the inferences are said to be subjective. This subjectivity of Bayesian inference is often mistaken for a subjective treatment of truth. Not only is such a view of Bayesianism incorrect, it is diametrically opposed to Bayesian philosophy. The Bayesian approach represents a constructive attempt to deal with the dilemma that scientific laws and facts should not be treated as known with certainty, whereas classic deductive logic yields conclusions only when some law, fact, or connection is asserted with 100% certainty.

A common criticism of Bayesian philosophy is that it diverts attention away from the classic goals of science, such as the discovery of how the world works, toward psychologic states of mind called "certainties," "subjective probabilities," or "degrees of belief" (Popper, 1959). This criticism, however, fails to recognize the importance of a scientist's state of mind in determining what theories to test and what tests to apply, the consequent influence of those states on the store of data available for inference, and the influence of the data on the states of mind.

Another reply to this criticism is that scientists already use data to influence their degrees of belief, and they are not shy about expressing those degrees of certainty. The problem is that the conventional process is informal, intuitive, and ineffable, and therefore not subject to critical scrutiny; at its worst, it often amounts to nothing more than the experts announcing that they have seen the evidence and here is how certain they are. How they reached this certainty is left unclear, or, put another way, is not "transparent." The problem is that no one, even an expert, is very good at informally and intuitively formulating certainties that predict facts and future events well (Kahneman et al., 1982; Gilovich, 1993; Piattelli-Palmarini, 1994; Gilovich et al., 2002). One reason for this problem is that biases and prior prejudices can easily creep into expert judgments. Bayesian methods force experts to "put their cards on the table" and specify explicitly the strength of their prior beliefs and why they have such beliefs, defend those specifications against arguments and evidence, and update their degrees of certainty with new evidence in ways that do not violate probability logic.

In any research context, there will be an unlimited number of hypotheses that could explain an observed phenomenon. Some argue that progress is best aided by severely testing (empirically challenging) those explanations that seem most probable in light of past research, so that short-comings of currently "received" theories can be most rapidly discovered. Indeed, much research in certain fields takes this form, as when theoretical predictions of particle mass are put to ever more precise tests in physics experiments. This process does not involve mere improved repetition of past studies. Rather, it involves tests of previously untested but important predictions of the theory. Moreover, there is an imperative to make the basis for prior beliefs criticizable and defensible. That prior probabilities can differ among persons does not mean that all such beliefs are based on the same information, nor that all are equally tenable.

Probabilities of auxiliary hypotheses are also important in study design and interpretation. Failure of a theory to pass a test can lead to rejection of the theory more rapidly when the auxiliary hypotheses on which the test depends possess high probability. This observation provides a rationale for preferring "nested" case-control studies (in which controls are selected from a roster of the source population for the cases) to "hospital-based" case-control studies (in which the controls are "selected" by the occurrence or diagnosis of one or more diseases other than the case-defining disease), because the former have fewer mechanisms for biased subject selection and hence are given a higher probability of unbiased subject selection.

Even if one disputes the above arguments, most epidemiologists desire some way of expressing the varying degrees of certainty about possible values of an effect measure in light of available data. Such expressions must inevitably be derived in the face of considerable uncertainty about methodologic details and various events that led to the available data and can be extremely sensitive to the reasoning used in its derivation. For example, as we shall discuss at greater length in Chapter 19, conventional confidence intervals quantify only random error under often questionable assumptions and so should not be interpreted as measures of total uncertainty, particularly for nonexperimental studies. As noted earlier, most people, including scientists, reason poorly in the face of uncertainty. At the very least, subjective Bayesian philosophy provides a methodology for sound reasoning under uncertainty and, in particular, provides many warnings against being overly certain about one's conclusions (Greenland 1998a, 1988b, 2006a; see also Chapters 18 and 19).

Such warnings are echoed in refutationist philosophy. As Peter Medawar (1979) put it, "I cannot give any scientist of any age better advice than this: the intensity of the conviction that a hypothesis is true has no bearing on whether it is true or not." We would add two points. First, the intensity of conviction that a hypothesis is false has no bearing on whether it is false or not. Second, Bayesian methods do not mistake beliefs for evidence. They use evidence to modify beliefs, which scientists routinely do in any event, but often in implicit, intuitive, and incoherent ways.

IMPOSSIBILITY OF SCIENTIFIC PROOF

Vigorous debate is a characteristic of modern scientific philosophy, no less in epidemiology than in other areas (Rothman, 1988). Can divergent philosophies of science be reconciled? Haack (2003) suggested that the scientific enterprise is akin to solving a vast, collective crossword puzzle. In areas in which the evidence is tightly interlocking, there is more reason to place confidence in the answers, but in areas with scant information, the theories may be little better than informed guesses. Of the scientific method, Haack (2003) said that "there is less to the 'scientific method' than meets the eye. Is scientific inquiry categorically different from other kinds? No. Scientific inquiry is continuous with everyday empirical inquiry—only more so."

Perhaps the most important common thread that emerges from the debated philosophies is that proof is impossible in empirical science. This simple fact is especially important to observational epidemiologists, who often face the criticism that proof is impossible in epidemiology, with the implication that it is possible in other scientific disciplines. Such criticism may stem from a view that experiments are the definitive source of scientific knowledge. That view is mistaken on at least two counts. First, the nonexperimental nature of a science does not preclude impressive scientific discoveries; the myriad examples include plate tectonics, the evolution of species, planets orbiting other stars, and the effects of cigarette smoking on human health. Even when they are possible, experiments (including randomized trials) do not provide anything approaching proof and in fact may be controversial, contradictory, or nonreproducible. If randomized clinical trials provided proof, we would never need to do more than one of them on a given hypothesis. Neither physical nor experimental science is immune to such problems, as demonstrated by episodes such as the experimental "discovery" (later refuted) of cold fusion (Taubes, 1993).

Some experimental scientists hold that epidemiologic relations are only suggestive and believe that detailed laboratory study of mechanisms within single individuals can reveal cause–effect relations with certainty. This view overlooks the fact that *all* relations are suggestive in exactly the manner discussed by Hume. Even the most careful and detailed mechanistic dissection of individual events cannot provide more than associations, albeit at a finer level. Laboratory studies often involve a degree of observer control that cannot be approached in epidemiology; it is only this control, not the level of observation, that can strengthen the inferences from laboratory studies. And again, such control is no guarantee against error. In addition, neither scientists nor decision makers are often highly persuaded when only mechanistic evidence from the laboratory is available.

All of the fruits of scientific work, in epidemiology or other disciplines, are at best only tentative formulations of a description of nature, even when the work itself is carried out without mistakes. The tentativeness of our knowledge does not prevent practical applications, but it should keep us skeptical and critical, not only of everyone else's work, but of our own as well. Sometimes etiologic hypotheses enjoy an extremely high, universally or almost universally shared, degree of certainty. The hypothesis that cigarette smoking causes lung cancer is one of the best-known examples. These hypotheses rise above "tentative" acceptance and are the closest we can come to "proof." But even these hypotheses are not "proved" with the degree of absolute certainty that accompanies the proof of a mathematical theorem.

CAUSAL INFERENCE IN EPIDEMIOLOGY

Etiologic knowledge about epidemiologic hypotheses is often scant, making the hypotheses themselves at times little more than vague statements of causal association between exposure and disease, such as "smoking causes cardiovascular disease." These vague hypotheses have only vague consequences that can be difficult to test. To cope with this vagueness, epidemiologists usually focus on testing the negation of the causal hypothesis, that is, the null hypothesis that the exposure does *not* have a causal relation to disease. Then, any observed association can potentially refute the hypothesis, subject to the assumption (auxiliary hypothesis) that biases and chance fluctuations are not solely responsible for the observation.

TESTS OF COMPETING EPIDEMIOLOGIC THEORIES

If the causal mechanism is stated specifically enough, epidemiologic observations can provide crucial tests of competing, non-null causal hypotheses. For example, when toxic-shock syndrome was first studied, there were two competing hypotheses about the causal agent. Under one hypothesis, it was a chemical in the tampon, so that women using tampons were exposed to the agent directly from the tampon. Under the other hypothesis, the tampon acted as a culture medium for staphylococci that produced a toxin. Both hypotheses explained the relation of toxic-shock occurrence to tampon use. The two hypotheses, however, led to opposite predictions about the relation between the frequency of changing tampons and the rate of toxic shock. Under the hypothesis of a chemical agent, more frequent changing of the tampon would lead to more exposure to the agent and possible absorption of a greater overall dose. This hypothesis predicted that women who changed tampons more frequently would have a higher rate than women who changed tampons infrequently. The culture-medium hypothesis predicts that women who change tampons frequently would have a lower rate than those who change tampons less frequently, because a short duration of use for each tampon would prevent the staphylococci from multiplying enough to produce a damaging dose of toxin. Thus, epidemiologic research, by showing that infrequent changing of tampons was associated with a higher rate of toxic shock, refuted the chemical theory in the form presented. There was, however, a third hypothesis that a chemical in some tampons (e.g., oxygen content) improved their performance as culture media. This chemical-promotor hypothesis made the same prediction about the association with frequency of changing tampons as the microbial toxin hypothesis (Lanes and Rothman, 1990).

Another example of a theory that can be easily tested by epidemiologic data relates to the observation that women who took replacement estrogen therapy had a considerably elevated rate of endometrial cancer. Horwitz and Feinstein (1978) conjectured a competing theory to explain the association: They proposed that women taking estrogen experienced symptoms such as bleeding that induced them to consult a physician. The resulting diagnostic workup led to the detection of endometrial cancer at an earlier stage in these women, as compared with women who were not taking estrogens. Horwitz and Feinstein argued that the association arose from this detection bias, claiming that without the bleeding-induced workup, many of these cancers would not have been detected at all. Many epidemiologic observations were used to evaluate these competing hypotheses. The detection-bias theory predicted that women who had used estrogens for only a short time would have the greatest elevation in their rate, as the symptoms related to estrogen use that led to the medical consultation tended to appear soon after use began. Because the association of recent estrogen use and endometrial cancer was the same in both long- and short-term estrogen users, the detection-bias theory was refuted as an explanation for all but a small fraction of endometrial cancer cases occurring after estrogen use. Refutation of the detection-bias theory also depended on many other observations. Especially important was the theory's implication that there must be a huge reservoir of undetected endometrial cancer in the typical population of women to account for the much greater rate observed in estrogen users, an implication that was not borne out by further observations (Hutchison and Rothman, 1978).

The endometrial cancer example illustrates a critical point in understanding the process of causal inference in epidemiologic studies: Many of the hypotheses being evaluated in the interpretation of epidemiologic studies are auxiliary hypotheses in the sense that they are independent of the presence, absence, or direction of any causal connection between the study exposure and the disease. For example, explanations of how specific types of bias could have distorted an association between exposure and disease are the usual alternatives to the primary study hypothesis. Much of the interpretation of epidemiologic studies amounts to the testing of such auxiliary explanations for observed associations.

CAUSAL CRITERIA

In practice, how do epidemiologists separate causal from noncausal explanations? Despite philosophic criticisms of inductive inference, inductively oriented considerations are often used as criteria for making such inferences (Weed and Gorelic, 1996). If a set of necessary and sufficient causal criteria could be used to distinguish causal from noncausal relations in epidemiologic studies, the job of the scientist would be eased considerably. With such criteria, all the concerns about the logic or lack thereof in causal inference could be subsumed: It would only be necessary to consult the checklist of criteria to see if a relation were causal. We know from the philosophy reviewed earlier that a set of sufficient criteria does not exist. Nevertheless, lists of causal criteria have become popular, possibly because they seem to provide a road map through complicated territory, and perhaps because they suggest hypotheses to be evaluated in a given problem.

A commonly used set of criteria was based on a list of considerations or "viewpoints" proposed by Sir Austin Bradford Hill (1965). Hill's list was an expansion of a list offered previously in the landmark U.S. Surgeon General's report *Smoking and Health* (1964), which in turn was anticipated by the inductive canons of John Stuart Mill (1862) and the rules given by Hume (1739). Subsequently, others, especially Susser, have further developed causal considerations (Kaufman and Poole, 2000).

Hill suggested that the following considerations in attempting to distinguish causal from noncausal associations that were already "perfectly clear-cut and beyond what we would care to attribute to the play of chance": (1) strength, (2) consistency, (3) specificity, (4) temporality, (5) biologic gradient, (6) plausibility, (7) coherence, (8) experimental evidence, and (9) analogy. Hill emphasized that causal inferences cannot be based on a set of rules, condemned emphasis on statistical significance testing, and recognized the importance of many other factors in decision making (Phillips and Goodman, 2004). Nonetheless, the misguided but popular view that his considerations should be used as criteria for causal inference makes it necessary to examine them in detail.

Strength

Hill argued that strong associations are particularly compelling because, for weaker associations, it is "easier" to imagine what today we would call an unmeasured confounder that might be responsible for the association. Several years earlier, Cornfield et al. (1959) drew similar conclusions. They concentrated on a single hypothetical confounder that, by itself, would explain entirely an observed association. They expressed a strong preference for ratio measures of strength, as opposed to difference measures, and focused on how the observed estimate of a risk ratio provides a minimum for the association that a completely explanatory confounder must have with the exposure (rather than a minimum for the confounder–disease association). Of special importance, Cornfield et al. acknowledged that having only a weak association does not rule out a causal connection (Rothman and Poole, 1988). Today, some associations, such as those between smoking and cardiovascular disease or between environmental tobacco smoke and lung cancer, are accepted by most as causal even though the associations are considered weak.

Counterexamples of strong but noncausal associations are also not hard to find; any study with strong confounding illustrates the phenomenon. For example, consider the strong relation between Down syndrome and birth rank, which is confounded by the relation between Down syndrome and maternal age. Of course, once the confounding factor is identified, the association is diminished by controlling for the factor.

These examples remind us that a strong association is neither necessary nor sufficient for causality, and that weakness is neither necessary nor sufficient for absence of causality. A strong association bears only on hypotheses that the association is entirely or partially due to unmeasured confounders or other source of modest bias.

Consistency

To most observers, consistency refers to the repeated observation of an association in different populations under different circumstances. Lack of consistency, however, does not rule out a causal association, because some effects are produced by their causes only under unusual circumstances. More precisely, the effect of a causal agent cannot occur unless the complementary component causes act or have already acted to complete a sufficient cause. These conditions will not always be met. Thus, transfusions can cause infection with the human immunodeficiency virus, but they do not always do so: The virus must also be present. Tampon use can cause toxic-shock syndrome, but only rarely, when certain other, perhaps unknown, conditions are met. Consistency is apparent only after all the relevant details of a causal mechanism are understood, which is to say very seldom. Furthermore, even studies of exactly the same phenomena can be expected to yield different results simply because they differ in their methods and random errors. Consistency serves only to rule out hypotheses that the association is attributable to some factor that varies across studies.

One mistake in implementing the consistency criterion is so common that it deserves special mention. It is sometimes claimed that a literature or set of results is inconsistent simply because some results are "statistically significant" and some are not. This sort of evaluation is completely fallacious even if one accepts the use of significance testing methods. The results (effect estimates) from a set of studies could all be identical even if many were significant and many were not, the difference in significance arising solely because of differences in the standard errors or sizes of the studies. Conversely, the results could be significantly in conflict even if all were all were nonsignificant individually, simply because in aggregate an effect could be apparent in some subgroups but not others (see Chapter 33). The fallacy of judging consistency by comparing P-values or statistical significance is not eliminated by "standardizing" estimates (i.e., dividing them by the standard deviation of the outcome, multiplying them by the standard deviation of the exposure, or both); in fact it is worsened, as such standardization can create differences where none exists, or mask true differences (Greenland et al., 1986, 1991; see Chapters 21 and 33).

Specificity

The criterion of specificity has two variants. One is that a cause leads to a single effect, not multiple effects. The other is that an effect has one cause, not multiple causes. Hill mentioned both of them. The former criterion, specificity of effects, was used as an argument in favor of a causal interpretation of the association between smoking and lung cancer and, in an act of circular reasoning, in favor of ratio comparisons and not differences as the appropriate measures of strength. When ratio measures were examined, the association of smoking to diseases looked "quantitatively specific" to lung cancer. When difference measures were examined, the association appeared to be nonspecific, with several diseases (other cancers, coronary heart disease, etc.) being at least as strongly associated with smoking as lung cancer was. Today we know that smoking affects the risk of many diseases and that the difference comparisons were accurately portraying this lack of specificity. Unfortunately, however, the historical episode of the debate over smoking and health is often cited today as justification for the specificity criterion and for using ratio comparisons to measure strength of association. The proper lessons to learn from that episode should be just the opposite.

Weiss (2002) argued that specificity can be used to distinguish some causal hypotheses from noncausal hypotheses, when the causal hypothesis predicts a relation with one outcome but no relation with another outcome. His argument is persuasive when, in addition to the causal hypothesis, one has an alternative noncausal hypothesis that predicts a nonspecific association. Weiss offered the example of screening sigmoidoscopy, which was associated in case-control studies with a 50% to 70% reduction in mortality from distal tumors of the rectum and tumors of the distal colon, within the reach of the sigmoidoscope, but no reduction in mortality from tumors elsewhere in the colon. If the effect of screening sigmoidoscopy were not specific to the distal colon tumors, it would lend support not to all noncausal theories to explain the association, as Weiss suggested, but only to those noncausal theories that would have predicted a nonspecific association. Thus, specificity can come into play when it can be logically deduced from the causal hypothesis in question and when nonspecificity can be logically deduced from one or more noncausal hypotheses.

Temporality

Temporality refers to the necessity that the cause precede the effect in time. This criterion is inarguable, insofar as any claimed observation of causation must involve the putative cause C preceding the putative effect D. It does *not,* however, follow that a reverse time order is evidence against the hypothesis that C can cause D. Rather, observations in which C followed D merely show that C could not have caused D in these instances; they provide no evidence for or against the hypothesis that C can cause D in those instances in which it precedes D. Only if it is found that C cannot precede D can we dispense with the causal hypothesis that C *could* cause D.

Biologic Gradient

Biologic gradient refers to the presence of a dose–response or exposure–response curve with an expected shape. Although Hill referred to a "linear" gradient, without specifying the scale, a linear gradient on one scale, such as the risk, can be distinctly nonlinear on another scale, such as the log risk, the odds, or the log odds. We might relax the expectation from linear to strictly monotonic (steadily increasing or decreasing) or even further merely to monotonic (a gradient that never changes direction). For example, more smoking means more carcinogen exposure and more tissue damage, hence more opportunity for carcinogenesis. Some causal associations, however, show a rapid increase in response (an approximate threshold effect) rather than a strictly monotonic trend. An example is the association between DES and adenocarcinoma of the vagina. A possible explanation is that the doses of DES that were administered were all sufficiently great to produce the maximum effect from DES. Under this hypothesis, for all those exposed to DES, the development of disease would depend entirely on other component causes.

The somewhat controversial topic of alcohol consumption and mortality is another example. Death rates are higher among nondrinkers than among moderate drinkers, but they ascend to the highest levels for heavy drinkers. There is considerable debate about which parts of the J-shaped dose–response curve are causally related to alcohol consumption and which parts are noncausal artifacts stemming from confounding or other biases. Some studies appear to find only an increasing relation between alcohol consumption and mortality, possibly because the categories of alcohol consumption are too broad to distinguish different rates among moderate drinkers and nondrinkers, or possibly because they have less confounding at the lower end of the consumption scale.

Associations that do show a monotonic trend in disease frequency with increasing levels of exposure are not necessarily causal. Confounding can result in a monotonic relation between a noncausal risk factor and disease if the confounding factor itself demonstrates a biologic gradient in its relation with disease. The relation between birth rank and Down syndrome mentioned earlier shows a strong biologic gradient that merely reflects the progressive relation between maternal age and occurrence of Down syndrome.

These issues imply that the existence of a monotonic association is neither necessary nor sufficient for a causal relation. A nonmonotonic relation only refutes those causal hypotheses specific enough to predict a monotonic dose–response curve.

Plausibility

Plausibility refers to the scientific plausibility of an association. More than any other criterion, this one shows how narrowly systems of causal criteria are focused on epidemiology. The starting point is an epidemiologic association. In asking whether it is causal or not, one of the considerations we take into account is its plausibility. From a less parochial perspective, the entire enterprise of causal inference would be viewed as the act of determining how plausible a causal *hypothesis* is. One of the considerations we would take into account would be epidemiologic associations, if they are available. Often they are not, but causal inference must be done nevertheless, with inputs from toxicology, pharmacology, basic biology, and other sciences.

Just as epidemiology is not essential for causal inference, plausibility can change with the times. Sartwell (1960) emphasized this point, citing remarks of Cheever in 1861, who had been commenting on the etiology of typhus before its mode of transmission (via body lice) was known:

> It could be no more ridiculous for the stranger who passed the night in the steerage of an emigrant ship to ascribe the typhus, which he there contracted, to the vermin with which bodies of the sick might be infested. An adequate cause, one reasonable in itself, must correct the coincidences of simple experience.

What was to Cheever an implausible explanation turned out to be the correct explanation, because it was indeed the vermin that caused the typhus infection. Such is the problem with plausibility: It is too often based not on logic or data, but only on prior beliefs. This is not to say that biologic knowledge should be discounted when a new hypothesis is being evaluated, but only to point out the difficulty in applying that knowledge.

The Bayesian approach to inference attempts to deal with this problem by requiring that one quantify, on a probability (0 to 1) scale, the certainty that one has in prior beliefs, as well as in new hypotheses. This quantification displays the dogmatism or open-mindedness of the analyst in a public fashion, with certainty values near 1 or 0 betraying a strong commitment of the analyst for or against a hypothesis. It can also provide a means of testing those quantified beliefs against new evidence (Howson and Urbach, 1993). Nevertheless, no approach can transform plausibility into an objective causal criterion.

Coherence

Taken from the U.S. Surgeon General's *Smoking and Health* (1964), the term *coherence* implies that a cause-and-effect interpretation for an association does not conflict with what is known of the natural history and biology of the disease. The examples Hill gave for coherence, such as the histopathologic effect of smoking on bronchial epithelium (in reference to the association between smoking and lung cancer) or the difference in lung cancer incidence by sex, could reasonably be considered examples of plausibility, as well as coherence; the distinction appears to be a fine one. Hill emphasized that the absence of coherent information, as distinguished, apparently, from the presence of conflicting information, should not be taken as evidence against an association being considered causal. On the other hand, the presence of conflicting information may indeed refute a hypothesis, but one must always remember that the conflicting information may be mistaken or misinterpreted. An example mentioned earlier is the "inhalation anomaly" in smoking and lung cancer, the fact that the excess of lung cancers seen among smokers seemed to be concentrated at sites in the upper airways of the lung. Several observers interpreted this anomaly as evidence that cigarettes were not responsible for the excess. Other observations, however, suggested that cigarette-borne carcinogens were deposited preferentially where the excess was observed, and so the anomaly was in fact consistent with a causal role for cigarettes (Wald, 1985).

Experimental Evidence

To different observers, experimental evidence can refer to clinical trials, to laboratory experiments with rodents or other nonhuman organisms, or to both. Evidence from human experiments, however, is seldom available for epidemiologic research questions, and animal evidence relates to different species and usually to levels of exposure very different from those that humans experience. Uncertainty in extrapolations from animals to humans often dominates the uncertainty of quantitative risk assessments (Freedman and Zeisel, 1988; Crouch et al., 1997).

To Hill, however, experimental evidence meant something else: the "experimental, or semi-experimental evidence" obtained from reducing or eliminating a putatively harmful exposure and seeing if the frequency of disease subsequently declines. He called this the strongest possible evidence of causality that can be obtained. It can be faulty, however, as the "semi-experimental" approach is nothing more than a "before-and-after" time trend analysis, which can be confounded or otherwise biased by a host of concomitant secular changes. Moreover, even if the removal of exposure does causally reduce the frequency of disease, it might not be for the etiologic reason hypothesized. The draining of a swamp near a city, for instance, would predictably and causally reduce the rate of yellow fever or malaria in that city the following summer. But it would be a mistake to call this observation the strongest possible evidence of a causal role of miasmas (Poole, 1999).

Analogy

Whatever insight might be derived from analogy is handicapped by the inventive imagination of scientists who can find analogies everywhere. At best, analogy provides a source of more elaborate hypotheses about the associations under study; absence of such analogies reflects only lack of imagination or experience, not falsity of the hypothesis.

We might find naive Hill's examples in which reasoning by analogy from the thalidomide and rubella tragedies made it more likely to him that other medicines and infections might cause other birth defects. But such reasoning is common; we suspect most people find it more credible that smoking might cause, say, stomach cancer, because of its associations, some widely accepted as causal, with cancers in other internal and gastrointestinal organs. Here we see how the analogy criterion can be at odds with either of the two specificity criteria. The more apt the analogy, the less specific are the effects of a cause or the less specific the causes of an effect.

Summary

As is evident, the standards of epidemiologic evidence offered by Hill are saddled with reservations and exceptions. Hill himself was ambivalent about their utility. He did not use the word *criteria* in the speech. He called them "viewpoints" or "perspectives." On the one hand, he asked, "In what circumstances can we pass from this observed *association* to a verdict of *causation*?" (emphasis in original). Yet, despite speaking of verdicts on causation, he disagreed that any "hard-and-fast rules of evidence" existed by which to judge causation: "None of my nine viewpoints can bring indisputable evidence for or against the cause-and-effect hypothesis and none can be required as a sine qua non" (Hill, 1965).

Actually, as noted above, the fourth viewpoint, temporality, is *a sine qua non* for causal explanations of observed associations. Nonetheless, it does not bear on the hypothesis that an exposure is capable of causing a disease in situations as yet unobserved (whether in the past or the future). For suppose every exposed case of disease ever reported had received the exposure after developing the disease. This reversed temporal relation would imply that exposure had not caused disease among these reported cases, and thus would refute the hypothesis that it had. Nonetheless, it would *not* refute the hypothesis that the exposure is *capable* of causing the disease, or that it had caused the disease in unobserved cases. It would mean only that we have no worthwhile epidemiologic evidence relevant to that hypothesis, for we had not yet seen what became of those exposed before disease occurred relative to those unexposed. Furthermore, what appears to be a causal sequence could represent reverse causation if preclinical symptoms of the disease lead to exposure, and then overt disease follows, as when patients in pain take analgesics, which may be the result of disease that is later diagnosed, rather than a cause.

Other than temporality, there is no necessary or sufficient criterion for determining whether an observed association is causal. Only when a causal hypothesis is elaborated to the extent that one can predict from it a particular form of consistency, specificity, biologic gradient, and so forth, can "causal criteria" come into play in evaluating causal hypotheses, and even then they do not come into play in evaluating the general hypothesis per se, but only some specific causal hypotheses, leaving others untested.

This conclusion accords with the views of Hume and many others that causal inferences cannot attain the certainty of logical deductions. Although some scientists continue to develop causal considerations as aids to inference (Susser, 1991), others argue that it is detrimental to cloud the inferential process by considering checklist criteria (Lanes and Poole, 1984). An intermediate, refutationist approach seeks to transform proposed criteria into deductive tests of causal hypotheses (Maclure, 1985; Weed, 1986). Such an approach helps avoid the temptation to use causal criteria simply to buttress pet theories at hand, and instead allows epidemiologists to focus on evaluating competing causal theories using crucial observations. Although this refutationist approach to causal inference may seem at odds with the common implementation of Hill's viewpoints, it actually seeks to answer the fundamental question posed by Hill, and the ultimate purpose of the viewpoints he promulgated:

> What [the nine viewpoints] can do, with greater or less strength, is to help us to make up our minds on the fundamental question—is there any other way of explaining the set of facts before us, is there any other answer equally, or more, likely than cause and effect? (Hill, 1965)

The crucial phrase "equally or more likely than cause and effect" suggests to us a subjective assessment of the certainty, or probability of the causal hypothesis at issue relative to another hypothesis. Although Hill wrote at a time when expressing uncertainty as a probability was unpopular in statistics, it appears from his statement that, for him, causal inference is a subjective matter of degree of personal belief, certainty, or conviction. In any event, this view is precisely that of subjective Bayesian statistics (Chapter 18).

It is unsurprising that case studies (e.g., Weed and Gorelick, 1996) and surveys of epidemiologists (Holman et al., 2001) show, contrary to the rhetoric that often attends invocations of causal criteria, that epidemiologists have *not* agreed on a set of causal criteria or on how to apply them. In one study in which epidemiologists were asked to employ causal criteria to fictional summaries of epidemiologic literatures, the agreement was only slightly greater than would have been expected by chance (Holman et al., 2001). The typical use of causal criteria is to make a case for a position for or against causality that has been arrived at by other, unstated means. Authors pick and choose among the criteria they deploy, and define and weight them in *ad hoc* ways that depend only on the exigencies of the discussion at hand. In this sense, causal criteria appear to function less like standards or principles and more like values (Poole, 2001b), which vary across individual scientists and even vary within the work of a single scientist, depending on the context and time. Thus universal and objective causal criteria, if they exist, have yet to be identified.

CHAPTER 3

Measures of Occurrence

Sander Greenland and Kenneth J. Rothman

Incidence Times 33
Incidence Rates 34
Person-Time and Population Time 34
Population and Individual Rates 34
Proper Interpretation of Incidence Rates 35
Rates of Recurrent Events 36
Types of Populations 36
Closed Populations 36
Open Populations 38
Populations versus Cohorts 38
Steady State 38
Relation of Incidence Rates to Incidence Times in Special Populations 39
Other Types of Rates 39
Incidence Proportions and Survival Proportions 40
Relations among Incidence Measures 41
Product-Limit Formula 42
Exponential Formula 43
Applications with Competing Risks 44
Relation of Survival Proportion to Average Incidence Time 45
Summary 45
Limitations and Generalizations of Basic Occurrence Measures 45
Prevalence 46
Use of Prevalence in Etiologic Research 46
Prevalence, Incidence, and Mean Duration 47
Average Age at Event 48
Standardization 49

In this chapter, we begin to address the basic elements, concepts, and tools of epidemiology. A good starting point is to define epidemiology. Unfortunately, there seem to be more definitions of epidemiology than there are epidemiologists. Some have defined it in terms of its methods. Although the methods of epidemiology may be distinctive, it is more typical to define a branch of science in terms of its subject matter rather than its tools. MacMahon and Pugh (1970) gave a widely cited definition, which we update slightly: Epidemiology is the study of the distribution and determinants of disease frequency in human populations. A similar subject-matter definition has been attributed to Gaylord Anderson (Cole, 1979), who defined epidemiology simply as the study of the *occurrence* of illness. Although reasonable distinctions can be made between the terms *disease* and *illness,* we shall treat them as synonyms here.

Recognizing the broad scope of epidemiology today, we may define epidemiology as the study of the distribution of health-related states and events in populations. With this definition we intend to capture not only disease and illness, but physiologic states such as blood pressure, psychologic measures such as depression score, and positive outcomes such as disease immunity. Other sciences, such as clinical medicine, are also directed toward the study of health and disease, but in epidemiology the focus is on population distributions.

The objective of much epidemiologic research is to obtain a valid and precise estimate of the effect of a potential cause on the occurrence of disease, which is often a binary (either/or) outcome such as "dead/alive." To achieve this objective, an epidemiologist must be able to measure the frequency of disease occurrence, either in absolute or in relative terms. We will focus on four basic measures of disease frequency. *Incidence times* are simply the times, after a common reference event, at which new cases of disease occur among population members. *Incidence rate* measures the occurrence of new cases of disease per unit of person-time. *Incidence proportion* measures the proportion of people who develop new disease during a specified period of time. *Prevalence,* a measure of status rather than of newly occurring disease, measures the proportion of people who have disease at a specific time. We will also discuss how these measures generalize to outcomes measured on a more complex scale than a dichotomy, such as lung function, lymphocyte count, or antibody titer. Finally, we will describe how measures can be *standardized* or averaged over population distributions of health-related factors to obtain summary occurrence measures.

INCIDENCE TIMES

In the attempt to measure the frequency of disease occurrence in a population, it is insufficient merely to record the number of people or the proportion of the population that is affected. It is also necessary to take into account the time elapsed before disease occurs, as well as the period of time during which events are counted. Consider the frequency of death. Because all people are eventually affected, the time from birth to death becomes the determining factor in the rate of occurrence of death. If, on average, death comes earlier to the members of one population than to members of another population, it is natural to say that the first population has a higher death rate than the second. Time is the factor that differentiates between the two situations shown in Figure 3–1.

In an epidemiologic study, we may measure the time of events in a person's life relative to any one of several reference events. Using age, for example, the reference event is birth, but we might instead use the start of a treatment or the start of an exposure as the reference event. The reference event may occur at a time that is unique to each person, as is the case with birth, but it could also be set to a common value, such as a day chosen from the calendar. The time of the reference event determines the time origin or *zero time* for measuring the timing of events.

Given an outcome event or "incident" of interest, a person's *incidence time* for this outcome is defined as the time span from zero time to the time at which the outcome event occurs, if it occurs. Synonyms for incidence time include *event time, failure time,* and *occurrence time.* A man who experienced his first myocardial infarction in 2000 at age 50 years has an incidence time of 2000 in (Western) calendar time and an incidence time of 50 in age time. A person's incidence time is undefined if that person never experiences the outcome event. There is a convention that classifies such a person as having an incidence time that is not specified exactly but is known to exceed the last time that the person could have experienced the outcome event. Under this convention, a woman who had a hysterectomy at age 45 years without ever having had endometrial cancer is classified as having an endometrial cancer incidence time that is unspecified but greater than age 45. It is then said that the hysterectomy *censored* the woman's endometrial cancer incidence at age 45 years.

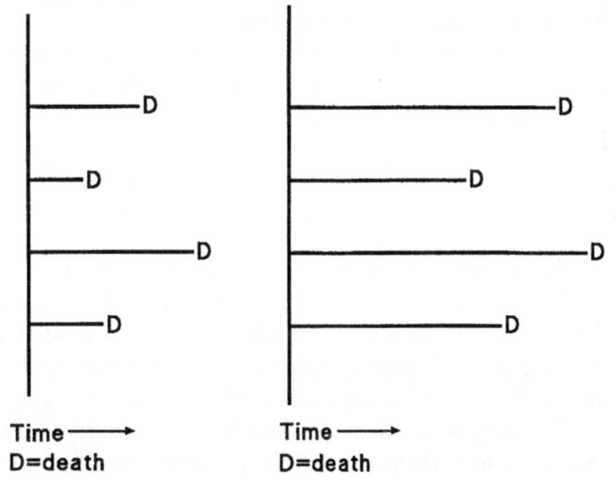

FIGURE 3–1 • Two different patterns of mortality.

There are many ways to summarize the distribution of incidence times in populations if there is no censoring. For example, one could look at the mean time, median time, and other summaries. Such approaches are commonly used with time to death, for which the average, or *life expectancy,* is a popular measure for comparing the health status of populations. If there is censoring, however, the summarization task becomes more complicated, and epidemiologists have traditionally turned to the concepts involving *person-time at risk* to deal with this situation.

The term *average age at death* deserves special attention, as it is sometimes used to denote life expectancy but is often used to denote an entirely different quantity, namely, the average age of those dying at a particular point in time. The latter quantity is more precisely termed the *cross-sectional* average age at death. The two quantities can be very far apart. Comparisons of cross-sectional average age at an event (such as death) can be quite misleading when attempting to infer causes of the event. We shall discuss these problems later on in this chapter.

INCIDENCE RATES

PERSON-TIME AND POPULATION TIME

Epidemiologists often study outcome events that are not inevitable or that may not occur during the period of observation. In such situations, the set of incidence times for a specific event in a population will not all be precisely defined or observed. One way to deal with this complication is to develop measures that account for the length of time each individual was in the *population at risk* for the event, that is, the period of time during which the event was a possibility and would have been counted as an event in the population, had it occurred. This length or span of time is called the *person-time* contribution of the individual.

The sum of these person-times over all population members is called the total *person-time at risk* or the *population-time at risk*. This total person-time should be distinguished from clock time in that it is a summation of time that occurs simultaneously for many people, whereas clock time is not. The total person-time at risk merely represents the total of all time during which disease onsets could occur and would be considered events occurring in the population of interest.

POPULATION AND INDIVIDUAL RATES

We define the *incidence rate* of the population as the number of new cases of disease (incident number) divided by the person-time over the period:

$$\text{Incidence rate} = \frac{\text{number of disease onsets}}{\sum_{\text{persons}} \text{time spent in population}}$$

This rate has also been called the *person-time rate, incidence density, force of morbidity* (or *force of mortality* in reference to deaths), *hazard rate,* and *disease intensity,* although the latter three terms are more commonly used to refer to the theoretical limit approached by an incidence rate as the unit of time measure approaches zero.

When the risk period is of fixed length Δt, the proportion of the period that a person spends in the population at risk is their amount of person-time divided by Δt. It follows that the average size of the population over the period is

$$\overline{N} = \sum_{\text{persons}} \frac{\text{time spent in population}}{\Delta t}$$

Hence, the total person-time at risk over the period is equal to the product of the average size of the population over the period, $\overline{N}$, and the fixed length of the risk period, Δt. If we denote the incident number by A, it follows that the incidence rate equals $A/(\overline{N} \cdot \Delta t)$. This formulation shows that the incidence rate has units of inverse time (per year, per month, per day, etc.). The units attached to an incidence rate can thus be written as year^{-1}, month^{-1}, or day^{-1}.

The only outcome events eligible to be counted in the numerator of an incidence rate are those that occur to persons who are contributing time to the denominator of the incidence rate at the time that the disease onset occurs. Likewise, only time contributed by persons eligible to be counted in the numerator if they suffer such an event should be counted in the denominator.

Another way of expressing a population incidence rate is as a time-weighted average of individual rates. An individual rate is either 0/(time spent in population) = 0, if the individual does not experience the event, or else 1/(time spent in the population) if the individual does experience the event. We then have that the number of disease onsets A is

$$A = \sum_{\text{persons}} (\text{time spent in poplation})\,(\text{individual rate})$$

and so

$$\text{Incidence rate} = \sum_{\text{persons}} (\text{time spent in population})\,(\text{individual rate}) \Big/ \sum_{\text{persons}} \text{time spent in population}$$

This formulation shows that the incidence rate ignores the distinction between individuals who do not contribute to the incident number A because they were in the population only briefly, and those who do not contribute because they were in the population a long time but never got the disease (e.g., immune individuals). In this sense, the incidence rate deals with the censoring problem by ignoring potentially important distinctions among those who do *not* get the disease.

Although the notion of an incidence rate is a central one in epidemiology, the preceding formulation shows it cannot capture all aspects of disease occurrence. This limitation is also shown by noting that a rate of 1 case/(100 years) = 0.01 year^{-1} could be obtained by following 100 people for an average of 1 year and observing one case, but it could also be obtained by following two people for 50 years and observing one case, a very different scenario. To distinguish these situations, more detailed measures of occurrence are also needed, such as incidence time.

PROPER INTERPRETATION OF INCIDENCE RATES

Apart from insensitivity to important distinctions, incidence rates have interpretational difficulties insofar as they are often confused with risks (probabilities). This confusion arises when one fails to account for the dependence of the numeric portion of a rate on the units used for its expression.

The numeric portion of an incidence rate has a lower bound of zero and no upper bound, which is the range for the ratio of a non-negative quantity to a positive quantity. The two quantities are the number of events in the numerator and the person-time in the denominator. It may be surprising that an incidence rate can exceed the value of 1, which would seem to indicate that more than 100% of a population is affected. It is true that at most 100% of persons in a population can get a disease, but the incidence rate does not measure the proportion of a population that gets disease, and in fact it is not a proportion at all. Recall that incidence rate is measured in units of the reciprocal of time. Among 100 people, no more than 100 deaths can occur, but those 100 deaths can occur in 10,000 person-years, in 1,000 person-years, in 100 person-years, or in 1 person-year (if the 100 deaths occur after an average of 3.65 days each, as in a military engagement). An incidence rate of 100 cases (or deaths) per 1 person-year might be expressed as

$$100\,\frac{\text{cases}}{\text{person-year}}$$

It might also be expressed as

$$10{,}000\,\frac{\text{cases}}{\text{person-century}}$$

$$8.33\,\frac{\text{cases}}{\text{person-month}}$$

$$1.92\,\frac{\text{cases}}{\text{person-week}}$$

$$0.27\,\frac{\text{cases}}{\text{person-day}}$$

The numeric value of an incidence rate in itself has no interpretability because it depends on the selection of the time unit. It is thus essential in presenting incidence rates to give the time unit used to calculate the numeric portion. That unit is usually chosen to ensure that the minimum rate has at least one digit to the left of the decimal place. For example, a table of incidence rates of 0.15, 0.04, and 0.009 cases per person-year might be multiplied by 1,000 to be displayed as 150, 40, and 9 cases per 1,000 person-years. One can use a unit as large as 1,000 person-years regardless of whether the observations were collected over 1 year of time, over 1 week of time, or over a decade, just as one can measure the speed of a vehicle in terms of kilometers per hour even if the speed is measured for only a few seconds.

RATES OF RECURRENT EVENTS

Incidence rates often include only the first occurrence of disease onset as an eligible event for the numerator of the rate. For the many diseases that are irreversible states, such as multiple sclerosis, cirrhosis, or death, there is at most only one onset that a person can experience. For some diseases that do recur, such as rhinitis, we may simply wish to measure the incidence of "first" occurrence, or first occurrence after a prespecified disease-free period, even though the disease can occur repeatedly. For other diseases, such as cancer or heart disease, the first occurrence is often of greater interest for etiologic study than subsequent occurrences in the same person, because the first occurrence or its medical therapies affect the rate of subsequent occurrences. Therefore, it is typical that the events in the numerator of an incidence rate correspond to the first occurrence of a particular disease, even in those instances in which it is possible for a person to have more than one occurrence. In this book, we will assume we are dealing with first occurrences, except when stated otherwise. As explained later on, the approaches for first occurrences extend naturally to subsequent occurrences by restricting the population at risk based on past occurrence.

When the events tallied in the numerator of an incidence rate are first occurrences of disease, then the time contributed by each person in whom the disease develops should terminate with the onset of disease. The reason is that the person is no longer eligible to experience the event (the first occurrence can occur only once per person), so there is no more information about first occurrence to obtain from continued observation of that person. Thus, each person who experiences the outcome event should contribute time to the denominator until the occurrence of the event, but not afterward. Furthermore, for the study of first occurrences, the number of disease onsets in the numerator of the incidence rate is also a count of people experiencing the event, because only one event can occur per person.

An epidemiologist who wishes to study both first and subsequent occurrences of disease may decide not to distinguish between first and later occurrences and simply count all the events that occur among the population under observation. If so, then the time accumulated in the denominator of the rate would not cease with the occurrence of the outcome event, because an additional event might occur in the same person. Usually, however, there is enough of a biologic distinction between first and subsequent occurrences to warrant measuring them separately. One approach is to define the "population at risk" differently for each occurrence of the event: The population at risk for the first event would consist of persons who have not experienced the disease before; the population at risk for the second event (which is the first recurrence) would be limited to those who have experienced the event once and only once, etc. Thus, studies of second cancers are restricted to the population of those who survived their first cancer. A given person should contribute time to the denominator of the incidence rate for first events only until the time that the disease first occurs. At that point, the person should cease contributing time to the denominator of that rate and should now begin to contribute time to the denominator of the rate measuring the second occurrence. If and when there is a second event, the person should stop contributing time to the rate measuring the second occurrence and begin contributing to the denominator of the rate measuring the third occurrence, and so forth.

TYPES OF POPULATIONS

CLOSED POPULATIONS

Given a particular time scale for displaying incidence, we may distinguish populations according to whether they are *closed* or *open* on that scale. A closed population adds no new members over

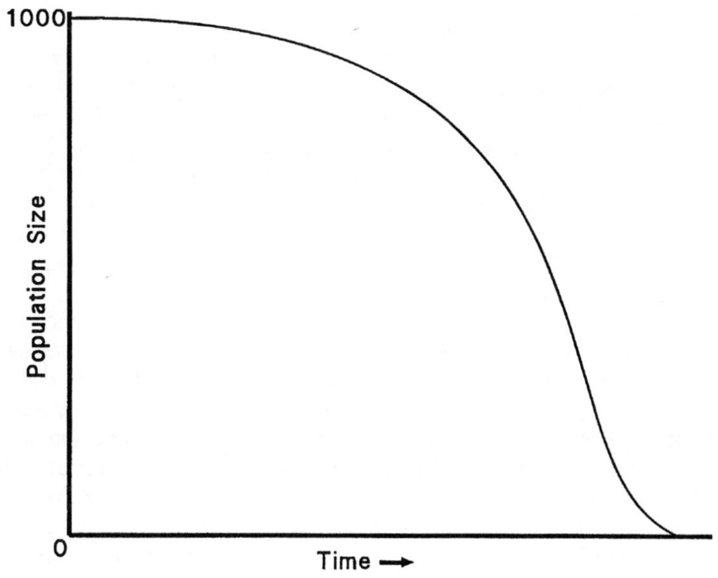

FIGURE 3–2 • Size of a closed population of 1,000 people, by time.

time and loses members only to death, whereas an open population may gain members over time, through immigration or birth, or lose members who are still alive through emigration, or both. (Some demographers and ecologists use a broader definition of a closed population in which births, but not immigration or emigration, are allowed.) Members of the population can leave this population only by dying.

Suppose we graph the survival experience of a closed population that starts with 1,000 people. Because death eventually claims everyone, after a period of sufficient time the original 1,000 will have dwindled to zero. A graph of the size of the population with time might approximate that in Figure 3–2. The curve slopes downward because as the 1,000 persons in the population die, the population at risk of death is reduced. The population is closed in the sense that we consider the fate of only the 1,000 persons present at time zero. The person-time experience of these 1,000 persons is represented by the area under the curve in the diagram. As each person dies, the curve notches downward; that person no longer contributes to the person-time denominator of the death (mortality) rate. Each person's contribution is exactly equal to the length of time that person is followed from start to finish. In this example, because the entire population is followed until death, the finish is the person's death. In other instances, the contribution to the person-time experience would continue until either the onset of disease or some arbitrary cutoff time for observation, whichever came sooner.

Suppose we added up the total person-time experience of this closed population of 1,000 and obtained a total of 75,000 person-years. The death rate would be $(1{,}000/75{,}000) \times \text{year}^{-1}$, because the 75,000 person-years represent the experience of all 1,000 people until their deaths. Furthermore, if time is measured from start of follow-up, the average death time in this closed population would be 75,000 person-years/1,000 persons = 75 years, which is the inverse of the death rate.

A closed population experiencing a constant death rate over time would decline in size exponentially (which is what is meant by the term *exponential decay*). In practice, however, death rates for a closed population change with time, because the population is aging as time progresses. Consequently, the decay curve of a closed human population is never exponential. *Life-table methodology* is a procedure by which the death rate (or disease rate) of a closed population is evaluated within successive small age or time intervals, so that the age or time dependence of mortality can be elucidated. With any method, however, it is important to distinguish age-related effects from those related to other time axes, because each person's age increases directly with an increase along any other time axis. For example, a person's age increases with increasing duration of employment, increasing calendar time, and increasing time from start of follow-up.

OPEN POPULATIONS

An open population differs from a closed population in that the population at risk is open to new members who did not qualify for the population initially. An example of an open population is the population of a country. People can enter an open population through various mechanisms. Some may be born into it; others may migrate into it. For an open population of people who have attained a specific age, persons can become eligible to enter the population by aging into it. Similarly, persons can exit by dying, aging out of a defined age group, emigrating, or becoming diseased (the latter method of exiting applies only if first bouts of a disease are being studied). Persons may also exit from an open population and then re-enter, for example by emigrating from the geographic area in which the population is located, and later moving back to that area.

The distinction between closed and open populations depends in part on the time axis used to describe the population, as well as on how membership is defined. All persons who ever used a particular drug would constitute a closed population if time is measured from start of their use of the drug. These persons would, however, constitute an open population in calendar time, because new users might accumulate over a period of time. If, as in this example, membership in the population always starts with an event such as initiation of treatment and never ends thereafter, the population is closed along the time axis that marks this event as zero time for each member, because all new members enter only when they experience this event. The same population will, however, be open along most other time axes. If membership can be terminated by later events other than death, the population is an open one along any time axis.

By the above definitions, any study population with loss to follow-up is open. For example, membership in a study population might be defined in part by being under active surveillance for disease; in that case, members who are lost to follow-up have by definition left the population, even if they are still alive and would otherwise be considered eligible for study. It is common practice to analyze such populations using time from start of observation, an axis along which no immigration can occur (by definition, time zero is when the person enters the study). Such populations may be said to be "closed on the left," and are often called "fixed cohorts," although the term *cohort* is often used to refer to a different concept, which we discuss in the following.

POPULATIONS VERSUS COHORTS

The term *population* as we use it here has an intrinsically temporal and potentially dynamic element: One can be a member at one time, not a member at a later time, a member again, and so on. This usage is the most common sense of population, as with the population of a town or country. The term *cohort* is sometimes used to describe any study population, but we reserve it for a more narrow concept, that of a group of persons for whom membership is defined in a permanent fashion, or a population in which membership is determined entirely by a single defining event and so becomes permanent. An example of a cohort would be the members of the graduating class of a school in a given year. The list of cohort members is fixed at the time of graduation, and will not increase. Other examples include the cohort of all persons who ever used a drug, and the cohort of persons recruited for a follow-up study. In the latter case, the study population may begin with all the cohort members but may gradually dwindle to a small subset of that cohort as those initially recruited are lost to follow-up. Those lost to follow-up remain members of the initial-recruitment cohort, even though they are no longer in the study population. With this definition, the members of any cohort constitute a closed population along the time axis in which the defining event (e.g., birth with Down syndrome, or study recruitment) is taken as zero time. A *birth cohort* is the cohort defined in part by being born at a particular time, e.g., all persons born in Ethiopia in 1990 constitute the Ethiopian birth cohort for 1990.

STEADY STATE

If the number of people entering a population is balanced by the number exiting the population in any period of time within levels of age, sex, and other determinants of risk, the population is said to be *stationary,* or in a *steady state.* Steady state is a property that can occur only in open populations, not closed populations. It is, however, possible to have a population in steady state in which no immigration or emigration is occurring; this situation would require that births perfectly balance

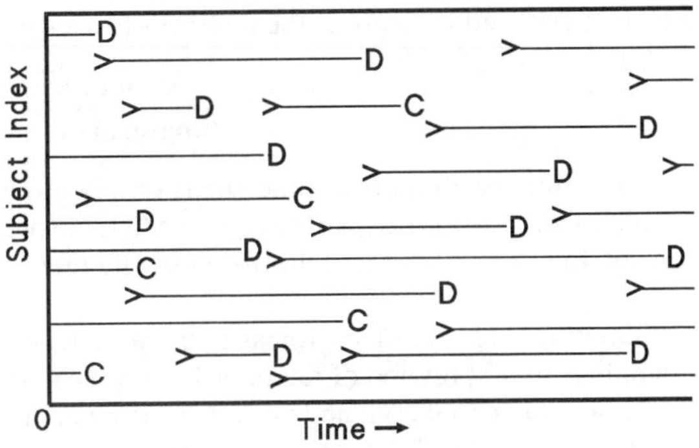

FIGURE 3–3 • Composition of an open population in approximate steady state, by time; > indicates entry into the population, D indicates disease onset, and C indicates exit from the population without disease.

deaths in the population. The graph of the size of an open population in steady state is simply a horizontal line. People are continually entering and leaving the population in a way that might be diagrammed as shown in Figure 3–3.

In the diagram, the symbol > represents a person entering the population, a line segment represents his or her person-time experience, and the termination of a line segment represents the end of his or her experience. A terminal D indicates that the experience ended because of disease onset, and a terminal C indicates that the experience ended for other reasons. In theory, any time interval will provide a good estimate of the incidence rate in a stationary population.

RELATION OF INCIDENCE RATES TO INCIDENCE TIMES IN SPECIAL POPULATIONS

The reciprocal of time is an awkward concept that does not provide an intuitive grasp of an incidence rate. The measure does, however, have a close connection to more interpretable measures of occurrence in closed populations. Referring to Figure 3–2, one can see that the area under the curve is equal to $N \times T$, where N is the number of people starting out in the closed population and T is the average time until death. The time-averaged death rate is then $N/(N \times T) = 1/T$; that is, the death rate equals the reciprocal of the average time until death.

In a stationary population with no migration, the crude incidence rate of an inevitable outcome such as death will equal the reciprocal of the average time spent in the population until the outcome occurs (Morrison, 1979). Thus, in a stationary population with no migration, a death rate of 0.04 year^{-1} would translate to an average time from entry until death of 25 years. Similarly, in stationary population with no migration, the cross-sectional average age at death will equal the life expectancy. The time spent in the population until the outcome occurs is sometimes referred to as the *waiting time* until the event occurs, and it corresponds to the incidence time when time is measured from entry into the population.

If the outcome of interest is not death but either disease onset or death from a specific cause, the average-time interpretation must be modified to account for *competing risks,* which are events that "compete" with the outcome of interest to remove persons from the population at risk. Even if there is no competing risk, the interpretation of incidence rates as the inverse of the average waiting time will usually not be valid if there is migration (such as loss to follow up), and average age at death will no longer equal the life expectancy. For example, the death rate for the United States in 1977 was 0.0088 year^{-1}. In a steady state, this rate would correspond to a mean lifespan, or expectation of life, of 114 years. Other analyses, however, indicate that the actual expectation of life in 1977 was 73 years (Alho, 1992). The discrepancy is a result of immigration and to the lack of a steady state. Note that the no-migration assumption cannot hold within specific age groups, for people are always "migrating" in and out of age groups as they age.

OTHER TYPES OF RATES

In addition to numbers of cases per unit of person-time, it is sometimes useful to examine numbers of events per other unit. In health services and infectious-disease epidemiology, epidemic curves are often depicted in terms of the number of cases per unit time, also called the *absolute rate,*

$$\frac{\text{no. of disease onsets}}{\text{time span of observation}}$$

or $A/\Delta t$. Because the person-time rate is simply this absolute rate divided by the average size of the population over the time span, or $A/(\overline{N} \cdot \Delta t)$, the person-time rate has been called the *relative rate* (Elandt-Johnson, 1975); it is the absolute rate relative to or "adjusted for" the average population size.

Sometimes it is useful to express event rates in units that do not involve time directly. A common example is the expression of fatalities by travel modality in terms of passenger-miles, whereby the safety of commercial train and air travel can be compared. Here, person-miles replace person-time in the denominator of the rate. Like rates with time in the denominator, the numerical portion of such rates is completely dependent on the choice of measurement units; a rate of 1.6 deaths per 10^6 passenger-miles equals a rate of 1 death per 10^6 passenger-kilometers.

The concept central to precise usage of the term *incidence rate* is that of expressing the change in incident number relative to the change in another quantity, so that the incidence rate always has a dimension. Thus, a person-time rate expresses the increase in the incident number we expect per unit increase in person-time. An absolute rate expresses the increase in incident number we expect per unit increase in clock time, and a passenger-mile rate expresses the increase in incident number we expect per unit increase in passenger miles.

INCIDENCE PROPORTIONS AND SURVIVAL PROPORTIONS

Within a given interval of time, we can also express the incident number of cases in relation to the size of the population at risk. If we measure population size at the start of a time interval and no one enters the population (immigrates) or leaves alive (emigrates) after the start of the interval, such a rate becomes the proportion of people who become cases among those in the population at the start of the interval. We call this quantity the *incidence proportion,* which may also be defined as the proportion of a closed population at risk that becomes diseased within a given period of time. This quantity is sometimes called the *cumulative incidence,* but that term is also used for another quantity we will discuss later. A more traditional term for incidence proportion is *attack rate,* but we reserve the term *rate* for person-time incidence rates.

If *risk* is defined as the probability that disease develops in a person within a specified time interval, then incidence proportion is a measure, or estimate, of average risk. Although this concept of risk applies to individuals whereas incidence proportion applies to populations, incidence proportion is sometimes called risk. This usage is consistent with the view that individual risks merely refer to the relative frequency of disease in a group of individuals like the one under discussion. *Average risk* is a more accurate synonym, one that we will sometimes use.

Another way of expressing the incidence proportion is as a simple average of the individual proportions. The latter is either 0 for those who do not have the event or 1 for those who do have the event. The number of disease onsets A is then a sum of the individual proportions,

$$A = \sum_{\text{persons}} \text{individual proportions}$$

and so

$$\text{Incidence proportion} = \frac{\sum_{\text{persons}} \text{individual proportions}}{\text{initial size of the population}} = A/N$$

If one calls the individual proportions the "individual risks," this formulation shows another sense in which the incidence proportion is also an "average risk." It also makes clear that the incidence proportion ignores the amount of person-time contributed by individuals and so ignores even more information than does the incidence rate, although it has a more intuitive interpretation.

Like any proportion, the value of an incidence proportion ranges from 0 to 1 and is dimensionless. It is not interpretable, however, without specification of the time period to which it applies. An incidence proportion of death of 3% means something very different when it refers to a 40-year period than when it refers to a 40-day period.

A useful complementary measure to the incidence proportion is the *survival proportion,* which may be defined as the proportion of a closed population at risk that does *not* become diseased within a given period of time. If R and S denote the incidence and survival proportions, then $S = 1 - R$. Another measure that is commonly used is the *incidence odds,* defined as $R/S = R/(1 - R)$, the ratio of the proportion getting the disease to the proportion not getting the disease. If R is small, $S \approx 1$ and $R/S \approx R$; that is, the incidence odds will approximate the incidence proportion when both quantities are small. Otherwise, because $S < 1$, the incidence odds will be greater than the incidence proportion and, unlike the latter, it may exceed 1.

For sufficiently short time intervals, there is a very simple relation between the incidence proportion and the incidence rate of a nonrecurring event. Consider a closed population over an interval t_0 to t_1, and let $\Delta t = t_1 - t_0$ be the length of the interval. If N is the size of the population at t_0 and A is the number of disease onsets over the interval, then the incidence and survival proportions over the interval are $R = A/N$ and $S = (N - A)/N$. Now suppose the time interval is short enough that the size of the population at risk declines only slightly over the interval. Then, $N - A \approx N$, $S \approx 1$, and so $R/S \approx R$. Furthermore, the average size of the population at risk will be approximately N, so the total person-time at risk over the interval will be approximately $N\Delta t$. Thus, the incidence rate (I) over the interval will be approximately $A/N\Delta t$, and we obtain

$$R = A/N = (A/N\Delta t)\Delta t \approx I\Delta t \quad \text{and} \quad R \approx R/S$$

In words, the incidence proportion, incidence odds, and the quantity $I\Delta t$ will all approximate one another if the population at risk declines only slightly over the interval. We can make this approximation hold to within an accuracy of $1/N$ by making Δt so short that no more than one person leaves the population at risk over the interval. Thus, given a sufficiently short time interval, one can simply multiply the incidence rate by the time period to approximate the incidence proportion. This approximation offers another interpretation for the incidence rate: It can be viewed as the limiting value of the ratio of the average risk to the duration of time at risk as the latter duration approaches zero.

A specific type of incidence proportion is the *case fatality rate,* or *case fatality ratio,* which is the incidence proportion of death among those in whom an illness develops (it is therefore not a rate in our sense, but a proportion). The time period for measuring the case fatality rate is often unstated, but it is always better to specify it.

RELATIONS AMONG INCIDENCE MEASURES

Disease occurrence in a population reflects two aspects of individual experiences: the amount of time the individual is at risk in the population, and whether the individual actually has the focal event (e.g., gets disease) during that time. Different incidence measures summarize different aspects of the distribution of these experiences. Average incidence time is the average time until an event and incidence proportion is the average "risk" of the event (where "risk" is 1 or 0 according to whether or not the event occurred in the risk period). Each is easy to grasp intuitively, but they are often not easy to estimate or even to define. In contrast, the incidence rate can be applied to the common situation in which the time at risk and the occurrence of the event can be unambiguously determined for everyone. Unfortunately, it can be difficult to comprehend correctly what the rate is telling us about the different dimensions of event distributions, and so it is helpful to understand its relation to incidence times and incidence proportions. These relations are a central component of the topics of survival analysis and failure-time analysis in statistics (Kalbfleisch and Prentice, 2002; Cox and Oakes, 1984).

There are relatively simple relations between the incidence proportion of an inevitable, nonrecurring event (such as death) and the incidence rate in a closed population. To illustrate them, we will consider the small closed population shown in Figure 3–4. The time at risk (risk history) of each member is graphed in order from the shortest on top to the longest at the bottom. Each history either ends with a D, indicating the occurrence of the event of interest, or ends at the end of the follow-up, at $t_5 = 19$. The starting time is denoted t_0 and is here equal to 0. Each time that one or more events occur is marked by a vertical dashed line, the unique event times are denoted by t_1 (the

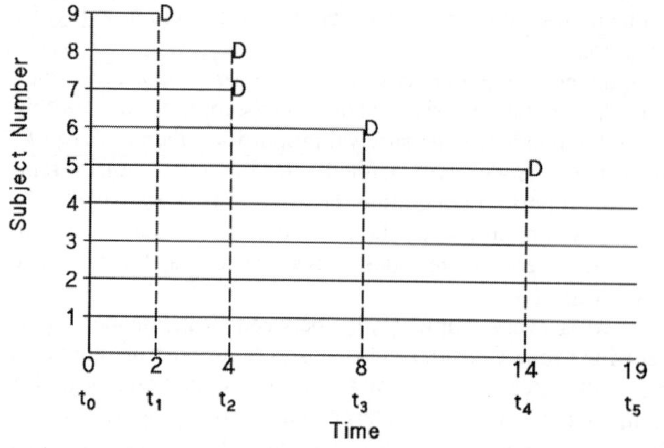

FIGURE 3–4 • Example of a small closed population with end of follow-up at 19 years.

earliest) to t_4, and the end of follow-up is denoted by t_5. We denote the number of events at time t_k by A_k, the total number of persons at risk at time t_k (including the A_k people who experience the event) by N_k, and the number of people alive at the end of follow-up by N_5.

PRODUCT-LIMIT FORMULA

Table 3–1 shows the history of the population over the 20-year follow-up period in Figure 3–4, in terms of t_k, A_k, and N_k. Note that because the population is closed and the event is inevitable, the number remaining at risk after t_k, N_{k+1}, is equal to $N_k - A_k$, which is the number at risk up to t_k minus the number experiencing the event at t_k. The proportion of the population remaining at risk up to t_k that also remains at risk after t_k is thus

$$s_k = \frac{N_k - A_k}{N_k} = \frac{N_{k+1}}{N_k}$$

We can now see that the proportion of the original population that remains at risk at the end of follow-up is

$$S = N_5/N_1 = (N_5/N_4)(N_4/N_3)(N_3/N_2)(N_2/N_1) = s_4 s_3 s_2 s_1$$

which for Table 3–1 yields

$$\text{S} = (4/5)(5/6)(6/8)(8/9) = 4/9$$

TABLE 3–1

Event Times and Intervals for the Closed Population in Figure 3–4

	Start	Outcome Event Times (t_k)				End
	0	**2**	**4**	**8**	**14**	**19**
Index (*k*)	0	1	2	3	4	5
No. of outcome events (A_k)	0	1	2	1	1	0
No. at risk (N_k)	9	9	8	6	5	4
Proportion surviving (S_k)		8/9	6/8	5/6	4/5	4/4
Length of interval (Δt_k)		2	2	4	6	5
Person-time ($N_k \Delta t_k$)		18	16	24	30	20
Incidence rate (I_k)		1/18	2/16	1/24	1/30	0/20

This multiplication formula says that the survival proportion over the whole time interval in Figure 3–4 is just the product of the survival proportions for every subinterval t_{k-1} to t_k. In its more general form,

$$S = \prod_{k=1}^{5} \frac{N_k - A_k}{N_k} \qquad [3\text{–}1]$$

This multiplication formula is called the *Kaplan-Meier* or *product-limit* formula (Kalbfleisch and Prentice, 2002; Cox and Oakes, 1984).

EXPONENTIAL FORMULA

Now let T_k be the total person-time at risk in the population over the subinterval from t_{k-1} to t_k, and let $\Delta t_k = t_k - t_{k-1}$ be the length of the subinterval. Because the population is of constant size N_k over this subinterval and everyone still present contributes Δt_k person-time units at risk, the total person-time at risk in the interval is $N_k \Delta t_k$, so that the incidence rate in the time following t_{k-1} up through (but not beyond) t_k is

$$I_k = \frac{A_k}{N_k \Delta t_k}$$

But the incidence proportion over the same subinterval is equal to $I_k \Delta t_k$, so the survival proportion over the subinterval is

$$s_k = 1 - I_k \Delta t_k$$

Thus, we can substitute $1 - I_k \Delta t_k$ for s_k in the earlier equation for S, the overall survival proportion, to get

$$\begin{aligned} S &= (1 - I_5\Delta t_5)(1 - I_4\Delta t_4)(1 - I_3\Delta t_3)(1 - I_2\Delta t_2)(1 - I_1\Delta t_1) \\ &= [1 - (0)5][1 - (1/30)6][1 - (1/24)4][1 - (2/16)2][1 - (1/18)2] \\ &= 4/9 \end{aligned}$$

as before.

If each of the subinterval incidence proportions $I_k \Delta t_k$ is small (<0.10 or so), we can simplify the last formula by using the fact that, for small x,

$$1 - x \approx \exp(-x)$$

Taking $x = I_k \Delta t_k$ in this approximation formula, we get $1 - I_k t_k \approx \exp(-I_k \Delta t_k)$, and so

$$\begin{aligned} S &\approx \exp(-I_5\Delta t_5)\exp(-I_4\Delta t_4)\cdots\exp(-I_1\Delta t_1) \\ &= \exp(-I_5\Delta t_5 - I_4\Delta t_4 - \cdots - I_1\Delta t_1) \\ &= \exp\left(-\sum_{k=1}^{5} I_k \Delta t_k\right) \end{aligned}$$

which for Table 3–1 yields

$$\exp[-0(5) - (1/30)6 - (1/24)4 - (2/16)2 - (1/18)2] = 0.483$$

not too far from the earlier value of $4/9 = 0.444$. Finally, we use the fact that the incidence proportion for the whole period is $1 - S$ to get

$$R = 1 - S \approx 1 - \exp\left(-\sum_{k=1}^{5} I_k \Delta t_k\right) \qquad [3\text{–}2]$$

The last formula is cited in many textbooks and is sometimes called the *exponential formula* for relating rates and incidence proportions. The sum in the exponent, $\sum_k I_k \Delta t_k$, is sometimes called the *cumulative incidence* (Breslow and Day, 1980) or *cumulative hazard* (Kalbfleisch and Prentice, 2002; Cox and Oakes, 1984). Confusingly, the term *cumulative incidence* is more often used to denote the incidence proportion. The cumulative hazard, although unitless, is *not* a proportion and will exceed 1.0 when the incidence proportion exceeds $1 - e^{-1} = 0.632$.

We wish to emphasize the assumptions we used to derive the exponential formula in equation 3–2:

1. The population is closed.
2. The event under study is inevitable (there is no competing risk).
3. The number of events A_k at each event time t_k is a small proportion of the number at risk N_k at that time (i.e., A_k/N_k is always small).

If the population is not very small, we can almost always force assumption 3 to hold by measuring time so finely that every event occurs at its own unique time (so that only one event occurs at each t_k). In Table 3–1, the discrepancy between the true R of $5/9 = 0.555$ and the exponential formula value of $1 - 0.483 = 0.517$ is rather small considering that A_k/N_k gets as large as $2/8 = 0.25$ (at t_2).

Assumptions 1 and 2 were also used to derive the product-limit formula in equation 3–1. These assumptions are rarely satisfied, yet they are often overlooked in presentations and applications of the formulas. Some form of the closed-population assumption (no. 1) is essential because the incidence proportion is defined only with reference to closed populations. A major use of the product-limit and exponential formulas is, however, in translating incidence-rate estimates from open populations into incidence-proportion estimates for a closed population of interest. By assuming that the incidence rates in the two populations are the same at each time, one can justify substituting the survival proportions $(N_k - A_k)/N_k$ or the incidence rates observed in the open population into the product-limit formula or the exponential formula. This assumption is often plausible when the open population one observes is a subset of the closed population of interest, as in a cohort study with losses to follow-up that are unrelated to risk.

APPLICATIONS WITH COMPETING RISKS

When competing risks remove persons from the population at risk, application of the product-limit and exponential formulas requires new concepts and assumptions. Consider the subinterval-specific incidence rates for our closed population of interest. When competing risks are present, the product-limit formula in equation 3–1 for the survival proportion S no longer holds, because competing risks may remove additional people between disease onset times, in which case N_{k+1} will be smaller than $N_k - A_k$. Also, when competing risks occur between t_{k-1} and t_k, the population size will not be constant over the subinterval. Consequently, the person-time in interval k will not equal $N_k \Delta t_k$ and $I_k \Delta t_k$ will not equal A_k/N_k. Thus, the exponential formula of equation 3–2 will not hold if competing risks occur. The amount of error will depend on the frequency of the events that are the competing risks.

We can, however, ask the following question: What would the incidence proportion over the total interval have been if no competing risk had occurred? This quantity is sometimes called the *conditional risk* of the outcome (conditioned on removal of competing risks). One minus the product-limit formula of equation 3–1 gives an estimate of this quantity under the assumption that the subinterval-specific incidence rates would not change if no competing risk occurred (*independent competing risks*). One minus the exponential formula of equation 3–2 remains an approximation to it if A_k/N_k is always small. The assumption that the rates would not change if competing risks were removed is made by almost all survival-analysis methods for estimating conditional risks, but it requires careful scrutiny. Under conditions that would eliminate competing risks, the incidence rates of the outcome under study may be likely to change. Suppose, for example, that the outcome of interest is colon cancer. Competing risks would include deaths from any causes other than colon cancer. Removal of so many risks would be virtually impossible, but an attempt to minimize them might involve dietary interventions to prevent deaths from other cancers and from heart disease. If these interventions were effective, they might also lower colon cancer rates, thus violating the assumption that the specific rates would not change if no competing risk occurred.

Because of the impracticality of removing competing risks without altering rates of the study disease, many authors caution against interpreting survival estimates based on statistical removal of competing risks as the incidence that would actually occur upon removal of competing risks (Cox and Oakes, 1984; Prentice and Kalbfleisch, 1988; Pepe and Mori, 1993; Kalbfleisch and Prentice, 2002; Greenland, 2002a, 2005a; Alberti et al., 2003). An arguably more practical approach is to focus on the risk (probability) of the outcome without removing competing risks, sometimes called the "unconditional risk." This quantity is estimable with no assumption about competing-risk removal (Benichou and Gail, 1990a; Pepe and Mori, 1993; Gooley et al., 1999; Kalbfleisch and Prentice, 2002).

A more defensible use of the product-limit formula is to estimate survival proportions in the presence of censoring (e.g., loss to follow-up); see Chapter 16 for details. For this usage, the assumption is made that the censoring is random (e.g., the experience of lost subjects differs only randomly from that of subjects not lost). This assumption is often questionable but is addressable in the design and analysis of a study via measurement and adjustment for factors that affect censoring and the outcome event (Kalbfleisch and Prentice, 2002).

RELATION OF SURVIVAL PROPORTION TO AVERAGE INCIDENCE TIME

Returning now to the simpler situation of an inevitable nonrecurring outcome in a closed population, we will derive an equation relating survival proportions to average incidence time. First, we may write the total person-time at risk over the total interval in Figure 3–4 as

$$N_1\Delta t_1 + \ldots + N_5\Delta t_5 = \sum_{k=1}^{5} N_k\Delta t_k = 18 + 16 + 24 + 30 + 20 = 108 \text{ person-years}$$

Thus, the average time at risk contributed by population members over the interval is

$$\frac{1}{N_0}\sum_{k=1}^{5} N_k\Delta t_k = \sum_{k=1}^{5}\left(\frac{N_k}{N_0}\right)\Delta t_k = \frac{1}{9}108 = 12 \text{ years}$$

Note that N_k/N_0 is just the proportion who remain at risk up to t_k, that is, the survival proportion from t_0 to t_k. If we denote this proportion N_k/N_0 by $S_{0,k}$ (to distinguish it from the subinterval-specific proportions s_k), the average time at risk can be written

$$\sum_{k=1}^{5} S_{0,k}\Delta t_k = \left(\frac{9}{9}\right)2 + \left(\frac{8}{9}\right)2 + \left(\frac{6}{9}\right)4 + \left(\frac{5}{9}\right)6 + \left(\frac{4}{9}\right)5 = 12 \text{ years}$$

as before. Now suppose that the interval is extended forward in time until the entire population has experienced the outcome of interest, as in Figure 3–2. The average time at risk will then equal the average incidence time, so the average incidence time will be computable from the survival proportions using the last formula. The survival proportions may in turn be computed from the subinterval-specific incidence rates, as described above.

SUMMARY

The three broad types of measures of disease frequency—incidence time, incidence rate, and incidence (and survival) proportion—are all linked by simple mathematical formulas that apply when one considers an inevitable nonrecurring event in a closed population followed until everyone has experienced the event. The mathematical relations become more complex when one considers events with competing risks, open populations, or truncated risk periods. Interpretations become particularly problematic when competing risks are present.

LIMITATIONS AND GENERALIZATIONS OF BASIC OCCURRENCE MEASURES

All the above measures can be viewed as types of arithmetic means, with possible weighting. Consequently, it is straightforward to extend these measures to outcomes that are more detailed than all-or-none. Consider, for example, antibody titer following vaccination of persons with no antibody for the target. We might examine the mean number of days until the titer reaches any given level L, or the proportion that reach L within a given number of days. We might also examine the rate at which persons reach L. To account for the fact that a titer has many possible levels, we could examine these measures for different values of L.

Means cannot capture all relevant aspects of a distribution and can even be misleading, except for some special distributions. For example, we have illustrated how—by itself—an incidence rate fails to distinguish among many people followed over a short period and a few people followed for a long period. Similarly, an incidence proportion of (say) 0.30 over 10 years fails to tell us whether the 30% of persons who had the event all had it within 2 years, or only after 8 years, or had events spread over the whole period. An average incidence time of 2 months among 101 people fails to tell us whether this average was derived from all 101 people having the event at 2 months, or from 100 people having the event at 1 month and 1 person having the event at 102 months, or something between these extremes.

One way to cope with these issues without making assumptions about the population distribution is to focus on how the distribution of the outcome event changes over time. We introduced this idea earlier by constructing survival proportions and incidence rates within time intervals (strata). By using short enough time intervals, we could see clearly how events are spread over time. For example, we could see whether our overall event rate reflects many people having the event early and a few people having it very late, or few having it early and many having it late, or anything between. We can also describe the distribution of event recurrences, such as asthma attacks.

We may generalize our notion of event to represent any transition from one state to another—not just from "no disease" to "diseased," but from (say) a diastolic blood pressure of 90 mm Hg in one time interval to 100 mm Hg in the next. We can examine these transitions on a scale as fine as our measurements allow, e.g., in studying the evolution of CD4 lymphocyte counts over time, we can imagine the rate of transitions from count x to count y per unit time for every sensible combination of x and y. Of course, this generalized viewpoint entails a much more complex picture of the population. Studying this complexity is the topic of *longitudinal data analysis*. Aside from some brief comments in Chapter 21, we will not discuss this important and vast field further. There are many textbooks devoted to different aspects of the topic; for example, Manton and Stallard (1988) provide a population-dynamics (demographic) approach, whereas Diggle et al. (2002) cover approaches based on statistical analysis of study cohorts, and van der Laan and Robins (2003) focus on longitudinal causal modeling.

PREVALENCE

Unlike incidence measures, which focus on new events or *changes* in health states, *prevalence* focuses on existing states. Prevalence of a state at a point in time may be defined as the proportion of a population in that state at that time; thus prevalence of a disease is the proportion of the population with the disease at the specified time. The terms *point prevalence, prevalence proportion,* and *prevalence rate* are sometimes used as synonyms. Prevalence generalizes to health states with multiple levels. For example, in considering cardiovascular health we could examine the prevalence of different levels of diastolic and systolic resting blood pressure; that is, we could examine the entire blood-pressure distribution, not just prevalence of being above certain clinical cutpoints.

The *prevalence pool* is the subset of the population in the given state. A person who dies with or from the state (e.g., from the disease under consideration) is removed from the prevalence pool; consequently, death decreases prevalence. People may also exit the prevalence pool by recovering from the state or emigrating from the population. Diseases with high incidence rates may have low prevalence if they are rapidly fatal or quickly cured. Conversely, diseases with very low incidence rates may have substantial prevalence if they are nonfatal but incurable.

USE OF PREVALENCE IN ETIOLOGIC RESEARCH

Seldom is prevalence of direct interest in etiologic applications of epidemiologic research. Because prevalence reflects both the incidence rate and the duration of disease, studies of prevalence or studies based on prevalent cases yield associations that reflect both the determinants of survival with disease and the causes of disease. The study of prevalence can be misleading in the paradoxical situation in which better survival from a disease and therefore a higher prevalence follow from the action of preventive agents that mitigate the disease once it occurs. In such a situation, the preventive agent may be positively associated with the prevalence of disease and so be misconstrued as a causative agent.

Nevertheless, for at least one class of diseases, namely, congenital malformations, prevalence is the measure usually employed. The proportion of babies born with some malformation is a prevalence proportion, not an incidence rate. The incidence of malformations refers to the occurrence of the malformations among the susceptible populations of embryos. Many malformations lead to early embryonic or fetal death that is classified, if recognized, as a miscarriage and not as a birth, whether malformed or not. Thus, malformed babies at birth represent only those fetuses who survived long enough with their malformations to be recorded as births. The frequency of such infants among all births is indeed a prevalence measure, the reference point in time being the moment of birth. The measure classifies the population of newborns as to their disease status, malformed or not, at the time of birth. This example illustrates that the reference time for prevalence need not be a point in calendar time; it can be a point on another time scale, such as age or time since treatment.

To study causes, it would be more useful to measure the incidence than the prevalence of congenital malformations. Unfortunately, it is seldom possible to measure the incidence rate of malformations, because the population at risk—young embryos—is difficult to ascertain, and learning of the occurrence and timing of the malformations among the embryos is equally problematic. Consequently, in this area of research, incident cases are not usually studied, and most investigators settle for the theoretically less desirable but much more practical study of prevalence at birth.

Prevalence is sometimes used to measure the occurrence of degenerative diseases with no clear moment of onset. It is also used in seroprevalence studies of the incidence of infection, especially when the infection has a long asymptomatic (silent) phase that can only be detected by serum testing. Human immunodeficiency virus (HIV) infection is a prime example (Brookmeyer and Gail, 1994). Here, incidence of infection may be back-calculated from incidence of symptom onset (acquired immune deficiency syndrome, or AIDS) and prevalence of infection using assumptions and data about the duration of the asymptomatic phase. Of course, in epidemiologic applications outside of etiologic research, such as planning for health resources and facilities, prevalence may be a more relevant measure than incidence.

PREVALENCE, INCIDENCE, AND MEAN DURATION

Often, the study of prevalence in place of incidence is rationalized on the basis of the simple relation between the two measures that obtains under certain very special conditions. We will examine these conditions carefully, with the objective of explaining why they rarely if ever provide a secure basis for studying prevalence as a proxy for incidence.

Recall that a stationary population has an equal number of people entering and exiting during any unit of time. Suppose that both the population at risk and the prevalence pool are stationary and that everyone is either at risk or has the disease. Then the number of people entering the prevalence pool in any time period will be balanced by the number exiting from it:

$$\text{Inflow (to prevalence pool)} = \text{outflow (from prevalence pool)}$$

People can enter the prevalence pool from the nondiseased population and by immigration from another population while diseased. Suppose there is no immigration into or emigration from the prevalence pool, so that no one enters or leaves the pool except by disease onset, death, or recovery. If the size of the population is N and the size of the prevalence pool is P, then the size of the population at risk that feeds the prevalence pool will be $N - P$. Also, during any time interval of length Δt, the number of people who enter the prevalence pool will be

$$I(N - P)\Delta t$$

where I is the incidence rate, and the outflow from the prevalence pool will be

$$I'P\Delta t$$

where I' represents the incidence rate of exiting from the prevalence pool, that is, the number who exit divided by the person-time experience of those in the prevalence pool. Therefore, in the absence of migration, the reciprocal of I' will equal the mean duration of the disease, $\overline{D}$, which is the mean time until death or recovery. It follows that

$$\text{Inflow} = I(N - P)\Delta t = \text{outflow} = (1/\overline{D})P\Delta t$$

which yields

$$\frac{P}{N - P} = I \cdot D$$

$P/(N - P)$ is the ratio of diseased to nondiseased people in the population or, equivalently, the ratio of the prevalence proportion to the nondiseased proportion. (We could call those who are nondiseased healthy except that we mean they do not have a specific illness, which does not imply an absence of all illness.)

The ratio $P/(N - P)$ is called the *prevalence odds;* it is the ratio of the proportion of a population that has a disease to the proportion that does not have the disease. As shown above, the prevalence odds equals the incidence rate times the mean duration of illness. If the prevalence is small, say <0.1, then

$$\text{Prevalence proportion} \approx I \cdot \overline{D}$$

because the prevalence proportion will approximate the prevalence odds for small values of prevalence. Under the assumption of stationarity and no migration in or out of the prevalence pool (Freeman and Hutchison, 1980),

$$\text{Prevalence proportion} = \frac{I \cdot \overline{D}}{1 + I \cdot \overline{D}}$$

which can be obtained from the above expression for the prevalence odds, $P/(N - P)$.

Like the incidence proportion, the prevalence proportion is dimensionless, with a range of 0 to 1. The above equations are in accord with these requirements, because in each of them the incidence rate, with a dimensionality of the reciprocal of time, is multiplied by the mean duration of illness, which has the dimensionality of time, giving a dimensionless product. Furthermore, the product $I \cdot \overline{D}$ has the range of 0 to infinity, which corresponds to the range of prevalence odds, whereas the expression

$$\frac{I \cdot \overline{D}}{1 + I \cdot \overline{D}}$$

is always in the range 0 to 1, corresponding to the range of a proportion.

Unfortunately, the above formulas have limited practical utility because of the no-migration assumption and because they do not apply to age-specific prevalence (Miettinen, 1976a). If we consider the prevalence pool of, say, diabetics who are 60 to 64 years of age, we can see that this pool experiences considerable immigration from younger diabetics aging into the pool, and considerable emigration from members aging out of the pool. More generally, because of the very strong relation of age to most diseases, we almost always need to consider age-specific subpopulations when studying patterns of occurrence. Under such conditions, proper analysis requires more elaborate formulas that give prevalence as a function of age-specific incidence, duration, and other population parameters (Preston, 1987; Manton and Stallard, 1988; Keiding, 1991; Alho, 1992).

AVERAGE AGE AT EVENT

Life expectancy is usually taken to refer to the mean age at death of a cohort or a closed population defined by a cohort, such as all persons born in a particular year. As such, life expectancy can only unfold over a time interval from cohort inception until the death of the final surviving cohort member (which may be more than a century). In contrast, average age at death usually refers to the average age of persons dying in a particular narrow time interval. For example, average age at death among people living in Vietnam as of 2010 represents experiences of persons born from roughly 1900 all the way up to 2010. It is heavily influenced by the size of the population in years that contribute to the calculation and by changes in life expectancy across the birth cohorts contributing to it. Thus, like prevalence, it is a cross-sectional (single-time point) attribute of a population, and the population may be open.

Had the population been in steady state for over a century and continued that way for another century or more, the life expectancy of those born today might resemble the average age at death today. The reality in many locales, however, is that the *number* of births per year increased dramatically over the 20th century, and thus the proportion in younger age groups increased. That change alone pulled the average age at death downward as it became more weighted by the increased number of deaths from younger age groups. Changes in actual life expectancy would exert other effects, possibly in the opposite direction. The net consequence is that the average age at death can differ considerably from life expectancy in any year.

These same forces and other similar forces also affect the average age of occurrence of other events, such as the occurrence of a particular disease. Comparisons among such cross-sectional averages mix the forces that affect the rate of disease occurrence with demographic changes that affect the age structure of the population. Such comparisons are therefore inherently biased as estimates of causal associations.

STANDARDIZATION

The notion of standardization is central to many analytic techniques in epidemiology, including techniques for control of confounding (Chapters 4 and 15) and for summarization of occurrence and effects (Chapters 20 and 21). Thus, standardized rates and proportions will arise at several points in this book, where they will be described in more detail. Standardization of occurrence measures is nothing more than weighted averaging of those measures. Proper use of the idea nonetheless requires careful attention to issues of causal ordering, which we will return to in later discussions. We also note that the term *standardization* has an entirely different definition in some branches of statistics, where it means re-expressing quantities in standard deviation units, a practice that can lead to severe distortions of effect estimates (Greenland et al., 1986, 1991; see Chapter 33).

To illustrate the basic idea of standardization, suppose we are given a distribution of person-time specific to a series of variables, for example, the person-years at risk experienced within age categories 50 to 59 years, 60 to 69 years, and 70 to 74 years, for men and women in Quebec in 2000. Let $T_1, T_2, \ldots, T_6$ be the distribution of person-years in the six age–sex categories in this example. Suppose also that we are given the six age–sex specific incidence rates $I_1, I_2, \ldots, I_6$ corresponding to the age–sex specific strata. From this distribution and set of rates, we can compute a weighted average of the rates with weights from the distribution,

$$I_s = \frac{I_1T_1 + \cdots + I_6T_6}{T_1 + \cdots + T_6} = \frac{\sum_{k=1}^{6} I_kT_k}{\sum_{k=1}^{6} T_k}$$

The numerator of I_s may be recognized as the number of cases one would see in a population that had the person-time distribution $T_1, T_2, \ldots, T_6$ and these stratum-specific rates. The denominator of I_s is the total person-time in such a population. Therefore, I_s is the rate one would see in a population with distribution $T_1, T_2, \ldots, T_6$ and specific rates $I_1, I_2, \ldots, I_6$.

I_s is traditionally called a *standardized rate*, and $T_1, T_2, \ldots, T_6$ is called the *standard distribution* on which I_s is based. I_s represents the overall rate that would be observed in a population whose person-time follows the standard distribution and whose specific rates are $I_1, I_2, \ldots, I_6$.

The standardization process can also be conducted with incidence or prevalence proportions. Suppose, for example, we have a distribution $N_1, N_2, \ldots, N_6$ of persons rather than person-time at risk and a corresponding set of stratum-specific incidence proportions $R_1, R_2, \ldots, R_6$. From this distribution and set of proportions, we can compute the weighted average risk

$$R_s = \frac{R_1N_1 + \cdots + R_6N_6}{N_1 + \cdots + N_6} = \frac{\sum_{k=1}^{6} R_kN_k}{\sum_{k=1}^{6} N_k}$$

which is a *standardized risk* based on the standard distribution $N_1, N_2, \ldots, N_6$. Standardization can also be applied using other measures (such as mean incidence times or mean blood pressures) in place of the rates or proportions.

Because the rates that apply to a population can affect the person-time distribution, the standardized rate is not necessarily the rate that would describe what would happen to a population with the standard distribution $T_1, \ldots, T_6$ if the specific rates $I_1, I_2, \ldots, I_6$ were applied to it. An analogous discrepancy can arise for standardized odds. This problem can distort inferences based on comparing standardized rates and odds, and will be discussed further in the next chapter. The problem does not arise when considering standardized risks because the initial distribution $N_1, \ldots, N_6$ cannot be affected by the subsequent risks $R_1, \ldots, R_6$.

CHAPTER 4

Measures of Effect and Measures of Association

Sander Greenland, Kenneth J. Rothman, and Timothy L. Lash

Measures of Effect 51
Difference Measures 52
Ratio Measures 53
Relative Excess Measures 53
Dependence of the Null State on the Effect Measure 54
The Theoretical Nature of Effect Measures 54
Defining Exposure in Effect Measures 55
Effects Mediated by Competing Risks 55
Association and Confounding 56
Measures of Association 57
Confounding 57
Confounders 58
A Simple Model That Distinguishes Causation from Association 59
Relations among Measures of Effect 60
Relations among Relative Risks 60
Effect-Measure Modification (Heterogeneity) 61
Relation of Stratum-Specific Measures to Overall Measures 62
Attributable Fractions 62
Excess Fractions 63
Etiologic Fractions 63
Probability of Causation and Susceptibility to Exposure 64
A Note on Terminology 65
Generalizing Definitions of Effect 66
Population-Attributable Fractions and Impact Fractions 67
Standardized Measures of Association and Effect 67
Standardized Morbidity Ratios (SMRs) 68
Prevalence Ratios 69
Other Measures 69

Suppose we wish to estimate the effect of an exposure on the occurrence of a disease. For reasons explained below, we cannot observe or even estimate this effect directly. Instead, we observe an association between the exposure and disease among study subjects, which estimates a population association. The observed association will be a poor substitute for the desired effect if it is a poor estimate of the population association, or if the population association is not itself close to the effect of interest. Chapters 9 through 12 address specific problems that arise in connecting observed associations to effects. The present chapter defines effects and associations in populations, and the basic concepts needed to connect them.

MEASURES OF EFFECT

Epidemiologists use the term *effect* in two senses. In one sense, any case of a given disease may be the effect of a given cause. *Effect* is used in this way to mean the endpoint of a causal mechanism, identifying the type of outcome that a cause produces. For example, we may say that human immunodeficiency virus (HIV) infection is an effect of sharing needles for drug use. This use of the term *effect* merely identifies HIV infection as one consequence of the activity of sharing needles. Other effects of the exposure, such as hepatitis B infection, are also possible.

In a more epidemiologic sense, an *effect* of a factor is a change in a population characteristic that is caused by the factor being at one level versus another. The population characteristics of traditional focus in epidemiology are disease-frequency measures, as described in Chapter 3. If disease frequency is measured in terms of incidence rate or proportion, then the effect is the change in incidence rate or proportion brought about by a particular factor. We might say that for drug users, the effect of sharing needles compared with not sharing needles is to increase the average risk of HIV infection from 0.001 in 1 year to 0.01 in 1 year. Although it is customary to use the definite article in referring to this second type of effect (*the* effect of sharing needles), it is not meant to imply that this is the only effect of sharing needles. An increase in risk for hepatitis or other diseases remains possible, and the increase in risk of HIV infection may differ across populations and time.

In epidemiology, it is customary to refer to potential causal characteristics as *exposures*. Thus, *exposure* can refer to a behavior (e.g., needle sharing), a treatment or other intervention (e.g., an educational program about hazards of needle sharing), a trait (e.g., a genotype), an exposure in the ordinary sense (e.g., an injection of contaminated blood), or even a disease (e.g., diabetes as a cause of death).

Population effects are most commonly expressed as effects on incidence rates or incidence proportions, but other measures based on incidence times or prevalences may also be used. Epidemiologic analyses that focus on survival time until death or recurrence of disease are examples of analyses that measure effects on incidence times. *Absolute effect measures* are differences in occurrence measures, and *relative effect measures* are ratios of occurrence measures. Other measures divide absolute effects by an occurrence measure.

For simplicity, our basic descriptions will be of effects in cohorts, which are groups of individuals. As mentioned in Chapter 3, each cohort defines a closed population starting at the time the group is defined. Among the measures we will consider, only those involving incidence rates generalize straightforwardly to open populations.

DIFFERENCE MEASURES

Consider a cohort followed over a specific time or age interval—say, from 2000 to 2005 or from ages 50 to 69 years. If we can imagine the experience of this cohort over the same interval under two different conditions—say, exposed and unexposed—then we can ask what the incidence rate of any outcome would be under the two conditions. Thus, we might consider a cohort of smokers and an exposure that consisted of mailing to each cohort member a brochure of current smoking-cessation programs in the cohort member's county of residence. We could then ask what the lung cancer incidence rate would be in this cohort if we carry out this treatment and what it would be if we do not carry out this treatment. These treatment histories represent mutually exclusive alternative histories for the cohort. The two incidence rates thus represent alternative *potential outcomes* for the cohort.

The difference between the two rates we call the absolute effect of our mailing program on the incidence rate, or the *causal rate difference.* To be brief, we might refer to the causal rate difference as the excess rate due to the program (which would be negative if the program prevented some lung cancers).

In a parallel manner, we might ask what the incidence proportion would be if we carry out this treatment and what it would be if we do not carry out this treatment. The difference between the two proportions we call the *absolute effect* of our treatment on the incidence proportion, or *causal risk difference,* or *excess risk* for short. Also in a parallel fashion, the difference in the average lung cancer–free years of life lived over the interval under the treated and untreated conditions is another absolute effect of treatment.

To illustrate the above measures in symbolic form, suppose we have a cohort of size N defined at the start of a fixed time interval and that anyone alive without the disease is at risk of the disease. Further, suppose that if every member of the cohort is exposed throughout the interval, A_1 cases will occur and the total time at risk will be T_1, but if no member of the same cohort is exposed during the interval, A_0 cases will occur and the total time at risk will be T_0. Then the causal rate difference will be

$$\frac{A_1}{T_1} - \frac{A_0}{T_0}$$

the causal risk difference will be

$$\frac{A_1}{N} - \frac{A_0}{N}$$

and the causal difference in average disease-free time will be

$$\frac{T_1}{N} - \frac{T_0}{N} = \frac{T_1 - T_0}{N}$$

When the outcome is death, the negative of the average time difference, $T_0/N - T_1/N$, is often called the *years of life lost* as a result of exposure. Each of these measures compares disease occurrence by taking differences, so they are called *difference* measures, or absolute measures. They are expressed in units of their component measures: cases per unit person-time for the rate difference, cases per person starting follow-up for the risk difference, and time units for the average-time difference.

RATIO MEASURES

Most commonly, effect measures are calculated by taking ratios. Examples of such ratio (or relative) measures are the *causal rate ratio,*

$$\frac{A_1/T_1}{A_0/T_0} = \frac{I_1}{I_0}$$

where $I_j = A_j/T_j$ is the incidence rate under condition j (1 = exposed, 0 = unexposed); the *causal risk ratio,*

$$\frac{A_1/N}{A_0/N} = \frac{A_1}{A_0} = \frac{R_1}{R_0}$$

where $R_i = A_j/N$ is the incidence proportion (average risk) under condition j; and the *causal ratio of disease-free time,*

$$\frac{T_1/N}{T_0/N} = \frac{T_1}{T_0}$$

In contrast to difference measures, ratio measures are dimensionless because the units cancel out upon division.

The rate ratio and risk ratio are often called *relative risks*. Sometimes this term is applied to odds ratios as well, although we would discourage such usage. "Relative risk" may be the most common term in epidemiology. Its usage is so broad that one must often look closely at the details of study design and analysis to discern which ratio measure is being estimated or discussed.

The three ratio measures are related by the formula

$$\frac{R_1}{R_0} = \frac{R_1 N}{R_0 N} = \frac{A_1}{A_0} = \frac{I_1 T_1}{I_0 T_0}$$

which follows from the fact that the number of cases equals the disease rate times the time at risk. A fourth relative measure can be constructed from the incidence odds. If we write $S_1 = 1 - R_1$ and $S_0 = 1 - R_0$, the *causal odds ratio* is then

$$\frac{R_1/S_1}{R_0/S_0} = \frac{A_1/(N - A_1)}{A_0/(N - A_0)}$$

RELATIVE EXCESS MEASURES

When a relative risk is greater than 1, reflecting an average effect that is causal, it is sometimes expressed as an *excess relative risk*, which may refer to the excess causal rate ratio,

$$IR - 1 = \frac{I_1}{I_0} - 1 = \frac{I_1 - I_0}{I_0}$$

where $IR = I_1/I_0$ is the causal rate ratio. Similarly, the excess causal risk ratio is

$$RR - 1 = \frac{R_1}{R_0} - 1 = \frac{R_1 - R_0}{R_0}$$

where $RR = R_1/R_0$ is the causal risk ratio. These formulas show how excess relative risks equal the rate or risk difference divided by (relative to) the unexposed rate or risk (I_0 or R_0), and so are sometimes called relative difference or relative excess measures.

More often, the excess rate is expressed relative to I_1, as

$$\frac{I_1 - I_0}{I_1} = \frac{I_1/I_0 - 1}{I_1/I_0} = \frac{IR - 1}{IR} = 1 - \frac{1}{IR}$$

where $IR = I_1/I_0$ is the causal rate ratio. Similarly, the excess risk is often expressed relative to R_1, as

$$\frac{R_1 - R_0}{R_1} = \frac{R_1/R_0 - 1}{R_1/R_0} = \frac{RR - 1}{RR} = 1 - \frac{1}{RR}$$

where $RR = R_1/R_0$ is the causal risk ratio. In both these measures the excess rate or risk attributable to exposure is expressed as a fraction of the total rate or risk under exposure; hence, $(IR - 1)/IR$ may be called the *rate fraction* and $(RR - 1)/RR$ the *risk fraction*. Both these measures are often called *attributable fractions*.

A number of other measures are also referred to as attributable fractions. Especially, the rate and risk fractions just defined are often confused with a distinct quantity called the *etiologic fraction*, which cannot be expressed as a simple function of the rates or risks. We will discuss these problems in detail later, where yet another relative excess measure will arise.

Relative excess measures were intended for use with exposures that have a net causal effect. They become negative and hence difficult to interpret with a net preventive effect. One expedient modification for dealing with preventive exposures is to interchange the exposed and unexposed quantities in the measures. The measures that arise from interchanging I_1 with I_0 and R_1 with R_0 in attributable fractions have been called *preventable fractions* and are easily interpreted. For example, $(R_0 - R_1)/R_0 = 1 - R_1/R_0 = 1 - RR$ is the fraction of the risk under nonexposure that could be prevented by exposure. In vaccine studies this measure is also known as the *vaccine efficacy*.

DEPENDENCE OF THE NULL STATE ON THE EFFECT MEASURE

If the occurrence measures being compared do not vary with exposure, the measure of effect will equal 0 if it is a difference or relative difference measure and will equal 1 if it is a ratio measure. In this case we say that the effect is *null* and that the exposure has no effect on the occurrence measure. This null state does not depend on the way in which the occurrence measure is compared (difference, ratio, etc.), but it may depend on the occurrence measure. For example, the 150-year average risk of death is always 100%, and so the 150-year causal risk difference is always 0 for any known exposure; nothing has been discovered that prevents death by age 150. Nonetheless, many exposures (such as tobacco use) will change the risk of death by age 60 relative to nonexposure, and so will have a nonzero 60-year causal risk difference; those exposures will also change the death rate and the average death time.

THE THEORETICAL NATURE OF EFFECT MEASURES

The definitions of effect measures given above are sometimes called *counterfactual* or *potential-outcome* definitions. Such definitions may be traced back to the writings of Hume in the 18th century. Although they received little explication until the latter third of the 20th century, they were being used by scientists (including epidemiologists and statisticians) long before; see Lewis (1973), Rubin (1990a), Greenland (2000a, 2004a), and Greenland and Morgenstern (2001) for early references.

They are called counterfactual measures because at least one of the two conditions in the definitions of the effect measures must be contrary to fact. The cohort may be exposed or treated (e.g., every member sent a mailing) or untreated (no one sent a mailing). If the cohort is treated, then the untreated condition will be counterfactual, and if it is untreated, then the treated condition will be counterfactual. Both conditions may be counterfactual, as would occur if only part of the cohort is sent the mailing. The outcomes of the conditions (e.g., I_1 and I_0, or R_1 and R_0, or T_1/N and T_0/N) remain potentialities until a treatment is applied to the cohort (Rubin, 1974, 1990a; Greenland, 2000a, 2004a).

One important feature of counterfactually defined effect measures is that they involve two distinct conditions: an index condition, which usually involves some exposure or treatment, and a reference condition—such as no treatment—against which this exposure or treatment will be evaluated. To ask for *the* effect of exposure is meaningless without reference to some other condition. In the preceding example, the effect of one mailing is defined only in reference to no mailing. We could have asked instead about the effect of one mailing relative to four mailings; this comparison is very different from one versus no mailing.

Another important feature of effect measures is that they are never observed separately from some component measure of occurrence. If in the mailing example we send the entire population one mailing, the rate difference comparing the outcome to no mailing, $I_1 - I_0$, is not observed directly; we observe only I_1, which is the sum of that effect measure and the (counterfactual) rate under no mailing, I_0: $I_1 = (I_1 - I_0) + I_0$. Therefore the researcher faces the problem of separating the effect measure $I_1 - I_0$ from the unexposed rate I_0 upon having observed only their sum, I_1.

DEFINING EXPOSURE IN EFFECT MEASURES

Because we have defined effects with reference to a *single* cohort under two distinct conditions, one must be able to describe meaningfully each condition for the one cohort (Rubin, 1990a; Greenland, 2002a, 2005a; Hernán, 2005; Maldonado and Greenland, 2002). Consider, for example, the effect of sex (male vs. female) on heart disease. For these words to have content, we must be able to imagine a cohort of men, their heart disease incidence, and what their incidence would have been had the very same men been women instead. The apparent ludicrousness of this demand reveals the vague meaning of sex effect. To reach a reasonable level of scientific precision, sex effect could be replaced by more precise mechanistic concepts, such as hormonal effects, discrimination effects, and effects of other sex-associated factors, which explain the association of sex with incidence. With such concepts, we can imagine what it means for the men to have their exposure changed: hormone treatments, sex-change operations, and so on.

The preceding considerations underscore the need to define the index and reference conditions in substantial detail to aid interpretability of results. For example, in a study of smoking effects, a detailed definition of the index condition for a current smoker might account for frequency of smoking (cigarettes per day), the duration of smoking (years), and the age at which smoking began. Similarly, definition of the absence of exposure for the reference condition—with regard to dose, duration, and induction period—ought to receive as much attention as the definition of the presence of exposure. While it is common to define all persons who fail to satisfy the current-smoker definition as unexposed, such a definition might dilute the effect by including former and occasional smokers in the reference group.

Whether the definitions of the index and reference conditions are sufficiently precise depends in part on the outcome under study. For example, a study of the effect of current smoking on lung cancer occurrence would set minimums for the frequency, duration, and induction period of cigarette smoking to define the exposed group and would set maximums (perhaps zero) for these same characteristics to define the unexposed group. Former smokers would not meet either the index or reference conditions. In contrast, a study of the effect of current smoking on the occurrence of injuries in a residential fire might allow any current smoking habit to define the exposed group and any current nonsmoking habit to define the unexposed group, even if the latter group includes former smokers (presuming that ex-smokers and never-smokers have the same household fire risk).

EFFECTS MEDIATED BY COMPETING RISKS

As discussed in Chapter 3, the presence of competing risks leads to several complications when interpreting incidence measures. The complexities carry over to interpreting effect measures. In particular, the interpretation of simple comparisons of incidence proportions must be tempered by the fact that they reflect exposure effects on competing risks as well as individual occurrences of the study disease. One consequence of these effects is that exposure can affect time at risk for the study disease. To take an extreme example, suppose that exposure was an antismoking treatment and the "disease" was being hit by a drunk driver. If the antismoking treatment was even moderately effective in reducing tobacco use, it would likely lead to a reduction in deaths, thus leading to more time alive, which would increase the opportunity to be struck by a drunk driver. The result would be more hits from drunk drivers for those exposed and hence higher risk under exposure.

This elevated risk of getting hit by a drunk driver is a genuine effect of the antismoking treatment, albeit an indirect and unintended one. The same sort of effect arises from any exposure that changes time at risk of other outcomes. Thus, smoking can reduce the average risk of accidental death simply by reducing the time at risk for an accident. Similarly, and quite apart from any direct biologic effect, smoking could reduce the average risk of Alzheimer's disease, Parkinson's disease, and other diseases of the elderly, simply by reducing the chance of living long enough to get these diseases. This indirect effect occurs even if we look at a narrow time interval, such as 2-year risk rather than lifetime risk: Even within a 2-year interval, smoking could cause some deaths and thus reduce the population time at risk, leading to fewer cases of these diseases.

Although the effects just described are real exposure effects, investigators typically want to remove or adjust away these effects and focus on more direct effects of exposure on disease. Rate measures account for the changes in time at risk produced by exposure in a simple fashion, by measuring number of disease events relative to time at risk. Indeed, if there is no trend in the disease rate over time and the only effect of the exposure on disease occurrence is to alter time at risk, the rate ratio and difference will be null (1 and 0, respectively). If, however, there are time trends in disease, then even rate measures will incorporate some exposure effects on time at risk; when this happens, time-stratified rate comparisons (survival analysis; see Chapter 16) are needed to account for these effects.

Typical risk estimates attempt to "adjust" for competing risks, using methods that estimate the counterfactual risk of the study disease if the competing risks were removed. As mentioned in Chapter 3, one objection to these methods is that the counterfactual condition is not clear: How are the competing risks to be removed? The incidence of the study disease would depend heavily on the answer. The problems here parallel problems of defining exposure in effect measures: How is the exposure to be changed to nonexposure, or vice versa? Most methods make the implausible assumptions that the exposure could be completely removed without affecting the rate of competing risks, and that competing risks could be removed without affecting the rate of the study disease. These assumptions are rarely if ever justified. A more general approach treats the study disease and the competing risks as parts of a *multivariate* or *multidimensional* outcome. This approach can reduce the dependence on implausible assumptions; it also responds to the argument that an exposure should not be considered in isolation, especially when effects of exposure and competing risks entail very different costs and benefits (Greenland, 2002a, 2005a).

Owing to the complexities that ensue from taking a more general approach, we will not delve further into issues of competing risks. Nonetheless, readers should be alert to the problems that can arise when the exposure may have strong effects on diseases other than the one under study.

ASSOCIATION AND CONFOUNDING

Because the single population in an effect definition can only be observed under one of the two conditions in the definition (and sometimes neither), we face a special problem in effect estimation: We must predict accurately the magnitude of disease occurrence under conditions that did not or will not in fact occur. In other words, we must predict certain outcomes under what are or will become counterfactual conditions. For example, we may observe $I_1 = 50$ deaths per 100,000 person-years in a target cohort of smokers over a 10-year follow-up and ask what rate reduction would have been achieved had these smokers quit at the start of follow-up. Here, we observe I_1, and need I_0 (the rate that would have occurred under complete smoking cessation) to complete $I_1 - I_0$.

Because I_0 is not observed, we must predict what it would have been. To do so, we would need to refer to data on the outcomes of nonexposed persons, such as data from a cohort that was not exposed. From these data, we would construct a prediction of I_0. Neither these data nor the prediction derived from them is part of the effect measure; they are only ingredients in our estimation process.

We use them to construct a measure of *association* that we hope will equal the effect measure of interest.

MEASURES OF ASSOCIATION

Consider a situation in which we contrast a measure of occurrence in *two* different populations. For example, we could take the ratio of cancer incidence rates among males and females in Canada. This cancer rate ratio comparing the male and female subpopulations is *not* an effect measure because its two component rates refer to different groups of people. In this situation, we say that the rate ratio is a *measure of association;* in this example, it is a measure of the association of sex with cancer incidence in Canada.

As another example, we could contrast the incidence rate of dental caries in children within a community in the year before and in the third year after the introduction of fluoridation of the water supply. If we take the difference of the rates in these before and after periods, this difference is *not* an effect measure because its two component rates refer to two different subpopulations, one before fluoridation and one after. There may be considerable or even complete overlap among the children present in the before and after periods. Nonetheless, the experiences compared refer to different time periods, so we say that the rate difference is a measure of association. In this example, it is a measure of the association between fluoridation and dental caries incidence in the community.

We can summarize the distinction between measures of effect and measures of association as follows: A measure of effect compares what would happen to *one* population under two possible but distinct life courses or conditions, of which at most only one can occur (e.g., a ban on all tobacco advertising vs. a ban on television advertising only). It is a theoretical (some would say "metaphysical") concept insofar as it is logically impossible to observe the population under both conditions, and hence it is logically impossible to see directly the size of the effect (Maldonado and Greenland, 2002). In contrast, a measure of association compares what happens in two distinct populations, although the two distinct populations may correspond to one population in different time periods. Subject to physical and social limitations, we can observe both populations and so can directly observe an association.

CONFOUNDING

Given the observable nature of association measures, it is tempting to substitute them for effect measures (perhaps after making some adjustments). It is even more natural to give causal explanations for observed associations in terms of obvious differences between the populations being compared. In the preceding example of dental caries, it is tempting to ascribe a decline in incidence following fluoridation to the act of fluoridation itself. Let us analyze in detail how such an inference translates into measures of effect and association.

The effect we wish to measure is that which fluoridation had on the rate. To measure this effect, we must contrast the actual rate under fluoridation with the rate that would have occurred *in the same time period* had fluoridation *not* been introduced. We cannot observe the latter rate, for fluoridation was introduced, and so the nonfluoridation rate in that time period is counterfactual. Thus, we substitute in its place, or exchange, the rate in the time period before fluoridation. In doing so, we substitute a measure of association (the rate difference before and after fluoridation) for what we are really interested in: the difference between the rate with fluoridation and what that rate would have been without fluoridation in the one postfluoridation time period.

This substitution will be misleading to the extent that the rate before fluoridation does not equal—so should not be exchanged with—the counterfactual rate (i.e., the rate that would have occurred in the postfluoridation period if fluoridation had not been introduced). If the two are not equal, then the measure of association will not equal the measure of effect for which it is substituted. In such a circumstance, we say that the measure of association is *confounded* (for our desired measure of effect). Other ways of expressing the same idea is that the before–after rate difference is confounded for the causal rate difference or that *confounding* is present in the before–after difference (Greenland and Robins, 1986; Greenland et al., 1999b; Greenland and Morgenstern, 2001). On the other hand, if the rate before fluoridation does equal the postfluoridation counterfactual rate, then the measure of association equals our desired measure of effect, and we say that the before–after difference is *unconfounded* or that no confounding is present in this difference.

The preceding definitions apply to ratios as well as differences. Because ratios and differences contrast the same underlying quantities, confounding of a ratio measure implies confounding of the corresponding difference measure and vice versa. If the value substituted for the counterfactual rate or risk does not equal that rate or risk, both the ratio and difference will be confounded.

The above definitions also extend immediately to situations in which the contrasted quantities are average risks, incidence times, odds, or prevalences. For example, one might wish to estimate the effect of fluoridation on caries prevalence 3 years after fluoridation began. Here, the needed but unobserved counterfactual is what the caries prevalence would have been 3 years after fluoridation began, had fluoridation not in fact begun. We might substitute for that counterfactual the prevalence of caries at the time fluoridation began. It is possible (though perhaps rare in practice) for one effect measure to be confounded but not another, if the two effect measures derive from different underlying measures of disease frequency (Greenland et al., 1999b). For example, there could in theory be confounding of the rate ratio but not the risk ratio, or of the 5-year risk ratio but not the 10-year risk ratio.

One point of confusion in the literature is the failure to recognize that incidence odds are risk-based measures, and hence incidence odds ratios will be confounded under exactly the same circumstances as risk ratios (Miettinen and Cook, 1981; Greenland and Robins, 1986; Greenland, 1987a; Greenland et al., 1999b). The confusion arises because of the peculiarity that the causal odds ratio for a whole cohort can be closer to the null than any stratum-specific causal odds ratio. Such *noncollapsibility* of the causal odds ratio is sometimes confused with confounding, even though it has nothing to do with the latter phenomenon; it will be discussed further in a later section.

CONFOUNDERS

Consider again the fluoridation example. Suppose that within the year after fluoridation began, dental-hygiene education programs were implemented in some of the schools in the community. If these programs were effective, then (other things being equal) some reduction in caries incidence would have occurred as a consequence of the programs. Thus, even if fluoridation had not begun, the caries incidence would have declined in the postfluoridation time period. In other words, the programs alone would have caused the counterfactual rate in our effect measure to be lower than the prefluoridation rate that substitutes for it. As a result, the measure of association (which is the before–after rate difference) must be larger than the desired measure of effect (the causal rate difference). In this situation, we say the programs *confounded* the measure of association or that the program effects are confounded with the fluoridation effect in the measure of association. We also say that the programs are *confounders* of the association and that the association is confounded by the programs.

Confounders are factors (exposures, interventions, treatments, etc.) that explain or produce all or part of the difference between the measure of association and the measure of effect that would be obtained with a counterfactual ideal. In the present example, the programs explain why the before–after association overstates the fluoridation effect: The before–after difference or ratio includes the effects of programs as well as the effects of fluoridation. For a factor to explain this discrepancy and thus confound, the factor must affect or at least predict the risk or rate in the unexposed (reference) group, and not be affected by the exposure or the disease. In the preceding example, we assumed that the presence of the dental hygiene programs in the years after fluoridation entirely accounted for the discrepancy between the prefluoridation rate and the (counterfactual) rate that would have occurred 3 years after fluoridation, if fluoridation had not been introduced.

A large portion of epidemiologic methods are concerned with avoiding or adjusting (controlling) for confounding. Such methods inevitably rely on the gathering and proper use of confounder measurements. We will return repeatedly to this topic. For now, we simply note that the most fundamental adjustment methods rely on the notion of *stratification* on confounders. If we make our comparisons within appropriate levels of a confounder, that confounder cannot confound the comparisons. For example, we could limit our before–after fluoridation comparisons to schools in states in which no dental hygiene program was introduced. In such schools, program introductions could not have had an effect (because no program was present), so effects of programs in those schools could not explain any decline following fluoridation.

A SIMPLE MODEL THAT DISTINGUISHES CAUSATION FROM ASSOCIATION

We can clarify the difference between measures of effect and measures of association, as well as the role of confounding and confounders, by examining risk measures under a simple potential-outcome model for a cohort of individuals (Greenland and Robins, 1986).

Table 4–1 presents the composition of two cohorts, cohort 1 and cohort 0. Suppose that cohort 1 is uniformly exposed to some agent of interest, such as one mailing of smoking-cessation material, and that cohort 0 is not exposed, that is, receives no such mailing. Individuals in the cohorts are classified by their outcomes when exposed and when unexposed:

1. Type 1 or "doomed" persons, for whom exposure is irrelevant because disease occurs with or without exposure
2. Type 2 or "causal" persons, for whom disease occurs if and only if they are exposed
3. Type 3 or "preventive" persons, for whom disease occurs if and only if they are unexposed
4. Type 4 or "immune" persons, for whom exposure is again irrelevant because disease does *not* occur, with or without exposure

Among the exposed, only type 1 and type 2 persons get the disease, so the incidence proportion in cohort 1 is $p_1 + p_2$. If, however, exposure had been absent from this cohort, only type 1 and type 3 persons would have gotten the disease, so the incidence proportion would have been $p_1 + p_3$. Therefore, the absolute change in the incidence proportion in cohort 1 caused by exposure, or the causal risk difference, is $(p_1 + p_2) - (p_1 + p_3) = p_2 - p_3$, while the relative change, or causal risk ratio, is $(p_1 + p_2)/(p_1 + p_3)$. Similarly, the incidence odds is $(p_1 + p_2)/[1 - (p_1 + p_2)] = (p_1 + p_2)/(p_3 + p_4)$ but would have been $(p_1 + p_3)/[1 - (p_1 + p_3)] = (p_1 + p_3)/(p_2 + p_4)$ if exposure had been absent; hence the relative change in the incidence odds (the causal odds ratio) is

$$\frac{(p_1 + p_2)/(p_3 + p_4)}{(p_1 + p_3)/(p_2 + p_4)}$$

Equal numbers of causal types (type 2) and preventive types (type 3) in cohort 1 correspond to $p_2 = p_3$. Equality of p_2 and p_3 implies that the causal risk difference $p_2 - p_3$ will be 0, and the causal risk and odds ratios will be 1. Thus, these values of the causal effect measures do *not* correspond to no effect, but instead correspond to a balance between causal and preventive effects.

TABLE 4–1

An Elementary Model of Causal Types and Their Distribution in Two Distinct Cohorts

	Response[a] under			Proportion of types in	
Type	Exposure	Nonexposure	Description	Cohort 1 (Exposed)	Cohort 0 (Unexposed)
1	1	1	Doomed	p_1	q_1
2	1	0	Exposure is causal	p_2	q_2
3	0	1	Exposure is preventive	p_3	q_3
4	0	0	Immune	p_4	q_4

[a] 1, gets disease; 0, does not get disease.

Source: Reprinted from Greenland S, Robins JM. Identifiability, exchangeability and epidemiological confounding. *Int J Epidemiol.* 1986;15:413–419.

The hypothesis of no effect at all is sometimes called the sharp null hypothesis, and here corresponds to $p_2 = p_3 = 0$. The sharp null is a special case of the usual null hypothesis that the risk difference is zero or the risk ratio is 1, which corresponds to causal and preventive effects balancing one another to produce $p_2 = p_3$. Only if we can be sure that one direction of effect does not happen (either $p_2 = 0$ or $p_3 = 0$) can we say that a risk difference of 0 or a risk ratio of 1 corresponds to no effect; otherwise we can only say that those values correspond to no *net* effect. More generally, population effect measures correspond only to net effects: A risk difference represents only the net change in the average risk produced by the exposure.

Among the unexposed, only type 1 and type 3 persons get the disease, so the incidence proportion in cohort 0 is $q_1 + q_3$ and the incidence odds is $(q_1 + q_3)/(q_2 + q_4)$. Therefore, the difference and ratio of the incidence proportions in the cohorts are $(p_1 + p_2) - (q_1 + q_3)$ and $(p_1 + p_2)/(q_1 + q_3)$, while the ratio of incidence odds is

$$\frac{(p_1 + p_2)/(p_3 + p_4)}{(q_1 + q_3)/(q_2 + q_4)}$$

These measures compare two different cohorts, the exposed and the unexposed, and so are associational rather than causal measures. They equal their causal counterparts only if $q_1 + q_3 = p_1 + p_3$, that is, only if the incidence proportion for cohort 0 equals what cohort 1 would have experienced if exposure were absent. If $q_1 + q_3 \neq p_1 + p_3$, then the quantity $q_1 + q_3$ is not a valid substitute for $p_1 + p_3$. In that case, the associational risk difference, risk ratio, and odds ratio are confounded by the discrepancy between $q_1 + q_3$ and $p_1 + p_3$, so we say that confounding is present in the risk comparisons.

Confounding corresponds to the difference between the desired counterfactual quantity $p_1 + p_3$ and the observed substitute $q_1 + q_3$. This difference arises from differences between the exposed and unexposed cohorts with respect to other factors that affect disease risk, the confounders. Control of confounding would be achieved if we could stratify the cohorts on a sufficient set of these confounders, or on factors associated with them, to produce strata within which the counterfactual and its substitute were equal, i.e., within which no confounding occurs.

Confounding depends on the cohort for which we are estimating effects. Suppose we are interested in the relative effect that exposure would have on risk in cohort 0. This effect would be measured by the causal ratio for cohort 0: $(q_1 + q_2)/(q_1 + q_3)$. Because cohort 0 is not exposed, we do not observe $q_1 + q_2$, the average risk it would have if exposed; that is, $q_1 + q_2$ is counterfactual. If we substitute the actual average risk from cohort 1, $p_1 + p_2$, for this counterfactual average risk in cohort 0, we obtain the same associational risk ratio used before: $(p_1 + p_2)/(q_1 + q_3)$. Even if this associational ratio equals the causal risk ratio for cohort 1 (which occurs only if $p_1 + p_3 = q_1 + q_3$), it will not equal the causal risk ratio for cohort 0 unless $p_1 + p_2 = q_1 + q_2$. To see this, suppose $p_1 = p_2 = p_3 = q_1 = q_3 = 0.1$ and $q_2 = 0.3$. Then $p_1 + p_3 = q_1 + q_3 = 0.2$, but $p_1 + p_2 = 0.2 \neq q_1 + q_2 = 0.4$. Thus, there is no confounding in using the associational ratio $(p_1 + p_2)/(q_1 + q_3) = 0.2/0.2 = 1$ for the causal ratio in cohort 1, $(p_1 + p_2)/(p_1 + p_3) = 0.2/0.2 = 1$, yet there is confounding in using the associational ratio for the causal ratio in cohort 0, for the latter is $(q_1 + q_2)/(q_1 + q_3) = 0.4/0.2 = 2$. This example shows that the presence of confounding can depend on the population chosen as the target of inference (the target population), as well as on the population chosen to provide a substitute for a counterfactual quantity in the target (the reference population). It may also depend on the time period in question.

Causal diagrams (graphical models) provide visual models for distinguishing causation from association, and thus for defining and detecting confounding (Pearl, 1995, 2000; Greenland et al., 1999a; Chapter 12). Potential-outcome models and graphical models can be linked via a third class of causal models, called *structural equations*, and lead to the same operational criteria for detection and control of confounding (Greenland et al., 1999a; Pearl, 2000; Greenland and Brumback, 2002).

RELATIONS AMONG MEASURES OF EFFECT

RELATIONS AMONG RELATIVE RISKS

Recall from Chapter 3 that in a closed population over an interval of length Δt, the incidence proportion R, the rate I, and the odds R/S (where $S = 1 - R$) will be related by $R \approx I\Delta t \approx R/S$

if the size of the population at risk declines only slightly over the interval (which implies that R must be small and $S = 1 - R \approx 1$). Suppose now we contrast the experience of the population over the interval under two conditions, exposure and no exposure, and that the size of the population at risk would decline only slightly under either condition. Then, the preceding approximation implies that

$$\frac{R_1}{R_0} \approx \frac{I_1/\Delta t}{I_0/\Delta t} = \frac{I_1}{I_0} \approx \frac{R_1/S_1}{R_0/S_0}$$

where $S_1 = 1 - R_1$ and $S_0 = 1 - R_0$. In other words, the ratios of the risks, rates, and odds will be approximately equal under suitable conditions. The condition that both R_1 and R_0 are small is sufficient to ensure that both S_1 and S_0 are close to 1, in which case the odds ratio will approximate the risk ratio (Cornfield, 1951). For the rate ratio to approximate the risk ratio, we must have $R_1/R_0 \approx I_1T_1/I_0T_0 \approx I_1/I_0$, which requires that exposure only negligibly affects the person-time at risk (i.e., that $T_1 \approx T_0$). Both conditions are satisfied if the size of the population at risk would decline by no more than a few percent over the interval, regardless of exposure status.

The order of the three ratios (risk, rate, and odds) in relation to the null is predictable. When $R_1 > R_0$, we have $S_1 = 1 - R_1 < 1 - R_0 = S_0$, so that $S_0/S_1 > 1$ and

$$1 < \frac{R_1}{R_0} < \frac{R_1}{R_0}\frac{S_0}{S_1} = \frac{R_1/S_1}{R_0/S_0}$$

On the other hand, when $R_1 < R_0$, we have $S_1 > S_0$, so that $S_0/S_1 < 1$ and

$$1 > \frac{R_1}{R_0} > \frac{R_1}{R_0}\frac{S_0}{S_1} = \frac{R_1/S_1}{R_0/S_0}$$

Thus, when exposure affects average risk, the risk ratio will be closer to the null (1) than the odds ratio.

Now suppose that, as we would ordinarily expect, the effect of exposure on the person-time at risk is in the opposite direction of its effect on risk, so that $T_1 < T_0$ if $R_1 > R_0$ and $T_1 > T_0$ if $R_1 < R_0$. Then, if $R_1 > R_0$, we have $T_1/T_0 < 1$ and so

$$1 < \frac{R_1}{R_0} = \frac{I_1T_1}{I_0T_0} < \frac{I_1}{I_0}$$

and if $R_1 < R_0$, we have $T_1/T_0 > 1$ and so

$$1 > \frac{R_1}{R_0} = \frac{I_1T_1}{I_0T_0} > \frac{I_1}{I_0}$$

Thus, when exposure affects average risk, we would ordinarily expect the risk ratio to be closer to the null than the rate ratio. Under further conditions, the rate ratio will be closer to the null than the odds ratio (Greenland and Thomas, 1982). Thus, we would usually expect the risk ratio to be nearest to the null, the odds ratio to be furthest from the null, and the rate ratio to fall between the risk ratio and the odds ratio.

EFFECT-MEASURE MODIFICATION (HETEROGENEITY)

Suppose we divide our population into two or more categories or strata. In each stratum, we can calculate an effect measure of our choosing. These stratum-specific effect measures may or may not equal one another. Rarely would we have any reason to suppose that they would equal one another. If they are not equal, we say that the effect measure is *heterogeneous* or *modified* or *varies* across strata. If they are equal, we say that the measure is *homogeneous, constant,* or *uniform* across strata.

A major point about effect-measure modification is that, if effects are present, it will usually be the case that no more than one of the effect measures discussed above will be uniform across strata. In fact, if the exposure has any effect on an occurrence measure, at most one of the ratio or difference measures of effect can be uniform across strata. As an example, suppose that among men the average risk would be 0.50 if exposure was present but 0.20 if exposure was absent, whereas among women the average risk would be 0.10 if exposure was present but 0.04 if exposure was absent. Then the causal risk difference for men is 0.50 – 0.20 = 0.30, five times the difference for women of 0.10 – 0.04 = 0.06. In contrast, for both men and women, the causal risk ratio is

$0.50/0.20 = 0.10/0.04 = 2.5$. Now suppose we change this example to make the risk differences uniform, say, by making the exposed male risk 0.26 instead of 0.50. Then, both risk differences would be 0.06, but the male risk ratio would be $0.26/0.20 = 1.3$, much less than the female risk ratio of 2.5. Finally, if we change the example by making the exposed male risk 0.32 instead of 0.50, the male risk difference would be 0.12, double the female risk difference of 0.06, but the male ratio would be 1.6, less than two thirds the female ratio of 2.5. Thus, the presence, direction, and size of effect-measure modification can be dependent on the choice of measure (Berkson, 1958; Brumback and Berg, 2008).

RELATION OF STRATUM-SPECIFIC MEASURES TO OVERALL MEASURES

The relation of stratum-specific effect measures to the effect measure for an entire cohort can be subtle. For causal risk differences and ratios, the measure for the entire cohort must fall somewhere in the midst of the stratum-specific measures. For the odds ratio, however, the causal odds ratio for the entire cohort can be closer to the null than any of the causal odds ratios for the strata (Miettinen and Cook, 1981; Greenland, 1987a; Geenland et al., 1999b). This bizarre phenomenon is sometimes referred to as *noncollapsibility* of the causal odds ratio. The phenomenon has led some authors to criticize the odds ratio as a measure of effect, except as an approximation to risk and rate ratios (Miettinen and Cook, 1981; Greenland, 1987a; Greenland et al., 1999b; Greenland and Morgenstern, 2001).

As an example, suppose we have a cohort that is 50% men, and among men the average risk would be 0.50 if exposure was present but 0.20 if exposure was absent, whereas among women the average risk would be 0.08 if exposure was present but 0.02 if exposure was absent. Then the causal odds ratios are

$$\frac{0.50/(1-0.50)}{0.20/(1-0.20)} = 4.0 \text{ for men} \quad \text{and} \quad \frac{0.08/(1-0.08)}{0.02/(1-0.02)} = 4.3 \text{ for women}$$

For the total cohort, the average risk if exposure was present would be just the average of the male and female average risks, $0.5(0.50) + 0.5(0.08) = 0.29$; similarly, the average risk exposure was absent would be $0.5(0.20) + 0.5(0.02) = 0.11$. Thus, the causal odds ratio for the total cohort is

$$\frac{0.29/(1-0.29)}{0.11/(1-0.11)} = 3.3$$

which is less than both the male and female odds ratios. This noncollapsibility can occur because, unlike the risk difference and ratio, the causal odds ratio for the total cohort is not a weighted average of the stratum-specific causal odds ratios (Greenland, 1987a). It should not be confused with the phenomenon of confounding (Greenland et al., 1999b), which was discussed earlier. Causal rate ratios and rate differences can also display noncollapsibility without confounding (Greenland, 1996a). In particular, the causal rate ratio for a total cohort can be closer to the null than all of the stratum-specific causal rate ratios. To show this, we extend the preceding example as follows. Suppose that the risk period in the example was the year from January 1, 2000, to December 31, 2000, that all persons falling ill would do so on January 1, and that no one else was removed from risk during the year. Then the rates would be proportional to the odds, because none of the cases would contribute a meaningful amount of person-time. As a result, the causal rate ratios for men and women would be 4.0 and 4.3, whereas the causal rate ratio for the total cohort would be only 3.3.

As discussed earlier, risk, rate, and odds ratios will approximate one another if the population at risk would decline only slightly in size over the risk period, regardless of exposure. If this condition holds in all strata, the rate ratio and odds ratio will approximate the risk ratio in the strata, and hence both measures will be approximately collapsible when the risk ratio is collapsible.

ATTRIBUTABLE FRACTIONS

One often sees measures that attempt to assess the public health impact of an exposure by measuring its contribution to the total incidence under exposure. For convenience, we will refer to the entire family of such fractional measures as *attributable fractions*. The terms *attributable risk percent* or just *attributable risk* are often used as synonyms, although "attributable risk" is also used to denote the risk difference (MacMahon and Pugh, 1970; Szklo and Nieto, 2000; Koepsell and Weiss, 2003). Such fractions may be divided into two broad classes, which we shall term *excess fractions* and *etiologic fractions*.

A fundamental difficulty is that the two classes are usually confused, yet excess fractions can be much smaller than etiologic fractions, even if the disease is rare or other reasonable conditions are met. Another difficulty is that etiologic fractions are not estimable from epidemiologic studies alone, even if those studies are perfectly valid: Assumptions about the underlying biologic mechanism must be introduced to estimate etiologic fractions, and the estimates will be very sensitive to those assumptions.

EXCESS FRACTIONS

One family of attributable fractions is based on recalculating an incidence difference as a proportion or fraction of the total incidence under exposure. One such measure is $(A_1 - A_0)/A_1$, the excess caseload due to exposure, which has been called the *excess fraction* (Greenland and Robins, 1988). In a cohort, the fraction of the exposed incidence proportion $R_1 = A_1/N$ that is attributable to exposure is exactly equal to the excess fraction:

$$\frac{R_1 - R_0}{R_1} = \frac{A_1/N - A_0/N}{A_1/N} = \frac{A_1 - A_0}{A_1}$$

where $R_0 = A_0/N$ is what the incidence proportion would be with no exposure. Comparing this formula to the earlier formula for the risk fraction $(R_1 - R_0)/R_1 = (RR - 1)/RR$, we see that in a cohort the excess caseload and the risk fraction are equal.

The rate fraction $(I_1 - I_0)/I_1 = (IR - 1)/IR$ is often mistakenly equated with the excess fraction $(A_1 - A_0)/A_1$. To see that the two are not equal, let T_1 and T_0 represent the total time at risk that would be experienced by the cohort under exposure and nonexposure during the interval of interest. The rate fraction then equals

$$\frac{A_1/T_1 - A_0/T_0}{A_1/T_1}$$

If exposure has any effect and the disease removes people from further risk (as when the disease is irreversible), then T_1 will be less than T_0. Thus, the last expression cannot equal the excess fraction $(A_1 - A_0)/A_1$ because $T_1 \neq T_0$, although if the exposure effect on total time at risk is small, T_1 will be close to T_0 and so the rate fraction will approximate the excess fraction.

ETIOLOGIC FRACTIONS

Suppose that all sufficient causes of a particular disease were divided into two sets, those that contain exposure and those that do not, and that the exposure is never preventive. This situation is summarized in Figure 4–1. C and C' may represent many different combinations of causal components. Each of the two sets of sufficient causes represents a theoretically large variety of causal mechanisms for disease, perhaps as many as one distinct mechanism for every case that occurs. Disease can occur either with or without E, the exposure of interest. The causal mechanisms are grouped in the diagram according to whether or not they contain the exposure. We say that exposure can cause disease if exposure will cause disease under at least some set of conditions C. We say that the exposure E caused disease if a sufficient cause that contains E is the first sufficient cause to be completed.

At first, it seems a simple matter to ask what fraction of cases was caused by exposure. We will call this fraction the *etiologic fraction*. Because we can estimate the total number of cases,

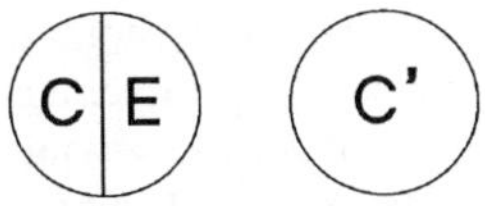

FIGURE 4–1 • Two types of sufficient causes of a disease.

we could estimate the etiologic fraction if we could estimate the number of cases that were caused by E. Unfortunately, this number is not estimable from ordinary incidence data, because the observation of an exposed case does not reveal the mechanism that caused the case. In particular, people who have the exposure can develop the disease from a mechanism that does not include the exposure. For example, a smoker may develop lung cancer through some mechanism that does not involve smoking (e.g., one involving asbestos or radiation exposure, with no contribution from smoking). For such lung cancer cases, smoking was incidental; it did not contribute to the cancer causation. There is no general way to tell which factors are responsible for a given case. Therefore, exposed cases include some cases of disease caused by the exposure, if the exposure is indeed a cause, and some cases of disease that occur through mechanisms that do not involve the exposure.

The observed incidence rate or proportion among the exposed reflects the incidence of cases in both sets of sufficient causes represented in Figure 4–1. The incidence of sufficient causes containing E could be found by subtracting the incidence of the sufficient causes that lack E. The latter incidence cannot be estimated if we cannot distinguish cases for which exposure played an etiologic role from cases for which exposure was irrelevant (Greenland and Robins, 1988; Greenland, 1999a). Thus, if I_1 is the incidence rate of disease in a population when exposure is present and I_0 is the rate in that population when exposure is absent, the rate difference $I_1 - I_0$ does not necessarily equal the rate of disease arising from sufficient causes with the exposure as a component cause, and need not even be close to that rate.

To see the source of this difficulty, imagine a cohort in which, for every member, the causal complement of exposure, C, will be completed before the sufficient cause C' is completed. If the cohort is unexposed, every case of disease must be attributable to the cause C'. But if the cohort is exposed from start of follow-up, every case of disease occurs when C is completed (E being already present), so every case of disease must be attributable to the sufficient cause containing C and E. Thus, the incidence rate of cases caused by exposure is I_1 when exposure is present, not $I_1 - I_0$, and thus the fraction of cases caused by exposure is 1, or 100%, even though the rate fraction $(I_1 - I_0)/I_1$ may be very small.

Excess fractions and rate fractions are often incorrectly interpreted as etiologic fractions. The preceding example shows that these fractions can be far less than the etiologic fraction: In the example, the rate fraction will be close to 0 if the rate difference is small relative to I_1, but the etiologic fraction will remain 1, regardless of A_0 or I_0. Robins and Greenland (1989a, 1989b) and Beyea and Greenland (1999) give conditions under which the rate fraction and etiologic fraction are equal, but these conditions are not testable with epidemiologic data and rarely have any supporting evidence or genuine plausibility (Robins and Greenland, 1989a, 1989b). One condition sometimes cited is that exposure acts independently of background causes, which will be examined further in a later section. Without such assumptions, however, the most we can say is that the excess fraction provides a lower bound on the etiologic fraction.

One condition that is irrelevant yet is sometimes given is that the disease is rare. To see that this condition is irrelevant, note that the above example made no use of the absolute frequency of the disease; the excess and rate fractions could still be near 0 even if the etiologic fraction was near 1. Disease rarity only brings the case and rate fractions closer to one another, in the same way as it brings the risk and rate ratios close together (assuming exposure does not have a large effect on the person-time); it does not bring the rate fraction close to the etiologic fraction.

PROBABILITY OF CAUSATION AND SUSCEPTIBILITY TO EXPOSURE

To further illustrate the difference between excess and etiologic fractions, suppose that at a given time in a cohort, a fraction F of completions of C' was preceded by completions of C. Again, no case can be attributable to exposure if the cohort is unexposed. But if the cohort is exposed, a fraction F of the A_0 cases that would have occurred without exposure will now be caused by exposure. In addition, there may be cases caused by exposure for whom disease would never have occurred. Let A_0 and A_1 be the numbers of cases that would occur over a given interval when exposure is absent and present, respectively. A fraction $1 - F$ of A_0 cases would be unaffected by exposure; for these cases, completions of C' precede completions of C. The product $A_0(1 - F)$ is the number of cases unaffected by exposure. Subtracting this product from A_1 gives $A_1 - A_0(1 - F)$ for the number of cases in which exposure played an etiologic role. The fraction of A_1 cases attributable to C (a sufficient cause with exposure) is thus

$$\frac{A_1 - A_0(1 - F)}{A_1} = 1 - (1 - F)/RR \qquad [4\text{–}1]$$

If we randomly sample one case, this etiologic fraction formula equals the probability that exposure caused that case, or the *probability of causation* for the case. Although it is of great biologic and legal interest, this probability cannot be epidemiologically estimated if nothing is known about the fraction F (Greenland and Robins, 1988, 2000; Greenland, 1999a; Beyea and Greenland, 1999; Robins and Greenland, 1989a, 1989b). This problem is discussed further in Chapter 16 under the topic of attributable-fraction estimation.

For preventive exposures, let F now be the fraction of exposed cases A_1 for whom disease would have been caused by a mechanism requiring absence of exposure (i.e., nonexposure, or not-E), had exposure been absent. Then the product $A_1(1 - F)$ is the number of cases unaffected by exposure; subtracting this product from A_0 gives $A_0 - A_1(1 - F)$ for the number of cases in which exposure would play a preventive role. The fraction of the A_0 unexposed cases that were caused by nonexposure (i.e., attributable to a sufficient cause with nonexposure) is thus

$$[A_0 - A_1(1 - F)]/A_0 = 1 - RR(1 - F)$$

As with the etiologic fraction, this fraction cannot be estimated if nothing is known about F.

Returning to a causal exposure, it is commonly assumed, often without statement or supporting evidence, that completion of C and C' occur independently in the cohort, so that the probability of "susceptibility" to exposure, $\Pr(C)$, can be derived by the ordinary laws of probability for independent events. Now $\Pr(C') = A_0/N = R_0$; thus, under independence,

$$\begin{aligned}\Pr(C \text{ or } C') &= A_1/N = R_1 \\ &= \Pr(C) + \Pr(C') - \Pr(C)\Pr(C') \\ &= \Pr(C) + R_0 - \Pr(C)R_0 \qquad [4\text{–}2]\end{aligned}$$

Rearrangement yields

$$\Pr(C) = \frac{A_1/N - A_0/N}{1 - A_0/N} = \frac{R_1 - R_0}{1 - R_0} \qquad [4\text{–}3]$$

The right-hand expression is the causal risk difference divided by the proportion surviving under nonexposure. Hence the equation can be rewritten

$$\Pr(\mathrm{C}) = (R_1 - R_0)/S_0 = (S_0 - S_1)/S_0 = 1 - S_1/S_0$$

This measure was first derived by Sheps (1958), who referred to it as the *relative difference;* it was later proposed as an index of susceptibility to exposure effects by Khoury et al. (1989a) based on the independence assumption. But as with the independence condition, one cannot verify equation 4–3 from epidemiologic data alone, and it is rarely if ever plausible on biologic grounds.

A NOTE ON TERMINOLOGY

More than with other concepts, there is profoundly inconsistent and confusing terminology across the literature on attributable fractions. Levin (1953) used the term *attributable proportion* for his original measure of population disease impact, which in our terms is an excess fraction or risk fraction. Many epidemiologic texts thereafter used the term *attributable risk* to refer to the risk difference $R_1 - R_0$ and called Levin's measure an *attributable risk percent* (e.g., MacMahon and Pugh, 1970; Koepsell and Weiss, 2003). By the 1970s, however, portions of the biostatistics literature began calling Levin's measure an *attributable risk* (e.g., Walter, 1976; Breslow and Day, 1980), and unfortunately, part of the epidemiologic literature followed suit. Some epidemiologists struggled to keep the distinction by introducing the term *attributable fraction* for Levin's concept (Ouellet et al., 1979; Deubner et al., 1980); others adopted the term *etiologic fraction* for the same concept and thus confused it with the fraction of cases caused by exposure. The term *attributable risk* continues to be used for completely different concepts, such as the risk difference, the risk fraction, the rate fraction, and the etiologic fraction. Because of this confusion we recommend that the term *attributable risk* be avoided entirely, and that the term *etiologic fraction* not be used for relative excess measures.

GENERALIZING DEFINITIONS OF EFFECT

For convenience, we have given the above definitions for the situation in which we can imagine the cohort of interest subject to either of two distinct conditions, treatments, interventions, or exposure levels over (or at the start of) the time interval of interest. We ordinarily think of these exposures as applying separately to each cohort member. But to study public health interventions, we must generalize our concept of exposure to general populations, and allow variation in exposure effects across individuals and subgroups. We will henceforth consider the "exposure" of a population as referring to the *pattern* of exposure (or treatment) among the individuals in the population. That is, we will consider the subscripts 1 and 0 to denote different *distributions* of exposure across the population. With this view, effect measures refer to comparisons of outcome distributions under different pairs of exposure patterns across the population of interest (Greenland, 2002a; Maldonado and Greenland, 2002).

To illustrate this general epidemiologic concept of effect, suppose our population comprises just three members at the start of a 5-year interval, each of whom smokes one pack of cigarettes a day at the start of the interval. Let us give these people identifying numbers, 1, 2, and 3, respectively. Suppose we are concerned with the effect of different distributions (patterns) of mailed antismoking literature on the mortality experience of this population during the interval. One possible exposure pattern is

Person 1: Mailing at start of interval and quarterly thereafter
Person 2: Mailing at start of interval and yearly thereafter
Person 3: No mailing

Call this pattern 0, or the reference pattern. Another possible exposure pattern is

Person 1: No mailing
Person 2: Mailing at start of interval and yearly thereafter
Person 3: Mailing at start of interval and quarterly thereafter

Call this exposure pattern 1, or the index pattern; it differs from pattern 0 only in that the treatment of persons 1 and 3 are interchanged.

Under both patterns, one third of the population receives yearly mailings, one third receives quarterly mailings, and one third receives no mailing. Yet it is perfectly reasonable that pattern 0 may produce a different outcome from pattern 1. For example, suppose person 1 would simply discard the mailings unopened, and so under either pattern would continue smoking and die at year 4 of a smoking-related cancer. Person 2 receives the same treatment under either pattern; suppose that under either pattern person 2 dies at year 1 of a myocardial infarction. But suppose person 3 would continue smoking under pattern 0, until at year 3 she dies from a smoking-related stroke, whereas under pattern 1 she would read the mailings, successfully quit smoking by year 2, and as a consequence suffer no stroke or other cause of death before the end of follow-up.

The total deaths and time lived under exposure pattern 0 would be $A_0 = 3$ (all die) and $T_0 = 4 + 1 + 3 = 8$ years, whereas the total deaths and time lived under exposure pattern 1 would be $A_1 = 2$ and $T_1 = 4 + 1 + 5 = 10$ years. The effects of pattern 1 versus pattern 0 on this population would thus be to decrease the incidence rate from $3/8 = 0.38$ per year to $2/10 = 0.20$ per year, a causal rate difference of $0.20 - 0.38 = -0.18$ per year and a causal rate ratio of $0.20/0.38 = 0.53$; to decrease the incidence proportion from $3/3 = 1.00$ to $2/3 = 0.67$, a causal risk difference of $0.67 - 1.00 = -0.33$ and a causal risk ratio of $0.67/1.00 = 0.67$; and to increase the total years of life lived from 8 to 10. The fraction of deaths under pattern 0 that is preventable by pattern 1 is $(3 - 2)/3 = 0.33$, which equals the fraction of deaths under pattern 0 for whom change to pattern 1 would have etiologic relevance. In contrast, the fraction of the rate "prevented" (removed) by pattern 1 relative to pattern 0 is $(0.38 - 0.20)/0.38 = 1 - 0.53 = 0.47$ and represents only the rate reduction under pattern 1; it does not equal an etiologic fraction.

This example illustrates two key points that epidemiologists should bear in mind when interpreting effect measures:

1. Effects on incidence rates are not the same as effects on incidence proportions (average risks). Common terminology, such as "relative risk," invites confusion among effect measures. Unless the outcome is uncommon for all exposure patterns under study during the interval of interest, the type of relative risk must be kept distinct. In the preceding example, the rate ratio was 0.53, whereas the risk ratio was 0.67. Likewise, the type of attributable fraction must be kept distinct. In the preceding example, the preventable fraction of deaths was 0.33, whereas the preventable fraction of the rate was 0.47.
2. Not all individuals respond alike to exposures or treatments. Therefore, it is not always sufficient to distinguish exposure patterns by simple summaries, such as "80% exposed" versus "20% exposed." In the preceding example, both exposure patterns had one third of the population given quarterly mailings and one third given yearly mailings, so the patterns were indistinguishable based on exposure prevalence. The effects were produced entirely by the differences in responsiveness of the persons treated.

POPULATION-ATTRIBUTABLE FRACTIONS AND IMPACT FRACTIONS

One often sees *population-attributable risk percent* or *population-attributable fraction* defined as the reduction in incidence that would be achieved if the population had been entirely unexposed, compared with its current (actual) exposure pattern. This concept, due to Levin (1953, who called it an *attributable proportion*), is a special case of the definition of attributable fraction based on exposure pattern. In particular, it is a comparison of the incidence (either rate or number of cases, which must be kept distinct) under the observed pattern of exposure with the incidence under a counterfactual pattern in which exposure or treatment is entirely absent from the population.

Complete removal of an exposure is often very unrealistic, as with smoking and with air pollution; even with legal restrictions and cessation or clean-up programs, many people will continue to expose themselves or to be exposed. A measure that allows for these realities is the *impact fraction* (Morgenstern and Bursic, 1982), which is a comparison of incidence under the observed exposure pattern with incidence under a counterfactual pattern in which exposure is only partially removed from the population. Again, this is a special case of our definition of attributable fraction based on exposure pattern.

STANDARDIZED MEASURES OF ASSOCIATION AND EFFECT

Consider again the concept of standardization as introduced at the end of Chapter 3. Given a standard distribution $T_1, \ldots, T_K$ of person-times across K categories or strata defined by one or more variables and a schedule $I_1, \ldots, I_K$ of incidence rates in those categories, we have the standardized rate

$$I_s = \frac{\sum_{k=1}^{K} T_k I_k}{\sum_{k=1}^{K} T_k}$$

which is the average of the I_k weighted by the T_k. If $I_1{}^*, \ldots, I_K{}^*$ represents another schedule of rates for the same categories, and

$$I_s{}^* = \frac{\sum_{k=1}^{K} T_k I_k{}^*}{\sum_{k=1}^{K} T_k}$$

is the standardized rate for this schedule, then

$$IR_s = \frac{I_s}{I_s^*} = \sum T_k I_k \Big/ \sum T_k I_k^*$$

is called a *standardized rate ratio.* The defining feature of this ratio is that the same standard distribution is used to weight the numerator and denominator rate. Similarly,

$$ID_s = \sum T_k I_k - \sum T_k I_k^* = \sum T_k (I_k - I_k^*)$$

is called the *standardized rate difference*; note that it is not only a difference of standardized rates, but is also a weighted average of the stratum-specific rate differences $I_k - I_k^*$ using the same weights as were used for the standardization (the T_k).

Suppose that $I_1, \ldots, I_K$ represent the rates observed or predicted for strata of a given target population if it is exposed to some cause or preventive of disease, $T_1, \ldots, T_K$ are the observed person-time in strata of that population, and $I_1^*, \ldots, I_K^*$ represent the rates predicted or observed for strata of the population if it is not exposed. The presumption is then that $IR_s = I_s/I_s^*$ and ID_s are the effects of exposure on this population, comparing the overall (crude) rates that would occur under distinct exposure conditions. This interpretation assumes, however, that the relative distribution of person-times would be unaffected by exposure.

If $I_1^*, \ldots, I_K^*$ represent counterfactual rather than actual rates, say, because the population was actually exposed, then I_s^* need not represent the overall rate that would occur in the population if exposure were removed. For instance, the change in rates from the I_k to the I_k^* could shift the person-time distribution $T_1, \ldots, T_K$ to $T_1^*, \ldots, T_K^*$. In addition, as discussed earlier, the exposure could affect competing risks, and this effect could also shift the person-time distribution. If this shift is large, the standardized rate ratio and difference will not properly reflect the actual effect of exposure on the rate of disease (Greenland, 1996a).

There are a few special conditions under which the effect of exposure on person-time will not affect the standardized rate ratio. If the stratum-specific ratios I_k/I_k^* are constant across categories, the standardized rate ratio will equal this constant stratum-specific ratio. If the exposure has only a small effect on person-time, then, regardless of the person-time distribution used as the standard, the difference between a standardized ratio and the actual effect will also be small. In general, however, one should be alert to the fact that a special assumption is needed to allow one to interpret a standardized rate ratio as an effect measure, even if there is no methodologic problem with the observations. Analogously, the standardized rate difference will not be an effect measure except when exposure does not affect the person-time distribution or when other special conditions exist, such as constant rate differences $I_k - I_k^*$ across categories.

Incidence proportions have denominators $N_1, \ldots, N_K$ that are not affected by changing rates or competing risks. Thus, if these denominators are used to create standardized risk ratios and differences, the resulting measures may be interpreted as effect measures without the need for the special assumptions required to interpret standardized rate ratios and differences.

STANDARDIZED MORBIDITY RATIOS (SMRs)

When the distribution of exposed person-time provides the standard, the standardized rate ratio takes on a simplified form. Suppose $T_1, \ldots, T_K$ are the exposed person time, $A_1, \ldots, A_K$ are the number of cases in the exposed, $I_1, \ldots, I_K$ are the rates in the exposed, and $I_1^*, \ldots, I_K^*$ are the rates that would have occurred in the exposed had they not been exposed. Then in each stratum we have $T_k I_k = A_k$, and so the standardized rate ratio becomes

$$\sum T_k I_k \Big/ \sum T_k I_k^* = \sum A_k \Big/ \sum T_k I_k^*$$

The numerator of this ratio is just the total number of exposed cases occurring in the population. The denominator is the number of cases that would be expected to occur in the absence of exposure if the exposure did not affect the distribution of person-time. This ratio of observed to expected cases is called the *standardized morbidity ratio* (SMR), *standardized incidence ratio* (SIR), or, when death is the outcome, the *standardized mortality ratio*. When incidence proportions are used in place of incidence rates, the same sort of simplification occurs upon taking the exposed distribution of persons as the standard: The standardized risk ratio reduces to a ratio of observed to expected cases.

Many occupational and environmental studies that examine populations of exposed workers attempt to estimate SMRs by using age–sex–race categories as strata, and then use age–sex–race specific rates from the general population in place of the desired counterfactual rates $I_1{}^*, \ldots, I_K{}^*$. A major problem with this practice is that of *residual confounding*. There will usually be many other differences between the exposed population and the general population besides their age, sex, and race distributions (differences in smoking, health care, etc.), and some of these differences will confound the resulting standardized ratio. This problem is an example of the more common problem of residual confounding in observational epidemiology, to which we will return in later chapters.

SMRs estimated across exposure categories or different populations are sometimes compared directly with one another to assess a dose–response trend, for example. Such comparisons are usually not fully standardized because each exposure category's SMR is weighted by the distribution of that category's person-time or persons, and these weights are not necessarily comparable across the exposure categories. The result is residual confounding by the variables used to create the strata as well as by unmeasured variables (Yule, 1934; Breslow and Day, 1987; Greenland, 1987e). There are, however, several circumstances under which this difference in weights will not lead to important confounding (beyond the residual confounding problem discussed earlier).

One circumstance is when the compared populations differ little in their distribution of person-time across strata (e.g., when they have similar age–sex–race distributions). Another circumstance is when the stratification factors have little effect on the outcome under study (which is unusual; age and sex are strongly related to most outcomes). Yet another circumstance is when the stratum-specific ratios are nearly constant across strata (no modification of the ratio by the standardization variables) (Breslow and Day, 1987). Although none of these circumstances may hold exactly, the first and last are often together roughly approximated; when this is so, the lack of mutual standardization among compared SMRs will lead to little distortion. Attention can then turn to the many other validity problems that plague SMR studies, such as residual confounding, missing data, and measurement error (see Chapters 9 and 19). If, however, one cannot be confident that the bias due to comparing SMRs directly is small, estimates should be based on a single common standard applied to the risks in all groups, or on a regression model that accounts for the differences among the compared populations and the effects of exposure on person-time (Chapter 20).

PREVALENCE RATIOS

In Chapter 3 we showed that the crude prevalence odds, PO, equals the crude incidence rate, I, times the average disease duration, $\overline{D}$, when both the population at risk and the prevalence pool are stationary and there is no migration in or out of the prevalence pool. Restating this relation separately for a single population under exposure and nonexposure, or one exposed and one unexposed population, we have

$$PO_1 = I_1\overline{D}_1 \quad \text{and} \quad PO_0 = I_0\overline{D}_0 \qquad [4\text{–}5]$$

where the subscripts 1 and 0 refer to exposed and unexposed, respectively. If the average disease duration is the same regardless of exposure, i.e., if $\overline{D}_1 = \overline{D}_0$, the crude prevalence odds ratio, POR, will equal the crude incidence rate ratio IR:

$$POR = \frac{PO_1}{PO_0} = \frac{I_1}{I_0} = IR \qquad [4\text{–}6]$$

Unfortunately, if exposure affects mortality, it will also alter the age distribution of the population. Thus, because older people tend to die sooner, exposure will indirectly affect average duration, so that $\overline{D}_1$ will not equal $\overline{D}_0$. In that, case equation 4–6 will not hold exactly, although it may still hold approximately (Newman, 1988).

OTHER MEASURES

The measures that we have discussed are by no means exhaustive of all those that have been proposed. Not all proposed measures of effect meet our definition of effect measure—that is, not all are a contrast of the outcome of a *single* population under two *different* conditions. Examples of measures that are *not* effect measures by our definition include correlation coefficients and related variance-reduction measures (Greenland et al., 1986, 1991). Examples of measures that are effect measures by our definition, but not discussed in detail here, include expected years of life lost (Murray et al., 2002), as well as risk and rate advancement periods (Brenner et al., 1993).

Years of life lost, $T_0/N - T_1/N$, and the corresponding ratio measure, T_0/T_1, have some noteworthy advantages over conventional rate and risk-based effect measures. They are not subject to the problems of inestimability that arise for etiologic fractions (Robins and Greenland, 1991), nor are they subject to concerns about exposure effects on time at risk. In fact, they represent the exposure effect on time at risk. They are, however, more difficult to estimate statistically from typical epidemiologic data, especially when only case-control data (Chapter 8) are available, which may in part explain their limited popularity thus far (Boshuizen and Greenland, 1997).

CHAPTER 5

Concepts of Interaction

Sander Greenland, Timothy L. Lash, and Kenneth J. Rothman

Statistical Interaction and Effect-Measure Modification 72
Scale Dependence of Effect-Measure Modification 72
Biologic Interactions 74
Potential Outcomes for Two Variables 75
Relation of Response-Type Distributions to Average Risks 77
Relation of Response-Type Distributions to Additivity 78
The Nonidentifiabilty of Interaction Response Types 79
Interactions under the Sufficient-Cause Model 80
Relation between the Potential-Outcome and Sufficient-Cause Models of Interaction 81
Biologic versus Statistical Interaction 82
Public Health Interactions 83

The concept of interaction centers on the idea that the effect of an exposure, compared with a reference unexposed condition, may depend on the presence of one or more other conditions. A well-known example concerns the effect of occupational exposure to asbestos dust on lung cancer risk, which depends on smoking status (Berry and Liddell, 2004). As a hypothetical illustration, suppose we examine the average 10-year risk of lung cancer in an occupational setting and find that, among nonsmoking male asbestos workers, this risk is 3/1,000, and the corresponding risk is 1/1,000 in comparable nonsmoking men who did not work with asbestos. Suppose also that the risk is 20/1,000 among male asbestos workers who smoked, and it is 10/1,000 in comparable men who smoked and did not work with asbestos. The risk ratio associating asbestos work with lung cancer risk is then $3/1 = 3$ in nonsmokers, greater than the risk ratio of $20/10 = 2$ in smokers. In contrast, the risk difference is $3 - 1 = 2/1{,}000$ among nonsmokers, less than the risk difference of $20 - 10 = 10/1{,}000$ among smokers. Thus, when using the ratio measure, it appears that the association between asbestos exposure and lung cancer risk is greater in nonsmokers than smokers. When using the difference measure, however, it appears that the association is considerably *less* for nonsmokers than for smokers.

The potential scale dependence of an assessment of interaction illustrates the kind of issue that complicates understanding of the concept. Indeed, the concept of interaction generated much debate when it first became a focus for epidemiologists, as seen in Rothman (1974, 1976a, 1976b), Koopman (1977), Kupper and Hogan (1978), Walter and Holford (1978), and Siemiatycki and Thomas (1981). The ensuing literature identified a number of distinctions and concepts whose delineation has helped shed light on the earlier disagreements and has pointed the way to further elaboration of concepts of interaction; for examples, see Blot and Day (1979), Rothman et al. (1980), Saracci (1980), Koopman (1981), Walker (1981), Miettinen (1982b), Weinberg (1986), Greenland and Poole (1988), Weed et al. (1988), Thompson (1991), Greenland (1993b), Darroch and Borkent (1994), Darroch (1997), and VanderWeele and Robins (2007a, 2008a).

In addition to scale dependence, another problem is the ambiguity of the term *interaction*, which has been used for a number of distinct statistical, biologic, and public health concepts. Failure to distinguish between these concepts was responsible for much of the early controversy (Blot and Day, 1979; Saracci, 1980; Rothman et al., 1980). Once these distinctions are made, there remains the question of what can be learned about interaction from epidemiologic data (Thompson, 1991).

The present chapter provides definitions and makes distinctions among concepts of interaction. Chapter 16 describes how stratified analysis methods can be used to study interactions and the limitations of such methods. We begin by discussing statistical interaction, a concept that refers to associations, whether causal or not. Statistical interaction is scale-dependent. When no bias is present, so that observed associations validly estimate causal effects of interest, statistical interaction corresponds to effect-measure modification. After discussing the relation of statistical interaction to effect modification, we discuss models for biologic interaction. We show that when effects are measured by causal risk differences and biologic interaction is defined as modification of potential-response types, biologic interaction is implied by departures from additivity of effects. We also show that biologic interaction may be present even if there is additivity of effects, when there are opposing types of interaction that cancel one another, leaving the net effect additive. We then contrast this potential-outcome model of biologic interaction to that based on the sufficient-component cause model introduced in Chapter 2. We conclude with a discussion of public health interaction.

STATISTICAL INTERACTION AND EFFECT-MEASURE MODIFICATION

When no bias is present, the definition of interaction that is often used in statistics books and software programs (particularly for analysis of variance) is logically equivalent to the definition of effect-measure modification or heterogeneity of effect. It is frequently described as "departure from additivity of effects on the chosen outcome scale." Thus, methods for analyzing statistical interactions can be viewed as methods for analyzing effect-measure modification under the assumption that all bias has been adequately controlled (see Chapter 15).

As seen in the above example of asbestos and smoking effects, the presence or absence of statistical interaction between two factors X and Z depends on the scale with which one chooses to measure their association. Suppose that both X and Z have effects, and the risk difference for one remains constant across levels of the other, so that there is no modification of the risk differences (i.e., there is homogeneity of the risk differences). If there is no bias (so that associations equal effects), this state of affairs corresponds to no statistical interaction *on the risk-difference scale* for the effect, because the combined effect of X and Z on risk can be computed simply by adding together the separate risk differences for X and Z. In the example of interaction between asbestos exposure and smoking, there was effect-measure modification, or statistical interaction, on the difference scale, because risk added by asbestos exposure was greater among smokers than among nonsmokers. There was also effect-measure modification, or statistical interaction, between asbestos and smoking on the risk-ratio scale for the effect, because the amount that asbestos multiplied the risk was less among smokers than among nonsmokers.

SCALE DEPENDENCE OF EFFECT-MEASURE MODIFICATION

As explained in Chapter 4, if both X and Z have effects and there is no modification (heterogeneity) of the risk differences for one factor by the other factor, there has to be modification of the risk ratios. Conversely, if X and Z have effects and there is no modification of the risk ratios, there has to be modification of the risk differences. Commonly, both the risk differences and risk ratios for one factor are heterogeneous across categories of the other. In that case, they may be modified in opposite directions, as seen in the example for asbestos and smoking.

To explain why homogeneity of the effect measure on one scale requires heterogeneity of the effect measure on the other scale when both factors have effects, we will first examine the case in which risk differences are homogeneous and risk ratios are heterogeneous. We will then examine the opposite case.

TABLE 5–1

Notation for Risks with Two Binary(1, 0) Exposure Variables

	$Z = 1$	$Z = 0$	Risk Difference	Risk Ratio
$X = 1$	R_{11}	R_{10}	$R_{11} - R_{10}$	R_{11}/R_{10}
$X = 0$	R_{01}	R_{00}	$R_{01} - R_{00}$	R_{01}/R_{00}
Risk difference	$R_{11} - R_{01}$	$R_{10} - R_{00}$		
Risk ratio	R_{11}/R_{01}	R_{10}/R_{00}		

To begin, write R_{ij} for the average risk (incidence proportion) when $X = i$ and $Z = j$, as in Table 5–1. Suppose the risk difference for $X = 1$ versus $X = 0$ when $Z = 0$ (which is $R_{10} - R_{00}$) equals the risk difference for $X = 1$ versus $X = 0$ when $Z = 1$ (which is $R_{11} - R_{01}$):

$$R_{11} - R_{01} = R_{10} - R_{00} \qquad [5\text{–}1]$$

By subtracting R_{00} from each side and rearranging, we can rewrite this equation as

$$R_{11} - R_{00} = (R_{10} - R_{00}) + (R_{01} - R_{00}) \qquad [5\text{–}2]$$

This equation shows that the risk difference for changing the exposure status from $X = Z = 0$ to $X = Z = 1$ can be found by simply *adding* the risk difference for $X = 1$ versus $X = 0$ when $Z = 0$ to the risk difference for $Z = 1$ versus $Z = 0$ when $X = 0$. If we divide both sides of equation 5–1 by R_{00} (the risk when $X = 0$, $Z = 0$), we get

$$\frac{R_{11}}{R_{00}} - \frac{R_{01}}{R_{00}} = \frac{R_{10}}{R_{00}} - 1 \qquad [5\text{–}3]$$

By subtracting 1 from each side and rearranging, we can rewrite this equation in terms of the excess risk ratios:

$$\frac{R_{11}}{R_{00}} - 1 = \left(\frac{R_{10}}{R_{00}} - 1\right) + \left(\frac{R_{01}}{R_{00}} - 1\right) \qquad [5\text{–}4]$$

If both X and Z have effects, the additivity of the excess risk ratio in equation 5–4 implies that $R_{11}/R_{01} \neq R_{10}/R_{00}$; that is, the risk ratio for $X = 1$ versus $X = 0$ when $Z = 1(R_{11}/R_{01})$ cannot equal the risk ratio for $X = 1$ versus $X = 0$ when $Z = 0(R_{10}/R_{00})$. We reach this conclusion because the equality

$$R_{11}/R_{01} = R_{10}/R_{00} \qquad [5\text{–}5]$$

implies *multiplicativity* of the risk ratios:

$$R_{11}/R_{00} = (R_{11}/R_{01})(R_{01}/R_{00}) = (R_{10}/R_{00})(R_{01}/R_{00}) \qquad [5\text{–}6]$$

which contradicts equation 5–4 unless $R_{10}/R_{00} = 1$ or $R_{01}/R_{00} = 1$. Neither of these risk ratios can equal 1, however, when X and Z both affect risk.

To show that homogeneity of the risk ratio requires heterogeneity of the risk difference, begin by assuming no modification of the risk ratio, so that equation 5–5 *does* hold. Then equation 5–6 must also hold, and we can take the logarithm of both sides to get the equation

$$\ln(R_{11}/R_{00}) = \ln(R_{10}/R_{00}) + \ln(R_{01}/R_{00}) \qquad [5\text{–}7]$$

or

$$\ln(R_{11}) - \ln(R_{00}) = \ln(R_{10}) - \ln(R_{00}) + \ln(R_{01}) - \ln(R_{00}) \qquad [5\text{–}8]$$

Equation 5–7 shows that the log risk ratio for changing the exposure status from $X = Z = 0$ to $X = Z = 1$ can be found by simply adding the log risk ratio for $X = 1$ versus $X = 0$ when $Z = 0$ to the log risk ratio for $Z = 1$ versus $Z = 0$ when $X = 0$. Thus, homogeneity (no modification) of the risk ratio corresponds to additivity (no statistical interaction) on the log-risk scale for the outcome (equation 5–8). Combined effects are simply the sum of effects on the log-risk scale. Furthermore, if both X and Z have nonzero effects and these effects are additive on the log-risk scale, the effects cannot be additive on the risk scale. That is, the absence of statistical interaction on the log-risk scale (equation 5–7) implies the presence of statistical interaction on the risk-difference scale, if both factors have effects and there is no bias.

Because the additive log-risk equation 5–7 is equivalent to the multiplicative risk-ratio equation 5–6, log risk-ratio additivity corresponds to risk-ratio multiplicativity. Thus, "no multiplicative interaction" is often described as "no statistical interaction on the log-risk ratio scale." Unfortunately, because most epidemiologic statistics are based on multiplicative models, there has developed a bad habit of dropping the word *multiplicative* and claiming that there is "no interaction" whenever one believes that the data are consistent with equation 5–5 or 5–6. Such loose usage invites confusion with other concepts of interaction. To avoid such confusion, we strongly advise that one should refer to the scale or measure that one is examining with more precise phrases, such as "no risk-ratio heterogeneity was evident," "no risk-difference heterogeneity was evident," "no departure from risk-ratio multiplicativity was evident," or "no departure from risk-difference additivity was evident," as appropriate. The term *effect modification* is also ambiguous, and we again advise more precise terms such as *risk-difference modification* or *risk-ratio modification,* as appropriate.

Another source of ambiguity is the fact that equations 5–1 through 5–8 can all be rewritten using a different type of outcome measure, such as rates, odds, prevalences, means, or other measures in place of risks R_{ij}. Each outcome measure leads to a different scale for statistical interaction and a corresponding concept of effect-measure modification and heterogeneity of effect. Thus, when both factors have effects, absence of statistical interaction on any particular scale necessarily implies presence of statistical interaction on many other scales.

Consider now relative measures of risk: risk ratios, rate ratios, and odds ratios. If the disease risk is low at all levels of the study variables (i.e., less than about 0.1), absence of statistical interaction for one of these ratio measures implies absence of statistical interaction for the other two measures. For larger risks, however, absence of statistical interaction for one ratio measure implies that there must be some modification of the other two ratio measures when both factors have effects. For example, the absence of modification of the odds ratio,

$$\frac{R_{11}/(1 - R_{11})}{R_{01}(1 - R_{01})} = \frac{R_{10}/(1 - R_{10})}{R_{00}/(1 - R_{00})} \qquad [5\text{–}9]$$

is equivalent to no multiplicative interaction on the odds scale. But, if X and Z have effects, then equation 5–9 implies that there must be modification of the risk ratio, so that equations 5–6 through 5–8 cannot hold unless all the risks are low. In a similar fashion, equation 5–9 also implies modification of the rate ratio. Parallel results apply for difference measures: If the disease risk is always low, absence of statistical interaction for one of the risk difference, rate difference, or odds difference implies absence of statistical interaction for the other two. Conversely, if disease risk is high, absence of statistical interaction for one difference measure implies that there must be some modification of the other two difference measures when both factors have effects.

The preceding examples and algebra demonstrate that statistical interaction is a phenomenon whose presence or absence, as well as magnitude, is usually determined by the scale chosen for measuring departures from additivity of effects. To avoid ambiguity, one must specify precisely the scale on which one is measuring such interactions. In doing so, it is undesirable to use a term as vague as *interaction,* because more precise phrases can always be substituted by using the equivalent concept of effect-measure modification or heterogeneity of the effect measure.

BIOLOGIC INTERACTIONS

There are two major approaches to the topic of biologic (causal) interaction. One approach is based on delineating specific mechanisms of interaction. The concept of *mechanistic interaction* is rarely given a precise definition, but it is meant to encompass the notion of direct physical or chemical reactions among exposures, their metabolites, or their reaction products within individuals or vectors of exposure transmission. Examples include the inhibition of gastric nitrosation of dietary amines and amides by ascorbic acid and the quenching of free radicals in tissues by miscellaneous antioxidants.

Description of a mechanism whereby such interactions take place does not lead immediately to precise predictions about epidemiologic observations. One reason is that rarely, if ever, is a mechanism proposed that can account for all observed cases of disease, or all effects of all risk factors, measured and unmeasured. Background noise, in the form of unaccounted-for effects and biologic interactions with other factors, can easily obliterate any pattern sought by the investigator. Nonetheless, efforts have been made to test hypotheses about biologic mechanisms and interactions using simplified abstract models. Such efforts have been concentrated largely in cancer epidemiology; for example, see Moolgavkar (1986, 2004).

A key limitation of these and other biologic modeling efforts is that any given data pattern can be predicted from a number of dissimilar mechanisms or models for disease development (Siemiatycki and Thomas, 1981; Thompson, 1991), even if no bias is present. In response to this limitation, a number of authors define biologic interactions within the context of a general causal model, so that it does not depend on any specific mechanistic model for the disease process. We describe two such definitions. The first definition, based on the *potential-outcome* or *counterfactual* causal model described in Chapter 4, has a long history in pharmacology (at least back to the 1920s) and is sometimes called the dependent-action definition of interaction. The second definition, based on the *sufficient-cause* model described in Chapter 2, has been more common in epidemiology. After providing these definitions, we will describe how they are logically related to one another.

POTENTIAL OUTCOMES FOR TWO VARIABLES

Consider the following example. Suppose we wish to study the effects of two fixed variables X and Z on 10-year mortality D in a closed cohort. If X and Z are binary indicators, there are four possible exposure combinations that each person in the cohort could have: $X = Z = 0$, $X = 1$ and $Z = 0$, $X = 0$ and $Z = 1$, or $X = Z = 1$. Furthermore, every person has one of two possible outcomes under each of the four combinations: They either survive the 10 years ($D = 0$) or they do not ($D = 1$). This means that there are $2 \cdot 2 \cdot 2 \cdot 2 = 2^4 = 16$ possible types of person in the cohort, according to how the person would respond to each of the four exposure combinations.

These 16 types of people are shown in Table 5–2. Columns 2 through 5 of the table show the outcome ($Y = 1$ if disease develops, 0 if not) for the type of person in the row under the exposure combination shown in the column heading. For each type, we can define the risk for that type under each combination of X and Z as the outcome Y under that combination. Thus for a given response type, R_{11} is 1 or 0 according to whether Y is 1 or 0 when $X = 1$ and $Z = 1$, and so on for the other combinations of X and Z. We can then define various risk differences for each type. For example, $R_{11} - R_{01}$ and $R_{10} - R_{00}$ give the effects of changing from $X = 0$ to $X = 1$, and $R_{11} - R_{10}$ and $R_{01} - R_{00}$ for the effects of changing from $Z = 0$ to $Z = 1$. These differences may be 1, 0, or -1, which correspond to causal effect, no effect, and preventive effect of the change.

We can also define the difference between these risk differences. A useful fact is that the difference of the risk differences for changing X is equal to the difference of the risk differences in changing Z:

$$(R_{11} - R_{01}) - (R_{10} - R_{00}) = (R_{11} - R_{10}) - (R_{01} - R_{00}) \qquad [5\text{–}10]$$

This equation tells us that the change in the effect of X when we move across levels of Z is the same as the change in the effect of Z when we move across levels of X. The equation holds for every response type. We will hereafter call the difference of risk differences in equation [5–10] the *interaction contrast*, or *IC*.

Note first that equation [5–10] and hence the interaction contrast equals $R_{11} - R_{10} - R_{01} + R_{00}$. The final column of Table 5–2 provides this interaction contrast for each response type, along with phrases describing the causal process leading to the outcome (disease or no disease) in each type of person. For six types—types 1, 4, 6, 11, 13, 16—at least one factor never has an effect, and so there can be no interaction, because both factors must have an effect for there to be an interaction. The interaction contrast equals 0 for these six types. The other 10 types (marked with an asterisk)

TABLE 5–2

Possible Response Types (Potential Outcomes) for Two Binary Exposure Variables *X* and *Z* and a Binary Outcome Variable *Y*

Type	Outcome (Risk) Y when Exposure Combination Is: $X = 1$, $Z = 1$	$X = 0$, $Z = 1$	$X = 1$, $Z = 0$	$X = 0$, $Z = 0$	Interaction Contrast (Difference in Risk Differences) $IC = R_{11} - R_{10} - R_{01} + R_{00}$ and Description of Causal Type	
1	1	1	1	1	0	no effect (doomed)
2*	1	1	1	0	−1	single plus joint causation by $X = 1$ and $Z = 1$
3*	1	1	0	1	1	$Z = 1$ blocks $X = 1$ effect (preventive antagonism)
4	1	1	0	0	0	$X = 1$ ineffective, $Z = 1$ causal
5*	1	0	1	1	1	$X = 1$ blocks $Z = 1$ effect (preventive antagonism)
6	1	0	1	0	0	$X = 1$ causal, $Z = 1$ ineffective
7*	1	0	0	1	2	mutual blockage (preventive antagonism)
8*	1	0	0	0	1	$X = 1$ plus $Z = 1$ causal (causal synergism)
9*	0	1	1	1	−1	$X = 1$ plus $Z = 1$ preventive (preventive synergism)
10*	0	1	1	0	−2	mutual blockage (causal antagonism)
11	0	1	0	1	0	$X = 1$ preventive, $Z = 1$ ineffective
12*	0	1	0	0	−1	$X = 1$ blocks $Z = 1$ effect (causal antagonism)
13	0	0	1	1	0	$X = 1$ ineffective, $Z = 1$ preventive
14*	0	0	1	0	−1	$Z = 1$ blocks $X = 1$ effect (causal antagonism)
15*	0	0	0	1	1	single plus joint prevention by $X = 1$ and $Z = 1$
16	0	0	0	0	0	no effect (immune)

*Defined as interaction response type in present discussion (types with a nonzero interaction contrast).

can be viewed as exhibiting some type of interaction (or interdependence) of the effects of the two factors (X and Z); for these 10 types, the interaction contrast is not 0.

The defining feature of these 10 interaction types is that we cannot say what the effect of X will be (to cause, prevent, or have no effect on disease) unless we know that person's value for Z (and conversely, we cannot know the effect of Z without knowing that person's value of X). In other words, for an interaction type, the effect of one factor depends on the person's status for the other factor. An equally apt description is to say that each factor modifies the effect of the other. Unfortunately, the term *effect modification* has often been used as a contraction of the term *effect-measure modification,* which we have showed is equivalent to statistical interaction and is scale-dependent, in contrast to the 10 interaction types in Table 5–2.

Some of the response types in Table 5–2 are easily recognized as interactions. For type 8, each factor causes the disease if and only if the other factor is present; thus both factors must be present for disease to occur. Hence, this type is said to represent synergistic effects. For type 10, each factor causes the disease if and only if the other factor is absent; thus each factor blocks the effect of the other. Hence, this type is said to represent mutually antagonistic effects.

Other interaction types are not always recognized as exhibiting interdependent effects. For example, type 2 has been described simply as one for which both factors can have an effect (Miettinen, 1982b). Note, however, that the presence of both factors can lead to a competitive interaction: For a type 2 person, each factor will cause disease when the other is absent, but neither factor can have an effect on the outcome under study ($D = 0$ or 1) once the other is present. Thus each factor affects the outcome under study only in the absence of the other, and so the two factors can be said to interact antagonistically for this outcome (Greenland and Poole, 1988).

RELATION OF RESPONSE-TYPE DISTRIBUTIONS TO AVERAGE RISKS

A cohort of more than a few people is inevitably a mix of different response types. To examine cohorts, we will return to using $R_{11}, R_{10}, R_{01}, R_{00}$ to denote the average risks (incidence proportions) in a cohort; these risks represent averages of the outcomes (risks) over the response types in the population under discussion. The risks shown in Table 5–2 can be thought of as special cases in which the cohort has just one member.

To compute the average risks, let p_k be the proportion of type k persons in the cohort (k = 1, . . . , 16). A useful feature of Table 5–2 is that we can compute the average risk of the cohort under any of the four listed combinations of exposure to X and Z by adding up the p_k for which there is a "1" in the column of interest. We thus obtain the following general formulas:

$$\begin{aligned} R_{11} &= \text{average risk if } X \text{ and } Z \text{ are } 1 \\ &= p_1 + p_2 + p_3 + p_4 + p_5 + p_6 + p_7 + p_8 \\ R_{01} &= \text{average risk if } X \text{ is } 0 \text{ and } Z \text{ is } 1 \\ &= p_1 + p_2 + p_3 + p_4 + p_9 + p_{10} + p_{11} + p_{12} \\ R_{10} &= \text{average risk if } X \text{ is } 1 \text{ and } Z \text{ is } 0 \\ &= p_1 + p_2 + p_5 + p_6 + p_9 + p_{10} + p_{13} + p_{14} \\ R_{00} &= \text{average risk if } X \text{ and } Z \text{ are } 0 \\ &= p_1 + p_3 + p_5 + p_7 + p_9 + p_{11} + p_{13} + p_{15} \end{aligned}$$

For a cohort in which none of the 10 interaction types is present, the additive-risk relation (equation 5–2) emerges among the average risks (incidence proportions) that would be observed under different exposure patterns (Greenland and Poole, 1988). With no interaction types, only p_1, p_4, p_6, p_{11}, p_{13}, and p_{16} are nonzero. In this situation, the incidence proportions under the four exposure patterns will be as follows:

$$\begin{aligned} R_{11} &= \text{average risk if } X \text{ and } Z \text{ are } 1 = p_1 + p_4 + p_6 \\ R_{01} &= \text{average risk if } X \text{ is } 0 \text{ and } Z \text{ is } 1 = p_1 + p_4 + p_{11} \\ R_{10} &= \text{average risk if } X \text{ is } 1 \text{ and } Z \text{ is } 0 = p_1 + p_6 + p_{13} \\ R_{00} &= \text{average risk if } X \text{ and } Z \text{ are } 0 = p_1 + p_{11} + p_{13} \end{aligned}$$

Then the separate risk differences for the effects of $X = 1$ alone and $Z = 1$ alone (relative to $X = Z = 0$) add to the risk difference for the effect of $X = 1$ and $Z = 1$ together:

$$R_{11} - R_{00} = p_4 + p_6 - (p_{11} + p_{13})$$

Rearranging the right side of the equation, we have

$$R_{11} - R_{00} = (p_6 - p_{13}) + (p_4 - p_{11})$$

Adding p_{13} to the left parenthetical and subtracting it from the right, and subtracting p_{11} from the left parenthetical and adding it to the right, we obtain

$$R_{11} - R_{00} = (p_6 + p_{13} - p_{11} - p_{13}) + (p_4 + p_{11} - p_{11} - p_{13}) \qquad [5\text{–}11]$$

Substituting from the definitions of incidence proportions with only noninteraction types, we have

$$R_{11} - R_{00} = (R_{10} - R_{00}) + (R_{01} - R_{00})$$

This equation is identical to equation 5–2 and so is equivalent to equation 5–1, which corresponds to no modification of the risk differences. There is a crucial difference in interpretation, however: Equation 5–2 is *descriptive* of the differences in risk among *different* study cohorts; in contrast, equation 5–10 is a *causal* relation among risks, because it refers to risks that would be observed in the *same* study cohort under different exposure conditions. The same cohort cannot be observed under different exposure conditions, so we must use the descriptive equation 5–2 as a substitute for the causal equation 5–11. This usage requires absence of confounding, or else standardization of the risks to adjust for confounding. The remainder of the present discussion will concern only the causal equation 5–11 and thus involves no concern regarding confounding or other bias. The discussion also applies to situations involving equation 5–2 in which either bias is absent or has been completely controlled (e.g., all confounding has been removed via standardization).

Four important points deserve emphasis. First, the preceding algebra shows that departures from causal additivity (equation 5–11) can occur only if interaction causal types are present in the cohort. Thus, *observation* of nonadditivity of risk differences (departures from equation 5–2) will imply the presence of interaction types in a cohort, provided the observed descriptive relations unbiasedly represent the causal relations in the cohort. Second, interaction types may be present and yet both the additive relations (equations 5–11 and 5–2) can still hold. This circumstance can occur because different interaction types could counterbalance each other's effect on the average risk. For example, suppose that, in addition to the noninteraction types, there were type 2 and type 8 persons in exactly equal proportions ($p_2 = p_8 > 0$). Then

$$R_{11} - R_{00} = p_2 + p_4 + p_6 + p_8 - (p_{11} + p_{13})$$

By rearranging, adding p_{13} to the left parenthetical and subtracting it from the right parenthetical, and adding p_{11} to the right parenthetical and subtracting it from the left parenthetical, we have

$$\begin{aligned} R_{11} - R_{00} &= (p_8 + p_6 + p_{13} - p_{11} - p_{13}) + (p_2 + p_4 + p_{11} - p_{11} - p_{13}) \\ &= (R_{10} - R_{00}) + (R_{01} - R_{00}) \end{aligned}$$

We may summarize these two points as follows: Departures from additivity imply the presence of interaction types, but additivity does not imply absence of interaction types.

The third point is that departure from risk additivity implies the presence of interaction types whether we are studying causal or preventive factors (Greenland and Poole, 1988). To see this, note that the preceding arguments made no assumptions about the absence of causal types (types 4 and 6 in the absence of interaction) or preventive types (types 11 and 13 in the absence of interaction). This point stands in contrast to earlier treatments, in which preventive interactions had to be studied using multiplicative models (Rothman, 1974; Walter and Holford, 1978).

The fourth point is that the definitions of response types (and hence interactions) given above are specific to the particular outcome under study. If, in our example, we switched to 5-year mortality, it is possible that many persons who would die within 10 years under some exposure combination (and so would be among types 1 through 15 in Table 5–2) would not die within 5 years. For instance, a person who was a type 8 when considering 10-year mortality could be a type 16 when considering 5-year mortality. In a similar fashion, it is possible that a person who would die within 10 years if and only if exposed to either factor would die within 5 years if and only if exposed to both factors. Such a person would be a type 2 (competitive action) for 10-year mortality but a type 8 (synergistic action) for 5-year mortality. To avoid the dependence of response type on follow-up time, one can base the definitions of response type on incidence time rather than risk (Greenland, 1993b).

RELATION OF RESPONSE-TYPE DISTRIBUTIONS TO ADDITIVITY

The interaction contrast $IC = R_{11} - R_{10} - R_{01} + R_{00}$ corresponds to departure of the risk difference contrasting $X = 1$ and $Z = 1$ to $X = 0$ and $Z = 0$ from what would be expected if no interaction types were present (i.e., if the risk difference for $X = Z = 1$ versus $X = Z = 0$ was just the sum of the risk difference for $X = 1$ versus $X = 0$ and the risk difference for $Z = 1$ versus $Z = 0$). In algebraic terms, we have

$$IC = (R_{11} - R_{00}) - (R_{10} - R_{00}) - (R_{01} - R_{00}) \qquad [5\text{–}12]$$

Substituting the proportions of response types for the risks in this formula and simplifying, we get

$$IC = (p_3 + p_5 + 2p_7 + p_8 + p_{15}) - (p_2 + p_9 + 2p_{10} + p_{12} + p_{14}) \qquad [5\text{–}13]$$

IC is thus composed of proportions of all 10 interaction types, and it will be zero if no interaction type is present. The proportions of types 7 and 10 weigh twice as heavily as the proportions of the other interaction types because they correspond to the types for which the effects of X reverse across strata of Z. Equation 5–13 illustrates the first two points above: Departure from additivity ($IC \neq 0$) implies the presence of interaction types, because $IC \neq 0$ requires some interaction types to be present; but additivity ($IC = 0$) does *not* imply absence of interaction types, because the *IC* can be zero even when some proportions within it are not zero. This phenomenon occurs when negative contributions to the *IC* from some interaction types balance out the positive contributions from other interaction types.

Departures from additivity may be separated into two classes. *Superadditivity* (also termed *transadditivity*) is defined as a "positive" departure, which for risks corresponds to $IC > 0$, or

$$R_{11} - R_{00} > (R_{10} - R_{00}) + (R_{01} - R_{00})$$

Subadditivity is a "negative" departure, which for risks corresponds to $IC < 0$, or

$$R_{11} - R_{00} < (R_{10} - R_{00}) + (R_{01} - R_{00})$$

Departures from risk additivity have special implications when we can assume that neither factor is ever preventive (neither factor will be preventive in the presence *or* absence of the other, which excludes types 3, 5, 7, and 9 through 15). Under this assumption, the interaction contrast simplifies to

$$IC = p_8 - p_2$$

Superadditivity ($IC > 0$) plus no prevention then implies that $p_8 > p_2$. Because $p_2 \geq 0$, superadditivity plus no prevention implies that synergistic responders (type 8 persons) must be present ($p_8 > 0$). The converse is false, however; that is, the presence of synergistic responders does *not* imply superadditivity, because we could have $p_2 > p_8 > 0$, in which case subadditivity would hold. Subadditivity plus no prevention implies that $p_8 < p_2$. Because $p_8 \geq 0$, subadditivity ($IC < 0$) plus no prevention implies that competitive responders (type 2 persons) must be present ($p_2 > 0$). Nonetheless, the converse is again false: The presence of competitive responders does *not* imply subadditivity, because we could have $p_8 > p_2 > 0$, in which case superadditivity would hold.

THE NONIDENTIFIABILTY OF INTERACTION RESPONSE TYPES

Epidemiologic data on risks or rates, even if perfectly valid, cannot alone determine the particular response types that are present or absent. In particular, one can never infer that a particular type of interaction in Table 5–2 is absent, and inference of presence must make untestable assumptions about absence of other response types. As a result, inferences about the presence of particular response types must depend on very restrictive assumptions about absence of other response types.

One cannot infer the presence of a particular response type even when *qualitative* statistical interactions are present among the actual effect measures, that is, when the actual effect of one factor entirely reverses direction across levels of another factor. Such reversals can arise from entirely distinct combinations of interaction types. Qualitative interaction demonstrates only that interaction types must be present.

Consider the example of the two cohorts shown in Table 5–3, for which the proportions of response types are different. In both cohorts, the risks at various combinations of X and Z are identical, and hence so are all the effect measures. For example, the risk difference for X when $Z = 1$ ($R_{11} - R_{01}$) equals 0.2 and when $Z = 0$ ($R_{10} - R_{00}$) equals −0.2, a qualitative statistical interaction. Thus, these two completely different cohorts produce identical interaction contrasts ($IC = 0.4$). In the first cohort, the two interaction types are those for whom X only has an effect in the presence of Z and this effect is causal (type 8) and those for whom X only has an effect in the absence of Z and this effect is preventive (type 15). In the second cohort, the only interaction type present is that in which the effect of X is causal when Z is present and preventive when Z is absent (type 7). In other words, even if we saw the actual effects, free of any bias or error, we could not

TABLE 5–3

Example of Two Cohorts with Different Proportions of Response Types that Yield the Same Interaction Contrast

Cohort #1						Cohort #2					
Response Type	Proportion	R_{11}	R_{10}	R_{01}	R_{00}	Response Type	Proportion	R_{11}	R_{10}	R_{01}	R_{00}
1	0.1	0.1	0.1	0.1	0.1	1	0.1	0.1	0.1	0.1	0.1
7	0	—	—	—	—	7	0.2	0.2	—	—	0.2
8	0.2	0.2	—	—	—	8	0	—	—	—	—
15	0.2	—	—	—	0.2	15	0	—	—	—	—
16	0.5	—	—	—	—	16	0.7	—	—	—	—
Total	1.0	0.3	0.1	0.1	0.3	Total	1.0	0.3	0.1	0.1	0.3

distinguish whether the qualitative statistical interaction arose because different people are affected by X in different Z strata ($p_8 = p_{15} = 0.2$, $p_{16} = 0.5$), or because the same people are affected but in these individuals the X effects reverse across Z strata ($p_7 = 0.2$, $p_{16} = 0.7$).

INTERACTIONS UNDER THE SUFFICIENT-CAUSE MODEL

In Chapter 2 we defined biologic interaction among two or more component causes to mean that the causes participate in the same sufficient cause. Here, a component cause for an individual is identical to a causal risk factor, or level of variable, the occurrence of which contributes to completion of a sufficient cause. Different causal mechanisms correspond to different sufficient causes of disease. If two component causes act to produce disease in a common sufficient cause, some cases of disease may arise for which the two component causes share in the causal responsibility. In the absence of either of the components, these cases would not occur. Under the sufficient-cause model, this coparticipation in a sufficient cause is defined as synergistic interaction between the components, causal coaction, or synergism.

There may also be mechanisms that require absence of one factor and presence of the other to produce disease. These correspond to a sufficient cause in which absence of one factor and presence of another are both component causes. Failure of disease to occur because both factors were present may be defined as an antagonistic interaction between the components, or antagonism.

If two factors never participate jointly in the same sufficient cause by synergism or antagonism, then no case of disease can be attributed to their coaction. Absence of biologic interaction, or independence of effects of two factors, thus means that no case of disease was caused or prevented by the joint presence of the factors.

We emphasize that two component causes can participate in the same causal mechanism without acting at the same time. Expanding an example from Chapter 2, contracting a viral infection can cause a person to have a permanent equilibrium disturbance. Years later, during icy weather, the person may slip and fracture a hip while walking along a path because the equilibrium disturbance has made balancing more difficult. The viral infection years before has interacted with the icy weather (and the choice of type of shoe, the lack of a handrail, etc.) to cause the fractured hip. Both the viral infection and the icy weather are component causes in the same causal mechanism, despite their actions being separated by many years.

We have said that two factors can "interact" by competing to cause disease, even if neither they nor their absence share a sufficient cause, because only one complete sufficient cause is required for disease to occur, and thus all sufficient causes compete to cause disease. Consider causes of death: Driving without seat belts can be a component cause of a fatal injury (the first completed sufficient cause), which prevents death from all other sufficient causes (such as fatal lung cancer) and their components (such as smoking). Driving without seat belts thus prevents deaths from smoking because it kills some people who would otherwise go on to die of smoking-related disease.

RELATION BETWEEN THE POTENTIAL-OUTCOME AND SUFFICIENT-CAUSE MODELS OF INTERACTION

There is a direct logical connection between the two definitions of biologic interaction discussed thus far, which can be exploited to provide a link between the sufficient-cause model (Chapter 2) and measures of incidence (Greenland and Poole, 1988). To build this connection, Figure 5–1 displays the nine sufficient causes possible when we can distinguish only two binary variables X and Z. The U_k in each circle represents all component causes (other than $X = 1$ or $X = 0$ and $Z = 1$ or $X = 0$) that are necessary to complete the sufficient cause. We say a person is at risk of, or susceptible to, sufficient cause k $(k = A, B, C, D, E, F, G, H, I)$ if U_k is present for that person, that is, if sufficient cause k is complete except for any necessary contribution from X or Z. Note that a person may

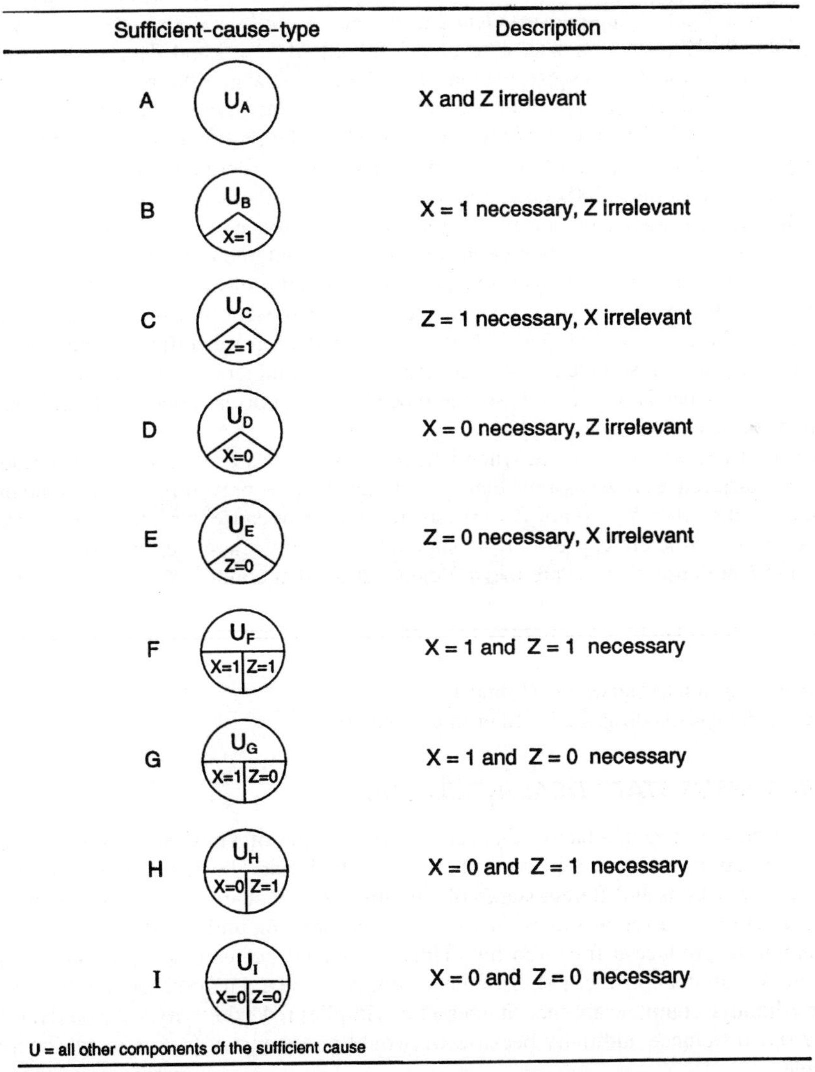

FIGURE 5–1 • Enumeration of the nine types of sufficient causes for two dichotomous exposure variables.

be at risk of none, one, or several sufficient causes. Of the nine types of sufficient causes in Figure 5–1, four (F, G, H, I) are examples of causal coaction (biologic interaction in the sufficient-cause sense).

We can deduce the causal response type of any individual given his or her risk status for sufficient causes. In other words, we can deduce the row in Table 5–2 to which an individual belongs if we know the sufficient causes for which he or she is at risk. For example, any person at risk of sufficient cause A is doomed to disease, regardless of the presence of X or Z, so that person is of response type 1 in Table 5–2. Also, a person at risk of sufficient causes B and C, but no other, will get the disease unless $X = Z = 0$, so is of type 2. Similarly, a person at risk of sufficient causes F, G, and H, but no other, will also get the disease unless $X = Z = 0$, so must be response type 2.

Several other combinations of sufficient causes will yield a type 2 person. In general, completely different combinations of susceptibilities to sufficient causes may produce the same response type, so that the sufficient-cause model is a "finer" or more detailed model than the potential-outcome (response-type) model of the effects of the same variables (Greenland and Poole, 1988; Greenland and Brumback, 2002; VanderWeele and Hernán, 2006; VanderWeele and Robins, 2007a). In other words, for every response type in a potential-outcome model we can construct at least one and often several sufficient-cause models that produce the response type. Nonetheless, there are a few response types that correspond to a unique sufficient cause. One example is the synergistic response type (type 8 in Table 5–2), for whom disease results if and only if $X = 1$ and $Z = 1$. The susceptibility pattern that results in such synergistic response is the one in which the person is at risk of only sufficient cause F. Sufficient cause F corresponds exactly to synergistic causation or causal coaction of $X = 1$ and $Z = 1$ in the sufficient-cause model. Thus, the presence of synergistic responders (type 8 in Table 5–2) corresponds to the presence of synergistic action (cause F in Fig. 5–1).

VanderWeele and Robins (2007a) show that the presence of interaction response type 7, 8, 10, 12, 14, or 15 implies the presence of causal coaction, i.e., the presence of a sufficient cause of the form F, G, H, or I (which they take as their definition of biologic interaction). In contrast, the other four response types defined as interactions above (2, 3, 5, 9) do not imply causal coaction, i.e., response types 2, 3, 5, and 9 can occur even if no causal coaction is present. For this reason, VanderWeele and Robins (2007a) define only types 7, 8, 10, 12, 14, and 15 as reflecting interdependent action, in order to induce a correspondence with coaction in the sufficient-cause model. The four types that they exclude (types 2, 3, 5, and 9) are the types for which disease occurs under 3 out of the 4 combinations of possible X and Z values.

As shown earlier, we can infer that synergistic response types are present from superadditivity of the causal risk differences if we assume that neither factor is ever preventive. Because no preventive action means that neither $X = 0$ nor $Z = 0$ acts in a sufficient cause, we can infer the presence of synergistic action (sufficient cause F) from superadditivity if we assume that sufficient causes D, E, G, H, and I are absent (these are the sufficient causes that contain $X = 0$ or $Z = 0$). Without assuming no preventive action, VanderWeele and Robins (2007a) show that if $R_{11} - R_{01} - R_{10} > 0$ (a stronger condition than superadditivity), then the sufficient cause F must be present—that is, there must be synergism between $X = 1$ and $Z = 1$. They also give analogous conditions for inferring the presence of sufficient causes G, H, and I.

Interaction analysis is described further in Chapter 16.

BIOLOGIC VERSUS STATISTICAL INTERACTION

Some authors have argued that factors that act in distinct stages of a multistage model are examples of independent actions with multiplicative effect (Siemiatycki and Thomas, 1981). By the definitions we use, however, actions at different stages of a multistage model are interacting with one another, despite their action at different stages, just as the viral infection and the slippery walk interacted in the example to produce a fractured hip. Thus, we would not call these actions independent. Furthermore, we do not consider risk-difference additivity to be a natural relation between effects that occur. Although complete absence of interactions implies risk additivity, we would rarely expect to observe risk-difference additivity because we would rarely expect factors to act independently in all people.

More generally, we reiterate that statistical interaction—effect-measure modification—should not be confused with biologic interaction. Most important, when two factors have effects, risk-ratio homogeneity—though often misinterpreted as indicating absence of biologic interaction—implies just the opposite, that is, *presence* of biologic interactions. This conclusion follows because, as shown earlier, homogeneity of a ratio measure implies heterogeneity (and hence nonadditivity) of the corresponding difference measure. This nonadditivity in turn implies the presence of some type of biologic interaction.

PUBLIC HEALTH INTERACTIONS

Assuming that costs or benefits of exposures or interventions are measured by the excess or reduction in case load they produce, several authors have proposed that departures from additivity of case loads (incident numbers) or incidences correspond to public health interaction (Blot and Day, 1979; Rothman et al., 1980; Saracci, 1980). The rationale is that, if the excess case loads produced by each factor are not additive, one must know the levels of all the factors in order to predict the public health impact of removing or introducing any one of them (Hoffman et al., 2006).

As an example, we can return to the interaction between smoking and asbestos exposure examined at the beginning of the chapter. Recall that in the hypothetical example the average 10-year mortality risk in a cohort of asbestos-exposed smokers was 0.020, but it would have been 0.003 if all cohort members quit smoking at the start of follow-up, it would have been 0.010 if only the asbestos exposure had been prevented, and it would have declined to 0.001 if everyone quit smoking *and* the asbestos exposure had been prevented. These effects are nonadditive, because

$$R_{11} - R_{00} = 0.020 - 0.001 = 0.019 > (R_{10} - R_{00}) + (R_{01} - R_{00})$$

$$= (0.003 - 0.001) + (0.010 - 0.001) = 0.011$$

If there were 10,000 exposed workers, prevention of asbestos exposure would have reduced the case load from (0.020)10,000 = 200 to (0.010)10,000 = 100 if smoking habits did not change, but it would have reduced the case load from 0.003(10,000) = 30 to 0.001(10,000) = 20 if everyone also quit smoking at the start of follow-up. Thus, the benefit of preventing asbestos exposure (in terms of mortality reduction) would have been five times greater if no one quit smoking than if everyone quit. Only if the risk differences were additive would the mortality reduction be the same regardless of smoking. Otherwise, the smoking habits of the cohort cannot be ignored when estimating the benefit of preventing asbestos exposure. As discussed in Chapter 2, complete removal of exposure is usually infeasible, but the same point applies to partial removal of exposure. The benefit of partial removal of one factor may be very sensitive to the distribution of other factors among those in whom the factor is removed, as well as being sensitive to the means of removal.

If public health benefits are not measured using case-load reduction, but instead are measured using some other benefit measure (for example, expected years of life gained or health care cost reduction), then public health interaction would correspond to nonadditivity for that measure, rather than for case load or risk differences. The general concept is that public health interactions correspond to a situation in which public health costs or benefits from altering one factor must take into account the prevalence of other factors. Because the presence and extent of public health interactions can vary with the benefit measure, the concept parallels algebraically certain types of statistical interaction or effect-measure modification, and so statistical methods for studying the latter phenomenon can also be used to study public health interaction. The study of public health interaction differs, however, in that the choice of the measure is dictated by the public health context, rather than by statistical convenience or biologic assumptions.

Section II

Study Design and Conduct

CHAPTER 6

Types of Epidemiologic Studies

Kenneth J. Rothman, Sander Greenland, and Timothy L. Lash

Experimental Studies 88
Randomization 88
Validity versus Ethical Considerations in Experiments on Human Subjects 89
Clinical Trials 89
Field Trials 92
Community Intervention and Cluster Randomized Trials 92

Nonexperimental Studies 93
Cohort Studies 94
Case-Control Studies 95
Prospective versus Retrospective Studies 95
Cross-Sectional Studies 97
Proportional Mortality Studies 97
Ecologic Studies 99
Hypothesis Generation versus Hypothesis Screening 99

Epidemiologic study designs comprise both experimental and nonexperimental studies. The experiment is emblematic of scientific activity. But what constitutes an experiment? In common parlance, an experiment refers to any trial or test. For example, a professor might introduce new teaching methods as an experiment. For many scientists, however, the term has a more specific meaning: An experiment is a set of observations, conducted under controlled circumstances, in which the scientist manipulates the conditions to ascertain what effect, if any, such manipulation has on the observations. Some might enlarge this definition to include controlled observations without manipulation of the conditions. Thus, the astronomical observations during the solar eclipse of 1919 that corroborated Einstein's general theory of relativity have often been referred to as an experiment. For epidemiologists, however, the word *experiment* usually implies that the investigator manipulates the exposure assigned to participants in the study. Experimental epidemiology is therefore limited by definition to topics for which the exposure condition can be manipulated. Because the subjects of these manipulations are human, experimental epidemiology is further limited ethically to studies in which all exposure assignments are expected to cause no harm.

When epidemiologic experiments meet minimal standards of feasibility and ethics, their design is guided by the objectives of reducing variation in the outcome attributable to extraneous factors and accounting accurately for the remaining extraneous variation. There are generally two or more forms of the intervention. Intervention assignments are ordinarily determined by the researcher by applying a randomized allocation scheme. The purpose of random allocation is to create groups that differ only randomly at the time of allocation with regard to subsequent occurrence of the study outcome. Epidemiologic experiments include clinical trials (with patients as subjects), field trials (with interventions assigned to individual community members), and community intervention trials (with interventions assigned to whole communities).

When experiments are infeasible or unethical, epidemiologists design nonexperimental (also known as observational) studies in an attempt to simulate what might have been learned had an experiment been conducted. In nonexperimental studies, the researcher is an observer rather than an agent who assigns interventions. The four main types of nonexperimental epidemiologic studies are cohort studies—in which all subjects in a source population are classified according to their exposure status and followed over time to ascertain disease incidence; case-control studies—in which cases arising from a source population and a sample of the source population are classified according to their exposure history; cross-sectional studies, including prevalence studies—in which one ascertains exposure and disease status as of a particular time; and ecologic studies—in which the units of observation are groups of people.

EXPERIMENTAL STUDIES

A typical experiment on human subjects creates experimental groups that are exposed to different treatments or agents. In a simple two-group experiment, one group receives a treatment and the other does not. Ideally, the experimental groups are identical with respect to extraneous factors that affect the outcome of interest, so that if the treatment had no effect, identical outcomes would be observed across the groups. This objective could be achieved if one could control all the relevant conditions that might affect the outcome under study. In the biologic sciences, however, the conditions affecting most outcomes are so complex and extensive that they are mostly unknown and thus cannot be made uniform. Hence there will be variation in the outcome, even in the absence of a treatment effect. This "biologic variation" reflects variation in the set of conditions that produces the effect.

Thus, in biologic experimentation, one cannot create groups across which only the study treatment varies. Instead, the experimenter may settle for creating groups in which the net effect of extraneous factors is expected to be small. For example, it may be impossible to make all animals in an experiment eat exactly the same amount of food. Variation in food consumption could pose a problem if it affected the outcome under study. If this variation could be kept small, however, it might contribute little to variation in the outcome across the groups.

The investigator would usually be satisfied if the net effect of extraneous factors across the groups were substantially less than the expected effect of the study treatment. Often not even that can be achieved, however. In that case, the experiment must be designed so that the variation in outcome due to extraneous factors can be measured accurately and thus accounted for in comparisons across the treatment groups.

RANDOMIZATION

In the early 20th century, R. A. Fisher and others developed a practical basis for experimental designs that accounts accurately for extraneous variability across experimental units (whether the units are objects, animals, people, or communities). This basis is called *randomization* (random allocation) of treatments or exposures among the units: Each unit is assigned treatment using a random assignment mechanism such as a coin toss. Such a mechanism is unrelated to the extraneous factors that affect the outcome, so any association between the treatment allocation it produces and those extraneous factors will be random. The variation in the outcome across treatment groups that is not due to treatment effects can thus be ascribed to these random associations and hence can be justifiably called chance variation.

A hypothesis about the size of the treatment effect, such as the null hypothesis, corresponds to a specific probability distribution for the potential outcomes under that hypothesis. This probability distribution can be compared with the observed association between treatment and outcomes. The comparison links statistics and inference, which explains why many statistical methods, such as analysis of variance, estimate random outcome variation within and across treatment groups. A study with random assignment of the treatment allows one to compute the probability of the observed association under various hypotheses about how treatment assignment affects outcome. In particular, if assignment is random and has no effect on the outcome except through treatment, any systematic (nonrandom) variation in outcome with assignment must be attributable to a treatment effect.

Scientists conducted experiments for centuries before the idea of random allocation crystallized, and experiments that have little extraneous outcome variation (as often occur in physical sciences) have no need of the method. Nonetheless, some social scientists and epidemiologists identify the term *experiment* with a randomized experiment only. Sometimes the term *quasi-experiment* is used to refer to controlled studies in which exposure was assigned by the investigator without using randomization (Cook and Campbell, 1979).

VALIDITY VERSUS ETHICAL CONSIDERATIONS IN EXPERIMENTS ON HUMAN SUBJECTS

In an experiment, those who are exposed to an experimental treatment are exposed only because the investigator has assigned the exposure to the subject. In a purely scientific experiment, the reason for assigning the specific exposure to the particular subject is only to maximize the validity of the study. The steps considered necessary to reach this goal are usually operationalized in a study protocol. The only reason for the assignment is to conform to the protocol rather than to meet the needs of the subject.

For example, suppose that a physician treating headache had prescribed a patented drug to her wealthy patients and a generic counterpart to her indigent patients, because the presumed greater reliability of the patented version was in her judgment not worth the greater cost for those of modest means. Should the physician want to compare the effects of the two medications among her patients, she could not consider herself to be conducting a valid experiment, despite the fact that the investigator herself had assigned the exposures. Because assignment was based in part on factors that could affect the outcome, such as wealth, one would expect there to be differences among the treatment groups even if the medications had the same effect on the outcome, i.e., one would expect there to be confounding (see Chapter 4). To conduct a valid experiment, she would have to assign the drugs according to a protocol that would not lead to systematic imbalance of extraneous causes of headache across the treatment groups. The assignment of exposure in experiments is designed to help the study rather than the individual subject. If it is done to help the subject, then a nonexperimental study is still possible, but it would not be considered an experiment because of the confounding that the treatment-assignment criterion might induce.

Because the goals of the study, rather than the subject's needs, determine the exposure assignment, ethical constraints limit severely the circumstances in which valid experiments on humans are feasible. Experiments on human subjects are ethically permissible only when adherence to the scientific protocol does not conflict with the subject's best interests. Specifically, there should be reasonable assurance that there is no known and feasible way a participating subject could be treated better than with the treatment possibilities that the protocol provides. From this requirement comes the constraint that any exposures or treatments given to subjects should be limited to potential preventives of disease. This limitation alone confines most etiologic research to the nonexperimental variety.

Among the more specific ethical implications is that subjects admitted to the study should not be thereby deprived of some preferable form of treatment or preventive that is not included in the study. This requirement implies that best available therapy should be included to provide a reference (comparison) for any new treatment. Another ethical requirement, known as *equipoise,* states that the treatment possibilities included in the trial must be equally acceptable given current knowledge. Equipoise severely restricts use of placebos: The Declaration of Helsinki states that it is unethical to include a placebo therapy as one of the arms of a clinical trial if an accepted remedy or preventive of the outcome already exists (World Medical Association, www.wma.net/e/policy/b3.htm; Rothman and Michels, 2002).

Even with these limitations, many epidemiologic experiments are conducted (some of which unfortunately ignore ethical principles such as equipoise). Most are clinical trials, which are epidemiologic studies evaluating treatments for patients who already have acquired disease (*trial* is used as a synonym for *experiment*). Epidemiologic experiments that aim to evaluate primary preventives (agents intended to prevent disease onset in the first place) are less common than clinical trials; these studies are either field trials or community intervention trials.

CLINICAL TRIALS

A clinical trial is an experiment with patients as subjects. The goal of most clinical trials is either to evaluate a potential cure for a disease or to find a preventive of disease sequelae such as death, disability, or a decline in the quality of life. The exposures in such trials are not primary preventives, because they do not prevent occurrence of the initial disease or condition, but they are preventives of the sequelae of the initial disease or condition. For example, a modified diet after an individual suffers a myocardial infarction may prevent a second infarction and subsequent death, chemotherapeutic agents given to cancer patients may prevent recurrence of cancer, and immunosuppressive drugs given to transplant patients may prevent transplant rejection.

Subjects in clinical trials of sequelae prevention must be diagnosed as having the disease in question and should be admitted to the study soon enough following diagnosis to permit the treatment assignment to occur in a timely fashion. Subjects whose illness is too mild or too severe to permit the form of treatment or alternative treatment being studied must be excluded. Treatment assignment should be designed to minimize differences between treatment groups with respect to extraneous factors that might affect the comparison. For example, if some physicians participating in the study favored the new therapy, they could conceivably influence the assignment of, say, their own patients or perhaps the more seriously afflicted patients to the new treatment. If the more seriously afflicted patients tended to get the new treatment, then confounding (see Chapter 4) would result and valid evaluation of the new treatment would be compromised.

To avoid this and related problems, it is desirable to assign treatments in clinical trials in a way that allows one to account for possible differences among treatment groups with respect to unmeasured "baseline" characteristics. As part of this goal, the assignment mechanism should deter manipulation of assignments that is not part of the protocol. It is almost universally agreed that randomization is the best way to deal with concerns about confounding by unmeasured baseline characteristics and by personnel manipulation of treatment assignment (Byar et al., 1976; Peto et al., 1976; Gelman et al., 2003). The validity of the trial depends strongly on the extent to which the random assignment protocol is the sole determinant of the treatments received. When this condition is satisfied, confounding due to unmeasured factors can be regarded as random, is accounted for by standard statistical procedures, and diminishes in likely magnitude as the number randomized increases (Greenland and Robins, 1986; Greenland, 1990). When the condition is not satisfied, however, unmeasured confounders may bias the statistics, just as in observational studies. Even when the condition is satisfied, the *generalizability* of trial results may be affected by selective enrollment. Trial participants do not often reflect the distribution of sex, age, race, and ethnicity of the target patient population (Murthy et al., 2004; Heiat et al., 2002). For reasons explained in Chapter 8, representative study populations are seldom scientifically optimal. When treatment efficacy is modified by sex, age, race, ethnicity, or other factors, however, and the study population differs from the population that would be receiving the treatment with respect to these variables, then the average study effect will differ from the average effect among those who would receive treatment. In these circumstances, extrapolation of the study results is tenuous or unwarranted, and one may have to restrict the inferences to specific subgroups, if the size of those subgroups permits.

Given that treatment depends on random allocation, rather than patient and physician treatment decision making, patients' enrollment into a trial requires their informed consent. At a minimum, informed consent requires that participants understand (a) that they are participating in a research study of a stated duration, (b) the purpose of the research, the procedures that will be followed, and which procedures are experimental, (c) that their participation is voluntary and that they can withdraw at any time, and (d) the potential risks and benefits associated with their participation.

Although randomization methods often assign subjects to treatments in approximately equal proportions, this equality is not always optimal. True equipoise provides a rationale for equal assignment proportions, but often one treatment is hypothesized to be more effective based on a biologic rationale, earlier studies, or even preliminary data from the same study. In these circumstances, equal assignment probabilities may be a barrier to enrollment. Adaptive randomization (Armitage, 1985) or imbalanced assignment (Avins, 1998) allows more subjects in the trial to receive the treatment expected to be more effective with little reduction in power.

Whenever feasible, clinical trials should attempt to employ blinding with respect to the treatment assignment. Ideally, the individual who makes the assignment, the patient, and the assessor of the outcome should all be ignorant of the treatment assignment. Blinding prevents certain biases that could affect assignment, assessment, or compliance. Most important is to keep the assessor blind, especially if the outcome assessment is subjective, as with a clinical diagnosis. (Some outcomes, such as death, will be relatively insusceptible to bias in assessment.) Patient knowledge of treatment assignment can affect adherence to the treatment regime and can bias perceptions of symptoms that might affect the outcome assessment. Studies in which both the assessor and the patient are blinded as to the treatment assignment are known as *double-blind studies*. A study in which the individual who makes the assignment is unaware which treatment is which (such as might occur if the treatments are coded pills and the assigner does not know the code) may be described as *triple-blind*, though this term is used more often to imply that the data analyst (in addition to the patient and the assessor) does not know which group of patients in the analysis received which treatment.

Depending on the nature of the intervention, it may not be possible or practical to keep knowledge of the assignment from all of these parties. For example, a treatment may have well-known side effects that allow the patients to identify the treatment. The investigator needs to be aware of and to report these possibilities, so that readers can assess whether all or part of any reported association might be attributable to the lack of blinding.

If there is no accepted treatment for the condition being studied, it may be useful to employ a placebo as the comparison treatment, when ethical constraints allow it. *Placebos* are inert treatments intended to have no effect other than the psychologic benefit of receiving a treatment, which itself can have a powerful effect. This psychologic benefit is called a *placebo response*, even if it occurs among patients receiving active treatment. By employing a placebo, an investigator may be able to control for the psychologic component of receiving treatment and study the nonpsychologic benefits of a new intervention. In addition, employing a placebo facilitates blinding if there would otherwise be no comparison treatment. These benefits may be incomplete, however, if noticeable side effects of the active treatment enhance the placebo response (the psychologic component of treatment) among those receiving the active treatment.

Placebos are not necessary when the objective of the trial is solely to compare different treatments with one another. Nevertheless, even without placebos, one should be alert to the possibility of a placebo effect, or of adherence differences, due to differences in noticeable side effects among the active treatments that are assigned.

Nonadherence to or noncompliance with assigned treatment results in a discrepancy between treatment assigned and actual treatment received by trial participants. Standard practice bases all comparisons on treatment assignment rather than on treatment received. This practice is called the intent-to-treat principle, because the analysis is based on the intended treatment, not the received treatment. Although this principle helps preserve the validity of tests for treatment effects, it tends to produce biased estimates of treatment effects; hence alternatives have been developed (Goetghebeur et al., 1998). Adherence may sometimes be measured by querying subjects directly about their compliance, by obtaining relevant data (e.g., by asking that unused pills be returned), or by biochemical measurements. These adherence measures can then be used to adjust estimates of treatment effects using special methods in which randomization plays the role of an *instrumental variable* (Sommer and Zeger, 1991; Angrist et al., 1996; Greenland, 2000b; Chapter 12).

Most trials are monitored while they are being conducted by a Data and Safety Monitoring Committee or Board (DSMB). The primary objective of these committees is to ensure the safety of the trial participants (Wilhelmsen, 2002). The committee reviews study results, including estimates of the main treatment effects and the occurrence of adverse events, to determine whether the trial ought to be stopped before its scheduled completion. The rationale for early stopping might be (a) the appearance of an effect favoring one treatment that is so strong that it would no longer be ethical to randomize new patients to the alternative treatment or to deny enrolled patients access to the favored treatment, (b) the occurrence of adverse events at rates considered to be unacceptable, given the expected benefit of the treatment or trial results, or (c) the determination that the reasonably expected results are no longer of sufficient value to continue the trial. The deliberations of the DSMB involve weighing issues of medicine, ethics, law, statistics, and costs to arrive at a decision about whether to continue a trial. Given the complexity of the issues, the membership of the DSMB must comprise a diverse range of training and experiences, and thus often includes clinicians, statisticians, and ethicists, none of whom have a material interest in the trial's result.

The frequentist statistical rules commonly used by DSMB to determine whether to stop a trial were developed to ensure that the chance of Type I error (incorrect rejection of the main null hypothesis of no treatment effect; see Chapter 10) would not exceed a prespecified level (the alpha level) during the planned interim analyses (Armitage et al., 1969). Despite these goals, DSMB members may misinterpret interim results (George et al., 2004), and strict adherence to these stopping rules may yield spurious results (Wheatley and Clayton, 2003). Stopping a trial early because of the appearance of an effect favoring one treatment will often result in an overestimate of the true benefit of the treatment (Pocock and Hughes, 1989). Furthermore, trials that are stopped early may not allow sufficient follow-up to observe adverse events associated with the favored treatment

(Cannistra, 2004), particularly if those events are chronic sequelae. Bayesian alternatives have been suggested to ameliorate many of these shortcomings (Berry, 1993; Carlin and Sargent, 1996).

FIELD TRIALS

Field trials differ from clinical trials in that their subjects are not defined by presence of disease or by presentation for clinical care; instead, the focus is on the initial occurrence of disease. Patients in a clinical trial may face the complications of their disease with high probability during a relatively short time. In contrast, the risk of incident disease among free-living subjects is typically much lower. Consequently, field trials usually require a much larger number of subjects than clinical trials and are usually much more expensive. Furthermore, because the subjects are not under active health care and thus do not come to a central location for treatment, a field trial often requires visiting subjects at work, home, or school, or establishing centers from which the study can be conducted and to which subjects are urged to report. These design features add to the cost.

The expense of field trials limits their use to the study of preventives of either extremely common or extremely serious diseases. Several field trials were conducted to determine the efficacy of large doses of vitamin C in preventing the common cold (Karlowski et al., 1975; Dykes and Meier, 1975). Paralytic poliomyelitis, a rare but serious illness, was a sufficient public health concern to warrant what may have been the largest formal human experiment ever attempted, the Salk vaccine trial, in which the vaccine or a placebo was administered to hundreds of thousands of school children (Francis et al., 1955). When the disease outcome occurs rarely, it is more efficient to study subjects thought to be at higher risk. Thus, the trial of hepatitis B vaccine was carried out in a population of New York City male homosexuals, among whom hepatitis B infection occurs with much greater frequency than is usual among New Yorkers (Szmuness, 1980). Similarly, the effect of cessation of vaginal douching on the risk of pelvic inflammatory disease was studied in women with a history of recent sexually transmitted disease, a strong risk factor for pelvic inflammatory disease (Rothman et al., 2003).

Analogous reasoning is often applied to the design of clinical trials, which may concentrate on patients at high risk of adverse outcomes. Because patients who had already experienced a myocardial infarction are at high risk for a second infarction, several clinical trials of the effect of lowering serum cholesterol levels on the risk of myocardial infarction were undertaken on such patients (Leren, 1966; Detre and Shaw, 1974). It is much more costly to conduct a trial designed to study the effect of lowering serum cholesterol on the first occurrence of a myocardial infarction, because many more subjects must be included to provide a reasonable number of outcome events to study. The Multiple Risk Factor Intervention Trial (MRFIT) was a field trial of several primary preventives of myocardial infarction, including diet. Although it admitted only high-risk individuals and endeavored to reduce risk through several simultaneous interventions, the study involved 12,866 subjects and cost $115 million (more than half a billion 2006 dollars) (Kolata, 1982).

As in clinical trials, exposures in field trials should be assigned according to a protocol that minimizes extraneous variation across the groups, e.g., by removing any discretion in assignment from the study's staff. A random assignment scheme is again an ideal choice, but the difficulties of implementing such a scheme in a large-scale field trial can outweigh the advantages. For example, it may be convenient to distribute vaccinations to groups in batches that are handled identically, especially if storage and transport of the vaccine is difficult. Such practicalities may dictate use of modified randomization protocols such as cluster randomization (explained later). Because such modifications can seriously affect the informativeness and interpretation of experimental findings, the advantages and disadvantages need to be weighed carefully.

COMMUNITY INTERVENTION AND CLUSTER RANDOMIZED TRIALS

The community intervention trial is an extension of the field trial that involves intervention on a community-wide basis. Conceptually, the distinction hinges on whether or not the intervention is implemented separately for each individual. Whereas a vaccine is ordinarily administered singly to individual people, water fluoridation to prevent dental caries is ordinarily administered to individual water supplies. Consequently, water fluoridation was evaluated by community intervention trials in which entire communities were selected and exposure (water treatment) was assigned on a community basis. Other examples of preventives that might be implemented on a community-wide basis include fast-response emergency resuscitation programs and educational programs conducted using mass media, such as Project Burn Prevention in Massachusetts (MacKay and Rothman, 1982).

Some interventions are implemented most conveniently with groups of subjects that are smaller than entire communities. Dietary intervention may be made most conveniently by family or household. Environmental interventions may affect an entire office, factory, or residential building. Protective sports equipment may have to be assigned to an entire team or league. Intervention groups may be army units, classrooms, vehicle occupants, or any other group whose members are exposed to the intervention simultaneously. The scientific foundation of experiments using such interventions is identical to that of community intervention trials. What sets all these studies apart from field trials is that the interventions are assigned to groups rather than to individuals.

Field trials in which the treatment is assigned randomly to groups of participants are said to be cluster randomized. The larger the size of the group to be randomized relative to the total study size, the less is accomplished by random assignment. If only two communities are involved in a study, one of which will receive the intervention and the other of which will not, such as in the Newburgh–Kingston water fluoridation trial (Ast et al., 1956), it cannot matter whether the community that receives the fluoride is assigned randomly or not. Differences in baseline (extraneous) characteristics will have the same magnitude and the same effect whatever the method of assignment—only the direction of the differences will be affected. It is only when the numbers of groups randomized to each intervention are large that randomization is likely to produce similar distributions of baseline characteristics among the intervention groups. Analysis of cluster randomized trials should thus involve methods that take account of the clustering (Omar and Thompson, 2000; Turner et al., 2001; Spiegelhalter, 2001), which are essential to estimate properly the amount of variability introduced by the randomization (given a hypothesis about the size of the treatment effects).

NONEXPERIMENTAL STUDIES

The limitations imposed by ethics and costs restrict most epidemiologic research to nonexperimental studies. Although it is unethical for an investigator to expose a person to a potential cause of disease simply to learn about etiology, people often willingly or unwillingly expose themselves to many potentially harmful factors. Consider the example of cigarettes (MacMahon, 1979):

> [People] choose a broad range of dosages of a variety of potentially toxic substances. Consider the cigarette habit to which hundreds of millions of persons have exposed themselves at levels ranging from almost zero (for those exposed only through smoking by others) to the addict's three or four cigarettes per waking hour, and the consequent two million or more deaths from lung cancer in the last half century in this country alone.

Beyond tobacco, people in industrialized nations expose themselves, among other things, to a range of exercise regimens from sedentary to grueling, to diets ranging from vegan to those derived almost entirely from animal sources, and to medical interventions for diverse conditions. Each of these exposures may have intended and unintended consequences that can be investigated by observational epidemiology.

Ideally, we would want the strength of evidence from nonexperimental research to be as high as that obtainable from a well-designed experiment, had one been possible. In an experiment, however, the investigator has the power to assign exposures in a way that enhances the validity of the study, whereas in nonexperimental research the investigator cannot control the circumstances of exposure. If those who happen to be exposed have a greater or lesser risk for the disease than those who are not exposed, a simple comparison between exposed and unexposed will be confounded by this difference and thus not reflect validly the sole effect of the exposure. The comparison will be confounded by the extraneous differences in risk across the exposure groups (i.e., differences that are not attributable to the exposure contrast under study).

Lack of randomization calls into question the standard practice of analyzing nonexperimental data with statistical methods developed for randomized studies. Without randomization, systematic variation is a composite of all uncontrolled sources of variation—including any treatment effect—but also including confounding factors and other sources of systematic error. As a result, in studies without randomization, the systematic variation estimated by standard statistical methods is not readily attributable to treatment effects, nor can it be reliably compared with the variation expected to occur by chance. Separation of treatment effects from the mixture of uncontrolled systematic variation in nonrandomized studies (or in randomized studies with noncompliance) requires additional hypotheses about the sources of systematic error. In nonexperimental studies, these hypotheses are usually no more than speculations, although they can be incorporated into the analysis as prior distributions in Bayesian analysis or as parameter settings in a bias analysis (Chapters 18 and 19). In this sense, causal inference in the absence of randomization is largely speculative. The validity of such inference depends on how well the speculations about the effect of systematic errors correspond with their true effect.

Because the investigator cannot assign exposure in nonexperimental studies, he or she must rely heavily on the primary source of discretion that remains: the selection of subjects. If the paradigm of scientific observation is the experiment, then the paradigm of nonexperimental epidemiologic research is the "natural experiment," in which nature emulates the sort of experiment the investigator might have conducted, but for ethical and cost constraints. By far the most renowned example is the elegant study of cholera in London conducted by John Snow. In London during the mid-19th century, there were several water companies that piped drinking water to residents, and these companies often competed side by side, serving similar clientele within city districts. Snow took advantage of this natural experiment by comparing the cholera mortality rates for residents subscribing to two of the major water companies: the Southwark and Vauxhall Company, which piped impure Thames River water contaminated with sewage, and the Lambeth Company, which in 1852 changed its collection point from opposite Hungerford Market to Thames Ditton, thus obtaining a supply of water that was free of the sewage of London. As Snow (1855) described it,

> . . . the intermixing of the water supply of the Southwark and Vauxhall Company with that of the Lambeth Company, over an extensive part of London, admitted of the subject being sifted in such a way as to yield the most incontrovertible proof on one side or the other. In the subdistricts. . . supplied by both companies, the mixing of the supply is of the most intimate kind. The pipes of each company go down all the streets, and into nearly all the courts and alleys. A few houses are supplied by one company and a few by the other, according to the decision of the owner or occupier at the time when the Water Companies were in active competition. In many cases a single house has a supply different from that on either side. Each company supplies both rich and poor, both large houses and small; there is no difference in either the condition or occupation of the persons receiving the water of the different companies. . . it is obvious that no experiment could have been devised which would more thoroughly test the effect of water supply on the progress of cholera than this.
>
> The experiment, too, was on the grandest scale. No fewer than three hundred thousand people of both sexes, of every age and occupation, and of every rank and station, from gentle folks down to the very poor, were divided into two groups without their choice, and, in most cases, without their knowledge; one group being supplied with water containing the sewage of London, and amongst it, whatever might have come from the cholera patients, the other group having water quite free from impurity.
>
> To turn this experiment to account, all that was required was to learn the supply of water to each individual house where a fatal attack of cholera might occur. . . .

There are two primary types of nonexperimental studies in epidemiology. The first, the *cohort study* (also called the follow-up study or incidence study), is a direct analog of the experiment. Different exposure groups are compared, but (as in Snow's study) the investigator only selects subjects to observe, and only classifies these subjects by exposure status, rather than assigning them to exposure groups. The second, the *incident case-control study,* or simply the *case-control study,* employs an extra step of sampling from the source population for cases: Whereas a cohort study would include all persons in the population giving rise to the study cases, a case-control study selects only a sample of those persons and chooses who to include in part based on their disease status. This extra sampling step can make a case-control study much more efficient than a cohort study of the same population, but it introduces a number of subtleties and avenues for bias that are absent in typical cohort studies.

More detailed discussions of both cohort and case-control studies and their variants, with specific examples, are presented in Chapters 7 and 8. We provide here brief overviews of the designs.

COHORT STUDIES

In the paradigmatic cohort study, the investigator defines two or more groups of people that are free of disease and that differ according to the extent of their exposure to a potential cause of disease.

These groups are referred to as the study cohorts. When two groups are studied, one is usually thought of as the exposed or index cohort—those individuals who have experienced the putative causal event or condition—and the other is then thought of as the unexposed, or reference cohort. There may be more than just two cohorts, but each cohort would represent a group with a different level or type of exposure. For example, an occupational cohort study of chemical workers might comprise cohorts of workers in a plant who work in different departments of the plant, with each cohort being exposed to a different set of chemicals. The investigator measures the incidence times and rates of disease in each of the study cohorts, and compares these occurrence measures.

In Snow's natural experiment, the study cohorts were residents of London who consumed water from either the Lambeth Company or the Southwark and Vauxhall Company and who lived in districts where the pipes of the two water companies were intermixed. Snow was able to estimate the frequency of cholera deaths, using households as the denominator, separately for people in each of the two cohorts (Snow, 1855):

> According to a return which was made to Parliament, the Southwark and Vauxhall Company supplied 40,046 houses from January 1 to December 31, 1853, and the Lambeth Company supplied 26,107 houses during the same period; consequently, as 286 fatal attacks of cholera took place, in the first four weeks of the epidemic, in houses supplied by the former company, and only 14 in houses supplied by the latter, the proportion of fatal attacks to each 10,000 houses was as follows: Southwark and Vauxhall 71, Lambeth 5. The cholera was therefore fourteen times as fatal at this period, amongst persons having the impure water of the Southwark and Vauxhall Company, as amongst those having the purer water from Thames Ditton.

Many cohort studies begin with but a single cohort that is heterogeneous with respect to exposure history. Comparisons of disease experience are made within the cohort across subgroups defined by one or more exposures. Examples include studies of cohorts defined from membership lists of administrative or social units, such as cohorts of doctors or nurses, or cohorts defined from employment records, such as cohorts of factory workers.

CASE-CONTROL STUDIES

Case-control studies are best understood and conducted by defining a source population at the outset, which represents a hypothetical study population in which a cohort study might have been conducted, and by identifying a single disease of interest. If a cohort study were undertaken, the primary tasks would be to identify the exposed and unexposed denominator experience, measured in person-time units of experience or as the number of people in each study cohort, and then to identify the number of cases occurring in each person-time category or study cohort. In a case-control study, these same cases are identified and their exposure status is determined just as in a cohort study, but denominators from which rates could be calculated are not measured. Instead, a control group of study subjects is sampled from the entire source population that gave rise to the cases.

The purpose of this control group is to determine the relative size of the exposed and unexposed denominators within the source population. Just as we can attempt to measure either risks or rates in a cohort, the denominators that the control series represents in a case-control study may reflect either the number of people in the exposed and unexposed subsets of the source population, or the amount of person-time in the exposed and unexposed subsets of the source population (Chapter 8). From the relative size of these denominators, the relative size of the incidence rates or incidence proportions can then be estimated. Thus, case-control studies yield direct estimates of relative effect measures. Because the control group is used to estimate the distribution of exposure in the source population, the cardinal requirement of control selection is that the controls must be sampled independently of their exposure status.

PROSPECTIVE VERSUS RETROSPECTIVE STUDIES

Studies can be classified further as either prospective or retrospective, although several definitions have been used for these terms. Early writers defined prospective and retrospective studies to denote cohort and case-control studies, respectively. Using the terms *prospective* and *retrospective* in this way conveys no additional information and fails to highlight other important aspects of a study for which the description prospective or retrospective might be illuminating, and therefore a different usage developed.

A central feature of study design that can be highlighted by the distinction between prospective and retrospective is the order in time of the recording of exposure information and the occurrence of disease. In some studies, in particular, those in which the exposure is measured by asking people about their history of exposure, it is possible that the occurrence of disease could influence the recording of exposure and bias the study results, for example, by influencing recall. A study based on such recall is one that merits the label retrospective, at least with respect to the recording of exposure information, and perhaps for the study as a whole. Assessing exposure by recall after disease has occurred is a feature of many case-control studies, which may explain why case-control studies are often labeled retrospective. A study with retrospective measurement in this sense is subject to the concern that disease occurrence or diagnosis has affected exposure evaluation.

Nevertheless, not all case-control studies involve recall. For example, case-control studies that evaluate drug exposures have prospective measurement if the information on the exposures and other risk factors is taken from medical records or exposure registries that predate disease development. These case-control studies may be more appropriately described as prospective, at least with respect to exposure measurement.

Not all study variables need be measured simultaneously. Some studies may combine prospective measurement of some variables with retrospective measurement of other variables. Such studies might be viewed as being a mixture of prospective and retrospective measurements. A reasonable rule might be to describe a study as prospective if the exposure measurement could not be influenced by the disease, and retrospective otherwise. This rule could lead to a study with a mixture of prospectively and retrospectively measured variables being described differently for different analyses, and appropriately so.

The access to data may affect study validity as much as the recording of the data. Historical ascertainment has implications for selection and missing-data bias insofar as records or data may be missing in a systematic fashion. For example, preserving exposure information that has been recorded in the past (that is, prospectively) may depend on disease occurrence, as might be the case if occupational records were destroyed except for workers who have submitted disability claims. Thus, prospectively recorded information might have a retrospective component to its inclusion in a study, if inclusion depends on disease occurrence. In determining whether the information in a study is prospectively or retrospectively obtained, the possibility that disease could influence either the recording of the data or its entry path into the study should be considered.

The terms *prospective* and *retrospective* have also been used to refer to the timing of the accumulated person-time with respect to the study's conduct. Under this usage, when the person-time accumulates before the study is conducted, it said to be a retrospective study, even if the exposure status was recorded before the disease occurred. When the person-time accumulates after the study begins, it is said to be a prospective study; in this situation, exposure status is ordinarily recorded before disease occurrence, although there are exceptions. For example, job status might be recorded for an occupational cohort at the study's inception and as workers enter the cohort, but an industrial hygienist might assign exposure levels to the job categories only after the study is completed and therefore after all cases of disease have occurred. The potential then exists for disease to influence the industrial hygienist's assignment.

Additional nuances can similarly complicate the classification of studies as retrospective or prospective with respect to study conduct. For example, cohort studies can be conducted by measuring disease events after the study begins, by defining cohorts as of some time in the past and measuring the occurrence of disease in the time before the study begins, or a combination of the two. Similarly, case-control studies can be based on disease events that occur after the study begins, or events that have occurred before the study begins, or a combination. Thus, either cohort or case-control studies can ascertain events either prospectively or retrospectively from the point of view of the time that the study begins. According to this usage, prospective and retrospective describe the timing of the events under study in relation to the time the study begins or ends: Prospective refers to events concurrent with the study, and retrospective refers to use of historical events.

These considerations demonstrate that the classification of studies as prospective or retrospective is not straightforward, and that these terms do not readily convey a clear message about the study. The most important study feature that these terms might illuminate would be whether the disease could influence the exposure information in the study, and this is the usage that we recommend. Prospective and retrospective will then be terms that could each describe some cohort studies and some case-control studies. Under the alternative definitions, studies labeled as "retrospective" might actually use methods that preclude the possibility that exposure information could have been influenced by disease, and studies labeled as "prospective" might actually use methods that do not exclude that possibility. Because the term *retrospective* often connotes an inherently less reliable design and the term *prospective* often connotes an inherently more reliable design, assignment of the classification under the alternative definitions does not always convey accurately the strengths or weaknesses of the design. Chapter 9 discusses further the advantages and drawbacks of concurrent and historical data and of prospective and retrospective measurement.

CROSS-SECTIONAL STUDIES

A study that includes as subjects all persons in the population at the time of ascertainment or a representative sample of all such persons, selected without regard to exposure or disease status, is usually referred to as a *cross-sectional study*. A cross-sectional study conducted to estimate prevalence is called a *prevalence study*. Usually, exposure is ascertained simultaneously with the disease, and different exposure subpopulations are compared with respect to their disease prevalence. Such studies need not have etiologic objectives. For example, delivery of health services often requires knowledge only of how many items will be needed (such as number of hospital beds), without reference to the causes of the disease. Nevertheless, cross-sectional data are so often used for etiologic inferences that a thorough understanding of their limitations is essential.

One problem is that such studies often have difficulty determining the time order of events (Flanders et al., 1992). Another problem, often called length-biased sampling (Simon, 1980a), is that the cases identified in a cross-sectional study will overrepresent cases with long duration and underrepresent those with short duration of illness. To see this, consider two extreme situations involving a disease with a highly variable duration. A person contracting this disease at age 20 and living until age 70 can be included in any cross-sectional study during the person's 50 years of disease. A person contracting the disease at age 40 and dying within a day has almost no chance of inclusion. Thus, if the exposure does not alter disease risk but causes the disease to be mild and prolonged when contracted (so that exposure is positively associated with duration), the prevalence of exposure will be elevated among cases. As a result, a positive exposure–disease association will be observed in a cross-sectional study, even though exposure has no effect on disease risk and would be beneficial if disease occurs. If exposure does not alter disease risk but causes the disease to be rapidly fatal if it is contracted (so that exposure is negatively associated with duration), then prevalence of exposure will be very low among cases. As a result, the exposure–disease association observed in the cross-sectional study will be negative, even though exposure has no effect on disease risk and would be detrimental if disease occurs. There are analytic methods for dealing with the potential relation of exposure to duration (e.g., Simon, 1980a). These methods require either the diagnosis dates of the study cases or information on the distribution of durations for the study disease at different exposure levels; such information may be available from medical databases.

Cross-sectional studies may involve sampling subjects differentially with respect to disease status to increase the number of cases in the sample. Such studies are sometimes called *prevalent case-control studies,* because their design is much like that of incident case-control studies, except that the case series comprises prevalent rather than incident cases (Morgenstern and Thomas, 1993).

PROPORTIONAL MORTALITY STUDIES

A proportional mortality study includes only dead subjects. The proportions of dead exposed subjects assigned to index causes of death are compared with the proportions of dead unexposed subjects assigned to the index causes. The resulting *proportional mortality ratio* (abbreviated PMR) is the traditional measure of the effect of the exposure on the index causes of death. Superficially, the comparison of proportions of subjects dying from a specific cause for an exposed and an unexposed group resembles a cohort study measuring incidence. The resemblance is deceiving, however, because a proportional mortality study does not involve the identification and follow-up of cohorts. All subjects are dead at the time of entry into the study.

The premise of a proportional mortality study is that if the exposure causes (or prevents) a specific fatal illness, there should be proportionately more (or fewer) deaths from that illness among dead people who had been exposed than among dead people who had not been exposed. This reasoning suffers two important flaws. First, a PMR comparison cannot distinguish whether exposure increases the occurrence of the index causes of death, prevents the occurrence of other causes of death, or some mixture of these effects (McDowall, 1983). For example, a proportional mortality study could find a proportional excess of cancer deaths among heavy aspirin users compared with nonusers of aspirin, but this finding might be attributable to a preventive effect of aspirin on cardiovascular deaths, which compose the great majority of noncancer deaths. Thus, an implicit assumption of a proportional mortality study of etiology is that the overall death rate for categories other than the index is not related to the exposure.

The second major problem in mortality comparisons is that they cannot determine the extent to which exposure causes the index causes of death or worsens the prognosis of the illnesses corresponding to the index causes. For example, an association of aspirin use with stroke deaths among all deaths could be due to an aspirin effect on the incidence of strokes, an aspirin effect on the severity of strokes, or some combination of these effects.

The ambiguities in interpreting a PMR are not necessarily a fatal flaw, because the measure will often provide insights worth pursuing about causal relations. In many situations, there may be only one or a few narrow causes of death that are of interest, and it may be judged implausible that an exposure would substantially affect either the prognosis or occurrence of any nonindex deaths. Nonetheless, many of the difficulties in interpreting proportional mortality studies can be mitigated by considering a proportional mortality study as a variant of the case-control study. To do so requires conceptualizing a combined population of exposed and unexposed individuals in which the cases occurred. The cases are those deaths, both exposed and unexposed, in the index category or categories; the controls are other deaths (Miettinen and Wang, 1981).

The principle of control series selection is to choose individuals who represent the source population from which the cases arose, to learn the distribution of exposure within that population. Instead of sampling controls directly from the source population, we can sample deaths occurring in the source population, provided that the exposure distribution among the deaths sampled is the same as the distribution in the source population; that is, the exposure should not be related to the causes of death among controls (McLaughlin et al., 1985). If we keep the objectives of control selection in mind, it becomes clear that we are not bound to select as controls all deaths other than index cases. We can instead select as controls a limited set of reference causes of death, selected on the basis of a presumed lack of association with the exposure. In this way, other causes of death for which a relation with exposure is known, suspected, or merely plausible can be excluded.

The principle behind selecting the control causes of death for inclusion in the study is identical to the principle of selecting a control series for any case-control study: The control series should be selected independently of exposure, with the aim of estimating the proportion of the source population experience that is exposed, as in density case-control studies (Chapter 8). Deaths from causes that are not included as part of the control series may be excluded from the study or may be studied as alternative case groups.

Treating a proportional mortality study as a case-control study can thus enhance study validity. It also provides a basis for estimating the usual epidemiologic measures of effect that can be derived from such studies (Wang and Miettinen, 1982). Largely for these reasons, proportional mortality studies are increasingly described and conducted as case-control studies. The same type of design and analysis has reappeared in the context of analyzing spontaneously reported adverse events in connection with pharmaceutical use. The U.S. Food and Drug Administration maintains a database of spontaneous reports, the Adverse Event Reporting System (AERS) (Rodriguez et al., 2001), which has been a data source for studies designed to screen for associations between drugs and previously unidentified adverse effects using empirical Bayes techniques (DuMouchel, 1999). Evans et al. (2001) proposed that these data should be analyzed in the same way that mortality data had been analyzed in proportional mortality studies, using a measure that they called the proportional reporting ratio, or PRR, which was analogous to the PMR in proportional mortality studies. This approach, however, is subject to the same problems that accompanied the PMR. As with the PMR, these problems can be mitigated by applying the principles of case-control studies to the task of surveillance of spontaneous report data (Rothman et al., 2004).

ECOLOGIC STUDIES

All the study types described thus far share the characteristic that the observations made pertain to individuals. It is possible, and sometimes necessary, to conduct research in which the unit of observation is a group of people rather than an individual. Such studies are called *ecologic* or *aggregate studies*. The groups may be classes in a school, factories, cities, counties, or nations. The only requirement is that information on the populations studied is available to measure the exposure and disease distributions in each group. Incidence or mortality rates are commonly used to quantify disease occurrence in groups. Exposure is also measured by an overall index; for example, county alcohol consumption may be estimated from alcohol tax data, information on socioeconomic status is available for census tracts from the decennial census, and environmental data (temperature, air quality, etc.) may be available locally or regionally. These environmental data are examples of exposures that are measured by necessity at the level of a group, because individual-level data are usually unavailable and impractical to gather.

When exposure varies across individuals within the ecologic groups, the degree of association between exposure and disease need not reflect individual-level associations (Firebaugh, 1978; Morgenstern, 1982; Richardson et al., 1987; Piantadosi et al., 1988; Greenland and Robins, 1994; Greenland, 2001a, 2002b; Chapter 25). In addition, use of proxy measures for exposure (e.g., alcohol tax data rather than consumption data) and disease (mortality rather than incidence) further distort the associations (Brenner et al., 1992b). Finally, ecologic studies usually suffer from unavailability of data necessary for adequate control of confounding in the analysis (Greenland and Robins, 1994). Even if the research goal is to estimate effects of group-level exposures on group-level outcomes, problems of data inadequacy as well as of inappropriate grouping can severely bias estimates from ecologic studies (Greenland, 2001a, 2002b, 2004a). All of these problems can combine to produce results of questionable validity on any level. Despite such problems, ecologic studies can be useful for detecting associations of exposure distributions with disease occurrence, because such associations may signal the presence of effects that are worthy of further investigation. A detailed discussion of ecologic studies is presented in Chapter 25.

HYPOTHESIS GENERATION VERSUS HYPOTHESIS SCREENING

Studies in which validity is less secure have sometimes been referred to as "hypothesis-generating" studies to distinguish them from "analytic studies," in which validity may be better. Ecologic studies have often been considered as hypothesis-generating studies because of concern about various biases. The distinction, however, between hypothesis-generating and analytic studies is not conceptually accurate. It is the investigator, not the study, that generates hypotheses, and any type of data may be used to test hypotheses. For example, international comparisons indicate that Japanese women have a much lower breast cancer rate than women in the United States. These data are ecologic and subject to the usual concerns about the many differences that exist between cultures. Nevertheless, the finding corroborates a number of hypotheses, including the theories that early menarche, high-fat diets, and large breast size (all more frequent among U.S. women than Japanese women) may be important determinants of breast cancer risk (e.g., see Trichopoulos and Lipman, 1992). The international difference in breast cancer rates is neither hypothesis-generating nor analytic, for the hypotheses arose independently of this finding. Thus, the distinction between hypothesis-generating and analytic studies is one that is best replaced by a more accurate distinction.

A proposal that we view favorably is to refer to preliminary studies of limited validity or precision as *hypothesis-screening studies*. In analogy with screening of individuals for disease, such studies represent a relatively easy and inexpensive test for the presence of an association between exposure and disease. If such an association is detected, it is subject to more rigorous and costly tests using a more valid study design, which may be called a confirmatory study. Although the screening analogy should not be taken to an extreme, it does better describe the progression of studies than the hypothesis-generating/analytic study distinction.

CHAPTER 7

Cohort Studies

Kenneth J. Rothman and Sander Greenland

Definition of Cohorts and Exposure Groups 100
Classifying Person-Time 102
Chronic Exposures 103
Unexposed Time in Exposed Subjects 104
Categorizing Exposure 105
Average Intensity and Alternatives 106
Immortal Person-Time 106
Postexposure Events 107
Timing of Outcome Events 107
Expense 108
Tracing of Subjects 109
Special-Exposure and General-Population Cohorts 109

The goal of a cohort study is to measure and usually to compare the incidence of disease in one or more study cohorts. As discussed in Chapter 3, the word *cohort* designates a group of people who share a common experience or condition. For example, a birth cohort shares the same year or period of birth, a cohort of smokers has the experience of smoking in common, and a cohort of vegetarians share their dietary habit. Often, if there are two cohorts in the study, one of them is described as the exposed cohort—those individuals who have experienced a putative causal event or condition—and the other is thought of as the unexposed, or reference, cohort. If there are more than two cohorts, each may be characterized by a different level or type of exposure.

The present chapter focuses on basic elements for the design and conduct of cohort studies. Further considerations for the design of cohort studies are given in Chapters 9 through 11, whereas analysis methods applicable to cohort studies are given in Chapters 14 through 21. Many special aspects of exposure assessment that are not covered here can be found in Armstrong et al. (1992).

DEFINITION OF COHORTS AND EXPOSURE GROUPS

In principle, a cohort study could be used to estimate average risks, rates, or occurrence times. Except in certain situations, however, average risks and occurrence times cannot be measured directly from the experience of a cohort. Observation of average risks or times of specific events requires that the whole cohort remain at risk and under observation for the entire follow-up period. Loss of subjects during the study period prevents direct measurements of these averages, because the outcome of lost subjects is unknown. Subjects who die from competing risks (outcomes other than the one of interest) likewise prevent the investigator from estimating conditional risks (risk of a specific outcome conditional on not getting other outcomes) directly. Thus, the only situation in which it is feasible to measure average risks and occurrence times directly is in a cohort study, in which there is little or no loss to follow-up and little competing risk. Although some clinical trials provide these conditions, many epidemiologic studies do not. When losses and competing risks do occur, one may still estimate the incidence rate directly, whereas average risk and occurrence time must be estimated using survival (life-table) methods (see Chapters 3 and 16).

Unlike average risks, which are measured with individuals as the unit in the denominator, incidence rates have person-time as the unit of measure. The accumulation of time rather than individuals in the denominator of rates allows flexibility in the analysis of cohort studies. Whereas studies that estimate risk directly are tied conceptually to the identification of specific cohorts of individuals, studies that measure incidence rates can, with certain assumptions, define the comparison groups in terms of person-time units that do not correspond to specific cohorts of individuals. A given individual can contribute person-time to one, two, or more exposure groups in a given study, because each unit of person-time contributed to follow-up by a given individual possesses its own classification with respect to exposure. Thus, an individual whose exposure experience changes with time can, depending on details of the study hypothesis, contribute follow-up time to several different exposure-specific rates. In such a study, the definition of each exposure group corresponds to the definition of person-time eligibility for each level of exposure.

As a result of this focus on person-time, it does not always make sense to refer to the members of an exposure group within a cohort study as if the same set of individuals were exposed at all points in time. The terms *open population* or *dynamic population* describe a population in which the person-time experience can accrue from a changing roster of individuals (see Chapter 3). (Sometimes the term *open cohort* or *dynamic cohort* is used, but this usage conflicts with other usage in which a cohort is a fixed roster of individuals.) For example, the incidence rates of cancer reported by the Connecticut Cancer Registry come from the experience of an open population. Because the population of residents of Connecticut is always changing, the individuals who contribute to these rates are not a specific set of people who are followed through time.

When the exposure groups in a cohort study are defined at the start of follow-up, with no movement of individuals between exposure groups during the follow-up, the groups are sometimes called *fixed cohorts*. The groups defined by treatment allocation in clinical trials are examples of fixed cohorts. If the follow-up of fixed cohorts suffers from losses to follow-up or competing risks, incidence rates can still be measured directly and used to estimate average risks and incidence times. If no losses occur from a fixed cohort, the cohort satisfies the definition of a *closed population* (see Chapter 3) and is often called a *closed cohort*. In such cohorts, unconditional risks (which include the effect of competing risks) and average survival times can be estimated directly.

In the simplest cohort study, the exposure would be a permanent and easily identifiable condition, making the job of assigning subjects to exposed and unexposed cohorts a simple task. Unfortunately, exposures of interest to epidemiologists are seldom constant and are often difficult to measure. Consider as an example the problems of identifying for study a cohort of users of a specific prescription drug. To identify the users requires a method for locating those who receive or who fill prescriptions for the drug. Without a record-keeping system of prescriptions, it becomes a daunting task. Even with a record system, the identification of those who receive or even those who fill a prescription is not equivalent to the identification of those who actually use the drug. Furthermore, those who are users of this drug today may not be users tomorrow, and vice versa. The definition of drug use must be tied to time because exposure can change with time. Finally, the effect of the drug that is being studied may be one that involves a considerable induction period. In that case, the exposure status at a given time will relate to a possible increase or decrease in disease risk only at some later time. Thus, someone who began to take the drug today might experience a drug-related effect in 10 years, but there might be no possibility of any drug-related effect for the first 5 years after exposure.

It is tempting to think of the identification of study cohorts as simply a process of identifying and classifying individuals as to their exposure status. The process can be complicated, however, by the need to classify the experience of a single individual in different exposure categories at different times. If the exposure can vary over time, at a minimum the investigator needs to allow for the time experienced by each study subject in each category of exposure in the definition of the study cohorts. The sequence or timing of exposure could also be important. If there can be many possible exposure sequences, each individual could have a unique sequence of exposure levels and so define a unique exposure cohort containing only that individual.

A simplifying assumption that is common in epidemiologic analysis is that the only aspect of exposure that determines current risk is some simple numeric summary of exposure history. Typical summaries include current level of exposure, average exposure, and cumulative exposure, that is, the sum of each exposure level multiplied by the time spent at that level. Often, exposure is *lagged* in the summary, which means that only exposure at or up to some specified time before the current time is counted. Although one has enormous flexibility in defining exposure summaries, methods based on assuming that only a single summary is relevant can be severely biased under certain conditions (Robins, 1987). For now, we will assume that a single summary is an adequate measure of exposure. With this assumption, cohort studies may be analyzed by defining the cohorts based on person-time rather than on persons, so that a person may be a member of different exposure cohorts at different times. We nevertheless caution the reader to bear in mind the single-summary assumption when interpreting such analyses.

The time that an individual contributes to the denominator of one or more of the incidence rates in a cohort study is sometimes called the *time at risk,* in the sense of being at risk for development of the disease. Some people and, consequently, all their person-time are not at risk for a given disease because they are immune or they lack the target organ for the study disease. For example, women who have had a hysterectomy and all men are by definition not at risk for uterine cancer, because they have no uterus.

CLASSIFYING PERSON-TIME

The main guide to the classification of persons or person-time is the study hypothesis, which should be defined in as much detail as possible. If the study addresses the question of the extent to which eating carrots will reduce the subsequent risk of lung cancer, the study hypothesis is best stated in terms of what quantity of carrots consumed over what period of time will prevent lung cancer. Furthermore, the study hypothesis should specify an induction time between the consumption of a given amount of carrots and the subsequent effect: The effect of the carrot consumption could take place immediately, begin gradually, or begin only after a delay, and it could extend beyond the time that an individual might cease eating carrots (Rothman, 1981).

In studies with chronic exposures (i.e., exposures that persist over an extended period of time), it is easy to confuse the time during which exposure occurs with the time at risk of exposure effects. For example, in occupational studies, time of employment is sometimes confused with time at risk for exposure effects. The time of employment is a time during which exposure accumulates. In contrast, the time at risk for exposure effects must logically come after the accumulation of a specific amount of exposure, because only after that time can disease be caused or prevented by that amount of exposure. The lengths of these two time periods have no constant relation to one another. The time at risk of effects might well extend beyond the end of employment. It is only the time at risk of effects that should be tallied in the denominator of incidence rates for that amount of exposure.

The distinction between time of exposure accrual and the time at risk of exposure effects is easier to see by considering an example in which exposure is very brief. In studies of the delayed effects of exposure to radiation emitted from the atomic bomb, the exposure was nearly instantaneous, but the risk period during which the exposure has had an effect has been very long, perhaps lifelong, although the risk for certain diseases did not increase immediately after exposure. Cancer risk after the radiation exposure increased only after a minimum induction period of several years, depending on the cancer. The incidence rates of cancer among those exposed to high doses of radiation from the bomb can be calculated separately for different times following exposure, so that one may detect elevations specific to the induction period addressed by the study hypothesis. Without stratification by time since exposure, the incidence rate measured among those exposed to the bomb would be an average rate reflecting periods of exposure effect and periods with no effect, because they would include in the denominator some experience of the exposed cohort that corresponds to time in which there was no increased risk from the radiation.

How should the investigator study hypotheses that do not specify induction times? For these, the appropriate time periods on which to stratify the incidence rates are unclear. There is no way to estimate exposure effects, however, without making some assumption, implicitly or explicitly, about the induction time. The decision about what time to include for a given individual in the denominator of the rate corresponds to the assumption about induction time. If in a study of delayed effects in survivors of the atomic bombs in Japan, the denominator of the rate included time experienced by study subjects beginning on the day after the exposure, the rate would provide a diluted effect estimate unless the induction period (including the "latent" period) had a minimum of only 1 day. It might be more appropriate to allow for a minimum induction time of some months or years after the bomb explosion.

What if the investigator does not have any basis for hypothesizing a specific induction period? It is possible to learn about the period by estimating effects according to categories of time since exposure. For example, the incidence rate of leukemia among atomic bomb survivors relative to that among those who were distant from the bomb at the time of the explosion can be examined according to years since the explosion. In an unbiased study, we would expect the effect estimates to rise above the null value when the minimum induction period has passed. This procedure works best when the exposure itself occurs at a point or narrow interval of time, but it can be used even if the exposure is chronic, as long as there is a model to describe the amount of time that must pass before a given accumulation of exposure would begin to have an effect. More sophisticated approaches for analyzing induction time are discussed in Chapter 16.

CHRONIC EXPOSURES

The definition of chronic exposure based on anticipated effects is more complicated than when exposure occurs only at a point in time. We may conceptualize a period during which the exposure accumulates to a sufficient extent to trigger a step in the causal process. This accumulation of exposure experience may be a complex function of the intensity of the exposure and time. The induction period begins only after the exposure has reached this hypothetical triggering point, and that point will likely vary across individuals. Occupational epidemiologists have often measured the induction time for occupational exposure from the time of first exposure, but this procedure involves the extreme assumption that the first contact with the exposure can be sufficient to produce disease. Whatever assumption is adopted, it should be made an explicit part of the definition of the cohort and the period of follow-up.

Let us consider the steps to take to identify study cohorts when exposure is chronic. First, the investigator must determine how many exposure groups will be studied and determine the definitions for each of the exposure categories. The definition of exposure level could be based on the maximum intensity of exposure experienced, the average intensity over a period of time, or some cumulative amount of exposure. A familiar measure of cigarette smoking is the measure "pack-years," which is the product of the number of packs smoked per day and the number of years smoked. This measure indexes the cumulative number of cigarettes smoked, with one pack-year equal to the product of 20 cigarettes per pack and 365 days, or 7,300 cigarettes. Cumulative indices of exposure and time-weighted measures of average intensity of exposure are both popular methods for measuring exposure in occupational studies. These exposure definitions should be linked to the time period of an exposure effect, according to the study hypothesis, by explicitly taking into account the induction period.

In employing cumulative or average exposure measures, one should recognize the composite nature of the measures and, if possible, separately analyze the components. For example, pack-years is a composite of duration and intensity of smoking: 20 pack-years might represent half a pack a day for 40 years, one pack a day for 20 years, or two packs a day for 10 years, as well as innumerable other combinations. If the biologic effects of these combinations differ to an important degree, use of pack-years would conceal these differences and perhaps even present a misleading impression of dose–response patterns (Lubin and Caporaso, 2006). Supplemental analyses of smoking as two exposure variables, duration (years smoked) and intensity (packs smoked per day), would provide a safeguard against inadequacies of the pack-years analysis. Other exposure variables that are not accounted for by duration and intensity, such as age at start of exposure, age at cessation of exposure, and timing of exposure relative to disease (induction or lag period), may also warrant separation in the analyses.

Let us look at a simplified example. Suppose the study hypothesis is that smoking increases the risk for lung cancer with a minimum induction time of 5 years. For a given smoking level, the time experienced by a subject is not "exposed" person-time until the individual has reached that level and then an additional 5 years have passed. Only then is the lung cancer experience of that individual related to smoking according to the study hypothesis. The definition of the study cohort with 20 pack-years of smoking will be the person-time experience of exposed individuals beginning 5 years after they have smoked 20 pack-years. Note that if the cohort study measures incidence rates, which means that it allocates the person-time of the individual study subjects, exposure groups are defined by person-time allocation rather than by rosters of individual subjects. Analysis of these rates depends on the assumption that only "current" exposure, defined as having smoked 20 pack-years as of 5 years ago, is relevant and that other aspects of exposure history, such as amount smoked after 5 years ago, are irrelevant.

UNEXPOSED TIME IN EXPOSED SUBJECTS

What happens to the time experienced by exposed subjects that does not meet the definition of time at risk of exposure effects according to the study hypothesis? Specifically, what happens to the time after the exposed subjects become exposed and before the minimum induction has elapsed, or after a maximum induction time has passed? Two choices are reasonable for handling this experience. One possibility is to consider any time that is not related to exposure as unexposed time and to apportion that time to the study cohort that represents no exposure. Possible objections to this approach would be that the study hypothesis may be based on guesses about the threshold for exposure effects and the induction period and that time during the exposure accumulation or induction periods may in fact be at risk of exposure effects. To treat the latter experience as not at risk of exposure effects may then lead to an underestimate of the effect of exposure (see Chapter 8 for a discussion of misclassification of exposure). Alternatively, one may simply omit from the study the experience of exposed subjects that is not at risk of exposure effects according to the study hypothesis. For this alternative to be practical, there must be a reasonably large number of cases observed among subjects with no exposure.

For example, suppose a 10-year minimum induction time is hypothesized. For individuals followed from start of exposure, this hypothesis implies that no exposure effect can occur within the first 10 years of follow-up. Only after the first 10 years of follow-up can an individual experience disease due to exposure. Therefore, under the hypothesis, only person-time occurring after 10 years of exposure should contribute to the denominator of the rate among exposed. If the hypothesis were correct, we should assign the first 10 years of follow-up to the denominator of the unexposed rate. Suppose, however, that the hypothesis were wrong and exposure could produce cases in less than 10 years. Then, if the cases and person-time from the first 10 years of follow-up were added to the unexposed cases and person-time, the resulting rate would be biased toward the rate in the exposed, thus reducing the apparent differences between the exposed and unexposed rates. If computation of the unexposed rate were limited to truly unexposed cases and person-time, this problem would be avoided.

The price of avoidance, however, would be reduced precision in estimating the rate among the unexposed. In some studies, the number of truly unexposed cases is too small to produce a stable comparison, and thus the early experience of exposed persons is too valuable to discard. In general, the best procedure in a given situation would depend on the decrease in precision produced by excluding the early experience of exposed persons and the amount of bias that is introduced by treating the early experience of exposed persons as if it were equivalent to that of people who were never exposed. An alternative that attempts to address both problems is to treat the induction time as a continuous variable rather than a fixed time, and model exposure effects as depending on the times of exposure (Thomas, 1983, 1988). This approach is arguably more realistic insofar as the induction time varies across individuals.

Similar issues arise if the exposure status can change from exposed to unexposed. If the exposure ceases but the effects of exposure are thought to continue, it would not make sense to put the experience of a formerly exposed individual in the unexposed category. On the other hand, if exposure effects are thought to be approximately contemporaneous with the exposure, which is to say that the induction period is near zero, then changes in exposure status should lead to corresponding changes in how the accumulating experience is classified with respect to exposure. For example, if individuals taking a nonsteroidal anti-inflammatory drug are at an increased risk for gastrointestinal bleeding only during the period that they take the drug, then only the time during exposure is equivalent to the time at risk for gastrointestinal bleeding as a result of the drug. When an individual stops using the drug, the bleeding events and person-time experienced by that individual should be reclassified from exposed to unexposed. Here, the induction time is zero and the definition of exposure does not involve exposure history.

CATEGORIZING EXPOSURE

Another problem to consider is that the study hypothesis may not provide reasonable guidance on where to draw the boundary between exposed and unexposed. If the exposure is continuous, it is not necessary to draw boundaries at all. Instead one may use the quantitative information from each individual fully either by using some type of smoothing method, such as moving averages (see Chapter 17), or by putting the exposure variable into a regression model as a continuous term (see Chapters 20 and 21). Of course, the latter approach depends on the validity of the model used for estimation. Special care must be taken with models of repeatedly measured exposures and confounders, which are sometimes called longitudinal-data models (see Chapter 21).

The simpler approach of calculating rates directly will require a reasonably sized population within categories of exposure if it is to provide a statistically stable result. To get incidence rates, then, we need to group the experience of individuals into relatively large categories for which we can calculate the incidence rates. In principle, it should be possible to form several cohorts that correspond to various levels of exposure. For a cumulative measure of exposure, however, categorization may introduce additional difficulties for the cohort definition. An individual who passes through one level of exposure along the way to a higher level would later have time at risk for disease that theoretically might meet the definition for more than one category of exposure.

For example, suppose we define moderate smoking as having smoked 50,000 cigarettes (equivalent to about 7 pack-years), and we define heavy smoking as having smoked 150,000 cigarettes (about 21 pack-years). Suppose a man smoked his 50,000th cigarette in 1970 and his 150,000th in 1980. After allowing for a 5-year minimum induction period, we would classify his time as moderate smoking beginning in 1975. By 1980 he has become a heavy smoker, but the 5-year induction period for heavy smoking has not elapsed. Thus, from 1980 to 1985, his experience is still classified as moderate smoking, but from 1985 onward his experience is classified as heavy smoking (Figure 7–1). Usually, the time is allocated only to the highest category of exposure that applies. This example illustrates the complexity of the cohort definition with a hypothesis that takes into account both the cumulative amount of exposure and a minimum induction time. Other apportionment schemes could be devised based on other hypotheses about exposure action, including hypotheses that allowed induction time to vary with exposure history.

One invalid allocation scheme would apportion to the denominator of the exposed incidence rate the unexposed experience of an individual who eventually became exposed. For example, suppose that in an occupational study exposure is categorized according to duration of employment in a

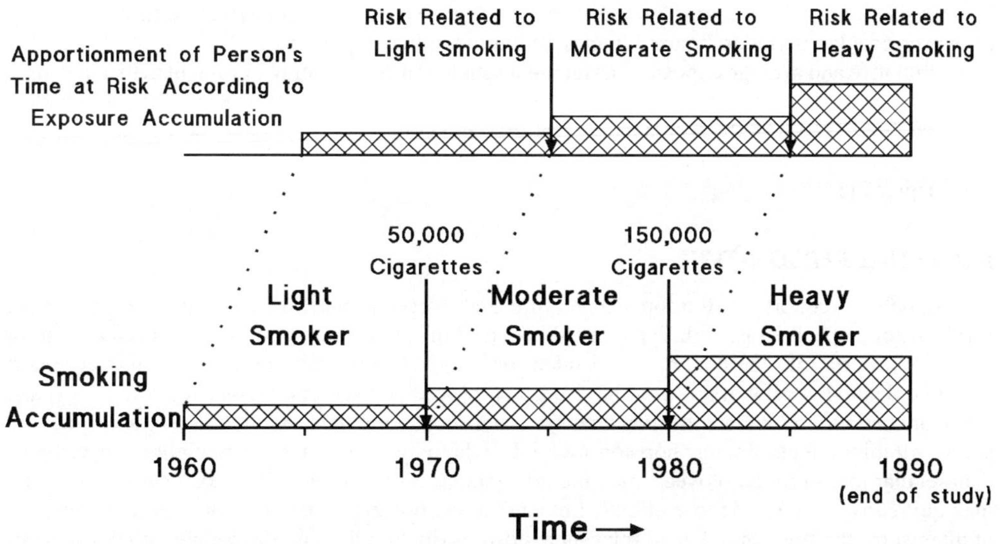

FIGURE 7–1 • Timeline showing how a smoker moves into higher categories of cumulative smoking exposure and how the time at risk that corresponds to these categories is apportioned to take into account a 5-year minimum induction period.

particular job, with the highest-exposure category being at least 20 years of employment. Suppose a worker is employed at that job for 30 years. It is a mistake to assign the 30 years of experience for that employee to the exposure category of 20 or more years of employment. The worker only reached that category of exposure after 20 years on the job, and only the last 10 years of his or her experience is relevant to the highest category of exposure. Note that if the worker had died after 10 years of employment, the death could not have been assigned to the 20-years-of-employment category, because the worker would have only had 10 years of employment.

A useful rule to remember is that the event and the person-time that is being accumulated at the moment of the event should both be assigned to the same category of exposure. Thus, once the person-time spent at each category of exposure has been determined for each study subject, the classification of the disease events (cases) follows the same rules. The exposure category to which an event is assigned is the same exposure category in which the person-time for that individual was accruing at the instant in which the event occurred. The same rule—that the classification of the event follows the classification of the person-time—also applies with respect to other study variables that may be used to stratify the data (see Chapter 15). For example, person-time will be allocated into different age categories as an individual ages. The age category to which an event is assigned should be the same age category in which the individual's person-time was accumulating at the time of the event.

AVERAGE INTENSITY AND ALTERNATIVES

One can also define current exposure according to the average (arithmetic or geometric mean) intensity or level of exposure up to the current time, rather than by a cumulative measure. In the occupational setting, the average concentration of an agent in the ambient air would be an example of exposure intensity, although one might also have to take into account any protective gear that affects the individual's exposure to the agent. Intensity of exposure is a concept that applies to a point in time, and intensity typically will vary over time. Studies that measure exposure intensity might use a time-weighted average of intensity, which would require multiple measurements of exposure over time. The amount of time that an individual is exposed to each intensity would provide its weight in the computation of the average.

An alternative to the average intensity is to classify exposure according to the maximum intensity, median intensity, minimum intensity, or some other function of the exposure history. The follow-up time that an individual spends at a given exposure intensity could begin to accumulate as soon as that level of intensity is reached. Induction time must also be taken into account. Ideally, the study hypothesis will specify a minimum induction time for exposure effects, which in turn will imply an appropriate lag period to be used in classifying individual experience.

Cumulative and average exposure-assignment schema suffer a potential problem in that they may make it impossible to disentangle exposure effects from the effects of time-varying confounders (Robins 1986, 1987). Methods that treat exposures and confounders in one period as distinct from exposure and confounders in other periods are necessary to avoid this problem (Robins et al., 1992; see Chapter 21).

IMMORTAL PERSON-TIME

Occasionally, a cohort's definition will require that everyone meeting the definition must have survived for a specified period. Typically, this period of immortality comes about because one of the entry criteria into the cohort is dependent on survival. For example, an occupational cohort might be defined as all workers who have been employed at a specific factory for at least 5 years. There are certain problems with such an entry criterion, among them that it will guarantee that the study will miss effects among short-term workers who may be assigned more highly exposed jobs than regular long-term employees, may include persons more susceptible to exposure effects, and may quit early because of those effects. Let us assume, however, that only long-term workers are of interest for the study and that all relevant exposures (including those during the initial 5 years of employment) are taken into account in the analysis.

The 5-year entry criterion will guarantee that all of the workers in the study cohort survived their first 5 years of employment, because those who died would never meet the entry criterion and so would be excluded. It follows that mortality analysis of such workers should exclude the first 5 years of employment for each worker. This period of time is referred to as *immortal person-time*. The workers at the factory were not immortal during this time, of course, because they could have died. The subset of workers that satisfy the cohort definition, however, is identified after the fact as those who have survived this period.

The correct approach to handling immortal person-time in a study is to exclude it from any denominator, even if the analysis does not focus on mortality. This approach is correct because including immortal person-time will downwardly bias estimated disease rates and, consequently, bias effect estimates obtained from internal comparisons. As an example, suppose that an occupational mortality study includes only workers who worked for 5 years at a factory, that 1,000 exposed and 1,000 unexposed workers meet this entry criterion, and that after the criterion is met we observe 200 deaths among 5,000 exposed person-years and 90 deaths among 6,000 unexposed person-years. The correct rate ratio and difference comparing the exposed and unexposed are then $(200/5{,}000)/(90/6{,}000) = 2.7$ and $200/5{,}000 - 90/6{,}000 = 25/1{,}000\ \text{year}^{-1}$. If, however, we incorrectly include the 5,000 exposed and 5,000 unexposed immortal person-years in the denominators, we get a biased ratio of $(200/10{,}000)/(90/11{,}000) = 2.4$ and a biased difference of $200/10{,}000 - 90/11{,}000 = 12/1{,}000\ \text{year}^{-1}$. To avoid this bias, if a study has a criterion for a minimum amount of time before a subject is eligible to be in a study, the time during which the eligibility criterion is met should be excluded from the calculation of incidence rates. More generally, the follow-up time allocated to a specific exposure category should exclude time during which the exposure-category definition is being met.

POSTEXPOSURE EVENTS

Allocation of follow-up time to specific categories should not depend on events that occur after the follow-up time in question has accrued. For example, consider a study in which a group of smokers is advised to quit smoking, with the objective of estimating the effect on mortality rates of quitting versus continuing to smoke. For a subject who smokes for a while after the advice is given and then quits later, the follow-up time as a quitter should only begin at the time of quitting, not at the time of giving the advice, because it is the effect of quitting that is being studied, not the effect of advice (were the effect of advice under study, follow-up time would begin with the advice). But how should a subject be treated who quits for a while and then later takes up smoking again?

When this question arose in an actual study of this problem, the investigators excluded anyone from the study who switched back to smoking. Their decision was wrong, because if the subject had died before switching back to smoking, the death would have counted in the study and the subject would not have been excluded. A subject's follow-up time was excluded if the subject switched back to smoking, something that occurred only *after* the subject had accrued time in the quit-smoking cohort. A proper analysis should include the experience of those who switched back to smoking up until the time that they switched back. If the propensity to switch back was unassociated with risk, their experience subsequent to switching back could be excluded without introducing bias. The incidence rate among the person-years while having quit could then be compared with the rate among those who continued to smoke over the same period.

As another example, suppose that the investigators wanted to examine the effect of being an ex-smoker for at least 5 years, relative to being an ongoing smoker. Then, anyone who returned to smoking within 5 years of quitting would be excluded. The person-time experience for each subject during the first 5 years after quitting should also be excluded, because it would be immortal person-time.

TIMING OF OUTCOME EVENTS

As may be apparent from earlier discussion, the time at which an outcome event occurs can be a major determinant of the amount of person-time contributed by a subject to each exposure category. It is therefore important to define and determine the time of the event as unambiguously and precisely as possible. For some events, such as death, neither task presents any difficulty. For other outcomes, such as human immunodeficiency virus (HIV) seroconversion, the time of the event can be defined in a reasonably precise manner (the appearance of HIV antibodies in the bloodstream), but measurement of the time is difficult. For others, such as multiple sclerosis and atherosclerosis, the very definition of the onset time can be ambiguous, even when the presence of the disease can be determined unambiguously. Likewise, time of loss to follow-up and other censoring events can be difficult to define and determine. Determining whether an event occurred by a given time is a special case of determining when an event occurred, because knowing that the event occurred by the given time requires knowing that the time it occurred was before the given time.

Addressing the aforementioned problems depends heavily on the details of available data and the current state of knowledge about the study outcome. We therefore will offer only a few general remarks on issues of outcome timing. In all situations, we recommend that one start with at least one written protocol to classify subjects based on available information. For example, seroconversion time may be measured as the midpoint between time of last negative and first positive test. For unambiguously defined events, any deviation of actual times from the protocol determination can be viewed as measurement error (which is discussed further in Chapter 9). Ambiguously timed diseases, such as cancers or vascular conditions, are often taken as occurring at diagnosis time, but the use of a minimum lag period is advisable whenever a long latent (undiagnosed or prodromal) period is inevitable. It may sometimes be possible to interview cases about the earliest onset of symptoms, but such recollections and symptoms can be subject to considerable error and between-person variability.

Some ambiguously timed events are dealt with by standard, if somewhat arbitrary, definitions. For example, in 1993, acquired immunodeficiency syndrome (AIDS) onset was redefined as occurrence of any AIDS-defining illnesses or clinical event (e.g., CD4 count $<200/\mu L$). As a second example, time of loss to follow-up is conventionally taken as midway between the last successful attempt to contact and the first unsuccessful attempt to contact. Any difficulty in determining an arbitrarily defined time of an event is then treated as a measurement problem, which can be addressed by the methods described in Chapter 19. One should recognize, however, that the arbitrariness of the definition for the time of an event represents another source of measurement error, with potential bias consequences that will be discussed in Chapter 9.

EXPENSE

Cohort studies are usually large enterprises. Most diseases affect only a small proportion of a population, even if the population is followed for many years. To obtain stable estimates of incidence requires a substantial number of cases of disease, and therefore the person-time giving rise to the cases must also be substantial. Sufficient person-time can be accumulated by following cohorts for a long span of time. Some cohorts with special exposures (e.g., Japanese victims of atomic bombs [Beebe, 1979]) or with detailed medical and personal histories (e.g., the Framingham, Massachusetts, study cohort [Kannel and Abbott, 1984]) have indeed been followed for decades. If a study is intended to provide more timely results, however, the requisite person-time can be attained by increasing the size of the cohorts. Of course, lengthy studies of large populations are expensive. It is not uncommon for cohort studies to cost millions of dollars, and expenses in excess of $100 million have occurred. Most of the expense derives from the need to establish a continuing system for monitoring disease occurrence in a large population.

The expense of cohort studies often limits feasibility. The lower the disease incidence, the poorer the feasibility of a cohort study, unless public resources devoted to health registries can be productively employed (see Chapter 23). Feasibility is further handicapped by a long induction period between the hypothesized cause and its effect. A long induction time contributes to a low overall incidence because of the additional follow-up time required to obtain exposure-related cases. To detect any effect, the study must span an interval at least as long as, and in practice considerably longer than, the minimum induction period. Cohort studies are poorly suited to study the effect of exposures that are hypothesized to cause rare diseases with long induction periods. Such cohort studies are expensive in relation to the amount of information returned, which is to say that they are not efficient.

The expense of cohort studies can be reduced in a variety of ways. One way is to use an existing system for monitoring disease occurrence (see Chapter 23). For example, a regional cancer registry may be used to ascertain cancer occurrence among cohort members. If the expense of case ascertainment is already being borne by the registry, the study will be considerably cheaper.

Another way to reduce cost is to rely on historical cohorts. Rather than identifying cohort members concurrently with the initiation of the study and planning to have the follow-up period occur during the study, the investigator may choose to identify cohort members based on records of previous exposure. The follow-up period until the occurrence of disease may be wholly or partially in the past. To ascertain cases occurring in the past, the investigators must rely on records to ascertain disease in cohort members. If the follow-up period begins before the period during which the study is conducted but extends into the study period, then active surveillance or a new monitoring system to ascertain new cases of disease can be devised.

To the extent that subject selection occurs after the follow-up period under observation (sometimes called retrospective cohort selection; see Chapter 6), the study will generally cost less than an equivalent study in which subject selection occurs before the follow-up period (sometimes called prospective). A drawback of retrospective cohort studies is their dependence on records, which may suffer from missing or poorly recorded information. Another drawback is that entire subject records may be missing. When such "missingness" is related to the variables under study, the study may suffer from selection biases similar to those that can occur in case-control studies (see Chapter 8). For example, if records are systematically deleted upon the death of a cohort member, then all of the retrospective person-time will be immortal, and should therefore be excluded.

A third way to reduce cost is to replace one of the cohorts, specifically the unexposed cohort, with general population information. Rather than collecting new information on a large unexposed population, existing data on a general population is used for comparison. This procedure has several drawbacks. For one, it is reasonable only if there is some assurance that only a small proportion of the general population is exposed to the agent under study, as is often the case with occupational exposures. To the extent that part of the general population is exposed, there is misclassification error that will introduce a bias into the comparison, which is ordinarily in the direction of underestimating the effect (see Chapter 9). Another problem is that information obtained for the exposed cohort may differ in quality from the existing data for the general population. If mortality data are used, the death certificate is often the only source of information for the general population. If additional medical information were used to classify deaths in an exposed cohort, the data thus obtained would not be comparable with the general population data. This noncomparability may reduce or increase bias in the resulting comparisons (Greenland and Robins, 1985a). Finally, the exposed cohort is likely to differ from the general population in many ways that are not measured, thus leading to uncontrollable confounding in the comparison. The classical "healthy worker effect" is one example of this problem, in which confounding arises because workers must meet a minimal criterion of health (they must be able to work) that the general population does not.

A fourth way to reduce the cost of a cohort study is to conduct a case-control study within the cohort, rather than including the entire cohort population in the study (Chapter 8). Such "nested" case-control studies can often be conducted at a fraction of the cost of a cohort study and yet produce the same findings with nearly the same precision.

TRACING OF SUBJECTS

Cohort studies that span many years present logistic problems that can adversely affect validity. Whether the study is retrospective or prospective, it is often difficult to locate people or their records many years after they have been enrolled into study cohorts. In prospective studies, it may be possible to maintain periodic contact with study subjects and thereby keep current information on their location. Such tracking adds to the costs of prospective cohort studies, yet the increasing mobility of society warrants stronger efforts to trace subjects. A substantial number of subjects lost to follow-up can raise serious doubts about the validity of the study. Follow-ups that trace less than about 60% of subjects are generally regarded with skepticism, but even follow-up of 70% or 80% or more can be too low to provide sufficient assurance against bias if there is reason to believe that loss to follow-up may be associated with both exposure and disease (Greenland, 1977).

SPECIAL-EXPOSURE AND GENERAL-POPULATION COHORTS

An attractive feature of cohort studies is the capability they provide to study a range of possible health effects stemming from a single exposure. A mortality follow-up can be accomplished just as easily for all causes of death as for any specific cause. Health surveillance for one disease endpoint can sometimes be expanded to include many or all endpoints without much additional work. A cohort study can provide a comprehensive picture of the health effect of a given exposure. Attempts to derive such comprehensive information about exposures motivate the identification of "special-exposure" cohorts, which are identifiable groups with exposure to agents of interest. Examples of such special-exposure cohorts include occupational cohorts exposed to workplace exposures, studies of fishermen or farmers exposed chronically to solar radiation, atomic bomb victims and the population around Chernobyl exposed to ionizing radiation, the population around Seveso, Italy, exposed to environmental dioxin contamination, Seventh-day Adventists who are "exposed" to vegetarian diets, and populations who are exposed to stress through calamities such as earthquakes and terrorist attacks. These exposures are not common and require the identification of exposed cohorts to provide enough information for study.

Common exposures are sometimes studied through cohort studies that survey a segment of the population that is identified without regard to exposure status. Such "general-population" cohorts have been used to study the effects of smoking, oral contraceptives, diet, and hypertension. It is most efficient to limit a general-population cohort study to exposures that a substantial proportion of people have experienced; otherwise, the unexposed cohort will be inefficiently large relative to the exposed cohort. A surveyed population can be classified according to smoking, alcoholic beverage consumption, diet, drug use, medical history, and many other factors of potential interest. A disadvantage is that the exposure information usually must be obtained by interviews with each subject, as opposed to obtaining information from records, as is often done with special-exposure cohorts.

CHAPTER 8

Case-Control Studies

Kenneth J. Rothman, Sander Greenland, and Timothy L. Lash

Common Elements of Case-Control Studies 113
Pseudo-frequencies and the Odds Ratio 113
Defining the Source Population 114
Case Selection 115
Control Selection 115
Common Fallacies in Control Selection 117
Sources for Control Series 117
Other Considerations for Subject Selection 120

Variants of the Case-Control Design 122
Nested Case-Control Studies 122
Case-Cohort Studies 123
Density Case-Control Studies 124
Cumulative ("Epidemic") Case-Control Studies 125
Case-Only, Case-Specular, and Case-Crossover Studies 125
Two-Stage Sampling 127
Proportional Mortality Studies 127
Case-Control Studies with Prevalent Cases 127

The use and understanding of case-control studies is one of the most important methodologic developments of modern epidemiology. Conceptually, there are clear links from randomized experiments to nonrandomized cohort studies, and from nonrandomized cohort studies to case-control studies. Case-control studies nevertheless differ enough from the scientific paradigm of experimentation that a casual approach to their conduct and interpretation invites misconception. In this chapter we review case-control study designs and contrast their advantages and disadvantages with cohort designs. We also consider variants of the basic case-control study design.

Conventional wisdom about case-control studies is that they do not yield estimates of effect that are as valid as measures obtained from cohort studies. This thinking may reflect common misunderstandings in conceptualizing case-control studies, which will be clarified later. It may also reflect concern about biased exposure information and selection in case-control studies. For example, if exposure information comes from interviews, cases will usually have reported the exposure information after learning of their diagnosis. Diagnosis may affect reporting in a number of ways, for example, by improving memory, thus enhancing sensitivity among cases, or by provoking more false memory of exposure, thus reducing specificity among cases. Furthermore, the disease may itself cloud memory and thus reduce sensitivity. These phenomena are examples of *recall bias*. Disease cannot affect exposure information collected before the disease occurred, however. Thus exposure information taken from records created before the disease occurs will not be subject to recall bias, regardless of whether the study is a cohort or a case-control design.

Conversely, cohort studies are not immune from problems often thought to be particular to case-control studies. For example, while a cohort study may gather information on exposure for an entire source population at the outset of the study, it still requires tracing of subjects to ascertain exposure variation and outcomes. If the success of this tracing is related to the exposure and the outcome, the resulting selection bias will behave analogously to that often raised as a concern in case-control studies (Greenland, 1977; Chapter 12). Similarly, cohort studies sometimes use recall to reconstruct or impute exposure history (retrospective evaluation) and are vulnerable to recall bias if this reconstruction is done after disease occurrence. Thus, although more opportunity for recall and selection bias may arise in typical case-control studies than in typical prospective cohort studies, each study must be considered in detail to evaluate its vulnerability to bias, regardless of its design.

Conventional wisdom also holds that cohort studies are useful for evaluating the range of effects related to a single exposure, whereas case-control studies provide information only about the one disease that afflicts the cases. This thinking conflicts with the idea that case-control studies can be viewed simply as more efficient cohort studies. Just as one can choose to measure more than one disease outcome in a cohort study, it is possible to conduct a set of case-control studies nested within the same population using several disease outcomes as the case series. The case-cohort study (see below) is particularly well suited to this task, allowing one control group to be compared with several series of cases. Whether or not the case-cohort design is the form of case-control study that is used, case-control studies do not have to be characterized as being limited with respect to the number of disease outcomes that can be studied.

For diseases that are sufficiently rare, cohort studies become impractical and case-control studies become the only useful alternative. On the other hand, if exposure is rare, ordinary case-control studies are inefficient, and one must use methods that selectively recruit additional exposed subjects, such as special cohort studies or two-stage designs. If both the exposure and the outcome are rare, two-stage designs may be the only informative option, as they employ oversampling of both exposed and diseased subjects.

As understanding of the principles of case-control studies has progressed, the reputation of case-control studies has also improved. Formerly, it was common to hear case-control studies referred to disparagingly as "retrospective" studies, a term that should apply to only some case-control studies and applies as well to some cohort studies (see Chapter 6). Although case-control studies do present more opportunities for bias and mistaken inference than cohort studies, these opportunities come as a result of the relative ease with which a case-control study can be mounted. Because it need not be extremely expensive or time-consuming to conduct a case-control study, many studies have been conducted by naive investigators who do not understand or implement the basic principles of valid case-control design. Occasionally, such haphazard research can produce valuable results, but often the results are wrong because basic principles have been violated. The bad reputation once suffered by case-control studies stems more from instances of poor conduct and overinterpretation of results than from any inherent weakness in the approach.

Ideally, a case-control study can be conceptualized as a more efficient version of a corresponding cohort study. Under this conceptualization, the cases in the case-control study are the same cases as would ordinarily be included in the cohort study. Rather than including all of the experience of the source population that gave rise to the cases (the study base), as would be the usual practice in a cohort design, controls are selected from the source population. Wacholder (1996) describes this paradigm of the case-control study as a cohort study with data missing at random and by design. The sampling of controls from the population that gave rise to the cases affords the efficiency gain of a case-control design over a cohort design. The controls provide an estimate of the prevalence of the exposure and covariates in the source population. When controls are selected from members of the population who were at risk for disease at the beginning of the study's follow-up period, the case-control odds ratio estimates the risk ratio that would be obtained from a cohort design. When controls are selected from members of the population who were noncases at the times that each case occurs, or otherwise in proportion to the person-time accumulated by the cohort, the case-control odds ratio estimates the rate ratio that would be obtained from a cohort design. Finally, when controls are selected from members of the population who were noncases at the end of the study's follow-up period, the case-control odds ratio estimates the incidence odds ratio that would be obtained from a cohort design. With each control-selection strategy, the odds-ratio calculation is the same, but the measure of effect estimated by the odds ratio differs. Study designs that implement each of these control selection paradigms will be discussed after topics that are common to all designs.

COMMON ELEMENTS OF CASE-CONTROL STUDIES

In a cohort study, the numerator and denominator of each disease frequency (incidence proportion, incidence rate, or incidence odds) are measured, which requires enumerating the entire population and keeping it under surveillance—or using an existing registry—to identify cases over the follow-up period. A valid case-control study observes the population more efficiently by using a control series in place of complete assessment of the denominators of the disease frequencies. The cases in a case-control study should be the same people who would be considered cases in a cohort study of the same population.

PSEUDO-FREQUENCIES AND THE ODDS RATIO

The primary goal for control selection is that the exposure distribution among controls be the same as it is in the source population of cases. The rationale for this goal is that, if it is met, we can use the control series in place of the denominator information in measures of disease frequency to determine the ratio of the disease frequency in exposed people relative to that among unexposed people. This goal will be met if we can sample controls from the source population such that the ratio of the number of exposed controls (B_1) to the total exposed experience of the source population is the same as the ratio of the number of unexposed controls (B_0) to the unexposed experience of the source population, apart from sampling error. For most purposes, this goal need only be followed within strata of factors that will be used for stratification in the analysis, such as factors used for restriction or matching (Chapters 11, 15, 16, and 21).

Using person-time to illustrate, the goal requires that B_1 has the same ratio to the amount of exposed person-time (T_1) as B_0 has to the amount of unexposed person-time (T_0), apart from sampling error:

$$\frac{B_1}{T_1} = \frac{B_0}{T_0}$$

Here B_1/T_1 and B_0/T_0 are the control sampling rates—that is, the number of controls selected per unit of person-time. Suppose that A_1 exposed cases and A_0 unexposed cases occur over the study period. The exposed and unexposed rates are then

$$I_1 = \frac{A_1}{T_1} \quad \text{and} \quad I_0 = \frac{A_0}{T_0}$$

We can use the frequencies of exposed and unexposed controls as substitutes for the actual denominators of the rates to obtain exposure-specific case-control ratios, or *pseudo-rates:*

$$\text{Pseudo-rate}_1 = \frac{A_1}{B_1}$$

and

$$\text{Pseudo-rate}_0 = \frac{A_0}{B_0}$$

These pseudo-rates have no epidemiologic interpretation by themselves. Suppose, however, that the control sampling rates B_1/T_1 and B_0/T_0 are equal to the same value r, as would be expected if controls are selected independently of exposure. If this common sampling rate r is known, the actual incidence rates can be calculated by simple algebra because, apart from sampling error, B_1/r should equal the amount of exposed person-time in the source population and B_0/r should equal the amount of unexposed person-time in the source population: $B_1/r = B_1/(B_1/T_1) = T_1$ and $B_0/r = B_0/(B_0/T_0) = T_0$. To get the incidence rates, we need only multiply each pseudo-rate by the common sampling rate, r.

If the common sampling rate is not known, which is often the case, we can still compare the sizes of the pseudo-rates by division. Specifically, if we divide the pseudo-rate for exposed by the pseudo-rate for unexposed, we obtain

$$\frac{\text{Pseudo-rate}_1}{\text{Pseudo-rate}_0} = \frac{A_1/B_1}{A_0/B_0} = \frac{A_1/[(B_1/T_1)T_1]}{A_0/[(B_0/T_0)T_0]} = \frac{A_1/(r \cdot T_1)}{A_0/(r \cdot T_0)} = \frac{A_1/T_1}{A_0/T_0}$$

In other words, the ratio of the pseudo-rates for the exposed and unexposed is an estimate of the ratio of the incidence rates in the source population, provided that the control sampling rate is independent of exposure. Thus, using the case-control study design, one can estimate the incidence rate ratio in a population without obtaining information on every subject in the population. Similar derivations in the following section on variants of case-control designs show that one can estimate the risk ratio by sampling controls from those at risk for disease at the beginning of the follow-up period (case-cohort design) and that one can estimate the incidence odds ratio by sampling controls from the noncases at the end of the follow-up period (cumulative case-control design). With these designs, the pseudo-frequencies correspond to the incidence proportions and incidence odds, respectively, multiplied by common sampling rates.

There is a statistical penalty for using a sample of the denominators rather than measuring the person-time experience for the entire source population: The precision of the estimates of the incidence rate ratio from a case-control study is less than the precision from a cohort study of the entire population that gave rise to the cases (the source population). Nevertheless, the loss of precision that stems from sampling controls will be small if the number of controls selected per case is large (usually four or more). Furthermore, the loss is balanced by the cost savings of not having to obtain information on everyone in the source population. The cost savings might allow the epidemiologist to enlarge the source population and so obtain more cases, resulting in a better overall estimate of the incidence-rate ratio, statistically and otherwise, than would be possible using the same expenditures to conduct a cohort study.

The ratio of the two pseudo-rates in a case-control study is usually written as A_1B_0/A_0B_1 and is sometimes called the *cross-product ratio*. The cross-product ratio in a case-control study can be viewed as the ratio of cases to controls among the exposed subjects (A_1/B_1), divided by the ratio of cases to controls among the unexposed subjects (A_0/B_0). This ratio can also be viewed as the odds of being exposed among cases (A_1/A_0) divided by the odds of being exposed among controls (B_1/B_0), in which case it is termed the *exposure odds ratio*. While either interpretation will give the same result, viewing this odds ratio as the ratio of case-control ratios shows more directly how the control group substitutes for the denominator information in a cohort study and how the ratio of pseudo-frequencies gives the same result as the ratio of the incidence rates, incidence proportion, or incidence odds in the source population, if sampling is independent of exposure.

One point that we wish to emphasize is that *nowhere* in the preceding discussion did we have to assume that the disease under study is "rare." In general, the rare-disease assumption is *not* needed in case-control studies. Just as for cohort studies, however, neither the incidence odds ratio nor the rate ratio should be expected to be a good approximation to the risk ratio or to be collapsible across strata of a risk factor (even if the factor is not a confounder) unless the incidence proportion is less than about 0.1 for every combination of the exposure and the factor (Chapter 4).

DEFINING THE SOURCE POPULATION

If the cases are a representative sample of all cases in a precisely defined and identified population and the controls are sampled directly from this source population, the study is said to be *population-based* or a *primary* base study. For a population-based case-control study, random sampling of controls may be feasible if a population registry exists or can be compiled. When random sampling from the source population of cases is feasible, it is usually the most desirable option.

Random sampling of controls does not necessarily mean that every person should have an equal probability of being selected to be a control. As explained earlier, if the aim is to estimate the incidence-rate ratio, then we would employ longitudinal (density) sampling, in which a person's control selection probability is proportional to the person's time at risk. For example, in a case-control study nested within an occupational cohort, workers on an employee roster will have been followed for varying lengths of time, and a random sampling scheme should reflect this varying time to estimate the incidence-rate ratio.

When it is not possible to identify the source population explicitly, simple random sampling is not feasible and other methods of control selection must be used. Such studies are sometimes called studies of *secondary* bases, because the source population is identified secondarily to the definition of a case-finding mechanism. A secondary source population or "secondary base" is therefore a source population that is defined from (secondary to) a given case series.

Consider a case-control study in which the cases are patients treated for severe psoriasis at the Mayo Clinic. These patients come to the Mayo Clinic from all corners of the world. What is the specific source population that gives rise to these cases? To answer this question, we would have to know exactly who would go to the Mayo Clinic if he or she had severe psoriasis. We cannot enumerate this source population, because many people in it do not know themselves that they would go to the Mayo Clinic for severe psoriasis, unless they actually developed severe psoriasis. This secondary source might be defined as a population spread around the world that constitutes those people who would go to the Mayo Clinic if they developed severe psoriasis. It is this secondary source from which the control series for the study would ideally be drawn. The challenge to the investigator is to apply eligibility criteria to the cases and controls so that there is good correspondence between the controls and this source population. For example, cases of severe psoriasis and controls might be restricted to those in counties within a certain distance of the Mayo Clinic, so that at least a geographic correspondence between the controls and the secondary source population could be assured. This restriction, however, might leave very few cases for study.

Unfortunately, the concept of a secondary base is often tenuously connected to underlying realities, and it can be highly ambiguous. For the psoriasis example, whether a person would go to the Mayo Clinic depends on many factors that vary over time, such as whether the person is encouraged to go by his regular physician and whether the person can afford to go. It is not clear, then, how or even whether one could precisely define, let alone sample from, the secondary base, and thus it is not clear that one could ensure that controls were members of the base at the time of sampling. We therefore prefer to conceptualize and conduct case-control studies as starting with a well-defined source population and then identify and recruit cases and controls to represent the disease and exposure experience of that population. When one instead takes a case series as a starting point, it is incumbent upon the investigator to demonstrate that a source population can be operationally defined to allow the study to be recast and evaluated relative to this source. Similar considerations apply when one takes a control series as a starting point, as is sometimes done (Greenland, 1985a).

CASE SELECTION

Ideally, case selection will amount to a direct sampling of cases within a source population. Therefore, apart from random sampling, all people in the source population who develop the disease of interest are presumed to be included as cases in the case-control study. It is not always necessary, however, to include all cases from the source population. Cases, like controls, can be randomly sampled for inclusion in the case-control study, so long as this sampling is independent of the exposure under study within strata of factors that will be used for stratification in the analysis. To see this, suppose we take only a fraction, f, of all cases. If this fraction is constant across exposure, and A_1 exposed cases and A_0 unexposed cases occur in the source population, then, apart from sampling error, the study odds ratio will be

$$\frac{A_1/B_1}{A_0/B_0} = \frac{fA_1/(r \cdot T_1)}{fA_0/(r \cdot T_0)} = \frac{A_1/T_1}{A_0/T_0}$$

as before. Of course, if fewer than all cases are sampled ($f < 1$), the study precision will be lower in proportion to f.

The cases identified in a single clinic or treated by a single medical practitioner are possible case series for case-control studies. The corresponding source population for the cases treated in a clinic is all people who would attend that clinic and be recorded with the diagnosis of interest if they had the disease in question. It is important to specify "if they had the disease in question" because clinics serve different populations for different diseases, depending on referral patterns and the reputation of the clinic in specific specialty areas. As noted above, without a precisely identified source population, it may be difficult or impossible to select controls in an unbiased fashion.

CONTROL SELECTION

The definition of the source population determines the population from which controls are sampled. Ideally, selection will involve direct sampling of controls from the source population. Based on the principles explained earlier regarding the role of the control series, many general rules for control selection can be formulated. Two basic rules are that:

1. Controls should be selected from the same population—the source population—that gives rise to the study cases. If this rule cannot be followed, there needs to be solid evidence that the population supplying controls has an exposure distribution identical to that of the population that is the source of cases, which is a very stringent demand that is rarely demonstrable.
2. Within strata of factors that will be used for stratification in the analysis, controls should be selected independently of their exposure status, in that the sampling rate for controls (r in the previous discussion) should not vary with exposure.

If these rules and the corresponding case rules are met, then the ratio of pseudo-frequencies will, apart from sampling error, equal the ratio of the corresponding measure of disease frequency in the source population. If the sampling rate is known, then the actual measures of disease frequency can also be calculated. (If the sampling rates differ for exposed and unexposed cases or controls, but are known, the measures of disease frequency and their ratios can still be calculated using special correction formulas; see Chapters 15 and 19.) For a more detailed discussion of the principles of control selection in case-control studies, see Wacholder et al. (1992a, 1992b, 1992c).

When one wishes controls to represent person-time, sampling of the person-time should be constant across exposure levels. This requirement implies that the sampling *probability* of any person as a control should be proportional to the amount of person-time that person spends at risk of disease in the source population. For example, if in the source population one person contributes twice as much person-time during the study period as another person, the first person should have twice the probability of the second of being selected as a control. This difference in probability of selection is automatically induced by sampling controls at a steady rate per unit time over the period in which cases are sampled (*longitudinal* or *density* sampling), rather than by sampling all controls at a point in time (such as the start or end of the follow-up period). With longitudinal sampling of controls, a population member present for twice as long as another will have twice the chance of being selected.

If the objective of the study is to estimate a risk or rate ratio, it should be possible for a person to be selected as a control and yet remain eligible to become a case, so that person might appear in the study as both a control and a case. This possibility may sound paradoxical or wrong, but it is nevertheless correct. It corresponds to the fact that in a cohort study, a case contributes to both the numerator and the denominator of the estimated incidence.

Suppose the follow-up period spans 3 years, and a person free of disease in year 1 is selected as a potential control at year 1. This person should in principle remain eligible to become a case. Suppose this control now develops the disease at year 2 and now becomes a case in the study. How should such a person be treated in the analysis? Because the person did develop disease during the study period, many investigators would count the person as a case but not as a control. If the objective is to have the case-control odds ratio estimate the incidence odds ratio, then this decision would be appropriate. Recall, however, that if a follow-up study were being conducted, each person who develops disease would contribute not only to the numerator of the disease risk or rate but also to the persons or person-time tallied in the denominator. We want the control group to provide estimates of the relative size of the denominators of the incidence proportions or incidence rates for the compared groups. These denominators include all people who later become cases. Therefore, each case in a case-control study should be eligible to be a control before the time of disease onset, each control should be eligible to become a case as of the time of selection as a control, and a person selected as a control who later does develop the disease and is selected as a case should be included in the study both as a control and as a case (Sheehe, 1962; Miettinen, 1976a; Greenland and Thomas, 1982; Lubin and Gail, 1984; Robins et al., 1986a). If the controls are intended to represent person time and are selected longitudinally, similar arguments show that a person selected as a control should remain eligible to be selected as a control again, and thus might be included in the analysis repeatedly as a control (Lubin and Gail, 1984; Robins et al., 1986a).

COMMON FALLACIES IN CONTROL SELECTION

In cohort studies, the study population is restricted to people at risk for the disease. Some authors have viewed case-control studies as if they were cohort studies done backwards, even going so far as to describe them as "trohoc" studies (Feinstein, 1973). Under this view, the argument was advanced that case-control studies ought to be restricted to those at risk for exposure (i.e., those with exposure opportunity). Excluding sterile women from a case-control study of an adverse effect of oral contraceptives and matching for duration of employment in an occupational study are examples of attempts to control for exposure opportunity. If the factor used for restriction (e.g., sterility) is unrelated to the disease, it will not be a confounder, and hence the restriction will yield no benefit to the validity of the estimate of effect. Furthermore, if the restriction reduces the study size, the precision of the estimate of effect will be reduced (Poole, 1986).

Another principle sometimes used in cohort studies is that the study cohort should be "clean" at start of follow-up, including only people who have never had the disease. Misapplying this principle to case-control design suggests that the control group ought to be "clean," including only people who are healthy, for example. Illness arising after the start of the follow-up period is not reason to exclude subjects from a cohort analysis, and such exclusion can lead to bias; similarly controls with illness that arose after exposure should not be removed from the control series. Nonetheless, in studies of the relation between cigarette smoking and colorectal cancer, certain authors recommended that the control group should exclude people with colon polyps, because colon polyps are associated with smoking and are precursors of colorectal cancer (Terry and Neugut, 1998). Such an exclusion actually reduces the prevalence of the exposure in the controls below that in the source population of cases and hence biases the effect estimates upward (Poole, 1999).

SOURCES FOR CONTROL SERIES

The following methods for control sampling apply when the source population cannot be explicitly enumerated, so random selection is not possible. All of these methods should only be implemented subject to the reservations about secondary bases described earlier.

Neighborhood Controls

If the source population cannot be enumerated, it may be possible to select controls through sampling of residences. This method is not straightforward. Usually, a geographic roster of residences is not available, so a scheme must be devised to sample residences without enumerating them all. For convenience, investigators may sample controls who are individually matched to cases from the same neighborhood. That is, after a case is identified, one or more controls residing in the same neighborhood as that case are identified and recruited into the study. If neighborhood is related to exposure, the matching should be taken into account in the analysis (see Chapter 16).

Neighborhood controls are often used when the cases are recruited from a convenient source, such as a clinic or hospital. Such usage can introduce bias, however, for the neighbors selected as controls may not be in the source population of the cases. For example, if the cases are from a particular hospital, neighborhood controls may include people who would not have been treated at the same hospital had they developed the disease. If being treated at the hospital from which cases are identified is related to the exposure under study, then using neighborhood controls would introduce a bias. As an extreme example, suppose the hospital in question were a U.S. Veterans Administration hospital. Patients at these hospitals tend to differ from their neighbors in many ways. One obvious way is in regard to service history. Most patients at Veterans Administration hospitals have served in the U.S. military, whereas only a minority of their neighbors will have done so. This difference in life history can lead to differences in exposure histories (e.g., exposures associated with combat or weapons handling). For any given study, the suitability of using neighborhood controls needs to be evaluated with regard to the study variables on which the research focuses.

Random-Digit Dialing

Sampling of households based on random selection of telephone numbers is intended to simulate sampling randomly from the source population. *Random-digit dialing,* as this method has been called (Waksberg, 1978), offers the advantage of approaching all households in a designated area, even those with unlisted telephone numbers, through a simple telephone call. The method requires considerable attention to details, however, and carries no guarantee of unbiased selection.

First, case eligibility should include residence in a house that has a telephone, so that cases and controls come from the same source population. Second, even if the investigator can implement a sampling method so that every telephone has the same probability of being called, there will not necessarily be the same probability of contacting each eligible control subject, because households vary in the number of people who reside in them, the amount of time someone is at home, and the number of operating phones. Third, making contact with a household may require many calls at various times of day and various days of the week, demanding considerable labor; many dozens of telephone calls may be required to obtain a control subject meeting specific eligibility characteristics (Wacholder et al., 1992b). Fourth, some households use answering machines, voicemail, or caller identification to screen calls and may not answer or return unsolicited calls. Fifth, the substitution of mobile telephones for land lines by some households further undermines the assumption that population members can be selected randomly by random-digit dialing. Finally, it may be impossible to distinguish accurately business from residential telephone numbers, a distinction required to calculate the proportion of nonresponders.

Random-digit-dialing controls are usually matched to cases on area code (in the United States, the first three digits of the telephone number) and exchange (the three digits following the area code). In the past, area code and prefix were related to residence location and telephone type (land line or mobile service). Thus, if geographic location or participation in mobile telephone plans was likely related to exposure, then the matching should be taken into account in the analysis. More recently, telephone companies in the United States have assigned overlaying area codes and have allowed subscribers to retain their telephone number when they move within the region, so the correspondence between assigned telephone numbers and geographic location has diminished.

Hospital- or Clinic-Based Controls

As noted above, the source population for hospital- or clinic-based case-control studies is not often identifiable, because it represents a group of people who would be treated in a given clinic or hospital if they developed the disease in question. In such situations, a random sample of the general population will not necessarily correspond to a random sample of the source population. If the hospitals or clinics that provide the cases for the study treat only a small proportion of cases in the geographic area, then referral patterns to the hospital or clinic are important to take into account in the sampling of controls. For these studies, a control series comprising patients from the same hospitals or clinics as the cases may provide a less biased estimate of effect than general-population controls (such as those obtained from case neighborhoods or by random-digit dialing). The source population does not correspond to the population of the geographic area, but only to the people who would seek treatment at the hospital or clinic were they to develop the disease under study. Although the latter population may be difficult or impossible to enumerate or even define very clearly, it seems reasonable to expect that other hospital or clinic patients will represent this source population better than general-population controls. The major problem with any nonrandom sampling of controls is the possibility that they are not selected independently of exposure in the source population. Patients who are hospitalized with other diseases, for example, may be unrepresentative of the exposure distribution in the source population, either because exposure is associated with hospitalization, or because the exposure is associated with the other diseases, or both. For example, suppose the study aims to evaluate the relation between tobacco smoking and leukemia using hospitalized cases. If controls are people who are hospitalized with other conditions, many of them will have been hospitalized for conditions associated with smoking. A variety of other cancers, as well as cardiovascular diseases and respiratory diseases, are related to smoking. Thus, a control series of people hospitalized for diseases other than leukemia would include a higher proportion of smokers than would the source population of the leukemia cases.

Limiting the diagnoses for controls to conditions for which there is no prior indication of an association with the exposure improves the control series. For example, in a study of smoking and hospitalized leukemia cases, one could exclude from the control series anyone who was hospitalized with a disease known to be related to smoking. Such an exclusion policy may exclude most of the potential controls, because cardiovascular disease by itself would represent a large proportion of hospitalized patients. Nevertheless, even a few common diagnostic categories should suffice to find enough control subjects, so that the exclusions will not harm the study by limiting the size of the control series. Indeed, in limiting the scope of eligibility criteria, it is reasonable to exclude categories of potential controls even on the suspicion that a given category might be related to the exposure. If wrong, the cost of the exclusion is that the control series becomes more homogeneous with respect to diagnosis and perhaps a little smaller. But if right, then the exclusion is important to the ultimate validity of the study.

On the other hand, an investigator can rarely be sure that an exposure is not related to a disease or to hospitalization for a specific diagnosis. Consequently, it would be imprudent to use only a single diagnostic category as a source of controls. Using a variety of diagnoses has the advantage of potentially diluting the biasing effects of including a specific diagnostic group that is related to the exposure, and allows examination of the effect of excluding certain diagnoses.

Excluding a diagnostic category from the list of eligibility criteria for identifying controls is intended simply to improve the representativeness of the control series with respect to the source population. Such an exclusion criterion does not imply that there should be exclusions based on disease history (Lubin and Hartge, 1984). For example, in a case-control study of smoking and hospitalized leukemia patients, one might use hospitalized controls but exclude any who are hospitalized because of cardiovascular disease. This exclusion criterion for controls does not imply that leukemia cases who have had cardiovascular disease should be excluded; only if the cardiovascular disease was a cause of the hospitalization should the case be excluded. For controls, the exclusion criterion should apply only to the cause of the hospitalization used to identify the study subject. A person who was hospitalized because of a traumatic injury and who is thus eligible to be a control would not be excluded if he or she had previously been hospitalized for cardiovascular disease. The source population includes people who have had cardiovascular disease, and they should be included in the control series. Excluding such people would lead to an underrepresentation of smoking relative to the source population and produce an upward bias in the effect estimates.

If exposure directly affects hospitalization (for example, if the decision to hospitalize is in part based on exposure history), the resulting bias cannot be remedied without knowing the hospitalization rates, even if the exposure is unrelated to the study disease or the control diseases. This problem was in fact one of the first problems of hospital-based studies to receive detailed analysis (Berkson, 1946), and is often called Berksonian bias; it is discussed further under the topics of selection bias (Chapter 9) and collider bias (Chapter 12).

Other Diseases

In many settings, especially in populations with established disease registries or insurance-claims databases, it may be most convenient to choose controls from people who are diagnosed with other diseases. The considerations needed for valid control selection from other diagnoses parallel those just discussed for hospital controls. It is essential to exclude any diagnoses known or suspected to be related to exposure, and better still to include only diagnoses for which there is some evidence indicating that they are unrelated to exposure. These exclusion and inclusion criteria apply only to the diagnosis that brought the person into the registry or database from which controls are selected. The history of an exposure-related disease should not be a basis for exclusion. If, however, the exposure directly affects the chance of entering the registry or database, the study will be subject to the Berksonian bias mentioned earlier for hospital studies.

Friend Controls

Choosing friends of cases as controls, like using neighborhood controls, is a design that inherently uses individual matching and needs to be evaluated with regard to the advantages and disadvantages of such matching (discussed in Chapter 11).

Aside from the complications of individual matching, there are further concerns stemming from use of friend controls. First, being named as a friend by the case may be related to the exposure status of the potential control (Flanders and Austin, 1986). For example, cases might preferentially name as friends their acquaintances with whom they engage in specific activities that might relate to the exposure. Physical activity, alcoholic beverage consumption, and sun exposure are examples of such exposures. People who are more reclusive may be less likely to be named as friends, so their exposure patterns will be underrepresented among a control series of friends. Exposures more common to extroverted people may become overrepresented among friend controls. This type of bias was suspected in a study of insulin-dependent diabetes mellitus in which the parents of cases identified the controls. The cases had fewer friends than controls, had more learning problems, and were more likely to dislike school. Using friend controls could explain these findings (Siemiatycki, 1989).

A second problem is that, unlike other methods of control selection, choosing friends as controls cedes much of the decision making about the choice of control subjects to the cases or their proxies (e.g., parents). The investigator who uses friend controls will usually ask for a list of friends and choose randomly from the list, but for the creation of the list, the investigator is completely dependent on the cases or their proxies. This dependence adds a potential source of bias to the use of friend controls that does not exist for other sources of controls.

A third problem is that using friend controls can introduce a bias that stems from the overlapping nature of friendship groups (Austin et al., 1989; Robins and Pike, 1990). The problem arises because different cases name groups of friends that are not mutually exclusive. As a result, people with many friends become overrepresented in the control series, and any exposures associated with such people become overrepresented as well (see Chapter 11).

In principle, matching categories should form a mutually exclusive and collectively exhaustive partition with respect to all factors, such as neighborhood and age. For example, if matching on age, bias due to overlapping matching groups can arise from *caliper matching,* a term that refers to choosing controls who have a value for the matching factor within a specified range of the case's value. Thus, if the case is 69 years old, one might choose controls who are within 2 years of age 69. Overlap bias can be avoided if one uses nonoverlapping age categories for matching. Thus, if the case is 69 years old, one might choose controls from within the age category 65 to 69 years. In practice, however, bias due to overlapping age and neighborhood categories is probably minor (Robins and Pike, 1990).

Dead Controls

A dead control cannot be a member of the source population for cases, because death precludes the occurrence of any new disease. Suppose, however, that the cases are dead. Does the need for comparability argue in favor of using dead controls? Although certain types of comparability are important, choosing dead controls will misrepresent the exposure distribution in the source population if the exposure causes or prevents death in a substantial proportion of people or if it is associated with an uncontrolled factor that does. If interviews are needed and some cases are dead, it will be necessary to use proxy respondents for the dead cases. To enhance comparability of information while avoiding the problems of taking dead controls, proxy respondents can also be used for those live controls matched to dead cases (Wacholder et al., 1992b). The advantage of comparable information for cases and controls is often overstated, however, as will be addressed later. The main justification for using dead controls is convenience, such as in studies based entirely on deaths (see the discussion of proportional mortality studies below and in Chapter 6).

OTHER CONSIDERATIONS FOR SUBJECT SELECTION

Representativeness

Some textbooks have stressed the need for representativeness in the selection of cases and controls. The advice has been that cases should be representative of all people with the disease and that controls should be representative of the entire nondiseased population. Such advice can be misleading. A case-control study may be restricted to any type of case that may be of interest: female cases, old cases, severely ill cases, cases that died soon after disease onset, mild cases, cases from Philadelphia, cases among factory workers, and so on. In none of these examples would the cases be representative of all people with the disease, yet perfectly valid case-control studies are possible in each one (Cole, 1979). The definition of a case can be quite specific as long as it has a sound rationale. The main concern is clear delineation of the population that gave rise to the cases.

Ordinarily, controls should represent the source population for cases (within categories of stratification variables), rather than the entire nondiseased population. The latter may differ vastly from the source population for the cases by age, race, sex (e.g., if the cases come from a Veterans Administration hospital), socioeconomic status, occupation, and so on—including the exposure of interest.

One of the reasons for emphasizing the similarities rather than the differences between cohort and case-control studies is that numerous principles apply to both types of study but are more evident in the context of cohort studies. In particular, many principles relating to subject selection apply identically to both types of study. For example, it is widely appreciated that cohort studies can be based on special cohorts rather than on the general population. It follows that case-control studies can be conducted by sampling cases and controls from within those special cohorts. The resulting controls should represent the distribution of exposure across those cohorts, rather than the general population, reflecting the more general rule that controls should represent the source population of the cases in the study, not the general population.

Comparability of Information Accuracy

Some authors have recommended that information obtained about cases and controls should be of comparable or equal accuracy, to ensure nondifferentiality (equal distribution) of measurement errors (Miettinen, 1985a; Wacholder et al., 1992a; MacMahon and Trichopoulos, 1996). The rationale for this principle is the notion that nondifferential measurement error biases the observed association toward the null, and so will not generate a spurious association, and that bias in studies with nondifferential error is more predictable than in studies with differential error.

The comparability-of-information (equal-accuracy) principle is often used to guide selection of controls and collection of data. For example, it is the basis for using proxy respondents instead of direct interviews for living controls whenever case information is obtained from proxy respondents. In most settings, however, the arguments for the principle are logically inadequate. One problem, discussed at length in Chapter 9, is that nondifferentiality of exposure measurement error is far from sufficient to guarantee that bias will be toward the null. Such guarantees require that the exposure errors also be *independent* of errors in other variables, including disease and confounders (Chavance et al., 1992; Kristensen, 1992), a condition that is not always plausible (Lash and Fink, 2003b). For example, it seems likely that people who conceal heavy alcohol use will also tend to understate other socially disapproved behaviors such as heavy smoking, illicit drug use, and so on.

Another problem is that the efforts to ensure equal accuracy of exposure information will also tend to produce equal accuracy of information on other variables. The direction of overall bias produced by the resulting nondifferential errors in confounders and effect modifiers can be larger than the bias produced by differential error from unequal accuracy of exposure information from cases and controls (Greenland, 1980; Brenner, 1993; Marshall and Hastrup, 1996; Marshall et al., 1999; Fewell et al., 2007). In addition, unless the exposure is binary, even independent nondifferential error in exposure measurement is not guaranteed to produce bias toward the null (Dosemeci et al., 1990). Finally, even when the bias produced by forcing equal measurement accuracy is toward the null, there is no guarantee that the bias is less than the bias that would have resulted from using a measurement with differential error (Greenland and Robins, 1985a; Drews and Greenland, 1990; Wacholder et al., 1992a). For example, in a study that used proxy respondents for cases, use of proxy respondents for the controls might lead to greater bias than use of direct interviews with controls, even if the latter results in greater accuracy of control measurements.

The comparability-of-information (equal accuracy) principle is therefore applicable only under very limited conditions. In particular, it would seem to be useful only when confounders and effect modifiers are measured with negligible error and when measurement error is reduced by using equally accurate sources of information. Otherwise, the bias from forcing cases and controls to have equal measurement accuracy may be as unpredictable as the effect of not doing so and risking differential error (unequal accuracy).

Number of Control Groups

Situations arise in which the investigator may face a choice between two or more possible control groups. Usually, there will be advantages for one group that are missing in the other, and vice versa. Consider, for example, a case-control study based on a hospitalized series of cases. Because they are hospitalized, hospital controls would be unrepresentative of the source population to the extent that exposure is related to hospitalization for the control conditions. Neighborhood controls would not suffer this problem, but might be unrepresentative of persons who would go to the hospital if they had the study disease. So which control group is better? In such situations, some have argued that more than one control group should be used, in an attempt to address the biases from each group (Ibrahim and Spitzer, 1979). For example, Gutensohn et al. (1975), in a case-control study of Hodgkin disease, used a control group of spouses to control for environmental influences during adult life but also used a control group of siblings to control for childhood environment and sex. Both control groups are attempting to represent the same source population of cases, but have different vulnerabilities to selection biases and match on different potential confounders.

Use of multiple control groups may involve considerable labor, so is more the exception than the rule in case-control research. Often, one available control source is superior to all practical alternatives. In such settings, effort should not be wasted on collecting controls from sources likely to be biased. Interpretation of the results will also be more complicated unless the different control groups yield similar results. If the two groups produced different results, one would face the problem of explaining the differences and attempting to infer which estimate was more valid. Logically, then, the value of using more than one control group is quite limited. The control groups can and should be compared, but a lack of difference between the groups shows only that both groups incorporate similar net bias. A difference shows only that at least one is biased, but does not indicate which is best or which is worst. Only external information could help evaluate the likely extent of bias in the estimates from different control groups, and that same external information might have favored selection of only one of the control groups at the design stage of the study.

Timing of Classification and Diagnosis

Chapter 7 discussed at length some basic principles for classifying persons, cases, and person-time units in cohort studies according to exposure status. The same principles apply to cases and controls in case-control studies. If the controls are intended to represent person-time (rather than persons) in the source population, one should apply principles for classifying person-time to the classification of controls. In particular, principles of person-time classification lead to the rule that controls should be classified by their exposure status as of their selection time. Exposures accrued after that time should be ignored. The rule necessitates that information (such as exposure history) be obtained in a manner that allows one to ignore exposures accrued after the selection time. In a similar manner, cases should be classified as of time of diagnosis or disease onset, accounting for any built-in lag periods or induction-period hypotheses. Determining the time of diagnosis or disease onset can involve all the problems and ambiguities discussed in the previous chapter for cohort studies and needs to be resolved by study protocol before classifications can be made.

As an example, consider a study of alcohol use and laryngeal cancer that also examined smoking as a confounder and possible effect modifier, used interviewer-administered questionnaires to collect data, and used neighborhood controls. To examine the effect of alcohol and smoking while assuming a 1-year lag period (a 1-year minimum induction time), the questionnaire would have to allow determination of drinking and smoking habits up to 1 year before diagnosis (for cases) or selection (for controls).

Selection time need not refer to the investigator's identification of the control, but instead may refer to an event analogous to the occurrence time for the case. For example, the selection time for controls who are cases of other diseases can be taken as time of diagnosis for that disease; the selection time of hospital controls might be taken as time of hospitalization. For other types of controls, there may be no such natural event analogous to the case diagnosis time, and the actual time of selection will have to be used.

In most studies, selection time will precede the time data are gathered. For example, in interview-based studies, controls may be identified and then a delay of weeks or months may occur before the interview is conducted. To avoid complicating the interview questions, this distinction is often ignored and controls are questioned about habits in periods dating back from the interview.

VARIANTS OF THE CASE-CONTROL DESIGN

NESTED CASE-CONTROL STUDIES

Epidemiologists sometimes refer to specific case-control studies as *nested* case-control studies when the population within which the study is conducted is a fully enumerated cohort, which allows formal random sampling of cases and controls to be carried out. The term is usually used in reference to a case-control study conducted within a cohort study, in which further information (perhaps from expensive tests) is obtained on most or all cases, but for economy is obtained from only a fraction of the remaining cohort members (the controls). Nonetheless, many population-based case-control studies can be thought of as nested within an enumerated source population. For example, when there is a population-based disease registry and a census enumeration of the population served by the registry, it may be possible to use the census data to sample controls randomly.

CASE-COHORT STUDIES

The *case-cohort study* is a case-control study in which the source population is a cohort and (within sampling or matching strata) every person in this cohort has an equal chance of being included in the study as a control, regardless of how much time that person has contributed to the person-time experience of the cohort or whether the person developed the study disease. This design is a logical way to conduct a case-control study when the effect measure of interest is the ratio of incidence proportions rather than a rate ratio, as is common in perinatal studies. The average risk (or incidence proportion) of falling ill during a specified period may be written

$$R_1 = \frac{A_1}{N_1}$$

for the exposed subcohort and

$$R_0 = \frac{A_0}{N_0}$$

for the unexposed subcohort, where R_1 and R_0 are the incidence proportions among the exposed and unexposed, respectively, and N_1 and N_0 are the initial sizes of the exposed and unexposed subcohorts. (This discussion applies equally well to exposure variables with several levels, but for simplicity we will consider only a dichotomous exposure.) Controls should be selected such that the exposure distribution among them will estimate without bias the exposure distribution in the source population. In a case-cohort study, the distribution we wish to estimate is among the $N_1 + N_0$ cohort members, not among their person-time experience (Thomas, 1972; Kupper et al., 1975; Miettinen, 1982a).

The objective is to select controls from the source cohort such that the ratio of the number of exposed controls (B_1) to the number of exposed cohort members (N_1) is the same as the ratio of the number of unexposed controls (B_0) to the number of unexposed cohort members (N_0), apart from sampling error:

$$\frac{B_1}{N_1} = \frac{B_0}{N_0}$$

Here, B_1/N_1 and B_0/N_0 are the control sampling fractions (the number of controls selected per cohort member). Apart from random error, these sampling fractions will be equal if controls have been selected independently of exposure.

We can use the frequencies of exposed and unexposed controls as substitutes for the actual denominators of the incidence proportions to obtain "pseudo-risks":

$$\text{Pseudo-risk}_1 = \frac{A_1}{B_1}$$

and

$$\text{Pseudo-risk}_0 = \frac{A_0}{B_0}$$

These pseudo-risks have no epidemiologic interpretation by themselves. Suppose, however, that the control sampling fractions are equal to the same fraction, f. Then, apart from sampling error, B_1/f should equal N_1, the size of the exposed subcohort; and B_0/f should equal N_0, the size of the unexposed subcohort: $B_1/f = B_1/(B_1/N_1) = N_1$ and $B_0/f = B_0/(B_0/N_0) = N_0$. Thus, to get the incidence proportions, we need only multiply each pseudo-risk by the common sampling fraction, f. If this fraction is not known, we can still compare the sizes of the pseudo-risks by division:

$$\frac{\text{Pseudo-risk}_1}{\text{Pseudo-risk}_0} = \frac{A_1/B_1}{A_0/B_0} = \frac{A_1/[(B_1/N_1)N_1]}{A_0/[(B_0/N_0)N_0]} = \frac{A_1/fN_1}{A_0/fN_0} = \frac{A_1/N_1}{A_0/N_0}$$

In other words, the ratio of pseudo-risks is an estimate of the ratio of incidence proportions (risk ratio) in the source cohort if control sampling is independent of exposure. Thus, using a case-cohort design, one can estimate the risk ratio in a cohort without obtaining information on every cohort member.

Thus far, we have implicitly assumed that there is no loss to follow-up or competing risks in the underlying cohort. If there are such problems, it is still possible to estimate risk or rate ratios from a case-cohort study, provided that we have data on the time spent at risk by the sampled subjects or we use certain sampling modifications (Flanders et al., 1990). These procedures require the usual assumptions for rate-ratio estimation in cohort studies, namely, that loss-to-follow-up and competing risks either are not associated with exposure or are not associated with disease risk.

An advantage of the case-cohort design is that it facilitates conduct of a set of case-control studies from a single cohort, all of which use the same control group. As a sample from the cohort at enrollment, the control group can be compared with any number of case groups. If matched controls are selected from people at risk at the time a case occurs (as in risk-set sampling, which is described later), the control series must be tailored to a specific group of cases. If common outcomes are to be studied and one wishes to use a single control group for each outcome, another sampling scheme must be used. The case-cohort approach is a good choice in such a situation.

Case-cohort designs have other advantages as well as disadvantages relative to alternative case-control designs (Wacholder, 1991). One disadvantage is that, because of the overlap of membership in the case and control groups (controls who are selected may also develop disease and enter the study as cases), one will need to select more controls in a case-cohort study than in an ordinary case-control study with the same number of cases, if one is to achieve the same amount of statistical precision. Extra controls are needed because the statistical precision of a study is strongly determined by the numbers of distinct cases and noncases. Thus, if 20% of the source cohort members will become cases, and all cases will be included in the study, one will have to select 1.25 times as many controls as cases in a case-cohort study to ensure that there will be as many controls who never become cases in the study. On average, only 80% of the controls in such a situation will remain noncases; the other 20% will become cases. Of course, if the disease is uncommon, the number of extra controls needed for a case-cohort study will be small.

DENSITY CASE-CONTROL STUDIES

Earlier, we described how case-control odds ratios will estimate rate ratios if the control series is selected so that the ratio of the person-time denominators T_1/T_0 is validly estimated by the ratio of exposed to unexposed controls B_1/B_0. That is, to estimate rate ratios, controls should be selected so that the exposure distribution among them is, apart from random error, the same as it is among the person-time in the source population or within strata of the source population. Such control selection is called *density sampling* because it provides for estimation of relations among incidence rates, which have been called *incidence densities*.

If a subject's exposure may vary over time, then a case's exposure history is evaluated up to the time the disease occurred. A control's exposure history is evaluated up to an analogous index time, usually taken as the time of sampling; exposure after the time of selection must be ignored. This rule helps ensure that the number of exposed and unexposed controls will be in proportion to the amount of exposed and unexposed person-time in the source population.

The time during which a subject is eligible to be a control should be the time in which that person is also eligible to become a case, if the disease should occur. Thus, a person in whom the disease has already developed or who has died is no longer eligible to be selected as a control. This rule corresponds to the treatment of subjects in cohort studies. Every case that is tallied in the numerator of a cohort study contributes to the denominator of the rate until the time that the person becomes a case, when the contribution to the denominator ceases. One way to implement this rule is to choose controls from the set of people in the source population who are at risk of becoming a case at the time that the case is diagnosed. This set is sometimes referred to as the *risk set* for the case, and this type of control sampling is sometimes called *risk-set sampling*. Controls sampled in this manner are matched to the case with respect to sampling time; thus, if time is related to exposure, the resulting data should be analyzed as matched data (Greenland and Thomas, 1982). It is also possible to conduct unmatched density sampling using probability sampling methods if one knows the time interval at risk for each population member. One then selects a control by sampling members with probability proportional to time at risk and then randomly samples a time to measure exposure within the interval at risk.

As mentioned earlier, a person selected as a control who remains in the study population at risk after selection should remain eligible to be selected once again as a control. Thus, although it is unlikely in typical studies, the same person may appear in the control group two or more times. Note, however, that including the same person at different times does not necessarily lead to exposure (or confounder) information being repeated, because this information may change with time. For example, in a case-control study of an acute epidemic of intestinal illness, one might ask about food ingested within the previous day or days. If a contaminated food item was a cause of the illness for some cases, then the exposure status of a case or control chosen 5 days into the study might well differ from what it would have been 2 days into the study.

CUMULATIVE ("EPIDEMIC") CASE-CONTROL STUDIES

In some research settings, case-control studies may address a risk that ends before subject selection begins. For example, a case-control study of an epidemic of diarrheal illness after a social gathering may begin after all the potential cases have occurred (because the maximum induction time has elapsed). In such a situation, an investigator might select controls from that portion of the population that remains after eliminating the accumulated cases; that is, one selects controls from among noncases (those who remain noncases at the end of the epidemic follow-up).

Suppose that the source population is a cohort and that a fraction f of both exposed and unexposed noncases is selected to be controls. Then the ratio of pseudo-frequencies will be

$$\frac{A_1/B_1}{A_0/B_0} = \frac{A_1/f(N_1 - A_1)}{A_0/f(N_0 - A_0)} = \frac{A_1/(N_1 - A_1)}{A_0/(N_0 - A_0)}$$

which is the incidence odds ratio for the cohort. This ratio will provide a reasonable approximation to the rate ratio, provided that the proportions falling ill in each exposure group during the risk period are low, that is, less than about 20%, and that the prevalence of exposure remains reasonably steady during the study period (see Chapter 4). If the investigator prefers to estimate the risk ratio rather than the incidence rate ratio, the study odds ratio can still be used (Cornfield, 1951), but the accuracy of this approximation is only about half as good as that of the odds-ratio approximation to the rate ratio (Greenland, 1987a). The use of this approximation in the cumulative design is the primary basis for the mistaken teaching that a rare-disease assumption is needed to estimate effects from case-control studies.

Before the 1970s, the standard conceptualization of case-control studies involved the cumulative design, in which controls are selected from noncases at the end of a follow-up period. As discussed by numerous authors (Sheehe, 1962; Miettinen, 1976a; Greenland and Thomas, 1982), density designs and case-cohort designs have several advantages outside of the acute epidemic setting, including potentially much less sensitivity to bias from exposure-related loss-to-follow-up.

CASE-ONLY, CASE-SPECULAR, AND CASE-CROSSOVER STUDIES

There are a number of situations in which cases are the only subjects used to estimate or test hypotheses about effects. For example, it is sometimes possible to employ theoretical considerations to construct a prior distribution of exposure in the source population and use this distribution in place of an observed control series. Such situations arise naturally in genetic studies, in which basic laws of inheritance may be combined with certain assumptions to derive a population or parental-specific distribution of genotypes (Self et al., 1991). It is also possible to study certain aspects of joint effects (interactions) of genetic and environmental factors without using control subjects (Khoury and Flanders, 1996); see Chapter 28 for details.

When the exposure under study is defined by proximity to an environmental source (e.g., a power line), it may be possible to construct a *specular* (hypothetical) control for each case by conducting a "thought experiment." Either the case or the exposure source is imaginarily moved to another location that would be equally likely were there no exposure effect; the case exposure level under this hypothetical configuration is then treated as the (matched) "control" exposure for the case (Zaffanella et al., 1998). When the specular control arises by examining the exposure experience of the case outside of the time in which exposure could be related to disease occurrence, the result is called a *case-crossover study*.

The classic *crossover* study is a type of experiment in which two (or more) treatments are compared, as in any experimental study. In a crossover study, however, each subject receives both treatments, with one following the other. Preferably, the order in which the two treatments are applied is randomly chosen for each subject. Enough time should be allocated between the two administrations so that the effect of each treatment can be measured and can subside before the other treatment is given. A persistent effect of the first intervention is called a *carryover effect*. A crossover study is only valid to study treatments for which effects occur within a short induction period and do not persist, i.e., carryover effects must be absent, so that the effect of the second intervention is not intermingled with the effect of the first.

The *case-crossover* study is a case-control analog of the crossover study (Maclure, 1991). For each case, one or more predisease or postdisease time periods are selected as matched "control" periods for the case. The exposure status of the case at the time of the disease onset is compared with the distribution of exposure status for that same person in the control periods. Such a comparison depends on the assumption that neither exposure nor confounders are changing over time in a systematic way.

Only a limited set of research topics are amenable to the case-crossover design. The exposure must vary over time within individuals rather than stay constant. Eye color or blood type, for example, could not be studied with a case-crossover design because both are constant. If the exposure does not vary within a person, then there is no basis for comparing exposed and unexposed time periods of risk within the person. Like the crossover study, the exposure must also have a short induction time and a transient effect; otherwise, exposures in the distant past could be the cause of a recent disease onset (a carryover effect).

Maclure (1991) used the case-crossover design to study the effect of sexual activity on incident myocardial infarction. This topic is well suited to a case-crossover design because the exposure is intermittent and is presumed to have a short induction period for the hypothesized effect. Any increase in risk for a myocardial infarction from sexual activity is presumed to be confined to a short time following the activity. A myocardial infarction is an outcome that is well suited to this type of study because it is thought to be triggered by events close in time. Other possible causes of a myocardial infarction that might be studied by a case-crossover study would be caffeine consumption, alcohol consumption, carbon monoxide exposure, drug exposures, and heavy physical exertion (Mittleman et al., 1993), all of which occur intermittently.

Each case and its control in a case-crossover study is automatically matched on all characteristics (e.g., sex and birth date) that do not change within individuals. Matched analysis of case-crossover data controls for all such fixed confounders, whether or not they are measured. Subject to special assumptions, control for measured time-varying confounders may be possible using modeling methods for matched data (see Chapter 21). It is also possible to adjust case-crossover estimates for bias due to time trends in exposure through use of longitudinal data from a nondiseased control group (case-time controls) (Suissa, 1995). Nonetheless, these trend adjustments themselves depend on additional no-confounding assumptions and may introduce bias if those assumptions are not met (Greenland, 1996b).

There are many possible variants of the case-crossover design, depending on how control time periods are selected. These variants offer trade-offs among potential for bias, inefficiency, and difficulty of analysis; see Lumley and Levy (2000), Vines and Farrington (2001), Navidi and Weinhandl (2002), and Janes et al. (2004, 2005) for further discussion.

TWO-STAGE SAMPLING

Another variant of the case-control study uses two-stage or two-phase sampling (Walker, 1982a; White, 1982b). In this type of study, the control series comprises a relatively large number of people (possibly everyone in the source population), from whom exposure information or perhaps some limited amount of information on other relevant variables is obtained. Then, for only a subsample of the controls, more detailed information is obtained on exposure or on other study variables that may need to be controlled in the analysis. More detailed information may also be limited to a subsample of cases. This two-stage approach is useful when it is relatively inexpensive to obtain the exposure information (e.g., by telephone interview), but the covariate information is more expensive to obtain (say, by laboratory analysis). It is also useful when exposure information already has been collected on the entire population (e.g., job histories for an occupational cohort), but covariate information is needed (e.g., genotype). This situation arises in cohort studies when more information is required than was gathered at baseline. As will be discussed in Chapter 15, this type of study requires special analytic methods to take full advantage of the information collected at both stages.

PROPORTIONAL MORTALITY STUDIES

Proportional mortality studies were discussed in Chapter 6, where the point was made that the validity of such studies can be improved if they are designed and analyzed as case-control studies. The cases are deaths occurring within the source population. Controls are not selected directly from the source population, which consists of living people, but are taken from other deaths within the source population. This control series is acceptable if the exposure distribution within this group is similar to that of the source population. Consequently, the control series should be restricted to categories of death that are not related to the exposure. See Chapter 6 for a more detailed discussion.

CASE-CONTROL STUDIES WITH PREVALENT CASES

Case-control studies are sometimes based on prevalent cases rather than incident cases. When it is impractical to include only incident cases, it may still be possible to select existing cases of illness at a point in time. If the prevalence odds ratio in the population is equal to the incidence-rate ratio, then the odds ratio from a case-control study based on prevalent cases can unbiasedly estimate the rate ratio. As noted in Chapter 4, however, the conditions required for the prevalence odds ratio to equal the rate ratio are very strong, and a simple general relation does not exist for age-specific ratios. If exposure is associated with duration of illness or migration out of the prevalence pool, then a case-control study based on prevalent cases cannot by itself distinguish exposure effects on disease incidence from the exposure association with disease duration or migration, unless the strengths of the latter associations are known. If the size of the exposed or the unexposed population changes with time or there is migration into the prevalence pool, the prevalence odds ratio may be further removed from the rate ratio. Consequently, it is always preferable to select incident rather than prevalent cases when studying disease etiology.

As discussed in Chapter 3, prevalent cases are usually drawn in studies of congenital malformations. In such studies, cases ascertained at birth are prevalent because they have survived with the malformation from the time of its occurrence until birth. It would be etiologically more useful to ascertain all incident cases, including affected abortuses that do not survive until birth. Many of these, however, do not survive until ascertainment is feasible, and thus it is virtually inevitable that case-control studies of congenital malformations are based on prevalent cases. In this example, the source population comprises all conceptuses, and miscarriage and induced abortion represent emigration before the ascertainment date. Although an exposure will not affect duration of a malformation, it may very well affect risks of miscarriage and abortion.

Other situations in which prevalent cases are commonly used are studies of chronic conditions with ill-defined onset times and limited effects on mortality, such as obesity, Parkinson's disease, and multiple sclerosis, and studies of health services utilization.

CHAPTER 9

Validity in Epidemiologic Studies

Kenneth J. Rothman, Sander Greenland, and Timothy L. Lash

Validity of Estimation 128
Confounding 129
Confounding as Mixing of Effects 129
Confounders and Surrogate Confounders 130
Properties of a Confounder 130
Confounders as Extraneous Risk Factors 131
Judging the Causal Role of a Potential Confounder 131
Criteria for a Confounding Factor 132
Selection Bias 134
Self-Selection Bias 134
Berksonian Bias 135
Distinguishing Selection Bias from Confounding 136
Information Bias 137
Measurement Error, Misclassification, and Bias 137
Differential Misclassification 138
Nondifferential Misclassification 139
Misclassification of Confounders 144
The Complexities of Simultaneous Misclassification 145
Generalizability 146

VALIDITY OF ESTIMATION

An epidemiologic estimate is the end product of the study design, the study conduct, and the data analysis. We will call the entire process leading to an estimate (study design, conduct, and analysis) the estimation process. The overall goal of an epidemiologic study can then usually be viewed as accuracy in estimation. More specifically, as described in previous chapters, the objective of an epidemiologic study is to obtain a valid and precise estimate of the frequency of a disease or of the effect of an exposure on the occurrence of a disease in the source population of the study. Inherent in this objective is the view that epidemiologic research is an exercise in measurement. Often, a further objective is to obtain an estimate that is generalizable to relevant target populations; this objective involves selecting a source population for study that either is a target or can be argued to experience effects similar to the targets.

Accuracy in estimation implies that the value of the parameter that is the object of measurement is estimated with little error. Errors in estimation are traditionally classified as either *random* or *systematic*. Although random errors in the sampling and measurement of subjects can lead to systematic errors in the final estimates, important principles of study design emerge from separate consideration of sources of random and systematic errors. Systematic errors in estimates are commonly referred to as *biases;* the opposite of bias is validity, so that an estimate that has little systematic error may be described as *valid*. Analogously, the opposite of random error is precision, and an estimate with little random error may be described as *precise*. Validity and precision are both components of accuracy.

The validity of a study is usually separated into two components: the validity of the inferences drawn as they pertain to the members of the source population (*internal validity*) and the validity of the inferences as they pertain to people outside that population (*external validity or generalizability*). Internal validity implies validity of inference for the source population of study subjects. In studies of causation, it corresponds to accurate measurement of effects apart from random variation. Under such a scheme, internal validity is considered a prerequisite for external validity.

Most violations of internal validity can be classified into three general categories: confounding, selection bias, and information bias, where the latter is bias arising from mismeasurement of study variables. Confounding was described in general terms in Chapter 4, while specific selection bias and measurement problems were described in Chapters 7 and 8. The present chapter describes the general forms of these problems in epidemiologic studies. Chapter 10 describes how to measure and limit random error, Chapter 11 addresses options in study design that can improve overall accuracy, and Chapter 12 shows how biases can be described and identified using causal diagrams. After an introduction to statistics in Chapters 13 and 14, Chapters 15 and 16 provide basic methods to adjust for measured confounders, while Chapter 19 introduces methods to adjust for unmeasured confounders, selection bias, and misclassification.

The dichotomization of validity into internal and external components might suggest that generalization is simply a matter of extending inferences about a source population to a target population. The final section of this chapter provides a different view of generalizability, in which the essence of scientific generalization is the formulation of abstract (usually causal) theories that relate the study variables to one another. The theories are abstract in the sense that they are not tied to specific populations; instead, they apply to a more general set of circumstances than the specific populations under study. Internal validity in a study is still a prerequisite for the study to contribute usefully to this process of abstraction, but the generalization process is otherwise separate from the concerns of internal validity and the mechanics of the study design.

CONFOUNDING

The concept of confounding was introduced in Chapter 4. Although confounding occurs in experimental research, it is a considerably more important issue in observational studies. Therefore, we will here review the concepts of confounding and confounders and then discuss further issues in defining and identifying confounders. As in Chapter 4, in this section we will presume that the objective is to estimate the effect that exposure had on those exposed in the source population. This effect is the actual (or realized) effect of exposure. We will indicate only briefly how the discussion should be modified when estimating counterfactual (or potential) exposure effects, such as the effect exposure might have on the unexposed. Chapter 12 examines confounding within the context of causal diagrams, which do not make these distinctions explicit.

CONFOUNDING AS MIXING OF EFFECTS

On the simplest level, confounding may be considered a confusion of effects. Specifically, the apparent effect of the exposure of interest is distorted because the effect of extraneous factors is mistaken for—or mixed with—the actual exposure effect (which may be null). The distortion introduced by a confounding factor can be large, and it can lead to overestimation or underestimation of an effect, depending on the direction of the associations that the confounding factor has with exposure and disease. Confounding can even change the apparent direction of an effect.

A more precise definition of confounding begins by considering the manner in which effects are estimated. Suppose we wish to estimate the degree to which exposure has changed the frequency of disease in an exposed cohort. To do so, we must estimate what the frequency of disease would have been in this cohort had exposure been absent and compare this estimate to the observed frequency under exposure. Because the cohort was exposed, this absence of exposure is *counterfactual* (contrary to the facts) and so the desired unexposed comparison frequency is unobservable. Thus, as a substitute, we observe the disease frequency in an unexposed cohort. But rarely can we take this unexposed frequency as fairly representing what the frequency would have been in the exposed cohort had exposure been absent, because the unexposed cohort may differ from the exposed cohort on many factors that affect disease frequency besides exposure. To express this problem, we say that the use of the unexposed as the referent for the exposed is *confounded,* because the disease frequency in the exposed differs from that in the unexposed as a result of a mixture of two or more effects, one of which is the effect of exposure.

CONFOUNDERS AND SURROGATE CONFOUNDERS

The extraneous factors that are responsible for difference in disease frequency between the exposed and unexposed are called *confounders*. In addition, factors associated with these extraneous causal factors that can serve as surrogates for these factors are also commonly called confounders. The most extreme example of such a surrogate is chronologic age. Increasing age is strongly associated with *aging*—the accumulation of cell mutations and tissue damage that leads to disease—but increasing age does not itself cause most such pathogenic changes (Kirkland, 1992), because it is just a measure of how much time has passed since birth.

Regardless of whether a confounder is a cause of the study disease or merely a surrogate for such a cause, one primary characteristic is that if it is perfectly measured it will be predictive of disease frequency within the unexposed (reference) cohort. Otherwise, the confounder cannot explain why the unexposed cohort fails to represent properly the disease frequency the exposed cohort would experience in the absence of exposure. For example, suppose that all the exposed were men and all the unexposed were women. If unexposed men have the same incidence as unexposed women, the fact that all the unexposed were women rather than men could not account for any confounding that is present.

In the simple view, confounding occurs only if extraneous effects become mixed with the effect under study. Note, however, that confounding can occur even if the factor under study has no effect. Thus, "mixing of effects" should not be taken to imply that the exposure under study has an effect. The mixing of the effects comes about from an association between the exposure and extraneous factors, regardless of whether the exposure has an effect.

As another example, consider a study to determine whether alcohol drinkers experience a greater incidence of oral cancer than nondrinkers. Smoking is an extraneous factor that is related to the disease among the unexposed (smoking has an effect on oral cancer incidence among alcohol abstainers). Smoking is also associated with alcohol drinking, because there are many people who are general "abstainers," refraining from alcohol consumption, smoking, and perhaps other habits. Consequently, alcohol drinkers include among them a greater proportion of smokers than would be found among nondrinkers. Because smoking increases the incidence of oral cancer, alcohol drinkers will have a greater incidence than nondrinkers, quite apart from any influence of alcohol drinking itself, simply as a consequence of the greater amount of smoking among alcohol drinkers. Thus, the apparent effect of alcohol drinking is distorted by the effect of smoking; the effect of smoking becomes mixed with the effect of alcohol in the comparison of alcohol drinkers with nondrinkers. The degree of bias or distortion depends on the magnitude of the smoking effect, the strength of association between alcohol and smoking, and the prevalence of smoking among nondrinkers who do not have oral cancer. Either absence of a smoking effect on oral cancer incidence or absence of an association between smoking and alcohol would lead to no confounding. Smoking must be associated with both oral cancer and alcohol drinking for it to be a confounding factor.

PROPERTIES OF A CONFOUNDER

In general, a variable must be associated with both the exposure under study and the disease under study to be a confounder. These associations do not, however, define a confounder, for a variable may possess these associations and yet not be a confounder. There are several ways this can happen. The most common way occurs when the exposure under study has an effect. In this situation, any correlate of that exposure will also tend to be associated with the disease as a consequence of its association with exposure. For example, suppose that frequent beer consumption is associated with the consumption of pizza, and suppose that frequent beer consumption is a risk factor for rectal cancer. Would consumption of pizza be a confounding factor? At first, it might seem that the answer is yes, because consumption of pizza is associated both with beer drinking and with rectal cancer. But if pizza consumption is associated with rectal cancer only because of its association with beer consumption, it would not be confounding; in fact, the association of pizza consumption with colorectal cancer would then be due entirely to confounding by beer consumption. A confounding factor must be associated with disease occurrence *apart* from its association with exposure. In particular, as explained earlier, the potentially confounding variate must be associated with disease among unexposed (reference) individuals. If consumption of pizza were associated with rectal cancer among nondrinkers of beer, then it could confound. Otherwise, if it were associated with rectal cancer only because of its association with beer drinking, it could not confound.

Analogous with this restriction on the association between a potential confounder and disease, the potential confounder must be associated with the exposure among the source population for cases, for this association with exposure is how the effects of the potential confounder become mixed with the effects of the exposure. In this regard, it should be noted that a risk factor that is independent of exposure in the source population can (and usually will) become associated with exposure among the cases; hence one cannot take the association among cases as a valid estimate of the association in the source population.

CONFOUNDERS AS EXTRANEOUS RISK FACTORS

It is also important to clarify what we mean by the term *extraneous* in the phrase "extraneous risk factor." This term means that the factor's association with disease arises from a causal pathway other than the one under study. Specifically, consider the causal diagram

$$\text{Smoking} \longrightarrow \text{elevated blood pressure} \longrightarrow \text{heart disease}$$

where the arrows represent causation. Is elevated blood pressure a confounding factor? It is certainly a risk factor for disease, and it is also correlated with exposure, because it can result from smoking. It is even a risk factor for disease among unexposed individuals, because elevated blood pressure can result from causes other than smoking. Nevertheless, it cannot be considered a confounding factor, because the effect of smoking is mediated through the effect of blood pressure. Any factor that represents a step in the causal chain between exposure and disease should not be treated as an extraneous confounding factor, but instead requires special treatment as an *intermediate* factor (Greenland and Neutra, 1980; Robins, 1989; see Chapter 12).

Finally, a variable may satisfy all of the preceding conditions but may not do so after control for some other confounding variable, and so may no longer be a confounder within strata of the second confounder. For example, it may happen that either (a) the first confounder is no longer associated with disease within strata of the second confounder, or (b) the first confounder is no longer associated with exposure within strata of the second confounder. In either case, the first confounder is only a surrogate for the second confounder. More generally, the status of a variable as a confounder may depend on which other variables are controlled when the evaluation is made; in other words, being a confounder is conditional on what else is controlled.

JUDGING THE CAUSAL ROLE OF A POTENTIAL CONFOUNDER

Consider the simple but common case of a binary exposure variable, with interest focused on the effect of exposure on a particular exposed population, relative to what would have happened had this population not been exposed. Suppose that an unexposed population is selected as the comparison (reference) group. A potential confounder is then a factor that is associated with disease among the unexposed, and is not affected by exposure or disease. We can verify the latter requirement if we know that the factor precedes the exposure and disease. Association with disease among the unexposed is a more difficult criterion to decide. Apart from simple and now obvious potential confounders such as age, sex, and tobacco use, the available epidemiologic data are often ambiguous as to predictiveness even when they do establish time order. Simply deciding whether predictiveness holds on the basis of a statistical test is usually far too insensitive to detect all important confounders and as a result may produce highly confounded estimates, as real examples demonstrate (Greenland and Neutra, 1980).

One answer to the ambiguity and insensitivity of epidemiologic methods to detect confounders is to call on other evidence regarding the effect of the potential confounder on disease, including nonepidemiologic (e.g., clinical or social) data and perhaps mechanistic theories about the possible effects of the potential confounders. Uncertainties about the evidence or mechanism can justify the handling of a potential confounding factor as both confounding and not confounding in different analyses. For example, in evaluating the effect of coffee on heart disease, it is unclear how to treat serum cholesterol levels. Elevated levels are a risk factor for heart disease and may be associated with coffee use, but serum cholesterol may mediate the action of coffee use on heart disease risk.

That is, elevated cholesterol may be an intermediate factor in the etiologic sequence under study. If the time ordering of coffee use and cholesterol elevation cannot be determined, one might conduct two analyses, one in which serum cholesterol is controlled (which would be appropriate if coffee does not affect serum cholesterol) and one in which it is either not controlled or is treated as an intermediate (which would be more appropriate if coffee affects serum cholesterol and is not associated with uncontrolled determinants of serum cholesterol). The interpretation of the results would depend on which of the theories about serum cholesterol were correct. Causal graphs provide a useful means for depicting these multivariable relations and, as will be explained in Chapter 12, allow identification of confounders for control from the structure of the graph.

CRITERIA FOR A CONFOUNDING FACTOR

We can summarize thus far with the observation that for a variable to be a confounder, it must have three necessary (but not sufficient or defining) characteristics, which we will discuss in detail. We will then point out some limitations of these characteristics in defining and identifying confounding.

1. *A confounding factor must be an extraneous risk factor for the disease.*

As mentioned earlier, a potential confounding factor need not be an actual cause of the disease, but if it is not, it must be a surrogate for an actual cause of the disease other than exposure. This condition implies that the association between the potential confounder and the disease must occur within levels of the study exposure. In particular, a potentially confounding factor must be a risk factor within the reference level of the exposure under study. The data may serve as a guide to the relation between the potential confounder and the disease, but it is the actual relation between the potentially confounding factor and disease, not the apparent relation observed in the data, that determines whether confounding can occur. In large studies, which are subject to less sampling error, we expect the data to reflect more closely the underlying relation, but in small studies the data are a less reliable guide, and one must consider other, external evidence ("prior knowledge") regarding the relation of the factor to the disease.

The following example illustrates the role that prior knowledge can play in evaluating confounding. Suppose that in a cohort study of airborne glass fibers and lung cancer, the data show more smoking and more cancers among the heavily exposed but no relation between smoking and lung cancer within exposure levels. The latter absence of a relation does not mean that an effect of smoking was not confounded (mixed) with the estimated effect of glass fibers: It may be that some or all of the excess cancers in the heavily exposed were produced solely by smoking, and that the lack of a smoking–cancer association in the study cohort was produced by an unmeasured confounder of that association in this cohort, or by random error.

As a converse example, suppose that we conduct a cohort study of sunlight exposure and melanoma. Our best current information indicates that, after controlling for age and geographic area of residence, there is no relation between Social Security number and melanoma occurrence. Thus, we would not consider Social Security number a confounder, regardless of its association with melanoma in the reference exposure cohort, because we think it is not a risk factor for melanoma in this cohort, given age and geographic area (i.e., we think Social Security numbers do not affect melanoma rates and are not markers for some melanoma risk factor other than age and area). Even if control of Social Security number would change the effect estimate, the resulting estimate of effect would be less accurate than one that ignores Social Security number, given our prior information about the lack of real confounding by social security number.

Nevertheless, because external information is usually limited, investigators often rely on their data to infer the relation of potential confounders to the disease. This reliance can be rationalized if one has good reason to suspect that the external information is not very relevant to one's own study. For example, a cause of disease in one population will be causally unrelated to disease in another population that lacks complementary component causes (i.e., susceptibility factors; see Chapter 2). A discordance between the data and external information about a suspected or known risk factor may therefore signal an inadequacy in the detail of information about interacting factors rather than an error in the data. Such an explanation may be less credible for variables such as age, sex, and smoking, whose joint relation to disease are often thought to be fairly stable across populations. In a parallel fashion, external information about the absence of an effect for a possible risk factor may be considered inadequate, if the external information is based on studies that had a considerable bias toward the null.

2. *A confounding factor must be associated with the exposure under study in the source population (the population at risk from which the cases are derived).*

To produce confounding, the association between a potential confounding factor and the exposure must be in the source population of the study cases. In a cohort study, the source population corresponds to the study cohort and so this proviso implies only that the association between a confounding factor and the exposure exists among subjects that compose the cohort. Thus, in cohort studies, the exposure–confounder association can be determined from the study data alone and does not even theoretically depend on prior knowledge if no measurement error is present.

When the exposure under study has been randomly assigned, it is sometimes mistakenly thought that confounding cannot occur because randomization guarantees exposure will be independent of (unassociated with) other factors. Unfortunately, this independence guarantee is only *on average* across repetitions of the randomization procedure. In almost any given single randomization (allocation), including those in actual studies, there will be random associations of the exposure with extraneous risk factors. As a consequence, confounding can and does occur in randomized trials. Although this random confounding tends to be small in large randomized trials, it will often be large within small trials and within small subgroups of large trials (Rothman, 1977). Furthermore, heavy nonadherence or noncompliance (failure to follow the assigned treatment protocol) or drop-out can result in considerable nonrandom confounding, even in large randomized trials (see Chapter 12, especially Fig. 12–5).

In a case-control study, the association of exposure and the potential confounder must be present in the source population that gave rise to the cases. If the control series is large and there is no selection bias or measurement error, the controls will provide a reasonable estimate of the association between the potential confounding variable and the exposure in the source population and can be checked with the study data. In general, however, the controls may not adequately estimate the degree of association between the potential confounder and the exposure in the source population that produced the study cases. If information is available on this population association, it can be used to adjust findings from the control series. Unfortunately, reliable external information about the associations among risk factors in the source population is seldom available. Thus, in case-control studies, concerns about the control group will have to be considered in estimating the association between the exposure and the potentially confounding factor, for example, via bias analysis (Chapter 19).

Consider a nested case-control study of occupational exposure to airborne glass fibers and the occurrence of lung cancer that randomly sampled cases and controls from cases and persons at risk in an occupational cohort. Suppose that we knew the association of exposure and smoking in the full cohort, as we might if this information were recorded for the entire cohort. We could then use the discrepancy between the true association and the exposure–smoking association observed in the controls as a measure of the extent to which random sampling had failed to produce representative controls. Regardless of the size of this discrepancy, if there were no association between smoking and exposure in the source cohort, smoking would not be a true confounder (even if it appeared to be one in the case-control data), and the unadjusted estimate would be the best available estimate (Robins and Morgenstern, 1987). More generally, we could use any information on the entire cohort to make adjustments to the case-control estimate, in a fashion analogous to two-stage studies (Chapters 8 and 15).

3. *A confounding factor must not be affected by the exposure or the disease. In particular, it cannot be an intermediate step in the causal path between the exposure and the disease.*

This criterion is automatically satisfied if the factor precedes exposure and disease. Otherwise, the criterion requires information outside the data. The investigator must consider evidence or theories that bear on whether the exposure or disease might affect the factor. If the factor is an intermediate step between exposure and disease, it should not be treated as simply a confounding factor; instead, a more detailed analysis that takes account of its intermediate nature is required (Robins, 1989; Robins and Greenland, 1992; Robins et al., 2000).

Although the above three characteristics of confounders are sometimes taken to define a confounder, it is a mistake to do so for both conceptual and technical reasons. Confounding is the confusion or mixing of extraneous effects with the effect of interest. The first two characteristics are simply logical consequences of the basic definition, properties that a factor must satisfy in order to confound. The third property excludes situations in which the effects cannot be disentangled in a straightforward manner (except in special cases). Technically, it is possible for a factor to possess all three characteristics and yet not have its effects mixed with the exposure, in the sense that a factor may produce no spurious excess or deficit of disease among the exposed, despite its association with exposure and its effect on disease. This result can occur, for example, when the factor is only one of several potential confounders and the excess of incidence produced by the factor among the exposed is perfectly balanced by the excess incidence produced by another factor in the unexposed.

The above discussion omits a number of subtleties that arise in qualitative determination of which variables are sufficient to control in order to eliminate confounding. These qualitative issues will be discussed using causal diagrams in Chapter 12. It is important to remember, however, that the degree of confounding is of much greater concern than its mere presence or absence. In one study, a rate ratio of 5 may become 4.6 after control of age, whereas in another study a rate ratio of 5 may change to 1.2 after control of age. Although age is confounding in both studies, in the former the amount of confounding is comparatively unimportant, whereas in the latter confounding accounts for nearly all of the crude association. Methods to evaluate confounding quantitatively will be described in Chapters 15 and 19.

SELECTION BIAS

Selection biases are distortions that result from procedures used to select subjects and from factors that influence study participation. The common element of such biases is that the relation between exposure and disease is different for those who participate and for all those who should have been theoretically eligible for study, including those who do not participate. Because estimates of effect are conditioned on participation, the associations observed in a study represent a mix of forces that determine participation and forces that determine disease occurrence.

Chapter 12 examines selection bias within the context of causal diagrams. These diagrams show that it is sometimes (but not always) possible to disentangle the effects of participation from those of disease determinants using standard methods for the control of confounding. To employ such analytic control requires, among other things, that the determinants of participation be measured accurately and not be affected by both exposure and disease. However, if those determinants are affected by the study factors, analytic control of those determinants will not correct the bias and may even make it worse.

Some generic forms of selection bias in case-control studies were described in Chapter 8. Those include use of incorrect control groups (e.g., controls composed of patients with diseases that are affected by the study exposure). We consider here some further types.

SELF-SELECTION BIAS

A common source of selection bias is *self-selection*. When the Centers for Disease Control investigated leukemia incidence among troops who had been present at the Smoky Atomic Test in Nevada (Caldwell et al., 1980), 76% of the troops identified as members of that cohort had known outcomes. Of this 76%, 82% were traced by the investigators, but the other 18% contacted the investigators on their own initiative in response to publicity about the investigation. This self-referral of subjects is ordinarily considered a threat to validity, because the reasons for self-referral may be associated with the outcome under study (Criqui et al., 1979).

In the Smoky Atomic Test study, there were four leukemia cases among the $0.18 \times 0.76 = 14\%$ of cohort members who referred themselves and four among the $0.82 \times 0.76 = 62\%$ of cohort members traced by the investigators, for a total of eight cases among the 76% of the cohort with known outcomes. These data indicate that self-selection bias was a small but real problem in the Smoky study. If the 24% of the cohort with unknown outcomes had a leukemia incidence like that of the subjects traced by the investigators, we should expect that only 4(24/62) = 1.5 or about one or two cases occurred among this 24%, for a total of only nine or 10 cases in the entire cohort. If instead we assume that the 24% with unknown outcomes had a leukemia incidence like that of subjects with known outcomes, we would calculate that 8(24/76) = 2.5 or about two or three cases occurred among this 24%, for a total of 10 or 11 cases in the entire cohort. It might be, however, that all cases among the 38% (= 24% + 14%) of the cohort that was untraced were among the self-reported, leaving no case among those with unknown outcome. The total number of cases in the entire cohort would then be only 8.

Self-selection can also occur before subjects are identified for study. For example, it is routine to find that the mortality of active workers is less than that of the population as a whole (Fox and Collier, 1976; McMichael, 1976). This "healthy-worker effect" presumably derives from a screening process, perhaps largely self-selection, that allows relatively healthy people to become or remain workers, whereas those who remain unemployed, retired, disabled, or otherwise out of the active worker population are as a group less healthy (McMichael, 1976; Wang and Miettinen, 1982). While the healthy-worker effect has traditionally been classified as a selection bias, one can see that it does not reflect a bias created by conditioning on participation in the study, but rather from the effect of another factor that influences both worker status and some measure of health. As such, the healthy-worker effect is an example of confounding rather than selection bias (Hernan et al, 2004), as explained further below.

BERKSONIAN BIAS

A type of selection bias that was first described by Berkson (1946) (although not in the context of a case-control study), which came to be known as *Berkson's bias* or *Berksonian bias,* occurs when both the exposure and the disease affect selection and specifically because they affect selection. It is paradoxical because it can generate a downward bias when both the exposure and the disease increase the chance of selection; this downward bias can induce a negative association in the study if the association in the source population is positive but not as large as the bias.

A dramatic example of Berksonian bias arose in the early controversy about the role of exogenous estrogens in causing endometrial cancer. Several case-control studies had reported a strong association, with about a 10-fold increase in risk for women taking estrogens regularly for a number of years (Smith et al., 1975; Ziel and Finkle, 1975; Mack et al., 1976; Antunes et al., 1979). Most investigators interpreted this increase in risk as a causal relation, but others suggested that estrogens were merely causing the cancers to be diagnosed rather than to occur (Horwitz and Feinstein, 1978). Their argument rested on the fact that estrogens induce uterine bleeding. Therefore, the administration of estrogens would presumably lead women to seek medical attention, thus causing a variety of gynecologic conditions to be detected. The resulting bias was referred to as detection bias.

The remedy for detection bias that Horwitz and Feinstein proposed was to use a control series of women with benign gynecologic diseases. These investigators reasoned that benign conditions would also be subject to detection bias, and therefore using a control series comprising women with benign conditions would be preferable to using a control series of women with other malignant disease, nongynecologic disease, or no disease, as earlier studies had done. The flaw in this reasoning was the incorrect assumption that estrogens caused a substantial proportion of endometrial cancers to be diagnosed that would otherwise have remained undiagnosed. Even if the administration of estrogens advances the date of diagnosis for endometrial cancer, such an advance in the time of diagnosis need not in itself lead to any substantial bias (Greenland, 1991a). Possibly, a small proportion of pre-existing endometrial cancer cases that otherwise would not have been diagnosed did come to attention, but it is reasonable to suppose that endometrial cancer that is not *in situ* (Horwitz and Feinstein excluded *in situ* cases) usually progresses to cause symptoms leading to diagnosis (Hutchison and Rothman, 1978). Although a permanent, nonprogressive early stage of endometrial cancer is a possibility, the studies that excluded such *in situ* cases from the case series still found a strong association between estrogen administration and endometrial cancer risk (e.g., Antunes et al., 1979).

The proposed alternative control group comprised women with benign gynecologic conditions that were presumed not to cause symptoms leading to diagnosis. Such a group would provide an overestimate of the proportion of the source population of cases exposed to estrogens, because administration of estrogens would indeed cause the diagnosis of a substantial proportion of the benign conditions. The use of a control series with benign gynecologic conditions would thus produce a bias that severely underestimated the effect of exogenous estrogens on risk of endometrial cancer. Another remedy that Horwitz and Feinstein proposed was to examine the association within women who had presented with vaginal bleeding or had undergone treatment for such bleeding. Because both the exposure (exogenous estrogens) and the disease (endometrial cancer) strongly increase bleeding risk, restriction to women with bleeding or treatment for bleeding results in a Berksonian bias so severe that it could easily diminish the observed relative risk by fivefold (Greenland and Neutra, 1981).

A major lesson to be learned from this controversy is the importance of considering selection biases quantitatively rather than qualitatively. Without appreciation for the magnitude of potential selection biases, the choice of a control group can result in a bias so great that a strong association is occluded; alternatively, a negligible association could as easily be exaggerated. Methods for quantitative consideration of biases are discussed in Chapter 19. Another lesson is that one runs the risk of inducing or worsening selection bias whenever one uses selection criteria (e.g., requiring the presence or absence of certain conditions) that are influenced by the exposure under study. If those criteria are also related to the study disease, severe Berksonian bias is likely to ensue.

DISTINGUISHING SELECTION BIAS FROM CONFOUNDING

Selection bias and confounding are two concepts that, depending on terminology, often overlap. For example, in cohort studies, biases resulting from differential selection at start of follow-up are often called selection bias, but in our terminology they are examples of confounding. Consider a cohort study comparing mortality from cardiovascular diseases among longshoremen and office workers. If physically fit individuals self-select into longshoreman work, we should expect longshoremen to have lower cardiovascular mortality than that of office workers, even if working as a longshoreman has no effect on cardiovascular mortality. As a consequence, the crude estimate from such a study could not be considered a valid estimate of the effect of longshoreman work relative to office work on cardiovascular mortality.

Suppose, however, that the fitness of an individual who becomes a lumberjack could be measured and compared with the fitness of the office workers. If such a measurement were done accurately on all subjects, the difference in fitness could be controlled in the analysis. Thus, the selection effect would be removed by control of the confounders responsible for the bias. Although the bias results from selection of persons for the cohorts, it is in fact a form of confounding.

Because measurements on fitness at entry into an occupation are generally not available, the investigator's efforts in such a situation would be focused on the choice of a reference group that would experience the same selection forces as the target occupation. For example, Paffenbarger and Hale (1975) conducted a study in which they compared cardiovascular mortality among groups of longshoremen who engaged in different levels of physical activity on the job. Paffenbarger and Hale presumed that the selection factors for entering the occupation were similar for the subgroups engaged in tasks demanding high or low activity, because work assignments were made after entering the profession. This design would reduce or eliminate the association between fitness and becoming a longshoreman. By comparing groups with different intensities of exposure within an occupation (internal comparison), occupational epidemiologists reduce the difference in selection forces that accompanies comparisons across occupational groups, and thus reduce the risk of confounding.

Unfortunately, not all selection bias in cohort studies can be dealt with as confounding. For example, if exposure affects loss to follow-up and the latter affects risk, selection bias occurs because the analysis is conditioned on a common consequence (remaining under follow-up is related to both the exposure and the outcome). This bias could arise in an occupational mortality study if exposure caused people to leave the occupation early (e.g., move from an active job to a desk job or retirement) and that in turn led both to loss to follow-up and to an increased risk of death. Here, there is no baseline covariate (confounder) creating differences in risk between exposed and unexposed groups; rather, exposure itself is generating the bias. Such a bias would be irremediable without further information on the selection effects, and even with that information the bias could not be removed by simple covariate control. This possibility underscores the need for thorough follow-up in cohort studies, usually requiring a system for outcome surveillance in the cohort. If no such system is in place (e.g., an insurance claims system), the study will have to implement its own system, which can be expensive.

In case-control studies, the concerns about choice of a control group focus on factors that might affect selection and recruitment into the study. Although confounding factors also must be considered, they can be controlled in the analysis if they are measured. If selection factors that affect case and control selection are themselves not affected by exposure (e.g., sex), any selection bias they produce can also be controlled by controlling these factors in the analysis. The key, then, to avoiding confounding and selection bias due to pre-exposure covariates is to identify in advance and measure as many confounders and selection factors as is practical. Doing so requires good subject-matter knowledge.

In case-control studies, however, subjects are often selected after exposure and outcome occurs, and hence there is an elevated potential for bias due to combined exposure and disease effects on selection, as occurred in the estrogen and endometrial cancer studies that restricted subjects to patients with bleeding (or to patients receiving specific medical procedures to treat bleeding). As will be shown using causal graphs (Chaper 12), bias from such joint selection effects usually cannot be dealt with by basic covariate control. This bias can also arise in cohort studies and even in randomized trials in which subjects are lost to follow-up. For example, in an occupational mortality study, exposure could cause people to leave the occupation early and that in turn could produce both a failure to locate the person (and hence exclusion from the study) and an increased risk of death. These forces would result in a reduced chance of selection among the exposed, with a higher reduction among cases.

In this example, there is no baseline covariate (confounder) creating differences in risk between exposed and unexposed groups; rather, exposure itself is helping to generate the bias. Such a bias would be irremediable without further information on the selection effects, and even with that information could not be removed by simple covariate control. This possibility underscores the need for thorough ascertainment of the outcome in the source population in case-control studies; if no ascertainment system is in place (e.g., a tumor registry for a cancer study), the study will have to implement its own system.

Because many types of selection bias cannot be controlled in the analysis, prevention of selection bias by appropriate control selection can be critical. The usual strategy for this prevention involves trying to select a control group that is subject to the same selective forces as the case group, in the hopes that the biases introduced by control selection will cancel the biases introduced by case selection in the final estimates. Meeting this goal even approximately can rarely be assured; nonetheless, it is often the only strategy available to address concerns about selection bias. This strategy and other aspects of control selection were discussed in Chapter 8.

To summarize, differential selection that occurs before exposure and disease leads to confounding, and can thus be controlled by adjustments for the factors responsible for the selection differences (see, for example, the adjustment methods described in Chapter 15). In contrast, selection bias as usually described in epidemiology (as well as the experimental-design literature) arises from selection affected by the exposure under study, and may be beyond any practical adjustment. Among these selection biases, we can further distinguish Berksonian bias in which both the exposure and the disease affect selection.

Some authors (e.g., Hernan et al., 2004) attempt to use graphs to provide a formal basis for separating selection bias from confounding by equating selection bias with a phenomenon termed *collider bias,* a generalization of Berksonian bias (Greenland, 2003a; Chapter 12). Our terminology is more in accord with traditional designations in which bias from pre-exposure selection is treated as a form of confounding. These distinctions are discussed further in Chapter 12.

INFORMATION BIAS

MEASUREMENT ERROR, MISCLASSIFICATION, AND BIAS

Once the subjects to be compared have been identified, one must obtain the information about them to use in the analysis. Bias in estimating an effect can be caused by measurement errors in the needed information. Such bias is often called *information bias.* The direction and magnitude depends heavily on whether the distribution of errors for one variable (e.g., exposure or disease) depends on the actual value of the variable, the actual values of other variables, or the errors in measuring other variables.

For discrete variables (variables with only a countable number of possible values, such as indicators for sex), measurement error is usually called *classification error* or *misclassification.* Classification error that depends on the actual values of other variables is called *differential misclassification.* Classification error that does not depend on the actual values of other variables is called *nondifferential misclassification.* Classification error that depends on the errors in measuring or classifying other variables is called *dependent error*; otherwise the error is called *independent* or *nondependent error. Correlated error* is sometimes used as a synonym for dependent error, but technically it refers to dependent errors that have a nonzero correlation coefficient.

Much of the ensuing discussion will concern misclassification of binary variables. In this special situation, the *sensitivity* of an exposure measurement method is the probability that someone who is truly exposed will be classified as exposed by the method. The *false-negative probability* of the method is the probability that someone who is truly exposed will be classified as unexposed; it equals 1 minus the sensitivity. The *specificity* of the method is the probability that someone who is truly unexposed will be classified as unexposed. The *false-positive probability* is the probability that someone who is truly unexposed will be classified as exposed; it equals 1 minus the specificity. The *predictive value positive* is the probability that someone who is classified as exposed is truly exposed. Finally, the *predictive value negative* is the probability that someone who is classified as unexposed is truly unexposed. All these terms can also be applied to descriptions of the methods for classifying disease or classifying a potential confounder or modifier.

DIFFERENTIAL MISCLASSIFICATION

Suppose a cohort study is undertaken to compare incidence rates of emphysema among smokers and nonsmokers. Emphysema is a disease that may go undiagnosed without special medical attention. If smokers, because of concern about health-related effects of smoking or as a consequence of other health effects of smoking (e.g., bronchitis), seek medical attention to a greater degree than nonsmokers, then emphysema might be diagnosed more frequently among smokers than among nonsmokers simply as a consequence of the greater medical attention. Smoking does cause emphysema, but unless steps were taken to ensure comparable follow-up, this effect would be overestimated: A portion of the excess of emphysema incidence would not be a biologic effect of smoking, but would instead be an effect of smoking on *detection* of emphysema. This is an example of differential misclassification, because underdiagnosis of emphysema (failure to detect true cases), which is a classification error, occurs more frequently for nonsmokers than for smokers.

In case-control studies of congenital malformations, information is sometimes obtained from interview of mothers. The case mothers have recently given birth to a malformed baby, whereas the vast majority of control mothers have recently given birth to an apparently healthy baby. Another variety of differential misclassification, referred to as *recall bias,* can result if the mothers of malformed infants recall or report true exposures differently than mothers of healthy infants (enhanced sensitivity of exposure recall among cases), or more frequently recall or report exposure that did not actually occur (reduced specificity of exposure recall among cases). It is supposed that the birth of a malformed infant serves as a stimulus to a mother to recall and report all events that might have played some role in the unfortunate outcome. Presumably, such women will remember and report exposures such as infectious disease, trauma, and drugs more frequently than mothers of healthy infants, who have not had a comparable stimulus. An association unrelated to any biologic effect will result from this recall bias.

Recall bias is a possibility in any case-control study that relies on subject memory, because the cases and controls are by definition people who differ with respect to their disease experience at the time of their recall, and this difference may affect recall and reporting. Klemetti and Saxen (1967) found that the amount of time lapsed between the exposure and the recall was an important indicator of the accuracy of recall; studies in which the average time since exposure was different for interviewed cases and controls could thus suffer a differential misclassification.

The bias caused by differential misclassification can either exaggerate or underestimate an effect. In each of the examples above, the misclassification ordinarily exaggerates the effects under study, but examples to the contrary can also be found.

NONDIFFERENTIAL MISCLASSIFICATION

Nondifferential exposure misclassification occurs when the proportion of subjects misclassified on exposure does not depend on the status of the subject with respect to other variables in the analysis, including disease. Nondifferential disease misclassification occurs when the proportion of subjects misclassified on disease does not depend on the status of the subject with respect to other variables in the analysis, including exposure.

Bias introduced by independent nondifferential misclassification of a binary exposure or disease is predictable in direction, namely, toward the null value (Newell, 1962; Keys and Kihlberg, 1963; Gullen et al., 1968; Copeland et al., 1977). Because of the relatively unpredictable effects of differential misclassification, some investigators go through elaborate procedures to ensure that the misclassification will be nondifferential, such as blinding of exposure evaluations with respect to outcome status, in the belief that this will guarantee a bias toward the null. Unfortunately, even in situations when blinding is accomplished or in cohort studies in which disease outcomes have not yet occurred, collapsing continuous or categorical exposure data into fewer categories can change nondifferential error to differential misclassification (Flegal et al., 1991; Wacholder et al., 1991). Even when nondifferential misclassification is achieved, it may come at the expense of increased total bias (Greenland and Robins, 1985a; Drews and Greenland, 1990).

Finally, as will be discussed, nondifferentiality alone does not guarantee bias toward the null. Contrary to popular misconceptions, nondifferential exposure or disease misclassification can sometimes produce bias away from the null if the exposure or disease variable has more than two levels (Walker and Blettner, 1985; Dosemeci et al., 1990) or if the classification errors depend on errors made in other variables (Chavance et al., 1992; Kristensen, 1992).

Nondifferential Misclassification of Exposure

As an example of nondifferential misclassification, consider a cohort study comparing the incidence of laryngeal cancer among drinkers of alcohol with the incidence among nondrinkers. Assume that drinkers actually have an incidence rate of 0.00050 $year^{-1}$, whereas nondrinkers have an incidence rate of 0.00010 $year^{-1}$, only one-fifth as great. Assume also that two thirds of the study population consists of drinkers, but only 50% of them acknowledge it. The result is a population in which one third of subjects are identified (correctly) as drinkers and have an incidence of disease of 0.00050 $year^{-1}$, but the remaining two thirds of the population consists of equal numbers of drinkers and nondrinkers, all of whom are classified as nondrinkers, and among whom the average incidence would be 0.00030 $year^{-1}$ rather than 0.00010 $year^{-1}$ (Table 9–1). The rate difference has been

TABLE 9–1

Effect of Nondifferential Misclassification of Alcohol Consumption on Estimation of the Incidence-Rate Difference and Incidence-Rate Ratio for Laryngeal Cancer (Hypothetical Data)

	Incidence Rate ($\times 10^5$ y)	Rate Difference ($\times 10^5$ y)	Rate Ratio
No misclassification			
1,000,000 drinkers	50	40	5.0
500,000 nondrinkers	10		
Half of drinkers classed with nondrinkers			
500,000 drinkers	50	20	1.7
1,000,000 "nondrinkers" (50% are actually drinkers)	30		
Half of drinkers classed with nondrinkers and one-third of nondrinkers classed with drinkers			
666,667 "drinkers" (25% are actually nondrinkers)	40	6	1.2
833,333 "nondrinkers" (60% are actually drinkers)	34		

reduced by misclassification from 0.00040 $year^{-1}$ to 0.00020 $year^{-1}$, while the rate ratio has been reduced from 5 to 1.7. This bias toward the null value results from nondifferential misclassification of some alcohol drinkers as nondrinkers.

Misclassification can occur simultaneously in both directions; for example, nondrinkers might also be incorrectly classified as drinkers. Suppose that in addition to half of the drinkers being misclassified as nondrinkers, one third of the nondrinkers were also misclassified as drinkers. The resulting incidence rates would be 0.00040 $year^{-1}$ for those classified as drinkers and 0.00034 $year^{-1}$ for those classified as nondrinkers. The additional misclassification thus almost completely obscures the difference between the groups.

This example shows how bias produced by nondifferential misclassification of a dichotomous exposure will be toward the null value (of no relation) if the misclassification is independent of other errors. If the misclassification is severe enough, the bias can completely obliterate an association and even reverse the direction of association (although reversal will occur only if the classification method is worse than randomly classifying people as "exposed" or "unexposed").

Consider as an example Table 9–2. The top panel of the table shows the expected data from a hypothetical case-control study, with the exposure measured as a dichotomy. The odds ratio is 3.0. Now suppose that the exposure is measured by an instrument (e.g., a questionnaire) that results in an exposure measure that has 100% specificity but only 80% sensitivity. In other words, all the truly

TABLE 9–2

Nondifferential Misclassification with Two Exposure Categories

	Exposed		Unexposed
Correct data			
Cases	240		200
Controls	240		600
		OR = 3.0	
Sensitivity = 0.8			
Specificity = 1.0			
Cases	192		248
Controls	192		648
		OR = 2.6	
Sensitivity = 0.8			
Specificity = 0.8			
Cases	232		208
Controls	312		528
		OR = 1.9	
Sensitivity = 0.4			
Specificity = 0.6			
Cases	176		264
Controls	336		504
		OR = 1.0	
Sensitivity = 0.0			
Specificity = 0.0			
Cases	200		240
Controls	600		240
		OR = 0.33	

OR, odds ratio.

unexposed subjects are correctly classified as unexposed, but there is only an 80% chance that an exposed subject is correctly classified as exposed, and thus a 20% chance an exposed subject will be incorrectly classified as unexposed. We assume that the misclassification is nondifferential, which means for this example that the sensitivity and specificity of the exposure measurement method is the same for cases and controls. We also assume that there is no error in measuring disease, from which it automatically follows that the exposure errors are independent of disease errors. The resulting data are given in the second panel of the table. With the reduced sensitivity in measuring exposure, the odds ratio is biased in that its approximate expected value decreases from 3.0 to 2.6.

In the third panel, the specificity of the exposure measure is assumed to be 80%, so that there is a 20% chance that someone who is actually unexposed will be incorrectly classified as exposed. The resulting data produce an odds ratio of 1.9 instead of 3.0. In absolute terms, more than half of the effect has been obliterated by the misclassification in the third panel: the excess odds ratio is $3.0 - 1 = 2.0$, whereas it is $1.9 - 1 = 0.9$ based on the data with 80% sensitivity and 80% specificity in the third panel.

The fourth panel of Table 9–2 illustrates that when the sensitivity and specificity sum to 1, the resulting expected estimate will be null, regardless of the magnitude of the effect. If the sum of the sensitivity and specificity is less than 1, then the resulting expected estimate will be in the opposite direction of the actual effect. The last panel of the table shows the result when both sensitivity and specificity are zero. This situation is tantamount to labeling all exposed subjects as unexposed and vice versa. It leads to an expected odds ratio that is the inverse of the correct value. Such drastic misclassification would occur if the coding of exposure categories were reversed during computer programming.

As seen in these examples, the direction of bias produced by independent nondifferential misclassification of a dichotomous exposure is toward the null value, and if the misclassification is extreme, the misclassification can go beyond the null value and reverse direction. With an exposure that is measured by dividing it into more than two categories, however, an exaggeration of an association can occur as a result of independent nondifferential misclassification (Walker and Blettner, 1985; Dosemeci et al., 1990). This phenomenon is illustrated in Table 9–3.

The correctly classified expected data in Table 9–3 show an odds ratio of 2 for low exposure and 6 for high exposure, relative to no exposure. Now suppose that there is a 40% chance that a person with high exposure is incorrectly classified into the low exposure category. If this is the only misclassification and it is nondifferential, the expected data would be those seen in the bottom panel of Table 9–3. Note that only the estimate for low exposure changes; it now contains a mixture of people who have low exposure and people who have high exposure but who have incorrectly been assigned to low exposure. Because the people with high exposure carry with them the greater

TABLE 9–3

Nondifferential Misclassification with Three Exposure Categories

	Unexposed	Low Exposure	High Exposure
Correct data			
Cases	100	200	600
Controls	100	100	100
		OR = 2	OR = 6
40% of high exposure → 4 low exposure			
Cases	100	440	360
Controls	100	140	60
		OR = 3.1	OR = 6

OR, odds ratio.

risk of disease that comes with high exposure, the resulting effect estimate for low exposure is biased upward. If some low-exposure individuals had incorrectly been classified as having had high exposure, then the estimate of the effect of exposure for the high-exposure category would be biased downward.

This example illustrates that when the exposure has more than two categories, the bias from nondifferential misclassification of exposure for a given comparison may be away from the null value. When exposure is polytomous (i.e., has more than two categories) and there is nondifferential misclassification between two of the categories and no others, the effect estimates for those two categories will be biased toward one another (Walker and Blettner, 1985; Birkett, 1992). For example, the bias in the effect estimate for the low-exposure category in Table 9–3 is toward that of the high-exposure category and away from the null value. It is also possible for independent nondifferential misclassification to bias trend estimates away from the null or to reverse a trend (Dosemeci et al., 1990). Such examples are unusual, however, because trend reversal cannot occur if the mean exposure measurement increases with true exposure (Weinberg et al., 1994d).

It is important to note that the present discussion concerns *expected* results under a particular type of measurement *method*. In a given study, random fluctuations in the errors produced by a method may lead to estimates that are further from the null than what they would be if no error were present, even if the method satisfies all the conditions that guarantee bias toward the null (Thomas, 1995; Weinberg et al., 1995; Jurek at al., 2005). Bias refers only to *expected* direction; if we do not know what the errors were in the study, at best we can say only that the observed odds ratio is probably closer to the null than what it would be if the errors were absent. As study size increases, the probability decreases that a particular result will deviate substantially from its expectation.

Nondifferential Misclassification of Disease

The effects of nondifferential misclassification of disease resemble those of nondifferential misclassification of exposure. In most situations, nondifferential misclassification of a binary disease outcome will produce bias toward the null, provided that the misclassification is independent of other errors. There are, however, some special cases in which such misclassification produces no bias in the risk ratio. In addition, the bias in the risk difference is a simple function of the sensitivity and specificity.

Consider a cohort study in which 40 cases actually occur among 100 exposed subjects and 20 cases actually occur among 200 unexposed subjects. Then, the actual risk ratio is $(40/100)/(20/200) = 4$, and the actual risk difference is $40/100 - 20/200 = 0.30$. Suppose that specificity of disease detection is perfect (there are no false positives), but sensitivity is only 70% in both exposure groups (that is, sensitivity of disease detection is nondifferential and does not depend on errors in classification of exposure). The expected numbers detected will then be $0.70(40) = 28$ exposed cases and $0.70(20) = 14$ unexposed cases, which yield an expected risk-ratio estimate of $(28/100)/(14/200) = 4$ and an expected risk-difference estimate of $28/100 - 14/200 = 0.21$. Thus, the disease misclassification produced no bias in the risk ratio, but the expected risk-difference estimate is only $0.21/0.30 = 70\%$ of the actual risk difference.

This example illustrates how independent nondifferential disease misclassification with perfect specificity will not bias the risk-ratio estimate, but will downwardly bias the absolute magnitude of the risk-difference estimate by a factor equal to the false-negative probability (Rodgers and MacMahon, 1995). With this type of misclassification, the odds ratio and the rate ratio will remain biased toward the null, although the bias will be small when the risk of disease is low (<10%) in both exposure groups. This approximation is a consequence of the relation of the odds ratio and the rate ratio to the risk ratio when the disease risk is low in all exposure groups (see Chapter 4).

Consider next the same cohort study, but now with perfect sensitivity of disease detection (no false negatives) and imperfect specificity of 80%. The expected number of apparent cases will then be $40 + (1 - 0.80)(100 - 40) = 52$ among the exposed and $20 + (1 - 0.80)(200 - 20) = 56$ among the unexposed. Under this formulation, the numerators yield an expected risk-ratio estimate of $(52/100)/(56/200) = 1.9$ and an expected risk-difference estimate of $52/100 - 56/200 = 0.24$. Both measures are biased toward the null, with the expected risk-difference estimate equal to $0.24/0.30 = 80\%$ of the actual value. This example illustrates how independent nondifferential disease misclassification with perfect sensitivity will bias both measures, with the absolute magnitude of the risk-difference estimate downwardly biased by a factor equal to the false-positive probability (Rodgers and MacMahon, 1995).

With imperfect sensitivity and specificity, the bias in the absolute magnitude of the risk difference produced by nondifferential disease misclassification that is independent of other errors will equal the sum of the false-negative and false-positive probabilities (Rodgers and MacMahon, 1995). The biases in relative effect measures do not have a simple form in this case.

We wish to emphasize that when both exposure and disease are nondifferentially misclassified but the classification errors are dependent, it is possible to obtain substantial bias away from the null (Chavance et al., 1992; Kristensen, 1992), and the simple bias relations just given will no longer apply. Dependent errors can arise easily in many situations, such as in studies in which exposure and disease status are both determined from interviews.

Pervasiveness of Misinterpretation of Nondifferential Misclassification Effects

The bias from independent nondifferential misclassification of a dichotomous exposure is always in the direction of the null value, so one would expect to see a larger estimate if misclassification were absent. As a result, many researchers are satisfied with achieving nondifferential misclassification in lieu of accurate classification. This stance may occur in part because some researchers consider it more acceptable to misreport an association as absent when it in fact exists than to misreport an association as present when it in fact does not exist, and regard nondifferential misclassification as favoring the first type of misreporting over the latter. Other researchers write as if positive results affected by nondifferential misclassification provide stronger evidence for an association than indicated by uncorrected statistics. There are several flaws in such interpretations, however.

First, many researchers forget that more than nondifferentiality is required to ensure bias toward the null. One also needs independence and some other constraints, such as the variable being binary. Second, few researchers seem to be aware that categorization of continuous variables (e.g., using quintiles instead of actual quantities of food or nutrients) can change nondifferential to differential error (Flegal et al., 1991; Wacholder et al., 1991), or that failure to control factors related to measurement can do the same even if those factors are not confounders.

Even if the misclassification satisfies all the conditions to produce a bias toward the null in the point estimate, it does not necessarily produce a corresponding upward bias in the P-value for the null hypothesis (Bross, 1954; Greenland and Gustafson, 2006). As a consequence, establishing that the bias (if any) was toward the null would not increase the evidence that a non-null association was present. Furthermore, bias toward the null (like bias away from the null) is still a distortion, and one that will vary across studies. In particular, it can produce serious distortions in literature reviews and meta-analyses, mask true differences among studies, exaggerate differences, or create spurious differences. These consequences can occur because differences in secondary study characteristics such as exposure prevalence will affect the degree to which misclassification produces bias in estimates from different strata or studies, even if the sensitivity and specificity of the classification do not vary across the strata or studies (Greenland, 1980). Typical situations are worsened by the fact that sensitivity and specificity as well as exposure prevalence will vary across studies (Begg, 1987).

Often, these differences in measurement performance arise from seemingly innocuous differences in the way variables are assessed or categorized, with worse performance arising from oversimplified or crude categorizations of exposure. For example, suppose that taking aspirin transiently reduces risk of myocardial infarction. The word "transiently" implies a brief induction period, with no preventive effect outside that period. For a given point in time or person-time unit in the history of a subject, the ideal classification of that time as exposed or unexposed to aspirin would be based on whether aspirin had been used before that time but within the induction period for its effect. By this standard, a myocardial infarction following aspirin use within the induction period would be properly classified as an aspirin-exposed case. On the other hand, if no aspirin was used within the induction period, the case would be properly classified as unexposed, even if the case had used aspirin at earlier or later times.

These ideal classifications reflect the fact that use outside the induction period is causally irrelevant. Many studies, however, focus on ever use (use at any time during an individual's life) or on any use over a span of several years. Such cumulative indices over a long time span augment possibly relevant exposure with irrelevant exposure, and can thus introduce a bias (usually toward the null) that parallels bias due to nondifferential misclassification.

Similar bias can arise from overly broad definition of the outcome. In particular, unwarranted assurances of a lack of any effect can easily emerge from studies in which a wide range of etiologically unrelated outcomes are grouped. In cohort studies in which there are disease categories with few subjects, investigators are occasionally tempted to combine outcome categories to increase the number of subjects in each analysis, thereby gaining precision. This collapsing of categories can obscure effects on more narrowly defined disease categories. For example, Smithells and Shepard (1978) investigated the teratogenicity of the drug Bendectin, a drug indicated for nausea of pregnancy. Because only 35 babies in their cohort study were born with a malformation, their analysis was focused on the single outcome, "malformation." But no teratogen causes all malformations; if such an analysis fails to find an effect, the failure may simply be the result of the grouping of many malformations not related to Bendectin with those that are. In fact, despite the authors' claim that "their study provides substantial evidence that Bendectin is not teratogenic in man," their data indicated a strong (though imprecise) relation between Bendectin and cardiac malformations.

Misclassification that has arguably produced bias toward the null is a greater concern in interpreting studies that seem to indicate the absence of an effect. Consequently, in studies that indicate little or no effect, it is crucial for the researchers to attempt to establish the direction of the bias to determine whether a real effect might have been obscured. Occasionally, critics of a study will argue that poor exposure data or poor disease classification invalidate the results. This argument is incorrect, however, if the results indicate a nonzero association and one can be sure that the classification errors produced bias toward the null, because the bias will be in the direction of underestimating the association. In this situation the major task will instead be in establishing that the classification errors were indeed of the sort that would produce bias toward the null.

Conversely, misclassification that has arguably produced bias away from the null is a greater concern in interpreting studies that seem to indicate an effect. The picture in this direction is clouded by the fact that forces that lead to differential error and bias away from the null (e.g., recall bias) are counterbalanced to an unknown extent (possibly entirely) by forces that lead to bias toward the null (e.g., simple memory deterioration over time). Even with only binary variables, a detailed quantitative analysis of differential recall may be needed to gain any idea of the direction of bias (Drews and Greenland, 1990), and even with internal validation data the direction of net bias may rarely be clear. We discuss analytic methods for assessing these problems in Chapter 19.

The importance of appreciating the likely direction of bias was illustrated by the interpretation of a study on spermicides and birth defects (Jick et al., 1981a, 1981b). This study reported an increased prevalence of several types of congenital disorders among women who were identified as having filled a prescription for spermicides during a specified interval before the birth. The exposure information was only a rough correlate of the actual use of spermicides during a theoretically relevant time period, but the misclassification that resulted was likely to be nondifferential and independent of errors in outcome ascertainment, because prescription information was recorded on a computer log before the outcome was known. One of the criticisms raised about the study was that inaccuracies in the exposure information cast doubt on the validity of the findings (Felarca et al., 1981; Oakley, 1982). These criticisms did not, however, address the direction of the resulting bias, and so are inappropriate if the structure of the misclassification indicates that the bias is downward, for then that bias could not explain the observed association (Jick et al., 1981b).

As an example, it is incorrect to dismiss a study reporting an association simply because there is independent nondifferential misclassification of a binary exposure, because without the misclassification the observed association would probably be even larger. Thus, the implications of independent nondifferential misclassification depend heavily on whether the study is perceived as "positive" or "negative." Emphasis on quantitative assessment instead of on a qualitative description of study results lessens the likelihood for misinterpretation, hence we will explore methods for quantitative assessment of bias in Chapter 19.

MISCLASSIFICATION OF CONFOUNDERS

If a confounding variable is misclassified, the ability to control confounding in the analysis is hampered (Greenland, 1980; Kupper, 1984; Brenner, 1993; Marshall and Hastrup, 1996; Marshall et al., 1999; Fewell et al., 2007). Independent nondifferential misclassification of a dichotomous confounding variable will reduce the degree to which the confounder can be controlled, and thus causes a bias in the direction of the confounding by the variable. The expected result will lie between the unadjusted association and the correctly adjusted association (i.e., the one that would have obtained if the confounder had not been misclassified). This problem may be viewed as one of residual confounding (i.e., confounding left after control of the available confounder measurements). The degree of residual confounding left within strata of the misclassified confounder will usually differ across those strata, which will distort the apparent degree of heterogeneity (effect modification) across strata (Greenland, 1980). Independent nondifferential misclassification of either the confounder or exposure can therefore give rise to the appearance of effect-measure modification (statistical interaction) when in fact there is none, or mask the appearance of such modification when in fact it is present.

If the misclassification is differential or dependent, the resulting adjusted association may not even fall between the crude and the correct adjusted associations. The problem then becomes not only one of residual confounding, but of additional distortion produced by differential selection of subjects into different analysis strata. Unfortunately, dependent errors among exposure variables are common, especially in questionnaire-based studies. For example, in epidemiologic studies of nutrients and disease, nutrient intakes are calculated from food intakes, and any errors in assessing the food intakes will translate into dependent errors among nutrients found in the same foods. Similarly, in epidemiologic studies of occupations and disease, chemical exposures are usually calculated from job histories, and errors in assessing these histories will translate into dependent errors among exposures found in the same jobs.

If the confounding is strong and the exposure–disease relation is weak or zero, misclassification of the confounder can produce extremely misleading results, even if the misclassification is independent and nondifferential. For example, given a causal relation between smoking and bladder cancer, an association between smoking and coffee drinking would make smoking a confounder of the relation between coffee drinking and bladder cancer. Because the control of confounding by smoking depends on accurate smoking information and because some misclassification of the relevant smoking information is inevitable no matter how smoking is measured, some residual confounding by smoking is inevitable (Morrison et al., 1982). The problem of residual confounding will be even worse if the only available information on smoking is a simple dichotomy such as "ever smoked" versus "never smoked," because the lack of detailed specification of smoking prohibits adequate control of confounding. The resulting residual confounding is especially troublesome because to many investigators and readers it may appear that confounding by smoking has been fully controlled.

THE COMPLEXITIES OF SIMULTANEOUS MISCLASSIFICATION

Continuing the preceding example, consider misclassification of coffee use as well as smoking. On the one hand, if coffee misclassification were nondifferential with respect to smoking and independent of smoking errors, the likely effect would be to diminish further the observed smoking–coffee association and so further reduce the efficacy of adjustment for smoking. The result would be even more upward residual confounding than when smoking alone were misclassified. On the other hand, if the measurements were from questionnaires, the coffee and smoking errors might be positively associated rather than independent, potentially counteracting the aforementioned phenomenon to an unknown degree. Also, if the coffee errors were nondifferential with respect to bladder cancer and independent of diagnostic errors, they would most likely produce a downward bias in the observed association.

Nonetheless, if the measurements were from a questionnaire administered after diagnosis, the nondifferentiality of both smoking or coffee errors with respect to bladder cancer would become questionable. If controls tended to underreport these habits more than did cases, the resulting differentiality would likely act in an upward direction for both the coffee and the smoking associations with cancer, partially canceling both the downward bias from the coffee misclassification and the upward bias from residual smoking confounding; but if cases tended to underreport these habits more than did controls, the differentiality would likely aggravate the downward bias from coffee misclassification and the upward bias from residual smoking confounding.

The net result of all these effects would be almost impossible to predict given the usual lack of accurate information on the misclassification rates. We emphasize that this unpredictability is over and above that of the random error assumed by conventional statistical methods; it is therefore not reflected in conventional confidence intervals, because the latter address only random variation in subject selection and actual exposure, and assume that errors in coffee and smoking measurement are absent.

GENERALIZABILITY

Physicists operate on the assumption that the laws of nature are the same everywhere, and therefore that what they learn about nature has universal applicability. In biomedical research, it sometimes seems as if we assume the opposite, that is, that the findings of our research apply only to populations that closely resemble those we study. This view stems from the experience that biologic effects can and do differ across different populations and subgroups. The cautious investigator is thus inclined to refrain from generalizing results beyond the circumstances that describe the study setting.

As a result, many epidemiologic studies are designed to sample subjects from a target population of particular interest, so that the study population is "representative" of the target population, in the sense of being a probability sample from that population. Inference to this target might also be obtained by oversampling some subgroups and then standardizing or reweighting the study data to match the target population distribution. Two-stage designs (Chapter 8 and 15) are simple examples of such a strategy.

Taken to an extreme, however, the pursuit of representativeness can defeat the goal of validly identifying causal relations. If the generalization of study results is literally limited to the characteristics of those studied, then causal inferences cannot be generalized beyond those subjects who have been studied and the time period during which they have been studied. On the other hand, even physicists acknowledge that what we consider to be universal physical laws could vary over time or under boundary conditions and therefore may not be truly universal. The process of generalization in science involves making assumptions about the domain in which the study results apply.

The heavy emphasis on sample representativeness in epidemiologic research probably derives from early experience with surveys, for which the inferential goal was only description of the surveyed population. Social scientists often perform and rely on probability-sample surveys because decisions about what is relevant for generalization are more difficult in the social sciences. In addition, the questions of interest to social scientists may concern only a particular population (e.g., voters in one country at one point in time), and populations are considerably more diverse in sociologic phenomena than in biologic phenomena.

In biologic laboratory sciences, however, it is routine for investigators to conduct experiments using animals with characteristics selected to enhance the validity of the experimental work rather than to represent a target population. For example, laboratory scientists conducting experiments with hamsters will more often prefer to study genetically identical hamsters than a representative sample of the world's hamsters, in order to minimize concerns about genetic variation affecting results. These restrictions may lead to concerns about generalizability, but this concern becomes important only after it has been accepted that the study results are valid for the restricted group that was studied.

Similarly, epidemiologic study designs are usually stronger if subject selection is guided by the need to make a valid comparison, which may call for severe restriction of admissible subjects to a narrow range of characteristics, rather than by an attempt to make the subjects representative, in a survey-sampling sense, of the potential target populations. Selection of study groups that are representative of larger populations in the statistical sense will often make it more difficult to make internally valid inferences, for example, by making it more difficult to control for confounding by factors that vary within those populations, more difficult to ensure uniformly high levels of cooperation, and more difficult to ensure uniformly accurate measurements.

To minimize the validity threats we have discussed, one would want to select study groups for homogeneity with respect to important confounders, for highly cooperative behavior, and for availability of accurate information, rather than attempt to be representative of a natural population. Classic examples include the British Physicians' Study of smoking and health and the Nurses' Health Study, neither of which were remotely representative of the general population with respect to sociodemographic factors. Their nonrepresentativeness was presumed to be unrelated to most of the effects studied. If there were doubts about this assumption, they would only become important once it was clear that the associations observed were valid estimates of effect within the studies themselves.

Once the nature and at least the order of magnitude of an effect are established by studies designed to maximize validity, generalization to other, unstudied groups becomes simpler. This generalization is in large measure a question of whether the factors that distinguish these other groups from studied groups somehow modify the effect in question. In answering this question, epidemiologic data will be of help and may be essential, but other sources of information such as basic pathophysiology may play an even larger role. For example, although most of the decisive data connecting smoking to lung cancer was derived from observations on men, no one doubted that the strong effects observed would carry over at least approximately to women, for the lungs of men and women appear to be similar if not identical in physiologic detail. On the other hand, given the huge sex differences in iron loss, it would seem unwise to generalize freely to men about the effects of iron supplementation observed in premenopausal women.

Such contrasting examples suggest that, perhaps even more than with (internal) inference about restricted populations, valid generalization must bring into play knowledge from diverse branches of science. As we have emphasized, representativeness is often a hindrance to executing an internally valid study, and considerations from allied science show that it is not always necessary for valid generalization. We thus caution that blind pursuit of representativeness will often lead to a waste of precious study resources.

CHAPTER 10

Precision and Statistics in Epidemiologic Studies

Kenneth J. Rothman, Sander Greenland, and Timothy L. Lash

Random Error and Statistical Precision 148
Study Size 149
Study Efficiency 150
Precision and Stratification 150
Approaches to Random Error 150
Significance Testing and Hypothesis Testing 151
Statistical Estimation 156
Conclusion 167

As described in Chapter 9, two types of error, systematic and random, detract from accuracy. Chapter 9 focused on understanding sources of systematic error. In this chapter we discuss methods to measure, limit, and account for random error in an epidemiologic study, and how to interpret these methods properly. In Chapter 11, we address options in study design that can reduce the amount of random error (i.e., improve precision) of a study within given cost and feasibility constraints.

RANDOM ERROR AND STATISTICAL PRECISION

What is random error? It is often equated with chance or random variation, which itself is rarely well defined. Many people believe that chance plays a fundamental role in all physical and, by implication, biologic phenomena. For some, the belief in chance is so dominant that it vaults random occurrences into an important role as component causes of all we experience. Others believe that causality may be viewed as deterministic, meaning that a full elaboration of the relevant factors in a given set of circumstances will lead unwaveringly, on sufficient analysis, to a perfect prediction of effects resulting from these causes. Under the latter view, all experience is predestined to unravel in a theoretically predictable way that follows inexorably from the previous pattern of actions. Even with this extreme deterministic view, however, one must face the fact that no one can acquire sufficient knowledge to predict effects perfectly for any but trivial cause–effect patterns. The resulting incomplete predictability of determined outcomes makes their residual variability indistinguishable from random occurrences.

A unifying description of incomplete predictability can thus be forged that equates random variation with ignorance about causes of our study outcomes, an ignorance that is inevitable whether or not physical chance is among the causes. For example, predicting the outcome of a tossed coin represents a physical problem, the solution of which is feasible through the application of physical laws. Whether the sources of variation that we cannot explain are actually chance phenomena makes little difference: We treat such variation as being random until we can explain it, and thereby reduce it, by relating it to known factors.

In an epidemiologic study, random variation has many components, but a major contributor is the process of selecting the specific study subjects. This process is usually referred to as *sampling*; the attendant random variation is known as *sampling variation* or *sampling error.* Case-control studies often involve a physical sampling process, whereas cohort studies often do not. Nevertheless, it is standard practice to treat all epidemiologic studies, including cohort studies, as having sampling error. In this view, the subjects in a study, whether physically sampled or not, are viewed as a figurative sample of possible people who could have been included in the study or of the different possible experiences the study subjects could have had. Even if all the individuals in a population were included in a study, the study subjects are viewed as a sample of the potential biologic experience of an even broader conceptual population. With this view, the statistical dictum that there is no sampling error if an entire population (as opposed to a sample of it) is studied does not apply to epidemiologic studies, even if an entire population is included in the study. Conceptually, the actual subjects are always considered a sample of a broader experience of interest—although they seldom actually satisfy the definition of a random sample that underpins the statistical tools ordinarily used to measure random variation (Greenland, 1990, 2005b).

Sampling is only one source of random error that contributes to unpredictable inaccuracies in epidemiologic studies. Another source is the unexplained variation in occurrence measures, such as observed incidence rates or prevalence proportions. For example, when exposure status is not randomly assigned, confounding (Chapter 4) may lead to deviations of estimated associations from target effects that far exceed what standard statistical models assume probable. Mismeasurement of key study variables also contributes to the overall inaccuracy, in both random and in systematic ways. As a result of these extra sources of variation, and because of the weak theoretical underpinnings for conceptualizing study subjects as a sample of a broader experience, the usual statistical tools that we use to measure random variation at best provide minimum estimates of the actual uncertainty we should have about the object of estimation (Greenland, 1990, 2005b). One elementary way to improve the quantification of our uncertainty is through *bias analysis,* which we discuss in Chapter 19.

A common measure of random variation in a measurement or estimation process is the *variance* of the process, which is discussed in Chapter 13. The *statistical precision of* (or *statistical information in*) a measurement or process is often taken to be the inverse of the variance of the measurements or estimates that the process produces. In this sense, precision is the opposite of random error. Precision of estimation can be improved (which is to say, variance can be reduced) by increasing the size of the study. Precision can also be improved by modifying the design of the study to decrease the variance given a fixed total number of subjects; this process is called improving the *statistical efficiency* of the study. It will be introduced here and discussed more fully in Chapter 13. Perhaps the most common epidemiologic example of such design improvement is the use of a case-control study rather than a cohort study, because for a fixed study size the variance of an effect estimate is heavily dependent on the proportion of subjects in the study that are cases.

STUDY SIZE

A common way to reduce random error in, or increase precision of, an epidemiologic estimate is to enlarge the size of the study. Practical constraints on resources inevitably limit study size, so one must plan accordingly. One method that is used to plan the size of a study is to calculate study size based on conventional statistical "sample-size" formulas (e.g., see Schlesselman, 1974; Rothman and Boice, 1982; Greenland, 1985b, 1988a). These formulas relate the size of a study to the study design, study population, and the desired power or precision.

Study-size formulas, being purely mathematical, do not account for anything that is not included as a variable in the formula. At best they serve only to provide rough guidelines, and in some situations they may be misleading from a broader perspective. For example, conventional formulas do not weigh the value of the information obtained from a study against its use of resources. Yet a focal problem in planning the study size is determining how to balance the value of greater precision in study results against the greater cost. Solving the problem thus involves a cost–benefit analysis of expending greater effort or funds to gain greater precision. Greater precision has a value to the beneficiaries of the research, but the value is indeterminate because it is always uncertain how many beneficiaries there will be. Furthermore, the potential benefits of the study involve intricacies of many social, political, and biologic factors that are almost never quantified. Consequently, only informal guesses as to a cost-efficient size for an epidemiologic study are feasible. Although study-size determination can be aided by conventional formulas, the final choice must also incorporate unquantified practical constraints and implications of various study sizes.

STUDY EFFICIENCY

Another way to reduce random error, or increase precision, in an epidemiologic estimate is to modify the design of the study. One feature that can often be manipulated by design is apportionment of subjects into study groups. When the study factor has no effect and no adjustment is needed, equal apportionment into exposure groups is the most efficient cohort design (Walter, 1977). For example, in the absence of an effect or confounding, a cohort study of 2,000 persons will be most efficient if it selects 1,000 exposed and 1,000 unexposed persons for study. Similarly, in a case-control study, in the absence of an effect or confounding it will be most statistically efficient to have an equal number of cases and controls. In the presence of an effect, the apportionment that is optimal for statistical efficiency differs from equal apportionment by an amount that is a function of the parameter being estimated (Walter, 1977). When (as is almost always the case) adjustments for confounding are needed, however, these results no longer apply strictly. Furthermore, these results assume that no effect is present—which is of course not known to be true in any real application (otherwise there would be no need for the study). Thus, these results should not be taken as anything more than rough guidelines for design.

PRECISION AND STRATIFICATION

In many epidemiologic analyses, the crude data are divided into strata to examine effects in subcategories of another variable or to control confounding. The efficiency of a study can be affected dramatically by stratifying the data. A study that has an overall apportionment ratio that is favorable for precision (which will be a ratio of 1.0 if there is no effect and no confounding) may nevertheless have apportionment ratios within strata that vary severely from low to high values. It is not uncommon to see some strata with the extreme apportionment ratios of 0 and infinity (e.g., no cases in some strata and no controls in others). The smaller the numbers within strata, the more extreme the variation in the apportionment ratio across strata is likely to be. The extreme values result from zero subjects or person-time units for one group in a stratum. Small numbers within strata result from having too few subjects relative to the number of strata created. This *sparse-data* problem can develop even with large studies, because the number of strata required in the analysis increases geometrically with the number of variables used for stratification. Indeed, sparse data are a major limitation of stratified analysis, although the same problem negatively affects regression modeling as well. Methods for dealing with sparsity are described in Chapters 15 and 21.

When comparisons within strata will be essential and much variation in the apportionment ratio is expected across strata, then *matching* on the stratification variables (Chapter 11) is one way to maintain an efficient apportionment ratio within strata and to reduce sparsity problems without increasing study size. When matching on all stratification variables is not feasible, increasing the overall number of subjects will at least reduce data sparsity and improve precision, even if only one group (e.g., the controls) can be expanded.

APPROACHES TO RANDOM ERROR

Statistics and its role in data analysis have undergone a gradual but profound transformation in recent times. There is an essential distinction between a qualitative study objective (to answer a question "yes" or "no") and a quantitative one (to measure something). The recent transformation reflects a growing preference for the latter objective and for statistical methods consistent with it. Until the 1970s, most applications of statistics in epidemiology focused on deciding whether "chance" or "random error" could be solely responsible for an observed association. The methods used for this decision were those of classical *significance testing*, predominant in British applications, and those of Neyman-Pearson *hypothesis testing*, predominant in American applications (Goodman, 1993; Gigerenzer, 2004). Because of their similarities, the term *significance testing* is often applied to both collections of methods.

These testing applications, which were subject to some early criticism (Boring, 1919; Berkson, 1938, 1942; Hogben, 1957), came under growing criticism by epidemiologists and statisticians throughout the 1970s and 1980s. The critics pointed out that most, if not all, epidemiologic applications need more than a decision as to whether chance alone could have produced an association. More important is estimation of the magnitude of the association, including an assessment of the precision of the estimation method. The estimation tool used by most authors is the confidence interval, which provides a range of values for the association, under the hypothesis that only random variation has created discrepancies between the true value of the association under study and the value observed in the data (Altman et al., 2000; see Chapters 13 through 16). Other authors, while favoring the move toward interval estimation, point out that confidence intervals suffer from some of the flaws associated with significance testing and favor other approaches to interval estimation (Goodman and Royall, 1988; Berger and Berry, 1988; Royall, 1997; Greenland, 2006a; Chapter 18).

SIGNIFICANCE TESTING AND HYPOTHESIS TESTING

Nearly 70 years ago, Berkson (1942) wrote:

> It is hardly an exaggeration to say that statistics, as it is taught at present in the dominant school, consists almost entirely of tests of significance, though not always presented as such, some comparatively simple and forthright, others elaborate and abstruse.

The ubiquitous use of P-values and references to "statistically significant" findings in the current medical literature demonstrates the dominant role that statistical hypothesis testing still plays in data analysis in some branches of biomedical sciences. Many researchers still believe that it would be fruitless to submit for publication any paper that lacks statistical tests of significance. Their belief is not entirely ill-founded, because many journal editors and referees still rely on tests of significance as indicators of sophisticated and meaningful statistical analysis as well as the primary means of assessing sampling variability in a study. *Statistical significance* is usually based on the P-value (described below): results are considered "significant" or "not significant" according to whether the P-value is less than or greater than an arbitrary cutoff value, usually 0.05, which is called the *alpha level* of the test.

The preoccupation with significance testing derives from the research interests of the statisticians who pioneered the development of statistical theory in the early 20th century. Their research problems were primarily industrial and agricultural, and they typically involved randomized experiments or random-sample surveys that formed the basis for a choice between two or more alternative courses of action. Such studies were designed to produce results that would enable a decision to be made, and the statistical methods employed were intended to facilitate decision making. The concepts that grew out of this heritage are today applied in clinical and epidemiologic research, and they strongly reflect this background of decision making.

Statistical significance testing of associations usually focuses on the *null hypothesis,* which is usually formulated as a hypothesis of no association between two variables in a *superpopulation,* the population from which the observed study groups were purportedly sampled in a random fashion. For example, one may test the hypothesis that the risk difference in the superpopulation is 0 or, equivalently, that the risk ratio is 1. Note that this hypothesis is about the superpopulation, *not* about the observed study groups. Testing may alternatively focus on any other specific hypothesis, e.g., that the risk difference is 0.1 or the risk ratio is 2. For non-null hypotheses, tests about one measure (e.g., a risk difference) are not usually equivalent to tests about another measure (e.g., a risk ratio), so one must choose a measure of interest to perform a non-null test.

A common misinterpretation of significance tests is to claim that there is no difference between two observed groups because the null test is not statistically significant, in that P is greater than the cutoff for declaring statistical significance (again, usually 0.05). This interpretation confuses a descriptive issue (whether the two observed groups differ) with an inference about the superpopulation. The significance test refers only to the superpopulation, not the observed groups. To say that the difference is not statistically significant means only that one cannot reject the null hypothesis that the superpopulation groups are different; it does *not* imply that the two observed groups are the same.

One need only look at the two observed groups to see whether they are different. Significance testing concerns instead whether the observed difference should lead one to infer that there is a difference between the corresponding groups in the superpopulation. Furthermore, even if the observed difference is not statistically significant, the superpopulation groups may be different (i.e., the result does not imply that the null is correct). Rather, the nonsignificant observed difference means only that one should not rule out the null hypothesis if one accepts the statistical model used to construct the test.

Conversely, it is a misinterpretation to claim that an association exists in the superpopulation because the observed difference is statistically significant. First, the test may be significant only because the model used to compute it is wrong (e.g., there may be many sources of uncontrolled bias). Second, the test may be significant because of chance alone; for example, even under perfect conditions, a test using a 0.05 alpha level will yield a statistically significant difference 5% of the time if the null hypothesis is correct.

As we emphasize, the alpha cutoff point is an arbitrary and questionable convention; it can be dispensed with simply by reporting the actual P-value from the test, which we now discuss in detail. We will then further explore and criticize the theory that led to widespread use of arbitrary testing cutoffs in research.

P-Values

There are two major types of P-values: one-tailed and two-tailed. Further, there are two types of one-tailed P-values: upper and lower. Accurate definitions and interpretations of these statistics are subtle and thus are rarely provided in epidemiologic texts. As a result, misinterpretation of P-values are common in epidemiology, as well as in other fields. We will thus devote much of this chapter and Chapter 13 to discussion of these statistics.

An *upper* one-tailed P-value is the probability that a corresponding quantity computed from the data, known as the *test statistic* (such as a t-statistic or a chi-square statistic), will be greater than or equal to its observed value, assuming that (a) the test hypothesis is correct and (b) there is no source of bias in the data collection or analysis processes. Similarly, a *lower* one-tailed P-value is the probability that the corresponding test statistic will be less than or equal to its observed value, again assuming that (a) the test hypothesis is correct and (b) there is no source of bias in the data collection or analysis processes (sometimes described by saying that the underlying statistical model is correct). The two-tailed P-value is usually defined as twice the smaller of the upper and lower P-values, although more complicated definitions have been used. Being a probability, a one-tailed P-value must fall between 0 and 1; the two-tailed P-value as just defined, however, may exceed 1. The following comments apply to all types of P-values. Some authors refer to P-values as "levels of significance" (Cox and Hinkley, 1974), but the latter term is best avoided because it has been used by other authors to refer to alpha levels.

In classical significance testing, small P-values are supposed to indicate that at least one of the assumptions used to derive it is incorrect, that is, either or both the test hypothesis (assumption 1) or the statistical model (assumption 2) is incorrect. All too often, the statistical model is taken as a given, so that a small P-value is taken as indicating a low degree of compatibility between the test hypothesis and the observed data. This incompatibility derives from the fact that a small P-value represents a low probability of getting a test statistic as extreme or more extreme than the observed statistic if the test hypothesis is true and no bias is operative. Small P-values, therefore, are supposed to indicate that the test hypothesis is not an acceptable explanation for the association observed in the data. This common interpretation has been extensively criticized because it does not account for alternative explanations and their acceptability (or lack thereof); for example, see Berkson (1942) and later epidemiologic criticisms by Goodman and Royall (1988), Greenland (1990), Goodman (1993), and Gigerenzer (2004). A less hypothetical and more cautious interpretation is then that a small P-value indicates that there is a problem with the test hypothesis or with the study, or with both (Fisher, 1943).

One of the most common naive misinterpretations of P-values is that they represent probabilities of test hypotheses. In many situations, one can compute a Bayesian probability, or credibility (see Chapter 18), for the test hypothesis, but it will almost always be far from the two-tailed P-value (Berger and Delampady, 1987; Berger and Sellke, 1987). A one-tailed P-value can be used to put a lower bound on the Bayesian probability of certain compound hypotheses (Casella and Berger, 1987), and under certain conditions will approximate the Bayesian probability that the true association is the opposite of the direction observed (Greenland and Gustafson, 2006). Nonetheless, a P-value for a simple test hypothesis (for example, that exposure and disease are unassociated) is not a probability of that hypothesis: That P-value is usually much smaller than such a Bayesian probability and so can easily mislead one into inappropriately rejecting the test hypothesis (Berger and Sellke, 1987; Goodman and Royall, 1988).

A common and blatantly incorrect interpretation is that the P-value is the probability of the observed data under the test hypothesis. This probability is known as the likelihood of the test hypothesis; see Goodman and Royall (1988), Royall (1997), Edwards (1992), and the following discussion. The likelihood of a hypothesis is usually much smaller than the P-value for the hypothesis, because the P-value includes not only the probability of the observed data under the test hypothesis, but also the probabilities for all other possible data configurations in which the test statistic was more extreme than that observed.

A subtle and common misinterpretation of a P-value for testing the null hypothesis is that it represents the probability that the data would show as strong an association as observed or stronger if the null hypothesis were correct. This misinterpretation can be found in many methodologic articles and textbooks. The nature of the misinterpretation can be seen in a study of a risk difference RD. The study might produce an estimate of RD of 0.33 with an estimated standard deviation of 0.20, which (from formulas in Chapter 14) would produce a standard normal test statistic of $z = 0.33/0.20 = 1.65$ and a two-tailed $P = 0.10$. The same study, however, might have instead estimated a RD of 0.30 and standard deviation of 0.15, which would produce a standard normal test statistic of $z = 0.30/0.15 = 2.00$ and $P = 0.05$. The result with the association nearer the null would then produce a smaller P-value. The point is that the P-value refers to the size of the test statistic (which in this case is the estimate divided by its estimated standard deviation), not to the strength or size of the estimated association.

It is crucial to remember that P-values are calculated from statistical models, which are assumptions about the form of study-to-study data variation. Every P-value, even "nonparametric" and "exact" P-values, depends on a statistical model; it is only the strength of the model assumptions that differ (Freedman, 1985; Freedman et al., 2007). A major problem with the P-values and tests in common use (including all commercial software) is that the assumed models make no allowance for sources of bias, apart from confounding by controlled covariates.

Neyman-Pearson Hypothesis Tests

A P-value is a continuous measure of the compatibility between a hypothesis and data. Although its utility as such a measure can be disputed (Goodman and Royall, 1988; Royall, 1997), a worse problem is that it is often used to force a qualitative decision about rejection of a hypothesis. As introduced earlier, a fixed cutoff point or alpha level, often denoted by the Greek letter α (alpha), is selected as a criterion by which to judge the P-value. This point is then used to classify the observation either as "significant at level α " if $P \leq \alpha$, in which case the test hypothesis is rejected, or "not significant at level α" if $P > \alpha$, in which case the test hypothesis is accepted (or, at least, not rejected).

The use of a fixed cutoff α is a hallmark of the Neyman-Pearson form of statistical hypothesis testing. Both the alpha level (Lehmann, 1986) and the P-value (Goodman, 1992, 1993) have been called the "significance level" of the test. This usage has led to misinterpretation of the P-value as the alpha level of a statistical hypothesis test. To avoid the error, one should recall that the P-value is a quantity computed from the data, whereas the alpha level is a fixed cutoff (usually 0.05) that can be specified without even seeing the data. (As a technical aside, Neyman and Pearson actually avoided use of P-values in their formulation of hypothesis tests, and instead defined their tests based on whether the value of the test statistic fell within a "rejection region" for the test.)

An incorrect rejection is called a *Type I error,* or alpha error. A hypothesis testing procedure is said to be *valid* if, whenever the test hypothesis is true, the probability of rejection (i.e., the probability that $P \leq \alpha$) does not exceed the alpha level (provided there is no bias and all test assumptions are satisfied). For example, a valid test with $\alpha = 0.01$ (a 1% alpha level) will lead to a Type I error with no more than 1% probability, provided there is no bias or incorrect assumption.

If the test hypothesis is false but is not rejected, the incorrect decision not to reject is called a *Type II,* or beta error. If the test hypothesis is false, so that rejection is the correct decision, the probability (over repetitions of the study) that the test hypothesis is rejected is called the *power* of the test. The probability of a Type II error is related to the power by the equation Pr (Type II error) = 1 − power.

There is a trade-off between the probabilities of a Type I and a Type II error. This trade-off depends on the chosen alpha level. Reducing the Type I error when the test hypothesis is true requires a smaller alpha level, for with a smaller alpha level a smaller P-value will be required to reject the test hypothesis. Unfortunately, a lower alpha level increases the probability of a Type II error if the test hypothesis is false. Conversely, increasing the alpha level reduces the probability of Type II error when the test hypothesis is false, but increases the probability of Type I error if it is true.

The concepts of alpha level, Type I error, Type II error, and power stem from a paradigm in which data are used to decide whether to reject the test hypothesis, and therefore follow from a qualitative study objective. The extent to which decision making dominates research thinking is reflected in the frequency with which the P-value, a continuous measure, is reported or interpreted only as an inequality (such as $P < 0.05$ or $P > 0.05$) or else not at all, with the evaluation focusing instead on "statistical significance" or its absence.

When a single study forms the sole basis for a choice between two alternative actions, as in industrial quality-control activities, a decision-making mode of analysis may be justifiable. Even then, however, a rational recommendation about which of two actions is preferable will require consideration of the costs and benefits of each action. These considerations are rarely incorporated into statistical tests. In most scientific and public health settings, it is presumptuous if not absurd for an investigator to act as if the results of his or her study will form the sole basis for a decision. Such decisions are inevitably based on results from a collection of studies, and proper combination of the information from the studies requires more than just a classification of each study into "significant" or "not significant" (see Chapter 33). Thus, degradation of information about an effect into a simple dichotomy is counterproductive, even for decision making, and can be misleading.

In a classic review of 71 clinical trials that reported no "significant" difference between the compared treatments, Freiman et al. (1978) found that in the great majority of such trials the data either indicated or at least were consistent with a moderate or even reasonably strong effect of the new treatment (Fig. 10–1). In all of these trials, the original investigators interpreted their data as indicative of no effect because the P-value for the null hypothesis was not "statistically significant." The misinterpretations arose because the investigators relied solely on hypothesis testing for their statistical analysis rather than on estimation. On failing to reject the null hypothesis, the investigators in these 71 trials inappropriately accepted the null hypothesis as correct, which probably resulted in Type II error for many of these so-called negative studies.

Type II errors result when the magnitude of an effect, biases, and random variability combine to give results that are insufficiently inconsistent with the null hypothesis to reject it. This failure to reject the null hypothesis can occur because the effect is small, the observations are too few, or both, as well as from biases. More to the point, however, is that Type I and Type II errors arise because the investigator has attempted to dichotomize the results of a study into the categories "significant" or "not significant." Because this degradation of the study information is unnecessary, an "error" that results from an incorrect classification of the study result is also unnecessary.

Why has such an unsound practice as Neyman-Pearson (dichotomous) hypothesis testing become so ingrained in scientific research? Undoubtedly, much of the popularity of hypothesis testing stems from the apparent objectivity and definitiveness of the pronouncement of significance. Declarations of significance or its absence can supplant the need for more refined interpretations of data; the declarations can serve as a mechanical substitute for thought, promulgated by the inertia of training and common practice. The neatness of an apparent clear-cut result may appear more gratifying to investigators, editors, and readers than a finding that cannot be immediately pigeonholed.

The unbridled authority given to statistical significance in the social sciences has also been attributed to the apparent objectivity that the pronouncement of significance can convey (Atkins and Jarrett, 1979):

> 'Let's look and see what's significant' is not too far from the approach of some researchers, and when the data involve perhaps several hundred variables the practical temptations to use a ready-made decision rule are enormous. . . . [T]he pressure to *decide,* in situations where the very use of probability models admits the uncertainty of the inference, has certain consequences for the presentation of knowledge. The significance test appears to guarantee the objectivity of the

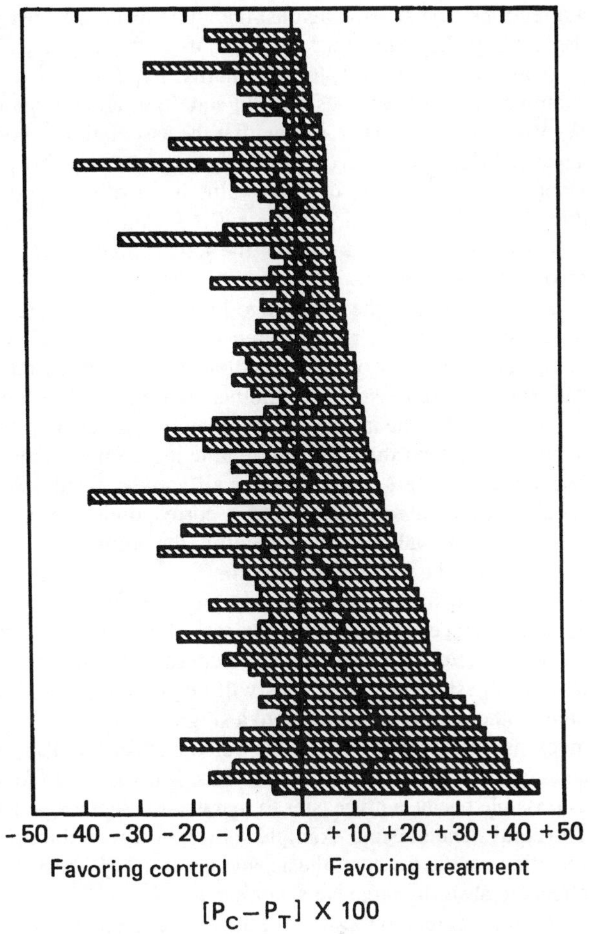

FIGURE 10–1 • Ninety percent confidence limits for the true percentage difference for the 71 trials. The vertical bar at the center of each interval indicates the observed difference, $P_C - P_T$, for each trial. (Reproduced with permission from Freiman JA, Chalmers TC, Smith H, et al. The importance of beta, the type II error and sample size in the design and interpretation of the randomized control trial. Survey of 71 "negative" trials. *N Engl J Med.* 1978;299:690–694.)

researcher's conclusions, and may even be presented as providing crucial support for the whole theory in which the research hypothesis was put forward. As we have seen, tests of significance cannot do either of these things—but it is not in the interests of anyone involved to admit this too openly.

The origin of the nearly universal acceptance of the 5% cutoff point for significant findings is tied to the abridged form in which the chi-square table was originally published (Freedman et al., 2007). Before computers and calculators could easily give quick approximations to the chi-square distribution, tables were used routinely. Because there is a different chi-square distribution corresponding to every possible value for the degrees of freedom, the tables could not give many points for any one distribution. The tables typically included values at 1%, 5%, and a few other levels, encouraging the practice of checking the chi-squared statistic calculated from one's data to see if it exceeded the cutoff levels in the table. In Neyman and Pearson's original formulation of hypothesis testing, the alpha level was supposed to be determined from contextual considerations, especially the cost of Type I and Type II errors. This thoughtful aspect of their theory was rapidly lost when the theory entered common scientific use.

The Alternative Hypothesis

Another hallmark of Neyman-Pearson hypothesis testing, and perhaps one that most distinguishes it from earlier significance-testing paradigms, is that if the test hypothesis is rejected, it is supposed to be rejected in favor of some alternative hypothesis. The alternative hypothesis may be very specific, but more often it is implicit and very broad. For example, if the test hypothesis postulates that there is no association, then the usual (implicit) alternative hypothesis is that there is an association. Such nonspecific alternatives lead to nondirectional tests based on comparing a two-tailed P-value from a directional test statistic against the alpha level. Because this P-value is sensitive to violations of the test hypothesis in either direction, it is often called a *two-sided* P-value.

Nonetheless, the test and alternative hypotheses can instead be one-sided (directional). For example, the test hypothesis could state that an association is not positive (that is, either null or negative). The alternative is then that the association is positive. Such an alternative leads to use of a *one-sided* test based on comparing an *upper-tailed* P-value from a directional test statistic against alpha. Because this one-tailed P-value is sensitive to violations of the test hypothesis in only one direction, it is often called a *one-sided* P-value. An analogous one-sided test that the association was not negative would employ the lower-tailed P-value; the alternative for this test is that the association is negative.

Another form of the alternative hypothesis is a finite interval of "equivalence" about the null, for example, that the risk difference RD is between -0.1 and $+0.1$. This alternative is found in comparisons of two treatments (so that the "exposed" are those given one treatment and the "unexposed" are those given another treatment). The bounds of the interval are selected so that any value within the interval is considered close enough to the null for practical purposes. The test hypothesis is then that the two treatments are not equivalent (RD is outside the interval), and is rejected if P is less than alpha for all values outside the interval of equivalence. This approach is called *equivalence testing*, and it corresponds to rejecting the test hypothesis when the $1 - \alpha$ confidence interval falls entirely within the equivalence interval (Blackwelder, 1998).

Note that the alternative hypothesis in all these examples comprises a range of values. For a two-sided test, the alternative comprises every possible value except the one being tested. For epidemiologic effect measures, this two-sided alternative hypothesis will range from absurdly large preventive effects to absurdly large causal effects, and include everything in between except the test hypothesis. This hypothesis will be compatible with any observed data. The test hypothesis, on the other hand, corresponds to a single value of effect and therefore is readily consistent with a much narrower range of possible outcomes for the data. Statistical hypothesis testing amounts to an attempt to falsify the test hypothesis. It is natural to focus on a test hypothesis that is as specific as possible because it is easier to marshal evidence against a specific hypothesis than a broad one. The equivalence-testing example shows, however, that in some cases the alternative may be more specific than the test hypothesis, and the test hypothesis may range from absurdly large preventive effects to absurdly large causal effects.

A major defect in the way all the above alternatives are usually formulated is that they assume the statistical model is correct. Because the model is never exactly correct and is often grossly incorrect, a scientifically more sound formulation of the alternative to the null hypothesis (for example) would be "either the null is false or else the statistical model is wrong" (Fisher, 1943). By adding the warning "or else the statistical model is wrong" to the alternative, we allow for the possibility that uncontrolled systematic errors were responsible for the rejection.

STATISTICAL ESTIMATION

If Neyman-Pearson hypothesis testing is misleading, how should results be interpreted and presented? In keeping with the view that science is based on measurement—which leads in turn to quantitative study objectives—the analysis of epidemiologic data can be conceptualized as a measurement problem rather than as a problem in decision making. Measurement requires more detailed statistics than the simple dichotomy produced by statistical hypothesis testing. Whatever the parameter that is the target of inference in an epidemiologic study—usually an effect measure, such as a ratio of rates or risks, but it can also be an incidence rate or any other epidemiologic measure—it will be measured on a continuous scale, with a theoretically infinite number of possible values.

The data from a study can be used to generate an estimate of the target parameter. An estimate may be presented as a single value on the measurement scale of the parameter; this value is referred to as a *point estimate*. A point estimate may be viewed as a measure of the extent of the association, or (in causal analyses) the magnitude of effect under study. There will be many forces that will determine the final data values, such as confounding, measurement error, selection biases, and "random" error. It is thus extremely unlikely that the point estimate will equal the true parameter.

Confidence Intervals and Confidence Limits

One way to account for random error in the estimation process is to compute P-values for a broad range of possible parameter values (in addition to the null value). If the range is broad enough, we will be able to identify an interval of parameter values for which the test P-value exceeds a specified alpha level (typically 0.05). All parameter values within the range are compatible with the data under the standard interpretation of significance tests. The range of values is called a *confidence interval,* and the endpoints of that interval are called *confidence limits*. The process of calculating the confidence interval is an example of the process of *interval estimation*.

The width of a confidence interval depends on the amount of random variability inherent in the data-collection process (as estimated from the underlying statistical model and the data). It also depends on an arbitrarily selected alpha level that specifies the degree of compatibility between the limits of the interval and the data. One minus this alpha level (0.95 if alpha is 0.05) is called the *confidence level* of the interval and is usually expressed as a percentage.

If the underlying statistical model is correct and there is no bias, a confidence interval derived from a valid test will, over unlimited repetitions of the study, contain the true parameter with a frequency no less than its confidence level. This definition specifies the coverage property of the method used to generate the interval, not the probability that the true parameter value lies within the interval. For example, if the confidence level of a valid confidence interval is 90%, the frequency with which the interval will contain the true parameter will be at least 90%, if there is no bias. Consequently, under the assumed model for random variability (e.g., a binomial model, as described in Chapter 14) and with no bias, we should expect the confidence interval to include the true parameter value in at least 90% of replications of the process of obtaining the data. Unfortunately, this interpretation for the confidence interval is based on probability models and sampling properties that are seldom realized in epidemiologic studies; consequently, it is preferable to view the confidence limits as only a rough estimate of the uncertainty in an epidemiologic result due to random error alone. Even with this limited interpretation, the estimate depends on the correctness of the statistical model, which may be incorrect in many epidemiologic settings (Greenland, 1990).

Relation of Confidence Intervals to Significance Tests and Hypothesis Tests

Consider now the relation between the confidence level and the alpha level of hypothesis testing. The confidence level equals 1 minus the alpha level $(1 - \alpha)$ of the test used to construct the interval. To understand this relation, consider the diagram in Figure 10–2. Suppose that we performed a test of the null hypothesis with $\alpha = 0.10$. The fact that the 90% confidence interval does not include the null point indicates that the null hypothesis would be rejected for $\alpha = 0.10$. On the other hand, the fact that the 95% confidence interval includes the null point indicates that the null hypothesis would not be rejected for $\alpha = 0.05$. Because the 95% interval includes the null point and the 90% interval does not, it can be inferred that the two-sided P-value for the null hypothesis is greater than 0.05 and less than 0.10.

The point of the preceding example is not to suggest that confidence limits should be used as surrogate tests of significance. Although they can be and often are used this way, doing so defeats all the advantages that confidence intervals have over hypothesis tests. An interval-estimation procedure

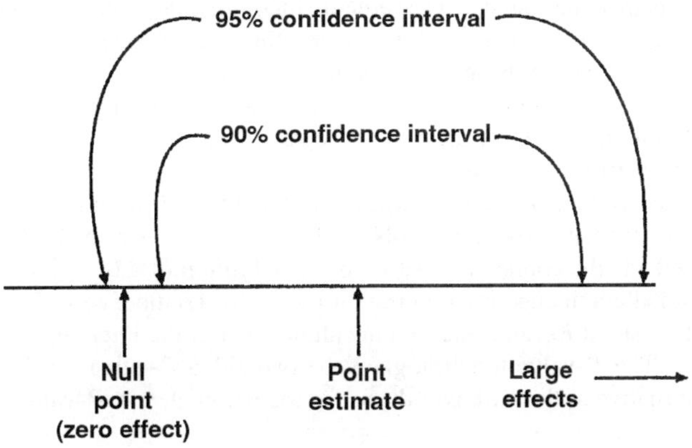

FIGURE 10–2 • Two nested confidence intervals, with the wider one including the null hypothesis.

TABLE 10–1

Hypothetical Data from a Cohort Study, Corresponding to the P-Value Function in Figure 10–3

	Exposure	
	Yes	No
Cases	9	2
Person-years	186	128

does much more than assess the extent to which a hypothesis is compatible with the data. It provides simultaneously an idea of the likely direction and magnitude of the underlying association and the random variability of the point estimate. The two-sided P-value, on the other hand, indicates only the degree of consistency between the data and a single hypothesis, and thus reveals nothing about the magnitude or even the direction of the association, or the random variability of the point estimate (Bandt and Boen, 1972).

For example, consider the data in Table 10–1. An exact test of the null hypothesis that the exposure is not associated with the disease gives a two-sided P-value of 0.14. (The methods used to calculate this P-value are described in Chapter 14.) This result might be reported in several ways. The least informative way is to report that the observed association is not significant. Somewhat more information can be given by reporting the actual P-value; to express the P-value as an inequality such as $P > 0.05$ is not much better than reporting the results as not significant, whereas reporting $P = 0.14$ at least gives the P-value explicitly rather than degrading it into a dichotomy. An additional improvement is to report $P_2 = 0.14$, denoting the use of a two-sided rather than a one-sided P-value.

Any one P-value, no matter how explicit, fails to convey the descriptive finding that exposed individuals had about three times the rate of disease as unexposed subjects. Furthermore, exact 95% confidence limits for the true rate ratio are 0.7–13. The fact that the null value (which, for the rate ratio, is 1.0) is within the interval tells us the outcome of the significance test: The estimate would not be statistically significant at the $1 - 0.95 = 0.05$ alpha level. The confidence limits, however, indicate that these data, although statistically compatible with no association, are even more compatible with a strong association—assuming that the statistical model used to construct the limits is correct. Stating the latter assumption is important because confidence intervals, like P-values, do nothing to address biases that may be present.

P-Value Functions

Although a single confidence interval can be much more informative than a single P-value, it is subject to the misinterpretation that values inside the interval are equally compatible with the data, and all values outside it are equally incompatible. Like the alpha level of a test, however, the specific level of confidence used in constructing a confidence interval is arbitrary; values of 95% or, less often, 90% are those most frequently used.

A given confidence interval is only one of an infinite number of ranges nested within one another. Points nearer the center of these ranges are more compatible with the data than points farther away from the center. To see the entire set of possible confidence intervals, one can construct a *P-value function* (Birnbaum, 1961; Miettinen, 1985b; Poole, 1987a). This function, also known as a consonance function (Folks, 1981) or confidence-interval function (Sullivan and Foster, 1990), reflects the connection between the definition of a two-sided P-value and the definition of a two-sided confidence interval (i.e., a two-sided confidence interval comprises all points for which the two-sided P-value exceeds the alpha level of the interval).

The P-value function gives the two-sided P-value for the null hypothesis, as well as every alternative to the null hypothesis for the parameter. A P-value function from the data in Table 10–1

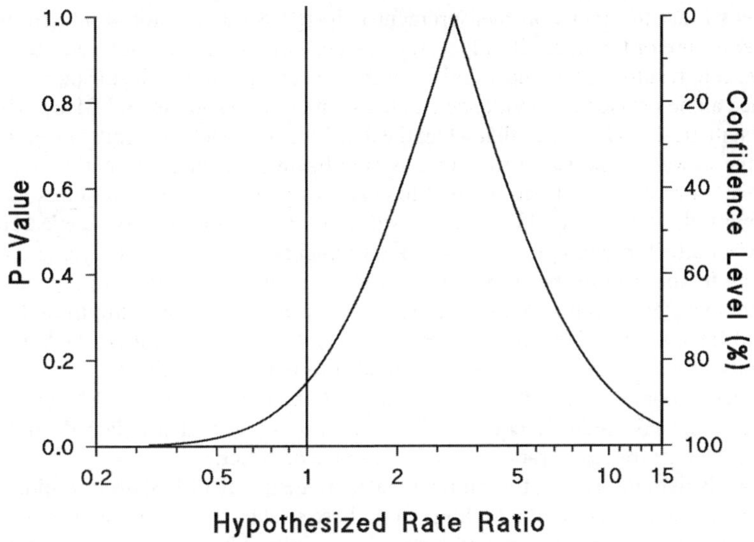

FIGURE 10–3 • *P*-value function, from which one can find all confidence limits, for a hypothetical study with a rate ratio estimate of 3.1 (see Table 10–1).

is shown in Figure 10–3. Figure 10–3 also provides confidence levels on the right, and so indicates all possible confidence limits for the estimate. The point at which the curve reaches its peak corresponds to the point estimate for the rate ratio, 3.1. The 95% confidence interval can be read directly from the graph as the function values where the right-hand ordinate is 0.95, and the 90% confidence interval can be read from the graph as the values where the right-hand ordinate is 0.90. The *P*-value for any value of the parameter can be found from the left-hand ordinate corresponding to that value. For example, the null two-sided *P*-value can be found from the left-hand ordinate corresponding to the height where the vertical line drawn at the hypothesized rate ratio = 1 intersects the *P*-value function.

A *P*-value function offers a visual display that neatly summarizes the two key components of the estimation process. The peak of the curve indicates the point estimate, and the concentration of the curve around the point estimate indicates the precision of the estimate. A narrow *P*-value function would result from a large study with high precision, and a broad *P*-value function would result from a small study that had low precision.

A confidence interval represents only one possible horizontal slice through the *P*-value function, but the single slice is enough to convey the two essential messages: Confidence limits usually provide enough information to locate the point estimate and to indicate the precision of the estimate. In large-sample epidemiologic statistics, the point estimate will usually be either the arithmetic or geometric mean of the lower and upper limits. The distance between the lower and upper limits indicates the spread of the full *P*-value function.

The message of Figure 10–3 is that the example data are more compatible with a moderate to strong association than with no association, assuming the statistical model used to construct the function is correct. The confidence limits, when taken as indicative of the *P*-value function, summarize the size and precision of the estimate (Poole, 1987b, Poole, 2001c). A single *P*-value, on the other hand, gives no indication of either the size or precision of the estimate, and, if it is used merely as a hypothesis test, might result in a Type II error if there indeed is an association between exposure and disease.

Evidence of Absence of Effect

Confidence limits and *P*-value functions convey information about size and precision of the estimate simultaneously, keeping these two features of measurement in the foreground. The use of a single *P*-value—or (worse) dichotomization of the *P*-value into significant or not significant—obscures these features so that the focus on measurement is lost. A study cannot be reassuring about the safety of an exposure or treatment if only a statistical test of the null hypothesis is reported. As we have already seen, results that are not significant may be compatible with substantial effects. Lack of significance alone provides no evidence against such effects (Altman and Bland, 1995).

Standard statistical advice states that when the data indicate a lack of significance, it is important to consider the power of the study to detect as significant a specific alternative hypothesis. The power of a test, however, is only an indirect indicator of precision, and it requires an assumption about the magnitude of the effect. In planning a study, it is reasonable to make conjectures about the magnitude of an effect to compute study-size requirements or power. In analyzing data, however, it is always preferable to use the information in the data about the effect to estimate it directly, rather than to speculate about it with study-size or power calculations (Smith and Bates, 1992; Goodman and Berlin, 1994; Hoenig and Heisey, 2001). Confidence limits and (even more so) *P*-value functions convey much more of the essential information by indicating the range of values that are reasonably compatible with the observations (albeit at a somewhat arbitrary alpha level), assuming the statistical model is correct. They can also show that the data do not contain the information necessary for reassurance about an absence of effect.

In their reanalysis of the 71 negative clinical trials, Freiman et al. (1978) used confidence limits for the risk differences to reinterpret the findings from these studies. These confidence limits indicated that probably many of the treatments under study were indeed beneficial, as seen in Figure 10–1. The inappropriate interpretations of the authors in most of these trials could have been avoided by focusing their attention on the confidence limits rather than on the results of a statistical test.

For a study to provide evidence of lack of an effect, the confidence limits must be near the null value and the statistical model must be correct (or, if wrong, only in ways expected to bias the interval away from the null). In equivalence-testing terms, the entire confidence interval must lie within the zone about the null that would be considered practically equivalent to the null. Consider Figure 10–4, which depicts the *P*-value function from Figure 10–3 on an expanded scale, along with another *P*-value function from a study with a point estimate of 1.05 and 95% confidence limits of 1.01 and 1.10.

The study yielding the narrow *P*-value function must have been large to generate such precision. The precision enables one to infer that, absent any strong biases or other serious problems with the statistical model, the study provides evidence against a strong effect. The upper confidence limit (with any reasonable level of confidence) is near the null value, indicating that the data are not readily compatible with large or even moderate effects. Or, as seen from the *P*-value function, the

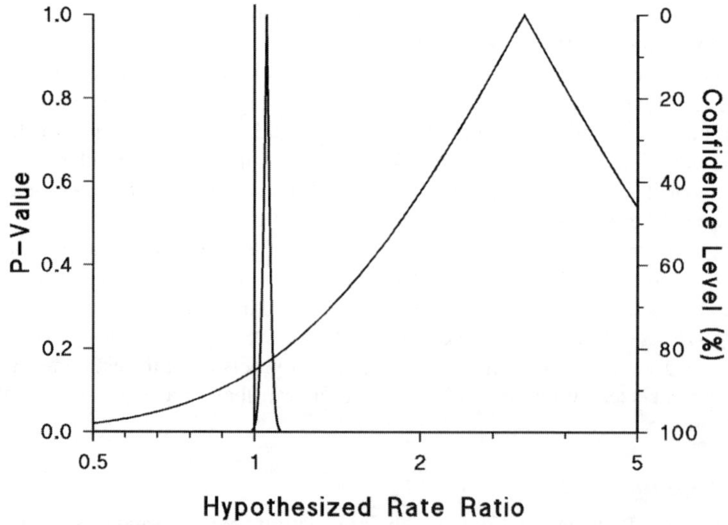

FIGURE 10–4 • A *P*-value function from a precise study with a relative risk estimate of 1.05 and the *P*-value function from Figure 10–3.

curve is a narrow spike close to the null point. The spike is not centered exactly on the null point, however, but slightly above it. In fact, the data from this large study would be judged as statistically significant by conventional criteria, because the (two-sided) P-value testing the null hypothesis is about 0.03. In contrast, the other P-value function in Figure 10–4 depicts data that, as we have seen, are readily compatible with large effects but are not statistically significant by conventional criteria.

Figure 10–4 illustrates the dangers of using statistical significance as the primary basis for inference. Even if one assumes no bias is present (i.e., that the studies and analyses are perfectly valid), the two sets of results differ in that one result indicates there may be a large effect, while the other offers evidence against a large effect. The irony is that it is the statistically significant finding that offers evidence *against* a large effect, while it is the finding that is not statistically significant that raises concern about a possibly large effect. In these examples, statistical significance gives a message that is opposite of the appropriate interpretation. Focusing on interval estimation and proper interpretation of the confidence limits avoids this problem.

Numerous real-world examples demonstrate the problem of relying on statistical significance for inference. One such example occurred in the interpretation of a large randomized trial of androgen blockade combined with the drug flutamide in the treatment of advanced prostate cancer (Eisenberger et al., 1998). This trial had been preceded by 10 similar trials, which in aggregate had found a small survival advantage for patients given flutamide, with the pooled results for the 10 studies producing a summary odds ratio of 0.88, with a 95% confidence interval of 0.76–1.02 (Rothman et al., 1999; Prostate Cancer Trialists' Collaborative Group, 1995). In their study, Eisenberger et al. reported that flutamide was ineffective, thus contradicting the results of the 10 earlier studies, despite their finding an odds ratio of 0.87 (equivalent in their study to a mortality rate ratio of 0.91), a result not very different from that of the earlier 10 studies. The P-value for their finding was above their predetermined cutoff for 'significance', which is the reason that the authors concluded that flutamide was an ineffective therapy. But the 95% confidence interval of 0.70–1.10 for their odds ratio showed that their data were readily compatible with a meaningful benefit for patients receiving flutamide. Furthermore, their results were similar to those from the summary of the 10 earlier studies. The P-value functions for the summary of the 10 earlier studies, and the study by Eisenberger et al., are shown in Figure 10–5. The figure shows how the findings of

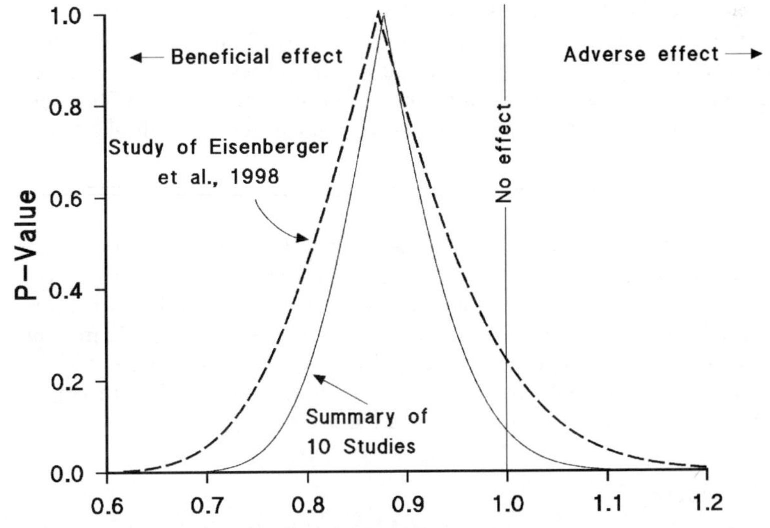

FIGURE 10–5 • P-value functions based on 10 earlier trials of flutamide (solid line) and the trial by Eisenberger et al. (dashed line), showing the similarity of results, and revealing the fallacy of relying on statistical significance to conclude, as did Eisenberger et al., that flutamide has no meaningful effect.

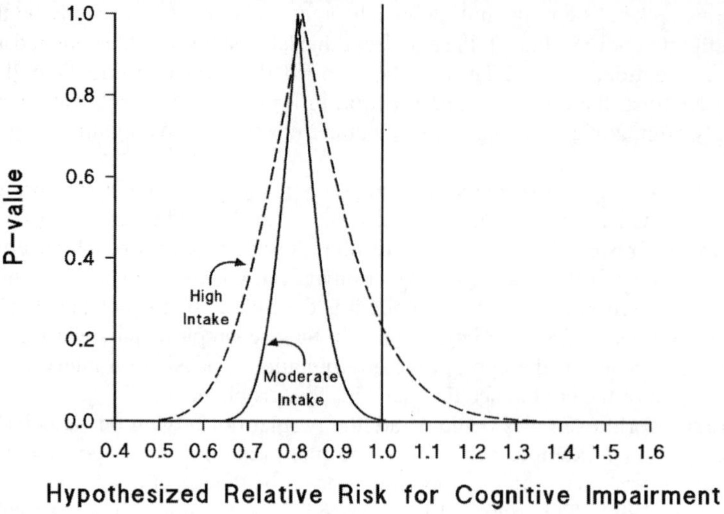

FIGURE 10–6 • *P*-value functions for moderate and heavier drinkers of alcohol showing essentially identical negative associations with decline in cognitive function. The authors incorrectly reported that there was an association with moderate drinking, but not with heavier drinking, because only the finding for moderate drinking was statistically significant (Reproduced with permission from Stampfer MJ, Kang JH, Chen J, et al. Effects of moderate alcohol consumption on cognitive function in women. *N Engl J Med.* 2005;352:245–253.)

Eisenberger et al. reinforce rather than refute the earlier studies. They misinterpreted their findings because of their focus on statistical significance.

Another example was a headline-generating study reporting that women who consumed moderate amounts of alcohol retained better cognitive function than nondrinkers (Stampfer et al., 2005). For moderate drinkers (up to 15 g of alcohol per day), the authors reported a risk ratio for impaired cognition of 0.81 with 95% confidence limits of 0.70 and 0.93, indicating that moderate drinking was associated with a benefit with respect to cognition. In contrast, the authors reported that "There were no significant associations between higher levels of drinking (15 to 30 g per day) and the risk of cognitive impairment or decline," implying no benefit for heavy drinkers, an interpretation repeated in widespread news reports. Nevertheless, the finding for women who consumed larger amounts of alcohol was essentially identical to the finding for moderate drinkers, with a risk-ratio estimate of 0.82 instead of 0.81. It had a broader confidence interval, however, with limits of 0.59 and 1.13. Figure 10–6 demonstrates how precision, rather than different effect size, accounted for the difference in statistical significance for the two groups. From the data, there is no basis to infer that the effect size differs for moderate and heavy drinkers; in fact, the hypothesis that is most compatible with the data is that the effect is about the same in both groups. Furthermore, the lower 95% confidence limit for the ratio of the risk ratio in the heavy drinkers to the risk ratio in the moderate drinkers is 0.71, implying that the data are also quite compatible with a much lower (more protective) risk ratio in the heavy drinkers than in the moderate drinkers.

Guidelines for Practice

Good data analysis does not demand that *P*-value functions be calculated routinely. It is usually sufficient to use conventional confidence limits to generate the proper mental visualization for the underlying *P*-value function. In fact, for large studies, only one pair of limits and their confidence level is needed to sketch the entire function, and one can easily learn to visualize the function that corresponds to any particular pair of limits. If, however, one uses the limits only to determine whether the null point lies inside or outside the confidence interval, one is only performing a significance test. It is lamentable to go to the trouble to calculate confidence limits and then use them for nothing more than classifying the study finding as statistically significant or not. One should instead remember that the precise locations of confidence limits are not important for proper interpretation. Rather, the limits should serve to give one a mental picture of the location and spread of the entire P-value function.

The main thrust of the preceding sections has been to argue the inadequacy of statistical significance testing. The view that estimation is preferable to testing has been argued by many scientists in a variety of disciplines, including, for example, economics, social sciences, environmental science, and accident research. There has been a particularly heated and welcome debate in psychology. In the overall scientific literature, hundreds of publications have addressed the concerns about statistical hypothesis testing. Some selected references include Rozeboom (1960), Morrison and Henkel (1970), Wulff (1973), Cox and Hinkley (1974), Rothman (1978a), Salsburg (1985), Simon and Wittes (1985), Langman (1986), Gardner and Altman (1986), Walker (1986), Oakes (1990), Ware et al. (1986), Pocock et al. (1987), Poole (1987a, 1987b), Thompson (1987), Evans et al. (1988), Anscombe (1990), Oakes (1990), Cohen (1994),), Hauer (2003), Gigerenzer (2004), Ziliak and McCloskey (2004), Batterham and Hopkins (2006), and Marshall (2006). To quote Atkins and Jarrett (1979):

> Methods of estimation share many of the problems of significance tests—being likewise based on probability model assumptions and requiring "arbitrary" limits of precision. But at least they do not require irrelevant null hypotheses to be set up nor do they force a decision about "significance" to be made—the estimates can be presented and evaluated by statistical *and other* criteria, by the researcher or the reader. In addition the estimates of one investigation can be compared with others. While it is often the case that different measurements or methods of investigation or theoretical approaches lead to "different" results, this is not a disadvantage; these differences reflect important theoretical differences about the meaning of the research and the conclusions to be drawn from it. And it is precisely those differences which are obscured by simply reporting the significance level of the results.

Indeed, because statistical hypothesis testing promotes so much misinterpretation, we recommend avoiding its use in epidemiologic presentations and research reports. Such avoidance requires that P-values (when used) be presented without reference to alpha levels or "statistical significance," and that careful attention be paid to the confidence interval, especially its width and its endpoints (the confidence limits) (Altman et al., 2000; Poole, 2001c).

Problems with Confidence Intervals

Because they can be derived from P-values, confidence intervals and P-value functions are themselves subject to some of the same criticisms as significance tests (Goodman and Royall, 1988; Greenland, 1990, 2006a). One problem that confidence intervals and P-value functions share with statistical hypothesis tests is their very indirect interpretations, which depend on the concept of "repetition of the study in a manner identical in all respects except for random error." Interpretations of statistics that appeal to such a concept are called repeated-sampling or *frequentist* interpretations, because they refer to the frequency of certain events (rejection by a test, or coverage by a confidence interval) in a series of repeated experiments.

An astute investigator may properly ask what frequency interpretations have to do with the single study under analysis. It is all very well to say that an interval estimation procedure will, in 95% of repetitions, produce limits that contain the true parameter. But in analyzing a given study, the relevant scientific question is this: Does the single pair of limits produced from this one study contain the true parameter? The ordinary (frequentist) theory of confidence intervals does not answer this question. The question is so important that many (perhaps most) users of confidence intervals mistakenly interpret the confidence level of the interval as the probability that the answer to the question is "yes." It is quite tempting to say that the 95% confidence limits computed from a study contain the true parameter with 95% probability. Unfortunately, this interpretation can be correct only for Bayesian interval estimates (discussed later and in Chapter 18), which often diverge from ordinary confidence intervals.

There are several alternative types of interval estimation that attempt to address these problems. We will discuss two of these alternatives in the next two subsections.

Likelihood Intervals

To avoid interpretational problems, a few authors prefer to replace confidence intervals with likelihood intervals, also known as support intervals (Goodman and Royall, 1988; Edwards, 1992; Royall, 1997). In ordinary English, "likelihood" is just a synonym for "probability." In likelihood theory, however, a more specialized definition is used: The *likelihood* of a specified parameter value given observed data is defined as the probability of the observed data given that the true parameter equals the specified parameter value. This concept is covered in depth in many statistics textbooks; for example, see Berger and Wolpert (1988), Clayton and Hills (1993), Edwards (1992), and Royall (1997). Here, we will describe the basic definitions of likelihood theory; more details are given in Chapter 13.

To illustrate the definition of likelihood, consider again the population in Table 10–1, in which 186/(186 + 128) = 59% of person-years were exposed. Under standard assumptions, it can be shown that, if there is no bias and the true rate ratio is 10, there will be a 0.125 chance of observing nine exposed cases given 11 total cases and 59% exposed person-years. (The calculation of this probability is beyond the present discussion.) Thus, by definition, 0.125 is the likelihood for a rate ratio of 10 given the data in Table 10–1. Similarly, if there are no biases and the true ratio is 1, there will be a 0.082 chance of observing nine exposed cases given 11 total and 59% exposed person-years; thus, by definition, 0.082 is the likelihood for a rate ratio of 1 given Table 10–1.

When one parameter value makes the observed data more probable than another value and hence has a higher likelihood, it is sometimes said that this parameter value has higher support from the data than the other value (Edwards, 1992; Royall, 1997). For example, in this special sense, a rate ratio of 10 has higher support from the data in Table 10–1 than a rate ratio of 1, because those data have a greater chance of occurring if the rate ratio is 10 than if it is 1.

For most data, there will be at least one possible parameter value that makes the chance of getting those data highest under the assumed statistical model. In other words, there will be a parameter value whose likelihood is at least as high as that of any other parameter value, and so has the maximum possible likelihood (or maximum support) under the assumed model. Such a parameter value is called a *maximum-likelihood estimate* (MLE) under the assumed model. For the data in Table 10–1, there is just one such value, and it is the observed rate ratio (9/186)/(2/128) = 3.1. If there are no biases and the true rate ratio is 3.1, there will be a 0.299 chance of observing nine exposed cases given 11 total and 59% exposed person-years, so 0.299 is the likelihood for a rate ratio of 3.1 given Table 10–1. No other value for the rate ratio will make the chance of these results higher than 0.299, and so 3.1 is the MLE. Thus, in the special likelihood sense, a rate ratio of 3.1 has the highest possible support from the data.

As has been noted, Table 10–1 yields a likelihood of 0.125 for a rate ratio of 10; this value (0.125) is 42% of the likelihood (of 0.299) for 3.1. Similarly, Table 10–1 yields a likelihood of 0.082 for a rate ratio of 1; this value (0.082) is 27% of the likelihood for 3.1. Overall, a rate ratio of 3.1 maximizes the chance of observing the data in Table 10–1. Although rate ratios of 10 and 1 have less support (lower likelihood) than 3.1, they are still among values that likelihoodists regard as having enough support to warrant further consideration; these values typically include all values with a likelihood above one-seventh of the maximum (Goodman and Royall, 1988; Edwards, 1992; Royall, 1997). Under a normal model for random errors, such one-seventh likelihood intervals are approximately equal to 95% confidence intervals (Royall, 1997).

The maximum of the likelihood is the height of the likelihood function at the MLE. A likelihood interval for a parameter (here, the rate ratio) is the collection of all possible values whose likelihood is no less than some specified fraction of this maximum. Thus, for Table 10–1, the collection of all rate ratio values with a likelihood no less than 0.299/7 = 0.043 (one-seventh of the highest likelihood) is a likelihood interval based on those data. Upon computing this interval, we find that all rate ratios between 0.79 and 20 imply a probability for the observed data at least one-seventh of the probability of the data when the rate ratio is 3.1 (the MLE). Because the likelihoods for rate ratios of 1 and 10 exceed 0.299/7 = 0.043, 1 and 10 are within this interval.

Analogous to confidence limits, one can graph the collection of likelihood limits for all fractions of the maximum (1/2, 1/4, 1/7, 1/20, etc.). The resulting graph has the same shape as one would obtain from simply graphing the likelihood for each possible parameter value. The latter graph is called the *likelihood function* for the data. Figure 10–7 gives the likelihood function for the data in Table 10–1, with the ordinate scaled to make the maximum (peak) at 3.1 equal to 1 rather than

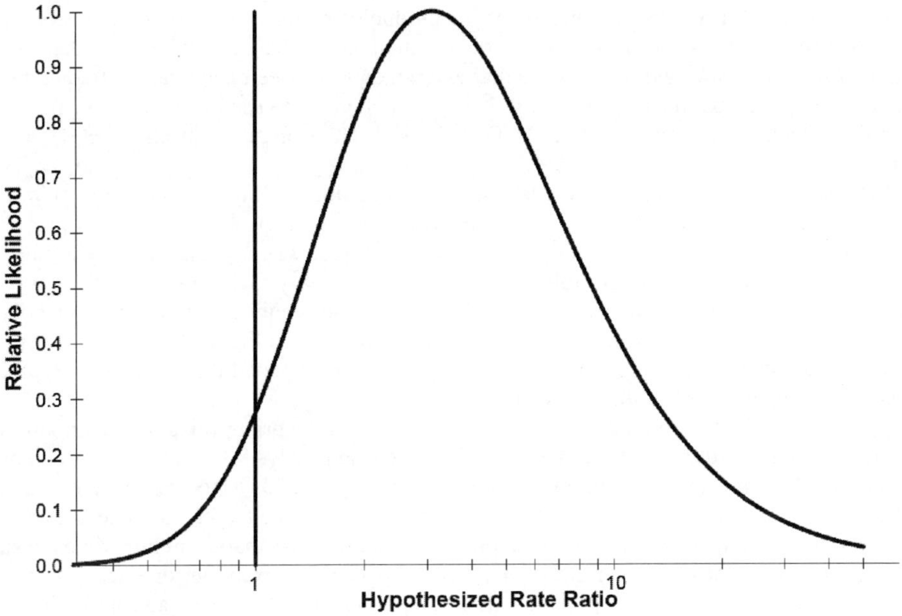

FIGURE 10–7 • Relative likelihood function based on Table 10–1.

0.299 (this is done by dividing all the likelihoods by the maximum, 0.299). Thus, Figure 10–6 provides all possible likelihood limits within the range of the figure.

The function in Figure 10–7 is proportional to

$$\left(\frac{86\,(IR)}{86\,(IR)+128}\right)^9 \left(\frac{128}{86\,(IR)+128}\right)^2$$

where IR is the hypothesized incidence rate ratio (the abscissa). Note that this function is broader and less sharply peaked than the P-value function in Figure 10–3, reflecting the fact that, by likelihood standards, P-values and confidence intervals tend to give the impression that the data provide more evidence against the test hypothesis than they actually do (Goodman and Royall, 1988). For larger data sets, however, there is a simple approximate relation between confidence limits and likelihood limits, which we discuss in Chapter 13.

Some authors prefer to use the natural logarithm of the likelihood function, or *log-likelihood function,* to compare the support given to competing hypotheses by the data (Goodman and Royall, 1988; Edwards, 1992; Royall, 1997). These authors sometimes refer to the log-likelihood function as the support function generated by the data. Although we find log-likelihoods less easily interpretable than likelihoods, log-likelihoods can be useful in constructing confidence intervals (Chapter 13).

Bayesian Intervals

As with confidence limits, the interpretation of likelihood limits is indirect, in that it does not answer the question: "Is the true value between these limits?" Unless the true value is already known (in which case there is no point in gathering data), it can be argued that the only rational answer to the question must be a *subjective* probability statement, such as "I am 95% sure that the true value is between these limits" (DeFinetti, 1974; Howson and Urbach, 1993; see Chapter 18). Such subjective probability assessments, or *certainties,* are common in everyday life, as when a weather forecaster predicts 80% chance of rain tomorrow, or when one is delayed while traveling and thinks that there is a 90% chance of arriving between 1 and 2 hours after the scheduled arrival time. If one is *sure* that the true arrival time will be between these limits, this sureness represents a subjective assessment of 100% probability (complete certainty) that arrival will be 1 to 2 hours late. In reality, however, there is always a chance (however small) that one will be delayed longer or may never arrive, so complete certainty is never warranted.

Subjective Bayesian analysis is concerned with producing realistic and rationally coherent probability assessments, and it is especially concerned with updating these assessments as data become available. *Rationally coherent* means only that assessments are free of logical contradictions and do not contradict the axioms of probability theory (which are also used as axioms for frequentist probability calculations) (Savage, 1972; DeFinetti, 1974; Howson and Urbach, 1993; Greenland, 1998b).

All statistical methods require a model for data probabilities. Bayesian analysis additionally requires a *prior probability distribution*. In theory, this means that one must have a probability assessment available for every relevant interval; for example, when trying to study a rate ratio, before seeing the data one must be able to specify one's certainty that the rate ratio is between 1 and 2, and between ½ and 4, and so on. This prior-specification requirement demands that one has a probability distribution for the rate ratio that is similar in shape to Figure 10–3 *before* seeing the data. This is a daunting demand, and it was enough to have impeded the use and acceptance of Bayesian methods for most of the 20th century.

Suppose, however, that one succeeds in specifying in advance a prior probability distribution that gives prespecified certainties for the target parameter. Bayesian analysis then proceeds by combining this prior distribution with the likelihood function (such as in Fig. 10–7) to produce a new, updated set of certainties, called the *posterior probability distribution* for the target parameter based on the given prior distribution and likelihood function. This posterior distribution in turn yields posterior probability intervals (posterior certainty intervals). Suppose, for example, one accepts the prior distribution as a good summary of previous information about the parameter, and similarly accepts the likelihood function as a good summary of the data probabilities given various possible values for the parameter. The resulting 95% posterior interval is then a range of numbers that one can be 95% certain contains the true parameter.

The technical details of computing exact posterior distributions can be quite involved and were also an obstacle to widespread adoption of Bayesian methods. Modern computing advances have all but eliminated this obstacle as a serious problem; also, the same approximations used to compute conventional frequentist statistics (Chapters 14 through 17) can be used to compute approximate Bayesian statistics (see Chapter 18).

Another obstacle to Bayesian methods has been that the intervals produced by a Bayesian analysis refer to subjective probabilities rather than objective frequencies. Some argue that, because subjective probabilities are just one person's opinion, they should be of no interest to objective scientists. Unfortunately, in nonexperimental studies there is (by definition) no identified random mechanism to generate objective frequencies over study repetitions; thus, in such studies, so-called objective frequentist methods (such as significance tests and confidence intervals) lack the objective repeated-sampling properties usually attributed to them (Freedman, 1985, 1987; Greenland, 1990, 1998b, 2005b, 2006a; Freedman et al., 2007). Furthermore, scientists do routinely offer their opinions and are interested in the opinions of colleagues. Therefore, it can be argued that a rational (if subjective) certainty assessment may be the only reasonable inference we can get out of a statistical analysis of observational epidemiologic data. Some argue that this conclusion applies even to perfect randomized experiments (Berger and Berry, 1988; Howson and Urbach, 1993; Spiegelhalter et al., 2004).

At the very least, Bayesian statistics provide a probabilistic answer to questions as "Does the true rate ratio lie between 1 and 4?" (to which one possible Bayesian answer is "In light of the data and my current prior information, I can be 90% certain that it does."). A more general argument for the use of Bayesian methods is that they can provide point and interval estimates that have better objective frequency (repeated-sampling) properties than ordinary frequentist estimates. These calibrated Bayesian statistics include Bayesian confidence intervals that are narrower (more precise) than ordinary confidence intervals with the same confidence level. Because the advantages of procedures with Bayesian justification can be so dramatic, some authors argue that only methods with a clear Bayesian justification should be used, even though repeated-sampling (objective frequency) properties are also desirable (such as proper coverage frequency for interval estimates) (Rubin, 1984, 1991; Gelman et al., 2003).

In addition to providing improved analysis methods, Bayesian theory can be used to evaluate established or newly proposed statistical methods. For example, if a new confidence interval is proposed, we may ask: "What prior distribution do we need to get this new interval as our Bayesian posterior probability interval?" It is often the case that the prior distribution one would need to justify a conventional confidence interval is patently absurd; for example, it would assign equal probabilities to rate ratios of 1 and 1,000,000 (Greenland, 1992a, 1998b, 2006a; Chapter 18). In such cases it can be argued that one should reject the proposed interval because it will not properly reflect any rational opinion about the parameter after a careful data analysis (Rubin, 1984; Greenland, 2006a).

Under certain conditions, ordinary (frequentist) confidence intervals and one-sided P-values can be interpreted as approximate posterior (Bayesian) probability intervals (Cox and Hinkley, 1974; Greenland and Gustafson, 2006). These conditions typically arise when little is known about the associations under study. Frequentist intervals cease to have Bayesian utility when much is already known or the data under analysis are too limited to yield even modestly precise estimates. The latter situation arises not only in small studies, but also in large studies that must deal with many variables at once, or that fail to measure key variables with sufficient accuracy.

Chapter 18 provides further discussion of these issues, and shows how to do basic Bayesian analysis of categorical (tabular) data using ordinary frequentist software. Similar Bayesian methods for epidemiologic regression analysis are given by Greenland (2007ab).

CONCLUSION

Statistics can be viewed as having a number of roles in epidemiology. Data description is one role, and statistical inference is another. The two are sometimes mixed, to the detriment of both activities, and are best distinguished from the outset of an analysis.

Different schools of statistics view statistical inference as having different roles in data analysis. The hypothesis-testing approach treats statistics as chiefly a collection of methods for making decisions, such as whether an association is present in a source population or "superpopulation" from which the data are randomly drawn. This approach has been declining in the face of criticisms that estimation, not decision making, is the proper role for statistical inference in science. Within the latter view, frequentist approaches derive estimates by using probabilities of data (either P-values or likelihoods) as measures of compatibility between data and hypotheses, or as measures of the relative support that data provide hypotheses. In contrast, the Bayesian approach uses data to improve existing (prior) estimates in light of new data. Different approaches can be used in the course of an analysis. Nonetheless, proper use of any approach requires more careful interpretation of statistics than has been common in the past.

CHAPTER 11

Design Strategies to Improve Study Accuracy

Kenneth J. Rothman, Sander Greenland, and Timothy L. Lash

Design Options to Control Confounding 168
Experiments and Randomization 168
Restriction 169
Apportionment Ratios to Improve Study Efficiency 169
Matching 171
Purpose and Effect of Matching 171
Matching in Cohort Studies 174
Matching in Case-Control Studies 175
Overmatching 179
Matching on Indicators of Information Accuracy 181
Alternatives to Traditional Matched Designs 182

This chapter covers a number of topics specific to the design of cohort and case-control studies. These topics pertain to the overlapping goals of efficient control of confounding and efficient subject selection. We use *efficiency* to refer to both the statistical precision and the cost-effectiveness of the study design.

DESIGN OPTIONS TO CONTROL CONFOUNDING

Various methods are used to help control confounding in the design of epidemiologic studies. One, randomization, is applicable only in experiments. In contrast, restriction is applicable to all study designs. Matching is often treated as another option for control of confounding, but this view is not accurate. The primary benefits of matching (when they arise) are more in the realm of improved *efficiency* in confounder control—that is, an increase in the precision of the confounder-adjusted estimate, for a given study size. Matching is therefore covered in its own section.

EXPERIMENTS AND RANDOMIZATION

When it is practical and ethical to assign exposure to subjects, one can in theory create study cohorts that would have equal incidences of disease in the absence of the assigned exposure and so eliminate the possibility of confounding. If only a few factors determine incidence and if the investigator knows of these factors, an ideal plan might call for exposure assignment that would lead to identical, balanced distributions of these causes of disease in each group. In studies of human disease, however, there are always unmeasured (and unknown) causes of disease that cannot be forced into balance among treatment groups. Randomization is a method that allows one to limit confounding by unmeasured factors probabilistically and to account quantitatively for the potential residual confounding produced by these unmeasured factors.

As mentioned in Chapter 6, randomization does not lead to identical distributions of all factors, but only to distributions that tend, on repeated trials, to be similar for factors that are not affected by treatment. The tendency increases as the sizes of the study groups increase. Thus, randomization works very well to prevent substantial confounding in large studies but is less effective for smaller studies (Rothman, 1977). In the extreme case in which only one randomization unit is included in each group (as in the community fluoridation trial described in Chapters 4 and 6, in which there was only one community in each group), randomization is completely ineffective in preventing confounding. As compensation for its unreliability in small studies, randomization has the advantage of providing a firm basis for calculating confidence limits that allow for confounding by unmeasured, and hence uncontrollable, factors. Because successful randomization allows one to account quantitatively for uncontrollable confounding, randomization is a powerful technique to help ensure valid causal inferences from studies, large or small (Greenland, 1990). Its drawback of being unreliable in small studies can be mitigated by measuring known risk factors before random assignment and then making the random assignments within levels of these factors. Such a process is known as *matched randomization* or *stratified* randomization.

RESTRICTION

A variable cannot produce confounding if it is prohibited from varying. Restricting the admissibility criteria for subjects to be included in a study is therefore an extremely effective method of preventing confounding. If the potentially confounding variable is measured on a nominal scale, such as race or sex, restriction is accomplished by admitting into the study as subjects only those who fall into specified categories (usually just a single category) of each variable of interest. If the potentially confounding variable is measured on a continuous scale such as age, restriction is achieved by defining a range of the variable that is narrow enough to limit confounding by the variable. Only individuals within the range are admitted into the study as subjects. If the variable has little effect within the admissible range, then the variable cannot be an important confounder in the study. Even if the variable has a non-negligible effect in the range, the degree of confounding it produces will be reduced by the restriction, and this remaining confounding can be controlled analytically.

Restriction is an excellent technique for preventing or at least reducing confounding by known factors, because it is not only extremely effective but also inexpensive, and therefore it is very efficient if it does not hamper subject recruitment. The decision about whether to admit a given individual to the study can be made quickly and without reference to other study subjects (as is required for matching). The main disadvantage is that restriction of admissibility criteria can shrink the pool of available subjects below the desired level. When potential subjects are plentiful, restriction can be employed extensively, because it improves validity at low cost. When potential subjects are less plentiful, the advantages of restriction must be weighed against the disadvantages of a diminished study group.

As is the case with restriction based on risk or exposure, one may be concerned that restriction to a homogeneous category of a potential confounder will provide a poor basis for generalization of study results. This concern is valid if one suspects that the effect under study will vary in an important fashion across the categories of the variables used for restriction. Nonetheless, studies that try to encompass a "representative" and thus heterogeneous sample of a general population are often unable to address this concern in an adequate fashion, because in studies based on a "representative" sample, the number of subjects within each subgroup may be too small to allow estimation of the effect within these categories. Depending on the size of the subgroups, a representative sample often yields unstable and hence ambiguous or even conflicting estimates across categories, and hence provides unambiguous information only about the average effect across all subgroups. If important variation (modification) of the effect exists, one or more studies that focus on different subgroups may be more effective in describing it than studies based on representative samples.

APPORTIONMENT RATIOS TO IMPROVE STUDY EFFICIENCY

As mentioned in Chapter 10, one can often apportion subjects into study groups by design to enhance study efficiency. Consider, for example, a cohort study of 100,000 men to determine the magnitude of the reduction in cardiovascular mortality resulting from daily aspirin consumption. A study this large might be thought to have good precision. The frequency of exposure, however, plays a crucial role in precision: If only 100 of the men take aspirin daily, the estimates of effect from the study will be imprecise because very few cases will likely occur in the mere 100 exposed subjects. A much more precise estimate could be obtained if, instead of 100 exposed and 99,900 unexposed subjects, 50,000 exposed and 50,000 unexposed subjects could be recruited instead.

The frequency of the outcome is equally crucial. Suppose the study had 50,000 aspirin users and 50,000 nonusers, but all the men in the study were between the ages of 30 and 39 years. Whereas the balanced exposure allocation enhances precision, men of this age seldom die of cardiovascular disease. Thus, few events would occur in either of the exposure groups, and as a result, effect estimates would be imprecise. A much more precise study would use a cohort at much higher risk, such as one comprising older men. The resulting study would not have the same implications unless it was accepted that the effect measure of interest changed little with age. This concern relates not to precision, but to generalizability, which we discussed in Chapter 9.

Consideration of exposure and outcome frequency must also take account of other factors in the analysis. If aspirin users were all 40 to 49 years old but nonusers were all over age 50, the age discrepancy might severely handicap the study, depending on how these nonoverlapping age distributions were handled in the analysis. For example, if one attempted to stratify by decade of age to control for possible age confounding, there would be no information at all about the effect of aspirin in the data, because no age stratum would have information on both users and nonusers.

Thus, we can see that a variety of design aspects affect study efficiency and in turn affect the precision of study results. These factors include the proportion of subjects exposed, the disease risk of these subjects, and the relation of these study variables to other analysis variables, such as confounders or effect modifiers.

Study efficiency can be judged on various scales. One scale relates the total information content of the data to the total number of subjects (or amount of person-time experience) in the study. One valid design is said to be more statistically efficient than another if the design yields more precise estimates than the other when both are performed with the same number of subjects or person-time (assuming proper study conduct).

Another scale relates the total information content to the costs of acquiring that information. Some options in study design, such as individual matching, may increase the information content per subject studied, but only at an increased cost. Cost efficiency relates the precision of a study to the cost of the study, regardless of the number of subjects in the study. Often the cost of acquiring subjects and obtaining data differs across study groups. For example, retrospective cohort studies often use a reference series from population data because such data can be acquired for a price that is orders of magnitude less than the information on the exposed cohort. Similarly, in case-control studies, eligible cases may be scarce in the source population, whereas those eligible to be controls may be plentiful. In such situations, more precision might be obtained per unit cost by including all eligible cases and then expanding the size of the reference series rather than by expanding the source population to obtain more cases. The success of this strategy depends on the relative costs of acquiring information on cases versus controls and the cost of expanding the source population to obtain more cases—the latter strategy may be very expensive if the study cannot draw on an existing case-ascertainment system (such as a registry).

In the absence of an effect and if no adjustment is needed, the most cost-efficient apportionment ratio is approximately equal to the reciprocal of the square root of the cost ratio (Miettinen, 1969). Thus, if C_1 is the cost of each case and C_0 is the cost of each control, the most cost-efficient apportionment ratio of controls to cases is $(C_1/C_0)^{1/2}$. For example, if cases cost four times as much as controls and there is no effect and no need for adjustments, the most cost-efficient design would include two times as many controls as cases. The square-root rule is applicable only for small or null effects. A more general approach to improving cost efficiency takes into account the conjectured magnitude of the effect and the type of data (Morgenstern and Winn, 1983). These formulas enable the investigator to improve the precision of the estimator of effect in a study for a fixed amount of resources.

Occasionally, one of the comparison groups cannot be expanded, usually because practical constraints limit the feasibility of extending the study period or area. For such a group, the cost of acquiring additional subjects is essentially infinite, and the only available strategy for acquiring more information is to expand the other group. As the size of one group increases relative to the other group, statistical efficiency does not increase proportionally. For example, if there are m cases, no effect, and no need to stratify on any factor, the proportion of the maximum achievable precision that can be obtained by using a control group of size n is $n/(m+n)$, often given as $r/(r+1)$, where

$r = n/m$. This relation implies that, if only 100 cases were available in a case-control study and no stratification was needed, a design with 400 controls could achieve 400/(100 + 400) = 80% of the maximum possible efficiency.

Unfortunately, the formulas we have just described are misleading when comparisons across strata of other factors are needed or when there is an effect. In either case, expansion of just one group may greatly improve efficiency (Breslow et al., 1983). Furthermore, study design formulas that incorporate cost constraints usually treat the costs per subject as fixed within study groups (Meydrech and Kupper, 1978; Thompson et al., 1982). Nonetheless, the cost per subject may change as the number increases; for example, there may be a reduction in cost if the collection time can be expanded and there is no need to train additional interviewers, or there may be an increase in cost if more interviewers need to be trained.

MATCHING

Matching refers to the selection of a reference series—unexposed subjects in a cohort study or controls in a case-control study—that is identical, or nearly so, to the index series with respect to the distribution of one or more potentially confounding factors. Early intuitions about matching were derived from thinking about experiments (in which exposure is assigned by the investigator). In epidemiology, however, matching is applied chiefly in case-control studies, where it represents a very different process from matching in experiments. There are also important differences between matching in experiments and matching in nonexperimental cohort studies.

Matching may be performed subject by subject, which is known as *individual matching,* or for groups of subjects, which is known as *frequency matching*. Individual matching involves selection of one or more reference subjects with matching-factor values equal to those of the index subject. In a cohort study, the index subject is exposed, and one or more unexposed subjects are matched to each exposed subject. In a case-control study, the index subject is a case, and one or more controls are matched to each case. Frequency matching involves selection of an entire stratum of reference subjects with matching-factor values equal to that of a stratum of index subjects. For example, in a case-control study matched on sex, a stratum of male controls would be selected for the male cases, and, separately, a stratum of female controls would be selected for the female cases.

One general observation applies to all matched studies: Matching on a factor may necessitate its control in the analysis. This observation is especially important for case-control studies, in which failure to control a matching factor can lead to biased effect estimates. With individual matching, often each matched set is treated as a distinct stratum if a stratified analysis is conducted. When two or more matched sets have identical values for all matching factors, however, the sets can and for efficiency should be coalesced into a single stratum in the analysis (Chapter 16). Given that strata corresponding to individually matched sets can be coalesced in the analysis, there is no important difference in the proper analysis of individually matched and frequency-matched data.

PURPOSE AND EFFECT OF MATCHING

To appreciate the different implications of matching for cohort and case-control studies, consider the hypothetical target population of 2 million individuals given in Table 11–1. Both the exposure and male sex are risk factors for the disease: Within sex, exposed have 10 times the risk of the unexposed, and within exposure levels, men have five times the risk of women. There is also substantial confounding, because 90% of the exposed individuals are male and only 10% of the unexposed are male. The crude risk ratio in the target population comparing exposed with unexposed is 33, considerably different from the sex-specific value of 10.

Suppose that a cohort study draws an exposed cohort from the exposed target population and matches the unexposed cohort to the exposed cohort on sex. If 10% of the exposed target population is included in the cohort study and these subjects are selected independently of sex, we have approximately 90,000 men and 10,000 women in the exposed cohort. If a comparison group of unexposed subjects is drawn from the 1 million unexposed individuals in the target population independently of sex, the cohort study will have the same confounding as exists in the target population (apart from sampling variability), because the cohort study is then a simple 10% sample of the target population. It is possible, however, to assemble the unexposed cohort so that its proportion

TABLE 11–1

Hypothetical Target Population of 2 Million People, in Which Exposure Increases the Risk 10-Fold, Men Have Five Times the Risk of Women, and Exposure Is Strongly Associated with Being Male

	Men		Women	
	Exposed	Unexposed	Exposed	Unexposed
No. of cases in 1 y	4,500	50	100	90
Total	900,000	100,000	100,000	900,000
1-y risk	0.005	0.0005	0.001	0.001

$$\text{Crude risk ratio} = \frac{(4{,}500 + 100)\,/1{,}000{,}000}{(50 + 90)\,/1{,}000{,}000} = 33$$

of men matches that in the exposed cohort. This matching of the unexposed to the exposed by sex will prevent an association of sex and exposure in the study cohort. Of the 100,000 unexposed men in the target population, suppose that 90,000 are selected to form a matched comparison group for the 90,000 exposed men in the study, and of the 900,000 unexposed women, suppose that 10,000 are selected to match the 10,000 exposed women.

Table 11–2 presents the expected results (if there is no sampling error) from the matched cohort study we have described. The expected risk ratio in the study population is 10 for men and 10 for women and is also 10 in the crude data for the study. The matching has apparently accomplished its purpose: The point estimate is not confounded by sex because matching has prevented an association between sex and exposure in the study cohort.

The situation differs considerably, however, if a case-control study is conducted instead. Consider a case-control study of all 4,740 cases that occur in the source population in Table 11–1 during 1 year. Of these cases, 4,550 are men. Suppose that 4,740 controls are sampled from the source population, matched to the cases by sex, so that 4,550 of the controls are men. Of the 4,740 cases, we expect

TABLE 11–2

Expected Results of a Matched 1-Year Cohort Study of 100,000 Exposed and 100,000 Unexposed Subjects Drawn from the Target Population Described in Table 10–1

	Men		Women	
	Exposed	Unexposed	Exposed	Unexposed
Cases	450	45	10	1
Total	90,000	90,000	10,000	10,000
Approximate expected	RR = 10		RR = 10	

$$\text{Crude risk ratio} = \frac{(450 + 10)\,/100{,}000}{(45 + 1)\,/100{,}000} = 10$$

RR, risk ratio.

TABLE 11–3

Expected Results of Case-Control Study with 4,740 Controls Matched on Sex When the Source Population Is Distributed as in Table 10–1

	Exposed	Unexposed
Cases	4,600	140
Controls	4,114	626

$$\text{Approximate expected crude OR} = \frac{4{,}600\,(626)}{4{,}114\,(140)} = 5.0$$

OR, odds ratio.

4,500 + 100 = 4,600 to be exposed and 4,740 − 4,600 = 140 to be unexposed. Of the 4,550 male controls, we expect about 90%, or 4,095, to be exposed, because 90% of the men in the target population are exposed. Of the 4,740 − 4,550 = 190 female controls, we expect about 10%, or 19, to be exposed, because 10% of the women in the target population are exposed. Hence, we expect 4,095 + 19 = 4,114 controls to be exposed and 4,740 − 4,114 = 626 to be unexposed. The expected distribution of cases and controls is shown in Table 11–3. The crude odds ratio (OR) is much less than the true risk ratio (RR) for exposure effect. Table 11–4 shows, however, that the case-control data give the correct result, RR = 10, when stratified by sex. Thus, unlike the cohort matching, the case-control matching has not eliminated confounding by sex in the crude point estimate of the risk ratio.

The discrepancy between the crude results in Table 11–3 and the stratum-specific results in Table 11–4 results from a bias that is introduced by selecting controls according to a factor that is related to exposure, namely, the matching factor. The bias behaves like confounding, in that the crude estimate of effect is biased but stratification removes the bias. This bias, however, is not a reflection of the original confounding by sex in the source population; indeed, it differs in direction from that bias.

The examples in Tables 11–1 through 11–4 illustrate the following principles: In a cohort study without competing risks or losses to follow-up, no additional action is required in the analysis to control for confounding of the point estimate by the matching factors, because matching unexposed to exposed prevents an association between exposure and the matching factors. (As we will discuss

TABLE 11–4

Expected Results of a Case Control Study of 4,740 Cases and 4,740 Matched Controls When the Source of Subjects Is the Target Population Described in Table 10–1 and Sampling Is Random within Sex

	Men		Women	
	Exposed	Unexposed	Exposed	Unexposed
Cases	4,500	50	100	90
Controls	4,095	455	19	171
Approximate expected	OR = 10		OR = 10	

OR, odds ratio.

later, however, competing risks or losses to follow-up may necessitate control of the matching factors.) In contrast, if the matching factors are associated with the exposure in the source population, matching in a case-control study requires control by matching factors in the analysis, even if the matching factors are not risk factors for the disease.

What accounts for this discrepancy? In a cohort study, matching is of *unexposed* to *exposed* on characteristics ascertained at the start of follow-up, so is undertaken without regard to events that occur during follow-up, including disease occurrence. By changing the distribution of the matching variables in the unexposed population, the matching shifts the risk in this group toward what would have occurred among the actual exposed population if they had been unexposed. In contrast, matching in a case-control study involves matching *nondiseased* to *diseased,* an entirely different process from matching unexposed to exposed. By selecting controls according to matching factors that are associated with exposure, the selection process will be differential with respect to both exposure and disease, thereby resulting in a selection bias that has no counterpart in matched cohort studies. The next sections, on matching in cohort and case-control designs, explore these phenomena in more detail.

MATCHING IN COHORT STUDIES

In cohort studies, matching unexposed to exposed subjects in a constant ratio can prevent confounding of the crude risk difference and ratio by the matched factors because such matching prevents an association between exposure and the matching factors among the study subjects at the start of follow-up. Despite this benefit, matched cohort studies are uncommon. Perhaps the main reason is the great expense of matching large cohorts. Cohort studies ordinarily require many more subjects than case-control studies, and matching is usually a time-consuming process. One exception is when registry data or other database information is used as a data source. In database studies, an unexposed cohort may be matched to an exposed cohort within the data source relatively easily and inexpensively. It also is possible to improve the poor cost efficiency in matched cohort studies by limiting collection of data on unmatched confounders to those matched sets in which an event occurs (Walker, 1982b), but this approach is rare in practice.

Another reason that matched cohort studies are rare may be that cohort matching does not necessarily eliminate the need to control the matching factors. If the exposure and the matching factors affect disease risk or censoring (competing risks and loss to follow-up), the original balance produced by the matching will not extend to the persons and person-time available for the analysis. That is, matching prevents an exposure-matching-factor association only among the original counts of persons at the start of follow-up; the effects of exposure and matching factors may produce an association of exposure and matching factors among the remaining persons and the observed person-time as the cohort is followed over time. Even if only pure-count data and risks are to be examined and no censoring occurs, control of any risk factors used for matching will be necessary to obtain valid standard-deviation estimates for the risk-difference and risk-ratio estimates (Weinberg, 1985; Greenland and Robins, 1985b).

Matching and Efficiency in Cohort Studies

Although matching can often improve statistical efficiency in cohort studies by reducing the standard deviation of effect estimates, such a benefit is not assured if exposure is not randomized (Greenland and Morgenstern, 1990). To understand this difference between nonexperimental and randomized cohort studies, let us contrast the matching protocols in each design. In randomized studies, matching is a type of *blocking*, which is a protocol for randomizing treatment assignment within groups (blocks). In *pairwise blocking,* a pair of subjects with the same values on the matching (blocking) factors is randomized, one to the study treatment and the other to the control treatment. Such a protocol almost invariably produces a statistically more precise (efficient) effect estimate than the corresponding unblocked design, although exceptions can occur (Youkeles, 1963).

In nonexperimental cohort studies, matching refers to a family of protocols for subject selection rather than for treatment assignment. In perhaps the most common cohort-matching protocol, unexposed subjects are selected so that their distribution of matching factors is identical to the distribution in the exposed cohort. This protocol may be carried out by individual or frequency matching. For example, suppose that the investigators have identified an exposed cohort for follow-up, and they tally the age and sex distribution of this cohort. Then, within each age–sex stratum, they may select for follow-up an equal number of unexposed subjects.

In summary, although matching of nonexperimental cohorts may be straightforward, its implications for efficiency are not. Classical arguments from the theory of randomized experiments suggest that matched randomization (blocking) on a risk factor will improve the precision of effect estimation when the outcome under study is continuous; effects are measured as differences of means, and random variation in the outcome can be represented by addition of an independent error term to the outcome. These arguments do not carry over to epidemiologic cohort studies, however, primarily because matched selection alters the covariate distribution of the entire study cohort, whereas matched randomization does not (Greenland and Morgenstern, 1990). Classical arguments also break down when the outcome is discrete, because in that case the variance of the outcome depends on the mean (expected) value of the outcome within each exposure level. Thus, in nonexperimental cohort studies, matching can sometimes harm efficiency, even though it introduces no bias.

MATCHING IN CASE-CONTROL STUDIES

In case-control studies, the selection bias introduced by the matching process can occur whether or not there is confounding by the matched factors in the source population (the population from which the cases arose). If there is confounding in the source population, as there was in the earlier example, the process of matching will superimpose a selection bias over the initial confounding. This bias is generally in the direction of the null value of effect, whatever the nature of the confounding in the source population, because matching selects controls who are more like cases with respect to exposure than would be controls selected at random from the source population. In the earlier example, the strong confounding away from the null in the source population was overwhelmed by stronger bias toward the null in the matched case-control data.

Let us consider more closely why matching in a case-control study introduces bias. The purpose of the control series in a case-control study is to provide an estimate of the distribution of exposure in the source population. If controls are selected to match the cases on a factor that is correlated with the exposure, then the crude exposure frequency in controls will be distorted in the direction of similarity to that of the cases. Matched controls are identical to cases with respect to the matching factor. Thus, if the matching factor were perfectly correlated with the exposure, the exposure distribution of controls would be identical to that of cases, and hence the crude odds ratio would be 1.0.

The bias of the effect estimate toward the null value does not depend on the direction of the association between the exposure and the matching factor; as long as there is an association, positive or negative, the crude exposure distribution among controls will be biased in the direction of similarity to that of cases. A perfect negative correlation between the matching factor and the exposure will still lead to identical exposure distributions for cases and controls and a crude odds ratio of 1.0, because each control is matched to the identical value of the matching factor of the case, guaranteeing identity for the exposure variable as well.

If the matching factor is not associated with the exposure, then matching will not influence the exposure distribution of the controls, and therefore no bias is introduced by matching. If the matching factor is indeed a confounder, however, the matching factor and the exposure will be associated. (If there were no association, the matching factor could not be a confounder, because a confounding factor must be associated with both the exposure and the disease in the source population.)

Thus, although matching is usually intended to control confounding, it does not attain that objective in case-control studies. Instead, it superimposes over the confounding a selection bias. This selection bias behaves like confounding, because it can be controlled in the analysis by the methods used to control for confounding. In fact, matching can introduce bias when none previously existed: If the matching factor is unrelated to disease in the source population, it would not be a confounder; if it is associated with the exposure, however, matching for it in a case-control study will introduce a controllable selection bias.

This situation is illustrated in Table 11–5, in which the exposure effect corresponds to a risk ratio of 5 and there is no confounding in the source population. Nonetheless, if the cases are selected for a case-control study, and a control series is matched to the cases by sex, the expected value for the crude estimate of effect from the case-control study is 2 rather than the correct value of 5.

TABLE 11–5

Source Population with No Confounding by Sex and a Case-Control Study Drawn from the Source Population, Illustrating the Bias Introduced by Matching on Sex

	Men		Women	
	Exposed	**Unexposed**	**Exposed**	**Unexposed**
A. Source Population				
Disease	450	10	50	90
Total	90,000	10,000	10,000	90,000
	RR = 5		RR = 5	

$$\text{Crude risk ratio} = \frac{(450 + 50)/100{,}000}{(10 + 1)90/100{,}000} = 5$$

	Men		Women	
	Exposed	**Unexposed**	**Exposed**	**Unexposed**
B. Case-Control Study Drawn from Source Population and Matched on Sex				
Cases	450	10	50	90
Controls	414	46	14	126
	OR = 5		OR = 5	

$$\text{Approximate expected crude OR} = \frac{(450 + 50)/(46 + 126)}{(10 + 90)/(414 + 14)} = 2.0$$

RR = risk ratio; OR, odds ratio.

In the source population, sex is not a risk factor because the incidence proportion is 0.001 in both unexposed men and unexposed women. Nevertheless, despite the absence of association between sex and disease within exposure levels in the source population, an association between sex and disease within exposure levels is introduced into the case-control data by matching. The result is that the crude estimate of effect seriously underestimates the correct value.

The bias introduced by matching in a case-control study is by no means irremediable. In Tables 11–4 and 11–5, the stratum-specific estimates of effect are valid; thus, both the selection bias introduced by matching and the original confounding can be dealt with by treating the matching variable as a confounder in the data analysis. Table 11–5 illustrates that, once case-control matching is undertaken, it may prove necessary to stratify on the matching factors, even if the matching factors were not confounders in the source population. Chapter 16 discusses guidelines and methods for control of matching factors.

Matching and Efficiency in Case-Control Studies

It is reasonable to ask why one might consider matching at all in case-control studies. After all, it does not prevent confounding and often introduces a bias. The utility of matching derives not from an ability to prevent confounding, but from the enhanced efficiency that it sometimes affords for the control of confounding. Suppose that one anticipates that age will confound the exposure–disease relation in a given case-control study and that stratification in the analysis will be needed. Suppose further that the age distribution for cases is shifted strongly toward older ages, compared with the age distribution of the entire source population. As a result, without matching, there may be some age strata with many cases and few controls, and others with few cases and many controls. If controls are matched to cases by age, the ratio of controls to cases will instead be constant over age strata.

Suppose now that a certain fixed case series has been or can be obtained for the study and that the remaining resources permit selection of a certain fixed number of controls. There is a most efficient ("optimal") distribution for the controls across the strata, in that selecting controls according to this distribution will maximize statistical efficiency, in the narrow sense of minimizing the variance of a common odds-ratio estimator (such as those discussed in Chapter 15). This "optimal" control distribution depends on the case distribution across strata. Unfortunately, it also depends on the unknown stratum-specific exposure prevalences among cases and noncases in the source population. Thus, this "optimal" distribution cannot be known in advance and used for control selection. Also, it may not be the scientifically most relevant choice; for example, this distribution assumes that the ratio measure is constant across strata, which is never known to be true and may often be false (in which case a focus on estimating a common ratio measure is questionable). Furthermore, if the ratio measure varies across strata, the most efficient distribution for estimating that variation in the effect measure may be far from the most efficient distribution for estimating a uniform (homogeneous) ratio measure.

Regardless of the estimation goal, however, extreme inefficiency occurs when controls are selected that are in strata that have no case (infinite control/case ratio) or when no control is selected in strata with one or more cases (zero control/case ratio). Strata without cases or controls are essentially discarded by stratified analysis methods. Even in a study in which all strata have both cases and controls, efficiency can be considerably harmed if the subject-selection strategy leads to a case-control distribution across strata that is far from the one that is most efficient for the estimation goal.

Matching forces the controls to have the same distribution of matching factors across strata as the cases, and hence prevents extreme departures from what would be the optimal control distribution for estimating a uniform ratio measure. Thus, given a fixed case series and a fixed number of controls, matching often improves the efficiency of a stratified analysis. There are exceptions, however. For example, the study in Table 11–4 yields a less efficient analysis for estimating a uniform ratio than an unmatched study with the same number of controls, because the matched study leads to an expected cell count in the table for women of only 19 exposed controls, whereas in an unmatched study no expected cell count is smaller than 50. This example is atypical because it involves only two strata and large numbers within the cells. In studies that require fine stratification whether matched or not, and so yield sparse data (expected cell sizes that are small, so that zero cells are common within strata), matching will usually result in higher efficiency than what can be achieved without matching.

In summary, matching in case-control studies can be considered a means of providing a more efficient stratified analysis, rather than a direct means of preventing confounding. Stratification (or an equivalent regression approach; see Chapter 21) may still be necessary to control the selection bias and any confounding left after matching, but matching will often make the stratification more efficient. One should always bear in mind, however, that case-control matching on a nonconfounder will usually harm efficiency, for then the more efficient strategy will usually be neither to match nor to stratify on the factor.

If there is some flexibility in selecting cases as well as controls, efficiency can be improved by altering the case distribution, as well as the control distribution, to approach a more efficient case-control distribution across strata. In some instances in which a uniform ratio is assumed, it may turn out that the most efficient approach is restriction of all subjects to one stratum (rather than matching across multiple strata). Nonetheless, in these and similar situations, certain study objectives may weigh against use of the most efficient design for estimating a uniform effect. For example, in a study of the effect of occupational exposures on lung cancer risk, the investigators may wish to ensure that there are sufficient numbers of men and women to provide reasonably precise sex-specific estimates of these effects. Because most lung cancer cases in industrialized countries occur in men and most high-risk occupations are held by men, a design with equal numbers of men and women cases would probably be less efficient for estimating summary effects than other designs, such as one that matched controls to a nonselective series of cases.

Partial or incomplete matching, in which the distribution of the matching factor or factors is altered from that in the source population part way toward that of the cases, can sometimes improve efficiency over no matching and thus can be worthwhile when complete matching cannot be done (Greenland, 1986a). In some situations, partial matching can even yield more efficient estimates than complete matching (Stürmer and Brenner, 2001). There are a number of more complex schemes for control sampling to improve efficiency beyond that achievable by ordinary matching, such as countermatching; see citations at the end of this section.

Costs of Matching in Case-Control Studies

The statistical efficiency that matching provides in the analysis of case-control data often comes at a substantial cost. One part of the cost is a research limitation: If a factor has been matched in a case-control study, it is no longer possible to estimate the effect of that factor from the stratified data alone, because matching distorts the relation of the factor to the disease. It is still possible to study the factor as a modifier of relative risk (by seeing how the odds ratio varies across strata). If certain population data are available, it may also be possible to estimate the effect of the matching factor (Greenland, 1981; Benichou and Wacholder, 1994).

A further cost involved with individual matching is the possible expense entailed in the process of choosing control subjects with the same distribution of matching factors found in the case series. If several factors are being matched, it may be necessary to examine data on many potential control subjects to find one that has the same characteristics as the case. Whereas this process may lead to a statistically efficient analysis, the statistical gain may not be worth the cost in time and money.

If the efficiency of a study is judged from the point of view of the amount of information per subject studied (size efficiency), matching can be viewed as an attempt to improve study efficiency. Alternatively, if efficiency is judged as the amount of information per unit of cost involved in obtaining that information (cost efficiency), matching may paradoxically have the opposite effect of decreasing study efficiency, because the effort expended in finding matched subjects might be spent instead simply in gathering information for a greater number of unmatched subjects. With matching, a stratified analysis would be more size efficient, but without it the resources for data collection can increase the number of subjects, thereby improving cost efficiency. Because cost efficiency is a more fundamental concern to an investigator than size efficiency, the apparent efficiency gains from matching are sometimes illusory.

The cost objections to matching apply to cohort study (exposed/unexposed) matching as well as to case-control matching. In general, then, a beneficial effect of matching on overall study efficiency, which is the primary reason for employing matching, is not guaranteed. Indeed, the decision to match subjects can result in less overall information, as measured by the expected width of the confidence interval for the effect measure, than could be obtained without matching, especially if the expense of matching reduces the total number of study subjects. A wider appreciation for the costs that matching imposes and the often meager advantages it offers would presumably reduce the use of matching and the number of variables on which matching is performed.

Another underappreciated drawback of case-control matching is its potential to increase bias due to misclassification. This problem can be especially severe if one forms unique pair matches on a variable associated only with exposure and the exposure is misclassified (Greenland, 1982a).

Benefits of Matching in Case-Control Studies

There are some situations in which matching is desirable or even necessary. If the process of obtaining exposure and confounder information from the study subjects is expensive, it may be more efficient to maximize the amount of information obtained per subject than to increase the number of subjects. For example, if exposure information in a case-control study involves an expensive laboratory test run on blood samples, the money spent on individual matching of subjects may provide more information overall than could be obtained by spending the same money on finding more subjects. If no confounding is anticipated, of course, there is no need to match; for example, restriction of both series might prevent confounding without the need for stratification or matching. If confounding is likely, however, matching will ensure that control of confounding in the analysis will not lose information that has been expensive to obtain.

Sometimes one cannot control confounding efficiently unless matching has prepared the way to do so. Imagine a potential confounding factor that is measured on a nominal scale with many categories; examples are variables such as neighborhood, sibship, referring physician, and occupation. Efficient control of sibship is impossible unless sibling controls have been selected for the cases; that is, matching on sibship is a necessary prerequisite to obtain an estimate that is both unconfounded and reasonably precise. These variables are distinguished from other nominal-scale variables such as ethnicity by the inherently small number of potential subjects available for each category. This situation is called a *sparse-data* problem: Although many subjects may be available, any given category has little chance of showing up in an unmatched sample. Without matching, most strata in a stratified analysis will have only one subject, either a case or a control, and thus will supply no information about the effect when using elementary stratification methods (Chapters 15 and 16). Matching does not prevent the data from being sparse, but it does ensure that, after stratification by the matched factor, each stratum will have both cases and controls.

Although continuous variables such as age have a multitude of values, their values are either easily combined by grouping or they may be controlled directly as continuous variables, avoiding the sparse-data problem. Grouping may leave residual confounding, however, whereas direct control requires the use of explicit modeling methods. Thus, although matching is not essential for control of such variables, it does facilitate their control by more elementary stratification methods.

A fundamental problem with stratified analysis is the difficulty of controlling confounding by several factors simultaneously. Control of each additional factor involves spreading the existing data over a new dimension; the total number of strata required becomes exponentially large as the number of stratification variables increases. For studies with many confounding factors, the number of strata in a stratified analysis that controls all factors simultaneously may be so large that the situation mimics one in which there is a nominal-scale confounder with a multitude of categories: There may be no case or no control in many strata, and hardly any comparative information about the effect in any stratum. Consequently, if a large number of confounding factors is anticipated, matching may be desirable to ensure that an elementary stratified analysis is informative. But, as pointed out earlier, attempting to match on many variables may render the study very expensive or make it impossible to find matched subjects. Thus, the most practical option is often to match only on age, sex, and perhaps one or a few nominal-scale confounders, especially those with a large number of possible values. Any remaining confounders can be controlled along with the matching factors by stratification or regression methods.

We can summarize the utility of matching as follows: Matching is a useful means for improving study efficiency in terms of the amount of information per subject studied, in some but not all situations. Case-control matching is helpful for known confounders that are measured on a nominal scale, especially those with many categories. The ensuing analysis is best carried out in a manner that controls for both the matching variables and unmatched confounders. We will discuss principles for control of matching variables in Chapter 16.

OVERMATCHING

A term that is often used with reference to matched studies is *overmatching*. There are at least three forms of overmatching. The first refers to matching that harms statistical efficiency, such as case-control matching on a variable associated with exposure but not disease. The second refers to matching that harms validity, such as matching on an intermediate between exposure and disease. The third refers to matching that harms cost efficiency.

Overmatching and Statistical Efficiency

As illustrated in Table 11–5, case-control matching on a nonconfounder associated with exposure but not disease can cause the factor to behave like a confounder: control of the factor will be necessary if matching is performed, whereas no control would have been needed if it had not been matched. The introduction of such a variable into the stratification ordinarily reduces the efficiency relative to an unmatched design in which no control of the factor would be needed (Kupper et al., 1981; Smith and Day, 1981; Thomas and Greenland, 1983). To explore this type of overmatching further, consider a matched case-control study of a binary exposure, with one control matched to each case on one or more nonconfounders. Each stratum in the analysis will consist of one case and one control unless some strata can be combined. If the case and its matched control are either both exposed or both unexposed, one margin of the 2×2 table will be 0. As one may verify from the Mantel-Haenszel odds-ratio formula in Chapter 15, such a pair of subjects will not contribute any information to the analysis. If one stratifies on correlates of exposure, one will increase the chance that such tables will occur and thus tend to increase the information lost in a stratified analysis. This information loss detracts from study efficiency, reducing both information per subject studied and information per dollar spent. Thus, by forcing one to stratify on a nonconfounder, matching can detract from study efficiency. Because the matching was not necessary in the first place and has the effect of impairing study efficiency, matching in this situation can properly be described as overmatching.

This first type of overmatching can thus be understood to be matching that causes a loss of information in the analysis because the resulting stratified analysis would have been unnecessary without matching. The extent to which information is lost by matching depends on the degree of correlation between the matching factor and the exposure. A strong correlate of exposure that has no relation to disease is the worst candidate for matching, because it will lead to relatively few informative strata in the analysis with no offsetting gain. Consider, for example, a study of the relation between coffee drinking and bladder cancer. Suppose that matching for consumption of cream substitutes is considered along with matching for a set of other factors. Because this factor is strongly associated with coffee consumption, many of the individual strata in the matched analysis will be completely concordant for coffee drinking and will not contribute to the analysis; that is, for many of the cases, controls matched to that case will be classified identically to the case with regard to coffee drinking simply because of matching for consumption of cream substitutes. If cream substitutes have no relation to bladder cancer, nothing is accomplished by the matching except to burden the analysis with the need to control for use of cream substitutes. This problem corresponds to the unnecessary analysis burden that can be produced by attempting to control for factors that are related only to exposure or exposure opportunity (Poole, 1986), which is a form of *overadjustment* (Chapter 15).

These considerations suggest a practical rule for matching: Do not match on a factor that is associated only with exposure. It should be noted, however, that unusual examples can be constructed in which case-control matching on a factor that is associated only with exposure improves efficiency (Kalish, 1986). More important, in many situations the potential matching factor will have at least a weak relation to the disease, and so it will be unclear whether the factor needs to be controlled as a confounder and whether matching on the factor will benefit statistical efficiency. In such situations, considerations of cost efficiency and misclassification may predominate.

When matched and unmatched controls have equal cost and the potential matching factor is to be treated purely as a confounder, with only summarization (pooling) across the matching strata desired, we recommend that one avoid matching on the factor unless the factor is expected to be a strong disease risk factor with at least some association with exposure (Smith and Day, 1981; Howe and Choi, 1983; Thomas and Greenland, 1983). When costs of matched and unmatched controls differ, efficiency calculations that take account of the cost differences can be performed and used to choose a design strategy (Thompson et al., 1982). When the primary interest in the factor is as an effect modifier rather than confounder, the aforementioned guidelines are not directly relevant. Nonetheless, certain studies have indicated that matching can have a greater effect on efficiency (both positive and negative) when the matching factors are to be studied as effect modifiers, rather than treated as pure confounders (Smith and Day, 1984; Thomas and Greenland, 1985).

Overmatching and Bias

Matching on factors that are affected by the study exposure or disease is almost never warranted and is potentially capable of biasing study results beyond any hope of repair. It is therefore crucial to understand the nature of such overmatching and why it needs to be avoided.

Case-control matching on a factor that is affected by exposure but is unrelated to disease in any way (except possibly through its association with exposure) will typically reduce statistical efficiency. It corresponds to matching on a factor that is associated only with exposure, which was discussed at length earlier, and is the most benign possibility of those that involve matching for a factor that is affected by exposure. If, however, the potential matching factor is affected by exposure and the factor in turn affects disease (i.e., is an intermediate variable), or is affected by both exposure and disease, then matching on the factor will bias both the crude and the adjusted effect estimates (Greenland and Neutra, 1981). In these situations, case-control matching is nothing more than an irreparable form of selection bias (see Chapters 8 and 12).

To see how this bias arises, consider a situation in which the crude estimate from an unmatched study is unbiased. If exposure affects the potential matching factor and this factor affects or is affected by disease, the factor will be associated with both exposure and disease in the source population. As a result, in all but some exceptional situations, the associations of exposure with disease within the strata of the factor will differ from the crude association. Because the crude association is unbiased, it follows that the stratum-specific associations must be biased for the true exposure effect.

The latter bias will pose no problem if we do not match our study subjects on the factor, because then we need only ignore the factor and use the crude estimate of effect (which is unbiased in this example). If we (inappropriately) adjust for the factor, we will bias our estimate (sometimes called *overadjustment bias*; see Chapter 15), but we can avoid this bias simply by not adjusting for the factor. If, however, we match on the factor, we will shift the exposure prevalence among noncases toward that of the cases, thereby driving the crude effect estimate toward the null. The stratified estimates will remain biased. With matching, then, both the crude and stratum-specific estimates will be biased, and we will be unable to obtain an unbiased effect estimate from the study data alone.

It follows that, if (as usual) interest is in estimating the net effect of exposure on disease, one should never match on factors that are affected by exposure or disease, such as symptoms or signs of the exposure or the disease, because such matching can irreparably bias the study data. The only exceptions are when the relative selection probabilities for the subjects under the matched design are known and can be used to adjust the estimates back to their expected unmatched form (Chapter 19).

Overmatching and Cost Efficiency

Some methods for obtaining controls automatically entail matching. Examples include neighborhood controls, sibling controls, and friend controls (Chapter 8). One should consider the potential consequences of the matching that results from the use of such controls. As an example, in a case-control study it is sometimes very economical to recruit controls by asking each case to provide the names of several friends who might serve as controls, and to recruit one or more of these friends to serve as controls. As discussed in Chapter 8, use of friend controls may induce bias under ordinary circumstances. Even when this bias is negligible, however, friendship may be related to exposure (e.g., through lifestyle factors), but not to disease. As a result, use of such friend controls could entail a statistical efficiency loss because such use corresponds to matching on a factor that is related only to exposure. More generally, the decision to use convenient controls should weigh any cost savings against any efficiency loss and bias relative to the viable alternatives (e.g., general population controls). Ordinarily, one would prefer the strategy that has the lowest total cost among strategies that are expected to have the least bias.

The problem of choice of strategy can be reformulated for situations in which the number of cases can be varied and situations in which the numbers of cases and controls are both fixed (Thompson et al., 1982). Unfortunately, one rarely knows in advance the key quantities needed to make the best choice with certainty, such as cost per control with each strategy, the number of subjects that will be needed with each strategy, and the biases that might ensue with each strategy. The choice will be easy when the same bias is expected regardless of strategy, and the statistically most efficient strategy is also the cheapest per subject: One should simply use that strategy. But in other settings, one may be able to do no better than conduct a few rough, speculative calculations to guide the choice of strategy.

MATCHING ON INDICATORS OF INFORMATION ACCURACY

Matching is sometimes employed to achieve comparability in the accuracy of information collected. A typical situation in which such matching might be undertaken is a case-control study in which some or all of the cases have already died and surrogates must be interviewed for exposure and confounder information. Theoretically, controls for dead cases should be living, because the source population that gave rise to the cases contains only living persons. In practice, because surrogate interview data may differ in accuracy from interview data obtained directly from the subject, some investigators prefer to match dead controls to dead cases.

Matching on information accuracy is not necessarily beneficial, however. Whereas using dead controls can be justified in proportional mortality studies, essentially as a convenience (see Chapter 6), matching on information accuracy does not always reduce overall bias (see Chapter 8). Some of the assumptions about the accuracy of surrogate data, for example, are unproved (Gordis, 1982). Furthermore, comparability of information accuracy still allows bias from nondifferential misclassification, which can be more severe in matched than in unmatched studies (Greenland, 1982a), and more severe than the bias resulting from differential misclassification arising from noncomparability (Greenland and Robins, 1985a; Drews and Greenland, 1990).

ALTERNATIVES TO TRADITIONAL MATCHED DESIGNS

Conventional matched and unmatched designs represent only two points on a broad spectrum of matching strategies. Among potentially advantageous alternatives are partial and marginal matching (Greenland, 1986a), countermatching (Langholz and Clayton, 1994; Cologne et al., 2004), and other matching strategies for improving efficiency (Stürmer and Brenner, 2002). Some of these approaches can be more convenient, as well as more efficient, than conventional matched or unmatched designs. For example, partial matching allows selection of matched controls for some subjects, unmatched controls for others, and the use of different matching factors for different subjects, where the "controls" may be either the unexposed in a cohort study or the noncases in a case-control study. Marginal matching is a form of frequency matching in which only the marginal (separate) distributions of the matching factors are forced to be alike, rather than the joint distribution. For example, one may select controls so that they have the same age and sex distributions as cases, without forcing them to have the same age–sex distribution (e.g., the proportion of men could be the same in cases and controls, even though the proportion of 60- to 64-year-old men might be different).

For both partial and marginal matching, the resulting data can be analyzed by treating all matching factors as stratification variables and following the guidelines for matched-data analysis given in Chapter 16. An advantage of partial and marginal matching is that one need not struggle to find a perfect matched control for each case (in a case-control study) or for each exposed subject (in a cohort study). Thus partial matching may save considerable effort in searching for suitable controls.

CHAPTER 12

Causal Diagrams

M. Maria Glymour and Sander Greenland

Introduction 183

Preliminaries for Causal Graphs 184

Statistical Independence 184

Causation and Association 185

Collider Bias 185

Summary 186

Graphical Models 186

Terminology 186

Rules Linking Absence of Open Paths to Statistical Independencies 187

Assumptions and Intuitions Underlying the Rules 190

Graphical Representation of Bias and its Control 191

Sufficient and Minimally Sufficient Conditioning Sets 192

Choosing Conditioning Sets to Identify Causal Effects 192

Confounding and Selection Bias 192

Some Applications 194

Why Conventional Rules for Confounding Are Not Always Reliable 194

Graphical Analyses of Selection Bias 196

Bias from Intentional Selection 196

Survivor Bias 198

Residual Confounding and Bias Quantification 198

Bias from Use of Missing-Data Categories or Indicators 199

Adjusting for an Intermediate Does Not Necessarily Estimate a Direct Effect 200

Instrumental Variables 202

Bias from Conditioning on a Descendant of the Outcome 204

Selection Bias and Matching in Case-Control Studies 205

How Adjusting for Baseline Values Can Bias Analyses of Change 206

Caveats and Extensions 208

Conclusion 209

INTRODUCTION

Diagrams of causal pathways have long been used to visually summarize hypothetical relations among variables of interest. Modern causal diagrams, or causal graphs, were more recently developed from a merger of graphical probability theory with path diagrams. The resulting theory provides a powerful yet intuitive device for deducing the statistical associations implied by causal relations. Conversely, given a set of observed statistical relations, a researcher armed with causal graph theory can systematically characterize all causal structures compatible with the observations. The theory also provides a visual representation of key concepts in the more general theory of longitudinal causality of Robins (1997); see Chapter 21 for further discussion and references on the latter topic.

The graphical rules linking causal relations to statistical associations are grounded in mathematics. Hence, one way to think of causal diagrams is that they allow nonmathematicians to draw logically sound conclusions about certain types of statistical relations. Learning the rules for reading statistical associations from causal diagrams may take a little time and practice. Once these rules are mastered, though, they facilitate many tasks, such as understanding confounding and selection bias, choosing covariates for adjustment and for regression analyses, understanding analyses of direct effects and instrumental-variable analyses, and assessing "natural experiments." In particular, diagrams help researchers recognize and avoid common mistakes in causal analysis.

This chapter begins with the basic definitions and assumptions used in causal graph theory. It then describes construction of causal diagrams and the graphical separation rules linking the causal assumptions encoded in a diagram to the statistical relations implied by the diagram. The chapter concludes by presenting some examples of applications. Some readers may prefer to begin with the examples and refer back to the definitions and rules for causal diagrams as needed. The section on Graphical Models, however, is essential to understanding the examples. Full technical details of causal diagrams and their relation to causal inference can be found in Pearl (2000) and Spirtes et al. (2001), while Greenland and Pearl (2008) provide a short technical review. Less technical articles geared toward health scientists include Greenland et al. (1999a), Robins (2001), Greenland and Brumback (2002), Hernán et al. (2002), Jewell (2004), and Glymour (2006b).

PRELIMINARIES FOR CAUSAL GRAPHS

Consider two variables X and Y for which we wish to represent a causal connection from X to Y, often phrased as "X causes Y" or "X affects Y." Causal diagrams may be constructed with almost any definition of cause and effect in mind. Nonetheless, as emphasized in Chapter 4, it is crucial to distinguish causation from mere association. For this purpose we use the potential-outcome (counterfactual) concept of causation. We say that X affects Y in a population of units (which may be people, families, neighborhoods, etc.) if and only if there is at least one unit for which changing (intervening on) X will change Y (Chapter 4).

STATISTICAL INDEPENDENCE

Association of X and Y corresponds to statistical dependence of Y and X, whereby the distribution of Y differs across population strata defined by levels of X. When the distribution of Y does not differ across strata of X, we say that X and Y are statistically independent, or unassociated. If X and Y are unassociated (independent), knowing the value of X gives us no information about the value of Y. Association refers to differences in Y *between* units with different X values. Such between-unit differences do not necessarily imply that changing the value of X for any single unit will result in a change in Y (which is causation).

It is helpful to rephrase the above ideas more formally. Let $\Pr(Y = y)$ be the expected proportion of people in the population who have y for the value of Y; this expected proportion is more often called the probability that $Y = y$. If we examine the proportion who have $Y = y$ within levels or strata of a second variable X, we say that we are examining the probability of Y *given* or *conditional on* X. We use a vertical line "|" to denote "given" or "conditional on." For example, $\Pr(Y = y|X = x)$ denotes the proportion with $Y = y$ in the subpopulation with $X = x$. Independence of X and Y then corresponds to saying that for any pair of values x and y for X and Y,

$$\Pr(Y = y|X = x) = \Pr(Y = y) \qquad [12\text{–}1]$$

which means that the distribution of Y values does not differ across different subpopulations defined by the X values. In other words, the equation says that the distribution of Y given (or conditional on) a particular value of X always equals the total population (marginal or unconditional) distribution of Y. As stated earlier, if X and Y are independent, knowing the value of X and nothing more about a unit provides no information about the Y value of the unit.

Equation 12–1 involves no variable other than X and Y, and is the definition of *marginal* independence of X and Y. When we examine the relations between two variables within levels of a third variable—for example, the relation between income and mortality within levels of education—we say that we are examining the conditional relation. We examine conditional relationships in many contexts in epidemiology. We may intentionally condition on a variable(s) through features of study design such as restriction or matching, or analytic decisions, such as stratification or regression modeling. Conditioning may arise inadvertently as well, for example due to refusal to participate or loss to follow-up. These events essentially force conditioning on variables that determine participation and ascertainment. Informally, it is sometimes said that conditioning on a variable is "holding the variable constant," but this phrase is misleading because it suggests we are actively intervening on the value of the variable, when all we are doing is separating the data into groups based on observed values of the variable and estimating the effects within these groups (and then, in some cases, averaging these estimates over the groups, see Chapter 15).

To say that X and Y are independent given Z means that for any values x, y, z for X, Y, and Z,

$$\Pr(Y = y|X = x, Z = z) = \Pr(Y = y|Z = z) \quad [12\text{–}2]$$

which says that, within any stratum of Z, the distribution of Y does not vary with X. In other words, within any stratum defined in terms of Z alone, we should see no association between X and Y. If X and Y are independent given Z, then once one knows the Z value of a unit, finding out the value of X provides no further information about the value of Y.

CAUSATION AND ASSOCIATION

As explained in Chapter 4, causation and association are qualitatively different concepts. Causal relations are directed; associations are undirected (symmetric). Sample associations are directly observable, but causation is not. Nonetheless, our intuition tells us that associations are the result of causal forces. Most obviously, if X causes Y, this will generally result in an association between X and Y. The catch, of course, is that even if we observe X and Y without error, many other forces (such as confounding and selection) may also affect the distribution of Y and thus induce an association between X and Y that is not due to X causing Y. Furthermore, unlike causation, association is symmetric in time (nondirectional), e.g., an association of X and Y could reflect Y causing X rather than X causing Y.

A study of causation must describe plausible explanations for observed associations in terms of causal structures, assess the logical and statistical compatibility of these structures with the observations, and (in some cases) develop probabilities for those structures. Causal graphs provide schematic diagrams of causal structures, and the independencies predicted by a graph provide a means to assess the compatibility of each causal structure with the observations.

More specifically, when we see an association of X and Y, we will seek sound explanations for this observation. For example, logically, if X always precedes Y, we know that Y cannot be causing X. Given that X precedes Y, obvious explanations for the association are that X causes Y, that X and Y share a common cause (confounding), or some combination of the two (which can also lead to no association even though X affects Y). Collider bias is a third type of explanation that seems much less intuitive but is easily illustrated with graphs. We will first discuss focus on collider bias because it arises frequently in epidemiology.

COLLIDER BIAS

As described in Chapter 9, a potentially large source of bias in assessing the effect of X on Y arises when selection into the population under study or into the study sample itself is affected by both X and Y. Such selection is a source of bias even if X and Y are independent before selection. This phenomenon was first described by Joseph Berkson in 1938 (published in Berkson [1946]). *Berksonian bias* is an example of the more general phenomenon called *collider bias,* in which the association of two variables X and Y changes upon conditioning on a third variable Z if Z is affected by both X and Y. The effects of X and Y are said to "collide" somewhere along the way to producing Z.

As an example, suppose that X and Y are marginally independent and $Z = Y - X$, so Z is completely determined by X and Y. Then X and Y will exhibit perfect dependence given Z: If $Z = z$, then $Y = X + z$. As a more concrete example, body mass index (BMI) is defined as (weight in kg)/(height in meters)^2 and so is strongly affected by both height and weight. Height and weight are associated in any natural population, but not perfectly: We could not exactly tell a person's weight from his or her height. Suppose, however, we learn that the person has BMI = 25 kg/m^2;

then, upon being told (say) that the person is 2 m tall, we can compute his weight exactly, as BMI(height^2) = 25(4) = 100 kg.

Collider bias occurs even when the causal dependency of the collider Z on X and Y is not perfect, and when there are several intermediates between X and the collider or between Y and the collider. It can also be induced when X and Z (or Y and Z) are associated due to a common cause rather than because X influences Z.

Collider bias can result from sample selection, stratification, or covariate adjustment if X and Y affect selection or the stratifying covariates. It can be just as severe as confounding, as shown in the classic example in which X, Y, and Z were exogenous estrogen use, endometrial cancer, and uterine bleeding (Chapter 9). As discussed later, it can also can induce confounding.

SUMMARY

Four distinct causal structures can contribute to an association between X and Y: (a) X may cause Y; (b) Y may cause X; (c) X and Y may share a common cause that we have failed to condition on (confounding); or (d) we have conditioned or selected on a variable affected by X and Y, factors influenced by such a variable, or a variable that shares causes with X and Y (collider bias). Of course, the observed association may also have been affected by purely random events. As described in Part III of this book, conventional statistics focus on accounting for the resulting random variation. The remainder of this chapter focuses on the representation of causal structures via graphical models, and on the insights that these representations provide. Throughout, we focus on the causal structures underlying our observations, ignoring random influences.

GRAPHICAL MODELS

TERMINOLOGY

Causal diagrams visually encode an investigator's assumptions about causal relations among the exposure, outcomes, and covariates. We say that a variable X affects a variable Y *directly* (relative to the other variables in the diagram) if there is an arrow from X to Y. We say that X affects Y *indirectly* if there is a head-to-tail sequence of arrows (or "one-way street") from X to Y; such a sequence is called a *directed path* or *causal path*. Any variable along a causal path from X to Y is called an *intermediate variable* between X and Y. X may affect Y both directly and indirectly. In Figure 12–1, X affects Y directly and Z indirectly. The absence of a directed path between two variables represents the assumption that neither affects the other; in Figure 12–1, U and X do not affect each other.

Children of a variable X are variables that are affected directly by X (have an arrow pointing to them from X); conversely, *parents* of X are variables that directly affect X (have an arrow pointing from them to X). More generally, the *descendants* of a variable X are variables affected, either directly or indirectly, by X; conversely, the *ancestors* of X are all the variables that affect X directly or indirectly. In Figure 12–1, Y has parents U and X, and a child Z; X has one child (Y) and two descendants (Y and Z); and Z has a parent Y and three ancestors, Y, U, and X.

It is not necessary to include all causes of variables in the diagram. If two or more variables in a graph share a cause, however, then this cause must also be shown in the graph as an ancestor of those variables, or else the graph is not considered a causal graph. A variable with no parents in a causal graph is said to be *exogenous* in the graph; otherwise it is *endogenous*. Thus, all

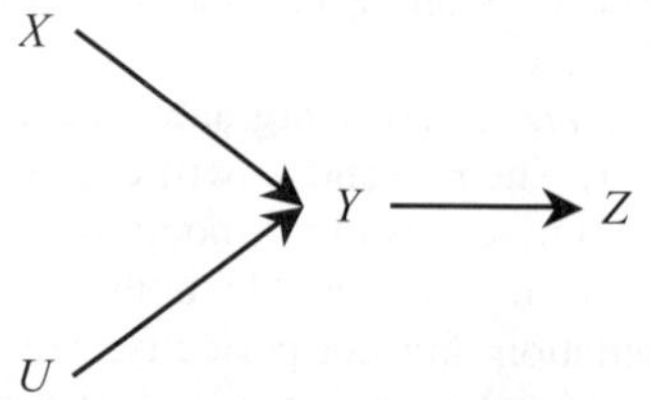

FIGURE 12–1 • A causal diagram with no confounding.

exogenous variables in the graph are assumed to share no cause with other variables in the graph. If unknown common causes of two variables may exist, a casual graph must show them; they may be represented as unspecified variables with arrows to the variables they are thought to influence. In a slight modification of these rules, some authors (e.g., Pearl, 2000) use a two-headed arrow between two variables as a shorthand to indicate that there is at least one unknown exogenous common cause of the two variables (e.g., $X \leftrightarrow Z$ means that there is at least one unknown exogenous variable U such that $X \leftarrow U \rightarrow Z$). We assume in the remainder of this chapter that unknown common causes are represented explicitly in causal diagrams, so there is no need for two-headed arrows.

All the graphs we will consider are *acyclic*, which means that they contain no feedback loops; this means that no variable is an ancestor or descendant of itself, so if X causes Y, Y cannot also cause X at the same moment. If a prior value of Y affects X, and then X affects a subsequent value of Y, these must each be shown as separate variables (e.g., $Y_0 \rightarrow X_1 \rightarrow Y_2$) (for discussions of extensions to causal structures including feedback, see Spirtes [1995], Pearl and Dechter [1996], and Lauritzen and Richardson [2002]). In most causal graphs the only connectors between variables are one-headed arrows ($\rightarrow$), although some graphs use an undirected dashed line (- - -) to indicate associations induced by collider bias. Connectors, whether arrows or dashed lines, are also known as *edges,* and variables are often called *nodes* or *vertices* of the graph. Two variables joined by a connector are said to be *adjacent* or *neighbors*. If the only connectors in the graph are one-headed arrows, the graph is called *directed.* A directed acyclic graph or DAG is thus a graph with only arrows between variables and with no feedback loops. The remainder of our discussion applies to DAGs and graphs that result from conditioning on variables in DAGs.

A *path* between X and Y is any noncrossing and nonrepeating sequence traced out along connectors (also called edges) starting with X and ending with Y, *regardless of the direction of arrowheads.* A variable along the path from X to Y is said to *intercept* the path. Directed paths are the special case in which all the connectors in the path flow head to tail. Any other path is an *undirected path.* In Figure 12–1, $U \rightarrow Y \leftarrow X$ is an undirected path from U to X, and Y intercepts the path.

When tracing out a path, a variable on the path where two arrowheads meet is called a *collider* on that path. In Figure 12–1, Y is a collider on the path $U \rightarrow Y \leftarrow X$ from U to X. Thus, a collider on a path is a direct effect (child) of both the variable just before it and the variable just after it on the path. A directed path cannot contain a collider. If a variable on a path has neighbors on both sides but is not a collider, then the variable must be either an intermediate ($X \rightarrow Y \rightarrow Z$ or $X \leftarrow Y \leftarrow Z$) or a cause ($X \leftarrow Y \rightarrow Z$) of its immediate neighbors on the path.

Being a collider is specific to a path. In the same DAG, a variable may be a collider on one path but an intermediate on another path; e.g., in Figure 12–1, Y is an intermediate rather than a collider on the path $X \rightarrow Y \rightarrow Z$. Nonetheless, a variable with two or more parents (direct causes) is called a collider in the graph, to indicate that it is a collider on at least one path. As we will see, paths with colliders can turn out to be sources of confounding and selection bias.

RULES LINKING ABSENCE OF OPEN PATHS TO STATISTICAL INDEPENDENCIES

Given a causal diagram, we can apply the *d-separation criteria* (or directed graph separation rules) to deduce independencies implied by the diagram. We first focus on rules for determining whether two variables are d-separated unconditionally, and then examine how conditioning on variables may d-separate or d-connect other variables in the graph. We emphasize that the deduced relations apply only "in expectation," meaning that they apply to the *expected* data distribution if the causal structure represented by the graph is correct. They do not describe the associations that may arise as a result of purely random events, such as those produced by randomization or random sampling.

Unconditional d-Separation

A path is said to be *open* or *unblocked* or *active* unconditionally if there is no collider on the path. Otherwise, if there is a collider on the path, it is said to be *closed* or *blocked* or *inactive,* and we say that the collider blocks the path. By definition a directed path has no collider, so every directed path is open, although not every open path is directed. Two variables X and Y are said to be *d-separated* if there is no open path between them; otherwise they are *d-connected.* In Figure 12–2, the only path from X to Y is open at Z_1 and Z_2 but closed at W, and hence it is closed overall; thus X and Y

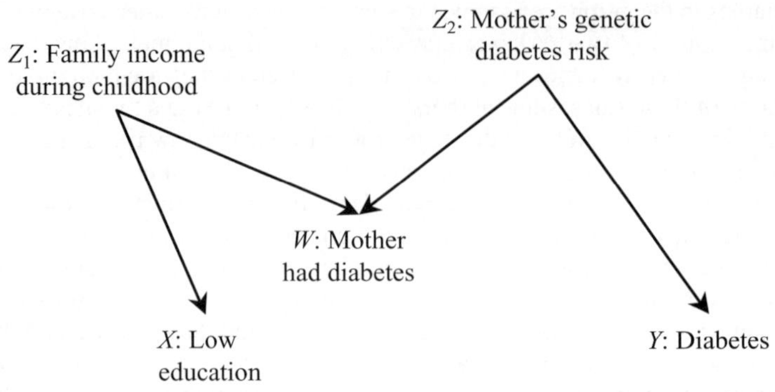

FIGURE 12–2 • A DAG under which traditional confounder-identification rules fail (an "*M* diagram").

are d-separated. When using these terms we will usually drop the "d-" prefix and just say that they are separated or connected as appropriate.

If X and Y are separated in a causal graph, then the causal assumptions encoded by the graph imply that X and Y will be unassociated. Thus, if every path from X to Y is closed, the graph predicts that X and Y will be marginally independent; i.e., for any values x and y of X and Y, $\Pr(Y = y|X = x) = \Pr(Y = y)$. More generally and informally we can say this: In a causal graph, the only sources of marginal association between variables are the open paths between them. Consider Table 12–1, which lists the causal assumptions represented by the diagram of Figure 12–1, and the associations implied by those causal assumptions. For example, the causal diagram implies that U and X are marginally independent because the only path between them passes through a collider, Y. This idea is formalized later when we define compatibility.

Conditional d-Separation

We also need the concept of graphical conditioning. Consider first conditioning on a noncollider Z on a path. Because it is a noncollider, Z must either be an intermediate between its neighbors on the path ($X \rightarrow Z \rightarrow Y$ or $X \leftarrow Z \leftarrow Y$) or a cause of its neighbors ($X \leftarrow Z \rightarrow Y$). In these cases the path is open at Z, but conditioning on Z closes the path and removes Z as a source of association between X and Y. These phenomena reflect the first criterion for blocking paths by conditioning on covariates:

- Conditioning on a noncollider Z on a path blocks the path at Z.

In contrast, conditioning on a collider requires reverse reasoning. If two variables X and Y are marginally independent, we expect them to become associated upon conditioning (stratifying) on a shared effect W. In particular, suppose we are tracing a path from X to Y and reach a segment on the path with a collider, $X \rightarrow W \leftarrow Y$. The path is blocked at W, so no association between X and Y passes through W. Nonetheless, conditioning on W or any descendant of W opens the path at W. In other words, we expect conditioning on W or any descendant to create an X–Y association via W. We thus come to the second criterion for blocking paths by conditioning on covariates:

- Conditioning on a collider W on a path, or any descendant of W, or any combination of W or its descendants, opens the path at W.

Combining these criteria, we see that conditioning on a variable reverses its status on a path: Conditioning closes noncolliders (which are open unconditionally) but opens colliders (which are closed unconditionally).

We say that a set of variables $\mathbf{S}$ *blocks a path* from X to Y if, after conditioning on $\mathbf{S}$, the path is closed (regardless of whether it was closed or open to begin with). Conversely, we say that a set of variables $\mathbf{S}$ unblocks a path if, after conditioning on $\mathbf{S}$, the path is open (regardless of whether it was closed or open to begin with). The criteria for a set of variables to block or unblock a path are summarized in Table 12–2.

TABLE 12–1

Assumptions Represented in the Directed Acyclic Graph in Figure 12–1, and Statistical Implications of These Assumptions

Causal Assumptions Represented in Figure 12–1	Independencies Implied by Figure 12–1	Marginal Associations Expected under Figure 12–1 (Assuming Faithfulness)	Conditional Associations Expected under Figure 12–1 (Assuming Faithfulness)
• X and U are each direct causes of Y (direct with respect to other variables in the diagram). • Y is a direct cause of Z. • X is not a direct cause of Z, but X is an indirect cause of Z via Y. • X is not a cause of U and U is not a cause of X. • U is not a direct cause of Z, but U is an indirect cause of Z via Y. • No two variables in the diagram (X, U, Y, or Z) share a prior cause not shown in the diagram, e.g., no variable causes both X and Y, or both X and U.	• X and U are independent (the only path between them is blocked by the collider Y). • X and Z are independent conditional on Y (conditioning on Y blocks the path between X and Z). • U and Z are independent conditional on Y.	• X and Y are associated. • U and Y are associated. • Y and Z are associated. • X and Z are associated. • U and Z are associated.	• X and U are associated conditional on Y (conditioning on a collider unblocks the path). • X and U are associated conditional on Z (Z is a descendant of the collider Y).

If **S** blocks every path from *X* to *Y*, we say that *X* and *Y* are *d-separated by* **S**, or that **S** *separates* *X* and *Y*. This definition of d-separation includes situations in which there was no open path before conditioning on **S**. For example, a set **S** may be sufficient to separate *X* and *Y* even if **S** includes no variables: if there is no open path between *X* and *Y* to begin with, the empty set separates them.

d-Separation and Statistical Independence

We have now specified the d-separation criteria and explained how to apply them to determine whether two variables in a graph are d-separated or d-connected, either marginally or conditionally. These concepts provide a link between the causal structure depicted in a DAG and the statistical associations we expect in data generated from that causal structure. The following two rules specify the relation between d-separation and statistical independence; these rules underlie the applications we will present.

Rule 1 (compatibility). Suppose that two variables *X* and *Y* in a causal graph are separated by a set of variables **S**. Then if the graph is correct, *X* and *Y* will be unassociated given **S**. In other

TABLE 12–2

Criteria for Determining Whether a Path is Blocked or Unblocked Conditional on a Set of Variables *S*

The Path from X to Y is Blocked Conditional on S if Either:	The Path from X to Y is Unblocked Conditional on S if Both:
A noncollider Z on the path is in $\mathbf{S}$ (because the path will be blocked by $\mathbf{S}$ at Z) OR There is a collider W on the path that is not in $\mathbf{S}$ and has no descendant in $\mathbf{S}$ (because W still blocks the path after conditioning on $\mathbf{S}$).	$\mathbf{S}$ contains no noncollider on the path (so conditioning on $\mathbf{S}$ blocks no noncollider) AND Every collider on the path is either in $\mathbf{S}$ or has a descendant in $\mathbf{S}$ (because conditioning on $\mathbf{S}$ opens every collider).

words, if $\mathbf{S}$ separates X from Y, we will have $\Pr(Y = y|X = x, \mathbf{S} = \mathbf{S}) = \Pr(Y = y|\mathbf{S} = \mathbf{S})$ for every possible value $x, y, \mathbf{S}$ of $X, Y, \mathbf{S}$.

Rule 2 (weak faithfulness). Suppose that $\mathbf{S}$ does not separate X and Y. Then, if the graph is correct, X and Y may be associated given $\mathbf{S}$. In other words, if X and Y are connected given $\mathbf{S}$, then without further information we should not assume that X and Y are independent given $\mathbf{S}$.

As an illustration, consider again Figure 12–1. U and X are unassociated. Because Y is a collider, however, we expect U and X to become associated after conditioning on Y or Z or both (that is, $\mathbf{S}$ unblocks the path whether $\mathbf{S} = \{Y\}$, $\mathbf{S} = \{Z\}$, or $\mathbf{S} = \{Y, Z\}$). In contrast, X and Z are marginally associated, but become independent after conditioning on Y or $\mathbf{S} = \{U, Y\}$.

ASSUMPTIONS AND INTUITIONS UNDERLYING THE RULES

Although informal diagrams of causal paths go back at least to the 1920s, the mathematical theory of graphs (including DAGs) developed separately and did not at first involve causal inference. By the 1980s, however, graphs were being used to represent the structure of joint probability distributions, with d-separation being used to encode "stable" conditional independence relations (Pearl, 1988). One feature of this use of graphs is that a given distribution will have more than one graph that encodes these relations. In other words, graphical representations of probability distributions are not unique. For example, in probabilistic (associational) terms, $A \rightarrow B$ and $B \rightarrow A$ have the same implication, that A and B are dependent. By the 1990s, however, several research groups had adapted these probability graphs to causal inference by letting the arrows represent cause–effect relations, as they had in path diagrams. Many graphical representations that are probabilistically equivalent are not causally equivalent. For example, if A precedes B temporally, then $B \rightarrow A$ can be ruled out as a representation for the relation of A and B.

The compatibility and faithfulness rules define what we mean when we say that a causal model for a set of variables is consistent with a probability model for the distribution of those variables. In practice, the rules are used to identify causal graphs consistent with the observed probability distributions of the graphed variables, and, conversely, to identify distributions that are consistent with a given causal graph. When the arrows in probability graphs represent causal processes, the compatibility rule above (rule 1) is equivalent to the *causal Markov assumption* (CMA), which formalizes the idea that (apart from chance) all unconditional associations arise from ancestral causal relations. Causal explanations of an association between two variables invoke some combination of shared common causes, collider bias, and one of the variables affecting the other. These relations form the basis for Rule 1.

Specifically, the CMA states that for any variable X, conditional upon its direct causes (parents), X is independent of all other variables that it does not affect (its nondescendants). This condition asserts that if we can hold constant the direct causes of X, then X will be independent of any other variable that is not itself affected by X. Thus, assuming X precedes Y temporally, in a DAG without conditioning there are only two sources of association between X and Y: Effects of X on Y (directed paths from X to Y), or common causes (shared ancestors) of X and Y, which introduce confounding. We will make use of this fact when we discuss control of bias.

The d-separation rule (Rule 1) and equivalent conditions such as the CMA codify common intuitions about how probabilistic relations (associations) arise from causal relations. We rely implicitly on these conditions in drawing causal inferences and predicting everyday events—ranging from assessments of whether a drug in a randomized trial was effective to predictions about whether flipping a switch on the wall will suffuse a room with light. In any sequence of events, holding constant both intermediate events and confounding events (common causes) will interrupt the causal cascades that produce associations. In both our intuition and in causal graph theory, this act of "holding constant" renders the downstream events independent of the upstream events. Conditioning on a set that d-separates upstream from downstream events corresponds to this act. This correspondence is the rationale for deducing the conditional independencies (features of a probability distribution) implied by a given causal graph from the d-separation rule.

The intuition behind Rule 2 is this: If, after conditioning on S, there is an open path between two variables, then there must be some causal relation linking the variables, and so they ought to be associated given S, apart from certain exceptions or special cases. An example of an exception occurs when associations transmitted along different open paths perfectly cancel each other, resulting in no association overall. Other exceptions can also occur. Rule 2 says only that we should not count on such special cases to occur, so that, in general, when we see an open path between two variables, we expect them to be associated, or at least we are not surprised if they are associated.

Some authors go beyond Rule 2 and assume that an open path between two variables means that they *must* be associated. This stronger assumption is called *faithfulness* or *stability* and says that if S does not d-separate X and Y, then X and Y will be associated given S. Faithfulness is thus the logical converse of compatibility (Rule 1). Compatibility says that if two variables are d-separated, then they must be independent; faithfulness says that if two variables are independent, then they must be d-separated. When both compatibility and faithfulness hold, we have *perfect compatibility,* which says that X and Y are independent given S if *and only if* S d-separates X and Y; faithfulness adds the "only if" part. For any given pattern of associations, the assumption of perfect compatibility rules out a number of possible causal structures (Spirtes et al., 2001). Therefore, when it is credible, perfect compatibility can help identify causal structures underlying observed data.

Nonetheless, because there are real examples of near-cancellation (e.g., when confounding obscures a real effect in a study) and other exceptions, faithfulness is controversial as a routine assumption, as are algorithms for inferring causal structure from observational data; see Robins (1997, section 11), Korb and Wallace (1997), Freedman and Humphreys (1999), Glymour et al. (1999), Robins and Wasserman (1999), and Robins et al. (2003). Because of this controversy, we discuss only uses of graphical models that do not rely on the assumption of faithfulness. Instead, we use Rule 2, which weakens the faithfulness condition by saying that the presence of open paths alerts us to the possibility of association, and so we should allow for that possibility.

The rules and assumptions just discussed should be clearly distinguished from the content-specific causal assumptions encoded in a diagram, which relate to the substantive question at hand. These rules serve only to link the assumed causal structure (which is ideally based on sound and complete contextual information) to the associations that we observe. In this fashion, they allow testing of those assumptions and estimation of the effects implied by the graph.

GRAPHICAL REPRESENTATION OF BIAS AND ITS CONTROL

A major use of causal graphs is to identify sources of bias in studies and proposed analyses, including biases resulting from confounding, selection, or overadjustment. Given a causal graph, we can use the definitions and rules we have provided to determine whether a set of measured variables $\boldsymbol{S}$ is sufficient to allow us to identify (validly estimate) the causal effect of X on Y.

Suppose that X precedes Y temporally and that the objective of a study is to estimate a measure of the effect of X on Y. We will call an undirected open path between X and Y a *biasing path* for the effect because such paths do not represent effects of X on Y, yet can contribute to the association of X and Y. The association of X and Y is *unconditionally unbiased* or *marginally unbiased* for the effect of X on Y if the only open paths from X to Y are the directed paths.

SUFFICIENT AND MINIMALLY SUFFICIENT CONDITIONING SETS

When there are biasing paths between X and Y, it may be possible to close these paths by conditioning on other variables. Consider a set of variables $\mathbf{S}$. The association of X and Y is *unbiased given* $\mathbf{S}$ if, after conditioning on $\mathbf{S}$, the open paths between X and Y are exactly (only and all) the directed paths from X to Y. In such a case we say that $\mathbf{S}$ is *sufficient* to control bias in the association of X and Y. Because control of colliders can open biasing paths, it is possible for a set $\mathbf{S}$ to be sufficient, and yet a larger set containing $\mathbf{S}$ and such colliders may be insufficient.

A sufficient set $\mathbf{S}$ is *minimally sufficient* to identify the effect of X on Y if no proper subset of $\mathbf{S}$ is sufficient (i.e., if removing any set of variables from $\mathbf{S}$ leaves an insufficient set). In practice, there may be several distinct sufficient sets and even several distinct minimally sufficient sets for bias control. Investigators may sometimes wish to adjust for more variables than are included in what appears as a minimally sufficient set in a graph (e.g., to allow for uncertainty about possible confounding paths). Identifying minimally sufficient sets can be valuable nonetheless, because adjusting for more variables than necessary risks introducing biases and reducing precision, and measuring extra variables is often difficult or expensive.

For example, the set of all parents of X is always sufficient to eliminate bias when estimating the effects of X in an unconditional DAG. Nonetheless, the set of parents of X may be far from *minimally* sufficient. Whenever X and Y share no ancestor and there is no conditioning or measurement error, the only open paths from X to Y are directed paths. In this case, there is no bias and hence no need for conditioning to prevent bias in estimating the effect of X on Y, no matter how many parents of X exist.

CHOOSING CONDITIONING SETS TO IDENTIFY CAUSAL EFFECTS

There are several reasons to avoid (where possible) including descendants of X in a set $\mathbf{S}$ of conditioning variables. First, conditioning on descendants of X that are intermediates will block directed (causal) paths that are part of the effect of interest, and thus create bias. Second, conditioning on descendants of X can unblock or create paths that are not part of the effect of X on Y and thus introduce another source of bias. For example, biasing paths can be created when one conditions on a descendant Z of both X and Y. The resulting bias is the Berksonian bias described earlier. Third, even when inclusion of a particular descendant of X induces no bias, it may still reduce precision in effect estimation.

Undirected paths from X to Y are termed *back-door* (relative to X) if they start with an arrow pointing into X (i.e., it leaves X from a "back door"). In Figure 12–2, the one path from X to Y is back-door because it starts with the back-step $X \leftarrow Z_1$. Before conditioning, all biasing paths in a DAG are open back-door paths, and all open back-door paths are biasing paths. Thus, to identify the causal effect of X on Y all the back-door paths between the two variables must be blocked. A set $\mathbf{S}$ satisfies the *back-door criterion* for identifying the effect of X on Y if $\mathbf{S}$ contains no descendant of X and there is no open back-door path from X to Y after conditioning on $\mathbf{S}$. If $\mathbf{S}$ satisfies the back-door criterion, then conditioning on $\mathbf{S}$ alone is sufficient to control bias in the DAG, and we say that the effect of X on Y is *identified* or *estimable* given $\mathbf{S}$ alone. We emphasize again, however, that further conditioning may introduce bias: Conditioning on a collider may create new biasing paths, and conditioning on an intermediate will block paths that are part of the effect under study.

CONFOUNDING AND SELECTION BIAS

The terms *confounding* and *selection bias* have varying and overlapping usage in different disciplines. The traditional epidemiologic concepts of confounding and selection bias both correspond to biasing paths between X and Y. The distinction between the two concepts is not consistent across the literature, however, and many phenomena can be reasonably described as both confounding and selection bias. We emphasize that the d-separation criteria are sufficient to identify structural sources of bias, and thus there is no need to categorize each biasing path as a confounding or selection-bias path. Nonetheless, the discussion below may help illustrate the correspondence between conventional epidemiologic terms and sources of bias in causal diagrams.

Traditionally, confounding is thought of as a source of bias arising from causes of Y that are associated with but not affected by X (Chapter 9). Thus we say that a biasing path from X to Y is

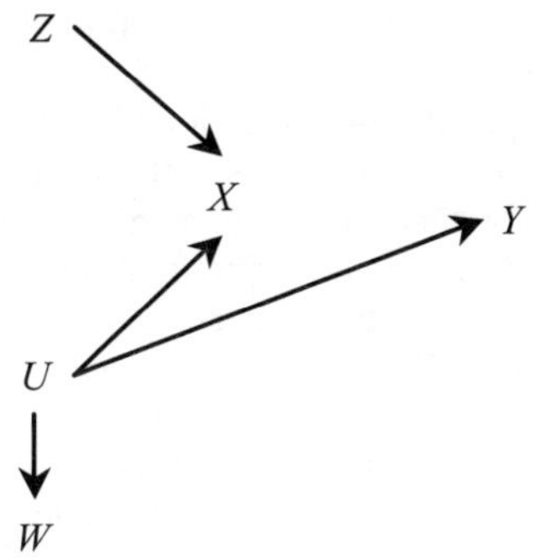

FIGURE 12–3 • A causal diagram with confounding of the X–Y association by U but not by Z.

a *confounding path* if it ends with an arrow into Y. Bias arising from a common cause of X and Y (and thus present in the unconditional graph, e.g., U in Figure 12–3) is sometimes called "classical confounding" (Greenland, 2003a) to distinguish it from confounding that arises from conditioning on a collider. Variables that intercept confounding paths between X and Y are *confounders*.

Often, only indirect measures of the variables that intercept a confounding path are available (e.g., W in Figure 12–3). In this case, adjusting for such surrogates or markers of proper confounders may help remediate bias (Greenland and Pearl, 2008). Such surrogates are often referred to informally as confounders. Caution is needed whenever adjusting for a surrogate in an effort to block a confounding path. To the extent that the surrogate is imperfectly related to the actual confounder, the path will remain partially open. Furthermore, if variables other than the actual confounder itself influence the surrogate, conditioning on the surrogate may open new paths and introduce collider bias. More generally, adjusting for an imperfect surrogate may increase bias under certain circumstances. Related issues will be discussed in the section on residual confounding.

If a confounding path is present, we say that the dependence of Y on X is *confounded,* and if no confounding path is present we say that the dependence is *unconfounded*. Note that an unconfounded dependency may still be biased because of biasing paths that are not confounding paths (e.g., if Berksonian bias is present). Thus, **S** may be sufficient for confounding control (in that it blocks all confounding paths), and yet may be insufficient to control other bias (such as Berksonian bias, which is often uncontrollable).

If W is a variable representing selection into the study sample (e.g., due to intentional selection, self-selection, or survival), all analyses are conditioned on W. Selection bias is thus sometimes defined as the collider bias that arises from conditioning on selection W. For example, in Figure 12–4, we would say that, before conditioning on W, the relation between X and Y is confounded by the path $X - Z_1 - W - Y$. Conditioning on W alone opens the confounding path $X - Z_1 - W - Z_2 - Y$; the bias that results is a collider bias because the bias arises from conditioning on W, a common

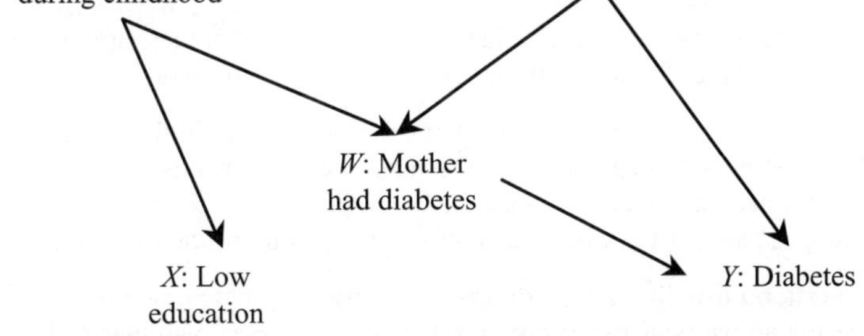

FIGURE 12–4 • A diagram under which control of W alone might increase bias even though W is a confounder.

effect of causes of X and Y. But it can also be called confounding, because the bias arises from a path that ends with an arrow into Y.

Econometricians and others frequently use "selection bias" to refer to any form of confounding. The motivation for this terminology is that some causes of Y also influence "selection for treatment," that is, selection of the level of X one receives, rather than selection into the study sample. This terminology is especially common in discussions of confounding that arises from self-selection, e.g., choosing to take hormone-replacement therapy. Other writers call any bias created by conditioning a "selection bias," thus using the term "selection bias" for what we have called collider bias (Hernán et al., 2004); they then limit their use of "confounding" to what we have defined as "classical confounding" (confounding from a common cause of X and Y).

Regardless of terminology, it is helpful to identify the potential sources of bias to guide both design and analysis decisions. Our examples show how bias can arise in estimating the effect of X on Y if selection is influenced either by X or by factors that influence X, and is also influenced by Y or factors that influence Y. Thus, to control the resulting bias, one will need good data on either the factors that influence both selection and X or the factors that influence both selection and Y. We will illustrate these concepts in several later examples, and provide further structure to describe biases due to measurement error, missing data, and model-form misspecification.

SOME APPLICATIONS

Causal diagrams help us answer causal queries under various assumed causal structures, or causal models. Consider Figure 12–3. If we are interested in estimating the effect of X on Y, it is evident that, under the model shown in the figure, our analysis should condition on U: There is a confounding path from X to Y, and U is the only variable on the path. On the other hand, suppose that we are interested in estimating the effect of Z on Y. Under the diagram in Figure 12–3, we need not condition on U, because the relation of Z to Y is unconfounded (as is the relation of X to Z), that is, there is no confounding path from Z to Y. Because Figure 12–3 is a DAG, we can rephrase these conditions by saying that there is an open back-door path from X to Y, but not from Z to Y.

We now turn to examples in which causal diagrams can be used to clarify methodologic issues. In some cases the diagrams simply provide a convenient way to express well-understood concepts. In other examples they illuminate points of confusion regarding the biases introduced by proposed analyses or study designs. In all these cases, the findings can be shown mathematically or seen by various informal arguments. The advantage of diagrams is that they provide flexible visual explanations of the problems, and the explanations correspond to logical relations under the definitions and rules given earlier.

WHY CONVENTIONAL RULES FOR CONFOUNDING ARE NOT ALWAYS RELIABLE

In both intuition and application, the graphical and conventional criteria for confounding overlap substantially. For example, in Chapter 9, confounding was informally described as a distortion in the estimated exposure effect that results from differences in risk between the exposed and unexposed that are not due to exposure. Similarly, Hennekens and Buring (1987, p. 35) say that confounding occurs when "an observed association. . . . is in fact due to a mixing of effects between the exposure, the disease, and a third factor. . . ."

Variations on the following specific criteria for identifying confounders are frequently suggested, although, as noted in Chapter 9, these criteria do not define a confounder:

1. A confounder must be associated with the exposure under study in the source population.
2. A confounder must be a "risk factor" for the outcome (i.e., it must predict who will develop disease), though it need not actually cause the outcome.
3. The confounding factor must not be affected by the exposure or the outcome.

These traditional criteria usually agree with graphical criteria; that is, one would choose the same set of covariates for adjustment using either set of criteria. For example, in Figure 12–3, both the graphical and intuitive criteria indicate that one should condition on U to derive an unbiased estimate of the effect of X on Y. Under the graphical criteria, U satisfies the back-door criterion for identifying the effect of X on Y: U is not an effect of X, and the only path between X and Y that contains an arrow into X can be blocked by conditioning on U. It fulfills the three traditional criteria because U and X will be associated, U will also predict Y, and U is not affected by X or Y.

Nonetheless, there are cases in which the criteria disagree, and when they diverge, it is the conventional criteria (1–3) that fail. Suppose that we are interested in whether educational attainment affects risk of type II diabetes. Figure 12–2 then depicts a situation under the causal null hypothesis in which education (X) has no effect on subject's diabetes (Y). Suppose that we have measured maternal diabetes status (W), but we do not have measures of family income during childhood (Z_1) or whether the mother had any genes that would increase risk of diabetes (Z_2). Should we adjust for W, maternal diabetes?

Figure 12–2 reflects the assumption that family income during childhood affects both educational attainment and maternal diabetes. The reasoning is that if a subject was poor as a child, his or her mother was poor as an adult, and this poverty also increased the mother's risk of developing diabetes (Robbins et al., 2005). Maternal diabetes will thus be associated with the subject's education, because under these assumptions they share a cause, family income. In Figure 12–2, this association is due entirely to confounding of the X–W (education-maternal diabetes) association. Figure 12–2 also reflects the assumption that a maternal genetic factor affects risk of both maternal diabetes and the subject's diabetes. Maternal diabetes will thus be associated with the subject's diabetes, because under these assumptions they share a cause, the genetic factor. In Figure 12–2, this association is purely confounding of the W–Y (maternal diabetes-subject's diabetes) association.

In Figure 12–2, maternal diabetes W is not affected by the subject's education level X or diabetes status Y. Thus, the mother's diabetes meets the three traditional criteria for a confounder, so these criteria could lead one to adjust for mother's diabetic status. Note, however, that both the associations on which the latter decision is based (traditional criteria 1 and 2) arise from confounding.

Turning to the graphical criteria, note first that there is only one undirected path between low education X and diabetes Y, and mother's diabetes W is a collider on that path. Thus this path is blocked at W and transmits no association between X and Y — that is, it introduces no bias. This structure means that we get an unbiased estimate if we do *not* adjust for the mother's diabetes. Because maternal diabetes is a collider, however, adjusting for it opens this undirected path, thus introducing a potential spurious association between low education and diabetes. The path opened by conditioning on W could be blocked by conditioning on either Z_1 or Z_2, but there is no need to condition on W in the first place. Therefore, under Figure 12–2, the graphical criteria show that one should not adjust for maternal diabetes, lest one introduce bias where none was present to begin with. In this sense, adjustment for W would be one form of overadjustment (Chapter 15), and the traditional criteria were mistaken to identify W as a confounder.

Figure 12–2 illustrates why in Chapter 9 it was said that the traditional criteria do not *define* a confounder: While every confounder will satisfy them, Figure 12–2 shows that some nonconfounders satisfy them as well. In some cases, adjusting for such nonconfounders is harmless, but in others, as in the example here, it introduces a bias. This bias may, however, be removed by adjustment for another variable on the newly opened path.

The situation in Figure 12–2 is analogous to Berksonian bias if we focus on the part of the graph (subgraph) in which $Z_1 \rightarrow W \leftarrow Z_2$: Conditioning on the collider W connects its parents Z_1 and Z_2, and thus connects X to Y. Another way to describe the problem is that we have a spurious appearance of confounding by W if we do not condition on Z_1 or Z_2, for then W is associated with X and Y. Because W temporally precedes X and Y, these associations may deceive one into thinking that W is a confounder. Nonetheless, the association between W and X is due solely to the effects of Z_1 on W and X, and the association between W and Y is due solely to the effects of Z_2 on W and Y. There is no common cause of X and Y, however, and hence no confounding if we do not condition on W.

To eliminate this sort of problem, traditional criterion 2 (here, that W is a "risk factor" for Y) is sometimes replaced by

2′. The variable must affect the outcome under study.

This substitution addresses the difficulty in examples like Figure 12–2 (for W will fail this revised criterion). Nonetheless, it fails to address the more general problem that conditioning may introduce bias. To see this failing, draw an arrow from W to Y in Figure 12–2, which yields Figure 12–4. W now affects the outcome, Y, and thus satisfies criterion 2′. This change is quite plausible, because having a mother with diabetes might lead some subjects to be more careful about their weight and diet, thus lowering their own diabetes risk. W is now a confounder: Failing to adjust for it leaves open a confounding path ($X \leftarrow Z_1 \rightarrow W \rightarrow Y$) that is closed by adjusting for W. But adjusting for W will open an undirected (and hence biasing) path from X to Y ($X \leftarrow Z_1 \rightarrow W \leftarrow Z_2 \rightarrow Y$), as just discussed. The only ways to block both biasing paths at once is to adjust for Z_1 (alone or in combination with any other variable) or both Z_2 and W together.

If neither Z_1 nor Z_2 is measured, then under Figure 12–4, we face a dilemma not addressed by the traditional criteria. As with Figure 12–2, if we adjust for W, we introduce confounding via Z_1 and Z_2; yet, unlike Figure 12–2, under Figure 12–4 we are left with confounding by W if we do not adjust for W. The question is, then, which undirected path is more biasing, that with adjustment for W or that without? Both paths are modulated by the same X–W connection ($X \leftarrow Z_1 \rightarrow W$), so we may focus on whether the connection of W to Y with adjustment ($W \leftarrow Z_2 \rightarrow Y$) is stronger than the connection without adjustment ($W \rightarrow Y$). If so, then we would ordinarily expect less bias when we don't adjust for W; if not, then we would ordinarily expect less bias if we adjust. The final answer will depend on the strength of the effect represented by each arrow, which is context-specific. Assessments of the likely relative biases (as well as their direction) thus depend on subject-matter information.

In typical epidemiologic examples with noncontagious events, the strength of association transmitted by a path attenuates rapidly as the number of variables through which it passes increases. More precisely, the longer the path, the more we would expect attenuation of the association transmitted by the path (Greenland, 2003a). In Figure 12–4, this means that the effects of Z_2 on W and Z_2 on Y would both have to be much stronger than the effect of W on Y in order for the unadjusted X–Y association to be less biased than the W-adjusted X–Y association. However, if the proposed analysis calls for stratifying or restricting on W (instead of adjusting for W), the bias within a single stratum of W can be larger than the bias when adjusting for W (which averages across all strata).

To summarize, expressing assumptions in a DAG provides a flexible and general way to identify "sufficient" sets under a range of causal structures, using the d-separation rules. For example, if we changed the structure in Fig 12–2 only slightly by reversing the direction of the relationship between Z_1 and W (so we have $X \leftarrow Z_1 \leftarrow W \leftarrow Z_2 \rightarrow Y$), then conditioning on W would be desirable, and any of Z_1, W, or Z_2 would provide a sufficient set for identifying the effect of X on Y. Modified versions of the conventional criteria for confounder identification have been developed that alleviate their deficiencies and allow them to identify sufficient sets, consistent with the graphical criteria (Greenland et al., 1999a). We do not present these here because they are rarely used and, in general, it is simpler to apply the graphical criteria.

GRAPHICAL ANALYSES OF SELECTION BIAS

Selection forces in a study may be part of the design (e.g., enrollment criteria, or hospitalization status in a hospital-based case-control study) or may be unintended (e.g., loss to follow-up in a cohort study, or refusals in any study). Selection forces can of course compromise generalizability (e.g., results for white men may mislead about risk factors in black women). As shown by the above examples and discussed in Chapters 7 through 9, they can also compromise the internal validity of a study.

Causal diagrams provide a unifying framework for thinking about well-known sources of bias and also illustrate how some intentional selection and analysis strategies result in bias in more subtle situations. To see these problems, we represent selection into a study as a variable, and then note that all analyses of a sample are conditioned on this variable. That is, we conceptualize selection as a variable with two values, 0 = not selected and 1 = selected; analyses are thus restricted to observations where selection = 1. Selection bias may occur if this selection variable (that is, entry into the study) depends on the exposure, the outcome, or their causes (whether shared or not).

BIAS FROM INTENTIONAL SELECTION

Even seemingly innocuous choices in dataset construction can induce severe selection bias. To take an extreme example, imagine a study of education (X) and Alzheimer's disease (Y) conducted

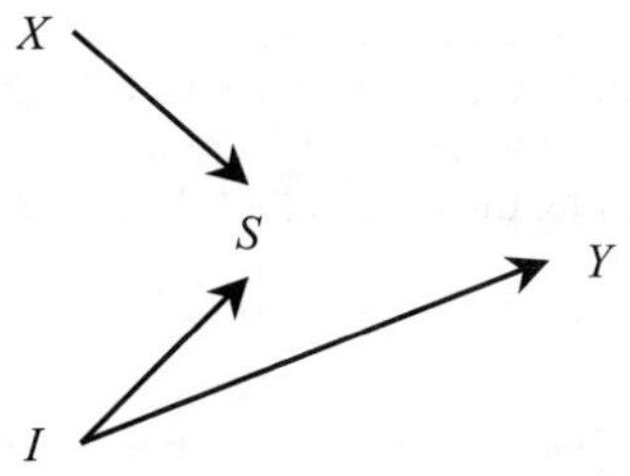

FIGURE 12–5 • A diagram with a selection indicator *S*.

by pooling two datasets, one consisting only of persons with college education (X = high), the other consisting only of persons diagnosed with impaired memory ($I = 1$). Within this pooled study, everyone without college education (X = low) has memory impairment ($I = 1$), which in turn is strongly associated with Alzheimer's disease because impairment is often a symptom of early, undiagnosed Alzheimer's disease (in fact, it is a precursor or prodrome). Likewise, any subject with no impairment ($I = 0$) has college education (X = high). Thus, in this study, college education is almost certainly negatively associated with Alzheimer's disease. This association would be completely spurious, induced by defining selection as an effect of both education (X) and memory impairment (I) as a result of pooling the two datasets. Graphing the relations in Figure 12–5, this association can be viewed as Berksonian bias: Selection S is strongly affected by both the exposure X and an independent cause of the outcome Y, hence is a collider between them. All analyses are conditioned on selection and the resulting collider bias will be large, greatly misrepresenting the population association between education and Alzheimer's disease.

This example parallels Berksonian bias in clinic-based and hospital-based studies, because selection was affected directly by exposure and outcome. Selection is often only indirectly related to exposure and outcome, however. Suppose we study how education affects risk for Alzheimer's disease in a study with selection based on membership in a high-prestige occupation. Achievement of high-prestige occupations is likely to be influenced by both education and intellect. Of course, many people obtain prestigious jobs by virtue of other advantages besides education or intelligence, but to keep our example simple, we will assume here that none of these other factors influence Alzheimer's disease.

There is evidence that intelligence protects against diagnosis of Alzheimer's disease (Schmand et al., 1997). Consider Figure 12–5 (relabeling the variables from the previous example), in which selection S (based on occupation) is influenced by education (X) and intellect (I), where the latter affects Alzheimer's disease (Y). Among the high-prestige job holders, people with less education (X = lower) are more likely to have high intellect (I = high), whereas those with lesser intellect (I = lower) are more likely to have advanced education (X = high), because most individuals had to have some advantage (at least one of X = high or I = high) to get their high-prestige job. In effect, X and I are compensatory, in that having more of one compensates somewhat for having less of the other, even if everyone in the study is above average on both.

The selection process thus biases the education–intellect association away from the association in the population as a whole. The strength of the spurious association will depend on the details of the selection process, that is, how strongly education and intellect each affect occupation and whether they interact in any way to determine occupation. Note, however, that if high-education subjects are less likely to have high intellect than low-education subjects, and high intellect protects against Alzheimer's disease, then high-education subjects will exhibit excess risk of Alzheimer's disease relative to low-education subjects even if education has no effect. In other words, whatever the true causal relation between education and Alzheimer's disease, in a study of high-prestige job holders, the association in the study will be biased downward, unless one can adjust for the effect of intellect on Alzheimer's disease.

Telling this story in words is complicated and prone to generating confusion, but analyzing a corresponding diagram is straightforward. In Figure 12–5, we can see that S is a collider between X and I, and so we should expect X and I to be associated conditional on S. Thus, conditional on S, we expect X and Y to be associated, even if X does not affect Y. Whether selection exacerbates or reduces bias in estimating a specific causal effect depends crucially on the causal relations among variables determining selection. If we added an arrow from I to X in Figure 12–5 (i.e. if intellect directly affects education), I would be a confounder and the X–Y association would be biased before selection. If the confounding produced by I were upward, the bias produced by selection on S might counteract it enough to lessen the overall (net) bias in the X–Y association.

SURVIVOR BIAS

Survivor bias, and more generally bias due to differential competing risks or loss to follow-up, can be thought of as a special case of selection bias. In life-course research on early life exposures and health in old age, a large fraction of the exposed are likely to die before reaching old age, so survivor bias could be large. Effect estimates for early life exposures often decline with age (Elo and Preston, 1996; Tate et al., 1998). An example is the black–white mortality crossover: Mortality is greater for blacks and other disadvantaged groups relative to whites at younger ages, but the pattern reverses at the oldest ages (Corti et al., 1999; Thornton, 2004). Do such phenomena indicate that the early life exposures become less important with age? Not necessarily. Selective survival can result in attenuated associations among survivors at older ages, even though the effects are undiminished (Vaupel and Yashin, 1985; Howard and Goff, 1998; Mohtashemi and Levins, 2002). The apparent diminution of the magnitude of effects can occur due to confounding by unobserved factors that conferred a survival advantage.

Apart from some special cases, such confounding should be expected whenever both the exposure under study and unmeasured risk factors for the outcome influence survival—even if the exposure and factors were unassociated at the start of life (and thus the factors are not initially confounders). Essentially, if exposure presents a disadvantage for survival, then exposed survivors will tend to have some other characteristic that helped them to survive. If that protective characteristic also influences the outcome, it creates a spurious association between exposure and the outcome. This result follows immediately from a causal diagram like Figure 12–5, interpreted as showing survival (S) affected by early exposure (X) and also by an unmeasured risk factor (I) that also affects the study outcome (Y).

RESIDUAL CONFOUNDING AND BIAS QUANTIFICATION

Ideally, to block a back-door path between X and Y by conditioning on a variable or set of variables Z, we would have sufficient data to create a separate analysis stratum for every observed value of Z and thus avoid making any assumptions about the form of the relation of Z to X or Y. Such complete stratification may be practical if Z has few observed values (e.g., sex). In most situations, however, Z has many levels (e.g., Z represents a set of several variables, including some, such as age, that are nearly continuous), and as a result we obtain cells with no or few persons if we stratify on every level of Z. The standard solutions compensate for small cell counts using statistical modeling assumptions (Robins and Greenland, 1986). Typically, these assumptions are collected in the convenient form of a regression model, as described in Chapter 20. The form of the model will rarely be perfectly correct, and to the extent that it is in error, the model-based analysis will not completely block confounding paths. The bias that remains as a result is an example of *residual confounding*, i.e., the confounding still present after adjustment.

Causal diagrams are nonparametric in that they make no assumption about the functional form of relationships among variables. For example, the presence of open paths between two variables leads us to expect they are associated in some fashion, but a diagram does not say how. The association between the variables could be linear, U-shaped, involve a threshold, or an infinitude of other forms. Thus the graphical models we have described provide no guidance on the form to use to adjust for covariates.

One aspect of the residual confounding problem, however, can be represented in a causal diagram, and that is the form in which the covariates appear in a stratified analysis or a regression model. Suppose Z is a covariate, that when uncontrolled induces a positive bias in the estimated relationship between the exposure and outcome of interest. Stratification or regression adjustment for a particular form of Z, say $g(Z)$, may eliminate bias; for example, there might be no bias if Z is entered in the analysis as its natural logarithm, $\ln(Z)$. But there might be considerable bias left if we enter Z in a different form $f(Z)$, e.g., as quartile categories, which in the lowest category combines persons

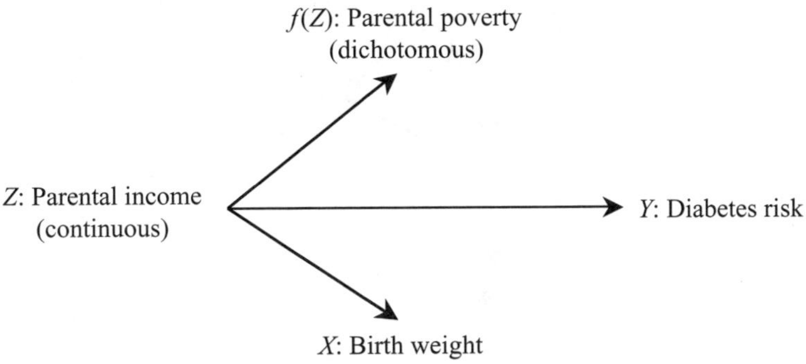

FIGURE 12–6 • Diagram with residual confounding of the X–Y association after control of $f(Z)$ alone.

with very different values of ln(Z). Similarly, use of measures $f(Z)$ of Z that suffer from substantial error could make it impossible to adjust accurately for Z.

"Blocking the path at Z" involves complete stratification on the variables in a sufficient set, or anything equivalent, even if the resulting estimate is too statistically unstable for practical use. We can thus represent our problem by adding to the diagram the possibly inferior functional form or measurement $f(Z)$ as a separate variable. This representation shows that, even if Z is sufficient to control confounding, $f(Z)$ may be insufficient.

To illustrate, suppose that we are interested in estimating the effect of birth weight on adult diabetes risk, and that Figure 12–6 shows the true causal structure. We understand that parental income Z is a potential confounder of the relationship between birth weight and diabetes risk because it affects both variables. Suppose further that this relationship is continuously increasing (more income is better even for parents who are well above the poverty line), but, unfortunately, our data set includes no measure of income. Instead, we have only an indicator $f(Z)$ for whether or not the parents were in poverty (a dichotomous variable); that is, $f(Z)$ is an indicator of very low income—e.g., $f(Z) = 1$ if $Z <$ poverty level, $f(Z) = 0$ otherwise. Poverty is an imperfect surrogate for income. Then the association between birth weight and diabetes may be confounded by parental income even conditional on $f(Z)$, because $f(Z)$ fails to completely block the confounding path between parental income and diabetes. The same phenomena will occur using a direct measure of income that incorporates substantial random error. In both cases, residual confounding results from inadequate control of income.

BIAS FROM USE OF MISSING-DATA CATEGORIES OR INDICATORS

Many methods for handling missing data are available, most of which are unbiased under some assumptions but biased under alternative scenarios (Robins et al., 1994; Greenland and Finkle, 1995; Little and Rubin, 2002; see Chapter 13). In handling missing data, researchers usually want to retain as many data records as possible to preserve study size and avoid analytic complexity. Thus, a popular approach to handling missing data on a variable Z is to treat "missing" as if it were just another value for Z. The idea is often implemented by adding a stratum for Z = "missing," which in questionnaires includes responses such as "unknown" and "refused." The same idea is implemented by adding an indicator variable for missingness to a regression model: We set Z to 0 when it is missing, and add an indicator $M_Z = 0$ if Z is observed, $M_Z = 1$ if Z is missing.

Missing indicators allow one to retain every subject in the analysis and are easy to implement, but they may introduce bias. This bias can arise even under the best-case scenario, that the data are missing completely at random (MCAR). MCAR means that missingness of a subject's value for Z is independent of every variable in the analysis, including Z. For example, if Z is sexual orientation, MCAR assumes that whether someone skips the question or refuses to answer has nothing to do with the person's age, sex, or actual preference. Thus MCAR is an exceedingly optimistic assumption, but it is often used to justify certain techniques.

Next, suppose that Figure 12–7 represents our study. We are interested in the effect of X on Y, and we recognize that it is important to adjust for the confounder Z. If Z is missing for some

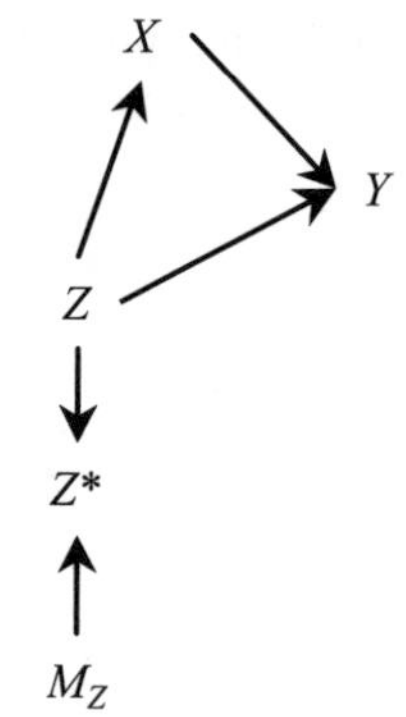

FIGURE 12–7 • Diagram with a missing-data indicator M_Z.

subjects, we add to the analysis the missing indicator M_Z. If Z is never zero, we also define a new variable, Z^*, that equals Z whenever Z is observed and equals 0 whenever Z is missing, that is, $Z^* = Z(1 - M_Z)$. There are no arrows pointing into M_Z in the diagram, implying that Z is unconditionally MCAR, but Z^* is determined by both Z and M_Z. Using the missing-indicator method, we enter both Z^* and M_Z in the regression model, and thus we condition on them both.

In Figure 12–7, the set $\{Z^*, M_Z\}$ does not block the back-door path from X to Y via Z, so control of Z^* and M_Z does not fully control the confounding by Z (and we expect this residual confounding to increase as the fraction with Z missing increases). Similarly, it should be clear from Figure 12–7 that conditioning only on Z* also fails to block the back-door path from X to Y. Now consider a complete-subject analysis, which uses only observations with Z observed—in other words, we condition on (restrict to) $M_Z = 0$. From Figure 12–7 we see that this conditioning creates no bias. Because we have Z on everyone with $M_Z = 0$, we can further condition on Z and eliminate all confounding by Z. So we see that instead of the biased missing-indicator approach, we have an unbiased (and even simpler) alternative: an analysis limited to subjects with complete data. The diagram can be extended to consider alternative assumptions about the determinants of missingness. Note, however, that more efficient and more broadly unbiased alternatives to complete-subject analysis (such as multiple imputation or inverse probability weighting) are available, and some of these methods are automated in commercial software packages.

ADJUSTING FOR AN INTERMEDIATE DOES NOT NECESSARILY ESTIMATE A DIRECT EFFECT

Once an effect has been established, attention often turns to questions of mediation. Is the effect of sex on depression mediated by hormonal differences between men and women or by differences in social conditions? Is the effect of prepregnancy body mass index on pre-eclampsia risk mediated by inflammation? Is the apparent effect of occupational status on heart disease attributable to psychologic consequences of low occupational status or to material consequences of low-paying jobs?

In considering exposure X and outcome Y with an intermediate (mediator) Z, a direct effect of X on Y (relative to Z) is an X effect on Y that is not mediated by Z. In a causal diagram, effects of X on Y mediated by Z, or "indirect effects," are those directed paths from X to Y that pass through Z. Direct effects are then represented by directed paths from X to Y that do not pass through Z. Nonetheless, because Z may modify the magnitude of a direct effect, the total effect of X on Y cannot necessarily be partitioned into nonoverlapping direct and indirect effects (Robins and Greenland, 1992).

The term *direct effect* may refer to either of two types of effects. The first type is the effect of X on Y in an experiment in which each individual's Z is held constant at the same value z. This has been termed the *controlled direct effect* because the intermediate is controlled. The magnitude of this direct effect may differ across each possible value of Z; thus there is a controlled direct effect defined for every possible value of Z. The second type is called a *pure* or *natural* direct effect and is the effect of X on Y when Z takes on the value it would "naturally" have under a single reference

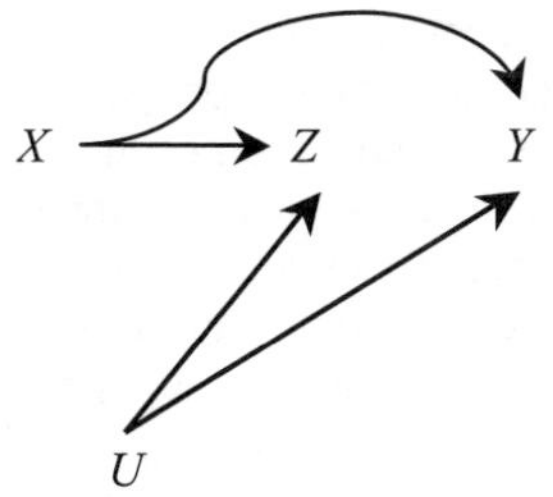

FIGURE 12–8 • Diagram with an unconfounded direct effect and no indirect effect of X on Y.

value x for X. Thus there is one of these effects for each possible value of X. For each direct effect of X on Y, we can also define a contrast between the total effect of X on Y and that direct effect. This contrast is sometimes referred to as the "indirect effect of X on Y" relative to the chosen direct effect. There will be one of these contrasts for every controlled direct effect (i.e., for every level of Z) and one for every pure direct effect (i.e., for every level of X).

A causal diagram can reveal pitfalls in naive estimation procedures, as well as additional data and assumptions needed to estimate direct effects validly. For example, a standard method of direct-effect estimation is to adjust for (condition on) Z in the analysis—e.g., by entering it in a regression of Y on X. The Z-adjusted estimate of the X coefficient is taken as an estimate of "the" direct effect of X on Y (without being clear about which direct effect is being estimated). The difference in the X coefficients with and without adjustment for Z is then taken as the estimate of the indirect effect of X on Y (with respect to Z).

The diagram in Figure 12–8 shows no confounding of the total effect of X on Y, and no effect of Z on Y at all, so no indirect effect of X on Y via Z (all the X effect on Y is direct). Z is, however, a collider on the closed path from X to Y via U; thus, if we adjust for Z, we will open this path and introduce bias. Consequently, upon adjusting for Z, we will see the X association with Y change, misleading us into thinking that the direct and total effects differ. This change, however, only reflects the bias we have created by adjusting for Z.

This bias arises because we have an uncontrolled variable U that confounds the Z–Y association, and that confounds the X–Y association upon adjustment for Z. The bias could be removed by conditioning on U. This example is like that in Figure 12–3, in which adjusting for a seeming confounder introduced confounding that was not there originally. After adjustment for the collider, the only remedy is to obtain and adjust for more covariates. Here, the new confounders may have been unassociated with X to begin with, as we would expect if (say) X were randomized, and so are not confounders of the total effect. Nonetheless, if they confound the association of Z with Y, they will confound any conventionally adjusted estimate of the direct effect of X on Y.

As an illustration of bias arising from adjustment for intermediates, suppose that we are interested in knowing whether the effect of education on systolic blood pressure (SBP) is mediated by adult wealth (say, at age 60). Unfortunately, we do not have any measure of occupational characteristics, and it turns out that having a high-autonomy job promotes the accumulation of wealth and also lowers SBP (perhaps because of diminished stress). Returning to Figure 12–8, now X represents education, Y represents SBP, Z represents wealth at age 60, and U represents job autonomy. To estimate the effect of education on SBP that is not mediated by wealth, we need to compare the SBP in people with high and low education if the value of wealth were not allowed to change in response to education. Thus we might ask, if we gave someone high education but intervened to hold her wealth to what she would have accumulated had she had low education (but changed no other characteristic), how would SBP change compared with giving the person less education?

We cannot conduct such an intervention. The naive direct-effect (mediation) analysis described above instead compares the SBP of people with high versus low education who happened to have the same level of adult wealth. On average, persons with high education tend to be wealthier than persons with low education. A high-education person with the same wealth as a low-education person is likely to have accumulated less wealth than expected for some other reason, such as a low-autonomy job. Thus, the mediation analysis will compare people with high education but low job autonomy to people with low education and average job autonomy. If job autonomy affects SBP, the high-education people will appear to be worse off than they would have been if they had average job autonomy, resulting in underestimation of the direct effect of education on SBP and hence overestimation of the indirect (wealth-mediated) effect.

The complications in estimating direct effects are a concern whether one is interested in mediator-controlled or pure (natural) direct effects. With a causal diagram, one can see that adjusting for a confounded intermediate will induce confounding of the primary exposure and outcome—even if that exposure is randomized. Thus confounders of the effect of the intermediate on the outcome must be measured and controlled. Further restrictions (e.g., no confounding of the X effect on Z) are required to estimate pure direct effects. For more discussion of estimation of direct effects, see Robins and Greenland (1992, 1994), Blakely (2002), Cole and Hernán (2002), Kaufman et al. (2004, 2005), Peterson et al. (2006), Peterson and van der Laan (2008), and Chapter 26.

INSTRUMENTAL VARIABLES

Observational studies are under constant suspicion of uncontrolled confounding and selection bias, prompting many to prefer evidence from randomized experiments. When noncompliance (nonadherence) and losses are frequent, however, randomized trials may themselves suffer considerable confounding and selection bias. Figure 12–9 illustrates both phenomena. In an observational study, U represents unmeasured confounders of the X–Y association. In a randomized trial, U represents variables that affect adherence to treatment assignment and thus influence received treatment X. In Figure 12–9, Z is called an *instrumental variable* (or *instrument*) for estimating the effect of X on Y.

Valid instruments for the effect of X on Y can be used to test the null hypothesis that X has no effect on Y. With additional assumptions, instrumental variable analyses can be exploited to estimate the magnitude of this effect within specific population subgroups. We will first review the assumptions under which a valid instrument can be used to test a null hypothesis of no causal effect, and then describe examples of additional assumptions under which an instrumental variable analysis identifies a specific causal parameter.

Under the assumptions in the DAG in Figure 12–9, assignment Z can be associated with Y only if Z affects X and X in turn affects Y, because the only open path from Z to Y is $Z \rightarrow X \rightarrow Y$. In other words, Z can be associated with Y only if the null hypothesis (that X does not affect Y) is false. Thus, if one rejects the null hypothesis for the Z–Y association, one must also reject the null hypothesis that X does not affect Y. This logical requirement means that, under Figure 12–9, a test of the Z–Y association will be a valid test of the X–Y null hypothesis, even if the X–Y association is confounded. The unconfoundedness of the Z–Y test, called the *intent-to-treat* test, is considered a "gold standard" in randomized trials: If Z represents the assigned treatment, Figure 12–9 holds if Z is truly randomized, even if the treatment received (X) is influenced by unmeasured factors that also affect the outcome Y.

In a DAG, a variable Z is an unconditionally valid instrument for the effect of X on Y if:

1. Z affects X (i.e., Z is an ancestor of X).
2. Z affects the outcome Y only through X (i.e., all directed paths from Z to Y pass through X).
3. Z and Y share no common causes.

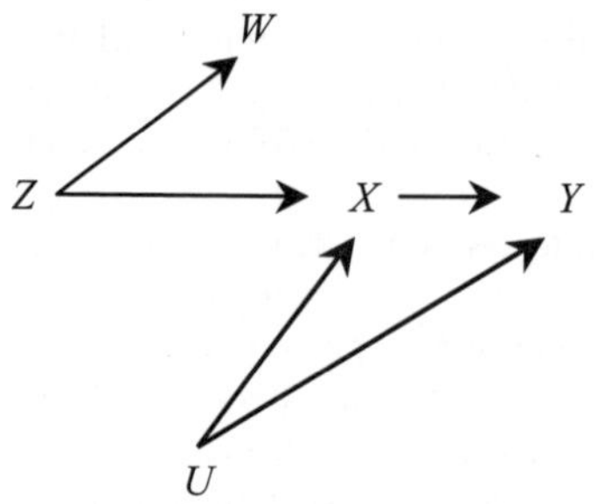

FIGURE 12–9 • Diagram with valid instruments Z, W for the X–Y effect.

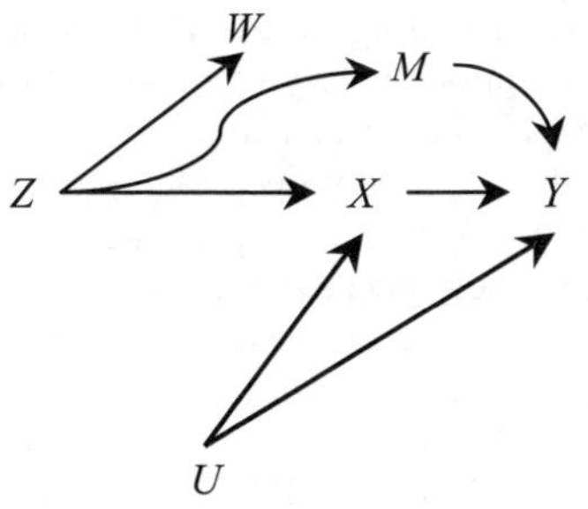

FIGURE 12–10 • Diagram for a confounded trial in which treatment assignment directly affects the outcome.

These assumptions are met in a well-conducted randomized trial in which Z is the randomized treatment-assignment variable. In Figure 12–10, assumption 2 is violated, and in Figure 12–11, assumption 3 is violated, and no unconditionally valid instrument is available in either case.

Most methods can be extended to allow use of certain descendants of Z (such as W in Figure 12–9) instead of Z itself to test whether X affects Y. Some authors extend the definition of instrumental variables to include such descendants. Note first that assumptions 2 and 3 imply that every open path from Z to Y includes an arrow pointing into X. This is a special case of a more general definition that W is an unconditional instrument for the $X \rightarrow Y$ effect in a DAG if (a) there is an open path from W to X, and (b) every open path from W to Y includes an arrow pointing into X. This definition extends to conditioning on a set of variables $\boldsymbol{S}$ that are unaffected by X: W is an instrument given $\boldsymbol{S}$ if, after conditioning on $\boldsymbol{S}$, (a) there is an open path from W to X, and (b) every open path from W to Y includes an arrow pointing into X (Pearl, 2000, section 7.4). For example, if W and Y share a common cause such as U_2 in Figure 12–11, but this common cause is included in $\boldsymbol{S}$, then W is a valid instrument for the effect of X on Y conditional on $\boldsymbol{S}$.

The assumptions for a valid instrument imply that, after conditioning on $\boldsymbol{S}$, the instrument–outcome association is mediated entirely through the X effect on Y. These assumptions require that $\boldsymbol{S}$ blocks all paths from W to Y not mediated by X. For example, conditioning on M in Figure 12–10 would render Z a valid instrument. Nonetheless, if $\boldsymbol{S}$ contains a descendant of W, there is a risk that conditioning on $\boldsymbol{S}$ may induce a W–Y association via collider bias, thus violating the conditional instrumental assumption (b). This collider bias might even result in an unconditionally valid instrument becoming conditionally invalid. Hence many authors exclude descendants of W (or Z) as well as descendants of X from $\boldsymbol{S}$.

Consider now a randomized trial represented by Figure 12–9. Although an association between Z and Y is evidence that X affects Y, the corresponding Z–Y (intent to treat or ITT) association will not equal the effect of X on Y if compliance is imperfect (i.e., if X does not always equal Z). In particular, the ITT (Z–Y) association will usually be attenuated relative to the desired $X \rightarrow Y$ effect because of the extra $Z \rightarrow X$ step. When combined with additional assumptions, however, the instrument Z may be used to estimate the effect of X on Y via special instrumental-variable (IV) estimation methods (Zohoori and Savitz, 1997; Newhouse and McClellan, 1998; Greenland, 2000b; Angrist and Krueger, 2001; Hernán and Robins, 2006; Martens et al., 2006) or related g-estimation methods (Robins and Tsiatis, 1991; Mark and Robins, 1993ab; White et al., 2002; Cole and Chu, 2005; Greenland et al., 2008; see also Chapter 21).

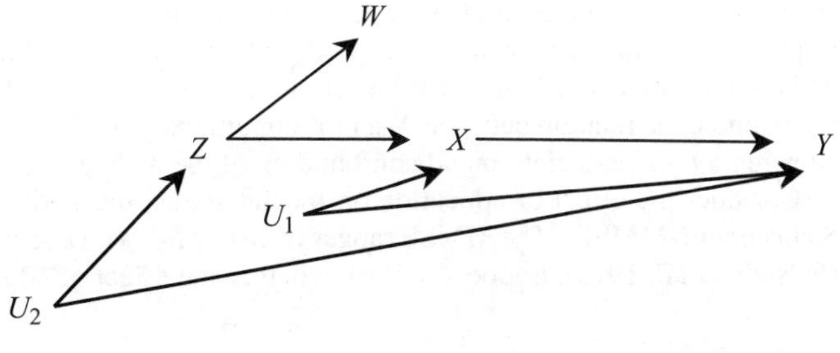

FIGURE 12–11 • Diagram for a confounded trial in which an unmeasured cause U_2 affects both treatment assignment Z and outcome Y.

Simple IV estimates are based on scaling up the Z–Y association in proportion to the Z–X association. An example of an assumption underlying these methods is *monotonicity* of the $Z \rightarrow X$ effect: For every member of the population, Z can affect X in only one direction (e.g., if increasing Z increases X for some people, then it cannot decrease X for anyone). Under monotonicity, IV estimates can be interpreted as the effect receiving the treatment had on those individuals who received treatment (got $X = 1$) precisely because they were assigned to do so (i.e., because they got $Z = 1$). Some methods use further assumptions, usually in the form of parametric models.

The causal structure in Figure 12–9 might apply even if the researcher did not assign Z. Thus, with this diagram in mind, a researcher might search for variables (such as Z or W) that are valid instruments and use these variables to calculate IV effect estimates (Angrist et al., 1996; Angrist and Krueger, 2001; Glymour, 2006a). Although it can be challenging to identify a convincing instrument, genetic studies (Chapter 28) and "natural experiments" may supply them:

- Day of symptom onset may determine the quality of hospital care received, but there is rarely another reason for day of onset to influence a health outcome. Day of symptom onset then provides a natural instrument for the effect of quality of hospital care on the outcome.
- Hour of birth may serve as an instrument for studying postpartum length of stay in relation to maternal and neonatal outcomes (Malkin et al., 2000).
- Mothers who deliver in hospitals with lactation counseling may be more likely to breast-feed. If being born in such a hospital has no other effect on child health, then hospital counseling (yes/no) provides an instrument for the effect of breastfeeding on child health.
- Women with relatives who had breast cancer may be unlikely to receive perimenopausal hormone therapy. If having relatives with breast cancer has no other connection to cardiovascular risk, having relatives with breast cancer is an instrument for the effect of hormone therapy on cardiovascular disease.

These examples highlight the core criteria for assessing proposed instruments (e.g., day of symptom onset, hour of birth). After control of measured confounders the instrument must have no association with the outcome except via the exposure of interest. In other words, if the exposure has no effect, the controlled confounders separate the instrument from the outcome.

A skeptical reader can find reason to doubt the validity of each of the above proposed instruments, which highlights the greatest challenge for instrumental variables analyses with observational data: finding a convincing instrument. Causal diagrams provide a clear summary of the hypothesized situation, enabling one to check the instrumental assumptions. When the instrument is not randomized, those assumptions (like common no-residual-confounding assumptions) are always open to question. For example, suppose we suspect that hospitals with lactation counseling tend to provide better care in other respects. Then the association of hospital counseling with child's outcome is in part not via breastfeeding, and counseling is not a valid instrument.

IV methods for confounding control are paralleled by IV methods for correcting measurement error in X. The latter methods, however, require only associational rather than causal assumptions, because they need not remove confounding (Carroll et al., 2006). For example, if Z is affected by X and is unassociated with Y given X, then Z may serve as an instrument to remove bias due to measurement error, even though Z will not be a valid instrument for confounding control.

BIAS FROM CONDITIONING ON A DESCENDANT OF THE OUTCOME

For various reasons, it may be appealing to examine relations between X and Y conditioning on a function or descendant Y^* of Y. For example, one might suspect that the outcome measurement available becomes increasingly unreliable at high values and therefore wish to exclude high-scoring respondents from the analysis. Such conditioning can produce bias, as illustrated in Figure 12–12. Although U affects Y, U is unassociated with X and so the X–Y association is unconfounded. If we examine the relation between X and Y conditional on Y^*, we open the $U \rightarrow Y \leftarrow X$ path, thus allowing a U–X association and confounding of the X–Y association by U.

Consider the effect of education on mental status, measuring the latter with the Mini-Mental Status Exam (MMSE). The MMSE ranges from 0 to 30, with a score below 24 indicating impairment (Folstein et al., 1975). Suppose we ask whether the effect of education on MMSE is the same for

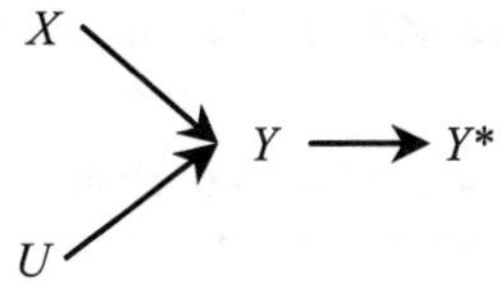

FIGURE 12–12 • Diagram illustrating effect of conditioning on an outcome variable.

respondents with MMSE $\geq$ 24 as for respondents with MMSE <24. If education does indeed affect MMSE score, we can apply Figure 12–12 with X = education, Y = MMSE score, and Y^* an indicator of MMSE score $\geq$24. U now represents unmeasured factors that affect MMSE score but do not confound the X–Y association. We should then expect to underestimate the association between education and MMSE score in both strata of Y^*. Among high-MMSE subjects, those with low education are more likely to have factors that raise MMSE scores, whereas among low-MMSE scorers, those with high education are less likely to have such factors. Thus, even if these unmeasured factors are not confounders to start, they will be negatively associated with education within strata of their shared effect, MMSE score.

This bias also occurs when there is an artificial boundary (ceiling or floor) on the measurement of Y and one deletes observations with these boundary values. It also can arise from deleting observations with extreme values of Y (outliers), although many might have to be deleted for the bias to become large. Such exclusions will condition the analysis on the value of Y and can thus introduce bias.

If X has no effect on Y, conditioning on Y^* will not open the $U \rightarrow Y \leftarrow X$ path in Figure 12–12. Thus, if there is no confounding of the X–Y relation and no effect of X on Y, the estimated effect of X on Y will remain unbiased after conditioning on Y^* (although precision of the estimate may be drastically reduced).

SELECTION BIAS AND MATCHING IN CASE-CONTROL STUDIES

Case-control studies are especially vulnerable to selection bias. By definition, case-control studies involve conditioning on a descendant of Y, specifically, the selection variable S. If we compute effect estimates from the case-control data as if there were no effect of Y on S—e.g., a risk difference—it will be severely biased. As discussed in Chapter 8, however, the bias produced by this conditioning will cancel out of the odds ratio from the study, provided S is associated with exposure only through Y (i.e., if Y separates S from X).

Suppose, however, that the situation is as in Figure 12–13. Here, W is not a confounder of the X–Y association if there is no conditioning, because it has no association with Y except through X. A case-control study, however, conditions on selection S. Because W is associated with exposure and affects selection, this conditioning results in a new association of W with Y via S. Thus $X \leftarrow W \rightarrow S \leftarrow Y$ is opened at S and so becomes a biasing path. To identify the effect of X on Y, this path must be blocked, for example, by conditioning on W. The same conclusion applies if Figure 12–13 is modified so that W is associated with X via a variable U with (say) $X \leftarrow U \rightarrow W$.

As discussed in Chapter 11, case-control matching on W means that W affects selection, and so Figure 12–13 can be taken to represent the situation in a case-control study matched on a nonconfounder associated with the exposure. Here, we see that the matching generated the W–S connection and thus necessitates control of W when no control would have been needed without matching. Thus, the figure illustrates a type of overmatching (Chapter 11).

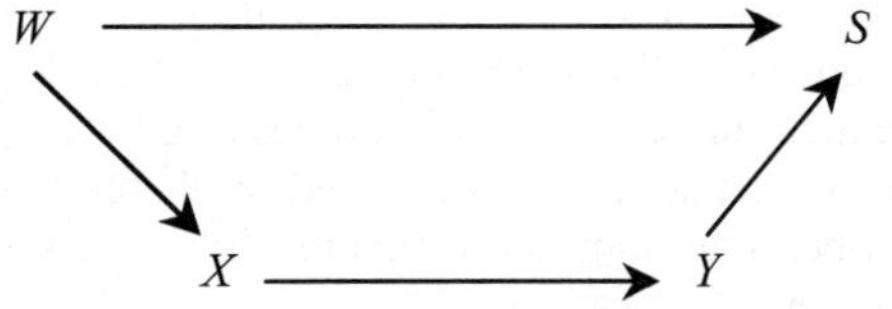

FIGURE 12–13 • Diagram showing potential selection bias in a case-control study with a cause of the exposure influencing selection into the study.

HOW ADJUSTING FOR BASELINE VALUES CAN BIAS ANALYSES OF CHANGE

Research often focuses on identifying determinants of change in a dynamic outcome, such as blood pressure, or depressive symptoms measured at start and end of follow-up, indicated by Y_1 and Y_2. Suppose we wish to estimate how much an exposure X, that was measured at baseline and preceded Y_1, affects the change in the outcome variable between times 1 and 2, measured with the *change score* $\Delta Y = Y_2 - Y_1$. An important issue is whether to adjust for (condition on) the baseline variable Y_1 when attempting to estimate the effect of X on change in the outcome. This conditioning may take the form of restriction or stratification on Y_1, or inclusion of Y_1 as a covariate in a regression of ΔY on X. Typically, X and Y_1 are associated. Indeed, this cross-sectional association may prompt researchers to investigate whether X similarly affects changes in Y.

A common rationale for baseline adjustment is that baseline "acts like a confounder" under the traditional confounder criteria: It is associated with X and likely affects the dependent variable (ΔY). This intuition can be misleading, however, in the common situation in which Y_1 and Y_2 are subject to measurement error (Glymour et al., 2005).

Suppose that our research question is whether graduating from college with honors affects changes in depressive symptoms after graduation. In a cohort of new college graduates, depressive symptoms are assessed with the Centers for Epidemiologic Studies—Depression scale at baseline (CES-D_1) and again after 5 years of follow-up (CES-D_2). The CES-D scale ranges from 0 to 60, with higher scores indicating worse depressive symptoms (Radloff, 1977). The dependent variable of interest is change in depressive symptoms, which we measure in our data using the CES-D change score ΔCES-D = CES-D_2 − CES-D_1. The CES-D is a common measure of depressive symptoms, but it is known to have considerable measurement error. In other words, the CES-D score is influenced both by actual underlying depression and by randomly fluctuating events such as the weather and the interviewer's rapport with the subject. In a causal diagram, we represent this by showing arrows into CES-D score from underlying depression and from a summary "error" variable. The error is not measured directly but is defined as the difference between the CES-D score and the latent variable "Depression," so that

$$\text{CES-D} = \text{Depression} + \text{Error}$$

Bear in mind that we are actually interested in change in Depression (ΔDepression), rather than change in CES-D (ΔCES-D).

Now suppose that, at baseline, graduating with honors (X) is associated with lower CES-D scores, that is, there is an inverse association between X and Y_1, perhaps because graduating with honors improves mood, at least temporarily. These assumptions are shown in a DAG in Figure 12–14. In this figure, there is an arrow from Error_1 to ΔCES-D. This arrow represents a deterministic (inverse) relationship between ΔCES-D and Error_1, because

$$\begin{aligned}\Delta\text{CES-D} &= \text{CES-D}_2 - \text{CES-D}_1\\ &= \text{Depression}_2 + \text{Error}_2 - (\text{Depression}_1 + \text{Error}_1)\\ &= \text{Depression}_2 - \text{Depression}_1 + \text{Error}_2 - \text{Error}_1\\ &= \Delta\text{Depression} + \text{Error}_2 - \text{Error}_1\end{aligned}$$

Another assumption in Figure 12–14 is that Error_1 and Error_2 are independent. Positive association of these errors reduces the magnitude of the bias we will discuss, but this bias is not eliminated unless the errors are identical (and so cancel out). Under the conditions of Figure 12–14, honors degree has no effect on change in depression. Correspondingly, honors degree and ΔCES-D are unconditionally independent under the null hypothesis because the only path in the diagram connecting honors degree and change score is blocked by the collider CES-D_1. Thus, when not adjusting for CES-D_1, we obtain an unbiased estimate of the overall (i.e., total) effect of honors degree on change in depression.

Conditional on CES-D_1, however, honors degree and ΔCES-D are associated, because conditioning on CES-D_1 unblocks the path. This result can be explained as follows. Anyone with a high

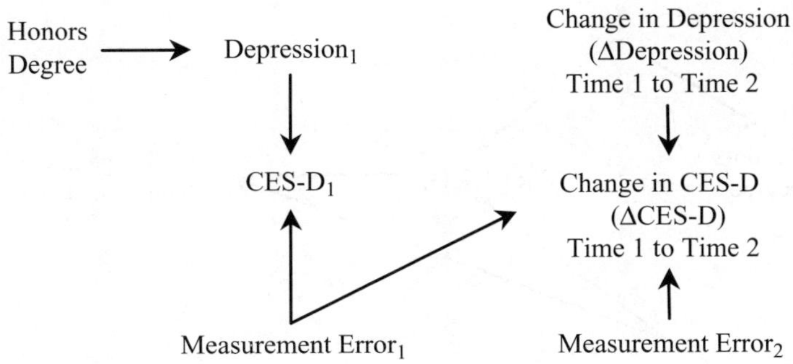

FIGURE 12–14 • An example in which baseline adjustment biases analyses of change.

CES-D_1 has either high Depression$_1$, or large positive measurement Error$_1$, or both. A nondepressed person with high CES-D_1 must have a positive Error$_1$, and a depressed person with low CES-D_1 must have a negative Error$_1$. Thus, *within levels of CES-D_1*, Depression$_1$ and Error$_1$ are inversely associated, and honors degree and Error$_1$ are therefore positively associated. Because Error$_1$ contributes negatively to ΔCES-D, ΔCES-D and Error$_1$ are negatively associated (this is an example of regression to the mean). Hence, conditional on CES-D_1, honors degree and ΔCES-D are inversely associated. Therefore the baseline-adjusted honors-degree association is inverse, making it appear that honors degrees predict declines in depression, even when receiving an honors degree does not affect changes in depression. The bias in the association is proportional to the error in the CES-D scores and the strength of the honors degree–Depression$_1$ association (Yanez et al., 1998).

To summarize the example, the unadjusted association of honors degree and ΔCES-D correctly reflects the effect of honors degree on change in actual depression (ΔDepression), whereas adjustment for baseline CES-D_1 biases the association downward in the direction of the cross-sectional association between CES-D_1 and honors degree.

Now consider baseline adjustment in a slightly different research question, in which we wish to estimate how much a baseline exposure X affects the change score ΔY over the follow-up period. In this case, we ignore measurement error and focus on identifying determinants of changes in CES-D score. We return to our example of the effect of graduating college with honors (X) and CES-D change scores. Figure 12–15 provides one model of the situation. There are confounding paths from X to ΔY via U and Y_1, which we can block by conditioning on baseline score Y_1. Thus, if U is unmeasured, it appears from this model that we ought to control for baseline score. This model for ΔY is fatally oversimplified, however, because there will always be other unmeasured factors that affect CES-D_1 (such as genetic risk factors), which influence both CES-D_1 and the rate of change.

If we expand Figure 12–15 to include such a factor, B, and B is unassociated with X, we obtain Figure 12–16. B does not appear to be a confounder, but it is a collider on a path between X and ΔY. Conditioning on baseline Y_1 opens the confounding path $X \leftarrow U \rightarrow Y_1 \leftarrow B \rightarrow \Delta Y$. Thus, adjusting for baseline is insufficient to eliminate bias in assessing the relation of X to the change score ΔY; after such adjustment, to ensure unbiasedness we would have to adjust for all shared causes of earlier and later scores—a daunting task to say the least.

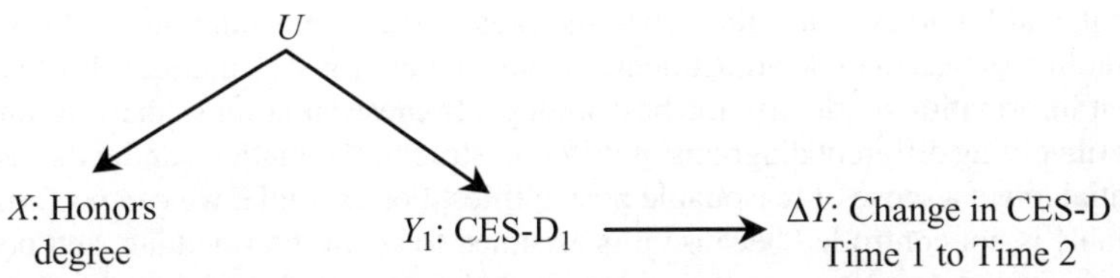

FIGURE 12–15 • An example in which baseline adjustment eliminates bias in analyses of change.

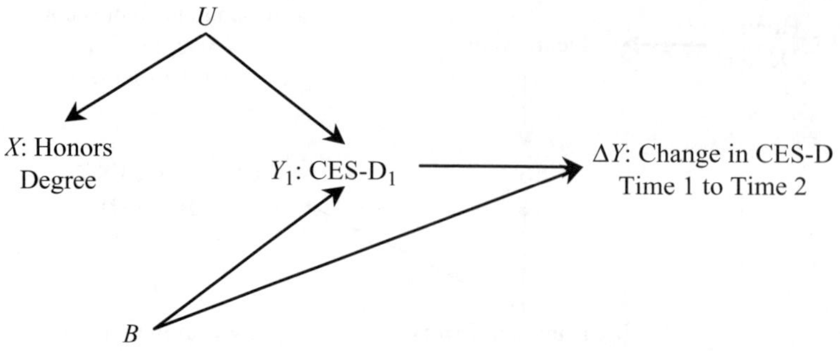

FIGURE 12–16 • An example in which baseline adjustment does not eliminate bias in analyses of change.

CAVEATS AND EXTENSIONS

For many if not most epidemiologic research questions, the data available or feasible to obtain are simply not adequate to identify the "right" answer. Given this reality, every method will be biased under conditions that we cannot rule out. Thus it is rarely enough to know that a particular approach is biased; we will want to estimate how biased it may be, especially relative to alternatives. Graphs alone, however, are silent with respect to the magnitude of likely biases.

Graphs can be augmented with signs on each arrow to indicate directions of effects, as is common with structural equation models (Duncan, 1975). Under the assumption of monotonic effects (causal monotonicity), the directions of associations and biases can be computed from these signs (VanderWeele and Robins, 2008b). More detail can be added to causal diagrams to indicate mechanism types under the sufficient-component cause model described in Chapters 2 and 5 (VanderWeele and Robins, 2007b). Nonetheless, causal diagrams as currently developed do not convey information about important aspects of causal relations and biases, such as the magnitudes or functional forms of the relations (e.g., effect size or effect-measure modification).

The g-computation algorithm or g-formula (Robins, 1986, 1987, 1997) can be used to quantify the size of effects and predict the consequences of interventions under an assumed causal structure (Pearl and Robins, 1995). The formula simplifies to ordinary standardization (Chapters 3 and 4) when the intervention variable is a fixed baseline characteristic (as opposed to a time-varying exposure) (Robins, 1987; Pearl, 1995, 2000). Applying the g-computation algorithm is often impractical, for the same reason that stratified analysis methods (Chapter 15) can be impractical with many covariates: There will rarely be enough observations for every combination of covariate levels. This problem is addressed by assuming parametric models for some or all of the relations among the covariates. This approach has a long history in the structural-equations literature (Duncan, 1975; Pearl, 2000). In the structural-equations model for a graph, each variable is represented as a function of its parents and a random error that represents effects of forces not shown in the graph. More advanced approaches such as *g-estimation* and *marginal structural modeling* estimate parameters using structural models only for the effect of interest, and use associational models to control confounding; see Chapter 21 for further description and references.

Modeling approaches allow comparison of bias magnitudes under various scenarios about causal relations. For example, assuming logistic models, Greenland (2003a) compared the bias left by failing to adjust for a variable that is both a collider and confounder, versus the bias introduced by adjusting for it, and found evidence that when the causal structure is unknown, adjustment is more likely to result in less bias than no adjustment. In many (if not most) situations, however, there will be insufficient information to identify the best strategy. In these situations, analyses under different assumptions (involving different diagrams or different structural equations under the same diagram) will be essential to get a sense of reasonable possibilities. For example, we can perform analyses in which a variable is not controlled because it is assumed to be an intermediate, and perform others in which it is treated as a confounder (Greenland and Neutra, 1980); and, in the latter case, we can vary the equations that relate the variable to exposure and disease. Such *sensitivity analyses* are described in Chapter 19.

A related difficulty is deciding whether a dubious causal relationship ought to be represented in a DAG. In typical epidemiologic examples, very weak relationships are unlikely to introduce large biases. Thus one heuristic for drawing DAGs would take the absence of an arrow between two variables to indicate that the direct causal relation between the variables is negligible. While such a heuristic can provide a useful perspective, we recommend starting with a DAG that shows all the arrows that cannot be ruled out based on available data or logic (like time order), to determine what assumptions are required in order to identify with certainty the causal parameter of interest with the available data.

CONCLUSION

Causal diagrams show how causal relations translate into associations. They provide a simple, flexible tool for understanding and discovering many problems, all using just a few basic rules. Rather than considering each type of bias as a new problem and struggling for the "right" answer, diagrams provide a unified framework for evaluating design and analysis strategies for any causal question under any set of causal assumptions. Nonetheless, drawing a diagram that adequately describes contextually plausible assumptions can be a challenge. To the extent that using diagrams forces greater clarity about assumptions, accepting the challenge can be beneficial. Although we may never know the "true" diagram, to the extent that we can specify the diagram, we will be able to identify key sources of bias and uncertainty in our observations and inferences.

Section III

Data Analysis

CHAPTER 13

Fundamentals of Epidemiologic Data Analysis

Sander Greenland and Kenneth J. Rothman

Elements of Data Analysis 213
Data Editing 214
Data Description and Summarization 216
Data Tabulation 216
Choice of Categories 217
Classification of Subjects and Person-Time 218
Handling of Missing Values 219
Methods of Testing and Estimation 219
Test Statistics and *P*-Values 220
Median-Unbiased Estimates 221
Sensitivity and Influence Analysis 221
Probability Distributions and Exact Statistics 222
Approximate Statistics: The Score Method 225
Approximate Statistics: The Wald Method 226
Likelihood Functions 227
Approximate Statistics: The Likelihood-Ratio Method 229
Likelihoods in Bayesian Analysis 230
Choice of Test Statistics 231
Continuity Corrections and Mid-*P*-Values 231
Computation and Interpretation of Two-Sided *P*-Values 234
Multiple Comparisons 234
Joint Confidence Regions 235
Problems with Conventional Approaches 236
Summary 237

ELEMENTS OF DATA ANALYSIS

In Chapter 9 we emphasized that a study may be thought of as a measurement exercise, in which the overall goal is accuracy in estimation. Data analysis is the step in this exercise in which the raw data are checked for accuracy, and estimates are then computed from the data, based on assumptions about the forces that led to those data. This chapter describes considerations in data preparation and then reviews the statistical theory that underpins conventional statistical methods, covering in more detail several of the topics introduced in Chapter 10.

By "conventional methods," we mean methods that assume all systematic errors are known and accounted for by the underlying statistical model. Such methods focus on accounting for random errors by familiar means such as standard deviations, *P*-values, confidence intervals, and hypothesis tests. These methods became the standard of analysis in the early to mid 20th century, in parallel with the ascendance of random sampling and randomization as the "gold standard" of study design. Because they remain the standard of presentation in the health and social science literature, Chapters 14 through 17 provide details of conventional methods for epidemiologic data analysis, and Chapter 18 presents their Bayesian analogs. Chapter 19 provides an introduction to methods that address the key shortcomings of conventional methods by examining the possible role of systematic errors (bias sources) in generating the observations.

A good data analysis has several distinct stages. In the first stage, the investigator should review the recorded data for accuracy, consistency, and completeness. This process is often referred to as *data editing*. Next, the investigator should summarize the data in a concise form for descriptive analysis, such as contingency tables that classify the observations according to key factors. This stage of the analysis is referred to as data reduction or *data summarization*. Finally, the summarized data are used to estimate the epidemiologic measures of interest, typically one or more measures of occurrence or effect (such as risk or relative-risk estimates), with appropriate confidence intervals. This estimation stage is usually based on smoothing or modeling the data, which can lead to many philosophical as well as technical issues (Greenland, 1993c); see Chapters 17–21.

The estimation stage of analysis usually includes statistical hypothesis testing. Chapter 10 explained why statistical hypothesis testing is undesirable in most epidemiologic situations. Nonetheless, because the statistical theory and methods of confidence intervals parallel those of statistical hypothesis testing, it is useful to study the theory and methods of statistical hypothesis testing as part of the foundation for understanding the estimation step of data analysis.

The final step of analysis involves properly interpreting the results from the summarization and estimation steps. This step requires consideration of unmeasured factors that may have influenced subject selection, measurement, and risk, as well as issues in statistical inference. These considerations are usually nothing more than description of possible factors, along with qualitative judgments about their possible importance. Chapter 19 describes ways in which these considerations can be given a more quantitative form.

DATA EDITING

The essential first task of data analysis is careful scrutiny of the raw data for errors and correction of such errors whenever possible (Chapter 24). Errors find their way into data in a variety of ways; some errors are detectable in editing and some are not.

The data in an epidemiologic study usually come from self-administered or interviewer-administered questionnaires, from existing records that are transcribed for research, or from electronic databases collected for purposes other than research (such as disease surveillance registries or administrative medical databases). The data from these sources may be transcribed from this primary form to a code form for machine entry, or they may be electronically loaded directly from one database to a research database. Coding of responses is often necessary. For example, occupational data obtained from interviews need to be classified into a manageable code, as does drug information, medical history, and many other types of data.

Data on continuous variables such as age, although often grouped into broad categories for reporting purposes, should be recorded in a precise form rather than grouped, because the actual values will allow greater flexibility later in the analysis. For example, different groupings may be necessary for comparisons with other studies. Year of birth may be preferable to age, because it tends to be reported more accurately and does not change with time.

Some nominal-scale variables that have only a limited number of possible values can be precoded on the primary forms by checking a designated box corresponding to the appropriate category. For nominal-scale variables with many possible categories, however, such as country of birth or occupation, precoded questions may not be practical if full detail is desired. If all data items can be precoded, it may be feasible to collect the data in a primary form that can be read directly by a machine, for example, by optical scanning. Otherwise, it will be necessary to translate the information on the primary data form before it is stored in a computer or in machine-readable form. Such translation may introduce errors, but it also provides an opportunity to check for errors on the primary form. Alternatively, respondents can be asked to answer questionnaires made available to them on a computer or via the Internet. These data will still need to be edited to code open-response items.

It is desirable to avoid rewriting the data onto a secondary data form during the coding process, which may generate additional transcription errors. The number of errors may be reduced by coding the data as part of the computer entry process. A computer program can be devised to prompt data entry item by item, displaying category codes on a terminal screen to assist in coding. If the data are coded and rewritten by hand, they will often require key entry anyway, unless they are coded onto optical-scanning sheets; consequently, direct data entry during coding reduces both costs and errors.

Whenever possible, data entry and data coding should be kept separate. Data entry should follow the original collection form as closely as possible. Computer algorithms should be used to code data from the entries, rather than relying on data-entry personnel to perform the coding. For example, if age information is collected as date of birth, it should be entered as date of birth and then age at the study date can be calculated by the computer. Similarly, with fewer rewriting operations between the primary record and the machine-stored version, fewer errors are likely to occur. If rewriting is unavoidable, it is useful to assess the extent of coding errors in the rewritten form by coding a proportion of the data forms twice, by two independent individuals. The information thus obtained can be used to judge the magnitude of bias introduced by misclassification from coding errors.

Basic editing of the data involves checking each variable for impossible or unusual values. For example, gender may be coded 1 for male and 2 for female, in which case any other recorded value for gender will represent an error or an unknown value. Usually a separate value, such as −1 or 9, is used to designate an unknown value. It is preferable not to use a code of 0 if it can be avoided, because non-numeric codes (such as special missing-value codes) may be interpreted by some programs as a 0. Not assigning 0 as a specific code, not even for unknown information, makes it easier to detect data errors and missing information. Any inadmissible values should be checked against the primary data forms. Unusual values such as unknown gender or unusual age or birth year should also be checked. A good data-entry program will provide for detection of such values.

The entire distribution of each variable should also be examined to see if it appears reasonable. In a typical residential population, one expects about half of the subjects to be male; if the subjects have, say, lung cancer, one might expect about 70% to be male; and if the subjects are a typical group of nurses, one might expect a few percent to be male. Deviations from expectations may signal important problems that might not otherwise come to light. For example, a programming error could shift all the data in each electronic record by one or more characters, thereby producing meaningless codes that might not be detected without direct visual inspection of data values. The potential for such errors heightens the need to check carefully the distribution of each variable during the editing of the data.

The editing checks described so far relate to each variable in the data taken singly. In addition to such basic editing, it is usually desirable to check the consistency of codes for related variables. It is not impossible, but it is unusual that a person who is 16 years of age will have three children. Men should not have been hospitalized for hysterectomy. People over 2 meters tall are unlikely to weigh less than 50 kg. Thorough editing will involve many such consistency and logic checks and is best accomplished by computer programs designed to flag such errors (MacLaughlin, 1980), although it can also be done by inspecting cross-tabulations. Occasionally, an apparently inconsistent result may appear upon checking to be correct, but many errors will turn up through such editing.

It is important, also, to check the consistency of various distributions. If exactly 84 women in a study are coded as "no menopause" for the variable "type of menopause" ("no menopause," surgical, drug-induced, natural), then it is reassuring that exactly 84 are likewise coded as having no menopause for the variable "age at menopause" (for such a variable, the code "no menopause" should take a different code number from that assigned to unknown—e.g., −1 for no menopause and −9 for unknown).

An important advantage of coding and entering data through a computer program is the ability to require all data forms to be entered twice. The data entered in the second pass are compared with the data entered on the first pass, and inconsistencies are flagged and resolved in real time. Double data entry reduces keystroke errors and other data-entry errors that affect data quality. A second advantage of entering data through a computer program is the ability to edit the data automatically during the entry process. Inadmissible or unusual values can be screened as they are entered. Inadmissible values can be rejected and corrected on the spot by programming the machine to display an error message on the screen and give an audible message as well to alert the operator about the error. Unlikely but possible values can be brought to the operator's attention in the same way.

A sophisticated data-entry program can also check for consistency between variables and can eliminate some potential inconsistencies by automatically supplying appropriate codes. For example, if a subject is premenopausal, the program can automatically supply the correct code for "age at menopause" and skip the question. On the other hand, it is safer to use the redundancy of the second question to guard against an error in the first. Nonetheless, even with sophisticated editing during data entry, it is still important to check the stored data for completeness and reasonableness of the distribution of each variable.

Even the most meticulous data-collection efforts can suffer from errors that are detectable during careful editing. If editing is planned as a routine part of handling the data, such errors need not cause serious problems. If editing is neglected, however, data errors may undermine subsequent analyses.

DATA DESCRIPTION AND SUMMARIZATION

Data analysis should begin with careful examination of the data distributions of the analysis variables (exposures, diseases, confounders, effect-measure modifiers). This examination can be done with tables, histograms, scatterplots, and any other visual aid. We wish to emphasize strongly, however, that these data descriptors do *not* include P-values, confidence intervals, or any other statistics designed for making inferences beyond the data. Unfortunately, many statistical packages automatically generate such inferential statistics with all descriptive statistics. This automation is hazardous for a number of reasons, not the least of which is that it invites one to treat inferential statistics as descriptions of one's data.

With few exceptions, inferential statistics should not be treated as data descriptors, because useful and correct interpretations of such statistics require some assumption or model about the relation of the data to some population or theoretical structure beyond the data. For example, interpretations of significance tests and confidence intervals refer to the true value of the association under study; this value does not exist in the data, but in some target population or some theoretical model relating disease to exposure. There are a few statistics that can be useful in both descriptive and inferential analyses; an example is the proportion getting disease in an observed cohort, which is both descriptive of the cohort and is also an estimate of the average risk of disease in cohorts exchangeable with the observed cohort. Nonetheless, attempts to claim a descriptive role for analytic statistics such as P-values and standard errors appear to be contrived and unnecessary.

If descriptive statistics are not for inference beyond the data, what are they for? First, they can help one spot data errors. There may be nothing unusual about having both women under age 40 and menopausal women in one's data, but if one sees a cross-tabulation of age and menopausal status (premenopausal, natural, surgical) in which there are women under age 40 who have had natural menopause, it behooves one to check the correctness of the age and menopausal status data.

Second, descriptive statistics can help one anticipate violations of assumptions required by inferential statistics. In epidemiology, most inferential statistics are *large-sample* (asymptotic) statistics, meaning that they require certain numbers of subjects to be "large" (where "large" may mean only "five or more"). For example, validity of the ordinary (Pearson) chi-square (χ^2) test of association for two categorical variables is usually said to require expected values of at least four or five per cell. Suppose, upon examining the observed data, one sees that there are fewer than eight subjects in some categories of an exposure. One should then immediately know that, in a complete table of exposure and disease, some cells will have fewer than four expected subjects and so will not have sufficiently large expected values for the Pearson χ^2 test to be valid. For such checking purposes, one will often want to return to the descriptive summaries after one has moved on to inferential statistics.

DATA TABULATION

In many fields, means, medians, and other continuous measures are common data summaries. In epidemiology, however, the most useful summaries are usually contingency tables in which the frequency of subjects (or units of observation) with specific combinations of variable values is tabulated for the key variables of interest. Such a table may contain essentially all the relevant information in the data. If so, the contingency table will be all the investigator needs for estimation.

Even if the table does not contain all relevant information, it can directly display relations among the main study variables. For variables (such as age and diastolic blood pressure) that are measured on continuous scales, scatterplots and other exploratory visual displays can provide further insights (Tukey, 1977).

Analysis of data in the form of a contingency table essentially assumes that there is at most only a small number of variables that might be confounders or effect-measure modifiers. If one must adjust simultaneously for a large number of variables, an analysis based on regression modeling may be necessary. Examination of contingency tables and scatterplots can reveal whether the number of subjects is adequate for certain types of regression models, and can also serve as a check on the validity of the regression analysis. Indeed, proceeding with an abridged analysis based on the contingency table data is essential even if one is certain that the final analysis will be based on a regression model.

CHOICE OF CATEGORIES

Collapsing the edited data into categories for the contingency table may necessitate some decision making. The process can be straightforward for nominal-scale variables such as religion or ethnicity, which are already categorized. Some categories may be collapsed together when data are sparse, provided these combinations do not merge groups that are very disparate with respect to the phenomena under study. For continuous variables, the investigator must decide how many categories to make and where the category boundaries should be. The number of categories will usually depend on the amount of data available. If the data are abundant, it is nearly always preferable to divide a variable into many categories. On the other hand, the purpose of data summarization is to present the data concisely and conveniently; creating too many categories will defeat this purpose.

For adequate control of confounding, about five categories may often suffice (Cochran, 1968), provided the boundaries are well chosen to reflect the size of the confounder effects expected across and within categories. As discussed later in this chapter and in Chapter 15, use of percentiles to create confounder categories (e.g., using quintiles as boundaries to create five equal-sized categories) may fail to control confounding adequately if the variable is a strong confounder and is unevenly distributed (highly nonuniform) across its range. In that case, one or a few of the resulting confounder-percentile categories are likely to be overly broad, resulting in large confounder effects within those categories (where they will be uncontrolled), and leaving the exposure-effect estimates seriously confounded within those categories.

Similarly, if an exposure variable is categorized to examine effect estimates for various levels of exposure, again about five categories may often suffice, provided the boundaries are well chosen to reflect the size of the effects expected across the range of exposure. As discussed later in this chapter and in Chapter 17, use of percentiles to create the exposure categories may fail to capture exposure effects adequately if the exposure distribution is quite uneven. In that case, one or a few of the resulting exposure-percentile categories are likely to be overly broad, resulting in exposure effects aggregated within those categories (where they may go undetected), and diminished estimates of exposure effects across categories.

All too often the data are so sparse that it will be impractical to use as many as five categories for a given variable. When the observations are stretched over too many categories, the numbers within categories become so small that patterns cannot be easily discerned in the resulting cross-tabulation. Even if the number of categories per variable is only two or three, a large body of data can be spread too thin if the contingency table involves many dimensions, that is, if many variables are used to classify the subjects.

Suppose that we create a separate two-way table (or stratum) of exposure and disease for each possible combination of levels for potentially confounding variables. With three confounders of three categories each, there will be $3^3 = 27$ strata, for a total of $27 \times 4 = 108$ table cells if both exposure and disease are dichotomous. With an additional two confounders of three categories each, there will be $3^5 = 243$ strata, for a total of $243 \times 4 = 972$ cells; this is enough to stretch even a considerable body of data quite thinly, because a study of 1,000 people will average only about one subject per cell of the multidimensional table. If five categories are used for the five confounders, there will be $5^5 = 3{,}125$ strata, for a total of $3{,}125 \times 4 = 12{,}500$ cells.

There is no generally accepted method to decide where to draw the boundary between categories. A frequently expressed concern is that boundaries might be "gerrymandered," that is, shifted after a preliminary examination of the effect estimates in such a way that the estimates are altered in a desired direction. Gerrymandering can occur even when the analyst is attempting to be honest, simply through failure to understand the problems it may engender. For example, conventional statistical methods assume that boundaries were chosen independently of the outcome. Nonetheless, there are legitimate reasons for inspecting the variable distributions when selecting category boundaries. For example, when the cells are large but the data patterns are sensitive to a small shift in the category boundaries, this sensitivity is a finding of potential interest, indicating some special feature of the data distribution. There may be natural categories if the distribution has more than one mode. Nonetheless, it is best to select exposure and outcome categories without regard to the resulting estimates and test statistics; otherwise, the estimates and P-values will be biased.

If meaningful category boundaries are inherent in the variable, these should be used whenever possible. For example, in categorizing subjects according to analgesic consumption, relevant categories will contrast the various therapeutic indications for analgesic use, for which the recommended doses can be specified in advance. It is often desirable, especially for an exposure variable, to retain extreme categories in the analysis without merging these with neighboring categories, because the extreme categories are often those that permit the most biologically informative contrasts, provided enough subjects fall into these categories.

As mentioned earlier, one common method for creating category boundaries is to set the boundaries at fixed percentiles (quantiles) of the variable. For example, quintile categories have boundaries at the 20th, 40th, 60th, and 80th percentiles of the variable distribution. Although this categorization is sometimes adequate, such an automatic procedure can lead to very misleading results in many situations. For example, for many occupational and environmental exposures, such as to electromagnetic fields, most people—over 90%—are exposed in a very narrow range. When this is so, there may be almost no difference in exposure among the first four of the five quintiles, and the fifth high-exposure quintile may itself contain many persons with exposure little different from the lower quintiles. As a result, a comparison of risk will reveal no effect across the first four quintiles, and a diluted effect comparing the fifth quintile to the fourth. The apparent absence of trend produced by such a quintile analysis may be taken as evidence against an effect, when in reality it is only an artifact of using quintiles rather than biologically or physically meaningful categories.

In a parallel fashion, use of percentiles to create confounder categories can leave serious residual confounding when most of the confounder distribution is concentrated in a very narrow range, but the confounder effect is considerable across its entire range. In that case, there might be almost no difference in the confounder across all but one of the categories, while the remaining category may contain persons with vastly different confounder values. As a consequence, that category may yield a highly confounded estimate of exposure effect and produce bias in any summary estimate of exposure effect.

Another problem in creating categories is how to deal with the ends of the scale. Open-ended categories can provide an opportunity for considerable residual confounding, especially if there are no theoretical bounds for the variable. For example, age categories such as 65+, with no upper limit, allow a considerable range of variability within which the desired homogeneity of exposure or risk may not be achieved. Another example is the study of the effects of alcohol consumption on the risk of oral cancer. Control of tobacco use is essential; within the highest category of tobacco use, it is likely that the heaviest alcohol users will also be the heaviest smokers (Rothman and Keller, 1972). When residual confounding from open-ended categories is considered likely, we recommend that one place strict boundaries on every category, including those at the extremes of the scale; if sparse categories result, one should use sparse-data analysis methods, such as Mantel-Haenszel methods (see Chapter 15) or modeling (Chapters 20–21).

A convenient method of assembling the final categories is to categorize the data initially much more finely than is necessary. A fine categorization will facilitate review of the distribution for each variable; fewer categories for subsequent analyses can then be created by combining adjacent categories. Combining adjacent strata of a confounding variable can be justified if no confounding is introduced by merging the categories. The advantage of starting with more categories than will ultimately be necessary is that the data can be used to help identify which mergings will not introduce confounding. Merging will generally not introduce confounding if the exposure distribution does not vary across strata of the study cohort (in a cohort study) or source population (in a case-control study). It will also not introduce confounding if average risk among the unexposed is constant across strata.

CLASSIFICATION OF SUBJECTS AND PERSON-TIME

Classification of subjects or person-time into categories of exposure and other covariates is rarely straightforward if the covariate is a time-varying subject characteristic such as an occupational exposure or medication. At the very least, the person-time experience classified as "exposed" needs to be defined according to a plausible model for induction time (see Chapters 7 and 16). Before a person becomes exposed, all of that person's time at risk is, naturally, unexposed person-time. If exposure occurs at a point in time and the induction-time model being evaluated calls for a minimum induction time of 5 years, then all the time at risk up to 5 years after the point of exposure for each individual should likewise be treated as unexposed person-time experience rather than exposed. The reason that this time following exposure should be treated as unexposed time is that, according to the induction-time model, any disease that occurs during the period just following exposure relates back to a period of time when exposure was absent.

Tallying persons or person-time units (time at risk) into the appropriate exposure categories must be done subject by subject. The assignment into categories may involve complicated rules if the exposure may vary. Incident cases are tallied into the same category to which the concurrent person-time units are being added. For example, if the induction-time model specified a minimum induction time of 5 years, an incident case occurring 4 years after exposure would not be tallied as an "exposed" case because the person-time for that individual at the time of diagnosis would not be contributing toward "exposed" person-time.

HANDLING OF MISSING VALUES

Frequently, some subject records in a data file are incomplete, in that values are missing from that record for some but not all values of study variables. A common way of dealing with such records is simply to delete them from any analyses that involve variables for which the records have missing values. This approach is called *complete-subject analysis.* It has the advantage of being easy to implement, and it is easy to understand when it is a valid approach. It will be valid (within the limits of the study) whenever subjects with complete data have been, in effect, been randomly sampled from all the subjects in the study; the missing data are then "missing completely at random." It will also be valid if these subjects are randomly sampled within levels of complete variables that are used for stratification (Little and Rubin, 2002).

A drawback of the complete-subject approach is that it is valid only under limited conditions compared with certain more complex approaches. It can also be very inefficient if many subjects have missing values, because it discards so much recorded data (it discards all the data in a record, even if only one study variable in the record has a missing value). For these reasons, many alternatives to complete-subject analysis have been developed, as can be found in more advanced statistics books (e.g., Allison, 2001; Little and Rubin, 2002; Tsiatis, 2006).

Most missing-data methods fall into one of two classes. Imputation methods predict and fill in the missing values based on the observed data and the missing-data pattern (the pattern of missing values seen among all records); multiple imputation is a common example (Little and Rubin, 2002). Inverse-probability weighted methods analyze directly only the complete records but assign special weights to those records based on estimated probabilities of completeness (Robins et al., 1994). All of these methods can be especially valuable when a high proportion of subjects are missing data on a study exposure or a strong confounder. Nonetheless, they assume that the probability that a variable is missing depends only on the observed portion of the data. This "missing at random" condition is weaker than the "missing completely at random" condition, but should not be assumed automatically, especially when the missing data are responses to sensitive personal questions.

Unfortunately, there are some methods commonly used in epidemiology that can be invalid even if data are missing completely at random. One such technique creates a special missing category for a variable with missing values, and then uses this category in the analysis as if it were just a special level of the variable. In reality, such a category is a mix of actual levels of the variable. As a result, the category can yield completely confounded results if the variable is a confounder (Vach and Blettner, 1991) and can thus lead to biased estimates of the overall effect of the study exposure. An equivalent method, sometimes recommended for regression analyses, is to create a special "missing-value" indicator variable for each variable with missing values. This variable equals 1 for subjects whose values are missing and 0 otherwise. This missing-indicator approach is just as biased as the "missing-category" approach (Greenland and Finkle, 1995). For handling ordinary missing-data problems, both the missing-category and missing-indicator approaches should be avoided in favor of other methods; even the complete-subject method is usually preferable, despite its limitations.

METHODS OF TESTING AND ESTIMATION

As indicated in Chapter 10, there is considerable controversy regarding what are the best or even proper approaches to statistical analysis. Most techniques currently used in epidemiology, however, can be derived from fairly standard methods of significance testing and interval estimation. All such methods require that the analyst (or, by default, the analyst's computer program) make assumptions about the probabilities of observing different data configurations. This is so even if one adopts a "nonparametric" or "distribution-free" approach to data analysis. "Distribution-free" methods involve assumptions (models) about data probabilities just as do other methods; they are distinguished only in that they require weaker assumptions than other methods to be valid. Because these weaker assumptions amount to assuming that sampling was random or exposure was randomized, and these assumptions are questionable in observational studies, analysis of epidemiologic data always requires critical examination of the models and assumptions underlying the statistical methods (Greenland, 1990; Chapter 19).

Two broad classes of methods can be distinguished. One comprises *small-sample* (or exact) methods, which are based on direct computation of data probabilities; the other comprises *large-sample* (or asymptotic) methods, which are based on approximations whose accuracy depends directly on the amount of data available. Approximate methods are used because exact methods can become computationally impractical when the analysis involves many subjects or many variables, and because exact methods are not available for all epidemiologic measures. These different approaches will be illustrated later in this chapter, but in most of this book we focus almost exclusively on simpler large-sample methods.

TEST STATISTICS AND P-VALUES

Recall from Chapter 10 that significance tests begin with a *test statistic.* Examples include the familiar Pearson or Mantel-Haenszel χ^2 statistic computed from a contingency table. Another common type of test statistic is the Wald statistic, which is the estimate of interest (such as an estimated rate difference, or estimated log rate ratio) divided by its estimated standard deviation; this statistic is also known as a *Z-ratio* or *Z-value.* Another common test statistic is the total number of exposed cases observed in the study, which is used in exact tests. A χ^2 statistic reflects only the absolute distance of the actual observations from the observation one would expect under the test hypothesis; it does not reflect direction of departure. In contrast, both the Z-ratio and the number of exposed cases reflect the direction of departure of the actual observations from the observation one would expect under the test hypothesis. For example, Wald statistics of -1.9 and 1.9 would represent equal but opposite departures of the actual observations from their expectations under the test hypothesis. One can compute an absolute (nondirectional) statistic by squaring or taking the absolute value of a directional statistic, provided the latter is 0 when the actual observations perfectly conform to what would be expected under the test hypothesis (as with Wald statistics).

To test a hypothesis with a given statistic, one must be able to compute the probability (frequency) distribution of the statistic over repetitions of the study when the test hypothesis is true. Such computations ordinarily assume the following *validity conditions:* (a) only chance produces differences between repetitions, (b) no biases are operating, and (c) the statistical model used to derive the distribution is correct. The *upper one-tailed P-value* for the observed test statistic is the probability that the statistic would be as high as observed or higher if the test hypothesis and validity conditions were correct; the *lower one-tailed P-value* for the statistic is the probability that the test statistic would be as low as observed or lower if the test hypothesis and validity conditions were correct. In the remainder of this chapter, we will refer to these P-values simply as *upper* and *lower.*

To interpret lower and upper P-values correctly, one must distinguish between absolute and directional test statistics. Consider an ordinary χ^2 statistic for a contingency table (Chapter 17). This absolute statistic ranges from 0 to extreme positive values. A very high value means that the observations are *far* from what would be expected under the test hypothesis, and a small upper P-value means the observations are unusually *far* from this expectation if the test hypothesis and validity conditions are correct. In contrast, a very low value is close to 0 and means that the observations are *close* to this expectation. A small lower P-value thus means the observations are unusually *close* to this expectation if the test hypothesis and validity conditions are correct.

Now consider an ordinary Wald statistic, or Z-score, computed from a point estimate and its standard error. This directional statistic ranges from extreme negative to extreme positive values. A very high value still means that the observations are far from this expectation, but in a positive direction. Now, however, a very low value is very negative, and means that the observations are *far* from what would be expected under the test hypothesis. A small lower P-value thus means that the observations are unusually *far* from this expectation if the test hypothesis and validity conditions are correct. Thus the meaning of a lower P-value is very different for absolute and directional statistics.

A questionable dual tradition regarding P-values and tests has become firmly established in statistical practice. First, it is traditional to use P-values that refer to absolute departures, regardless of whether the actual scientific, medical, or policy context would dictate concern with only one direction of departure (e.g., a positive direction). This practice is bad enough on contextual grounds. For example, in the legal arena it has led to use of absolute statistics to determine whether evidence of harm is "significant," even though by the very statement of the problem, the only concern is with a harmful direction of effect.

Suppose now, whether from context or tradition, one wishes to use an absolute test. Such a test logically dictates use of an absolute statistic. In a rather strange second tradition, however, it has become common first to compute a directional statistic, and from that to compute a nondirectional *two-sided* P-value for the test. This two-sided P-value is usually defined as twice the smaller of the upper and lower P-values. There is, however, a logical problem with two-sided P-values defined in this manner: Unlike one-tailed P-values, they are not necessarily probabilities, as can be seen by noting that they may exceed 1 (as will be shown in a later section). Several different proposals have been made to overcome this problem, one of which (mid-P-values) we discuss later. For now, we use the most common definitions of P-values, in which a one-tailed P-value is always a true probability, but a two-sided P-value is simply twice the smaller of two probabilities and so is not necessarily a probability.

These traditions have implications for interpreting confidence intervals. Recall that a two-sided 90% confidence interval is the set of all values for the measure of interest that have a two-sided P-value of at least 0.10. It follows that a point is inside the two-sided 90% confidence interval if and only if both its lower and upper P-values are greater than $0.10/2 = 0.05$. Similarly, a point is inside the two-sided 95% confidence interval if and only if both its lower and upper P-values are greater than $0.05/2 = 0.025$. Indeed, these conditions are equivalent to the definitions of 90% and 95% confidence intervals.

MEDIAN-UNBIASED ESTIMATES

An exact two-sided P-value reaches its maximum at the point where the lower and upper P-values are equal (the peak of the exact P-value function). This point may be taken as a point estimate of the measure of interest and is called the *median-unbiased estimate*. The name *median unbiased* suggests that the estimate has equal probability of being above the true value as below it. The median-unbiased estimate does not exactly satisfy this condition; rather, it is the point for which the test statistic would have equal probability of being above and below its observed value over repetitions of the study, as well as the peak (maximum) of the exact two-sided P-value function.

Under "large-sample" conditions that will be discussed later, the median-unbiased estimate tends to differ little from the far more common *maximum-likelihood* estimate, also discussed later. We thus focus on the latter estimate in the ensuing chapters of this book.

SENSITIVITY AND INFLUENCE ANALYSIS

Inferential statistics such as P-values and confidence limits must themselves be subjected to scrutiny to complete the statistical portion of the data analysis. Two broad components of this scrutiny are sensitivity and influence analysis.

As mentioned earlier, *all* statistical techniques, even so-called nonparametric or distribution-free methods, are based on assumptions that often cannot be checked with available data. For example, one may be concerned that the observed association (or lack thereof) was a consequence of an unmeasured confounder, or misclassification, or an undetected violation of the model used for analysis. One way to deal with the issue of possible assumption violations is to conduct a *sensitivity analysis,* in which the statistical analysis is systematically repeated, using different assumptions each time, to see how sensitive the statistics are to changes in the analysis assumptions. In sensitivity analysis, one may repeat the analysis with different adjustments for uncontrolled confounding, measurement errors, and selection bias, and with different statistical models for computing P-values and confidence limits. Chapter 19 provides an introduction to sensitivity analysis.

It is possible for analysis results to hinge on data from only one or a few key subjects, even when many subjects are observed. *Influence analysis* is a search for such problems. For example, the analysis may be repeated deleting each subject one at a time, or deleting each of several special subgroups of subjects, to see if the statistics change to an important extent upon such deletions. Statistical quantities that change little in response to such deletions are sometimes said to be *resistant* to the deletions. When the key estimates of interest are found to be strongly influenced by deletions, it will be necessary to report the influential observations and their degree of influence on the estimates.

PROBABILITY DISTRIBUTIONS AND EXACT STATISTICS

We will illustrate basic concepts in the context of a prevalence survey for human immunodeficiency virus (HIV). Suppose that we take as our test statistic the number of HIV-positive subjects observed in the sample. It is possible that among 1,000 sampled subjects, 10 would test positive; it is also possible that four would test positive; it may also be possible that 100 would test positive. If, however, our sample of 1,000 was drawn randomly from all U.S. Army enlistees, getting 100 positives would be highly improbable (in the sense that we would expect that result to occur very rarely), whereas getting four positives would not. The reasons are that the U.S. Army will not knowingly enlist high-risk or HIV-positive persons (so such persons tend to avoid enlistment), and HIV prevalence in the general U.S. population is less than a few percent.

A *probability distribution* for a test statistic is just a rule, model, or function that tells us the probability of each possible value for our test statistic. For the present example, our test statistic for testing hypotheses about HIV prevalence in the sampled population will be $Y =$ the number of HIV-positive sample subjects. Suppose that the survey sample is a simple random sample of the population, the true prevalence of HIV in the population is 0.004, and the sample size is no more than a fraction of a percent of the population size. Then the probability of getting $Y = 2$ (two positives) among 1,000 surveyed is given by

$$\Pr(Y = 2 \mid \text{HIV prev.} = 0.004) = 0.146$$

or about one chance in seven.

We can derive the preceding probability (of 0.146) as follows. Suppose the subjects are to be selected in sequence, from the first to the 1,000th subject. With our assumptions, the HIV status of each subject is approximately independent of the status of any other subject. Thus, the probability that the first and second subject are HIV-positive and the others are not is

$$0.004^2(1 - 0.004)^{1{,}000-2}$$

We obtain the same number for the probability that any two distinct subjects (e.g., first and third, or second and fourth) are positive and the others are not.

To find the total probability that exactly two subjects are positive, we must multiply the preceding number by the number of combinations (ways) in which exactly two of the 1,000 subjects are positive. To find this number of combinations, note that there are $1{,}000 \cdot 1{,}000$ pairs of orders of subjects (first, first), (first, second), (second, first), etc. However, in 1,000 of these pairs of orders the first and second entries are the same and so do not contain two subjects, i.e., the pairs (first, first), (second, second), and so on. Removing these one-subject pairs leaves

$$1{,}000 \cdot 1{,}000 - 1{,}000 = 1{,}000(1{,}000 - 1) = 1{,}000 \cdot 999$$

two-subject pairs of orders. However, each of these two-subject pairs has a companion pair that contains the same two subjects in reverse order, e.g., the pair (first, second) represents the same two subjects as (second, first). Therefore, the total number of unique combinations of two subjects among the 1,000 is $1{,}000 \cdot 999/2$. To finish, we multiply this number by the probability that a given pair is positive and the remaining subjects are not:

$$(1{,}000 \cdot 999/2)0.004^2(1 - 0.004)^{1{,}000-2} = 0.146$$

which is the probability that exactly two subjects are HIV-positive.

The preceding paragraph is an example of a *combinatorial argument.* Such arguments are often used to find sample probabilities when random sampling or randomization has been employed in selecting subjects for study. Such arguments also form the foundation of most small-sample statistical methods. The number of unique possible combinations of y subjects taken from N total is given by the formula $N!/y!(N - y)!$. (The exclamation point ! following a number y is read "factorial" and indicates that one should take the product of all numbers from 1 to y; that is, $y! = 1 \cdot 2 \cdot \cdots \cdot y$; by definition, $0!$ is set equal to 1.)

The number of combinations is so important in probability that it is usually expressed with a special notation defined by

$$\binom{N}{y} = \frac{N!}{y!(N-y)!}$$

The number of combinations $\binom{N}{y}$ is often read "N choose y" and is sometimes called the *combinatorial coefficient* or *binomial coefficient*. The latter term arises from the fact that $\binom{N}{y}$ appears in the general formula for the binomial distribution (see later). In the above example of finding the number of combinations of two subjects out of 1,000, we get

$$\binom{1{,}000}{2} = \frac{1{,}000!}{2!(1{,}000-2)!} = \frac{1{,}000 \cdot 999 \cdot 998 \cdot \cdots \cdot 2 \cdot 1}{2 \cdot 1(998 \cdot 997 \cdot \cdots \cdot 2 \cdot 1)} = 1{,}000 \cdot 999/2$$

which is what we deduced earlier.

Under the above assumptions, the probability of getting $Y = y$ (y positives) out of 1,000 subjects, given an HIV prevalence of 0.004, is

$$\Pr(Y = y \mid \text{HIV prevalence} = 0.004) = \binom{1{,}000}{y} 0.004^{y}(1-0.004)^{1{,}000-y} \qquad [13\text{–}1]$$

Equation 13–1 is an example of a probability distribution. Specifically, it is an example of a *binomial* distribution with a probability *parameter* of 0.004 and a sample size of 1,000.

Now suppose that we carry out the random-sample survey and observe only one positive among 1,000 sampled persons. From formula 13–1, we can compute the probability of observing $Y \leq 1$ (one or fewer positives) under the test hypothesis that the HIV prevalence is 0.004 in the sampled population. Because only $Y = 0$ and $Y = 1$ correspond to one or fewer positives, the probability of one or fewer positives is

$$\begin{aligned}
&\Pr(Y \leq 1 \mid \text{HIV prevalence} = 0.004) \\
&\quad = \Pr(Y = 0 \mid \text{HIV prevalence} = 0.004) \\
&\qquad + \Pr(Y = 1 \mid \text{HIV prevalence} = 0.004) \\
&\quad = \binom{1{,}000}{0} 0.004^{0}(1-0.004)^{1{,}000} + \binom{1{,}000}{1} 0.004^{1}(1-0.004)^{999} \\
&\quad = (1-0.004)^{1{,}000} + 1{,}000(0.004)(1-0.004)^{999} \\
&\quad = 0.091
\end{aligned}$$

This probability is P_{lower}, the traditional (Fisher) lower-tailed exact P-value for the test hypothesis. Here, the number of positives Y serves as the test statistic, and we compute the P-value directly from the exact distribution of Y as given by formula 13–1.

If we repeat our calculation under the test hypothesis that the HIV prevalence is 0.005, we have to use the following probability distribution to get P-values:

$$\begin{aligned}
&\Pr(Y = y \mid \text{HIV prevalence} = 0.005) \\
&\quad = \binom{1{,}000}{y} 0.005^{y}(1-0.005)^{1{,}000-y} \qquad [13\text{–}2]
\end{aligned}$$

The differences between formulas 13–1 and 13–2 illustrate how the probability distribution for the test statistic changes when the test hypothesis is changed, even though the test statistic Y does not. Formula 13–2 yields a lower P-value of

$$\begin{aligned}
P_{\text{lower}} &= \Pr(Y \leq 1 \mid \text{HIV prevalence} = 0.005) \\
&= \Pr(Y = 0 \mid \text{HIV prevalence} = 0.005) + \Pr(Y = 1 \mid \text{HIV prevalence} = 0.005) \\
&= (1-0.005)^{1{,}000} + 1{,}000(0.005)(1-0.005)^{999} = 0.040
\end{aligned}$$

By doubling the above P-values, we get two-sided P-values of 0.18 under the hypothesis that the HIV prevalence is 0.004, and 0.08 under the hypothesis that the HIV prevalence is 0.005. To illustrate, recall that a two-sided 90% confidence interval derived from a test comprises all points for which the two-sided P-value from the test is at least 0.10, and the 90% confidence limits are the two points at which the two-sided P-value is 0.10. Because a prevalence of 0.0040 yielded a two-sided P-value greater than 0.10, it must be inside the 90% interval. Because a prevalence of 0.0050 yielded a two-sided P-value less than 0.10, it must be outside the 90% interval. We can interpolate that the upper 90% limit must be roughly $(0.10 - 0.08)/(0.18 - 0.08) =$ one fifth of the way from 0.005 to 0.004, which corresponds to a prevalence of 0.0048. One way to check this interpolation is to compute the lower exact P-value for 0.0048:

$$P_{\text{lower}} = (1 - 0.0048)^{1,000} + 1{,}000(0.0048)(1 - 0.0048)^{999} = 0.0474$$

Doubling this lower exact P-value yields a two-sided P-value of 0.095. Because this P-value is just under 0.10, we may conclude that a prevalence of 0.0048 is just outside the 90% interval, and that the upper 90% confidence limit is a little under 0.0048 (the limit is in fact closer to 0.0047).

To obtain a point estimate of the HIV prevalence, we must find the test hypothesis at which the lower P-value and upper P-value equal one another. We must therefore also calculate the upper exact P-value, P_{upper}, which is the probability that Y is at least as big as the observed value of 1. It is often easier to work with 1 minus this probability, which is the probability that Y is less than its observed value. For example, if we wish to test the hypothesis that the HIV prevalence is 0.001, we use the relation

$$\begin{aligned} P_{\text{upper}} &= \Pr(Y \geq 1 \mid \text{HIV prevalence} = 0.001) \\ &= 1 - \Pr(Y < 1 \mid \text{HIV prevalence} = 0.001) \end{aligned}$$

Because 0 is the only possible Y value of less than 1, we have

$$\begin{aligned} P_{\text{upper}} &= 1 - \Pr(Y = 0 \mid \text{HIV prevalence} = 0.001) \\ &= 1 - (1 - 0.001)^{1,000} = 0.63 \end{aligned}$$

The lower P-value for the same test hypothesis is

$$\begin{aligned} P_{\text{lower}} &= \Pr(Y \leq 1 \mid \text{HIV prevalence} = 0.001) \\ &= (1 - 0.001)^{1,000} + 1{,}000(0.001)(1 - 0.001)^{999} = 0.74 \end{aligned}$$

Thus $P_{\text{upper}} < P_{\text{lower}}$ for an HIV prevalence of 0.001. If, however, we increase the test hypothesis to 0.0011 and recompute the P-values, we get

$$P_{\text{upper}} = 1 - (1 - 0.0011)^{1,000} = 0.67$$

and this equals

$$P_{\text{lower}} = (1 - 0.0011)^{1,000} + 1{,}000(0.0011)(1 - 0.0011)^{999} = 0.67$$

Thus, 0.0011 is the median-unbiased estimate of the HIV prevalence. Note that this estimate is not quite equal to the sample prevalence of $1/1{,}000 = 0.0010$. The sample prevalence, however, is not an ideal estimate in very small samples (Bishop et al., 1975; Chapter 12; Greenland, 2006b).

This process of repeated P-value computation typifies many computational approaches for exact analysis, as well as for various approximate methods such as *g-estimation* (Chapter 21). For the preceding simple example, there are formulas that give the exact limits in just one step, but for more complicated data one must turn to iterative computations (and hence computers) to get exact results.

In the preceding example, the most crucial statistical assumption underlying the applications of the binomial distribution was the assumption that the sampling of 1,000 participants from the target population was random. If the sampling was not random, then the above statistical analysis (and any inference based on it) would be open to question. Even if the sampling was random, further assumptions would be needed to make valid inferences about HIV prevalence in the sampled population, among them that the measurement technique (here, the test for HIV) used by the survey is error-free. Such an assumption is of course not realistic, but it could be assessed via sensitivity analysis (Chapter 19).

By computing P-values for many different test hypotheses, we are in effect drawing out the P-value function. Returning to the preceding example, we may continue to draw out the P-value function for the HIV prevalence based on our random-sampling model by writing a general form for the probability distributions. If we let the Greek letter π (pi) stand for the HIV prevalence in the sampled population, we can write the probability distribution for the number of HIV positives in our sample of 1,000 as

$$\Pr(Y = y \mid \text{HIV prevalence} = \pi) = \binom{1{,}000}{y} \pi^y (1 - \pi)^{1{,}000-y}$$

The earlier distributions are special cases of this formula, with π hypothesized to equal 0.004, 0.005, 0.0048, 0.001, and 0.0011, respectively. The number π in this formula is called a *parameter* of the distribution, because each different value for π produces a different probability distribution. In our example, π represents the true prevalence of HIV in the sampled population; in other examples, π will represent risk of disease or death.

We can be even more general by letting N represent the size of our random sample; then the last equation becomes

$$\binom{N}{y} \pi^y (1 - \pi)^{N-y} \qquad [13-3]$$

Given a fixed sample size N and parameter π, any probability distribution of this form is called a *binomial distribution.* Equations 13–1 and 13–2 are examples with $N = 1{,}000$ and $\pi = 0.004$ and 0.005, respectively.

APPROXIMATE STATISTICS: THE SCORE METHOD

Exact distributions such as the binomial can be unwieldy to work with if N is very large. This difficulty has led to extensive development of approximations to such distributions, which allow calculation of approximate P-values and estimates.

Some approximations to the binomial distribution are very accurate. Rather than display the most accurate, we focus on two approximate methods, the score method and the Wald method, that are simpler and are special cases of the most common methods. We present many examples of score and Wald statistics in later chapters. The reader has probably encountered examples in past reading, for most epidemiologic statistics are of one of these two types.

Suppose that we have a test statistic Y and formulas $E(Y|\pi)$ and $V(Y|\pi)$ that give us the exact mean and variance of Y when the true parameter value is π. We may then construct approximate tests of the parameter by treating Y as if it were normal with mean and variance computed from the formulas. In the HIV example, Y is binomial, and the formulas for its mean and variance are $N\pi$ and $N\pi(1 - \pi)$. We then test values of π by treating Y as if it were normal with mean $N\pi$ and standard deviation (SD) $[N\pi(1 - \pi)]^{1/2}$. This procedure implies that the *score statistic,* given by

$$\chi_{\text{score}} = (Y - N\pi)/[N\pi(1 - \pi)]^{1/2} \qquad [13-4]$$

has a "standard" normal distribution (that is, a normal distribution with a mean of 0 and a SD of 1). Thus, to find an approximate lower P-value when $Y = y$, we merely look up the probability that a standard normal variate would be less than or equal to χ_{score} with y substituted for Y. To find an approximate upper P-value, we look up the probability that a standard normal deviate would be greater than or equal to χ_{score} with y substituted for Y.

To illustrate this process, suppose that, in the HIV example, the test hypothesis is that the HIV prevalence π is 0.004. Because $N = 1{,}000$ subjects were observed and only $Y = 1$ was HIV-positive, we get

$$\chi_{\text{score}} = \frac{1 - 1{,}000(0.004)}{[1{,}000(0.004)(1 - 0.004)]^{1/2}} = -1.503$$

To get the lower P-value based on this statistic, we need only use a table of the standard normal distribution to find the probability that a standard normal variate would be less than or equal to -1.503; it is 0.067. This value is not particularly close to the exact lower P-value of 0.091 that we obtained earlier. The discrepancy is not surprising, considering that the approximation depends on both $N\pi$ and $N(1 - \pi)$ being "large" (5 or more), and that $N\pi$ is here only $1{,}000(0.004) = 4$. If, however, we next test $\pi = 0.005$, we get $N\pi = 5$, a score statistic of $\chi_{\text{score}} = -1.793$, and an approximate lower P-value of 0.036, practically the same as the exact lower P-value of 0.040 for

$\pi = 0.005$. As before, to get a two-sided P-value, we would just double the smaller of the upper and lower P-values.

This example illustrates that some care is needed when using approximate formulas such as formula 13–4. The criteria for valid approximation are usually summarized by saying that the sample size N must be "large." Unfortunately, a truly large sample is neither necessary nor sufficient for a close approximation. For example, a sample size of 10 can yield a useful approximation if $\pi = 0.5$, for then $N\pi = N(1 - \pi) = 5$. In contrast, a sample size of 100,000 is not big enough to test approximately an hypothesized prevalence of 0.00002, for then $N\pi$ is only 2.

We could, if we wished, find approximate 90% confidence limits for the HIV prevalence π just as before, by trying different hypothesized prevalences π in the score statistic until we found the pair of prevalences with approximate two-sided P-values of 0.10. From a table of the standard normal distribution, we can see that this pair of prevalences must be the pair that yields score statistics (χ_{score}) of -1.645 and 1.645, because a standard normal deviate has a 5% chance of falling below -1.645 and a 5% chance of falling above 1.645. For 95% limits, we would need to find the pair of prevalences that yield score statistics of -1.96 and 1.96. From trying different values for π in formula 13–4 with $N = 1{,}000$, we can see that a prevalence of 0.0045 yields a score statistic χ_{score} of -1.645. Thus, 0.0045 must be the approximate (upper) 90% confidence limit based on the score statistic given above. This value is not far from the exact limit of 0.0047, which we could have anticipated from the fact that $1{,}000(0.0045) = 4.5$ is close to 5.

The approximate point estimate corresponding to the score statistic is easy to find: The approximate upper and lower P-values can be equal only for the prevalence $\hat{\pi}$ that makes $\chi_{\text{score}} = 0$. The latter can happen only if the numerator of χ_{score} is zero, so that

$$Y - N\hat{\pi} = 0$$

Solving for $\hat{\pi}$ yields the approximate estimator $\hat{\pi} = Y/N$. This result shows that the score estimate equals the observed sample proportion. In our example, $\hat{\pi} = 1/1{,}000 = 0.0010$, corresponding to an HIV prevalence of 0.10%. This approximate estimate is remarkably close to the median-unbiased estimate of 0.0011, considering that the informal large-sample criterion $N\hat{\pi}$ equals $1{,}000(0.0010) = 1$, and so is nowhere near "large."

Summarizing and generalizing the above discussion, the score method is based on taking a test statistic Y for which we can compute the exact mean and variance $E(Y|\pi)$ and $V(Y|\pi)$, and creating from these quantities a *score statistic*

$$\chi_{\text{score}} = \frac{Y - E(Y|\pi)}{V(Y|\pi)^{1/2}} \qquad [13\text{–}5]$$

Approximate P-values are found by treating this score statistic as normal with a mean of 0 and a SD of 1. An approximate point estimate may be found by solving the score equation

$$Y - E(Y|\pi) = 0$$

to obtain the $\hat{\pi}$ that has a score statistic of 0 (and hence a two-sided score P-value of 1, the largest possible value).

Under the most commonly used probability models (such as those that assume the observed outcomes are independent and have a binomial, Poisson, or normal distribution), the point estimate $\hat{\pi}$ obtained from the score equation turns out to equal the *maximum-likelihood estimate* (see later). This equivalence arises because the numerator of the score statistic equals the derivative of the log-likelihood function produced by those models. A score statistic obtained by differentiating the log-likelihood function is sometimes called the *efficient score statistic* under the assumed probability model (Cox and Hinkley, 1974). Some statistics books drop the word *efficient* and use the term *score statistic* to refer only to the score statistic derived from the log-likelihood function.

APPROXIMATE STATISTICS: THE WALD METHOD

Although score statistics are much easier to use than exact statistics, they still require some modest computing to find confidence limits. This computational requirement arises because the SD in the denominator of a score statistic changes for each test hypothesis (prevalence). A simpler approximation, called the *Wald method,* replaces the SD in the score statistic (formula 13–5) by a single unchanging value, the SD when $\pi = \hat{\pi}$, the approximate point estimate. This substitution yields the *Wald statistic* based on Y,

$$\chi_{\text{Wald}} = \frac{Y - E(Y|\pi)}{V(Y|\pi = \hat{\pi})^{1/2}} \qquad [13\text{–}6]$$

In the HIV example, $\hat{\pi} = Y/N$, so

$$\begin{aligned}\chi_{\text{Wald}} &= \frac{Y - N\pi}{[N\hat{\pi}(1-\hat{\pi})]^{1/2}} \\ &= \frac{Y - N\pi}{[Y(N-Y)/N]^{1/2}} \qquad [13\text{–}7]\end{aligned}$$

If we replace χ_{Wald} by the value that a desired upper confidence limit π_{U} would yield, we could solve the resulting equation for this π_{U}. For example, to get the upper limit of a two-sided 90% interval, we need to find the prevalence π_{U} that solves

$$\chi_{\text{Wald}} = \frac{y - N\pi_{\text{U}}}{[y(N-Y)/N]^{1/2}} = -1.645$$

Solving for π_{U}, we get

$$\pi_{\text{U}} = Y/N + 1.645\,[Y(N-Y)/N]^{1/2}/N$$

In our HIV example,

$$\begin{aligned}\pi_{\text{U}} &= 1/1{,}000 + 1.645[1(999)/1{,}000]^{1/2}/1{,}000 \\ &= 0.0026\end{aligned}$$

This approximation is poor compared with the score limit. The score statistic yielded an upper limit of 0.0045, whereas the exact upper limit was 0.0047. Unfortunately, this result is typical: Simpler formulas usually yield poorer approximations.

In general, P-values and hence intervals from the Wald method are less accurate than those from the score method, because the Wald method is itself an approximation to the score method (in the above example, it replaces the varying denominator of the score statistic χ_{score}, which depends on π, with a single standard deviation). Because the score method is also an approximation, the Wald method is an approximation to an approximation, and so requires criteria more stringent—for binomial distributions, larger $N\pi$ and $N(1-\pi)$—than those required for the score method to be accurate. Nonetheless, because it is so simple, the Wald method is the most widely used approximation. Its accuracy can be improved by applying it to a function of the proportion, such as the logit transform, instead of to the proportion itself (see Chapter 14).

LIKELIHOOD FUNCTIONS

Likelihood functions play a central role in modern statistical theory. Consider again the general formula 13–3 for the binomial distribution with sample size N, number of observed cases y, and probability parameter π. Let us substitute into this formula the data values for N and y from our hypothetical HIV survey, 1,000 and 1. We get

$$\binom{1{,}000}{1}\pi^{1}(1-\pi)^{1{,}000-1} = 1{,}000\pi(1-\pi)^{999} \qquad [13\text{–}8]$$

Note carefully the following crucial point: Once we replace the data variables in the general binomial probability formula, equation 13–3, with actual data numbers, we are left with a formula, equation 13–8, that has only one variable, π, which is the unknown prevalence parameter that we are trying to estimate.

We can view equation 13–8 as representing a simple mathematical function of the parameter π. This function is called the *likelihood function* for π and is denoted by $L(\pi)$. That is,

$$L(\pi) = 1{,}000\pi(1-\pi)^{999} \qquad [13\text{–}9]$$

is the likelihood function for π given the hypothetical data in our example. This function has a number of applications in statistical analysis. First, it can be used to measure directly the relative support the data provide to various hypotheses. Second, it can supply approximate tests and estimates that have reasonable accuracy in large samples. Third, it can be used to compute Bayesian statistics.

The first two applications begin by finding the value for π, the unknown parameter, that makes the likelihood function $L(\pi)$ as large as it can be. In other words, we find the value of π that brings $L(\pi)$ to its *maximum* value. For example, with calculus we can show that the maximum of formula 13–9 occurs when π is $1/1{,}000 = 0.001$. This value for π is called the *maximum-likelihood estimate* (MLE) of π. More generally, with calculus we can show that the maximum-likelihood estimate for a binomial parameter π is equal to the number of cases divided by the number sampled, y/N. We denote this estimate by $\hat{\pi}_{\text{ml}}$ to distinguish it from the median-unbiased estimate, which was 0.0011 in our example.

Next, consider the maximum value of the likelihood function,

$$
\begin{aligned}
&= L(\hat{\pi}_{\text{ml}}) = L(0.001)\\
&\qquad = 1{,}000(0.001)(1 - 0.001)^{999} = 0.3681
\end{aligned}
$$

Suppose that we are interested in testing a particular hypothesized value for π, say 0.005. One way to do so would be to take the ratio of the likelihood function at $\pi = 0.005$ to the function at $\hat{\pi}_{\text{ml}} = 0.001$. We have

$$L(0.005) = 1{,}000(0.005)(1 - 0.005)^{999} = 0.0334$$

which is $0.0334/0.3681 = 0.0908$ (about 9%) of the maximum value. Some authors suggest using this likelihood ratio or its logarithm to measure directly the degree to which the data support the hypothesized value for π (Edwards, 1992; Goodman and Royall, 1988). Such direct use of likelihood ratios is sometimes called "pure likelihood inference."

In general terms, if we are given a hypothesized (test) value π, then we may measure the relative support the data give π by the *likelihood ratio*

$$LR(\pi) = L(\pi)/L(\hat{\pi}_{\text{ml}}) \qquad [13\text{–}10]$$

or its natural logarithm $\ln[LR(\pi)]$ (Goodman and Royall, 1988; Royall, 1997). In our example, if the test value is 0.005, then the likelihood ratio is

$$LR(0.005) = 0.0334/0.3681 = 0.0908$$

If the test value is 0.004, the likelihood ratio is

$$
\begin{aligned}
LR(0.004) &= L(0.004)/L(\hat{\pi}_{\text{ml}})\\
&= 1{,}000(0.004)(1 - 0.004)^{999}/0.3681 = 0.0730/0.3681 = 0.198
\end{aligned}
$$

or about 20%, more than twice the likelihood ratio for 0.005. Thus, in pure likelihood terms, we could say that a prevalence of 0.004 has twice as much relative support from the data as 0.005.

In likelihood theory, all support is measured relative to the maximum-likelihood estimate. Consequently, the maximum-likelihood estimate $\hat{\pi}_{\text{ml}}$ (0.001 in our example) always has the 100% relative support, because

$$LR(\hat{\pi}_{\text{ml}}) = L(\hat{\pi}_{\text{ml}})/L(\hat{\pi}_{\text{ml}}) = 1.00$$

Although there are no firm guidelines, it is sometimes implied that test values for the study parameter π that have likelihood ratios below $e^{-2} = 0.135$ (13.5% or about 1/7) of the maximum are not well supported by the data (Edwards, 1992). In our example, the upper-score 90% confidence limit of 0.0045 determined earlier has a likelihood ratio of

$$LR(0.0045) = 1{,}000(0.0045)(1 - 0.0045)^{999}/0.3681 = 0.135$$

and so by the 13.5% criterion is on the boundary in terms of relative support. The value 0.0045 is thus an example of a *pure likelihood limit* at the 13.5% relative support level. It is an upper limit, as can be seen from the fact that 0.004 has more relative support and 0.005 has less.

APPROXIMATE STATISTICS: THE LIKELIHOOD-RATIO METHOD

Although pure likelihood limits are not conceptually the same as confidence limits, 13.5% likelihood limits and 95% confidence limits tend to be close in value in large samples. The two types of limits are guaranteed to be close if the confidence limits are approximate ones calculated by the likelihood-ratio method, which we now describe.

As before, suppose that π is the test value of the parameter of interest. Then −2 times the natural log of the likelihood ratio,

$$\chi^2_{\mathrm{LR}} = -2 \cdot \ln[LR(\pi)] \qquad [13\text{–}11]$$

will have an approximately χ^2 distribution with one degree of freedom if π is the true value of the parameter (i.e., if the test hypothesis is true), provided all the usual validity conditions hold (absence of bias and the correct probability model is used to construct the likelihood function) and the sample is "large" in the sense described earlier ($N\pi$ and $N(1-\pi)$ both greater than 5) (Lehmann, 1986; Cox and Hinkley, 1974). The test statistic χ^2_{LR} in formula 13–11 is called the *likelihood-ratio statistic* or *deviance statistic* for testing the hypotheses that π is the true value, and the test of π based on it is called the *likelihood-ratio test* or *deviance test.*

Unlike the score and Wald statistics, the likelihood-ratio statistic bears no resemblance to the ordinary test statistics of elementary courses. It requires some calculus (specifically, the use of a Taylor-series expansion) to show the rather remarkable fact that χ^2_{score}, the score χ^2 based on taking the number of cases as the test statistic (formula 13–5), will approximate χ^2_{LR}, the likelihood-ratio statistic (formula 13–11), if the sample size is large enough and the test value has reasonably high support (Cox and Hinkley, 1974). Because the P-value from χ^2_{score} is two-sided, we can see that the P-value derived from χ^2_{LR} must also be two-sided.

How good are the likelihood-ratio statistics in our example? Because there is only one case among the 1,000 persons sampled, they appear very poor relative to the exact statistics. The likelihood ratio for an HIV prevalence of 0.004 was found earlier to be 0.198, so the likelihood-ratio statistic for this prevalence is $-2 \cdot \ln(0.198) = 3.24$. From a one-degree-of-freedom χ^2 table, we see that this statistic yields a two-sided P-value of 0.072. Contrast this result with the corresponding two-sided exact P-value of $2(0.091) = 0.18$, or the two-sided score P-value of $2(0.067) = 0.13$. Only the two-sided Wald P-value looks less accurate than the likelihood-ratio result in this example. The Wald statistic is

$$\frac{1 - 1{,}000(0.004)}{[1{,}000(0.001)(1 - 0.001)]^{1/2}} = -3.00$$

which yields a two-sided P-value of 0.003.

In this example, the large disparities among the statistics are due chiefly to the fact that the maximum-likelihood estimate of the expected number of cases is very far from the large-sample criterion: $N\hat{\pi}_{\mathrm{ml}} = 1{,}000(0.001) = 1$ in this example. If $\hat{\pi}_{\mathrm{ml}}$, $N\pi$, $N(1-\hat{\pi}_{\mathrm{ml}})$, and $N(1-\pi)$ were all at least 5, we would expect the likelihood-ratio statistic to be much closer to the score statistic.

Likelihood-ratio confidence limits are computed by finding the two parameter values that have likelihood-ratio P-values equal to 1 minus the confidence level. This calculation is equivalent to finding the two limits that have likelihood-ratio statistics equal to the desired percentile of a one-degree-of-freedom χ^2 distribution. Thus, to find 90% likelihood-ratio confidence limits, we find the two parameter values π_{L} and π_{U} that solve the equation

$$-2 \cdot \ln[LR(\pi)] = 2.71 \qquad [13\text{–}12]$$

because 2.71 is the 90th percentile of a χ^2 distribution with one degree of freedom. In the HIV example, we find the limits by solving

$$-2 \cdot \ln[1{,}000\pi(1-\pi)^{999}/0.3681] = 2.71$$

The solution for the upper limit π_U is 0.0036. This limit is not close to the exact limit of 0.0047 or the score limit of 0.0045, but it is still better than the Wald limit of 0.0030. Again, with more cases, the likelihood-ratio result would be much closer to the score result, and all the results would converge to one another.

If we had desired 95% limits instead, we would solve

$$-2 \cdot \ln[LR(\pi)] = 3.84 \qquad [13\text{–}13]$$

because 3.84 is the 95th percentile of a χ^2 distribution with one degree of freedom. This equation yields an upper 95% limit for π of 0.0044, very close to the 13.5% upper pure likelihood limit found earlier. This is no coincidence. Recall that the pure likelihood limit was the upper value for π such that $LR(\pi) = e^{-2}$. If we solve the confidence-limit equation 13–13 for the likelihood ratio $LR(\pi)$, we get

$$LR(\pi) = \exp[-\tfrac{1}{2}(3.84)] = e^{-1.92} = 0.147$$

Thus, the pure-likelihood equation for 13.5% limits and the likelihood-ratio equations for 95% confidence limits are almost the same, and so should yield almost the same interval estimates for π.

For more thorough discussions of the uses of likelihood functions in testing and estimation, and their relation to the score and Wald methods, see Clayton and Hills (1993) for a basic treatment oriented toward epidemiologic applications. Cox and Hinkley (1974) provide a classic treatment oriented toward general conceptual issues as well as mathematical details (the latter authors refer to the Wald statistic as the "maximum-likelihood test statistic").

LIKELIHOODS IN BAYESIAN ANALYSIS

The third application of likelihood ratios is in computing Bayesian statistics, which may be illustrated in its simplest form by combining likelihood ratios with prior odds of hypotheses to find posterior odds of hypotheses. Returning to the HIV survey, suppose that, *before seeing the data,* we think it twice as probable that the prevalence π is 0.004 as opposed to 0.005. That is, we would bet in favor of 0.004 over 0.005 with two-to-one (2/1) odds (perhaps because of previous survey results). How should we revise these betting odds upon seeing the data? More generally, given a prior odds (odds *before* seeing the data) for parameter value π_1 versus parameter value π_0, what should be the posterior odds (odds *after* seeing the data)?

The answer can be computed from elementary probability theory to be

$$\text{Odds after data} = \frac{\text{likelihood for } \pi_1}{\text{likelihood for } \pi_0}\ \text{odds before data}$$

or

$$\text{Posterior odds} = \frac{L(\pi_1)}{L(\pi_0)}\ \text{prior odds} \qquad [13\text{–}14]$$

Unlike the earlier applications, the likelihood ratio in formula 13–14 does *not* involve the maximum-likelihood estimate (the latter is often unnecessary for a Bayesian analysis). In our example, $\pi_1 = 0.004$, $\pi_0 = 0.005$, and our prior odds were $2/1 = 2$, so $L(\pi_1) = L(0.004) = 0.0730$, $L(\pi_0) = L(0.005) = 0.0334$, and

$$\text{Posterior odds} = \frac{0.0730}{0.0334}\frac{2}{1} = \frac{0.1460}{0.0334} = \frac{4.36}{1}$$

Thus, if we started out 2/1 in favor of $\pi = 0.004$ over $\pi = 0.005$, after seeing the data we should be 4.36/1 in favor of 0.004 over 0.005.

One must take care to note that the last answer applies only to the stated pair of hypotheses, $\pi_1 = 0.004$ and $\pi_0 = 0.005$. Even though we may favor 0.004 over 0.005 by a wide margin, it does *not* mean that 0.004 should be our most favored or 0.005 our least favored hypothesis when considering *other* hypotheses. Calculation of other posterior odds for other pairs of values for π would be needed to broaden the scope of our analysis.

Bayesian philosophy and elementary Bayesian methods will be covered in Chapter 18. There it is shown how Bayesian statistics can be computed from ordinary frequentist programs via the device of "prior data." There are now many books that give comprehensive treatments of Bayesian theory and methods for applied researchers, such as Gelman et al. (2003).

CHOICE OF TEST STATISTICS

So far, we have given no indication of how one should go about choosing a statistic Y on which to base testing and estimation. In any analysis there will be many possibilities. In the survey example we took the number of positives (cases) as our test statistic Y. If we let A stand for the number of cases, we can say we took $Y = A$. But we could have taken $Y = \ln(A)$ or $Y = \text{logit}(A/N) = \ln[A/(N - A)]$ as test statistics for normal approximation, to name only two of many possibilities. Why choose Y to be the number of cases?

This is a subtle issue, and we can only outline certain aspects of it here. Statisticians have used various criteria to choose test statistics in a given problem. The primary criterion, confidence validity, requires that the chosen statistic yield approximate confidence intervals with proper coverage: For reasonably sized samples and reasonable parameter values, an approximate interval should contain (cover) the true parameter with a frequency no less than its stated (nominal) confidence level (Rubin, 1996). For example, an approximate 95% confidence interval is valid if it will contain the true parameter with a frequency no less than 95% over study repetitions. To choose among valid approximate intervals, we may further impose a second criterion, which is precision. For reasonable-sized samples and reasonable parameter values, a valid and precise interval has an average width over the repetitions that is no greater than other valid intervals. Taken together, the two criteria of validity and precision are sometimes referred to as *accuracy* criteria.

Although we have stated these two criteria qualitatively, it is more practical to use them quantitatively and note the trade-off between validity and precision. For example, in a given setting, one approximate 95% confidence interval might cover 94% of the time while another might cover 95% of the time, but if the second interval were always 30% wider than the first, we should prefer the first interval for precision, even though it is not quite as valid as the second.

A third criterion in choosing a statistic Y is the ease or availability of computational formulas for its mean and variance. For most choices of Y, including logit(A/N) in the preceding example, one must use approximate means and variances. Worse, approximate intervals that use $\ln(A)$ or logit(A/N) directly as test statistics tend to be less valid than those based on $Y = A$, with little or no precision or computation advantage. On the other hand, taking $Y = \text{arcsine}[(A/N)^{1/2}]$ can produce more valid intervals than taking $Y = A$, but it also requires use of approximations to its mean and variance that become unwieldy in stratified analyses. We thus might view the choice $Y = A$, the number of cases, as representing a compromise between accuracy and simplicity. The choice $Y = A$ can also be derived from consideration of score statistics and likelihood functions (Gart and Tarone, 1983).

CONTINUITY CORRECTIONS AND MID-*P*-VALUES

As we saw in earlier sections, there can be some discrepancies between exact and approximate results. There are two major philosophies for dealing with these discrepancies, each with corresponding methods.

The traditional philosophy is based on the fact that only traditional exact confidence intervals are *conservatively calibrated*: If the underlying assumptions are correct, a traditional exact 90% interval is guaranteed to cover (contain) the true measure of occurrence or effect with a frequency *no less than 90%*. Parallel statements apply for other confidence levels. We emphasize the phrase "no less than 90%" because, although in some situations the actual frequency will be 90%, in others the traditional exact 90% interval will cover the true measure with a greater frequency—as much as 100% in some extreme examples.

The traditional philosophy maintains that overcoverage (coverage frequency above the stated confidence level) is always preferable to undercoverage (coverage frequency below the confidence level). Thus, because traditional exact intervals never suffer from undercoverage, the traditional philosophy would have us adjust our approximation methods so that our approximate P-values and intervals come close to the traditional exact P-values and intervals. In other words, it would have us take traditional exact results as the "gold standard."

Perhaps the simplest way to implement this philosophy is to adopt what are known as *continuity corrections* for approximate statistics (Yates, 1934). The score approximation uses a normal curve whose mean and SD are $E(Y|\pi)$ and $V(Y|\pi)^{1/2}$. In the preceding example, the lower P-value was taken as the area under the normal curve to the left of the observed Y value. A better approximation is obtained by taking the area under the normal curve to the left of the point *midway* between the observed Y and the next largest Y. That is, to get a better approximation to the traditional exact lower P-value, we should replace Y by $Y + 1/2$ in the score statistic χ_{score} (equation 13–5). Similarly, to get a better approximation to the traditional exact upper P-value, we should replace Y by $Y - 1/2$ in the score statistic.

The factors $1/2$ for P_{lower} and $-1/2$ for P_{upper} are examples of continuity corrections, and the statistics obtained when using them are said to be *continuity corrected.* In the HIV survey example, the continuity-corrected score statistic for getting a lower P-value to test a prevalence of 0.004 is

$$\frac{1 + 1/2 - 1{,}000(0.004)}{[1{,}000(0.004)(1 - 0.004)]^{1/2}} = -1.253$$

This statistic yields a continuity-corrected lower P-value of 0.105, which (as desired) is closer to the traditional exact value of 0.091 than the uncorrected value of 0.067 found earlier.

A second, alternative philosophy rejects the notions that traditional exact P-values should be taken as the "gold standard" and that overcoverage is always preferable to undercoverage. Instead, it maintains that we should seek procedures that produce the narrowest confidence intervals whose coverage is (in some average sense) as close as possible to the stated confidence level. In this view, a confidence interval with a stated confidence level of 90% that sometimes covered the truth with only 88% frequency would be preferable to a much wider interval that always covered with at least 90% frequency. In other words, some risk of moderate undercoverage is acceptable if worthwhile precision gains can be obtained.

One way of implementing this alternative philosophy is to replace traditional exact P-values with *mid-P*-values (Lancaster, 1949, 1961; Berry and Armitage, 1995). The lower mid-P-value is defined as the probability under the test hypothesis that the test statistic Y is less than its observed value, plus half the probability that Y equals its observed value. Thus, for the HIV survey example,

$$\begin{aligned}\text{mid-}P_{\text{lower}} &= \Pr(Y < 1 \mid \text{HIV prevalence} = 0.004) + \Pr(Y = 1 \mid \text{HIV prevalence} = 0.004)/2 \\ &= (1 - 0.004)^{1{,}000} + 1{,}000(0.004)(1 - 0.004)^{999}/2 = 0.055\end{aligned}$$

This mid-P-value is notably less than the traditional exact P-value of 0.091. For an HIV prevalence of 0.0041, the lower mid-P-value is 0.050, so 0.0041 is the upper mid-P 90% confidence limit for the HIV prevalence. This limit is notably less than the traditional exact upper limit of 0.0047, so it more precisely bounds the HIV prevalence.

To approximate the lower mid-P-value using a normal distribution, we should take the area under the normal curve to the left of the observed Y value. It follows that, if we wish to approximate the results from mid-P-values, we should *not* use continuity corrections (Miettinen, 1974a). This conclusion is very apparent in the HIV survey example, in which the mid-P-value and the uncorrected score P-value for a prevalence of 0.004 are 0.055 and 0.067, while the continuity corrected score P-value is 0.105.

Upper mid-P-values are defined analogously to lower mid-P-values: The upper mid-P-value is the probability under the test hypothesis that the test statistic Y is greater than its observed value, plus half the probability that Y equals its observed value. The two-sided mid-P-value is then just twice the smaller of the upper and lower mid-P-values. One pleasant property of the two-sided mid-P-value is that (unlike the traditional two-sided P-value) it cannot exceed 1. To see this, note that the upper and lower mid-P-values always sum to 1:

$$\begin{aligned}
\text{mid-}P_{\text{lower}} + \text{mid-}P_{\text{upper}} &= \Pr(Y \text{ less than observed} \mid \text{test hypothesis}) \\
&\quad + \Pr(Y \text{ equals observed} \mid \text{test hypothesis})/2 \\
&\quad + \Pr(Y \text{ greater than observed} \mid \text{test hypothesis}) \\
&\quad + \Pr(Y \text{ equals observed} \mid \text{test hypothesis})/2 \\
&= \Pr(Y \text{ less than observed} \mid \text{test hypothesis}) \\
&\quad + \Pr(Y \text{ equals observed} \mid \text{test hypothesis}) \\
&\quad + \Pr(Y \text{ greater than observed} \mid \text{test hypothesis}) \\
&= 1
\end{aligned}$$

This result implies that the smaller of mid-P_{lower} and mid-P_{upper} must be ½ or less, so twice this smaller value (the two-sided mid-P-value) cannot exceed 1.

The median-unbiased point estimate was earlier defined as the point for which the upper and lower traditional exact P-values are equal. This estimate is also the point for which the upper and lower mid-P-values are equal. Thus, use of mid-P-values in place of traditional exact P-values does not change the point estimate.

Mid-P-values are always smaller than traditional exact P-values. As a result, for a given confidence level, fewer points will fall inside the confidence interval produced from mid-P-values than the traditional exact interval; in other words, the mid-P interval will always be narrower than the traditional exact interval.

These advantages of mid-P-values do have a price. For example, in some situations involving small observed numbers, mid-P intervals can suffer from notable undercoverage, as can intervals based on normal approximations. Thus mid-P intervals, like the approximate intervals, are not guaranteed to perform well when the observed numbers are very small. They do, however, perform as well as or better than approximate methods such as the score or Wald method.

Another disadvantage of mid-P-values is that they cannot be interpreted as exact probabilities. Whereas upper and lower (but not two-sided) traditional exact P-values are exact frequency probabilities of certain events, mid-P-values have no such straightforward frequency interpretation. They do have useful Bayesian probability interpretations (Nurminen and Mutanen, 1987), but these are beyond our present discussion. In any case, it can be argued that this interpretational disadvantage of mid-P-values is of no practical concern if the P-values are used only to construct confidence intervals.

In sum, one position is that traditional exact P-values are the "gold standard" because confidence intervals based on them have coverage frequencies no less than the stated (nominal) confidence level (e.g., 95%). If one accepts this position, one should use continuity corrections with approximate statistics. The alternative position is that one should not ignore precision concerns, but instead seek the narrowest interval that is consistent with keeping coverage close to the stated confidence level of the interval. In particular, some risk of moderate undercoverage is tolerable. If one accepts this position, one should use mid-P-values in place of traditional exact P-values, and not use continuity corrections with approximate statistics.

Neither position is completely logically compelling, nor is either position dominant in statistics today. It may also be argued that the choice is of little practical importance, because any data set in which the choice makes a large numerical difference must have very little information on the measure of interest. It can be shown that, when the sample size is large, all the methods (traditional, mid-P, approximate with or without correction) will give similar results. The difference among them is marked only when the results are so statistically unstable that most inferences from the data are unwarranted, even in the absence of biases. For example, in the HIV survey example, the mid-P confidence limits are not close to the traditional exact limits, because only one case was observed and hence the results are imprecise.

For simplicity, in the remainder of this book we limit our discussion of approximate statistics to those without continuity corrections.

COMPUTATION AND INTERPRETATION OF TWO-SIDED P-VALUES

As we have mentioned, only traditional one-tailed P-values can be interpreted as probabilities in all circumstances (this is because they are defined as probabilities). Mid-P-values and two-sided P-values do not share this property except in special circumstances. Nonetheless, if the sample numbers are large enough so that the traditional, approximate, and mid-P-values are all nearly equal, the two-sided P-values will have an approximate probability interpretation. Specifically, in this situation the two-sided P-values will approximately equal the probability that the square of the score statistic is greater than or equal to its observed value.

For example, if Y has a binomial distribution (as in the HIV example), the square of the score statistic χ_{score} for testing π is

$$\chi^2_{\text{score}} = \frac{(Y - N\pi)^2}{N\pi(1-\pi)} \qquad [13\text{–}15]$$

In most of the statistics literature, χ^2_{score} rather than χ_{score} is called the score statistic. If both $N\pi$ and $N(1-\pi)$ are more than 5 or so, all the two-sided P-values discussed above (traditional, score, Wald, and mid-P) will approximate the probability that χ^2_{score} is greater than or equal to its observed value. In this large-sample situation, χ_{score} has approximately a normal distribution with a mean of 0 and a SD of 1, and so χ^2_{score} will have approximately a χ^2 distribution with one degree of freedom. Thus, if we are interested only in the two-sided P-value, we can simply compute χ^2_{score} and look up the probability that a χ^2 variate with one degree of freedom is this large or larger. Tables and functions for this purpose are widely available in statistics books and software.

A common misinterpretation of the two-sided P-value is that it represents the probability that the point estimate would be as far or farther from the test value as was observed. This interpretation is not even approximately correct for many epidemiologic estimates, particularly risk differences, because a P-value refers to the distribution of a test statistic, not a point estimate. As an example, consider again the HIV survey, this time taking the sample proportion of HIV-positives (which was 0.001) as the test statistic. Suppose our test hypothesis is that the HIV prevalence is 0.005. The distance between the observed sample proportion of 0.001 and the test value of 0.005 is 0.004. For the sample proportion to be as far or farther from the test value of 0.005 as was observed, it would have to be either less than or equal to $0.005 - 0.004 = 0.001$ or greater than or equal to $0.005 + 0.004 = 0.009$. If the true prevalence is 0.005, the probability of the sample proportion being less than 0.001 or more than 0.009 is 0.11. This probability is more than the traditional two-sided P-value of 0.080 computed earlier and more than twice the size of the two-sided mid-P-value of 0.047.

Again, the preceding interpretational obstacles need not concern us if we use two-sided P-values only to find confidence limits, rather than attempting to interpret them directly. This advantage is yet another reason to focus on confidence intervals and their coverage interpretation when analyzing data.

MULTIPLE COMPARISONS

Consider the following problem: We conduct a study in which we examine every exposure–disease association among 10 exposures and 10 diseases, for a total of $10 \times 10 = 100$ associations (exposure–disease pairs). To analyze each association, we use a "perfect" method to set 95% confidence limits—i.e., one that produces intervals containing the true association with exactly 95% frequency. If the coverage of each interval is independent of the coverage of every other interval, how many of the 100 resulting confidence intervals should we expect to contain their respective true value?

The answer to this question is simply 95% of the 100, or 95. This means that of the 100 independent confidence intervals we are to examine, we should expect five to miss their target (the corresponding true value). Of course, anywhere from 0 to 100 may actually miss their target, and five represents only an average over hypothetical repetitions of the study. But the point is that we should *expect* several of these intervals to miss their target, even if we use a perfectly valid 95% confidence-interval method.

Furthermore, we cannot identify the intervals that missed their targets. Suppose we are very uncomfortable with the idea of reporting five intervals that miss their targets completely, even if the other 95 intervals cover their targets. One alternative is to increase the confidence level of our intervals. For example, if we increase our confidence level to 99% we can then expect only one of the 100 intervals to miss their targets. Although this will widen every interval by a considerable factor (for Wald intervals, the factor will be 2.576/1.960 − 1, or 31%), the widening is an inevitable price of reducing the 5% miss rate to 1%.

The trade-off we have just described, between the width and the miss rate of the confidence interval, in no way affects the P-values computed for each association; we simply choose a lower alpha level and hence a lower slice through the P-value functions to get our interval estimates. There is, however, another perspective, which leads to an entirely different P-value function from the data. It is the result of a *multiple-comparisons* analysis, also known as simultaneous testing, joint testing, or multiple inference. In this view, we do *not* treat the 100 associations as 100 separate parameters to be estimated. Instead, we treat them as composing a *single* entity with 100 components, called the joint parameter or *vector* parameter for the associations. Here we provide an example for a conceptual introduction and discuss the issues further in Chapter 17.

Suppose that the true values of the 100 associations correspond to 100 risk ratios of 3.0, 2.1, 4.2, 0.6, 1.0, 1.5, and so on (up to 100 values). Then the single vector parameter representing these 100 true values is the ordered list of the values:

$$(3.0, 2.1, 4.2, 0.6, 1.0, 1.5, \ldots)$$

where the ellipsis represents the list of the remaining 94 risk ratios. Each number in this ordered list (vector) corresponds to one of the 100 associations of interest and is called a *component* of the list. In other words, every single association is only one component of the entire list.

With this simultaneous view of the 100 associations, we can formulate a *joint hypothesis* that the entire list of true associations equals a particular list of 100 specified numbers. Most commonly, this hypothesized list is a list of nothing but null values; for risk ratios this list would comprise 100 ones,

$$(1, 1, 1, 1, 1, 1, \ldots)$$

where the ellipsis represents 94 more ones. This null list or null vector corresponds to the *joint null hypothesis* that there is no association among all 100 exposure–disease pairs. It is also possible to test other joint hypotheses, for example, that all 100 risk ratios are equal to 2, or that the first 50 in the list equal 1 and the remaining 50 in the list equal 0.5.

For any joint hypothesis we can imagine, it is possible to construct a statistic for testing that the hypothesis is true, which yields a P-value and test for that hypothesis. Such a P-value and test are called a *joint P-value* and *joint test* (or simultaneous test) for the associations. In particular, we can perform a simultaneous test of the joint null hypothesis (that no exposure is associated with any disease). If the joint test is valid *and* the joint null hypothesis is correct—so that there really are no associations at all—there will be no more than a 5% chance that the joint P-value from the test will fall below 0.05.

JOINT CONFIDENCE REGIONS

We can consider the joint P-values for all possible vectors of values for the 100 associations. This collection of P-values is the multiple-comparisons analog of the P-value function. The collection of all vectors that have a joint P-value of at least 0.05 is called a 95% *joint confidence region* for the vector of parameter values. A 95% confidence region constructed from a valid testing method has the useful property that it will include the true parameter vector with a frequency no less than 95%, provided there is no bias and all assumptions underlying the method are satisfied.

How is this joint confidence region for the vector of 100 associations related to the 100 single-association confidence intervals that we usually compute? If the joint null hypothesis is indeed correct and single-association intervals are independent of one another, then on average we should expect about five of the single-association intervals to miss their target, which in every case is the null value (a risk ratio of 1). We should also expect a valid joint confidence region to include the null vector 95% of the time, because there is at least a 95% chance that $P > 0.05$ when the joint null hypothesis is correct. Thus, if there are no associations, we have this apparently paradoxical result: The joint confidence region will probably contain the null vector, apparently saying that the joint null hypothesis is compatible with the data; yet it is also probable that at least a few of the single 95% confidence intervals will miss the null, apparently saying that at least a few single null hypotheses are not compatible with the data. In other words, we expect the joint confidence region to indicate that every association may be null, and the single intervals to indicate that some associations are not null. In fact, if all the null hypotheses are correct, the single-interval coverage probabilities are exactly 95%, and the intervals are independent, then the probability that at least two of the single intervals will miss the null is 1 minus the binomial probability that only none or one of the intervals misses the null:

$$1 - 0.95^{100} - 100(0.05)0.95^{99} = 0.96$$

or 96%.

This apparent paradox has been the source of much confusion. Its resolution comes about by recognizing that the joint confidence region and the 100 single intervals are all addressing different questions and have different objectives. A single 95% interval addresses the question, "What is the value of this parameter?," where "this" means just one of the 100, ignoring the other 99. Its objective is to miss the correct value of that one parameter no more than 5% of the time, *without regard to whether any of the other intervals miss or not.* Thus, each single interval addresses only one of 100 distinct single-association questions and has only one of 100 distinct objectives. In contrast, the joint confidence region addresses the question, "What is the *vector* of parameter values?"; its objective is to miss the true *vector* of all 100 associations no more than 5% of the time.

If we are indeed trying to meet the latter objective, we must recognize that some misses by the single intervals are very likely to occur by chance even if no association is present. Thus, to meet the objective of joint estimation, we cannot naively combine the results from the single intervals. For example, suppose that we take as our confidence region the set of all vectors for which the first component (i.e., the first association in the list) falls within the single 95% interval for the first association, the second component falls within the single 95% interval for the second association, and so on for all 100 components. The chance that such a combined region will contain the true vector of associations is equal to the chance that *all* the single intervals will contain the corresponding components. If all the exposures and diseases are independent of one another, this probability will be 0.95^{100}, which is only 0.6%! These issues are discussed further in Chapter 17.

PROBLEMS WITH CONVENTIONAL APPROACHES

The preceding example illustrates how the tasks of joint testing and estimation are much more stringent than those of single one-at-a-time testing and estimation. One awful response to this stringency is to construct the single confidence intervals to have a confidence level that guarantees the naive combination method just described will yield a valid joint confidence region. This procedure is called the *Bonferroni* method for "adjusting for multiple comparisons." If we want a 95% confidence region from overlapping the single intervals, in the preceding example we will need a single-interval alpha level that is one-hundredth the desired joint alpha level. This value is $\alpha = 0.05/100 = 0.0005$, which corresponds to a single-interval confidence level of $1 - 0.0005 = 99.95\%$. This choice yields a $0.9995^{100} = 95\%$ chance that a naive combination of all the single 99.95% confidence intervals will produce a confidence region that includes the true vector of associations. Thus the Bonferroni method is valid, but the single intervals it produces are much too wide (conservative) for use in single-association estimation (e.g., Wald intervals have to be 70% wider to get a 95% joint Bonferroni region when there are 100 associations). Also, the joint Bonferroni confidence region is typically much larger (more imprecise) than it needs to be; that is, the Bonferroni region is also unnecessarily imprecise for joint estimation purposes. For hypothesis testing, a procedure that is equivalent to the Bonferroni adjustment, and equally bad, is to use a 0.05 alpha level but multiply all the single-association P-values by the number of associations before comparing them to the alpha level.

A deeper problem in the multiple-comparisons literature is that joint confidence regions have been recommended in situations in which the scientific objectives of the study call for single intervals. Typically, the different associations in a study are of interest on a purely one-at-a-time basis, often to different investigators with different interests. For example, a large health survey or cohort study may collect data pertaining to many possible associations, including data on diet and cancer, on exercise and heart disease, and perhaps many other distinct topics. A researcher can legitimately deny interest in any joint hypothesis regarding all of these diverse topics, instead wanting to focus on those few (or even one) pertinent to his or her specialties. In such situations, multiple-inference procedures such as we have outlined are irrelevant, inappropriate, and wasteful of information (because they will produce improperly imprecise single intervals) (Rothman, 1990a; Savitz and Olshan, 1995, 1998; Mayo and Cox, 2006).

Nevertheless, it is important to recognize that investigators frequently conduct data searches or "data dredging" in which joint hypotheses are of genuine interest (Greenland and Robins, 1991; Thompson, 1998a, 1998b). Such searches are usually done with multiple single-inference procedures, when special multiple-inference procedures should be used instead. Classic examples of such misuse of single-inference procedures involve selecting for further analysis only those associations or interactions that are "statistically significant." This approach is commonly used in attempts to identify harmful exposures, high-risk population subgroups, or subgroups that are selectively affected by study exposures. Such attempts represent multiple-inference problems, because the study question and objectives concern the vector of all the tested associations. For example, central questions that drive searches for harmful exposures may include "Which (if any) of these associations is positive?" or "Which of these associations is important in magnitude?"

Unfortunately, conventional approaches to multiple-inference questions (such as Bonferroni adjustments and stepwise regression) are poor choices for answering such questions, in part because they have low efficiency or poor accuracy (Greenland, 1993a). More modern procedures, such as hierarchical (empirical-Bayes) modeling, can offer dramatic performance advantages over conventional approaches and are well suited to epidemiologic data searches (Thomas et al., 1985; Greenland and Robins, 1991; Greenland, 1992a; Greenland and Poole, 1994; Steenland et al., 2000; Greenland, 2000c). We briefly describe these methods in Chapter 21.

SUMMARY

In any analysis involving testing or estimation of multiple parameters, it is important to clarify the research questions to discern whether multiple-inference procedures will be needed. Multiple-inference procedures will be needed if and only if joint hypotheses are of interest. Even if one is interested in a joint hypothesis, conventional or classical multiple-inference procedures will usually provide poor results, and many better procedures are now available.

When in doubt about the best strategy to pursue, most audiences will find acceptable a presentation of the results of all single-inference procedures (e.g., confidence intervals for all associations examined). When this is not possible, and one must select associations to present based on statistical criteria, one should at least take care to note the number and nature of the associations examined, and the probable effect of such selection on the final results (for example, the high probability that at least a few intervals have missed their target).

Chapter 17 provides further discussion of multiple-comparisons procedures, and a graphical illustration of the distinction between single- and multiple-comparison procedures.

CHAPTER 14

Introduction to Categorical Statistics

Sander Greenland and Kenneth J. Rothman

Sample-Size Considerations 239
Independence of Outcomes 239
Homogeneity Assumptions 239
Classification of Analysis Methods 240
Person-Time Data: Large-Sample Methods 240
Single Study Group 240
Two Study Groups 243
Pure Count Data: Large-Sample Methods 245
Single Study Group: Large-Sample Methods 245
Two Study Groups: Large-Sample Methods 247
Relations among the Ratio Measures 250
Case-Control Data 250
Case-Cohort Data 252
Small-Sample Statistics for Person-Time Data 253
Single Study Group 253
Two Study Groups 254
Small-Sample Statistics for Pure Count Data 255
Single Study Group 255
Two Study Groups 256
Application of Exact 2 × 2 Programs to Person-Time Data and Single-Group Data 257

In Chapter 13 we discussed the fundamentals of epidemiologic data analysis, focusing on methods used to estimate the proportion of a population with a disease. In this chapter we turn to comparisons of disease proportions, odds, or rates in two groups of people. We therefore present the basic structure of statistical techniques for cross-tabulations of person-counts and person-time. To do so, we focus almost exclusively on methods for unstratified (crude) data and then, in Chapter 15, extend these methods to stratified data. We also discuss only differences and ratios of risks, rates, and odds, and defer discussion of attributable fractions and survival-time comparisons until Chapter 16. Finally, we limit the present chapter to data with a dichotomized exposure and outcome variable. In Chapter 17, the methods given here and in Chapter 15 are extended to exposures and outcomes with multiple levels. Chapter 18 provides Bayesian analogs of the basic methods given here and in Chapter 15.

In order to discourage the use of confidence intervals as 0.05-level significance tests, we often use 90% or 99% intervals rather than the conventional 95% intervals in our examples. A large-sample 90% interval has the small technical advantage of more closely approximating the corresponding exact interval. The present chapter provides both approximate and exact intervals, so that the reader can obtain a feel for the difference between the two. In any event, the formulas allow one to choose one's own confidence level.

Although it is usually necessary to take into account factors beyond the exposure and the disease of interest, it is not unusual to see data analyzed and presented in crude form. Narrow restrictions on covariates in subject selection to prevent confounding can sometimes obviate the need for stratification. Results of large randomized trials may often be summarized adequately in unstratified form.

As is usually done in basic statistical presentations, we assume throughout this chapter that there is no source of bias in the study—no measurement error, selection bias, follow-up bias, or confounding. Confounding and some forms of selection bias due to measured covariates can be handled by stratification. Chapter 19 discusses analysis of confounding by unmeasured covariates, general selection bias, and misclassification. Several other statistical assumptions will be used in most of what we present: sufficiency of sample size, independence of subject outcomes, and homogeneity of risk within levels of exposure and stratification variables. Throughout, we point out the sample-size limitations of the large-sample methods.

SAMPLE-SIZE CONSIDERATIONS

For most applications, computation of small-sample statistics (such as exact and mid-P-values and confidence limits) are practical only if one has computer software that provides them, whereas for unstratified data one can quickly compute large-sample (approximate) statistics with a hand calculator. Therefore, we focus on large-sample methods. In the final sections of this chapter we present small-sample methods for unstratified data, without computational details. The formulas we present are intended only to illustrate the concepts underlying small-sample statistics. Good statistical programs employ more general and more efficient formulas; hence, we expect and recommend that users will obtain small-sample statistics from packaged software. After introducing exact methods for count data, we illustrate how to trick programs written to do exact analysis of 2×2 tables (which are used to compare two cohorts) into providing the corresponding analyses of single cohorts and of person-time data. Rothman and Boice (1982), Rothman (1986), and Hirji (2006) provide more formulas for small-sample analysis.

INDEPENDENCE OF OUTCOMES

Most of the methods discussed in this book assume that the outcomes of study subjects are *independent,* in the following narrow sense: Once you know the risk of a group (such as the exposed group), discovering the outcome status of one group member will tell you nothing about the outcome status of any other group member. This assumption has subtleties and is often misunderstood or overlooked. A straightforward practical consequence of this assumption, however, is that all the P-value and confidence-interval methods we present will usually not give valid results when the disease is contagious, or when the subjects under study can contribute multiple disease events to the total case count (as in studies of recurrent outcomes). A simple solution in the latter case is to count only the first event contributed by each subject, although this simplification will limit generalizability.

When dependence is present, many phenomena can arise that require special analytic attention. At the very least, the standard deviations (SDs) of conventional estimates are likely to be underestimated by conventional techniques, thus leading to underestimation of the uncertainty in the results. Therefore, we frequently remind the reader that conventional models implicitly assume independence. The independence assumption is plausible in most studies of first occurrences of chronic diseases (e.g., carcinomas, myocardial infarction) but is implausible in studies of contagious diseases. Note, however, that neither dependence nor contagiousness is synonymous with the disease having an infectious agent among its causes. First, some infectious diseases (such as Lyme disease) may have no transmission among humans. Second, some noninfectious conditions, such as drug use and other health-related behaviors may be transmitted socially among humans.

HOMOGENEITY ASSUMPTIONS

Implicit in comparisons of observed incidence rates is the concept that a given amount of person-time, say 100 person-years, can be derived from observing many people for a short time or few people for a long time. That is, the experience of 100 persons for 1 year, 200 persons for 6 months, 50 persons for 2 years, or 1 person for 100 years are assumed to be equivalent. Most statistical methods assume that, within each analysis subgroup defined by exposure and confounder levels, the probability (risk) of an outcome event arising within a unit of person-time is identical for all person-time units in the stratum. For example, the methods based on the Poisson distribution that we present are based on this *homogeneity* assumption. Because risk almost inevitably changes over time, the homogeneity assumption is only an unmet idealization. Although the assumption may be a useful approximation in many applications, it is inadvisable in extreme situations. For example, observing one individual for 50 years to obtain 50 person-years would rarely approximate the assumption, whereas observing 100 similar people for an average of 6 months each may sometimes do so. Usually the units of person-time in the denominator of a rate are restricted by age and the amount of calendar time over which person-time has been observed, which together prevent the within-stratum heterogeneity that aging could produce.

In a similar fashion, most statistical methods for pure count data assume that, within each analysis subgroup, subjects have identical risks. Another way of stating this assumption is that the probability of experiencing an outcome event is identical for all persons in a given subgroup. For example, the methods based on the binomial and hypergeometric distributions presented in this chapter are based on this homogeneity assumption.

For both person-time and pure-count data, heterogeneity of risk (violation of the homogeneity assumption) will invalidate the standard-deviation formulas based on that assumption, and so will lead to erroneous uncertainty assessments.

CLASSIFICATION OF ANALYSIS METHODS

Epidemiologists often group basic types of epidemiologic studies into cohort, case-control, or cross-sectional studies (Chapter 6). Classification according to the probability model underlying the statistics leads to a different categorization, according to whether or not the data include person-time (time-at-risk) measurements among the basic observations. Although person-time observations pertain only to cohort studies, not all analyses of cohorts make use of such data. If there is no loss-to-follow-up or late entry in any study group, the study groups form closed populations (Chapter 3). It may then be convenient to present the data in terms of proportions experiencing the outcome, that is, incidence proportions (which serve as risk estimates). For these closed-cohort studies, the number of cases can be measured relative to person counts (cohort sizes), as well as relative to person-time experience. Clinical trials are often presented in this manner. Person-count cohort data are also common in perinatal research, for example, in studies in which neonatal death is the outcome.

It can be shown that, under conventional assumptions of independence and identical risk of persons within exposure levels and analysis strata (along with absence of bias), many of the statistical methods developed for cohort data can also be applied to analysis of case-control data and prevalence (cross-sectional) data (Anderson, 1972; Mantel, 1973; Prentice and Breslow, 1978; Farewell, 1979; Prentice and Pyke, 1979; Thomas, 1981b; Greenland, 1981; Weinberg and Wacholder, 1993). As discussed in Chapter 15, relatively minor modifications are required for basic analyses of two-stage data. These facts greatly reduce the number of analytic methods needed in epidemiology. Slightly more complicated methods are needed for estimating risk ratios from case-cohort data.

In studies that involve extended follow-up, some subjects may leave observation before the study disease occurs or the risk period of interest ends (e.g., because of loss to follow-up or competing risks). For such studies, methods that stratify on follow-up time will be needed; these methods are given in Chapter 16.

PERSON-TIME DATA: LARGE-SAMPLE METHODS

SINGLE STUDY GROUP

The simplest statistics arise when the data represent incidence in a single study group. Examples are common in occupational and environmental epidemiology, especially in the initial analysis of excess morbidity or mortality in a single workplace, community, or neighborhood. In such studies, the analysis proceeds in two steps: First, an expected number of cases, E, is calculated; second, the number of cases observed in the study group, A, is compared with this expected number.

Usually, E is calculated by applying stratum-specific incidence rates obtained from a large reference population (such as vital statistics data for a state or country) to the stratum-specific person-time experience of the study group. The process by which this is done is an example of *standardization,* which in this situation involves taking a weighted sum of the reference rates, using the stratum-specific person-time from the study group as weights (see Chapter 3). For example, if we are studying the stomach cancer rates in a group consisting of persons aged 51 to 75 years divided into three age categories (ages 51 to 60 years, 61 to 70 years, 71 to 75 years), two sexes, and two ethnicity categories, there are a total of 3(2)2 = 12 possible age–sex–ethnicity categories. Suppose that the person-times observed in each subgroup are $T_1, T_2, \ldots, T_{12}$, and the corresponding age–sex–ethnicity specific rates in the reference population are known to be $I_1, \ldots, I_{12}$. Then, for a cohort that had the same age–sex–ethnicity specific rates as the reference population and the same person-time distribution as that observed in the study group, the number of cases we should expect is

$$E = T_1 I_1 + T_2 I_2 + \cdots + T_{12} I_{12}$$

The quantity E is generally not precisely equal to the number of cases one should expect in the study group if it had experienced the rates of the reference population (Keiding and Vaeth, 1986). This inequality arises because an alteration of the person-time rates in the study group will usually alter the distribution of person-time in the study group (see Chapters 3 and 4). Nonetheless, the quantity E has several valid statistical uses, which involve comparing A with E.

The ratio A/E is sometimes called the *standardized morbidity ratio* (or standardized mortality ratio, if the outcome is death), usually abbreviated as SMR. Let T be the total person-time observed in the study group; that is, $T = \sum_k T_k$. Then A/T is the observed crude rate in the study group, and E/T is the rate that would be expected in a population with the specific rates of the reference population and the person-time distribution of the study group. The ratio of these rates is

$$\frac{A/T}{E/T} = \frac{A}{E}$$

which shows that the SMR is a rate ratio.

Boice and Monson (1977) reported $A = 41$ breast cancer cases out of 28,010 person-years at risk in a cohort of women treated for tuberculosis with x-ray fluoroscopy. Only $E = 23.3$ cases were expected based on the age-year specific rates among women in Connecticut, so $A/E = 41/23.3 = 1.76$ is the ratio of the rate observed in the treated women to that expected in a population with the age-year specific rates of Connecticut women and the person-time distribution observed in the treated women.

To account for unknown sources of variation in the single observed rate A/T, we must specify a probability model for the random variability in the observed number of cases A. If the outcome under study is not contagious, the conventional probability model for a single observed number of cases A is the *Poisson distribution.* Define I to be the average rate we would observe if we could repeat the study over and over again under the same conditions with the same amount of person-time T observed each time (the latter condition could be imposed by ending follow-up upon reaching T units). The Poisson model specifies that the probability of observing $A = a$ (that is, the probability that the number of cases observed equals a), given that T person-time units were observed in the study group, is

$$\Pr(A = a) = \exp(-I \cdot T)(I \cdot T)^a / a! \qquad [14\text{–}1]$$

The Poisson model arises as a distribution for the number of cases occurring in a stationary population of size N followed for a fixed time span T/N. It also arises as an approximation to the binomial distribution (see Chapter 13) when N is very large and risk is very low (Clayton and Hills, 1993). The latter view of the Poisson distribution reveals that underlying use of this distribution are assumptions of homogeneity of risk and independence of outcomes described earlier, because these assumptions are needed to derive the binomial distribution.

In data analysis, the average rate I is an unknown quantity called the *rate parameter,* whereas A and T are known quantities. The function of I that results when the observed number of cases and person-time units are put into equation 14–1 is called the Poisson likelihood for I based on the data.

We state without proof the following facts. Under the Poisson model (equation 14–1),

1. A/T is the maximum-likelihood estimator (MLE) of I (for a discussion of maximum-likelihood estimation, see Chapter 13).
2. $I \cdot T$ is the average value of A that we would observe over study repetitions in which T person-time units were observed, and so $I \cdot T/E$ is the average value of the SMR over those repetitions ($I \cdot T/E$ is sometimes called the SMR parameter); $I \cdot T$ is also the variance of A over those repetitions.

It follows from the second fact that a large-sample statistic for testing the null hypothesis that the unknown rate parameter I equals the expected rate E/T is the score statistic

$$\chi_{\text{score}} = \frac{A - E}{E^{1/2}}$$

because if $I = E/T$, the mean and variance of A are both $(E/T)T = E$.

For the Boice and Monson (1977) study of breast cancer, the Poisson likelihood is

$$\exp(-I \cdot 28{,}010)(I \cdot 28{,}010)^{41}/41!,$$

the MLE of I is $41/28{,}010 = 146$ cases/100,000 person-years, and the score statistic for testing whether $I = 23.3/28{,}010 = 83$ cases/100,000 person-years is

$$\chi_{\text{score}} = \frac{A - E}{E^{1/2}} = \frac{41 - 23.3}{23.3^{1/2}} = 3.67$$

From a standard normal table, this yields an upper-tailed P-value of 0.0001. Thus a score statistic as large or larger than that observed would be very improbable under the Poisson model if no bias was present and the specific rates in the cohort were equal to the Connecticut rates.

Let IR be the ratio of the rate parameter of the study group I and the expected rate based on the reference group E/T:

$$IR = \frac{I}{E/T}$$

Because A/T is the MLE of I,

$$\widehat{IR} = \frac{A/T}{E/T} = \frac{A}{E}$$

is the MLE of IR. To set approximate Wald confidence limits for IR, we first set limits for the natural logarithm of IR, $\ln(IR)$, and then take the antilogs of these limits to get limits for IR. To do so, we use the fact that an estimate of the approximate SD of $\ln(\widehat{IR})$ is

$$\widehat{SD}[\ln(\widehat{IR})] = \frac{1}{A^{1/2}}$$

Let γ be the desired confidence percentage for interval estimation, and let Z_γ be the number such that the chance that a standard normal variable falls between $-Z_\gamma$ and Z_γ is $\gamma\%$ (for example, $Z_{90} = 1.65$, $Z_{95} = 1.96$, and $Z_{99} = 2.58$). Then $\gamma\%$ Wald confidence limits for IR are given by

$$\underline{IR}, \overline{IR} = \exp[\ln(\widehat{IR}) \pm Z_\gamma(1/A^{1/2})]$$

For the Boice and Monson (1977) comparison, the 90% and 95% limits are

$$\underline{IR}, \overline{IR} = \exp[\ln(41/23.3) \pm 1.65(1/41^{1/2})] = 1.36, 2.28$$

and

$$\underline{IR}, \overline{IR} = \exp[\ln(41/23.3) \pm 1.96(1/41^{1/2})] = 1.30, 2.39$$

These results suggest that, if the Poisson model is correct, if the variability in E is negligible, and if there is no bias, there is a nonrandom excess of breast cancers among fluoroscoped women relative to the Connecticut women, but do not indicate very precisely just how large this excess might be.

TABLE 14–1

Format for Unstratified Data with Person-Time Denominators

	Exposed	Unexposed	Total
Cases	A_1	A_0	M_1
Person-time	T_1	T_0	T

Under the Poisson model (equation 14–1), the score statistic provides an adequate approximate P-value when E exceeds 5, whereas the Wald limits will be adequate if $\underline{IR} \cdot E$ and $\overline{IR} \cdot E$ exceed 5. If these criteria are not met, then, as illustrated later in this chapter, one can compute small-sample statistics directly from the Poisson distribution.

TWO STUDY GROUPS

Now suppose that we wish to compare observations from two study groups, which we shall refer to as "exposed" and "unexposed" groups. The crude data can be displayed in the format shown in Table 14–1.

Unlike the notation in Chapter 4, A_1 and A_0 now represent cases from two distinct populations. As for a single group, if the outcome is not contagious, one conventional probability model for the observed numbers of cases A_1 and A_0 is the Poisson model. If I_1 and I_0 are the rate parameters for the exposed and unexposed groups, this model specifies that the probability of observing $A_1 = a_1$ and $A_0 = a_0$ is

$$\begin{aligned}\Pr(A_1 = a_1, A_0 = a_0) &= \Pr(A_1 = a_1)\Pr(A_0 = a_0)\\ &= \exp(-I_1T_1)\frac{(I_1T_1)^{a_1}}{a_1!}\exp(-I_0T_0)\frac{(I_0T_0)^{a_0}}{a_0!}\end{aligned} \quad [14\text{–}2]$$

which is just the product of the probabilities for the two single groups (exposed and unexposed).

In data analysis, I_1 and I_0 are unknown parameters, whereas A_1, T_1, A_0, and T_0 are observed quantities. The function of I_1 and I_0 that results when the observed data numbers are put into equation 14–2 is called the Poisson likelihood for I_1 and I_0, based on the data.

Under the Poisson model (equation 14–2):

1. A_1/T_1 and A_0/T_0 are the maximum-likelihood estimates (MLEs) of I_1 and I_0.
2. The MLE of the rate ratio $IR = I_1/I_0$ is

$$\widehat{IR} = \frac{A_1/T_1}{A_0/T_0}$$

3. The MLE of the rate difference $ID = I_1 - I_0$ is $\widehat{ID} = A_1/T_1 - A_0/T_0$.
4. Suppose that $I_1 = I_0$ (no difference in the rates). Then $E = M_1T_1/T$ is the average number of exposed cases A_1 one would observe over study repetitions in which M_1 total cases were observed out of T_1 exposed and T_0 unexposed person-time totals. Also, the variance of A_1 over the same repetitions would be

$$V = \frac{ET_0}{T} = \frac{M_1T_1T_0}{T^2}$$

It follows from the last fact that a large-sample statistic for testing the null hypothesis $I_1 = I_0$ (which is the same hypothesis as $IR = 1$ and $ID = 0$) is

$$\chi_{\text{score}} = \frac{A_1 - E}{V^{1/2}}$$

(Oleinick and Mantel, 1970).

TABLE 14–2

Breast Cancer Cases and Person-Years of Observation for Women with Tuberculosis Who Are Repeatedly Exposed to Multiple x-Ray Fluoroscopies, and Unexposed Women with Tuberculosis

	Radiation Exposure		
	Yes	No	Total
Breast cancer cases	41	15	56
Person-years	28,010	19,017	47,027

From Boice JD, Monson RR. Breast cancer in women after repeated fluoroscopic examinations of the chest. *J Natl Cancer Inst.* 1977;59:823–832.

Table 14–2 gives both study groups from the Boice and Monson (1977) study of breast cancer and x-ray fluoroscopy among women with tuberculosis. For these data, we have

$$\widehat{IR} = \frac{41/28{,}010}{15/19{,}017} = 1.86$$

$$\widehat{ID} = \frac{41}{28{,}010\text{ y}} - \frac{15}{19{,}017\text{ y}} = \frac{68}{100{,}000\text{ y}}$$

$$E = \frac{56(28{,}010)}{47{,}047} = 33.35$$

$$V = \frac{33.35(19{,}017)}{47{,}047} = 13.49$$

and

$$\chi_{\text{score}} = \frac{41 - 33.35}{(13.49)^{1/2}} = 2.08$$

which, from a standard normal table, corresponds to an upper-tailed P-value of 0.02. The rate ratio is similar to the value of 1.76 found using Connecticut women as a reference group, and it is improbable that as large a score statistic or larger would be observed (under the Poisson model) if no bias were present and exposure had no effect on incidence.

To set approximate confidence intervals for the rate ratio IR and the rate difference ID, we use the facts that an estimate of the approximate SD of $\ln(IR)$ is

$$\widehat{SD}[\ln(\widehat{IR})] = \left(\frac{1}{A_1} + \frac{1}{A_0}\right)^{1/2}$$

and an estimate of the SD of ID is

$$\widehat{SD}(\widehat{ID}) = \left(\frac{A_1}{T_1^2} + \frac{A_0}{T_0^2}\right)^{1/2}$$

We obtain $\gamma\%$ Wald limits for $\ln(IR)$ and then take antilogs to get limits for IR:

$$\underline{IR}, \overline{IR} = \exp\{\ln(\widehat{IR}) \pm Z_\gamma \widehat{SD}[\ln(\widehat{IR})]\}$$

We obtain Wald limits for ID directly:

$$\underline{ID}, \overline{ID} = \widehat{ID} \pm Z_\gamma \widehat{SD}(\widehat{ID})$$

From the data of Table 14–2 we get

$$\widehat{SD}[\ln(\widehat{IR})] = \left(\frac{1}{41} + \frac{1}{15}\right)^{1/2} = 0.302$$

and

$$\widehat{SD}(\widehat{ID}) = \left[\frac{41}{(28{,}010\text{ y})^2} + \frac{15}{(19{,}017\text{ y})^2}\right]^{1/2} = \frac{31}{100{,}000\text{ y}}$$

Hence, 90% Wald limits for *IR* and *ID* are

$$\underline{IR}, \overline{IR} = \exp[\ln(1.86) \pm 1.645(0.302)] = 1.13, 3.06$$

and

$$\underline{ID}, \overline{ID} = \frac{68}{100{,}000\text{ y}} \pm 1.645\left(\frac{31}{100{,}000\text{ y}}\right) = 17, 119 \text{ per } 10^5\text{ y}$$

The corresponding 95% limits are 1.03, 3.35 for *IR*, and 7.5, 128 per 10^5 years for *ID*. Thus, although the results suggest a nonrandom excess of breast cancers among fluoroscoped women, they are very imprecise about just how large this excess might be.

Under the two-Poisson model, the score statistic should provide an adequate approximate *P*-value when both E and $M_1 - E$ exceed 5, whereas the Wald limits for *IR* will be adequate if both

$$\frac{M_1 T_0}{(\overline{IR})T_1 + T_0} \quad \text{and} \quad \frac{M_1(\underline{IR})T_0}{(\underline{IR})T_1 + T_0}$$

exceed 5. These numbers are the expected values for the A_0 cell and the A_1 cell assuming that $IR = \overline{IR}$ and $IR = \underline{IR}$, respectively. For the above 95% limits, these numbers are

$$\frac{56(19{,}017)}{3.35(28{,}010) + 19{,}017} = 9.4 \quad \text{and} \quad \frac{56(1.03)28{,}010}{1.03(28{,}010) + 19{,}017} = 33.8,$$

both well above 5.

If the preceding criteria are not met, small-sample methods are recommended. The last section of this chapter illustrates how programs that do exact analysis of 2 × 2 tables can be used to compute small-sample *P*-values and rate-ratio confidence limits from person-time data in the format of Table 14–1. Unfortunately, at this time there is no widely distributed small-sample method for the rate difference, *ID*, although approximations better than the Wald limits have been developed (Miettinen, 1985).

PURE COUNT DATA: LARGE-SAMPLE METHODS

Most cohort studies suffer from losses of subjects to follow-up and to competing risks. Studies in which these losses are not negligible should be analyzed using survival methods. Such methods in effect stratify on follow-up time, so they are properly viewed as stratified analysis methods. They are discussed in Chapter 16. Here we assume that we have cohort data with no loss to follow-up and no competing risk. Such data can be analyzed as pure count data, with denominators consisting of the number of persons at risk in the study, rather than person-time. They can also be analyzed using person-time if times of events are available and relevant.

SINGLE STUDY GROUP: LARGE-SAMPLE METHODS

It is sometimes necessary to analyze an incidence proportion arising from a single occupational, geographic, or patient group, such as the proportion of infants born with malformations among women living near a toxic waste site, or the proportion of patients who go into anaphylactic shock when treated with a particular drug. If A cases are observed out of N persons at risk and the outcome is not contagious, the conventional model used to analyze the incidence proportion A/N is the binomial distribution (introduced in Chapter 13).

Define R as the probability that a subject will experience the outcome. If we assume that this probability is the same for all the subjects, and that the subject outcomes are independent, we obtain the *binomial model,* which specifies that the probability of observing $A = a$ cases out of N persons is

$$\Pr(A = a) = \binom{N}{a} R^a (1 - R)^{N-a} \qquad [14\text{–}3]$$

In data analysis, R is an unknown quantity called the *risk parameter,* whereas A and N are known quantities. The function of R that results when the observed data numbers are put into equation 14–3 is called the *binomial likelihood* for R, based on the data.

Under the binomial model (equation 14–3):

1. $\hat{R} = A/N$ is the maximum-likelihood estimator (MLE) of R.
2. $N \cdot R$ is the average value of A that we would observe over study repetitions, and $N \cdot R(1 - R)$ is the variance of A over the repetitions.

It follows from the last fact that a large-sample statistic for testing the null hypothesis that R equals some expected risk R_E is the score statistic

$$\chi_{\text{score}} = \frac{A - E}{[E(N - E)/N]^{1/2}}$$

where $E = N \cdot R_E$ is the expected number of cases.

It is common practice to use the Wald method to set approximate confidence limits for the *logit* of R (the natural logarithm of the odds):

$$L = \text{logit}(R) = \ln\left(\frac{R}{1 - R}\right)$$

One then transforms the limits $\underline{L}$, $\overline{L}$ for the logit back to the risk scale by means of the *logistic transform,* which is defined by

$$R = \text{expit}(L) \equiv \frac{e^L}{1 + e^L} = \frac{1}{1 + e^{-L}}$$

Wald limits use the fact that an estimate of the approximate SD of logit($\hat{R}$) is

$$\widehat{SD}[\text{logit}(\hat{R})] = (1/A + 1/B)^{1/2}$$

where $B = N - A$ is the number of noncases. Approximate γ% limits for R are then

$$\underline{R}, \overline{R} = \text{expit}\{\text{logit}(\hat{R}) \pm Z_\gamma \widehat{SD}[\text{logit}(\hat{R})]\}$$

If we want γ% limits for the risk ratio $RR = R/R_E$, we use $\underline{R}/R_E$, $\overline{R}/R_E$.

Lancaster (1987) observed six infants with neural tube defects in a cohort of 1,694 live births conceived through in vitro fertilization, an incidence proportion of $\hat{R} = 6/1{,}694 = 0.00354$. He cited a general population risk of 1.2 per 1,000, so $R_E = 0.0012$. This risk yields an expected number of cases of 0.0012(1,694) = 2.0, and a score statistic of

$$\chi_{\text{score}} = \frac{6 - 2.0}{[2.0(1{,}694 - 2.0)/1{,}694]^{1/2}} = 2.83$$

which, from a standard normal table, yields an upper-tailed P-value of 0.002. Also, SD[logit($\hat{R}$)] = $(1/6 + 1/1{,}688)^{1/2} = 0.409$, so the 90% limits for the risk R based on the Wald method are

$$\underline{R}, \overline{R} = \text{expit}[\text{logit}(0.00354) \pm 1.645(0.409)] = 0.0018, 0.0070$$

which yield 90% limits for the risk ratio RR of $\underline{RR}$, $\overline{RR} = \underline{R}/0.0012$, $\overline{R}/0.0012 = 1.5, 5.8$. The corresponding 95% limits are 1.3, 6.6. The results suggest that if the binomial model is correct, either a bias is present or there is an elevated rate of defects in the study cohort, but the magnitude of elevation is very imprecisely estimated.

TABLE 14–3

Notation for a Crude 2 × 2 Table

	Exposed	Unexposed	Total
Cases	A_1	A_0	M_1
Noncases	B_1	B_0	M_0
Total	N_1	N_0	N

Another concern is that the study size is probably too small for these approximate statistics to be accurate. As with the person-time statistics, the score statistic will be adequate when E and $N - E$ exceed 5, and the Wald limits will be adequate when both $N\underline{R}$ and $N(1 - \overline{R})$ exceed 5. In the Lancaster study, E is only 2 and $N\underline{R} = 1{,}694(0.0016) = 2.7$, so exact methods are needed.

TWO STUDY GROUPS: LARGE-SAMPLE METHODS

When comparing two study groups, the data can be displayed in a 2 × 2 table of counts. The four cells of the table are the numbers of subjects classified into each combination of presence or absence of exposure and occurrence or nonoccurrence of disease. The notation we will use is given in Table 14–3.

Superficially, Table 14–3 resembles Table 14–1 except for the addition of a row for noncases. The denominators in Table 14–3, however, are frequencies (counts) of subjects rather than person-time accumulations. Conveniently, crude data from a case-control study has a form identical to Table 14–3 and can be analyzed using the same probability model as used for pure-count cohort data.

For a noncontagious outcome, one conventional probability model for the observed numbers of cases A_1 and A_0 is the binomial model. If R_1 and R_0 are the risk parameters for exposed and unexposed cohorts, this model specifies that the probability of observing $A_1 = a_1$ and $A_0 = a_0$ is

$$\Pr(A_1 = a_1, A_0 = a_0) = \Pr(A_1 = a_1)\Pr(A_0 = a_0)$$
$$= \binom{N_1}{a_1} R_1{}^{a_1}(1 - R_1)^{N_1 - a_1} \binom{N_0}{a_0} R_0{}^{a_0}(1 - R_0)^{N_0 - a_0} \quad [14\text{–}4]$$

which is just the product of the probabilities for the two cohorts.

In data analysis, R_1 and R_0 are unknown parameters, whereas A_1, N_1, A_0, and N_0 are known quantities. The function of the unknowns R_1 and R_0 obtained when actual data values are put into equation 14–4 is called the *binomial likelihood* of R_1 and R_0, based on the data.

Under the two-binomial model (equation 14–4):

1. A_1/N_1 and A_0/N_0 are the maximum-likelihood estimators of R_1 and R_0.
2. The MLE of the risk ratio $RR = R_1/R_0$ is

$$\widehat{RR} = \frac{A_1/N_1}{A_0/N_0}$$

3. The MLE of the risk difference $RD = R_1 - R_0$ is

$$\widehat{RD} = \frac{A_1}{N_1} - \frac{A_0}{N_0}$$

4. The MLE of the risk-odds ratio

$$OR = \frac{R_1/(1 - R_1)}{R_0/(1 - R_0)}$$

TABLE 14–4

Diarrhea During a 10-Day Follow-Up Period in 30 Breast-Fed Infants Colonized with *Vibrio cholerae* 01, According to Antipolysaccharide Antibody Titers in the Mother's Breast Milk

	Antibody Level		
	Low	High	Total
Diarrhea	12	7	19
No diarrhea	2	9	11
Totals	14	16	30

From Glass RI, Svennerholm AM, Stoll BJ, et al. Protection against cholera in breast-fed children by antibiotics in breast milk. *N Engl J Med.* 1983;308:1389–1392.

is the observed incidence-odds ratio

$$\widehat{OR} = \frac{A_1/B_1}{A_0/B_0} = \frac{A_1 B_0}{A_0 B_1}$$

5. If $R_1 = R_0$ (no difference in risk), $E = M_1 N_1 / N$ is the average number of exposed cases A_1 that one would observe over the subset of study repetitions in which M_1 total cases were observed, and

$$V = \frac{E M_0 N_0}{N(N-1)} = \frac{M_1 N_1 M_0 N_0}{N^2(N-1)}$$

is the variance of A_1 over the same subset of repetitions.

It follows from the last fact that a large-sample statistic for testing the null hypothesis $R_1 = R_0$ (the same hypothesis as $RR = 1, RD = 0$, and $OR = 1$) is

$$\chi_{\text{score}} = \frac{A_1 - E}{V^{1/2}}$$

This score statistic has the same form as the score statistic for person-time data. Nonetheless, the formula for V, the variance of A_1, has the additional multiplier $M_0/(N-1)$. This multiplier reflects the fact that we are using a different probability model for variation in A_1.

Table 14–4 presents data from a cohort study of diarrhea in breast-fed infants colonized with *Vibrio cholerae* 01, classified by level of antibody titers in their mother's breast milk (Glass et al., 1983). A low titer confers an elevated risk and so is taken as the first column of Table 14–4. From these data, we obtain

$$\widehat{RR} = (12/14)/(7/16) = 1.96$$
$$\widehat{RD} = 12/14 - 7/16 = 0.42$$
$$\widehat{OR} = 12(9)/7(2) = 7.71$$
$$E = 19(14)/30 = 8.87$$
$$V = 8.87(11)16/30(30-1) = 1.79$$

and

$$\chi_{\text{score}} = \frac{12 - 8.87}{1.79^{1/2}} = 2.34$$

The latter yields an upper-tailed P-value of 0.01. Thus a score statistic as large or larger than that observed has low probability in the absence of bias or an antibody effect.

There are at least two cautions to consider in interpreting the statistics just given. First, infant diarrhea is usually infectious in origin, and causative agents could be transmitted between subjects if there were contact between the infants or their mothers. Such phenomena would invalidate the score test given above. Second, there are only two low-antibody noncases, raising the possibility that the large-sample statistics ($\widehat{RR}$, $\widehat{OR}$, χ_{score}) are not adequate. We expect χ_{score} to be adequate when all four expected cells, E, $M_1 - E$, $N_1 - E$, and $M_0 - N_1 + E$ exceed 5; $\widehat{RR}$ to be adequate when N_1R_1 and N_0R_0 exceed 5; and $\widehat{OR}$ to be adequate when N_1R_1, N_0R_0, $N_1(1 - R_1)$, and $N_0(1-R_0)$ all exceed 5. In the diarrhea example, the smallest of the expected cells is $N_1 - E = 5.13$, just above the criterion. Because B_1 is an estimate of $N_1(1 - R_1)$ and is only 2, $\widehat{OR}$ seems less trustworthy.

Turning now to interval estimation, a SD estimate for $\widehat{RD}$ is

$$\widehat{SD}(\widehat{RD}) = \left[\frac{A_1B_1}{N_1^2(N_1 - 1)} + \frac{A_0B_0}{N_0^2(N_0 - 1)}\right]^{1/2}$$

which yields the $\gamma\%$ Wald confidence limits

$$\widehat{RD} \pm Z_\gamma \widehat{SD}(\widehat{RD})$$

This formula can produce quite inaccurate limits when the expected cell sizes are small, as evidenced by limits that may fall below -1 or above 1. Improved approximate confidence limits for the risk difference can be found from

$$\underline{RD}, \overline{RD} = \frac{e^{\pm s} - d}{e^{\pm s} + d}$$

where

$$s = \frac{2Z_\gamma \widehat{SD}(\widehat{RD})}{1 - \widehat{RD}^2}$$

and

$$d = \frac{1 - \widehat{RD}}{1 + \widehat{RD}}$$

(Zou and Donner, 2004). When $\widehat{RD} = 1$ or -1 this formula fails, but then the upper limit should be set to 1 if $\widehat{RD} = 1$, or to -1 if $\widehat{RD} = -1$.

Approximate SD estimates for $\ln(\widehat{RR})$ and $\ln(\widehat{OR})$ are

$$\widehat{SD}[\ln(\widehat{RR})] = \left(\frac{1}{A_1} - \frac{1}{N_1} + \frac{1}{A_0} - \frac{1}{N_0}\right)^{1/2}$$

and

$$\widehat{SD}[\ln(\widehat{OR})] = \left(\frac{1}{A_1} + \frac{1}{B_1} + \frac{1}{A_0} + \frac{1}{B_0}\right)^{1/2}$$

which yield $\gamma\%$ Wald limits of

$$\underline{RR}, \overline{RR} = \exp\{\ln(\widehat{RR}) \pm Z_\gamma \widehat{SD}[\ln(\widehat{RR})]\}$$

and

$$\underline{OR}, \overline{OR} = \exp\{\ln(\widehat{OR}) \pm Z_\gamma \widehat{SD}[\ln(\widehat{OR})]\}$$

For the data of Table 14–4,

$$\widehat{SD}(\widehat{RD}) = \left[\frac{12(2)}{14^2 13} + \frac{7(9)}{16^2 15}\right]^{1/2} = 0.161$$

$$\widehat{SD}[\ln(\widehat{RR})] = \left(\frac{1}{12} - \frac{1}{14} + \frac{1}{7} - \frac{1}{16}\right)^{1/2} = 0.304$$

and

$$\widehat{SD}[\ln(\widehat{OR})] = \left(\frac{1}{12} + \frac{1}{2} + \frac{1}{7} + \frac{1}{9}\right)^{1/2} = 0.915$$

which yield 90% Wald limits of

$$\underline{RD}, \overline{RD} = 0.42 \pm 1.645(0.161) = 0.16, 0.68$$

$$\underline{RR}, \overline{RR} = \exp[\ln(1.96) \pm 1.645(0.304)] = 1.2, 3.2$$

and

$$\underline{OR}, \overline{OR} = \exp[\ln(7.71) \pm 1.645(0.915)] = 1.7, 35$$

The improved approximate 90% limits for *RD* are 0.13, 0.65, which are slightly shifted toward the null compared with the simple Wald limits. The simple 95% Wald limits are 0.10, 0.73 for *RD*, 1.1, 3.6 for *RR*, and 1.3, 46 for *OR*. Thus, although the data show a positive association, the measures are imprecisely estimated, especially the odds ratio.

Under the two-binomial model, we expect the Wald limits for the risk difference and ratio to be adequate when the limits for the odds ratio are adequate. The Wald limits for the odds ratio should be adequate when all four cell expectations given the lower odds-ratio limit *and* all four cell expectations given the upper odds-ratio limit exceed 5. This rather unwieldy criterion takes much labor to apply, however. Instead, we recommend that, if there is any doubt about the adequacy of the study size for Wald methods, one should turn to more accurate methods. There are more accurate large-sample approximations than the Wald method for setting confidence limits (see Chapter 13), but only the odds ratios have widely available small-sample methods; these methods are described at the end of this chapter.

RELATIONS AMONG THE RATIO MEASURES

As discussed in Chapter 4, *OR* is always further from the null value of 1 than *RR*. In a parallel fashion, $\widehat{OR}$ is always further from 1 than $\widehat{RR}$ in an unstratified study; therefore, use of $\widehat{OR}$ from a cohort study as an estimate for *RR* tends to produce estimates that are too far from 1. The disparity between *OR* and *RR* increases with both the size of the risks R_1 and R_0 and the strength of the association (as measured by *OR* or *RR*). A parallel relation holds for $\widehat{OR}$ and $\widehat{RR}$. The disparity increases as both the size of the incidence proportions A_1/N_1 and A_0/N_0 and the strength of the observed association increases. For Table 14–4, $RR = 2.0$ and $OR = 7.7$ are far apart because both observed proportions exceed 40% and the association is strong.

One often sees statements that the odds ratio approximates the risk ratio when the disease is "rare." This statement can be made more precise in a study of a closed population: If both risk odds $R_1/(1-R_1)$ and $R_0/(1-R_0)$ are under 10%, then the disparity between *OR* and *RR* will also be under 10% (Greenland, 1987a). In a parallel fashion, if the observed incidence odds A_1/B_1 and A_0/B_0 are under 10%, then the disparity between $\widehat{OR}$ and $\widehat{RR}$ will be under 10%.

The relation of the odds ratio and risk ratio to the rate ratio *IR* is more complex. Nonetheless, if the incidence rates change only slightly across small subintervals of the actual follow-up period (i.e., the incidence rates are nearly constant across small time strata), *IR* will be further from the null than *RR* and closer to the null than *OR* (Greenland and Thomas, 1982). It follows that, given constant incidence rates over time, $\widehat{OR}$ as an estimate of *IR* tends to be too far from the null, and $\widehat{IR}$ as an estimate of *RR* tends to be too far from the null. Again, however, the disparity among the three measures will be small when the incidence is low.

CASE-CONTROL DATA

Assuming that the underlying source cohort is closed, the odds-ratio estimates given earlier can be applied directly to cumulative case-control data. Table 14–5 provides data from a case-control study of chlordiazepoxide use in early pregnancy and congenital heart defects. For testing $OR = 1$

TABLE 14–5

History of Chlordiazepoxide Use in Early Pregnancy for Mothers of Children Born with Congenital Heart Defects and Mothers of Normal Children

	Chlordiazepoxide Use		
	Yes	No	Total
Case mothers	4	386	390
Control mothers	4	1,250	1,254
Totals	8	1,636	1,644

From Rothman KJ, Fyler DC, Goldblatt A, et al. Exogenous hormones and other drug exposures of children with congenital heart disease. *Am J Epidemiol.* 1979;109:433–439.

(no association), we have

$$E = \frac{390(8)}{1{,}644} = 1.90$$

$$V = \frac{1.90(1{,}254)(1{,}636)}{1{,}644(1{,}643)} = 1.44$$

and

$$\chi_{\text{score}} = \frac{4 - 1.90}{1.44^{1/2}} = 1.75$$

which yields an upper-tailed P-value of 0.04. Also,

$$\widehat{OR} = \frac{4(1{,}250)}{4(386)} = 3.24$$

and

$$\widehat{SD}[\ln(\widehat{OR})] = \left(\frac{1}{4} + \frac{1}{4} + \frac{1}{386} + \frac{1}{1{,}250}\right)^{1/2} = 0.710$$

which yield 90% Wald limits of

$$\exp[\ln(3.24) \pm 1.65(0.710)] = 1.00,\ 10.5$$

and 95% Wald limits of 0.81, 13. Thus, the data exhibit a positive association but do so with little precision, indicating that, even in the absence of bias, the data are reasonably compatible with effects ranging from little or nothing up through more than a 10-fold increase in risk.

If the exposure prevalence does not change over the sampling period, the above odds-ratio formulas can also be used to estimate rate ratios from case-control studies done with density sampling (see Chapter 8). Because controls in such studies represent person-time, persons may at different times be sampled more than once as controls, and may be sampled as a case after being sampled as a control. Data from such a person must be entered repeatedly, just as if the person had been a different person at each sampling time. If a person's exposure changes over time, the data entered for the person at each sampling time will differ. For example, in a study of smoking, it is conceivable (though extremely unlikely in practice) that a single person could first be sampled as a smoking control, then later be sampled as a nonsmoking control (if the person quit between the sampling times); if the person then fell ill, he or she could be sampled a third time as a case (smoking or nonsmoking, depending on whether the person resumed or not between the second and third sampling times).

TABLE 14–6

Notation for Crude Case-Cohort Data When All Cases in the Cohort Are Selected

	Exposed	Unexposed	Total
Case but not control	A_{11}	A_{01}	M_{11}
Case and control	A_{10}	A_{00}	M_{10}
Noncase control	B_1	B_0	M_0
Total	N_1	N_0	N

The repeated-use rule may at first appear odd, but it is no more odd than the use of multiple person-time units from the same person in a cohort study. One caution should be borne in mind, however: If exposure prevalence changes over the course of subject selection, and risk changes over time or subjects are matched on sampling time, one should treat sampling time as a potential confounder and thus stratify on it (see Chapters 15 and 16) (Greenland and Thomas, 1982). With fine enough time strata, no person will appear twice in the same time stratum. Such fine stratification should also be used if one desires a small-sample (exact) analysis of density-sampled data.

CASE-COHORT DATA

Case-cohort data differ from cumulative case-control data in that some of the controls may also be cases, because controls in case-cohort data are a sample of the entire cohort, whereas controls in cumulative case-control data are a sample of noncases only. We limit our discussion of methods to the common special case in which every case in the source cohort is ascertained and selected for study. We further stipulate that the source cohort is closed and that the cohort sample was selected by simple random sampling. We may then use the notation given in Table 14–6 for case-cohort data.

Table 14–6 resembles Table 14–3 except that the cases are now split into cases that were not also selected as controls and cases that were. Data in the form of Table 14–6 can be collapsed into the form of Table 14–3 by adding together the first two rows, so that

$$A_1 = A_{11} + A_{10} \quad A_0 = A_{01} + A_{00} \quad M_1 = M_{11} + M_{10}$$

With the data collapsed in this fashion, the odds ratio can be tested and estimated using the same large- and small-sample methods as given in previous sections for case-control data. In other words, we can obtain P-values from the score statistic or from the hypergeometric formula below (equation 14–8), and Wald-type limits for OR as before. As in cohort studies and in case-control studies of a cohort, if the source cohort for the case-cohort study suffers meaningful losses to follow-up or from competing risks, it will be important to analyze the data with stratification on time (see Chapter 16).

One can estimate the risk ratio directly from the case-cohort data using large-sample formulas that generalize the risk-ratio methods for full-cohort data. To describe the maximum-likelihood estimator of the risk ratio in case-cohort data (Sato, 1992a), we first must define the "pseudo-denominators"

$$N_1^* = \frac{A_1 M_{10}}{M_1} + B_1$$

and

$$N_0^* = \frac{A_0 M_{10}}{M_1} + B_0$$

M_{10} is the number of cases among the controls, M_1 is the total number of cases, and M_{10}/M_1 is the proportion of cases that are controls. The ratio N_1^*/N_0^* is a more stable estimate of the ratio of exposed to unexposed in the source cohort than the intuitive estimate $(A_{10} + B_1)/(A_{00} + B_0)$ obtained from the controls alone. Thus we take as our case-cohort risk-ratio estimate

$$\widehat{RR} = \frac{A_1/N_1^*}{A_0/N_0^*} = \frac{A_1/A_0}{N_1^*/N_0^*}$$

The approximate variance of $\ln(\widehat{RR})$ is estimated as

$$\hat{V}[\ln(\widehat{RR})] =$$

$$\frac{1}{A_1} + \frac{1}{A_0} + \left(\frac{M_{11} - M_{10}}{M_1}\right)\left(\frac{1}{N_1^*} + \frac{1}{N_0^*}\right) - \left(\frac{1}{A_1} + \frac{1}{A_0}\right)\left(\frac{1}{N_1^*} + \frac{1}{N_0^*}\right)^2\left(\frac{M_{11}M_{10}}{M_1^2}\right)$$

so that 95% confidence limits for the risk ratio can be computed from

$$\underline{RR}, \overline{RR} = \exp[\ln(\widehat{RR}) \pm 1.96\, \widehat{SD}]$$

where $\widehat{SD}$ is the square root of $\hat{V}[\ln(\widehat{RR})]$.

If the disease is so uncommon that no case appears in the control sample, then $M_{10} = 0$, $M_{11} = M_1$, $N_1^* = B_1$, $N_0^* = B_0$, and so

$$\widehat{RR} = \frac{A_1 B_0}{A_0 B_1} = \widehat{OR}$$

and

$$\hat{V}[\ln(\widehat{RR})] = \left(\frac{1}{A_1} + \frac{1}{A_0} + \frac{1}{B_1} + \frac{1}{B_0}\right)$$

which are identical to the odds-ratio point and variance estimates for case-control data. On the other hand, if every cohort member is selected as a control, then $M_{11} = 0$ and these formulas become identical to the risk-ratio formulas for closed cohort data.

SMALL-SAMPLE STATISTICS FOR PERSON-TIME DATA

SINGLE STUDY GROUP

Consider again a study in which A cases occur in observation of T person-time units, and E cases would be expected if reference-population rates applied. The mean value of A, which is $I \cdot T$ in the Poisson distribution (equation 14–1), is equal to $IR \cdot E$:

$$I \cdot T = \left[\frac{I}{(E/T)}\right]\left(\frac{E}{T}\right) \cdot T = IR \cdot E$$

Using this relation, we can compute the mid-P-value functions for IR directly from the Poisson distribution with $IR \cdot E$ in place of $I \cdot T$:

$$\begin{aligned} P_{\text{lower}} &= \frac{1}{2}\Pr(A = a) + \Pr(A < a) \\ &= \frac{1}{2}\exp(-IR \cdot E)(IR \cdot E)^a/a! + \sum_{k=0}^{a-1}\exp(-IR \cdot E)(IR \cdot E)^k/k! \\ &= 1 - P_{\text{upper}} = 1 - \left[\frac{1}{2}\Pr(A = a) + \Pr(A > a)\right] \end{aligned}$$

To get the median-unbiased estimate of IR we find that value of IR for which $P_{\text{lower}} = P_{\text{upper}}$ (which exists only if $A > 0$) (Birnbaum, 1964). This value of IR will have lower and upper mid-P-values equal to 0.5. To get a two-sided $(1 - \alpha)$-level mid-P confidence interval for IR, we take the lower limit to be the value $\underline{IR}$ for IR for which $P_{\text{upper}} = \alpha/2$, and take the upper limit to be the value $\overline{IR}$ for IR for which $P_{\text{lower}} = \alpha/2$. To get limits for I, we multiply $\underline{IR}$ and $\overline{IR}$ by E/T.

Waxweiler et al. (1976) observed $A = 7$ deaths from liver and biliary cancer in a cohort of workers who were exposed for at least 15 years to vinyl chloride. Only $E = 0.436$ deaths were expected based on general population rates. The mid-P-value functions are given by

$$P_{\text{lower}} = \frac{1}{2}\Pr(A = 7) + \Pr(A < 7)$$

$$= \frac{1}{2}\exp[-IR(0.436)][IR(0.436)]^7/7! + \sum_{k=0}^{6}\exp[-IR(0.436)][IR(0.436)]^k/k!$$

$$= 1 - P_{\text{upper}} = 1\left[\frac{1}{2}\Pr(A = 7) + \Pr(A > 7)\right]$$

The lower mid-P-value for the hypothesis $IR = 1$ is under 0.00001. The value of IR for which $P_{\text{lower}} = P_{\text{upper}} = 0.5$ is 16.4, which is the median-unbiased estimate. The value of IR for which $P_{\text{lower}} = 0.10/2 = 0.05$ is $\underline{IR} = 8.1$, the lower limit of the $1 - 0.10 = 90\%$ mid-P confidence interval. The value of IR for which $P_{\text{upper}} = 0.10/2 = 0.05$ is $\overline{IR} = 29$, the upper limit of the 90% mid-P confidence interval. The 95% limits are 6.9 and 32, and the 99% limits are 5.1 and 38. The number of cases observed is clearly far greater than we would expect under the Poisson model with $IR = 1$. Thus it appears that this null model is wrong, as would occur if biases are present or there is a rate elevation in the study cohort ($IR > 1$).

For comparison, the MLE of IR in this example is $IR = 7/0.436 = 16.1$, the score statistic is $(7 - 0.436)/0.436^{1/2} = 9.94$, the upper P-value less than 0.00001, the 90% Wald limits are

$$\underline{IR}, \overline{IR} = \exp[\ln(7/0.436) \pm 1.65(1/7^{1/2})] = 8.6, 30$$

and the 95% and 99% Wald limits are 7.7, 34 and 6.1, 43. As may be apparent, the 90% Wald limits provide better approximations than the 95% limits, and the 95% provide better approximations than the 99% limits.

The simple examples we have given illustrate the basic principles of small-sample analysis: Compute the upper and lower P-value functions directly from the chosen probability model, and then use these functions to create equations for point and interval estimates, as well as to compute P-values.

TWO STUDY GROUPS

Consider again a study in which A_1 cases occur in observation of T_1 exposed person-time, and A_0 cases occur in observation of T_0 unexposed person-time. The expectation E and variance V for the exposed-case cell A_1 in the score statistic were computed only for study repetitions in which the total number of cases M_1 was equal to its observed value. Another way of putting this restriction is that M_1 was treated as *fixed* in the computation of E and V. In more technical and general terms, we say that computation of E and V was done *conditional* on M_1, the observed case margin.

The philosophy behind fixing M_1 is based on a statistical concept called *conditionality* (Cox and Hinkley, 1974; Little, 1989). One useful consequence of this step is that it greatly simplifies small-sample statistics. By treating M_1 as fixed, we can compute exact and mid-P-values and limits for the incidence rate ratio IR using the following *binomial* probability model for the number of exposed cases, A_1, given the total number of cases observed, M_1:

$$\Pr(A_1 = a_1 | M_1 = m_1) = \binom{m_1}{a_1} s^{a_1}(1 - s)^{m_1 - a_1} \qquad [14\text{–}5]$$

where s is the probability that a randomly sampled case is exposed. It turns out that s is a simple function of the incidence rate ratio IR and the observed person-time:

$$s = \frac{\text{average number of exposed cases}}{\text{average total number of cases}}$$

$$= \frac{I_1 T_1}{I_1 T_1 + I_0 T_0} = \frac{(I_1/I_0)T_1}{(I_1/I_0)T_1 + T_0} = \frac{IR \cdot T_1}{IR \cdot T_1 + T_0} \qquad [14\text{–}6]$$

where the averages are over repetitions of the study (keeping T_1 and T_0 fixed). We can set small-sample confidence limits $\underline{s}$, $\overline{s}$ for s by computing directly from the binomial equation 14–5. We can then convert these limits to rate-ratio limits $\underline{IR}$, $\overline{IR}$ by solving equation 14–6 for IR and then substituting $\underline{s}$ and $\overline{s}$ into the resulting formula,

$$IR = \frac{s}{1-s}\left(\frac{T_0}{T_1}\right) \qquad [14\text{–}7]$$

(Rothman and Boice, 1982). Computing directly from the binomial distribution (equation 14–5) the mid-P-value functions are

$$P_{\text{lower}} = \frac{1}{2}\binom{m_1}{a_1} s^{a_1}(1-s)^{m_1-a_1} + \sum_{k=0}^{a_1-1}\binom{m_1}{k} s^k(1-s)^{M_1-k} = 1 - P_{\text{upper}}$$

The median-unbiased estimate of s is the value of s at which $P_{\text{lower}} = P_{\text{upper}}$, the lower limit of the $1-\alpha$ mid-P interval is the value of s at which $P_{\text{upper}} = \alpha/2$, and the upper limit of the $1-\alpha$ mid-P interval is the value of s at which $P_{\text{lower}} = \alpha/2$. These can be converted to a point estimate and confidence limits for IR using equation 14–7. If we have a particular value of IR we wish to test, we can convert to a test value of s using equation 14–6; the resulting mid-P-values apply to the original test value of IR as well as to the derived test value of s.

For the data in Table 14–2,

$$P_{\text{lower}} = \frac{1}{2}\Pr(A_1 = 41) + \Pr(A_1 < 41)$$

$$= \frac{1}{2}\binom{56}{41} s^{41}(1-s)^{15} + \sum_{k=0}^{40}\binom{56}{k} s^k(1-s)^{56-k} = 1 - P_{\text{upper}}$$

where

$$s = \frac{IR(28{,}010)}{IR(28{,}010) + 19{,}017}$$

and

$$IR = \frac{s}{1-s}\left(\frac{19{,}017}{28{,}010}\right)$$

For $IR = 1$, we get $s = 28{,}010/47{,}027 = 0.596$, which has a lower mid-$P$-value of 0.02; this is also the lower mid-P-value for the hypothesis $IR = 1$. The lower and upper 90% mid-P limits for s are 0.626 and 0.8205, which translate into limits for IR of

$$\frac{0.626}{1-0.626}\cdot\frac{19{,}017}{28{,}010} = 1.14 \quad \text{and} \quad \frac{0.8205}{1-0.8205}\cdot\frac{19{,}017}{28{,}010} = 3.10$$

The corresponding 95% limits are 1.04, 3.45. Because the numbers of cases in the study are large, these small-sample statistics are close to the large-sample statistics obtained earlier.

SMALL-SAMPLE STATISTICS FOR PURE COUNT DATA

SINGLE STUDY GROUP

Consider again a study in which A cases occur among N persons observed at risk. Computing directly from the binomial distribution (equation 14–5), the mid-P-value functions are

$$P_{\text{lower}} = \frac{1}{2}\binom{N}{a} R^a(1-R)^{N-a} + \sum_{k=0}^{a-1}\binom{N}{k} R^k(1-R)^{N-k} = 1 - P_{\text{upper}}$$

The median-unbiased estimate of R is the value at which $P_{\text{lower}} = P_{\text{upper}}$, the lower limit of the $1-\alpha$ mid-P interval is the value $\underline{R}$ at which $P_{\text{upper}} = \alpha/2$, and the upper limit of the $1-\alpha$ mid-P interval is the value $\overline{R}$ at which $P_{\text{lower}} = \alpha/2$. If the expected risk derived from an external reference population is R_E, we obtain estimates of the risk ratio $RR = R/R_E$ by substituting $R_E \cdot RR$ for R in the formula.

For the Lancaster data, $A = 6$, $N = 1{,}694$, and $R_E = 0.0012$, which yield the mid-P-value function

$$P_{\text{lower}} = \frac{1}{2}\binom{1{,}694}{6}(0.0012RR)^6(1 - 0.012RR)^{1{,}688}$$

$$+ \sum_{k=0}^{5}\binom{1{,}694}{6}(0.0012RR)^k(1 - 0.0012RR)^{1{,}694-k}$$

Substituting 0.5 for P_{lower} and solving for RR yields a median-unbiased risk-ratio estimate of 3.1. Other substitutions yield 90% mid-P limits for the risk ratio of 1.4 and 5.7, 95% mid-P limits of 1.2 and 6.4, and a lower mid-P-value for testing $RR = 1$ ($R = R_E = 0.0012$) of 0.01. Despite the small number of cases, these confidence limits are very similar to the large-sample limits (which were 1.5, 5.8 at 90% confidence and 1.3, 6.6 at 95% confidence).

TWO STUDY GROUPS

Consider again a study in which A_1 cases occur among N_1 exposed persons at risk and A_0 cases occur among N_0 unexposed persons at risk. As in person-time data, the expectation E and variance V in the score statistic for Table 14–3 are computed as if all the margins (M_1, M_0, N_1, N_0) were fixed. In reality, none of the designs we have described has both margins fixed: In a cohort study, the case total M_1 is free to vary; in a case-control study, the exposed total N_1 is free to vary; and in a prevalence survey, all the margins may be free to vary.

The philosophy behind treating all the margins in a two-way table as fixed is even more abstract than in the person-time situation (Fisher, 1935; for more modem perspectives, see Little, 1989, and Greenland, 1991b). Although it is mildly controversial, the practice is virtually universal in epidemiologic statistics. It originated in the context of testing the null hypothesis in randomized experiments. Consider the sharp (strong) null hypothesis, that exposure has no effect on anyone, in the context of an experiment that will assign exactly N_1 out of N persons to exposure. Then, under the potential-outcome model of Chapter 4, no causal "type 2" or preventive "type 3" persons are in the study, and the total number of cases M_1 is just the number of doomed "type 1" persons in the study. Once persons are chosen for the study, M_1 is unaffected by exposure and so in this sense is fixed, given the cohort. In particular, if only exposure status may vary (e.g., via experimental assignment), and the number exposed N_1 is also predetermined, then under the sharp null hypothesis, the only quantities left to vary are the internal table cells. Furthermore, given one cell and the fixed margins, we can compute all the other cells by subtraction, e.g., given A_1 we get $A_0 = M_1 - A_1$ and $B_1 = N_1 - A_1$. If exposure is assigned by simple randomization, the resulting distribution for A_1 is the null hypergeometric distribution

$$\Pr(A_1 = a_1 | M_1 = m_1, M_0 = m_0, N_1 = n_1, N_0 = n_0, \text{ null hypothesis}) = \frac{\binom{n_1}{a_1}\binom{n_0}{m_1 - a_1}}{\binom{n}{m_1}}$$

Fisher's exact test computes P-values for the null hypothesis directly from this distribution.

In the non-null situation the rationale for computing statistics by fixing the margins is less straightforward and applies only to inference on odds ratios. For this purpose, it has the advantage of reducing small-sample bias in estimation even if the margins are not actually fixed (Mantel and Hankey, 1975; Pike et al., 1980). Those who remain uncomfortable with the use of fixed margins for a table in which the margins are not truly fixed may find comfort in the fact that the fixed-margins assumption makes little difference compared with statistical methods that do not assume fixed margins when the observed table cells are large enough to give precise inferences.

When treating all margins as fixed, we can compute exact and mid-P-values and limits for the odds ratio using only the noncentral (non-null) *hypergeometric* distribution for the number of exposed cases, A_1, given the margins:

$$\Pr(A_1 = a_1 | M_1 = m_1, M_0 = m_0, N_1 = n_1, N_0 = n_0) = \frac{\binom{n_1}{a_1}\binom{n_0}{m_1 - a_1} OR^{a_1}}{\sum_k \binom{n_1}{k}\binom{n_0}{m_1 - k} OR^k} \qquad [14\text{–}8]$$

where k ranges over all possible values for A_1 (Breslow and Day, 1980; McCullagh and Nelder, 1989). Under the null hypothesis, $OR = 1$ and this distribution reduces to the null hypergeometric. One can compute median-unbiased estimates, exact P-values, and mid-P-values from the hypergeometric equation 14–8 in the manner illustrated earlier for other models.

Upon entering data values a_1, m_1, n_1, n_0 into equation 14–8 only one unknown remains, the odds ratio OR, and so the formula becomes an odds-ratio function. This odds-ratio function is called the *conditional-likelihood function* for the odds ratio based on the data, and the value of OR that makes it largest is called the *conditional maximum-likelihood estimate* (CMLE) of OR. This CMLE does *not* equal the familiar unconditional maximum-likelihood estimate $\widehat{OR} = a_1b_1/a_0b_0$ given earlier, and in fact it has no explicit formula. It is always closer to the null and tends to be closer to the true odds ratio than the unconditional MLE $\widehat{OR}$, although for unstratified samples in which all cells are "large" (>4) it will be very close to $\widehat{OR}$ and the median-unbiased estimate of OR.

For the data in Table 14–4 on infant diarrhea, equation 14–8 yields the mid-P-value function

$$P_{\text{lower}} = \frac{\frac{1}{2}\binom{14}{12}\binom{16}{7} OR^{12}}{\sum_{k=3}^{14}\binom{14}{k}\binom{16}{19-k} OR^k} + \frac{\sum_{k=3}^{11}\binom{14}{k}\binom{16}{19-k} OR^k}{\sum_{k=3}^{14}\binom{14}{k}\binom{16}{19-k} OR^k} = 1 - P_{\text{upper}}$$

This function yields a lower mid-P-value of 0.01 for the hypothesis $OR = 1$, and a median-unbiased odds-ratio estimate (the OR for which mid-P_{lower} = mid-P_{upper} = 0.5) of 6.9. The conditional maximum-likelihood estimate is 7.2, whereas the unconditional (ordinary) maximum-likelihood estimate is $12(9)/7(2) = 7.7$. The mid-P 90% limits (the values of OR at which $P_{\text{upper}} = 0.05$ and $P_{\text{lower}} = 0.05$, respectively) are 1.6 and 40, whereas the mid-P 95% limits are 1.3 and 61. The lower mid-P limits are close to the approximate lower limits (of 1.7 and 1.3) obtained earlier, but the upper mid-P limits are somewhat greater than the approximate upper limits (which were 35 and 46).

APPLICATION OF EXACT 2 × 2 PROGRAMS TO PERSON-TIME DATA AND SINGLE-GROUP DATA

The results in the last example were obtained from a public-domain program for exact analysis of one or more 2 × 2 tables (Martin and Austin, 1996). Although this and some other exact programs also provide exact analyses of 1 × 2 tables like Table 14–1, many do not. For such programs, one can analyze person-time data as follows: First, multiply the person-time denominators T_1 and T_0 by a number h so large that $hT_1 > 1{,}000A_1$ and $hT_0 > 1{,}000A_0$; second, enter the data into the 2 × 2 program as if it were person-count data with $N_l = hT_1$ and $N_0 = hT_0$. The resulting odds-ratio statistics from the 2 × 2 program will, to within about 0.1%, equal the corresponding rate-ratio statistics obtained from a person-time analysis. For the data in Table 14–2, $h = 2$ will do. The theoretical basis for this trick is the fact that the hypergeometric probability (equation 14–8) approximates the binomial probability (equation 14–3) when one substitutes RR for OR and T_1 and T_0 for N_1 and N_0, provided T_1 and T_0 are numerically much greater than A_1 and A_0.

If the outcome is uncommon, a similar trick can be used to compare a single-group proportion to an expected E/N using the 2 × 2 table program. First, enter A and N as the "exposed" column of the table; second, find a number h such that $hE > 1{,}000A$ and $h(N - E) > 1{,}000(N - A)$; and third, enter hE and hN as the "unexposed" column of the table. The resulting P-values will be correct for comparing A with E, and if the risk parameter R is small (as in the Lancaster example), the resulting odds-ratio limits will be accurate risk-ratio limits.

CHAPTER 15

Introduction to Stratified Analysis

Sander Greenland and Kenneth J. Rothman

Heterogeneity versus Confounding 259
Assessment of Confounding 260
Selecting Confounders for Control 261
Statistical Biases in Variable Selection 263
Selecting Confounder Categories 263
Examining Stratum-Specific Estimates 264
Standardization 265
Standardized Differences 266
Standardized Ratios 267
Confidence Intervals 267
Standardized Case-Control Estimates 269
Estimation Assuming Homogenity Across Strata 270
Rationale 270
Estimates of a Homogenous Measure 271
Maximum-Likelihood Estimators 271
Unconditional versus Conditional Analysis 272
Mantel-Haenszel Estimation: Person-Time Data 273
Mantel-Haenszel Estimation: Pure Count Data 274
Small-Sample Methods 276
***P*-Values for the Stratified Null Hypothesis 277**
P-Values for Stratified Person-Time Data 277
P-Values for Stratified Pure Count Data 278
Testing Homogeneity 279
Case-Cohort Data 280
Two-Stage Data 281

Stratification is the mainstay of epidemiologic analyses. Even with studies that ultimately require more complicated analyses, stratification is an important intermediate step. It familiarizes the investigator with distributions of key variables and patterns in the data that are less transparent when using other methods.

Several analytic concerns motivate stratification. Most prominent are evaluation and control of confounding and certain forms of selection bias, such as the bias produced by case-control matching. Another is the need to evaluate effect-measure modification, or heterogeneity of measures, as we will refer to it here. Stratification on follow-up time is also used in cohort studies to address problems of loss to follow-up and competing risks. Finally, stratification on times between exposure and disease may be used to begin analyses of latency and induction.

This chapter presents elementary stratified-analysis methods for dealing with confounding and heterogeneity of a measure. We first review the distinctions between these concepts, which were introduced in Chapter 4. We then discuss the assessment of confounding via stratification. The remainder of the chapter gives methods for executing a sequence of steps that an investigator might reasonably take in analyzing stratified data:

1. Examine stratum-specific estimates.
2. If the examination indicates heterogeneity is present, report the stratum-specific estimates. In addition, one may use regression analysis to further study and describe the heterogeneity. One

may also estimate standardized measures to evaluate the overall effect of exposure on a population having a specific "standard" distribution of the stratifying factors.

3. If the data are reasonably consistent with homogeneity, then obtain a single summary estimate across strata that is statistically efficient (or nearly so); if this summary *and* its confidence limits are negligibly altered by ignoring a particular stratification variable, one may (but need not) simplify presentation by noting this fact and giving only results that ignore the variable.
4. Obtain a P-value for the null hypothesis of no stratum-specific association of exposure with disease.

Chapter 16 discusses how basic stratified methods can be applied to analysis of matched data, attributable fractions, induction time, and cohort studies in which losses or competing risks occur. The latter application is usually referred to as *survival analysis* (Cox and Oakes, 1984) or *failure-time analysis* (Kalbfleisch and Prentice, 2002). Chapter 17 extends basic stratified methods to exposures and diseases with multiple levels, and Chapter 18 shows how these methods can be used to construct Bayesian analyses.

Regardless of our best efforts, there is likely to be some residual confounding and other bias within our analysis strata. Thus, the quantities we are actually estimating with the methods in this chapter are stratum-specific and summary *associations* of exposure with disease, which may differ considerably from the stratum-specific and summary *effects* of exposure on disease. Chapter 19 introduces methods for estimating the latter effects, after allowing for residual bias.

HETEROGENEITY VERSUS CONFOUNDING

As discussed in Chapter 4, *effect-measure modification* refers to variation in the magnitude of a measure of exposure effect across levels of another variable. As discussed in Chapter 5, this concept is often confused with biologic interaction, but it is a distinct concept. The variable across which the effect-measure varies is called an *effect modifier*. Effect-measure modification is also known as heterogeneity of effect, nonuniformity of effect, and effect variation. *Absence* of effect-measure modification is also known as homogeneity of effect, uniformity of effect, and commonality of effect across strata. In most of this chapter we will use the more general phrase, *heterogeneity of a measure,* to refer to variation in any measure of effect or association across strata.

Effect-measure modification differs from confounding in several ways. The most central difference is that, whereas confounding is a bias that the investigator hopes to prevent or remove from the effect estimate, effect-measure modification is a property of the effect under study. Thus, effect-measure modification is a finding to be reported rather than a bias to be avoided. In epidemiologic analysis one tries to eliminate confounding, but one tries to detect and estimate effect-measure modification.

Confounding originates from the interrelation of the confounders, exposure, and disease in the source population from which the study subjects are selected. By changing the source population that will be studied, design strategies such as restriction can prevent a variable from becoming a confounder and thus eliminate the burden of adjusting for the variable. Unfortunately, the same design strategies may also impair the ability to study effect-measure modification by the variable. For example, restriction of subjects to a single level of a variable will prevent it from being a confounder in the study, but will also prevent one from examining whether the exposure effect varies across levels of the variable.

Epidemiologists commonly use at least two different types of measures, ratios and differences. As discussed in Chapter 4, the degree of heterogeneity of a measure depends on the measure one uses. In particular, ratios and differences can vary in opposite directions across strata. Consider stratifying by age. Suppose that the outcome measure varies both within age strata (with exposure) and across age strata (e.g., the exposure-specific rates or risks vary across strata). Then at least one of (and usually both) the difference and ratio must vary across the age strata (i.e., they cannot both be homogeneous over age). In contrast to this measure dependence, confounding can be defined without reference to a particular measure of effect (although its apparent severity may differ according to the chosen measure).

ASSESSMENT OF CONFOUNDING

As discussed in Chapters 4 and 9, confounding is a distortion in the estimated exposure effect that results from differences in risk between the exposed and unexposed that are not due to exposure. When estimating the effect of exposure on those exposed, two necessary criteria for a variable to explain such differences in risk (and hence explain some or all of the confounding) are

1. It must be a risk factor for the disease among the unexposed (although it need not be a cause of disease).
2. It must be associated with the exposure variable in the source population from which the subjects arise.

In order to avoid bias due to inappropriate control of variables, the following criterion is traditionally added to the list:

3. It must *not* be affected by exposure or disease (although it may affect exposure or disease).

The three criteria were discussed in Chapter 9 and are more critically evaluated in Greenland et al. (1999a), Pearl (2000), and Chapter 12. Adjustment for variables that violate any of these criteria is sometimes called *overadjustment* and is the analytic parallel of the design error of overmatching (Chapter 11).

If a variable violates any of these criteria, its use in conventional stratified analysis (as covered in this chapter) can reduce the efficiency (increase the variance) of the estimation process, without reducing bias. If the variable violates the third criterion, such use can even increase bias (Chapters 9 and 12). Among other things, the third criterion excludes variables that are intermediate on the causal pathway from exposure to disease. This exclusion can be relaxed under certain conditions, but in doing so special analytic techniques must be applied (Robins, 1989, 1997, 1999; Robins et al., 1992a, 2000; Chapter 21). In the remainder of this chapter we will assume that variables being considered for use in stratification have been prescreened to meet the above criteria, for example, using causal diagrams (Chapter 12).

The data in Table 15–1 are from a large multicenter clinical trial that examined the efficacy of tolbutamide in preventing the complications of diabetes. Despite the fact that subjects were randomly assigned to treatment groups, the subjects in the tolbutamide group tended to be older than the placebo group. A larger proportion of subjects who were assigned to receive tolbutamide were in the age category 55+ years. As a result, the crude risk difference falls outside the ranges of the stratum-specific measures: The stratum-specific risk differences are 0.034 and 0.036, whereas the crude is 0.045. The presence of confounding is not as obvious for the risk ratio: The stratum-specific risk ratios are 1.81 and 1.19, whereas the crude is 1.44.

TABLE 15–1

Age-Specific Comparison of Deaths from All Causes for Tolbutamide and Placebo Treatment Groups, University Group Diabetes Program (1970)

	Stratum 1, Age <55 y		Stratum 2, Age 55+ y		Total (Crude)	
	Tolbutamide	Placebo	Tolbutamide	Placebo	Tolbutamide	Placebo
Dead	8	5	22	16	30	21
Surviving	98	115	76	69	174	184
Total	106	120	98	85	204	205
Average risk	0.076	0.042	0.224	0.188	0.147	0.102
RD	0.034		0.036		0.045	
RR	1.81		1.19		1.44	

From University Group Diabetes Program. A study of the effects of hypoglycemic agents on vascular complications in patients with adult onset diabetes. *Diabetes.* 1970;19:747 830.

The variable "age 55+" in Table 15–1 satisfies the traditional criteria for a confounding factor. First, it is a risk factor for the outcome, death, and this relation holds within levels of the exposure, tolbutamide. In Table 15–1, the proportion dying of the unexposed (placebo) group was $5/120 = 0.042$ among those under age 55, but was $16/85 = 0.19$ (over four times higher) among those age 55+. Second, age is associated with exposure in the source population (which is the entire randomized cohort): the proportion under age 55 was $106/204 = 0.52$ among the tolbutamide-treated, but was $120/205 = 0.59$ among the placebo-treated. Finally, we know with certainty that being assigned to take tolbutamide does *not* alter a person's age.

It is possible to detect confounding by examining whether, in the source population, a potentially confounding factor is associated with exposure, and with disease conditional on exposure. Nonetheless, the magnitude of the confounding is difficult to assess in this way, because it is a function of both of these component associations. Further, when several factors are being examined, the component associations should ideally be examined conditional on the other confounding factors, thereby complicating the problem (Chapter 12).

More direct methods for confounder assessment compare the estimates of effect obtained with and without control of each potential confounder (assuming that the potential confounder is not affected by exposure). The magnitude of confounding is estimated by the degree of discrepancy between the two estimates. For example, the unadjusted risk difference in Table 15–1 is $0.147 - 0.102 = 0.045$. If we adjust for age confounding by standardizing (averaging) the age-specific risks in Table 15–1 using the total cohort as the standard (see Chapter 4), we obtain a standardized risk-difference of

$$\frac{226(0.076) + 183(0.224)}{226 + 183} - \frac{226(0.042) + 183(0.0188)}{226 + 183} = 0.142 - 0.107 = 0.035$$

Thus, the relatively crude age adjustments obtained by treating age as a dichotomy has reduced the estimated risk difference produced by tolbutamide from 4.5% to 3.5%. Similarly, the unadjusted risk ratio in Table 15–1 is $0.147/0.102 = 1.44$, whereas the age-standardized risk ratio is $0.142/0.107 = 1.33$.

SELECTING CONFOUNDERS FOR CONTROL

Having computed estimates both with and without adjustment for the age dichotomy (under age 55 vs. age 55+), the analyst must now decide whether it is important to adjust for this variable when presenting results. It may be important to do so simply because many readers would not trust results that are not adjusted for age, despite the fact that tolbutamide was randomized. This distrust stems from knowledge that age is strongly related to disease and mortality rates, and thus could confound any comparison if it were imbalanced between the tolbutamide and placebo groups (even if this imbalance were random).

In Table 15–1, $98/204 = 48\%$ of the tolbutamide group is age 55+, versus $85/205 = 41\%$ of the placebo group. Although this difference is small, it is still worrisome given the strong relation of age to mortality (about 3 times the mortality among those age 55+ vs. those under age 55 in each group). Note that a significance test of the null hypothesis of no age difference would be useless in evaluating this observed age difference: The study was randomized, and so we know that the null hypothesis is true and the difference is purely random. Whether random or not, the older age of the tolbutamide group should lead us to expect a higher mortality in that group, even if tolbutamide had no effect. Thus age is a confounder and adjustment may be warranted, even if the age difference is not "statistically significant" (Miettinen, 1976b; Rothman, 1977; Greenland and Neutra, 1980; Robins and Morgenstern, 1987).

Suppose, however, we wish to apply a quantitative criterion to see whether it is contextually important to control for age and other variables. To do so, the analyst must choose a cutoff for what constitutes an important change in the estimate. In Table 15–1 the unadjusted risk ratio is $(1.44 - 1.33)/1.33 = 8\%$ larger than the adjusted (although the effect component of the measure, RR – 1, is 33% greater). If only changes of greater than 10% in the RR are considered important, then this 8% change is not important; but if changes of greater than 5% are considered important, then this change is important and indicates that age should not be ignored in further analyses.

The exact cutoff for importance is somewhat arbitrary but is limited in range by the subject matter. For example, a 5% change in the risk ratio would be considered ignorable in most contexts, but rarely if ever would a 50% change. Similar observations apply when considering confidence limits. Changes might instead be expressed in units of standard deviation of the difference on the log(RR) scale (Greenland and Mickey, 1988), although then it may be more difficult to specify contextually meaningful changes. For example, a change of 1.96 standard deviations or more (corresponding to $P > 0.05$) is often contextually erroneous as a criterion, usually because it is too large. The most important point, however, is that one should report the criterion used to select confounders for adjustment so that the reader may critically evaluate the criterion.

Although many have argued against the practice (Miettinen, 1976b; Breslow and Day, 1980; Greenland and Neutra, 1980; Greenland, 1989a, b), one often sees statistical tests used to select confounders (as in stepwise regression), rather than the change-in-estimate criterion just discussed. Usually, the tests are of the confounder–disease association, although sometimes the difference between the unadjusted and adjusted estimates are tested (the latter approach is often termed *collapsibility testing*). It has been argued that these testing approaches will perform adequately if the tests have high enough power to detect any important confounder effects. One way to ensure adequate power is to raise the α level for rejecting the null (of no confounding) to 0.20 or even more, instead of using the traditional 0.05 level (Dales and Ury, 1978). Limited simulation studies indicate that this approach is reasonable, in that use of a 0.20 or higher α level instead of a 0.05 level for confounder selection can make the difference between acceptable and poor performance of statistical testing for confounder selection (Mickey and Greenland, 1989; Maldonado and Greenland, 1993a).

Several important subtleties must be considered when more than one potential confounder must be examined. First, it can make a big difference in the observed change in estimate whether one evaluates the change with or without adjustment for other confounders. For example, suppose that we have to consider adjustment for age and sex. To evaluate age, we could compare the estimates without and with age adjustment, ignoring sex in both instances. Or we could compare the estimate with age and sex adjustment to that with only sex adjustment. In other words, we could evaluate age confounding without or with background adjustment for sex. Furthermore, we could evaluate sex confounding with or without background adjustment for age. Our decision about importance could be strongly influenced by the strategy we choose.

To cope with this complexity, several authors have suggested the following "backward deletion" strategy (Miettinen, 1976b; Kleinbaum et al., 1984): First, one adjusts for all the potential confounders one can. Then, if one would like to use fewer confounders in further analyses, one deletes the confounders from adjustment one by one in a stepwise fashion, at each step deleting that confounder that makes the smallest change in the exposure effect estimate upon deletion. One stops deleting confounders when the *total* change in the estimate and confidence limits accrued from the start of the process (with all confounders controlled) would exceed the chosen limit of importance. One often sees analogous stepwise confounder-selection strategies based on testing the confounder coefficients and deleting in sequence the least statistically significant coefficient; again, such strategies can produce extremely confounded results unless the α levels for deletion and retention are set much higher than 0.05 (Dales and Ury, 1978; Maldonado and Greenland, 1993a).

Sometimes not a single confounder can be deleted without producing important changes, but more often at least a few will appear to be ignorable if others are controlled. Sometimes, however, it is impossible to control all the confounders (at least by stratification), because the data become too thinly spread across strata to yield any estimate at all (this occurs when no stratum contains both a case and a noncase, as well as in other situations). When this problem occurs, the pure "backwards deletion" strategy just described cannot be implemented. One approach proposed for this situation is to use a "forward selection" strategy, in which one starts with the exposure-effect estimate from the simplest acceptable stratification (e.g., one involving only age and sex), then stratifies on the confounder that makes the most difference in the estimate, then adds confounders one by one to the stratification, at each step adding the confounder that makes the most difference among those not yet added. The process stops when addition of variables ceases to make an "important" difference.

Certain methods such as hierarchical and exposure-probability regression can handle far more confounders than traditional stratification and regression methods. Use of these methods can avoid the need for selection among variables identified as potential confounders. These methods are discussed in Chapter 21.

STATISTICAL BIASES IN VARIABLE SELECTION

If the data become very thin when all or most confounders are used for stratification or regression, all confounder-selection strategies based on approximate statistics can suffer from certain statistical artefacts that lead to very biased final results. No conventional approach to confounding (based on change-in-estimate or more traditional significance testing) can wholly address this problem, and the artefacts can appear even when only a few confounders are involved (Robins and Greenland, 1986; Greenland et al., 2000). Although hierarchical and exposure-probability modeling can cope with these situations, a more transparent stratified analysis is usually a desirable preliminary to such techniques, and may often suffice. For this reason, epidemiologists often resort to some sort of forward selection strategy when data are sparse.

There is a hallmark symptom of the bias that arises when stratification has exceeded the limits of the data: The estimates of exposure–disease association get further and further from the null as more variables are added to the stratification or regression model. For example, one might observe only estimates of modest size as one moves from adjustment for the strongest confounder alone to adjustment for the two or three strongest confounders. Then, with further adjustment, the estimate becomes very large (e.g., odds ratios above 5 or under 0.20) as more confounders are controlled. This inflation is often interpreted as evidence of confounding, but in our experience it more often reflects bias due to applying large-sample methods to excessively sparse data.

Another problem with all variable-selection approaches, whether based on change-in-estimate or statistical testing, is their potential to distort P-values and confidence intervals away from their nominal behavior. For example, conventional 95% confidence intervals computed after using the data to select variables can have true coverage much less than 95% because the computation of such intervals assumes that no selection of variables has been done (Greenland, 1989a, 1993a; Hurvich and Tsai, 1990). This distortion arises because the intervals produced after selection do not reflect the uncertainty about confounder effects and thus are too narrow. The limited studies performed thus far suggest that the distortion produced by typical confounder-selection strategies need not be large in practice if very high α levels (0.20 or more) are used for selection (Mickey and Greenland, 1989; Maldonado and Greenland, 1993b). The alternative is to use methods that can operate with a large number of confounders and so require no selection, such as hierarchical or shrinkage regression (Greenland, 2008; Chapter 21).

One way to reduce distortion due to confounder selection is to insist that the confidence limits do not change to an important degree if a confounder is to be deleted from control. If one uses confidence limits rather than the point estimate to monitor the change produced by adding or deleting control of a confounder, one can use exact confidence limits rather than the usual large-sample approximate limits produced by Mantel-Haenszel or maximum-likelihood methods. With exact limits, the sparse-data bias discussed earlier will not occur. Unfortunately, exact intervals can become excessively wide if they are computed from traditional exact P-values, which is the default method in most software; mid-P methods do not suffer from this problem (see Chapter 13).

Selection of confounders can lead to complex problems, especially if there are many confounders from which to choose. Strategies based on examining changes in the exact confidence limits seem to be the best that can be carried out with standard software, although if enough data are available one may instead use approximate limits to monitor the changes. Most important, if selection is done, one should report the strategy used to select potential confounders for control in the methods section of the research report. In addition, one may have to include certain potential confounders on subject-matter grounds, even if they do not meet the quantitative criteria for inclusion. For example, a study of lung cancer might be well advised to adjust for smoking whenever possible, as well as age and sex, because of the known strong relations of these variables to lung cancer rates.

SELECTING CONFOUNDER CATEGORIES

An issue that is closely related to selection of confounders is selection of confounder categories. Some aspects of this issue are discussed in Chapter 13. In particular, we want to choose categories such that no important confounding by the confounder can occur within the categories. In the tolbutamide example, one might well question whether the age dichotomy (under age 55 vs. age 55+) is adequate, for, within the broad category of "age 55+," age has a profound association with death risk.

To address such concerns, one can examine whether use of a finer categorization (such as under age 55, age 55 to 64, age 65 to 74, age 75+) appreciably alters the point and interval estimates. In doing so, all the issues raised earlier should be considered, including problems with the criteria and statistics used to determine "appreciably." A strategy based on examining exact limits seems best, given current software; approximate limits can be used instead if the sample size is adequate, as in the tolbutamide example. As always, we caution that category boundaries are best chosen to ensure that risk will not change profoundly within categories, and that percentile categories can do poorly in this regard if the variable is a strong confounder and is unevenly distributed across its range, e.g., if it is highly skewed (see Chapter 13).

EXAMINING STRATUM-SPECIFIC ESTIMATES

In its simplest form, stratified analysis involves computing a separate estimate from each stratum, so that the single crude estimate is replaced with a set of estimates, one per stratum. In most stratified analyses there is some variation in the estimates across the strata. One must then determine (a) whether the variation in the stratum-specific estimates is of any scientific or public health importance and (b) whether the variation is compatible with random statistical fluctuation. The answers to these questions determine what analytic methods are used to present the results of the stratified analysis.

Consider the coronary death-rate ratio for smokers relative to nonsmokers in the data in Table 15–2. The crude mortality-rate ratio is 1.7, which may be confounded by age. Age confounding is much reduced within the 10-year age categories by which the data have been stratified. In addition to removing most of the age confounding, stratification has revealed that the rate-ratio estimates decline with age (although the risk differences increase until the oldest category). One often sees such a decline in ratio estimates across categories of a variable as the risk of disease among the unexposed increases, an example of what is sometimes called modification by baseline risk. This pattern of variation in the estimates is a key result of the analysis.

This example illustrates the importance of examining stratum-specific estimates whenever it is feasible to do so. It is not always feasible to do so by simple stratification, however. Some variables have too many categories to examine each separately. For example, studies may be conducted with potential confounding by family or neighborhood, for which there are too few subjects to produce stable estimates from each stratum. Instead, one can only treat such variables as confounders when

TABLE 15–2

Age-Specific Coronary Disease Deaths, Person-Years Observed, and Coronary Death Rates among British Male Doctors by Cigarette Smoking

	Cigarette Smokers			Nonsmokers			
Age (y)	Deaths	Years	Rate[a]	Deaths	Years	Rate[a]	Rate Ratio
35–44	32	52,407	6.1	2	18,790	1.1	5.7
45–54	104	43,248	24.0	12	10,673	11.2	2.1
55–64	206	28,612	72.0	28	5,710	49.0	1.5
65–74	186	12,663	146.9	28	2,585	108.3	1.4
75–84	102	5,317	191.8	31	1,462	212.0	0.9
Total	630	142,247	—	101	39,220	—	—

[a] Deaths per 10,000 person-years.
From Doll R, Hill AB. Mortality of British doctors in relation to smoking; observations on coronary thrombosis. In: Haenszel W, ed. *Epidemiological approaches to the study of cancer and other chronic diseases. Monogr Natl Cancer Inst.* 1966;19:205–268.

analyzing heterogeneity across other variables. For example, if neighborhood is a confounder, then to examine heterogeneity of a risk ratio across age, one will have to create and compare neighborhood-adjusted estimates for each age stratum.

When there are adequate numbers to examine stratum-specific estimates, however, it may be desirable to report findings separately for each stratum. These stratum-specific estimates may themselves be adjusted for other variables. For example, we might infer that the rate ratio differs for males and females and so report sex-specific estimates, each adjusted for age and perhaps other confounding variables.

In addition to the stratum-specific presentation of results, the investigator might choose to fit a regression model to the pattern of estimates and use the model to describe heterogeneity. A regression model, for example, could be used to model the variation in the stratum-specific rate ratios. We discuss such models in Chapter 20. Regression methods, however, are not as easily understood as stratum-specific results. Furthermore, a regression model can summarize a set of stratum-specific estimates parsimoniously only if each stratum can be assigned a meaningful numeric value. For example, a model for the variation of the risk difference across age strata can be greatly simplified by making use of the natural ordering of age; the same simplification is not available when examining variation across strata of religion.

STANDARDIZATION

As discussed in Chapters 3 and 4, epidemiologic measures can be summarized across strata by standardization. Standardization involves taking weighted averages of the stratum-specific outcome measure (rates, risks, prevalences, or means). Summary ratios and differences can then be obtained as the ratios and differences of the standardized incidences or prevalences. A *standard* is a set of weights that is used in taking the weighted average. For example, if the only stratification variable is age, a standard might be the amount of person-time or number of persons in a standard population that fall into each of the age categories.

If the stratum-specific incidences of a population are standardized to that population's distribution, then the standardized incidence will be equal to the crude incidence for that population. Thus, a crude incidence is an average weighted by the distribution of the study population itself. A standardized incidence can be interpreted as the crude incidence in a population that has the same stratum-specific incidences as those of the observed population, but in which the distribution of the stratification variables is given by the standard.

The formula we will use for a standardized rate is

$$I_w = \frac{\sum_i w_i I_i}{\sum_i w_i} \qquad [15\text{–}1]$$

where w_i is the weight for stratum i and I_i is the rate in stratum i; w_i is usually the amount of person-time observed in stratum i of a standard population. Similarly, the standardized risk formula we will use is

$$R_w = \frac{\sum_i w_i R_i}{\sum_i w_i}, \qquad [15\text{–}2]$$

where w_i is the weight for stratum i and R_i is the risk in stratum i; w_i is usually the number of persons in stratum i of a standard population. Standardized prevalences or standardized means can be constructed using the same formulas, substituting stratum-specific prevalences or means for the stratum-specific rates or risks.

As mentioned in Chapter 4, if exposure affects the distribution used to construct the standardization weights, comparisons of standardized incidences will not properly reflect the net exposure effect on the population incidence if the same standard weights are used to construct each standardized incidence. This problem will occur, for example, when exposure alters the person-time distribution of the population, and the weights are person-times (Greenland, 1996a). If exposure has an effect, it will alter not only the rates but also the distribution of person-time over the follow-up period.

If one wishes to estimate the total effect of exposure when exposure affects the weighting distribution, it will be necessary to use weights that change with exposure in a manner that reflects the exposure effect. Inverse-probability-of-exposure weighting (Chapter 21) provides examples of such exposure-dependent weighting. For the present chapter we will assume that exposure has negligible effects on the weights. This assumption would be satisfied in risk standardization when the standard is the baseline (starting) distribution of confounders in a cohort study, and exposure occurs only at baseline. An example of risk estimation in which this assumption is violated will be given in the attributable-fraction discussion in the next chapter.

STANDARDIZED DIFFERENCES

If I_{1i} is the rate among the exposed in stratum i and I_{0i} is the rate among the unexposed in stratum i, then the standardized rate difference is $ID_w = I_{1w} - I_{0w}$, the difference between the standardized rates for exposed and unexposed. The following algebra shows that a standardized rate difference is the weighted average of the stratum-specific rate differences $ID_i = I_{1i} - I_{0i}$ using the same standard weights:

$$ID_w = \frac{\sum_i w_i I_{1i}}{\sum_i w_i} - \frac{\sum_i w_i I_{0i}}{\sum_i w_i} = \frac{\sum_i w_i (I_{1i} - I_{0i})}{\sum_i w_i} = \frac{\sum_i w_i ID_i}{\sum_i w_i} \qquad [15\text{–}3]$$

Similarly, the standardized risk difference $RD_w = R_{1w} - R_{0w}$ is the weighted average of the stratum-specific risk differences $RD_i = R_{1i} - R_{0i}$ based on the standard weights:

$$RD_w = \frac{\sum_i w_i RD_i}{\sum_i w_i} \qquad [15\text{–}4]$$

The standard should be chosen to facilitate interpretation of the results. For some applications, there may be a conventional standard, such as the world age–sex distribution in a given year, or a national age–sex distribution from a specific census, that facilitates comparisons with other data. For most analyses, however, the standard should be derived from the specific population for which one wants to estimate exposure effect.

From data in Table 15–1, suppose that we wish to estimate what the effect of tolbutamide would have been if every patient in the study (not just those randomized to tolbutamide) had received tolbutamide. To adjust for age, we should use the distribution of the entire cohort as the standard, which corresponds to weights of $106 + 120 = 226$ for the "under age 55" stratum and $98 + 85 = 183$ for the "age 55+" stratum. These yield standardized risk estimates of

$$\hat{R}_{0w} = \frac{226(5/120) + 183(16/85)}{226 + 183} = 0.107$$

$$\hat{R}_{1w} = \frac{226(8/106) + 183(22/98)}{226 + 183} = 0.142$$

which yield a standardized risk difference estimate of $0.142 - 0.107 = 0.035$.

For the British doctors' data in Table 15–2, using the age distribution of smoking subjects as the standard yields an estimated standardized coronary death rate for smoking doctors ($\hat{I}_{1w}$) that is the same as the crude rate for this group, 630/142,247 years = 44.3 cases per 10^4 person-years. The corresponding standardized rate for the nonsmoking British doctors is estimated by taking a weighted average of the age-specific rates for the nonsmoking doctors using the number of person-years in each age category of the smoking doctors as the weights:

$$\hat{I}_{0w} = \frac{52{,}407\left(\dfrac{2}{18{,}790}\right) + \cdots + 5{,}317\left(\dfrac{31}{1{,}462}\right)}{52{,}407 + \cdots + 5{,}317}$$

$$= 444.41/142{,}247 \text{ years} = 31.2 \text{ cases per } 10^4 \text{ person-years}$$

The estimated standardized rate difference is the difference between these two standardized rate estimates, which is about 13 cases per 10^4 person-years. This value can also be obtained by taking a weighted average of the stratum-specific rate differences, weighting by the number of person-years among smoking doctors in each age category.

STANDARDIZED RATIOS

A standardized risk ratio is the ratio of two standardized risks,

$$RR_w = \frac{\sum_i w_i R_{1i} \Big/ \sum_i w_i}{\sum_i w_i R_{0i} \Big/ \sum_i w_i} = \frac{\sum_i w_i R_{1i}}{\sum_i w_i R_{0i}} = \frac{\sum_i w_i R_{0i} RR_i}{\sum_i w_i R_{0i}} \qquad [15\text{–}5]$$

where RR_i is the stratum-specific risk ratio, R_{1i}/R_{0i}. Similarly, a standardized rate ratio is the ratio of two standardized rates,

$$IR_w = \frac{\sum_i w_i I_{1i} \Big/ \sum_i w_i}{\sum_i w_i I_{0i} \Big/ \sum_i w_i} = \frac{\sum_i w_i I_{1i}}{\sum_i w_i I_{0i}} = \frac{\sum_i w_i I_{0i} IR_i}{\sum_i w_i I_{0i}} \qquad [15\text{–}6]$$

where IR_i is the stratum-specific rate ratio, I_{1i}/I_{0i}. Note that both RR_w and IR_w are weighted averages of stratum-specific ratios, but the weights for this averaging are not the weights for standardization; they are instead the products of the weights for standardization and the risks or rates among the unexposed in each stratum.

We can estimate a standardized risk ratio from the tolbutamide data in Table 15–1 as $0.142/0.107 = 1.33$ when the total cohort is used as the standard. Similarly, we estimate a standardized rate ratio from the data in Table 15–2 by dividing the standardized rate estimate among the smokers by the standardized rate estimate among the nonsmokers. Using smokers as the standard, this gives $44.3/31.2 = 1.42$.

A standardized ratio that is standardized to the distribution of an exposed group (the group in the numerator of the standardized ratio) is traditionally referred to as a *standardized morbidity ratio* (SMR), or SMR estimate. These were introduced in Chapter 14 as observed/expected (A/E) case ratios. The estimate of 1.42 from Table 15–2 is another example. Note that a standardized ratio will not be an SMR if it does not use the exposed group as a standard. As explained in Chapter 4, if the stratum-specific ratios are heterogeneous and there is confounding across the strata, a comparison of two or more SMR estimates will remain confounded by the stratifying factors, because the SMRs are standardized to different exposure groups.

CONFIDENCE INTERVALS

Confidence intervals for standardized measures can be calculated from the stratified data and from the weights used for standardization. Suppose that A_i cases are observed out of T_i person-time units or N_i persons in stratum i. The variance for a standardized rate can then be estimated from

$$\widehat{\text{Var}}(\hat{I}_w) = \frac{\sum w_i^2 \,\widehat{\text{Var}}(\hat{I}_i)}{\left(\sum_i w_i\right)^2} \qquad [15\text{–}7]$$

$\widehat{\text{Var}}(\hat{I}_i)$, the estimated variance of the rate in each stratum i, depends on the probability model assumed for the number of cases A_i in each stratum. For person-time data and a Poisson model for the A_i,

$$\widehat{\text{Var}}(\hat{I}_i) = A_i/T_i^2 = \hat{I}_i/T_i \qquad [15\text{–}8]$$

For pure count data from a closed cohort and a binomial model for the A_i, we use formula 15–7 to obtain $\widehat{\text{Var}}(\hat{R}_w)$, but with

$$\widehat{\text{Var}}(\hat{R}_i) = \frac{A_i(N_i - A_i)}{N_i^2(N_i - 1)} = \frac{\hat{R}_i(1 - \hat{R}_i)}{N_i - 1} \qquad [15\text{–}9]$$

in place of $\widehat{\text{Var}}(\hat{I}_i)$. As noted in Chapter 14, the Poisson and binomial models assume no contagion or other sources of dependence among outcomes. Less restrictive models lead to more generally applicable variance formulas (Carriere and Roos, 1994; Stukel et al., 1994).

Suppose now that the data are divided into two exposure groups, distinguished by a subscript that is either 1 (for exposed) or 0 (for unexposed). Confidence intervals for a standardized rate difference and a standardized rate ratio can be calculated using the variance estimates

$$\widehat{\text{Var}}(\widehat{ID}_w) = \widehat{\text{Var}}(\hat{I}_{1w}) + \widehat{\text{Var}}(\hat{I}_{0w}) \qquad [15\text{–}10]$$

$$\widehat{\text{Var}}[\ln(\widehat{IR}_w)] = \widehat{\text{Var}}(\hat{I}_{1w})/\hat{I}_{1w}^2 + \widehat{\text{Var}}(\hat{I}_{0w})/\hat{I}_{0w}^2 \qquad [15\text{–}11]$$

Both these formulas assume that the standardized rate in the exposed varies independently of the standardized rate in the unexposed. Parallel formulas can be applied to estimate risk differences $\widehat{RD}_w$, risk ratios $\widehat{RR}_w$, and standard deviations of $\widehat{RD}_w$ and $\ln(\widehat{RR}_w)$ using $\hat{R}_{1w}$ and $\hat{R}_{0w}$ in place of $\hat{I}_{1w}$ and $\hat{I}_{0w}$. For setting confidence limits on the standardized risk difference, we recommend using the improved formula given in the preceding chapter (Zou and Donner, 2004).

For the data in Table 15–2, taking the person-years for smokers as the stratum-specific weights, we use formulas 15–7, 15–8, and 15–10 to obtain a variance estimate for $\widehat{ID}_w$. Intermediate calculations are given in Table 15–3. We get

$$\widehat{\text{Var}}(\hat{I}_{1w}) = \frac{630}{142{,}247^2} = \frac{3.114}{(10^4\ \text{y})^2}$$

$$\widehat{\text{Var}}(\hat{I}_{0w}) = \frac{1{,}997.56}{142{,}247^2} = \frac{9.872}{(10^4\ \text{y})^2}$$

$$\widehat{\text{Var}}(\widehat{ID}_w) = \frac{3.114}{(10^4\ \text{y})^2} = \frac{9.872}{(10^4\ \text{y})^2} + \frac{12.99}{(10^4\ \text{y})^2}$$

Taking the square root, we get a standard deviation (SD) of 3.60×10^4 years, which yields transformed 90% confidence limits for the standardized rate difference of 7.1 and 19.0 per 10^4 years.

TABLE 15–3

Intermediate Calculations for Estimating the Variance of Standardized Estimates from the Data in Table 15–2

Age (y)	w_i	$w_i \hat{I}_{1i}$	$w_i \hat{I}_{0i}$	$w_i^2 \text{Var}(\hat{I}_{1i})$	$w_i^2 \text{Var}(\hat{I}_{0i})$
35–44	52,407	32	5.58	32	15.56
45–54	43,248	104	48.63	104	197.03
55–64	28,612	206	140.30	206	703.04
65–74	12,663	186	137.16	186	671.91
75–84	5,317	102	112.74	102	410.02
Total	142,247	630	444.41	630	1,997.56

For the standardized rate ratio, using the smokers in Table 15–2 as the standard gives the SMR. From formula 15–11, the estimated variance of ln(SMR) is

$$\widehat{\text{Var}}[\ln(\widehat{\text{SMR}})] = \frac{3.114(10^4\text{ y})^2}{(44.29/10^4\text{ y})^2} + \frac{9.872(10^4\text{ y})^2}{(31.24/10^4\text{ y})^2}$$
$$= 0.00159 + 0.01012 = 0.0117$$

The estimated SD is therefore $(0.0117)^{1/2} = 0.1082$, and a 90% confidence interval for the SMR is

$$\exp[\ln(1.42) \pm 1.645(0.1082)] = 1.19, 1.70$$

STANDARDIZED CASE-CONTROL ESTIMATES

Without external information, case-control studies do not provide stratum-specific rate or rate-difference estimates, but can provide standardized rate-ratio estimates under density sampling schemes or a rare-disease assumption (Chapter 8). Use of external information to estimate other measures is discussed in Chapter 21. Let A_{1i} and A_{0i} be the numbers of exposed and unexposed cases and B_{1i} and B_{0i} be the numbers of exposed and unexposed controls in stratum i, and suppose the source population experiences T_{1i} and T_{0i} person-time units at risk during the study period. Recall from Chapter 8 that, in the absence of biases, B_{1i}/B_{0i} estimates the ratio of exposed to unexposed person-time in the source population, T_{1i}/T_{0i}. It follows that $B_{1i}(A_{0i}/B_{0i}) = E_{1i} = A_{0i}B_{1i}/B_{0i}$ estimates the number of exposed cases one should expect in stratum i of the study *if* the exposed population in that stratum experienced the unexposed rate and T_{1i} person-time units. Furthermore, $\widehat{\text{SMR}} = A_{1+}/E_{1+}$ is then an estimator of the SMR for case-control data, where $A_{1+} = \sum_i A_{1i}$ and $E_{1+} = \sum_i E_{1i}$ (Miettinen, 1972). Under the binomial model for case-control data, the logarithm of $\widehat{\text{SMR}}$ has a variance estimator

$$\widehat{\text{Var}}[\ln(\widehat{\text{SMR}})] = \frac{1}{A_{1+}} + \frac{\sum_i E_{1i}^2(1/A_{0i} + 1/B_{1i} + 1/B_{0i})}{E_{1+}^2} \qquad [15\text{–}12]$$

It is also possible to estimate a standardized rate ratio from case-control data using other standards (Miettinen, 1972). For example, in the absence of biases, $E_{0i} = A_{1i}B_{0i}/B_{1i}$ estimates the number of cases one should have expected among the unexposed in stratum i *if* they had experienced the exposed rate and T_{0i} person-time units; thus, an estimator of the standardized rate ratio using the unexposed population as the standard is $\widehat{\text{SRR}}_u = E_{0+}/A_{0+}$, where $A_{0+} = \sum_i A_{0i}$ and $E_{0+} = \sum_i E_{0i}$. The logarithm of $\widehat{\text{SRR}}_u$ has a variance estimator

$$\widehat{\text{Var}}[\ln(\widehat{\text{SRR}}_u)] = \frac{\sum_i E_{0i}^2(1/A_{1i} + 1/B_{1i} + 1/B_{0i})}{E_{0+}^2} + \frac{1}{A_{0+}} \qquad [15\text{–}13]$$

Similarly, an estimator of the standardized rate ratio using the total population as the standard is $\widehat{\text{SRR}}_t = (A_{1+} + E_{0+})/(E_{1+} + A_{0+})$. The logarithm of $\widehat{\text{SRR}}_t$ has a variance estimator

$$\widehat{\text{Var}}[\ln(\widehat{\text{SRR}}_t)] = [A_{1+} + \Sigma_i E_{0i}^2(1/A_{1i} + 1/B_{1i} + 1/B_{0i})]/(A_{1+} + E_{0+})^2$$
$$+ [\Sigma_i E_{1i}^2(1/A_{0i} + 1/B_{1i} + 1/B_{0i}) + A_{0+}]/(E_{1+} + A_{0+})^2 \qquad [15\text{–}14]$$

The standardized estimators presented above assume that the expected values of the stratum-specific numbers (A_{1+}, B_{1i}, A_{0i}, B_{0i}) are "large" (at least 5). If the data are sparse, as is often the case in matched case-control studies, one should instead use estimators based on homogeneity assumptions or regression models. Such estimators need not assume homogeneity over all stratification variables; for example, see Flanders and Rhodes (1987) and Greenland (1986b,1987b, 1991c).

ESTIMATION ASSUMING HOMOGENITY ACROSS STRATA

RATIONALE

Standardization summarizes measures across strata without assuming that the measures are homogenous across strata. Use of methods that do invoke a homogeneity assumption need not require that one actually believes that assumption. Use of the homogeneity assumption can instead be viewed as a decision to simplify analysis and reporting, based on the idea that such heterogeneity that is present cannot be accurately analyzed given the study's size. This rationale is reasonable as long as the homogeneity assumption is not clearly contradicted by the data or other evidence. The assumption should thus be viewed as a potentially useful approximation.

Given that one can never be sure of homogeneity, how should one interpret estimates based on such an assumption? When the ratios do not vary much across strata, the homogeneous risk and rate ratio estimates discussed here appear to provide good estimates of risk and rate ratios standardized using the total population (exposed plus unexposed) as the standard (Greenland and Maldonado, 1994). This is also true of homogeneous odds-ratio estimators derived from unmatched case-control studies, provided the stratum-specific odds ratios approximate the stratum-specific risk or rate ratios. These approximations provide a straightforward interpretation of homogeneous ratio estimators and so justify their use even when some ratio heterogeneity is present (as is always the case). Nonetheless, they do not provide a rationale for failing to search for heterogeneity and report it when it appears likely to be of important magnitude.

There is no rigid criterion for deciding whether the homogeneity assumption can be used (although statistical tests of homogeneity are sometimes used to force this decision). The first step should be to inspect the stratum-specific estimates. Although one should expect some random variation in the stratum-specific estimates even when the underlying parameter is homogeneous, excessive variation (relative to that expected by chance) or obvious nonrandom patterns of variation may be evident. The investigator's judgment about heterogeneity should not be limited to the appearance of the data under analysis; if it is available, knowledge from previous studies or more general biologic insight should be integrated into the evaluation process.

Typically, outside knowledge is scant, and investigators desire a more formal statistical evaluation of the extent to which variation in the stratum-specific estimates is consistent with purely random behavior. Toward this end, a variety of statistical tests can be applied. Part of the variety derives from the fact that ratio and difference measures require separate evaluations, because homogeneity of the ratio measure usually implies heterogeneity of the difference measure and vice versa. In Chapter 10 we criticized the use of statistical tests, and especially criticized the concept of "statistical significance," which artificially forces a continuous measure (the P-value) into a dichotomy. The use of statistical tests is a bit more defensible, however, when an immediate decision rests on the outcome of a single statistical evaluation. Such may be the case if an investigator is attempting to decide whether the extent of variation in a set of stratum-specific estimates is consistent with probable random departures from a homogeneous measure, so that homogeneity is tenable in light of the data.

Statistical tests of homogeneity (i.e., tests of the hypothesis that the measure has a "common" or constant value across the strata) are based on comparisons of stratum-specific estimates against a summary estimate that assumes homogeneity, or of observed cell counts against cell counts expected under the homogeneity hypothesis. Thus, to test homogeneity we first conduct an analysis in which we assume homogeneity and derive an estimate of the homogeneous measure. The next section discusses analysis methods based on the homogeneity assumption. We will then present some basic methods for testing this assumption.

One should bear in mind that tests of the homogeneity assumption usually have very low power (Greenland, 1983). Studies are often designed to have "sufficient" power (e.g., 80%) to detect a crude association of a fixed plausible size. Tests of homogeneity require that the data be divided into strata, and that the stratum-specific estimates—each with its own variance estimate—are compared with one another. The power of tests of homogeneity is therefore reduced in two ways relative to the crude power: The study sample is divided into strata, which increases the total variance; and every stratum (some of much smaller size than the total) must be used to estimate its own measure for comparison to other strata.

ESTIMATES OF A HOMOGENOUS MEASURE

In Table 15–1, the point estimates of the risk difference were 0.034 and 0.036 in the two age strata, so that any estimate summarizing these differences should be between 0.034 and 0.036. Even if the true measure is identical across strata, however, it is reasonable to expect that estimates of the measure will vary across strata because of random error. Thus, even if one assumes homogeneity across strata, one must derive an overall estimate of association or effect from stratified data. A summary estimate derived under the homogeneity assumption is sometimes called a "pooled estimate."

Pooled estimates are usually weighted averages of stratum-specific estimates. Taking a weighted average of stratum-specific estimates describes standardization as well as pooling. The difference is that with standardization, the weights are derived from a standard distribution that may be external to the data, are applied to the estimated occurrence measures (or case-control ratios) rather than to association or effect measures, and the entire process does not assume homogeneity of the measure across strata. With pooling, the weights are applied to the estimated association or effect measure, are determined solely by the data and the homogeneity assumption, and are chosen to reduce the random variability of the summary estimate. In particular, if the measure is homogeneous across strata, each stratum provides an estimate of the same quantity, and the only question is then how to average these stratum-specific estimates in a manner to minimize variance.

A standardized estimate might assign relatively large weight to strata with little data, and little weight to strata with ample data. In contrast, pooling is designed to assign weights that reflect the amount of information in each stratum. If the measure is homogeneous, one way to minimize the variance of the overall weighted average without introducing bias is to assign weights to the stratum-specific values that are inversely proportional to the estimated variance of each stratum-specific estimate. Direct pooling, or precision weighting, involves first estimating the stratum-specific variances, then inverting these to get the weights, and finally averaging the stratum-specific estimates using these weights; this is sometimes known as the Woolf method or weighted least squares (Breslow and Day, 1980). To be valid, direct pooling requires large numbers within each cell in each stratum. Because many stratified analyses have sparse data, directly weighted approaches are not as broadly applicable as the alternatives we will discuss below (Breslow, 1981).

One alternative is to find the value of the measure that maximizes the probability of the data under the homogeneity assumption. This maximum-likelihood (ML) method (Chapter 13) produces the pooled estimate without explicitly determining stratum-specific weights; for example, see Breslow and Day (1980), Jewell (2004), or Newman (2001). ML estimates have certain desirable statistical properties (such as minimum large-sample variance among approximately unbiased estimators), and consequently ML methods are often considered the optimal large-sample estimating methods. Nonetheless, there are other relevant statistical criteria (such as mean-squared error) under which ML estimation is inferior to certain methods, such as penalized-likelihood estimation (Chapter 21).

Another approach to estimating a homogeneous measure is the Mantel-Haenszel method. Mantel-Haenszel estimators are easy to calculate, and in many applications are nearly as accurate as ML estimators. We will restrict our attention to maximum-likelihood and Mantel-Haenszel estimators for homogeneous measures, providing only citations for small-sample methods. Because likelihood computations can be complex and are invariably done by computers, we will omit formulas for ML estimates and instead focus on Mantel-Haenszel formulas. For a more detailed introduction to likelihood methods in epidemiologic analysis, see Clayton and Hills (1993), Jewell (2004), or Newman (2001).

MAXIMUM-LIKELIHOOD ESTIMATORS

Maximum-likelihood estimation of a homogeneous measure involves taking the data probabilities for each stratum and multiplying them together to produce a total data probability. For person-time data, the latter probability is a function of the stratum-specific rates in the exposed I_{1i}, and the unexposed I_{0i}. If no constraint is imposed on these rates, the maximum-likelihood estimates (MLEs) of the stratum-specific rates will simply be the observed rates,

$$\hat{I}_{1i} = A_{1i}/T_{1i} \quad \text{and} \quad \hat{I}_{0i} = A_{0i}/T_{0i}$$

If, however, we assume that one of the association measures is homogeneous across the strata, the MLEs of the stratum-specific rates and this homogeneous measure requires iterative computation, either with a spreadsheet or using software written for this purpose. Software is available when a homogeneous rate ratio is assumed, that is, when we assume that

$$I_{1i}/I_{0i} = IR$$

where *IR* is constant across strata. Most such software assumes a Poisson probability model for the stratum-specific counts A_{1i} and A_{0i} (Chapter 14), and that the counts are independent of one another within and across strata. Neither assumption is realistic when the disease under study is contagious, but they are reasonable for most other diseases.

Less frequently, a homogeneous rate difference may be assumed, that is,

$$I_{1i} - I_{0i} = ID$$

Finding the MLEs under this assumption usually requires converting the assumption into a regression model and using a maximum-likelihood Poisson regression program (Chapter 21).

For closed-cohort data with count denominators N_{1i} and N_{0i} in each stratum, the maximum-likelihood estimates of the stratum-specific average risks are the observed incidence proportions

$$\hat{R}_{1i} = A_{1i}/N_{1i} \quad \text{and} \quad \hat{R}_{0i} = A_{0i}/N_{0i}$$

if no constraint is imposed. If, however, we constrain either the risk ratio, odds ratio or risk difference measure to be homogeneous across the strata, then the MLEs of the stratum-specific risks and the ratio or difference measure must be found by iterative computation. Much software is available for estimating a homogeneous odds ratio, that is, assuming that the stratum-specific odds ratios

$$\frac{R_{1i}/(1 - R_{1i})}{R_{0i}/(1 - R_{0i})}$$

are the same across strata. Most such software assumes a binomial probability model for the counts A_{1i} and A_{0i} (Chapter 14), and that these counts are independent within and across strata. Assuming either a homogeneous risk difference $R_{1i} - R_{0i} = RD$ or homogeneous risk ratio $R_{1i}/R_{0i} = RR$ usually requires use of a maximum-likelihood binomial regression program (Chapter 21).

UNCONDITIONAL VERSUS CONDITIONAL ANALYSIS

Chapter 14 introduced two different probability models used for analyzing rate ratios: a two-Poisson model and a single-binomial model that was based on taking the observed number of cases (M_1) as given, or "fixed." It also introduced two different models for analysis of odds ratios in 2 × 2 tables: a two-binomial model and a single-hypergeometric model that was based on taking all the table margins (M_1, M_0, N_1, N_0) as fixed. The fixed-margin models are called conditional models, because they condition all data probabilities on the observed margins.

The hypergeometric likelihood statistics are more often called conditional-likelihood statistics, and the MLE of the common odds ratio derived from the hypergeometric model is called the conditional maximum-likelihood estimate (CMLE). The binomial-likelihood statistics are often called unconditional likelihood statistics, and the MLE of the common odds ratio derived from the two-binomial model is often called the unconditional maximum-likelihood estimate (UMLE). Usually, if a discussion does not specify which MLE is being considered, it is the unconditional estimate that is under discussion.

Stratified analysis of rate and odds ratios may also be conducted with or without conditioning on the stratum margins. For rate ratios, the difference is essentially only computational. For odds ratios, however, the choice of whether to model each stratum with two binomials or a single hypergeometric probability can have a profound effect on the resulting common odds-ratio analysis. Only conditional-likelihood methods (based on the hypergeometric model, conditioning on all stratum margins M_{1i}, M_{0i}, N_{0i}) and Mantel-Haenszel methods remain approximately valid in sparse data, that is, data in which the number of subjects per stratum is small. As discussed below, however, they require that the total number of subjects contributing to the estimates at each exposure–disease combination be adequate (Mantel and Fleiss, 1980; Greenland et al., 2000a; Greenland, 2000e).

Unconditional likelihood methods (based on the two-binomial model) additionally require that each binomial denominator in each stratum (N_{1i} and N_{0i} in a cohort study, M_{1i} and M_{0i} in a case-control study) be "large," meaning about 10 or more for odds-ratio analysis (Pike et al., 1980).

Only exact methods have no sample-size requirement. Because the unconditional odds-ratio MLE additionally requires large numbers *within* strata whereas the conditional MLE does not, one may well ask why the unconditional MLE is used at all. There are at least two reasons: First, the conditional MLE is computationally much more demanding, and when the numbers within strata are large ($N_{1i} > 10$ and $N_{0i} > 10$), the two estimators will usually be almost equal and so there will be no need to use the conditional MLE. Second, only the unconditional method is theoretically justifiable for estimation of quantities other than rate ratios and odds ratios, such as risks, risk differences, and risk ratios.

MANTEL-HAENSZEL ESTIMATION: PERSON-TIME DATA

It is possible to construct Mantel-Haenszel estimators of homogeneous rate differences, but such estimators can have much higher variances than the corresponding maximum-likelihood estimator (Greenland and Robins, 1985b). We therefore recommend maximum likelihood for estimating a homogeneous rate difference, subject to the caution that there be at least 10 cases per stratum. If, however, there are fewer than 10 cases per stratum, the maximum-likelihood rate difference can become excessively biased, whereas the Mantel-Haenszel rate difference remains unbiased. The Mantel-Haenszel rate difference is essentially a standardized rate difference with standard weights given by

$$w_{MHi} = T_{1i}T_{0i}/T_{+i}$$

where $T_{+i} = T_{1i} + T_{0i}$. This weighting yields

$$\widehat{ID}_{MH} = \frac{\sum_i w_{MHi}(\hat{I}_{1i} - \hat{I}_{0i})}{\sum_i w_{MHi}} = \frac{\sum_i (A_{1i}T_{0i} - A_{0i}T_{1i})/T_{+i}}{\sum_i T_{1i}T_{0i}/T_{+i}} \quad [15\text{–}15]$$

where $\hat{I}_{1i} = A_{1i}/T_{1i}$ and $\hat{I}_{0i} = A_{0i}/T_{0i}$ are the stratum-specific rate estimates. A variance estimator for $\widehat{ID}_{MH}$ that is appropriate even if the data are sparse is

$$\widehat{\text{Var}}(\widehat{ID}_{MH}) = \frac{\sum_i w_{MHi}^2(\hat{I}_{1i}/T_{1i} + \hat{I}_{0i}/T_{0i})}{\left(\sum_i w_{MHi}\right)^2} \quad [15\text{–}16]$$

(Greenland and Robins, 1985b). The variance of $\widehat{ID}_{MH}$ can be considerably reduced by using $T_{1i}T_{0i}/M_{1i}$ instead of w_{MHi} as the weight, but this change renders the estimator invalid for sparse data.

Unlike the Mantel-Haenszel rate difference, in most situations the Mantel-Haenszel rate ratio based on the weights w_{MHi} has a variance equal to or not much larger than that of the MLE (Greenland and Robins, 1985b; Walker, 1985). It reduces to an exceptionally simple form:

$$\widehat{IR}_{MH} = \frac{\sum_i w_{MHi}\hat{I}_{1i}}{\sum_i w_{MHi}\hat{I}_{0i}} = \frac{\sum_i A_{1i}T_{0i}/T_{+i}}{\sum_i A_{0i}T_{1i}/T_{+i}} \quad [15\text{–}17]$$

(Nurminen, 1981; Rothman and Boice, 1982). A variance estimator for the logarithm of the Mantel-Haenszel rate ratio is

$$\widehat{\text{Var}}[\ln(\widehat{IR}_{MH})] = \frac{\sum_i M_{1i}T_{1i}T_{0i}/T_{+i}^2}{\left(\sum_i A_{1i}T_{0i}/T_{+i}\right)\left(\sum_i A_{0i}T_{1i}/T_{+i}\right)} \quad [15\text{–}18]$$

TABLE 15–4

Intermediate Calculations for Mantel-Haenszel Analysis of the Smoking/Coronary Mortality Data in Table 15–2

Age (y)	$T_{1i}T_{0i}/T_{+i}$	$A_{1i}T_{0i}/T_{+i}$	$A_{0i}T_{1i}/T_{+i}$	$M_{1i}T_{1i}/T_{+i}$	$M_{1i}T_{1i}T_{0i}/T_{+i}^2$
35–44	13,831	8.45	1.47	25.05	6.60
45–54	8,560	20.59	9.62	93.04	18.42
55–64	4,760	34.27	23.34	195.07	32.45
65–74	2,147	31.53	23.25	177.72	30.13
75–84	1,147	22.00	24.31	104.32	22.50
Total	30,445	116.8	82.0	595.2	110.1

(Greenland and Robins, 1985b). Both these rate-ratio formulas remain valid even if the data are sparse. Nonetheless, like the MLEs, both are "large-sample" formulas, in that their validity requires adequate numbers of subjects observed at each exposure–disease combination. As a rough guide, one should use exact limits if either of the following expressions is less than 5:

$$\underline{A} = \sum_i \frac{M_{1i}\underline{IR} \cdot T_{1i}}{\underline{IR} \cdot T_{1i} + T_{0i}}, \quad \overline{A} = \sum_i \frac{M_{1i}T_{0i}}{\overline{IR} \cdot T_{1i} + T_{0i}}$$

where $\underline{IR}$, $\overline{IR}$ are the lower and upper confidence limits derived from the above formulas.

Table 15–4 gives the intermediate calculations for Mantel-Haenszel analysis of the coronary mortality data in Table 15–2. In units of deaths per 10^4 years,

$$\widehat{ID}_{\text{MH}} = \frac{13{,}831(6.1 - 1.1) + \cdots + 1{,}147(191.8 - 212.0)}{30{,}445^2} = 11.44$$

$$\widehat{\text{Var}}(\widehat{ID}_{\text{MH}}) = \frac{13{,}831^2(6.1/52{,}407 + 1.1/18{,}790) + \ldots}{30{,}445^2} = 9.57$$

which yield 90% limits for a common rate difference of $11.44 \pm 1.645(9.57)^{1/2} = 6.35, 16.53$ per 10^4 person-years.

If instead we assume a common rate ratio, we get

$$\widehat{IR}_{\text{MH}} = 116.8/82.0 = 1.42$$

$$\widehat{\text{Var}}[\ln(\widehat{IR}_{\text{MH}})] = \frac{110.1}{116.8(82.0)} = 0.01150$$

which yield 90% confidence limits of

$$\exp[\ln(1.424) \pm 1.645(0.01150)^{1/2}] = 1.19, 1.70$$

Maximum likelihood yields virtually the same point estimate and confidence limits for the rate ratio.

MANTEL-HAENSZEL ESTIMATION: PURE COUNT DATA

Suppose that our data come from a closed cohort. Mantel-Haenszel risk-difference and risk-ratio estimators are then standardized estimators based on the standard weights

$$w_{\text{MH}i} = N_{1i}N_{0i}/N_{+i}$$

where $N_{+i} = N_{1i} + N_{0i}$. These weights are direct analogs of the person-time weights. They yield the risk-difference estimator

$$\widehat{RD}_{\text{MH}} = \frac{\sum_i (A_{1i}N_{0i} - A_{0i}N_{1i})/N_{+i}}{\sum_i N_{1i}N_{0i}/N_{+i}} \qquad [15\text{–}19]$$

(Cochran, 1954) and risk-ratio estimator

$$\widehat{RR}_{\text{MH}} = \frac{\sum_i A_{1i}N_{0i}/N_{+i}}{\sum_i A_{0i}N_{1i}/N_{+i}} \qquad [15\text{–}20]$$

(Nurminen, 1981). As in the person-time situation, these Mantel-Haenszel estimators can have much higher variance than the maximum-likelihood estimators of the homogeneous risk difference or ratio. Unlike the corresponding MLEs, however, the Mantel-Haenszel estimators remain valid in sparse data (Greenland and Robins, 1985b). A variance estimator for $\widehat{RD}_{\text{MH}}$ that is valid for all types of data is given by Sato (1989). It is rather complex and so is omitted here. If every denominator (N_{1i} and N_{0i}) is greater than 1, one can use the variance estimator

$$\widehat{\text{Var}}(\widehat{RD}_{MH}) = \frac{\sum_i w_{MHi}^2 \left[\dfrac{A_{1i}B_{1i}}{N_{1i}^2(N_{1i}-1)} + \dfrac{A_{0i}B_{0i}}{N_{0i}^2(N_{0i}-1)}\right]}{\left(\sum_i w_{MHi}\right)^2} \qquad [15\text{–}21]$$

Unless all the cell counts are large, it is best to set limits using the improved approximation formula given for the crude *RD* in Chapter 14. A variance estimator for $\ln(\widehat{RR}_{\text{MH}})$ that is valid for all types of data is

$$\widehat{\text{Var}}[\ln(\widehat{RR}_{\text{MH}})] = \frac{\sum_i (M_{1i}N_{1i}N_{01}/N_{+i}^2 - A_{1i}A_{0i}/N_{+i})}{\left(\sum_i \dfrac{A_{1i}N_{0i}}{N_{+i}}\right)\left(\sum_i \dfrac{A_{0i}N_{1i}}{N_{+i}}\right)} \qquad [15\text{–}22]$$

Like the MLEs, $\widehat{RR}_{\text{MH}}$ and its variance estimator are "large-sample" estimators, but $\widehat{RR}_{\text{MH}}$ does not require the strata to be large. This issue will be discussed further in the testing section that follows.

The variance of $\widehat{RD}_{\text{MH}}$ can be greatly reduced by using $N_{1i}N_{0i}/M_{1i}$ instead of $w_{\text{MH}i}$ as the weight. Similarly, if $M_{0i} = N_{+i} - M_{1i}$ is the total number of noncases in stratum i, the variance of $\widehat{RR}_{\text{MH}}$ can be reduced by using $N_{1i}N_{0i}/M_{0i}$ instead of $w_{\text{MH}i}$ as the weight (Tarone, 1981). These modifications, however, render the estimates invalid for sparse data.

Consider again Table 15–1, comparing tolbutamide with placebo. From these data, we obtain a Mantel-Haenszel risk difference of 0.035 with an estimated SD of 0.032, which yield 90% confidence limits of $0.035 \pm 1.645(0.032) = -0.018$ and 0.088. These results suggest that those who received tolbutamide may have had a greater average risk of death during the study than those who received placebo, despite the fact that tolbutamide was intended to prevent death in these patients. For comparison, the maximum-likelihood estimate of the risk difference is 0.034 with an estimated SD of 0.028; these yield 90% confidence limits of −0.012 and 0.080, a bit narrower than the Mantel-Haenszel limits.

The Mantel-Haenszel risk-ratio estimate from Table 15–1 is 1.33, and the variance estimate for its logarithm is 0.0671. These yield approximate 90% confidence limits of

$$\exp[\ln(1.33) \pm 1.645(0.0671)^{1/2}] = 0.87, 2.0$$

For comparison, the maximum-likelihood estimate and 90% confidence limits are 1.31 and 0.86, 2.0.

TABLE 15–5

Infants with Congenital Heart Disease and Down Syndrome, and Healthy Controls, according to Maternal Spermicide Use before Conception and Maternal Age at Delivery

	Maternal Age <35 y, Spermicide Use			Maternal Age 35+ y, Spermicide Use		
	Yes	No	Total	Yes	No	Total
Down syndrome	3	9	12	1	3	4
Control	104	1,059	1,163	5	86	91
Total	107	1,068	1,175	6	89	95

From Rothman KJ. Spermicide use and Down syndrome. *Am J Public Health*, 1982;72:399–401.

For cohort, case-control, and cross-sectional data, one may wish to assume a homogeneous odds ratio, *OR*. The Mantel-Haenszel estimate of this parameter is

$$\widehat{OR}_{\text{MH}} = \frac{\sum_i A_{1i}B_{0i}/N_{+i}}{\sum_i A_{0i}B_{1i}/N_{+i}} = \frac{\sum_i G_i}{\sum_i H_i} \qquad [15\text{–}23]$$

where $G_i = A_{1i}B_{0i}/N_{+i}$ and $H_i = A_{0i}B_{1i}/N_{+i}$ (Mantel and Haenszel, 1959). For values of the odds ratio not far from 1, this estimator has a variance not much greater than the MLE, and it remains valid in sparse data (Breslow, 1981; Breslow and Liang, 1982). Nonetheless, it is a "large-sample" estimator in the sense explained below. A variance estimator for the logarithm of the Mantel-Haenszel estimator that is valid even if the data are sparse is

$$\widehat{\text{Var}}[\ln(\widehat{OR}_{MH})] = \frac{\sum_i G_i P_i}{2\left(\sum_i G_i\right)^2} + \frac{\sum_i (G_i Q_i + H_i P_i)}{2\sum_i G_i \sum_i H_i} + \frac{\sum_i H_i Q_i}{2\left(\sum_i H_i\right)^2} \qquad [15\text{–}24]$$

where $P_i = (A_{1i} + B_{0i})/N_{+i}$ and $Q_i = (A_{0i} + B_{1i})/N_{+i}$ (Robins et al., 1986b, 1986c).

Table 15–5 provides data from a case-control study of congenital heart disease, Down syndrome, and maternal spermicide use before conception. The Mantel-Haenszel estimate of the maternal-age stratified odds ratio relating maternal spermicide use to Down syndrome is

$$\widehat{OR}_{\text{MH}} = \frac{(3 \cdot 1059)/1{,}175 + (1 \cdot 86)/95}{(104 \cdot 9)/1{,}175 + (5 \cdot 3)/95} = 3.78$$

The estimated variance from the above formula is 0.349, which yields 90% confidence limits of 1.43, 10.0. For comparison, the unconditional MLE is 3.79, the conditional MLE is 3.76, and the mid-*P* 90% limits are 1.30, 9.78. In view of the small number of exposed cases, the differences are remarkably minor.

SMALL-SAMPLE METHODS

One can avoid approximations and conduct stratified analyses of a homogeneous measure by computing traditional exact or mid-*P*-values (and hence confidence limits) directly from an exact probability model for the data. These approaches are direct extensions of the small-sample methods discussed in Chapter 14. Although conceptually simple, the necessary formulas and computations become quite complex in stratified data, and are limited to rate-ratio and odds-ratio analyses (Breslow and Day, 1980, 1987). The chief advantage of such analyses is that no sample-size assumption is needed. For a description of these methods, see Hirji (2006) or Cytel (2006).

P-VALUES FOR THE STRATIFIED NULL HYPOTHESIS

Examples can be found in which a pooled estimate of a homogeneous rate difference shows a negative association whereas a pooled estimate of a homogeneous rate ratio shows a positive association for the same data. Such discrepancies stem from differences in the optimal weighting schemes for the different pooled estimators and reflect the fact that at most one of the measures can be homogeneous. For the purposes of testing the null hypothesis of no association in any stratum, however, the efficient (variance-minimizing) weightings are approximately equivalent for all measures. Consequently, only a single hypothesis test of no association need be considered, whatever the parameter used to measure the association.

Hypothesis testing is generally performed with respect to the overall departure of the data from the null value of no association. Even if the chosen measure varies substantially across strata, tests of the null that assume homogeneity can often outperform tests that do not. If the stratum-specific values of the rate ratio (in person-time data) or odds ratio (in pure count data) are in fact homogeneous, the tests described below are optimal under certain restrictive criteria (Gart and Tarone, 1983).

If the true values of the rate ratio or odds ratio vary across strata, specialized tests can be constructed that will be more powerful than the tests of overall departure from the null value described here. Even in this situation, the tests given below are still valid. More problematically, however, it is possible that estimates could be strongly positive in some strata and strongly negative in others. In such circumstances, the pooled estimate may be near the null value as a result of the balancing of the opposing estimates in individual strata. If the underlying stratum-specific measures change direction across strata, the tests given below may have little power to detect the presence of stratum-specific associations.

Test statistics for stratified data represent a straightforward extension of the corresponding statistics for unstratified data. The score tests for stratified data retain the general form of the score tests in Chapter 14; they extend the formulas for crude data by summing stratum-specific components for the test statistics (the observed number of exposed cases, the number expected under the null hypothesis, and the null variance).

P-VALUES FOR STRATIFIED PERSON-TIME DATA

As with unstratified data, the test statistic is the total number of exposed cases, $A_{1+} = \sum_i A_{1i}$. The expectations and variances for the number of exposed cases under the test hypothesis are calculated within each stratum and are summed over the strata. Conditional on the total numbers of cases M_{1i} in each stratum, and assuming the null hypothesis ($IR = 1$), the expectation for the total number of exposed cases is

$$E = E(A_{1+} \mid IR = 1) = \sum_i \frac{M_{1i} T_{1i}}{T_{+i}}$$

and the null variance is

$$V = \operatorname{Var}(A_{1+} \mid IR = 1) = \sum_i \frac{M_{1i} T_{1i} T_{0i}}{T_{+i}^2}$$

E and V yield the score statistic

$$\chi_{\text{score}} = \frac{A_{1+} - E}{V^{1/2}} \qquad [15\text{–}25]$$

(Shore et al., 1976). This statistic is perhaps better known as the Mantel-Haenszel statistic for person-time data; it is identical to the test statistic for unstratified person-time data, except that the three components of the test statistic are obtained by summing their stratum-specific contributions. It is valid in sparse data, but it requires large total numbers. As a rough guide, small-sample methods are recommended if either E or the quantity

$$\sum_i \frac{M_{1i} \widehat{IR}_{\text{MH}} T_{1i}}{\widehat{IR}_{\text{MH}} T_{1i} + T_{0i}}$$

is less than 5 or greater than $M_{1+} - 5$.

For the data in Table 15–2, the number of exposed cases, A_1, equals 630, whereas the expected value and variance of A_1 under the null hypothesis are seen from Table 15–4 to be $E = 595.2$ and $V = 110.1$. Hence,

$$\chi_{\text{score}} = \frac{630 - 595.2}{(110.1)^{1/2}} = 3.3$$

which corresponds to an upper-tailed P-value of 0.0005.

P-VALUES FOR STRATIFIED PURE COUNT DATA

The extension of the unstratified score test for pure count data to stratified 2×2 tables is analogous to the extension of the unstratified score test for person-time data. As before, the contributions to each of the three components of the test statistic (the number of exposed cases and the expectation and variance for the number of exposed cases) are derived separately for each stratum and then summed over the strata. Assuming that all stratum margins are fixed, the expectation and variance for the number of exposed cases under the null hypothesis ($OR = 1$) are

$$E = E(A_{1+} \mid OR = 1) = \sum_i \frac{M_{1i} N_{1i}}{N_{+i}}$$

and

$$V = \text{Var}(A_{+1} \mid OR = 1) = \sum_i \frac{M_{1i} M_{0i} N_{1i} N_{0i}}{N_{+i}^2 (N_{+i} - 1)}$$

E and V yield the score statistic

$$\chi_{\text{score}} = \frac{A_{1+} - E}{V^{1/2}} \qquad [15\text{–}26]$$

This test statistic, first derived by Cochran (1954) and later modified by Mantel and Haenszel (1959) to the above form, is now known as the Mantel-Haenszel statistic. It has been widely used in epidemiology and other fields. It is valid in sparse data but requires "large" numbers overall. The precise requirements are rather complex (Mantel and Fleiss, 1980) and so are not given here, but they imply that small-sample methods should be used if any of the crude totals (A_{1+}, A_{0+}, B_{1+}, B_{0+}) or their null expected values (E, $M_1 + -E$, $N_{1+} - E$, $N_{0+} - M_{1+} + E$) are less than 5, as well as in some other situations.

Consider the P-value for the hypothesis of no association between tolbutamide and death using the data in Table 15–1 and the Mantel-Haenszel statistic. The number of exposed cases A_{1+}, where "exposed" indicates tolbutamide therapy, equals $8 + 22 = 30$. The expected value and variance of A_1 under the null hypothesis are

$$E = \frac{(106)(13)}{226} + \frac{(98)(38)}{183} = 6.10 + 20.35 = 26.45$$

$$V = \frac{(106)(120)(13)(213)}{(226)^2(225)} + \frac{(98)(85)(38)(145)}{(183)^2(182)} = 3.06 + 7.53 = 10.60$$

so that the statistic is

$$\chi_{\text{score}} = \frac{30 - 26.45}{(10.60)^{1/2}} = 1.09$$

which gives a lower-tailed P-value of 0.86, or a two-sided P-value of 0.28. (Because tolbutamide was being studied as preventive of the complications of diabetes, departures from the null value were expected to occur in the direction of preventing death. Therefore, the relevant one-sided null hypothesis is that there is no inverse association, in which is tested by the lower-tailed P-value.)

Consider again the spermicide and Down syndrome data in Table 15–5. The Mantel-Haenszel (score) statistic is 2.41 with an upper-tailed P-value of 0.008, which is not close to the upper-tailed mid-P-value of 0.023. This discrepancy reflects the fact that the sample size is too small (only four exposed cases) for the Mantel-Haenszel P-value to approximate the mid-P-value.

TESTING HOMOGENEITY

The general form of a Wald statistic for testing the hypothesis that a measure U is homogeneous across strata is

$$\chi^2_{\text{Wald}} = \sum_i \frac{(\hat{U}_i - \hat{U})^2}{\hat{V}_i}$$

where $\hat{U}_i$ is the stratum-specific MLE of the measure, $\hat{V}_i$ is the estimated variance of $\hat{U}_i$, and $\hat{U}$ is the MLE of the hypothesized homogeneous (common) value of the measure. This homogeneity statistic will have a χ^2 distribution with degrees of freedom one less than the number of strata if the true measures U_i are homogeneous across strata. Thus, a P-value for the homogeneity hypothesis can be obtained by looking up the statistic in a χ^2 table. The stratum-specific estimates $\hat{U}_i$ may be adjusted for factors other than the modifier under study. For example, we may test homogeneity across age strata while adjusting for sex, so that i varies across age strata; $\hat{U}_i$ is then the MLE obtained by stratifying on sex within stratum i of age, and $\hat{U}$ is the overall MLE obtained by stratifying on age and sex.

One important caution in using χ^2_{Wald} is that, for ratio measures, U should be taken to be the *logarithm* of the ratio. Substitution of the logarithm of the Mantel-Haenszel rate or odds ratio for the logarithm of the corresponding MLE, though not theoretically correct, will usually make little difference in the result. If U is a rate or risk difference or a risk ratio, however, one should *not* use the Mantel-Haenszel estimate in place of a MLE, as this would invalidate the statistic.

Consider again the tolbutamide data in Table 15–1. Applying the unstratified formulas from Chapter 14 to each age stratum yields

Stratum 1: $\widehat{RR}_1 = 1.81$, $\widehat{\text{Var}}[\ln(\widehat{RR}_1)] = 0.3072$.
Stratum 2: $\widehat{RR}_2 = 1.19$, $\widehat{\text{Var}}[\ln(\widehat{RR}_2)] = 0.0860$.

Earlier, we mentioned that the MLE of a common RR for these data is 1.31. Thus

$$\chi^2_{\text{Wald}} = \frac{[\ln(1.81) - \ln(1.31)]^2}{0.3072} + \frac{[\ln(1.19) - \ln(1.31)]^2}{0.0860} = 0.45$$

Because there are only two strata, this statistic has $2 - 1 = 1$ degree of freedom and yields a P-value of 0.50. Thus, the data are compatible with the hypothesis of homogeneity of the risk ratio. Repeating the process for the risk difference, we get

Stratum 1: $\widehat{RD}_1 = 0.034$, $\widehat{\text{Var}}(\widehat{RD}_1) = 0.0010$.
Stratum 2: $\widehat{RD}_2 = 0.036$, $\widehat{\text{Var}}(\widehat{RD}_2) = 0.0036$.

Because the MLE of a common RD is 0.034, we get

$$\chi^2_{\text{Wald}} = \frac{(0.034 - 0.034)^2}{0.0010} + \frac{(0.036 - 0.034)^2}{0.0036} = 0.001$$

with one degree of freedom, which yields $P = 1.00$. Thus, as is evident from the point estimates, the same data are almost perfectly compatible with the hypothesis of homogeneity of the risk difference.

As mentioned earlier, if both the exposure and the stratifying variables are risk factors, then at most one of the risk ratio and risk difference can be homogeneous. Thus, if there is any stratum-specific association of tolbutamide with death, at least one of the above homogeneity hypotheses *must* be wrong. Yet the tests reject neither hypothesis. This result reflects a general problem of homogeneity testing mentioned earlier: The standard tests of homogeneity have very low power in typical epidemiologic settings. That is, there is often only a small probability that they will reject homogeneity, even if there is heterogeneity (Breslow and Day, 1980; Greenland, 1983). When there are more than two strata, it is often possible to use more powerful tests that make use of ordering of the strata with respect to the stratifying variables. Such tests are more easily described in the context of testing product terms in regression models (Chapters 20 and 21).

Even with such improved tests, one should always bear in mind that a high P-value from a homogeneity test does not show that the measure is homogeneous; it means only that heterogeneity was not detected by the test. When heterogeneity is detected, it is usually best to present and discuss stratum-specific estimates. Nonetheless, standardized summaries (as opposed to summaries that assume homogeneity) retain valid interpretations and can be used as measures of population effect (Miettinen, 1972; Greenland, 1982b).

Consider again the coronary death and smoking data in Table 15–2. We will test the homogeneity of the rate ratio using the Mantel-Haenszel estimate. Because the variances of the stratum-specific log rate-ratio estimates are $1/A_{1i} + 1/A_{0i}$ (Chapter 14), our test statistic is

$$\chi^2_{\text{Wald}} = \sum_i \frac{[\ln(\widehat{IR}_i) - \ln(\widehat{IR}_{\text{MH}})]^2}{1/A_{1i} + 1/A_{0i}}$$

$$= \frac{\ln[(6.1/1.1) - \ln(1.42)]^2}{1/32 + 1/2} + \cdots + \frac{[\ln(191.8/212.0) - \ln(1.42)]^2}{1/102 + 1/31} = 10.41$$

Because there are five age strata, this statistic has $5 - 1 = 4$ degrees of freedom, which yields a P-value of 0.03. Thus, it appears that homogeneity of the rate ratio is not a good assumption for analyzing the data. It also appears that the declining trend in ratios seen in Table 15–2 should be accounted for in the analysis and presentation of results. For a simple trend such as that in Table 15–2, a regression analysis may provide the most parsimonious complete summary, although the estimated SMR of 1.43 remains a valid (if incomplete) summary.

Most computer programs for stratified analysis provide an approximate test of homogeneity, such as a Wald test, score test, or likelihood-ratio test; a few packages, such as StatXact (Cytel, 2006), can supply an exact homogeneity P-value if the numbers are not too large. Tests for qualitative interaction (reversal of association) have also been developed (Gail and Simon, 1985).

Except for exact tests, basic homogeneity tests require the study numbers to be large within strata. It is possible to apply the sample-size criteria given in Chapter 14 on a stratum-by-stratum basis to determine whether unconditional maximum-likelihood estimates and unconditional homogeneity tests can be validly applied to stratified data. For example, if every stratum is large enough for the valid estimation of the stratum-specific rate ratio, the Wald test of rate-ratio homogeneity will usually be approximately valid as well. This stratum-by-stratum criterion is probably more strict than needed for score and likelihood-ratio tests of homogeneity. Nonetheless, if the criterion is not satisfied, it is unlikely that any of the standard homogeneity tests will yield a small P-value, and thus use of an exact test is unlikely to alter the inferences.

CASE-COHORT DATA

As for unstratified case-cohort data (Chapter 14), one can estimate a homogeneous odds ratio and compute a P-value from case-cohort data simply by combining all cases together (whether they come from the case sample or the cohort sample) and then analyzing the data as if they were case-control data. For risk-ratio estimation, however, we must distinguish cases that are not controls (i.e., not part of the cohort sample) and cases that are controls (i.e., are part of the cohort sample). We will use the notation in Table 15–6 to represent a stratum in the study.

TABLE 15–6

Notation for a Stratum in a Case-Cohort Study

	Exposed	Unexposed	Total
Case, not control	A_{11i}	A_{01i}	M_{11i}
Case and control	A_{10i}	A_{00i}	M_{10i}
Noncase control	B_{1i}	B_{0i}	M_{0i}
Total	N_{1i}	N_{0i}	N_{+i}

Also, let

$A_{1i} = A_{11i} + A_{10i}$ = exposed cases in stratum i
$A_{0i} = A_{01i} + A_{00i}$ = unexposed cases in stratum i
$M_{1i} = A_{1i} + A_{0i}$ = total cases in stratum i
$C_{1i} = A_{10i} + B_{1i}$ = exposed controls in stratum i
$C_{0i} = A_{00i} + B_{0i}$ = unexposed controls in stratum i

A Mantel-Haenszel risk-ratio estimator for case-cohort data is then

$$\widehat{RR}_{\mathrm{MH}} = \frac{\sum_i A_{1i}C_{0i}/N_{+i}}{\sum_i A_{0i}C_{1i}/N_{+i}} \qquad [15\text{–}27]$$

(Greenland, 1986c). A variance estimator for the logarithm of $\widehat{RR}_{\mathrm{MH}}$ is

$$\widehat{\mathrm{Var}}[\ln(\widehat{RR}_{MH})] = \frac{(A_{01i} + B_{0i})A_{1i}C_{1i} + (A_{11i} + B_{1i})A_{0i}C_{0i} + A_{11i}B_{0i} + A_{01i}B_{1i}]/N_{+i}^2}{\left(\sum_i A_{1i}C_{0i}/N_{+i}\right)\left(\sum_i A_{0i}C_{1i}/N_{+i}\right)}$$

[15–28]

(Sato, 1992a). Like the other Mantel-Haenszel estimators, both of these estimators remain valid for sparse data but require adequate numbers of subjects contributing to the estimate at each exposure–disease combination. The variance of the risk-ratio estimator $\widehat{RR}_{\mathrm{MH}}$ can be reduced by replacing N_i with $C_i = C_{1i} + C_{0i}$ throughout (including the variance formula), but then the estimator will no longer be valid for sparse data.

Maximum-likelihood analysis of stratified case-cohort data is also feasible (Sato, 1992b), but as in other designs the MLEs require iterative computation, and the MLE of the risk ratio will not be valid in sparse data.

TWO-STAGE DATA

In a two-stage (two-phase) study, the exposure and disease status of an entire study cohort is known, so a crude (unstratified) analysis can be computed for the entire cohort, but data on other variables are obtained only on subsamples from each of the four exposure–disease cells (Chapter 8). Maximum-likelihood analysis of two-stage data is possible, but rather complex (Breslow and Holubkov, 1997ab). We focus here on slightly less efficient but much simpler methods.

Let A_1^*, A_0^*, B_1^*, and B_0^* be the numbers of exposed and unexposed cases and exposed and unexposed noncases in the *entire* cohort. Suppose that simple random subsamples of size A_{1+}, A_{0+}, B_{1+}, and B_{0+} are selected from the four cohort cells A_1^*, A_0^*, B_1^*, and B_0^*, and we obtain covariate information only for the subjects in these subsamples. Estimates of the stratum-specific full-cohort numbers and measures are then

$$\begin{aligned}
\hat{A}_{1i}^* &= A_{1i}(A_1^*/A_{1+}) & \hat{A}_{0i}^* &= A_{0i}(A_0^*/A_{0+}) \\
\hat{B}_{1i}^* &= B_{1i}(B_1^*/B_{1+}) & \hat{B}_{0i}^* &= B_{0i}(B_0^*/B_{0+}) \\
\hat{N}_{1i}^* &= \hat{A}_{1i} + \hat{B}_{1i} & \hat{N}_{0i}^* &= \hat{A}_{0i} + \hat{B}_{0i} \\
\hat{R}_{1i} &= \hat{A}_{1i}^*/\hat{N}_{1i}^* & \hat{R}_{0i} &= \hat{A}_{0i}^*/\hat{N}_{0i}^* \\
\widehat{RD}_i &= \hat{R}_{1i} - \hat{R}_{0i} & \widehat{RR}_i &= \hat{R}_{1i}/\hat{R}_{0i}
\end{aligned}$$

and

$$\widehat{OR}_i = \hat{A}_{1i}^*\hat{B}_{0i}^*/\hat{A}_{0i}^*\hat{B}_{0i}^*$$

General variance formulas for two-stage estimators are much more complicated than those given earlier for unsampled cohort data. We will give only simple approximate formulas for estimating odds ratios under the condition that the subsample sizes are fixed by design. Let F be the crude odds ratio for the total cohort divided by the crude odds ratio for the sample:

$$F = \frac{(A_{0+}/A_0^*)(B_{1+}/B_1^*)}{(A_{1+}/A_1^*)(B_{0+}/B_0^*)} = \frac{A_1^* B_0^*}{A_0^* B_1^*}\left(\frac{A_{1+}B_{0+}}{A_{0+}B_{1+}}\right)^{-1} \qquad [15\text{–}29]$$

Then the stratum-specific odds-ratio estimator given above can be rewritten

$$\widehat{OR}_i = FA_{1i}B_{0i}/A_{0i}B_{1i}$$

Similarly, the Mantel-Haenszel estimator of the homogeneous odds ratio for two-stage data is

$$\widehat{OR}_{\text{MH}} = F\frac{\sum_i A_{1i}B_{0i}/N_{+i}}{\sum_i A_{0i}B_{1i}/N_{+i}} \qquad [15\text{–}30]$$

where the N_{+i} are the actual stratum-specific sampled number of subjects (Walker, 1982a). An approximate variance estimator for the two-stage $\ln(\widehat{OR}_{\text{MH}})$ can be computed by subtracting

$$1/A_1 + 1/A_{0+} + 1/B_{1+} + 1/B_{0+} - 1/A_1^* - 1/A_0^* - 1/B_1^* - 1/B_0^*$$

from the usual Mantel-Haenszel variance estimator given in formula 15–24; this variance correction was originally derived for the estimator given by Cain and Breslow (1988).

White (1982b) gives point and variance estimators for a homogeneous odds ratio, and homogeneity tests, for the situation in which the sampling fractions are random. Unfortunately, these estimators and tests are not valid with sparse data. It is possible to modify the usual Mantel-Haenszel (score) statistic to apply to two-stage data, but the forms of the null expectation and variance for A_{1+} when $F \neq 1$ are complex. For simplicity, Walker (1982a) and White (1982b) recommend using a Wald statistic. For example, one may use

$$\chi_{\text{Wald}} = \frac{\ln(\widehat{OR}_{\text{MH}})}{\widehat{\text{Var}}[\ln(\widehat{OR}_{\text{MH}})]^{1/2}} \qquad [15\text{–}31]$$

This is an approximately normal statistic for testing the hypothesis that there is no stratum-specific association of exposure and disease; it is slightly less powerful than the modified Mantel-Haenszel statistic.

CHAPTER 16

Applications of Stratified Analysis Methods

Sander Greenland

Analysis of Data from Matched Studies 283
Analysis of Matched-Pair Cohort Data 284
Analysis of Matched-Pair Case-Control Data 287
Analysis of Case-Crossover and Other Case-Only Designs 288
Basic Survival Analysis 289
Risk Estimation 290
Estimation of Average Survival Time 293
Comparison of Rates Over Time 294
Attributable Fraction Estimation 295
Adjusted Attributable Fraction Estimates 295
Etiologic Fraction and Probability of Causation 297
Analyses of Biologic Interactions 298
Biologic Interaction and Additivity Conditions 298
Limitations of Statistical Inferences about Interactions 299
Analyses of Induction Periods 300

This chapter describes how to apply basic stratified methods to analyses of matched data; to average risks and incidence times in censored cohort data (commonly known as survival analysis or failure-time analysis); to attributable fractions; and to biologic interactions. It also discusses fundamental problems in analyses of attributable and etiologic fractions, biologic interactions, and induction periods. The main sections in this chapter are independent of one another and thus may be read in any order.

ANALYSIS OF DATA FROM MATCHED STUDIES

Analysis of matched data involves the same statistical methods as are used for unmatched data. Even though many textbooks present special "matched-data" techniques, these techniques are just special cases of general stratified methods for sparse data. The evenly balanced nature of matched covariates, however, can result in great simplifications of more general formulas, especially when the data are pair-matched. We will illustrate this simplification by showing how the general Mantel-Haenszel formulas introduced in Chapter 15 reduce to simple matched-pair analysis formulas.

With modern computing resources, there is little practical need to consider other simplifications (e.g., for matched data with multiple controls). Instead, a general approach to matched data as stratified data may be used. There is, however, one important guideline to follow in such an approach: Each matching category should be treated as a unique stratum, at least in the initial stages of analysis. Exceptions occur only if one can demonstrate that such detailed stratification makes no difference in the study results. For example, suppose that subjects have been matched on sex (two levels) and age in four 5-year categories of age 60 to 64 years, age 65 to 69 years, age 70 to 74 years, and age 75 to 79 years. To account fully for the matched nature of subject selection, it is necessary to stratify on at least the eight composite matching strata formed by each sex–age category combination. In particular, broader age categories are not sufficient to remove the selection bias introduced by matching.

On the other hand, any stratification that is as fine as or finer than the original matching criteria will remove the bias induced by the matching. For example, given enough data, one could use 1-year age strata with 5-year age category matching; this additional stratification will adjust for any residual age confounding within the original 5-year matching strata. One could also include unmatched variables in the stratification process. The limitation of such extensions is that many strata could end up with only a single subject and thus contribute nothing to the estimation process. For this reason, many analysts turn to "matched" modeling methods such as conditional logistic regression, which allow use of regression terms to control residual confounding (the confounding left after stratification on the matching factors). These matched-regression methods are just special cases of general modeling methods for sparse data, which are discussed in Chapter 21. In some situations it may instead be possible to use the matching factors as regressors in an ordinary model. This use can lead to bias, however, if the factors are continuous and treated as such instead of being categorized to reflect the matching protocol (Greenland, 1986a, 1997a).

Sometimes care is needed in determining what constitutes sufficient stratification by the matching factors. It is not always necessary and can be inefficient to retain the original matches made in subject selection (Brookmeyer et al., 1986). For example, if two cases and their paired controls all have identical values for the matching factors (say, all four subjects have the same age, sex, and neighborhood), then combining these subjects into a single stratum will produce an estimator with lower variance and no less validity than that produced by an analysis in which the two pairs are kept separate. Another advantage of combining matched sets with identical matching values is that it can eliminate "double loss" of subjects. When one member of a pair has missing data, its corresponding match will be ignored by any paired analysis method that requires the missing information. If, however, the matched pair belongs to a larger stratum, the corresponding match can be retained as part of that stratum.

If a continuous variable is matched using caliper intervals rather than fixed categories, some ambiguity can arise in determining proper analysis strata, and a small amount of bias may be unavoidable, regardless of the analysis used (Austin et al., 1989). For example, matching "age $\pm$ 2 years" could yield two case-control pairs: one with case of age 65 and matched control age 63, and the other with a case age 63 and a matched control age 61. Among these four subjects, the first control and the second case are the best age match and should be in the same stratum. Nonetheless, combining all four subjects in the same age 61–65 stratum will yield a 4-year age range for the stratum, twice that specified by the 2-year caliper radius. A conservative approach is to form strata no wider than the caliper radius, but this might produce strata with only one subject from a pair. A more accurate result will likely be obtained by using a slightly biased but less variable estimator based on broader categories (such as 4-year or even 5-year categories). In general, however, there is no unambiguously best way to analyze caliper-matched data, because of the inherent bias in such matching (Austin et al., 1989). We view this ambiguity as constituting a minor but practical reason for preferring fixed-category matching over caliper matching.

To summarize, validity of the odds-ratio estimate in a matched case-control study may require that one stratify on any matching factors related to exposure in at least as much detail as was used for matching. In contrast, control of matching factors is not necessary for validity of point estimates of the risk difference or risk ratio in a cohort study. Nonetheless, stratification by matched risk factors is in principle necessary in cohort studies, because matching on risk factors affects the *variance* (and hence the confidence limits) of the risk difference and ratio estimators. This matching effect is accounted for by stratification on the matching factors (Greenland and Robins, 1985b; Weinberg, 1985).

The remainder of this section illustrates some special formulas that apply when each stratum contains one matched pair of subjects.

ANALYSIS OF MATCHED-PAIR COHORT DATA

Suppose that stratification of a cohort yields P uniquely matched pairs of exposed and unexposed subjects. Each stratum (pair) can then be one of only four possible types.

TABLE 16–1

General Form for Uniquely Pair-Matched Cohort Data

		Unexposed Pair Member		
		Disease	No Disease	Exposed Totals
Exposed	Disease	T	U	$T+U$
Pair Member	No disease	V	W	$V+W$
	Unexposed totals	$T+V$	$U+W$	P

1. Both exposed and unexposed get disease, so that (in the notation of Chapter 15) $A_{1i} = A_{0i} = 1$, $B_{1i} = B_{0i} = 0$.
2. Exposed get disease but unexposed does not, so that $A_{1i} = B_{0i} = 1$, $A_{0i} = B_{1i} = 0$.
3. Unexposed get disease but exposed does not, so that $A_{1i} = B_{0i} = 0$, $A_{0i} = B_{1i} = 1$.
4. Neither exposed nor unexposed get disease, so that $A_{1i} = A_{0i} = 0$, $B_{1i} = B_{0i} = 1$.

Note that, in every stratum, $N_{1i} = N_{0i} = 1$, so $N_{+i} = N_{1i} + N_{0i} = 2$. We can summarize the four types of strata in a cohort *matched-pair table,* given in a general form in Table 16–1.

In this notation, there are T, U, V, and W strata (or pairs) of types 1, 2, 3, and 4, respectively. Recall from Chapter 15 that the Mantel-Haenszel estimator of a common risk ratio is

$$\widehat{RR}_{\text{MH}} = \frac{\sum_i A_{1i} N_{0i}/N_{+i}}{\sum_i A_{0i} N_{1i}/N_{+i}} \qquad [16–1]$$

The T type-1 pairs and U type-2 pairs have $A_{1i} = 1$, so have $A_{1i}N_{0i}/N_{+i} = 1/2$, whereas the V type-3 and W type-4 pairs have $A_{1i} = 0$, so have $A_{1i}N_{0i}/N_{+i} = 0$. Similarly, the T type-1 and V type-3 pairs have $A_{0i} = 1$, so have $A_{0i}N_{1i}/N_{+i} = 1/2$ whereas the U type-2 and W type-4 pairs have $A_{0i} = 0$, so have $A_{0i}N_{1i}/N_{+i} = 0$. Hence, the Mantel-Haenszel risk ratio (equation 16–1) simplifies to

$$\widehat{RR}_{\text{MH}} = \frac{(T+U)/2}{(T+V)/2} = \frac{T+U}{T+V} \qquad [16–2]$$

Note that $T + U$ and $T + V$ are just the total (crude) numbers of exposed and unexposed cases. Because there are P pairs, there are exactly P exposed and P unexposed subjects total. Hence the crude risk ratio is

$$\frac{(T+U)/2}{(T+V)/2} = \frac{T+U}{T+V}$$

equal to the Mantel-Haenszel risk ratio. This equality illustrates how pair matching in a cohort study prevents confounding by the matching factors if no loss to follow-up occurs.

In a manner analogous to that just shown, formula 15–22 for the estimated variance of $\ln(\widehat{RR}_{\text{MH}})$ simplifies to

$$\frac{U+V}{(T+U)(T+V)} \qquad [16–3]$$

In contrast, the crude variance estimator is

$$\frac{1}{T+U} + \frac{1}{T+V} - \frac{2}{P} = \frac{2T+U+V}{(T+U)(T+V)} - \frac{2}{P}$$

$$= \frac{2T}{(T+U)(T+V)} + \frac{U+V}{(T+U)(T+V)} - \frac{2}{P} \qquad [16–4]$$

This quantity is larger than that in formula 16–3 if the pair outcomes are positively associated, i.e., if $TW > UV$, as is usually the case. In this case, the crude variance estimator is upwardly biased for the matched data, even though the crude point estimator is unbiased.

Although we forgo the details, one can similarly show that the Mantel-Haenszel risk difference for the matched pairs simplifies to the crude risk difference,

$$\frac{T+U}{P} - \frac{T+V}{P} = \frac{U-V}{P} \qquad [16\text{–}5]$$

but the (correct) Mantel-Haenszel variance estimate is smaller than the crude variance estimate if $TW > UV$. The Mantel-Haenszel odds ratio reduces to an even simpler form for matched-pair cohort data: It equals U/V, the ratio of discordant pairs. We show later that the same type of simplification occurs for matched-pair case-control data.

Another interesting simplification occurs for the Mantel-Haenszel statistic. Recall that it equals

$$\chi_{\text{score}} = \frac{A_{1+} - E}{V^{1/2}} \qquad [16\text{–}6]$$

where $A_{1+} = \sum_i A_{1i}$, $E = \sum_i M_{1i}N_{1i}/N_{+i}$, and $V = \sum_i M_{1i}M_{0i}N_{1i}N_{0i}/N_{+i}{}^2(N_{+i} - 1)$. For type-1 pairs, $M_{1i} = 2, M_{0i} = 0$; for type-2 and type-3 pairs, $M_{1i} = M_{0i} = 1$; and for type-4 pairs, $M_{1i} = 0$, $M_{0i} = 2$. After substituting these values as appropriate and using $N_{1i} = N_{0i} = 1, N_{+i} = 2$, we find that $A_{1+} = T + U$ (as before), $E = (2T + U + V)/2$, and $V = (U + V)/4$. Thus, for pairs,

$$\chi_{\text{score}} = \frac{T + U - (2T + U + V)/2}{[(U+V)/4]^{1/2}} = \frac{U - V}{(U+V)^{1/2}} \qquad [16\text{–}7]$$

This expression is better known as the McNemar matched-pair test statistic (McNemar, 1947) and has been a mainstay of matched-pair analysis. Under the null hypothesis of no exposure–disease association, it has an approximately normal distribution with a mean of 0 and a standard deviation (SD) of 1. The test statistic calculated from the crude table does not simplify to this form.

A useful fact about the matched-cohort risk-ratio and test statistic is that they do not depend on any matched sets with no disease. This fact implies that one can estimate risk ratios from a population by using only case surveillance (population registry) data, as long as the data are naturally matched and the exposure status of cases and their matches can be ascertained. Examples of such naturally matched sets include twins, siblings, spouses, and vehicle riders. As an illustration, consider the problem of estimating the risk ratio comparing accident fatalities of motorcycle drivers and passengers. The Fatal Accident Reporting System (FARS) of the U.S. National Highway Safety Administration attempts to register all U.S. motor vehicle accidents that report a fatality, and obtains basic data on the accidents and persons involved. Evans and Frick (1988) reported from these data that, among two-rider motorcycle crashes in which both driver and passenger were male and neither wore a helmet, in $T = 226$ both died, in $U = 546$ only the driver died, and in $V = 378$ only the passenger died. Because accidents without a fatality are not reported to the FARS, we do not know W = number of two-rider crashes in which neither died. Nonetheless, we can estimate the death-risk ratio for drivers versus passengers as

$$\widehat{RR}_{\text{MH}} = (226 + 546)/(226 + 378) = 1.278$$

The logarithm of this ratio has an estimated SD of

$$\{(546 + 378)/[(226 + 546)(226 + 378)]\}^{1/2} = 0.0445$$

which yields 95% limits of

$$\exp[\ln(1.278) \pm 1.96(0.0445)] = 1.17, 1.39$$

The Mantel-Haenszel statistic is

$$(546 - 378)/(546 + 378)^{1/2} = 5.53$$

which yields $P < 0.0001$. Thus, in two-rider motorcycle crashes in the United States in which both riders are men and neither is helmeted, it appears that the driver is at moderately higher risk of death than the passenger.

Basic analysis of matched cohort data may proceed by stratifying on the matching factors (and by other factors, if deemed necessary) and employing appropriate stratified analysis methods. We nonetheless caution that one should examine the strata visually and use sparse-data methods (such as Mantel-Haenszel methods) if most within-stratum numerators (A_{1i} and A_{0i}) are small. If the number of exposed cases is small or the number of unexposed cases is small, small-sample ("exact") methods should be used. As a rough guide, "small" may be taken as "under 5."

For person-time analyses of follow-up data, the analysis formulas do not simplify as extensively as do the formulas for count data, so we do not present them. Similar to count data, matched person-time data may be analyzed using ordinary stratified-analysis formulas.

ANALYSIS OF MATCHED-PAIR CASE-CONTROL DATA

Suppose that stratification of a case-control data set yields P uniquely matched pairs of case and control subjects. Each stratum (pair) can then be one of only four possible types:

1. Both the case and control are exposed, so that (in the notation of Chapter 15) $A_{1i} = B_{1i} = 1$, $A_{0i} = B_{0i} = 0$.
2. The case is exposed, but the control is not, so that $A_{1i} = B_{0i} = 1$, $A_{0i} = B_{1i} = 0$.
3. The control is exposed, but the case is not, so that $A_{1i} = B_{0i} = 0$, $A_{0i} = B_{1i} = 1$.
4. Neither case nor control are exposed, so that $A_{1i} = B_{1i} = 0$, $A_{0i} = B_{0i} = 1$.

Note that, in every stratum, $M_{1i} = M_{0i} = 1$ and $N_{+i} = M_{1i} + M_{0i} = 2$. We can summarize the four types of strata in a case-control matched-pair table, given in general form in Table 16–2. In this notation, there are, respectively, T, U, V, and W strata (pairs) of type 1, 2, 3, and 4 listed above.

Recall from Chapter 15 that the Mantel-Haenszel estimator of a common odds ratio is

$$\widehat{OR}_{\text{MH}} = \frac{\sum_i A_{1i} B_{0i} / N_{+i}}{\sum_i A_{0i} B_{1i} / N_{+i}}. \qquad [16\text{–}8]$$

The T type-1 and W type-4 pairs have $A_{1i} B_{0i}/N_{+i} = A_{0i} B_{1i}/N_{+i} = 0$ and so contribute nothing to $\widehat{OR}_{\text{MH}}$. The U type-2 pairs have $A_{1i} B_{0i}/N_{+i} = 1(1)/2 = 1/2$ and $A_{0i} B_{1i}/N_{+i} = 0$, whereas the V type-3 pairs have $A_{1i} B_{0i}/N_{+i} = 0$ and $A_{0i} B_{1i}/N_{+i} = 1(1)/2 = 1/2$. Hence, the Mantel-Haenszel odds ratio (equation 16–8) simplifies to

$$\widehat{OR}_{\text{MH}} = \frac{U(1/2)}{V(1/2)} = \frac{U}{V} \qquad [16\text{–}9]$$

This formula may be recognized as the classical matched-pair odds-ratio estimator (Kraus, 1960), which is the ratio of the two types of exposure-discordant pairs. It is also identical to the conditional maximum-likelihood (CML) estimator of the common odds ratio across strata (pairs) (Breslow and Day, 1980). In a similar fashion, the SD estimator of Robins et al. (1986b, c) for $\ln(\widehat{OR}_{\text{MH}})$ given in Chapter 15 simplifies to $(1/U + 1/V)^{1/2}$ for matched-pair data. The latter expression is just the usual approximate SD estimator for $\ln(U/V)$ (Breslow and Day, 1980). Finally,

TABLE 16–2

General Form for Uniquely Pair-Matched Case-Control Data

		Control Pair Member		
		Exposed	Unexposed	Case Totals
Case	Exposed	T	U	$T+U$
Pair Member	Unexposed	V	W	$V+W$
	Control totals	$T+V$	$U+W$	P

using essentially the same derivation as given earlier for matched-pair cohort data, one can show that the Mantel-Haenszel test statistic applied to case-control pairs simplifies to the McNemar statistic $(U - V)/(U + V)^{1/2}$.

The crude counts obtained by ignoring the matching are $A_{1+} = T + U$, $A_{0+} = V + W$, $B_{1+} = T + V$, and $B_{0+} = U + W$. The crude odds ratio is thus

$$\widehat{OR}_c = \frac{(T + U)(U + W)}{(T + V)(V + W)}$$

The degree to which the case and control exposures are associated can be measured by the difference in diagonal products $TW - UV$. This quantity is positive if the case and control exposures are positively associated, and negative if these exposures are negatively associated. In general, the crude odds ratio $\widehat{OR}_c$ will be closer to 1.0 than $\widehat{OR}_{MH} = U/V$ if the case and control exposures are positively associated, and will be farther from 1.0 than $\widehat{OR}_{MH}$ if the case and control exposures are negatively associated. Typically, we expect matching to make cases and controls more alike on exposure, and thus to induce a positive association of the case and control exposures. Thus, ordinarily we expect the crude odds ratio to be closer to the null (1.0) than the matched odds ratio. Exceptions occur, however.

As an illustration of the above points and formulas, we consider data from a matched-pair study of risk factors for adenomatous polyps of the colon (Witte et al., 1996). In this study, both cases and controls had undergone sigmoidoscopy screening, and controls were matched to cases on time of screening (3-month categories), clinic (two clinics), age (50 to 54 years, 55 to 59 years, 60 to 64 years, 65 to 69 years, 70+ years; 76 years maximum age), and sex. Of major interest is the possible effect of low fruit and vegetable consumption; here, low consumption (exposure) is defined as two or fewer servings per day. There were $U = 45$ pairs in which the case but not the control reported low consumption, and $V = 24$ pairs in which the control but not the case reported low consumption. Thus, the Mantel-Haenszel odds ratio is $45/24 = 1.875$, whose logarithm has an estimated standard error of $(1/45 + 1/24)^{1/2} = 0.253$. These yield 95% limits of

$$\exp[\ln(1.875) \pm 1.96(0.253)] = 1.14, 3.08$$

The McNemar (Mantel-Haenszel) test statistic is $(45 - 24)/(45 + 24)^{1/2} = 2.53$, $P = 0.011$. These results can be contrasted to those obtained from the crude data. In $T = 4$ pairs, both the case and control reported low consumption, while in $W = 415$ pairs, neither reported low consumption. The crude counts are thus $A_{1+} = 4 + 45 = 49$, $A_{0+} = 24 + 415 = 439$, $B_{1+} = 4 + 24 = 28$, and $B_{0+} = 415 + 45 = 460$, which yield a crude odds ratio of 1.83 with 95% limits of 1.13, 2.97, and a X_{score} statistic of 2.49, $P = 0.013$. These are very similar to the matched results, indicating that the matching factors were not closely related to exposure (low consumption).

Many authors have noted, with some discomfort, that the matched-pair estimator U/V makes no use of the $T + W$ concordant pairs (which often compose most of the pairs). It is possible to derive odds-ratio estimators that make use of the concordant pairs, and which as a result have smaller variance than U/V (Kalish, 1990). The cost of this variance reduction is the introduction of some bias, although the bias is considered worth the increase in accuracy afforded by the variance reduction. Because the formulas for these estimators are not simple, we do not present them here.

For more complex matched case-control data, analysis may proceed by stratifying on the matching factors and employing appropriate stratified analysis methods. As always, however, one should examine the strata and use sparse-data methods (such as Mantel-Haenszel or conditional maximum likelihood) if most of the within-stratum case or control counts are small. If the total numbers of exposed and unexposed cases and controls are also small, small-sample (exact) methods should be used.

ANALYSIS OF CASE-CROSSOVER AND OTHER CASE-ONLY DESIGNS

Chapter 8 described several case-only designs related to case-control studies. When the exposure status of cases is known over the entire time period of a case-crossover study, and the exposure distribution of case time at risk is representative of the source population distribution, one may estimate the rate ratio from the data as if it were person-time data from a cohort study (Maclure,

1991). Similarly, if case exposure status is known only at certain time points, and the exposure distribution of these points is representative of the time at risk in the source population, one may estimate the rate ratio from case-crossover data as if it were matched case-control data, with the data from a single case at different time points forming a matched set (Mittleman et al., 1995; Greenland, 1999c). This set comprises a "case" (the case record as of disease incidence time) and "controls" (the records from other time periods, which are used for reference).

The assumptions that permit such simple approaches to case-crossover data depend heavily on how the time points were sampled, as well on the disease process under study, and cannot be expected to hold in general. Sampling designs and analysis methods to address these issues are discussed by Lumley and Levy (2000), Vines and Farrington (2001), Navidi and Weinhandl (2002), and Janes et al. (2004, 2005).

Analysis of case-specular studies may be conducted by treating the case and specular as matched pairs (Zaffanella et al., 1998; Greenland, 1999c). See Chapter 28 and Thomas (2004) for discussions of the analysis of genetic case-only studies, as well as other genetic designs.

BASIC SURVIVAL ANALYSIS

Suppose that we wish to compare the average risk of disease in two cohorts, exposed and unexposed. Our discussion thus far has implicitly assumed that each cohort member is followed until either the event of interest occurs or the risk period of interest is over. In other words, the pure count methods given in Chapters 14 and 15 assume that there are no losses to follow-up or competing risks. Although this condition is usually met in some settings, such as perinatal mortality studies, it is often not met in others, especially when the follow-up period is very long.

Losses to follow-up can occur in many ways. If the study ends before the end of a subject's risk period, the subject is lost to follow-up; such losses are sometimes called "withdrawals from observation." Subjects or their physicians may refuse further participation in the study after some point in time and deny the investigator further contact. Subjects may move away and leave behind no means of further contact (true losses). If the outcome under study is not inevitable, subjects may suffer from a competing risk and so be removed from follow-up. For example, in a study of long-term risk of uterine cancer, many women will have hysterectomies or die from other causes during the risk period.

Most statistical methods for follow-up data treat losses to follow-up and losses to competing risks as forms of *censoring*. Nonetheless, these two forms of censoring are very different phenomena, and usually have very different relations to the study variables. For example, consider a cohort study of fat intake and colon cancer. Over the very long follow-up period of such a study, people will drop out of the study or move away and be lost for a variety of reasons. We expect few if any of these losses to be related both to fat intake and colon cancer risk. But people will also be censored (lost to observation) as a result of competing risks. For example, many will die of coronary heart disease (CHD), which we expect to be related both to fat intake and also to colon cancer risk (through mutual risk factors such as sedentary lifestyle and poor diet). As a result of these relations, we expect that prevention of the competing risk of fatal CHD via improvements in diet and exercise habits will lower the risk of colon cancer as well. This assumption implies that projecting risk outward from the followed subjects to those lost to CHD death will overestimate what the colon cancer risk of the latter subjects would have been if their CHD had been prevented.

The last point is particularly important, because all standard risk-estimation methods, including the basic procedures we now present, assume that all censoring (whether due to loss to follow-up or competing risks) is unrelated to risk of the disease under study. In other words, we assume that, within every stratum and exposure level and over any time interval within the study, the average risk of the study disease among subjects not lost to follow-up or competing risks is the same as what the average risk would be if no such censoring occurred. We will call this the *independent-censoring* assumption, for it demands that censoring be unrelated to risks within stratum-specific exposure levels.

If competing risks are present, the independent-censoring assumption *defines* the risks being estimated as "conditional risks," that is, the disease risks that would apply if all competing risks were absent. These are purely hypothetical quantities. As just discussed, actual prevention of competing risks may alter the subsequent risk of the study disease, as when it involves changing exposures that are risk factors for both the competing risks and the study disease. Stratification on such exposures will, however, produce a conditional-risk estimate that assumes no alteration is made. Thus, stratified comparisons of conditional-risk estimates assume that (somehow) competing risks can be removed without altering the distribution of risk factors, which is an unrealistic assumption (Kalbfleisch and Prentice, 1980; Greenland, 2005a).

An alternative answer to the competing-risks problem is to focus attention on estimating "unconditional risks" of the study disease, that is, average risks in the presence of the competing risks, also known as absolute or marginal risks (Benichou and Gail, 1990a). Other alternatives are also possible (Pepe and Mori, 1993). These alternatives avoid much of the ambiguity inherent in standard methods, but they are somewhat more complex than adaptation of the basic stratification methods given earlier. We will thus confine our discussion of survival analysis to standard methods, with the caveat that unambiguous interpretation of the estimates may require an unrealistic assumption about the independence of the study disease and its competing risks.

RISK ESTIMATION

Basic survival analysis involves stratification on follow-up time and is traditionally known as *life-table analysis.* As discussed in Chapter 3, the overall survival proportion (proportion of subjects not getting disease) in a cohort with no competing risk is simply the product of survival proportions over the time strata. A parallel relation holds for probabilities (which are expected proportions). Suppose that we have K time strata indexed by $k = 1, \ldots, K$, each with an upper boundary t_k, and with the lower boundary of the first interval being the start of follow-up. Imagine that there is a certain probability s_k of getting *through* time interval k without disease if one gets *to* the interval without the disease. The probability of getting through all the intervals without disease is then

$$S = s_1 \times s_2 \times \cdots \times s_K = \prod_k s_k \qquad [16\text{–}10]$$

and the overall risk of disease is $R = 1 - S$.

To estimate the overall risk up to a given time t_{end}, we may construct the intervals so that the incidence times of study disease occurring up to t_{end} form the upper interval boundaries $t_1, \ldots, t_k$, where t_k is the last incidence time up to t_{end} (so $t_k \geq t_{\text{end}}$). We then define A_k to be the number of cohort members observed to get disease at t_k, B_k to be the number observed at risk at t_k who do *not* get disease at t_k, and N_k to be $A_k + B_k$, the total still under follow-up at t_k. Then, provided censoring is independent of study disease risk,

$$\hat{S}_{\text{KM}} = \prod_k \hat{s}_k = \prod_k B_k/N_k \qquad [16\text{–}11]$$

will be a valid estimate of S, the probability of surviving past time t_{end} without disease if no competing risk occurs, and $\hat{R}_{\text{KM}} = 1 - \hat{S}_{\text{KM}}$ will be a valid estimate of R, the probability of getting disease by t_{end} if no competing risk occurs. $\hat{S}_{\text{KM}}$ is known as the *Kaplan-Meier* or *product-limit* estimate of survival probability (Chapter 3).

An estimator for the large-sample variance of the logit of $\hat{S}_{\text{KM}}$, $\ln(\hat{S}_{\text{KM}}/\hat{R}_{\text{KM}})$, based on *Greenwood's formula* (Cox and Oakes, 1984), is

$$\widehat{\text{Var}}[\text{logit}(\hat{S}_{\text{KM}})] = \widehat{\text{Var}}[\ln(\hat{S}_{\text{KM}}/\hat{R}_{\text{KM}})] = \frac{1}{\hat{R}^2_{\text{KM}}}\sum_k\left(\frac{1}{B_k} - \frac{1}{N_k}\right) \qquad [16\text{–}12]$$

which is also an estimate of the variance of the logit of $\hat{R}_{\text{KM}}$, $\ln(\hat{R}_{\text{KM}}/\hat{S}_{\text{KM}})$. This estimate can be used to set confidence limits for S and R,

$$\underline{S}, \overline{S} = \text{expit}\{\text{logit}(\hat{S}_{\text{KM}}) \pm Z_\gamma \widehat{\text{Var}}[\text{logit}(\hat{S}_{\text{KM}})]^{1/2}\}$$

where Z_γ is 1.645 for 90% limits and 1.960 for 95% limits, with limits $\underline{R} = 1 - \overline{S}$ and $\overline{R} = 1 - \underline{S}$ for R. Because these are large-sample limits, we recommend there be at least five cases observed and at least five survivors under observation at the end of the study period (i.e., $A_+ \geq 5$ and $B_k \geq 5$); other formulas are available that produce more accurate limits, especially in small samples

TABLE 16–3

Death Times (in weeks) in a Cohort of 26 Leukemia Patients with Baseline White Blood Counts of <50,000

Time Index (k)	Death Time (t_k)	Interval Length (Δt_k)	AG-Negative Deaths (A_{1k})	AG-Negative Survivors (B_{1k})	AG-Negative Total (N_{1k})	AG-Positive Deaths (A_{0k})	AG-Positive Survivors (B_{0k})	AG-Positive Total (N_{0k})
1	2	2	1	12	13	0	13	13
2	3	1	3	9	12	0	13	13
3	4	1	2	7	9	1	12	13
4	7	3	1	6	7	0	12	12
5	8	1	1	5	6	0	12	12
6	16	8	1	4	5	1	11	12
7	17	1	1	3	4	0	11	11
8	22	5	1	2	3	1	10	11
9	26	4	0	2	2	1	9	10

From Feigl P, Zelen M. Estimation of exponential survival probabilities with concomitant information. *Biometrics*. 1965;21:826–838.

(Rothman, 1978b; Anderson et al., 1982). If censoring occurs, it is best that time be measured finely enough so that censoring and disease times are distinct (so that no censoring occurs at an interval boundary t_k). Finally, accuracy will be enhanced if time is measured finely enough so that few incidence times are equal to one another (so that A_k is only infrequently greater than 1).

In a study of leukemia patients (Feigl and Zelen, 1965), the 13 AG-negative patients (patients with no Auer rods or significant granulature) whose white blood count (WBC) was under 50,000 at baseline ($t = 0$) had death times at weeks 2, 3, 3, 3, 4, 4, 7, 8, 16, 17, 22, 56, and 65 (Table 16–3). Suppose that we are interested in the probability of surviving 13 weeks among such patients. There are $N = 5$ distinct death times in the first 13 weeks: $t_1 = 2, t_2 = 3, t_3 = 4, t_4 = 7, t_5 = 8$ weeks. The numbers of subjects surviving up *to* each time are $N_1 = 13$, $N_2 = 12$, $N_3 = 9$, $N_4 = 7$, and $N_5 = 6$. The numbers surviving *past* each time are $B_1 = 12$, $B_2 = 9$, $B_3 = 7$, $B_4 = 6$, $B_5 = 5$. The product-limit estimate is thus

$$\hat{S}_{\mathrm{KM}} = (12/13)(9/12)(7/9)(6/7)(5/6) = 0.385$$

$$\hat{R}_{\mathrm{KM}} = 1 - 0.385 = 0.615$$

Because there is no censoring, $\hat{S}_{\mathrm{KM}}$ equals the simple survival proportion $5/13 = 0.385$. The estimated variance of logit($\hat{S}_{\mathrm{KM}}$) and logit($\hat{R}_{\mathrm{KM}}$) is

$$\frac{1}{0.615^2}\left(\frac{1}{12} - \frac{1}{13} + \frac{1}{9} - \frac{1}{12} + \frac{1}{7} - \frac{1}{9} + \frac{1}{6} - \frac{1}{7} + \frac{1}{5} - \frac{1}{6}\right) = 0.325$$

which yields 90% limits for S and R of

$$\underline{S}, \overline{S} = \mathrm{expit}\left[\ln\left(\frac{0.385}{0.615}\right) \pm 1.645(0.325)^{1/2}\right] = 0.20, 0.62$$

$$\underline{R}, \overline{R} = 1 - 0.62, 1 - 0.20 = 0.38, 0.80$$

Thus, S and R are very imprecisely estimated.

A simple alternative to the product-limit estimator, the *Nelson-Aalen* estimator, is based on the exponential formula:

$$\hat{S}_{NA} = \exp\left(-\sum_k A_k/N_k\right), \hat{R}_{NA} = 1 - \hat{S}_{NA} \qquad [16\text{–}13]$$

where $A_k = N_k - B_k$ is the number of cases occurring at time t_k. This estimator has about the same performance as the product-limit estimator, as it is a good approximation to it in large samples (see Chapter 3). An approximate variance estimator for the logits of $\hat{S}_{NA}$ and $\hat{R}_{NA}$ is

$$\widehat{\text{Var}}[\text{logit}(\hat{S}_{NA})] = \frac{1}{\hat{R}^2_{NA}} \sum_k \frac{A_k B_k}{N_k^2(N_k - 1)} \qquad [16\text{–}14]$$

For the Feigl and Zelen (1965) data, the exponential formula (Nelson-Aalen) estimates are

$$\hat{S}_{NA} = \exp\left(-\frac{1}{13} - \frac{3}{12} - \frac{2}{9} - \frac{1}{7} - \frac{1}{6}\right) = 0.424$$

$$\hat{R}_{NA} = 1 - 0.424 = 0.576$$

These are not too far from the product-limit estimates of 0.385 and 0.615 considering the very small numbers and the great imprecision involved. The estimated variance of logit($\hat{S}_{NA}$) and logit($\hat{R}_{NA}$) is

$$\frac{1}{0.576^2}\left(\frac{1 \cdot 12}{13^2 12} + \frac{3 \cdot 9}{12^2 11} + \frac{2 \cdot 7}{9^2 8} + \frac{1 \cdot 6}{7^2 6} + \frac{1 \cdot 5}{6^2 5}\right) = 0.279$$

which yields 90% limits for S of 0.24 and 0.63.

Suppose now that we have independent survival risk estimates $\hat{S}_1$, $\hat{R}_1$ and $\hat{S}_0$, $\hat{R}_0$, for exposed and unexposed cohorts with variance estimates $\hat{V}_1$ and $\hat{V}_0$ for their logits, such as the product-limit estimates given above. Approximate variance estimates for the risk-difference estimator $\hat{R}_1 - \hat{R}_0$ and the log risk-ratio estimator $\ln(\hat{R}_1 / \hat{R}_0)$ are then

$$\widehat{\text{Var}}(\hat{R}_1 - \hat{R}_0) = \hat{R}_1^2 \hat{S}_1^2 \hat{V}_1 + \hat{R}_0^2 \hat{S}_0^2 \hat{V}_0 \qquad [16\text{–}15]$$

and

$$\widehat{\text{Var}}[\ln(\hat{R}_1/\hat{R}_0)] = \hat{S}_1^2 \hat{V}_1 + \hat{S}_0^2 \hat{V}_0 \qquad [16\text{–}16]$$

These formulas can be used to set confidence limits for the risk difference and risk ratio.

Table 16–3 summarizes death times for 13 AG-negative and 13 AG-positive patients in the first 26 weeks (6 months) of a study of leukemia patients described earlier (only patients with white blood cell counts of <50,000 are presented). Because there is no censoring in these data, the product-limit 6-month survival estimates are $\hat{S}_1 = 2/13$ and $\hat{S}_0 = 9/13$, with $\hat{R}_1 = 11/13$ and $\hat{R}_0 = 4/13$. The variance estimates for the logits of $\hat{R}_1$ and $\hat{R}_0$ simplify to

$$\hat{V}_1 = \frac{1}{(11/13)^2}\left(\frac{1}{2} - \frac{1}{13}\right) = \frac{13}{22}$$

and

$$\hat{V}_0 = \frac{1}{(4/13)^2}\left(\frac{1}{9} - \frac{1}{13}\right) = \frac{13}{36}$$

These yield variance estimates for the risk difference and log risk-ratio estimates of

$$\left(\frac{2}{13}\right)^2\left(\frac{11}{13}\right)^2\frac{13}{22} + \left(\frac{4}{13}\right)^2\left(\frac{9}{13}\right)^2\frac{13}{36} = 0.0264$$

and

$$\left(\frac{2}{13}\right)^2\frac{13}{22} + \left(\frac{9}{13}\right)^2\frac{13}{36} = 0.187$$

and 90% limits for the risk difference and risk ratio of

$$\frac{11}{13} - \frac{4}{13} \pm 1.645(0.0264)^{1/2} = 0.27, 0.81$$

and

$$\exp\left[\ln\left(\frac{11/13}{4/13}\right) \pm 1.645(0.187)^{1/2}\right] = 1.35, 5.60$$

Because there is no censoring, these results are identical to what would be obtained by applying the unstratified methods of Chapter 14 to the data, ignoring (collapsing over) time. If censoring were present, however, the unstratified and stratified results would differ.

It is possible to reduce the variances of risk estimators through use of survival models (Cox and Oakes, 1984). Chapter 20 discusses such models.

ESTIMATION OF AVERAGE SURVIVAL TIME

Suppose that we are studying an inevitable outcome, such as death. To estimate the average (expected) survival or incidence time experienced from a start time until a specific end time t_{end}, we extend the relation of survival proportions to average incidence time outlined in Chapter 3, using survival probability estimates (e.g., product-limit estimates) in place of the proportions. Suppose that $t_1, \ldots, t_k$ are the incidence times and $\hat{S}_{\text{KM}_1}, \ldots, \hat{S}_{\text{KM}_K}$ are the product-limit estimates of the probabilities of surviving past each time. Then an estimator of the average survival time up to t_{end} is

$$\begin{aligned}\overline{T} &= \sum_k \hat{S}_{\text{KM}_{k-1}}(t_k - t_{k-1}) + \hat{S}_{\text{KM}_K}(t_{\text{end}} - t_K) \\ &= \sum_k (\hat{S}_{\text{KM}_{k-1}} - \hat{S}_{\text{KM}_k})t_k + \hat{S}_{\text{KM}_K} t_{\text{end}}\end{aligned} \qquad [16\text{–}17]$$

where the sums are from $k = 1$ to K, t_0 is defined to be 0, and S_0 is defined to be 1. Other survival-probability estimates (such as Nelson-Aalen estimates) may be used in place of product-limit estimates in this formula. If one uses product-limit estimators, however, the formula simplifies to

$$\overline{T} = \sum_k \frac{A_k}{N_k} t_k + \hat{S}_{\text{KM}_K} t_{\text{end}}. \qquad [16\text{–}18]$$

If we have two groups with estimates T_1 and T_0, we can compare the groups using the difference or ratio of these estimates. When death is the outcome and time is age, the difference $T_0 - T_1$ is commonly known as the estimated expected years of life lost up to age t_{end}. For chronic diseases, T_1 and T_0 are known as the average ages at first occurrence among the exposed and unexposed, and for irreversible diseases $T_0 - T_1$ is the estimated expected years of disease-free life lost.

We will estimate the average survival time up to $t_{\text{end}} = 28$ weeks for AG-positive patients, using the data in Table 16–3. The death times for this group are weeks 4, 16, 22, and 26, and the estimated probabilities of surviving past these times are 12/13, 11/13, 10/13, and 9/13. (Because there is no censoring, we can use the observed survival proportions as estimates, rather than the Kaplan-Meier or Nelson-Aalen estimates.) These values yield an estimate for the average survival time of

$$\begin{aligned}\overline{T} &= 1(4-0) + \frac{12}{13}(16-4) + \frac{11}{13}(22-16) + \frac{10}{13}(26-22) + \frac{9}{13}(28-26) \text{ weeks} \\ &= \left(1 - \frac{12}{13}\right)4 + \left(\frac{12}{13} - \frac{11}{13}\right)16 + \left(\frac{11}{13} - \frac{10}{13}\right)22 + \left(\frac{10}{13} - \frac{9}{13}\right)26 + \frac{9}{13}28 \text{ weeks} \\ &= \frac{1}{13}4 + \frac{1}{13}16 + \frac{1}{13}22 + \frac{1}{13}26 + \frac{9}{13}28 = 24.6 \text{ weeks}\end{aligned}$$

In contrast, the estimate for the AG-negative group is 11.2 weeks. Thus, these data indicate that AG-positive patients experience 24.6 − 11.2 = 13.4 more weeks or about 3 more months of life, on average, during a 28-week follow-up.

Differences and ratios of average survival times often provide more useful measures of harm than differences and ratios of average risks or rates (Robins and Greenland, 1991; Boshuizen and Greenland, 1997). Nonetheless, because survival-time comparisons can become rather complicated when losses to follow-up occur, comparisons of incidence and survival times are most easily conducted using incidence-time (survival) models, as discussed in Chapter 20.

COMPARISON OF RATES OVER TIME

Suppose that we wish to compare disease rates in an exposed and an unexposed cohort. Let $t_1, \ldots, t_K$ represent (in order) *all* the distinct disease incidence times, whether among exposed or unexposed subjects. For the purposes of estimating and testing a uniform rate difference or ratio, we need only consider time as one more stratification variable, along with other variables, and include it among the factors defining the analysis strata. For example, suppose that death is the outcome and time is measured from assignment to one of the two alternative drug therapies, with "exposed" = new therapy assigned and "unexposed" = standard therapy assigned. If age at assignment and sex are the other stratifying factors, each stratum in the analysis will contain the number of deaths and subjects remaining alive at a specific death time among patients of a specific age and sex.

A stratification that places a boundary at every incidence time will produce sparse strata, because each stratum will contain only those cases that occurred at that time in that stratum. If there is no stratification variable other than time, there will be only one or two cases in most strata; if there are other stratification variables, many strata will contain no case. Thus, one should use only sparse-data methods (exact, conditional maximum-likelihood, or Mantel-Haenszel) for the analysis.

Having stratified the data on incidence time, and perhaps other variables, one may tally the exposed and unexposed person-time within strata and apply standard methods for stratified person-time data. Consider again the data in Table 16–3. The AG-negative and AG-positive person-times at risk observed in each time interval are

$$T_{1k} = N_{1k}\Delta t_k \quad \text{and} \quad T_{0k} = N_{0k}\Delta t_k$$

For example, the times at risk for $k = 4$ are 3(7) = 21 negative weeks and 3(12) = 36 positive weeks. From the formulas given in Chapter 15, the Mantel-Haenszel estimate of a uniform rate ratio comparing AG-negative patients to AG-positive patients is 6.24, with a log rate-ratio variance estimate of 0.445, which yields 90% confidence limits of 2.08 and 18.7. The Mantel-Haenszel person-time χ (score statistic) is 3.14 (two-sided $P = 0.0017$). We note, however, that these data do not quite fulfill the large-sample criteria given earlier: There are only four deaths among the positives (i.e., $A_{0+} = 4$). Thus, use of small-sample methods is preferable.

Use of person-times (as in the preceding example) implicitly assumes that the rates are homogeneous (constant) over the time intervals between disease times. This assumption can be avoided, at a small increase in variance, by using a simpler and more common approach in which one forms a 2 × 2 table for each stratum. Each table contains the number of cases occurring in that stratum's time interval and the number of subjects (noncases) remaining at risk through the end of the stratum's time interval. One then analyzes the odds ratios in the resulting set of 2 × 2 tables using any of the large-sample or small-sample (exact) methods given in Chapter 15.

A simple rationale for the odds-ratio approach is as follows: Suppose that one adheres to our earlier recommendations and measures incidence time on a scale fine enough so that no tied incidence time occurs (that is, only one case occurs at each time-interval boundary t_k), and one does not attempt to analyze follow-up beyond the point at which five survivors remain under observation in each exposure group. Then, within each exposure group and time interval, the proportion observed to get disease will be low (mostly less than $1/5 = 0.20$, and often 0). As a consequence, we expect the uniform odds ratio estimate obtained from analyzing the data as a series of 2 × 2 tables to be close to the uniform rate-ratio estimate obtained from a person-time analysis (which involves slightly more labor and one extra assumption).

Consider again Table 16–3. Using only the counts to form 2 × 2 tables (A_{1k}, B_{1k}, N_{1k}, and A_{0k}, B_{0k}, N_{0k} in each table's columns), instead of the person-times, we obtain a Mantel-Haenszel odds-ratio estimate comparing negatives to positives of 7.58 (which is here being used to approximate a rate ratio), with a log odds-ratio variance estimate of 0.461. These yield 90% limits of 2.48 and 23.2. From the formula in Chapter 15, the Mantel-Haenszel χ statistic for these count data is 3.24

(two-sided $P = 0.0012$). These results are close to the direct person-time results (rate ratio = 6.24, 90% limits = 2.08, 18.7), considering that none of the criteria for a good approximation is met: There are only four positive cases; only two negative subjects survived the whole period (i.e., $B_{0K} = 2$); and there are several tied death times (in four of the nine strata there is more than 1 death, so it would have been better to measure time in days, not weeks).

Using more sophisticated arguments, it is possible to show that in large enough samples and with time measured finely enough (essentially, as a continuous variable), the conditional maximum-likelihood and Mantel-Haenszel odds-ratio estimates from the time-stratified 2 × 2 tables will provide valid estimates of a rate-ratio parameter that is constant (uniform) over time (Cox and Oakes, 1984). Furthermore, the Mantel-Haenszel statistic for pure count data when applied to the tables will supply a valid test of the null hypothesis (that the incidence rates for the exposed and unexposed groups are equal within strata). When applied in this manner to survival analysis data, the Mantel-Haenszel test is often called the *log-rank test.*

In an approximate (large-sample) sense, the log-rank test is as powerful as any valid and unbiased test can be under the uniform rate-ratio model. There are, however, other simple models for exposure effect in which the log-rank test is generally inferior to alternatives (Kalbfleisch and Prentice, 2002; Cox and Oakes, 1984). Perhaps the most important of these is the accelerated-life (accelerated failure-time) model, which we will describe briefly in Chapter 20.

ATTRIBUTABLE FRACTION ESTIMATION

ADJUSTED ATTRIBUTABLE FRACTION ESTIMATES

Suppose that we study a closed cohort and a causal exposure. Recall from the results in Chapter 4 that the fraction of exposed cases that would not have occurred if exposure had not occurred (the attributable fraction among the exposed) is given by

$$AF_e = (RR - 1)/RR$$

where RR is the causal risk ratio (the proportionate increase in average risk among the exposed produced by exposure). If stratification has successfully removed all confounding and there is no bias, the risk ratio standardized to the exposed (the SMR parameter) will equal the causal risk ratio. Thus, we will get a valid estimate and confidence limits for AF_e from any valid estimate of the SMR:

$$\widehat{AF}_e = (\widehat{SMR} - 1)/\widehat{SMR} \qquad [16\text{–}19]$$

$$\underline{AF}_e,\ \overline{AF}_e = (\underline{SMR} - 1)/\underline{SMR},\ (\overline{SMR} - 1)/\overline{SMR}$$

The situation is not so simple if we wish to estimate the fraction of *all* cases (exposed and unexposed) that would not have occurred if exposure had not occurred, the population attributable fraction AF_p. Suppose that the numbers exposed and unexposed in the cohort are N_1 and N_0. If no adjustment is needed, we have the simple relation

$$AF_p = \frac{N_1(R_1 - R_0)}{N_1R_1 + N_0R_0} = \frac{p(RR - 1)}{p(RR - 1) - 1} \qquad [16\text{–}20]$$

where $p = N_1/(N_1 + N_0)$ is the proportion exposed in the entire cohort.

If adjustment is needed, the above simple formula (equation 16–20) for AF_p no longer holds (Greenland, 1984b). If the stratification successfully removes confounding, we still have the following simple formula, however:

$$AF_p = p_c AF_e = p_c \frac{SMR - 1}{SMR} \qquad [16\text{–}21]$$

where again the SMR is the risk ratio standardized to the exposed and p_c is exposure prevalence *among cases* (Miettinen, 1974b). Another useful decomposition of AF_p is as a weighted average of stratum-specific population attributable fractions AF_{pi}:

$$AF_p = \sum_i p_i AF_{pi} \qquad [16\text{–}22]$$

where p_i is the proportion of cases falling in stratum i (Walter, 1976).

In almost all situations, p_c and the p_i are not known. If, however, they can be validly estimated from the study data, we can use the simple point estimator

$$\widehat{AF}_p = \hat{p}_c \frac{\widehat{SMR} - 1}{\widehat{SMR}} = \sum_i \hat{p}_i \widehat{AF}_{pi} \qquad [16\text{–}23]$$

where

$$\hat{p}_c = A_{1+}/M_{1+} \qquad \hat{p}_i = M_{1i}/M_{1+} \qquad \widehat{AF}_{pi} = \frac{A_{1i}}{M_{1i}} \frac{\widehat{RR}_i - 1}{\widehat{RR}_i}$$

and $\widehat{SMR}$ is the estimate of the risk ratio standardized to the exposed. If the risk ratio is homogeneous across strata and the disease is uncommon, we can replace $\widehat{SMR}$ with any valid common rate-ratio or common odds-ratio estimator:

$$\widehat{AF}_p = \frac{A_{1+}}{M_{1+}} \frac{\widehat{RR} - 1}{\widehat{RR}} \qquad [16\text{–}24]$$

where $\widehat{RR}$ may be a maximum-likelihood or Mantel-Haenszel estimator of a common rate ratio IR or a common odds ratio OR.

For setting confidence limits, it helps to transform AF_p to $H = \ln(1 - AF_p)$. Then $\hat{H} = \ln(1 - \widehat{AF}_p)$ has variance estimator

$$\widehat{\text{Var}}(\hat{H}) = \widehat{\text{Var}}[\ln(1 - \widehat{AF}_p)] = \frac{\widehat{AF}_p{}^2}{(1 - \widehat{AF}_p)^2} \left[\frac{\hat{V}}{(\widehat{RR} - 1)^2} + \frac{2}{A_{1+}(\widehat{RR} - 1)} + \frac{A_{0+}}{A_{1+}M_{1+}} \right] \qquad [16\text{–}25]$$

where $\hat{V}$ is a variance estimator for $\ln(\widehat{RR})$, such as one of those given in Chapter 15, as appropriate (Greenland, 1987c). The limits $\underline{H}, \overline{H} = \hat{H} \pm Z_\alpha \widehat{\text{Var}}(\hat{H})^{1/2}$ found using equation 16–25 can then be transformed back to limits for $AF_p = 1 - \exp(-H)$. The point and interval estimators of AF_p obtained from 16–24 and 16–25 will be valid in sparse data if the *RR* and variance estimators used in the formulas are valid in sparse data (e.g., a Mantel-Haenszel or a conditional maximum-likelihood [CML] estimator).

To estimate the fraction of coronary deaths in the British Doctors Study (Chapter 15, Table 15–2) that could be attributable to smoking, we use the Mantel-Haenszel estimate computed from Chapter 15, Table 15–4, which was $\widehat{IR}_{MH} = 1.424$ with variance estimate for $\ln(\widehat{IR}_{MH}) = 0.01150$. These yield

$$\widehat{AF}_p = \frac{630}{731} \frac{1.424 - 1}{1.424} = 0.255$$

$$\widehat{\text{Var}}[\ln(1 - \widehat{AF}_p)] = \frac{0.255^2}{0.745^2} \left[\frac{0.01150}{0.424^2} + \frac{2}{630(0.424)} + \frac{101}{630(731)} \right]$$
$$= 0.008397$$

and 95% limits for $\ln(1 - AF_p)$ of $\ln(1 - 0.255) \pm 1.96(0.008397)^{1/2} = -0.4740, -0.1148$. The latter transform to AF_p limits of $1 - \exp(-0.1148)$, $1 - \exp(-0.4740) = 0.108, 0.377$. Using the SMR estimate instead yields almost the same $\widehat{AF}_p$ estimate,

$$\widehat{AF}_p = \frac{630}{731} \frac{1.43 - 1}{1.43} = 0.259$$

One might be tempted to interpret these estimates as indicating that on the order of 25% fewer coronary deaths would have occurred had these doctors not smoked. Of course, this interpretation assumes that biases are absent. The interpretation also assumes that absence of smoking would not expand the person-years at risk of coronary death by removing other (competing) risks for death, such as lung cancer. This assumption cannot be exactly true, because smoking does affect the rates of many other causes of death, particularly lung cancer.

The preceding example points out that the common public health interpretation of the attributable fraction (as potential caseload reduction) assumes that removing exposure will not affect the size of the population at risk. This assumption is not always correct, and it needs to be scrutinized in any discussion of an attributable-fraction estimate. For example, to estimate the excess of Down syndrome cases that could be attributable to spermicide exposure in the study in Chapter 15, Table 15–5, we might use the Mantel-Haenszel odds ratio of 3.78 as an approximate risk-ratio estimate (because Down syndrome is very uncommon). This odds ratio yields

$$\widehat{AF}_{\mathrm{p}} = \frac{4}{16}\,\frac{3.78 - 1}{3.78} = 0.18$$

which seems to suggest that on the order of 20% fewer cases would have occurred if no one had used spermicide. Again, this interpretation assumes that bias is absent. Even if the study were perfectly valid, however, this figure could not be interpreted as the effect of spermicide use on the number of Down syndrome cases, because this interpretation unrealistically assumes that absence of spermicide use would not lead to more pregnancies. In reality, absence of spermicide use would probably lead to more pregnancies, thus expanding the source cohort and increasing the number of cases.

ETIOLOGIC FRACTION AND PROBABILITY OF CAUSATION

As we have defined it, the attributable fraction is the excess caseload arising over a risk period due to the presence of exposure as opposed to its absence. This quantity sounds like and hence is often confused with the etiologic fraction, in which the latter is the fraction of cases for whom exposure was involved in the causal mechanism (or sufficient cause) that produced the disease. As discussed in Chapters 2 and 4, however, the latter quantity may be quite a bit larger than the attributable fraction, because it includes cases caused by exposure that would have occurred from other causes if exposure had been absent (Greenland and Robins, 1988; Robins and Greenland, 1989a). Thus, even for a purely causal exposure, it is logically possible for the attributable (excess) fraction to be 0% and the etiologic fraction to be 100%. This possibility would happen, for example, if exposure never affected anyone who would not get the disease if unexposed, but displaced another causal component among all those who would get the disease if unexposed. Note well that such phenomena can occur no matter how rare the outcome is or how short the time period under study is.

Like the risk ratio from which it is derived, the attributable fraction requires no biologic model for its estimation. Thus, it can be estimated from epidemiologic data using only the usual assumptions about study validity and that the exposure does not change the population at risk. In contrast, estimation of the etiologic fraction requires assumptions about the mechanism of exposure action, especially in relation to sufficient causes that act in the absence of exposure. At one extreme, mechanisms involving exposure would occur and act independently of other "background" mechanisms, in which case the attributable and etiologic fractions will be equal. At the other extreme, in which exposure advances the incidence time whenever a background mechanism is present, the attributable fraction can be tiny but the etiologic fraction will be 100% (Robins and Greenland, 1989a). Both extremes are rather implausible in typical settings, and there is rarely enough information to pin down the etiologic fraction, even if the attributable fraction is known accurately.

The distinction is of great social importance because of the equality between the etiologic fraction and the *probability of causation,* where the latter is the probability that the disease of a randomly selected case was produced by a mechanism involving exposure (and usually the population under discussion is restricted to the exposed only). The same arguments apply as with the etiologic fraction: The attributable fraction and the probability of causation may be very far apart, and to estimate the probability of causation one must make strong assumptions about the mechanism of exposure action (Robins and Greenland, 1989b; Beyea and Greenland, 1999; Greenland and Robins, 2000).

The confusion between the attributable fraction and the probability of causation has led to serious distortions in regulatory and legal decision criteria (Greenland, 1999a; Robins and Greenland, 2000). The distortions arise when criteria based solely on epidemiologic evidence (such as estimated relative risks) are used to determine whether the probability of causation meets some threshold. The most common mistake is to infer that the probability of causation is below 50% when the relative risk is inferred to be below 2. The reasoning is that $(RR - 1)/RR$ represents the probability of causation, and that this quantity is below 50% unless RR is at least 2. This reasoning is fallacious, however, because $(RR - 1)/RR$ is the attributable fraction among the exposed. It thus may understate the probability of causation to an arbitrarily large degree, in the same manner as it understates the etiologic fraction, even if the RR estimate is highly valid and precise (Robins and Greenland, 1989b; Greenland, 1999a; Greenland and Robins, 2000).

ANALYSES OF BIOLOGIC INTERACTIONS

BIOLOGIC INTERACTION AND ADDITIVITY CONDITIONS

A number of basic relations among risks and rates can be derived under various assumptions regarding biologic interactions (e.g., Koopman, 1981; Walker, 1981; Miettinen, 1982b; Weinberg, 1986; Greenland and Poole, 1988; Robins and Greenland, 1989a; Koopman and Weed, 1990; VanderWeele and Robins, 2007a, 2008a). As described in Chapter 5 for two binary variables, absence of interaction response types will lead to an additive pattern among the causal risk differences. This relation means that the sum of the differences comparing the risks given each factor alone to the risk in absence of both factors will equal the difference comparing risk given both factors to risk absent both factors. Suppose that X and Z are binary variables equal to 1 or 0, and let R_{xz} be the average risk in a given cohort when factor $X = x$ and factor $Z = z$. Additivity corresponds to

$$R_{11} - R_{00} = R_{10} - R_{00} + R_{01} - R_{00}$$

If we define RD_{xz} to be $R_{xz} - R_{00}$, then additivity is $RD_{11} = RD_{10} + RD_{01}$.

Assuming that neither factor is ever preventive, superadditivity ($RD_{11} > RD_{10} + RD_{01}$, also known as transadditivity) can occur only if synergistic response types (type 8 in Table 5–2) are present; subadditivity ($RD_{11} < RD_{10} + RD_{01}$) can occur only if competitive (type 2 in Table 5–2) or antagonistic response types are present. We also have that the "interaction contrast" $IC = RD_{11} - RD_{10} - RD_{01}$ is zero if and only if the risk differences for X are constant across Z and the risk differences for Z are constant across X, that is,

$$IC = RD_{11} - RD_{10} - RD_{01} = R_{11} - R_{10} - R_{01} + R_{00} = 0$$

if and only if $R_{11} - R_{10} = R_{01} - R_{00}$ and $R_{11} - R_{01} = R_{10} - R_{00}$.

Recall that R_{11}, R_{01}, R_{10}, and R_{00} refer to only *one* target cohort under *four* different exposure conditions. Unfortunately, we can only observe different cohorts under different exposure conditions, and we must adjust for any difference of these cohorts from the target cohort via standardization or some other technique. Suppose that we have four adjusted estimates $\hat{R}_{11}$, $\hat{R}_{01}$, $\hat{R}_{10}$, $\hat{R}_{00}$ of average risk in the target cohort under the four possible exposure conditions (these estimates may be obtained in a manner that accounts for losses to follow-up, as in survival analysis). Then if $\widehat{RD}_{jk} = \hat{R}_{jk} - \hat{R}_{00}$, our estimate of the interaction contrast is

$$\widehat{IC} = \widehat{RD}_{11} - \widehat{RD}_{10} - \widehat{RD}_{01} = \hat{R}_{11} - \hat{R}_{01} - \hat{R}_{10} - \hat{R}_{00}$$

Because additivity (an interaction contrast of zero) corresponds to homogeneity (uniformity) of the risk differences, we can use any test of risk-difference homogeneity as a test of additivity (Hogan et al., 1978). If the average-risk estimates $\hat{R}_{xz}$ are standardized based on weights from the target population, a variance estimate for $\widehat{IC}$ is the sum of the separate variance estimates for the $\hat{R}_{xz}$. These separate variance estimates can be computed as described in Chapter 15. On the other hand, if the risks are estimated using a homogeneity assumption (for example, that the risk or odds ratios are constant across the confounder strata), then more complex variance estimates must be used, and it is easier to recast the problem as one of testing and estimating product terms in additive-risk models (Chapters 20 and 21).

The risk differences RD_{xz} cannot be estimated from case-control data without an estimate of sampling fractions or incidence in the source population for the study. Absent such an estimate, one can still test the additivity hypothesis from case-control data if the observed odds ratios can be used to estimate the risk ratios. To see this, let $RR_{xz} = R_{xz}/R_{00}$ and let

$$\begin{aligned} ICR &= IC/R_{00} = R_{11}/R_{00} - R_{10}/R_{00} - R_{01}/R_{00} + R_{00}/R_{00} \\ &= RR_{11} - RR_{10} - RR_{01} + 1 \end{aligned}$$

Then $ICR = 0$ if and only if the interaction contrast IC equals 0. Thus, any P-value for the hypothesis $ICR = 0$ provides a P-value for the additivity hypothesis. Furthermore, because ICR and IC must have the same sign (direction), we can infer superadditivity (or subadditivity) if we can infer that $ICR > 0$ (or $ICR < 0$). One can construct a P-value for $ICR = 0$ from stratified case-control data alone. It is, however, much easier to recast the problem as one of examining product terms in additive odds-ratio models (Chapters 20 and 21). ICR has previously been labeled the "relative excess risk for interaction" or RERI (Rothman, 1986). Several interaction measures besides IC and ICR have been proposed that reflect the presence of interaction types under certain assumptions (Rothman 1976b, 1986; Walker, 1981; Hosmer and Lemeshow, 1992).

Suppose now that all the risk differences contrasting level 1 to level 0 are positive, i.e., $RD_{11} > \max(RD_{10}, RD_{01})$ and $\min(RD_{10}, RD_{01}) > 0$ or, equivalently, $RR_{11} > \max(RR_{10}, RR_{01})$ and $\min(RR_{10}, RR_{01}) > 1$. We then have that risk-ratio multiplicativity or beyond, $RR_{11} \geq RR_{10}(RR_{01})$, implies superadditivity $RD_{11} > RD_{10} + RD_{01}$ or, equivalently, $RR_{11} > RR_{10} + RR_{01} - 1$ or $IC > 0$. Thus, by assuming a multiplicative model with positive risk differences, we are forcing superadditivity to hold. Parallel results involving negative differences follow from recoding X or Z or both (switching 1 and 0 as the codes) to make all the differences positive.

Next, suppose that $R_{11} > R_{10} + R_{01}$ or, equivalently, $RR_{11} > RR_{10} + RR_{01}$. VanderWeele and Robins (2007a, 2008a) show that these conditions imply the presence of causal co-action (co-participation in a sufficient cause, or interaction in a sufficient-cause model). They also show how to test these conditions and adjust for confounders when substituting estimates for the risks, and extend these results to co-action among three or more variables. Again, parallel results with protective (negative) net effects follow from recoding X or Z or both. These conditions imply superadditivity but can coexist with submultiplicative or supermultiplicative relations. In particular, if both $RR_{10} < 2$ and $RR_{01} < 2$ (both effects "weakly positive"), then multiplicativity will imply that $RR_{11} < RR_{10} + RR_{01}$, but if both $RR_{10} > 2$ and $RR_{01} > 2$ (both effects are "not weak"), then multiplicativity will imply that $RR_{11} > RR_{10} + RR_{01}$. Thus, assuming a multiplicative model with positive effects does *not* by itself force $RR_{11} > RR_{10} + RR_{01}$, even though that model *does* force $RR_{11} > RR_{10} + RR_{01} - 1$ ("superadditive risks").

LIMITATIONS OF STATISTICAL INFERENCES ABOUT INTERACTIONS

Several arguments have been made that interaction relations and measures may have limited practical utility (e.g., Thompson, 1991). First, as described in Chapter 15, study size is usually set to address the average effect of a single exposure, which involves comparison across groups defined by a single variable. Interaction analyses require dividing the study population into smaller groups to create contrasts across subgroups defined by multiple variables. Interaction analyses are therefore handicapped in that they compare smaller subsets of study subjects and thus have less precision than the primary study analysis. For example, statistical tests of additivity (as well as tests for other statistical interactions) have very little power at typical study sizes, and the corresponding estimates of departures from additivity have little precision (Greenland, 1983; Breslow and Day, 1987; Lubin et al., 1990).

Another problem is that simple assumptions (such as no interaction) become difficult to justify when the two factors X and Z are replaced by continuous variables. For example, it can become impossible to separate assumptions about induction time and dose–response from those concerning interactions (Thomas, 1981; Greenland, 1993a). Even greater complexity arises when effects of other variables must be considered. Third, as shown in Chapter 5, one cannot infer that a particular interaction response type is absent, and inference of presence must make assumptions about absence of other response types. As a result, inferences about the presence of particular response types must depend on very restrictive assumptions about absence of other response types, even when *qualitative* statistical interactions are present, that is, when the epidemiologic measure of the effect of one factor entirely reverses direction across levels of another factor.

Regardless of these issues, it is important not to confuse statistical interaction (effect-measure modification) with biologic interaction. In particular, when two factors have effects and the study estimates are valid, risk-ratio homogeneity—though often misinterpreted as indicating absence of biologic interaction—in fact implies *presence* of interaction response types (as defined in Chapter 5), because homogeneity of the risk, rate, or odds ratio implies heterogeneity (and hence nonadditivity) of the risk differences.

ANALYSES OF INDUCTION PERIODS

Ideally, causal analyses should be longitudinal rather than cross-sectional, in that there should be an allowance for a time interval between exposure and disease onset that corresponds to a meaningful induction period. In cohort studies, the interval may be accommodated by restricting the accumulation of person-time experience in the denominator of incidence rates for the exposed to that period of time following exposure that corresponds to the limits of the possible induction period. In case-control studies, the interval may be accommodated by obtaining data on exposure status at a time that precedes the disease onset or control selection by an amount that corresponds to the limits of the possible induction period.

Suppose that one is studying whether exposure to canine distemper in one's pet causes multiple sclerosis, and the induction period (to the time of diagnosis) is assumed to be 10 to 25 years. Using the latter assumption in a cohort study, exposed individuals will not contribute to person-time at risk until 10 years from the time the pet had distemper. Such contribution to the risk experience begin at 10 years and last 15 years (the duration of the induction-time interval), or less if the subject is removed from follow-up (because he or she died, was lost, or was diagnosed with multiple sclerosis). Only if multiple sclerosis is diagnosed during this same interval will it be considered to be potentially related to exposure. In a case-control study, cases of multiple sclerosis would be classified as exposed if the patient's pet dog had distemper during the interval of 10 to 25 years before the diagnosis of multiple sclerosis. If exposure to distemper occurred outside this time window, the case would be considered unexposed. Controls would be questioned with reference to a comparable time period and similarly classified.

It is also possible to study and compare different possible induction periods. An example of this technique was a case-control study of pyloric stenosis that examined the role of Bendectin exposure during early gestation (Aselton et al., 1984). Different time windows of 1-week duration during early pregnancy were assumed. Exposure before week 6 of pregnancy or after week 12 led to a relative-risk estimate of less than 2, whereas an estimate greater than 3 was obtained for exposure to Bendectin during weeks 6 to 12. The largest effect estimate, a relative risk of 3.7, was obtained for exposure during weeks 8 and 9 after conception. This example illustrates how epidemiologic analyses have been used to estimate a narrow period of causal action. If only one analysis had been conducted using a single exposure period before or after the relevant one, little or no information about the time relation between exposure and disease would have resulted.

All analyses of exposure effects are based on some assumption about induction time. If a case-control study measures exposure from birth (or conception) until diagnosis, some period that is irrelevant to meaningful exposure is likely to be included, diluting the measurement of relevant exposure. If a cross-sectional study examines current exposure and disease (the onset of which may even have antedated the exposure), this too involves use of an irrelevant exposure, if only as a proxy for the unknown relevant exposure. Often the assumption about induction period is implicit and obscure. Good research practice dictates making such assumptions explicit and evaluating them to the extent possible.

If the wrong induction period is used, the resulting exposure measure may be thought of as a mismeasured version of the true exposure. Under certain assumptions (see Chapter 9) this mismeasurement would tend to reduce the magnitude of associations and underestimate effects: The smaller the overlap between the assumed induction period window in a given analysis and the actual induction times, the greater the amount of nondifferential misclassification and consequent bias toward the null. Ideally, a set of induction-time assumptions would produce a set of effect estimates that reach a peak for an induction-time assumption that corresponds more closely to the correct value than alternative assumptions. Rothman (1981) proposed that this phenomenon could be used to infer the induction period, as in the study on pyloric stenosis. By repeating the analysis of the data while varying the assigned limits (or "window") for the induction period, one could see whether a consistent pattern of effects emerged that reflected apparent nondifferential misclassification of exposure with various induction time assumptions. Rothman (1981) suggested that, if such a pattern is apparent, the middle of the assumed induction period that gives the largest effect estimate will estimate the average induction period.

A closely related and perhaps more common approach to induction-period analysis involves *exposure lagging,* in which only exposures preceding a certain cutoff time before disease occurrence (in cases) or sampling time (for controls in a case-control study) are used to determine exposure status. Similarly, the exposure of a person-time unit (such as a person-year) is determined only by the status of the contributing person before a given cutoff time (Checkoway et al., 1989, 1990). For example, to lag asbestos exposure by 5 years, only exposure up to 5 years before disease time would be used to classify cases; in a case-control study, only exposure up to 5 years before sampling time would be used to classify controls; and, in a cohort study, only a person's exposure up to 5 years before a given year at risk would be used to classify the exposure of the person-year contributed by that person in that year.

Lagged analysis may be repeated using different lag periods. One might then take the lag that yields the strongest association as an estimated induction period. Note that this use of induction period refers to a *minimum* time for pathogenesis and detection, rather than an average time as with the window method.

Unfortunately, there can be serious problems with "largest estimate" methods, whether based on windows or lags, especially if they are applied without regard to whether the data demonstrate a regular pattern of estimates. Without evidence of such a pattern, these approaches will tend to pick out induction periods whose estimate is large simply by virtue of large statistical variability. Estimates of effect derived in this way will be biased away from the null and will not serve well as a summary estimate of effect. To deal with these problems, Salvan et al. (1995) proposed taking the induction period that yields the highest likelihood-ratio (deviance) statistic for exposure effect as the estimated induction period. This approach is equivalent to taking the induction period that yields the lowest P-value and so corresponds to taking the most "statistically significant" estimate. The result will be that the final P-value will be biased downward, i.e., it will understate the probability of getting a statistic as extreme or more extreme than observed if there are no exposure effects.

Another problem is that the degree of bias resulting from exposure misclassification can vary across windows for reasons that are not related to the exposure effect. For example, the degree of misclassification bias depends in part on the exposure prevalence (Chapter 19). Hence, variation in exposure prevalence over time will lead to variation in misclassification bias over time, so it can distort the pattern of effect estimates across time windows.

A third problem in any approach based on separate analyses of windows is that they do not control for an exposure effect that appears in multiple windows (that is, an exposure effect that has a long and variable induction time, so that the exposure effect is reflected in several windows). Such "multiple effects" often (if not always) lead to mutual confounding among the estimates obtained using just one window at a time (Robins, 1987), because exposures tend to be highly associated across windows. Furthermore, the resulting confounding will almost certainly vary in magnitude across windows. For example, the association of exposures in adjacent windows will often be higher than those for nonadjacent windows. In that case, effect estimates for windows adjacent to those close to the true induction period will be more confounded than other estimates.

A first attempt to avoid the problems just mentioned would estimate the effects for each window while adjusting for the exposures from other windows (as well as other confounders). There are two problems with this approach. A major practical problem is that one may quickly run out of numbers when trying to examine one window while stratifying on other windows and confounders. In the Bendectin example, use of 1-week windows during 5 to 15 weeks would yield 11 windows, so that estimates for one window would have to control for 10 other window variables, plus other confounders. One could limit this problem by using just a few broad windows, at a cost of precision in the definitions.

A more subtle theoretical problem is that exposures in early windows can affect exposures in later windows. As a result, effect estimates for earlier windows will at best only reflect direct effects of exposures in those windows (Robins, 1987, 1989), and at worst may be more biased than the one-at-a-time estimates because of confounding generated by control of the intermediate windows (Robins and Greenland, 1992; Cole and Hernán, 2002; Chapter 12). To deal with the problems inherent in using all exposure windows in the same analysis, several authors have developed sophisticated modeling methods for analyses of longitudinal exposure data. These methods incorporate all exposure variables into a single model, which may have an explicit parameter for average induction time (Thomas, 1988) or may be based on parameters for disease time (Robins, 1997). The latter *g-estimation* methods will be discussed in Chapter 21.

Despite the potential for bias, we suggest a preliminary stratified analysis using windows broad enough to allow simultaneous control of other windows, as well as other confounders, which should then be followed by more sophisticated methods. We caution, however, that even with this approach, the overall pattern of estimates across the windows should be taken into account. Simply choosing the largest estimate will lead to a result that is biased away from the null as an estimate of the largest window effect; the smallest P-value will *not* provide a valid test of the null hypothesis of no exposure effect; and the induction times that define the windows with the largest effect estimate and smallest P-value will not provide an unbiased estimate of average induction time. Nonetheless, a table of estimates obtained from a simultaneous analysis of windows can provide an initial idea of the shape of the induction-time distribution, subject to restrictive assumptions that there is no measurement error and no confounding of any window when other windows are controlled.

CHAPTER 17

Analysis of Polytomous Exposures and Outcomes

Sander Greenland

Categorization of Ordered Variables 303
Basic Tabular Analysis 305
Dose–Response and Trend Analysis 308
Graphing a Trend 308
Plotting Confidence Limits 309
Vertical Scaling 310
Incremental (Slope) Plots 311
Horizontal Scaling and Category Scores 312
Smoothing the Graph 313
Trend Statistics 314
Special Handling of the Zero Level 316
Moving Averages 317
Variable-Span Smoothers 321
Categorical Estimates as Moving Averages 321
More General Smoothers 321
Basic Analysis of Multiple Outcomes 321
Simultaneous Statistics for Tabular Data 323
Joint Confidence Regions 324
Simultaneous Analysis of Multiple Outcomes 325
Relation between Simultaneous and Single Comparisons 326

This chapter introduces extensions of tabular analysis methods to polytomous data—that is, data in which the exposure or outcome has more than two levels. These extensions provide a conceptual bridge between simple tabular methods and more sophisticated regression analysis, as well as being useful in their own right. They also provide an initial approach to dose–response and trend analyses. Finally, they provide an important means of checking the results of regression analyses, to see if patterns suggested by regressions can be seen in the basic counts that summarize the data.

The primary focus in this chapter is on methods for analyzing an exposure with multiple levels and a binary disease outcome. It also shows how these methods extend to analyses of multiple outcomes, such as arise when multiple diseases are under study or when a case-control study employs multiple control groups. It begins, however, by reviewing issues in categorization of variables, because most of the methods discussed in this chapter assume that exposure is categorized.

CATEGORIZATION OF ORDERED VARIABLES

As discussed in Chapters 13 and 15, choice of categories for variables is an important step in data analysis. When the variable is measured on an ordered scale with many levels, one often sees this step disposed of by using percentile category boundaries. For example, quartiles correspond to four categories with boundaries at the 25th, 50th, and 75th percentiles, whereas quintiles correspond to five categories with boundaries at the 20th, 40th, 60th, and 80th percentiles. Such automatic procedures for category formation are suboptimal in most applications and can sometimes be quite harmful to power, precision, and confounder control (Lagakos, 1988; Zhao and Kolonel, 1992;

Greenland, 1995a, 1995b). Percentile boundaries also make it difficult to compare associations or effects across studies, because those boundaries will correspond to different exposure values in each study.

Most important, percentile categories rarely correspond to subject-matter knowledge. Instead, they blindly lump together disparate subgroups of subjects and may thereby hide important effects. For example, vitamin C levels are high enough in most Western diets that persons with borderline or deficient intakes will constitute less than 10% of a typical study group. As a result, these people will compose fewer than half of the subjects in the lowest quartile for vitamin C intake. If only this deficient minority suffers an elevated disease risk, this fact will be obscured by the quartile analysis. The elevated risk of the 10% minority is averaged with the normal risk of the 15% majority in the lowest quartile, and then compared with the normal risk in the three higher-intake quartiles. There will be only a limited elevation of risk in the lowest quartile, which might be difficult to detect in a categorical analysis.

As another example, in many occupational and environmental studies only a small percentage of subjects have a biologically important amount of exposure. Here again, use of quartiles or quintiles submerges these subjects among a larger mass of barely exposed (and thus unaffected) subjects, thereby reducing power and possibly inducing a biased impression of dose–response (Greenland 1995b, 1995c). Mixing persons of different risk in broad categories is also a problem when the categorized variable is a strong confounder. In this situation, broad categories of the confounder can result in stratum-specific estimates with substantial residual confounding.

Perhaps the most common alternative to percentiles is equally spaced boundaries. For example, vitamin C intake might be categorized in 10- or 20-mg increments of daily average intake. Such boundaries often make more subject-matter sense than percentiles, because they allow those with very low or very high intake to be put in separate categories and because the categories conform with familiar units of dose. Nonetheless, equally spaced boundaries are also generally suboptimal and, like percentile boundaries, can sometimes submerge high-risk groups and yield poor power and precision (Greenland, 1995b).

Ideally, categories should make sense based on external information. This guideline can be especially important and easiest to accomplish in categorization of confounders, because the prior information that led to their identification can also be used to create categories. To illustrate, consider maternal age as a potential confounder in perinatal studies. The relation of maternal age to risk can be poorly captured by either percentile or equally spaced categories, because most maternal-age effects tend to be concentrated at one or both extremes. For example, risk of neonatal death is highest when the mother is under 18 or over 40 years of age, whereas risk of Down syndrome is highest when the mother is over 40 years of age, with very little change in risk of either outcome during the peak reproductive ages of 20 to 35 years. Yet in typical U.S. or European populations, quartile or quintile boundaries would fall within this homogeneous-risk range, as would standard equally spaced maternal age category boundaries of, say, 20, 25, 30, and 35 years. Quartile categories, quintile categories, and these equally spaced categories would all fail to separate the heterogeneous mix of risks at the extremes of maternal age, and would instead focus attention on the intermediate age range, with its small differences in risk.

Ideal categories would be such that any important differences in risk will exist between them but not within them. Unfortunately, this scheme may result in some categories (especially end categories) with too few subjects to obtain a reasonably precise estimate of the outcome measure in that category. One way to cope with this problem is to broaden the categories gradually until there are adequate numbers in each one, while retaining meaningful boundaries. In doing so, however, it is important to avoid defining categories based on the size of the estimates obtained from the categorizations unless the shape of the trend is known (e.g., as for a well-studied confounder such as age). If category choice is based on the resulting estimates, the trend estimates and standard errors from the final categorization may be biased. For example, if we collapse together adjacent categories to maximize the appearance of a linear trend, the apparent trend in the final estimates will be biased toward a linear pattern, away from any true departures from linearity. Such a collapsing procedure might be justifiable, however, if it were known that the true trend was approximately linear.

Open-ended categories (e.g., "20+ years exposure") are particularly hazardous because they may encompass a broad range of exposure or confounder effects. We thus recommend that one make sure the single boundary of an open-ended category is not too far from the most extreme value in the category. For example, if having more than 10 additional years of exposure could have a large effect on risk, we would try to avoid using the "20+ years exposure" category if the largest exposure value in the data is >30 years. Another drawback of open-ended categories is the difficulty of assigning a point to the category against which its response might be plotted.

A consequence of using close to ideal categories is that the cell counts within strata may become small. One sometimes sees books that recommend adding ½ to each cell of a table in which the counts are small. Worse, some packaged programs automatically add ½ to all cells when one or more cell count equals 0. This practice is suboptimal because it can create distortions in certain statistics; for example, it artificially inflates the study size. More sophisticated methods for handling small counts have long been available (Chapter 12 of Bishop et al., 1975; Greenland, 2006b). For example, one may replace each cell count with an average of that count and the count expected under a simple hypothesis or model. A version of this approach will be described later, in the section on graphics. An alternative to such procedures is to employ methods that do not require large cells, such as Mantel-Haenszel methods, exact methods, moving averages, and running lines or curves.

We emphasize again that all the above problems of exposure categorization apply to confounder categorization (Greenland 1995a; Greenland 1995b; Brenner and Blettner 1997; Brenner, 1998; Austin and Brunner 2006). In particular, use of automated categorization methods such as percentile boundaries can easily lead to overly broad categories in which much residual confounding remains.

BASIC TABULAR ANALYSIS

Table 17–1 displays the notation we use for stratified person-time data with $J+1$ exposure levels and with strata indexed by i. In this table, the ellipses represent all the remaining exposure levels X_j, counts A_{ji}, and person-times T_{ji} between level X_J and level X_1. (If there are only three levels, $J=2$ and there is no level between X_J and X_1.) We will always take the rightmost (X_0) exposure column to be the reference level of exposure, against which the J nonreference levels will be compared. Usually, X_0 is an "unexposed" or "low exposure" level, such as when the levels X_0 to X_J correspond to increasing levels of exposure to a possibly harmful agent. Sometimes, however, X_0 is simply a commonly found level, such as when the levels X_0 to X_J are the range of an unordered variable such as religion or race. For preventive exposures, the highest exposure level is sometimes chosen for X_0.

The notation in Table 17–1 may be modified to represent person-count data by adding a row for noncase counts, $B_{Ji}, \ldots, B_{1i}, B_{0i}$ and then changing the person-times T_{ji} to column totals $N_{ji} = A_{ji} + B_{ji}$, as in Table 17–2. It may also be modified so that known expected values E_{ji} for the case-counts A_{ji} replace the person-times T_{ji}. The notations used in Chapter 15 were just the special cases of these notations in which X_1 = "exposed" and X_0 = "unexposed."

If the exposure variable is unordered or its ordering is ignored, analyses of polytomous data may proceed using computations identical in form to those given in Chapters 14 and 15. To start, we may use any and all of the binary-exposure techniques given earlier to compare any pair of exposure levels. As an example, Table 17–3 presents crude data from a study of the relation of fruit

TABLE 17–1

Notation for Stratified Person-Time Data with a Polytomous Exposure

	Exposure Level				
	X_J	...	X_1	X_0	
Cases	A_{Ji}	...	A_{1i}	A_{0i}	M_{1i}
Person-time	T_{Ji}	...	T_{1i}	T_{0i}	T_{+i}

TABLE 17–2

Notation for Stratified Count Data with a Polytomous Exposure

	Exposure Level				
	X_J	...	X_1	X_0	
Cases	A_{Ji}	...	A_{1i}	A_{0i}	M_{1i}
Noncases	B_{Ji}	...	B_{1i}	B_{0i}	M_{0i}
Totals	N_{Ji}	...	N_{1i}	N_{0i}	N_{+i}

and vegetable intake to colon polyps, divided into three index categories of equal width and a broad reference category. (These data are discussed in Chapter 16.) Also presented are the odds ratios and 95% confidence limits obtained from comparing each category below the highest intake level to the highest intake level, and each category to the next higher category. It appears that the odds ratios decline as intake increases, with the sharpest decline occurring among the lowest intakes. Stratification of the data on the matching factors and computation of Mantel-Haenszel statistics yield virtually the same results.

The number of possible comparisons grows rapidly as the number of exposure levels increases: The number of exposure-level pairs is $(J + 1)J/2$, which equals 3 when there are three exposure

TABLE 17–3

Data on Fruit and Vegetable Intake (Average Number of Servings per Day) in Relation to Colon Polyps, Odds Ratios, 95% Confidence Limits, and 2-Sided *P*-Values

	Servings of Fruit and Vegetables per Day				
	≤2	>2, ≤4	>4, ≤6	>6	Totals
Cases	49	125	136	178	488
Controls	28	111	140	209	488
Total	77	236	276	387	976
	Comparison to Highest (>6) Category				
Odds ratio	2.05	1.32	1.14	1.0 (referent)	
Lower limit	1.24	0.96	0.84		
Upper limit	3.41	1.83	1.55		
P-value	0.005	0.092	0.40		
	Incremental Comparisons to Next Higher Category				
Odds ratio	1.55	1.16	1.14		
Lower limit	0.91	0.82	0.84		
Upper limit	2.64	1.64	1.55		
P-value	0.10	0.41	0.40		

From Witte JS, Longnecker MP, Bird CL, et al. Relation of vegetable, fruit, and grain consumption to colorectal adenomatous polyps. *Am J Epidemiol.* 1996;144:1015–1025.

levels ($J = 2$) but rises to six when there are four exposure levels ($J = 3$, as in Table 17–3) and 10 when there are five exposure levels ($J = 4$). Pairwise analysis of a polytomous exposure thus raises an issue of multiple comparisons, which was discussed in general terms in Chapter 13. This issue can be addressed by using either a trend test or an unordered simultaneous test statistic. Both approaches provide P-values for the joint null hypothesis that there is no association between exposure and disease across all levels of exposure.

Several equivalent simultaneous test statistics can be used for unstratified data. The oldest and most famous such statistic is the *Pearson* χ^2 *statistic,* which for unstratified person-time data has the form

$$\chi^2_{\mathrm{P}} = \sum_j (A_j - E_j)^2 / E_j \qquad [17\text{–}1]$$

where the sum is from $j = 0$ to J, and $E_j = M_1 T_j / T_+$ is the expected value for A_j under the joint null hypothesis that there is no exposure–disease association. (The notation here is as in Table 17–1, but without the stratum subscript i.) If there are no biases and the joint null hypothesis H_{Joint} is correct, χ^2_{P} has approximately a χ^2 distribution with J degrees of freedom. For pure count data with exposure totals $N_j = A_j + B_j$ (where B_j is the observed number of noncases) and grand total $N_+ = \sum_j N_j$, the Pearson χ^2 equals

$$\chi^2_{\mathrm{P}} = \sum_j (A_j - E_j)^2 / V_j \qquad [17\text{–}2]$$

where $E_j = M_1 N_j / N_+$ and $V_j = E_j(N_j - E_j)/N_j$ are the mean and variance of A_j under the joint null hypothesis. Equation 17–2 is equivalent to the more familiar form

$$\chi^2_{\mathrm{P}} = \sum_j [(A_j - E_j)^2 / E_j + (B_j - F_j)^2 / F_j] \qquad [17\text{–}3]$$

where $F_j = M_0 N_j / N_+$ is the mean of B_j under the joint null hypothesis. For the data in Table 17–3, equation 17–3 yields

$$\chi^2_{\mathrm{P}} = \frac{[49 - 488(77)/976]^2}{488(77)/976} + \cdots + \frac{[209 - 488(387)/976]^2}{488(387)/976} = 9.1$$

which has three degrees of freedom and $P = 0.03$. Note that this simultaneous P-value is smaller than all but one of the pairwise P-values in Table 17–3.

We use the Pearson statistic here because it is very easy to compute. For unstratified data, the quantity $(N - 1)\chi^2_{\mathrm{P}}/N$ is identical to the generalized Mantel-Haenszel statistic for testing the joint null hypothesis (Breslow and Day, 1980; Somes, 1986). When it is extended to stratified data, the Pearson statistic requires that all stratum expected counts be "large" (usually taken to be more than four or five), whereas the generalized Mantel-Haenszel statistic can remain valid even if all the stratum counts are small (although the crude counts must be "large"). When stratification is needed, joint statistics can be more easily computed using regression programs, however, and so we defer presenting such statistics until Chapter 21. We discuss unordered statistics further in the section on simultaneous analysis.

Note that the pairwise P-values considered singly or together do *not* provide an appropriate P-value for the null hypothesis that there is no association of exposure and disease. As will be illustrated in the final section, it is possible to have all the pairwise P-values be much larger than the simultaneous P-value. Conversely, it is possible to have one or more of the pairwise P-values be much smaller than the simultaneous P-value. Thus, to evaluate a hypothesis that involves more than two exposure levels, one should compute a simultaneous test statistic.

For stratified data, the ordinary Mantel-Haenszel estimates can be somewhat inefficient when exposure is polytomous, because they do not make use of the fact that the product of the common ratios comparing level i with level j and level j with level k must equal the common ratio comparing level i with level k (the "common ratio" may be a risk, rate, or odds ratio). They can, however, be modified to use this information and so be made more efficient (Yanagawa and Fujii, 1994). Efficient estimates can also be obtained from regression analyses; see Chapter 20 for polytomous exposure models.

TABLE 17–4

Data on Fruit and Vegetable Intake and Colon Polyps, Including Mean Servings per Day, Mean Log Servings, and Case-Control Ratios in Each Category

Upper Category Boundary	Mean Servings	Mean Log Servings	No. of Cases	No. of Controls	Case-Control Ratio
1	0.68	−0.52	13	4	3.25
2	1.58	0.45	36	24	1.50
3	2.57	0.94	55	44	1.25
4	3.55	1.26	70	67	1.04
5	4.52	1.51	77	74	1.04
6	5.51	1.71	59	66	0.89
7	6.50	1.87	54	48	1.12
8	7.58	2.02	33	41	0.80
9	8.51	2.14	33	31	1.06
10	9.43	2.24	24	22	1.04
11	10.48	2.35	10	26	0.38
12	11.49	2.44	6	12	0.50
14	12.83	2.55	9	12	0.75
18	15.73	2.75	4	11	0.36
27	20.91	3.03	5	6	0.83
Totals	—	—	488	488	—

DOSE–RESPONSE AND TREND ANALYSIS

If the exposure levels have a natural ordering, a serious source of inefficiency in the pairwise and unordered analyses is that the statistics take no account of this ordering. Dose–response and trend analysis concerns the use of such ordering information.

Table 17–4 presents the data used in Table 17–3 in more detail, using the finest categories with integer boundaries that yield at least four cases and four controls per category. These data will be used in the examples that follow. (Subjects in this study often had fractional values of average servings per day, because servings per day were calculated from questions asking the consumption frequencies of individual fruits and vegetables, such as apples and broccoli.)

GRAPHING A TREND

Perhaps the simplest example of trend analyses is a plot of estimates against the exposure levels. Occurrence plots are straightforward. For example, given population data, one may plot estimates of the average risks $R_0, R_1, \ldots, R_J$ or the incidence rates $I_0, I_1, \ldots, I_J$ against the exposure levels $X_0, X_1, \ldots, X_J$. For unmatched case-control data, the case-control ratios $A_0/B_0, A_1/B_1, \ldots, A_J/B_J$ may substitute for the risk or rate estimates (Easton et al., 1991; Greenland et al., 1999c). If important confounding appears to be present, one may standardize the measures, or plot them separately for different confounder strata.

The pattern exhibited by plotted estimates is called a trend. A trend is *monotonic* or *monotone* if every change in the height of the plotted points is always in the same direction. A monotone trend never reverses direction, but it may have flat segments. A trend is *strictly monotone* if it is either always increasing or always decreasing. Such a trend never reverses and has no flat segments. One commonly sees phrases such as "the data exhibited a dose–response relation" used to indicate that

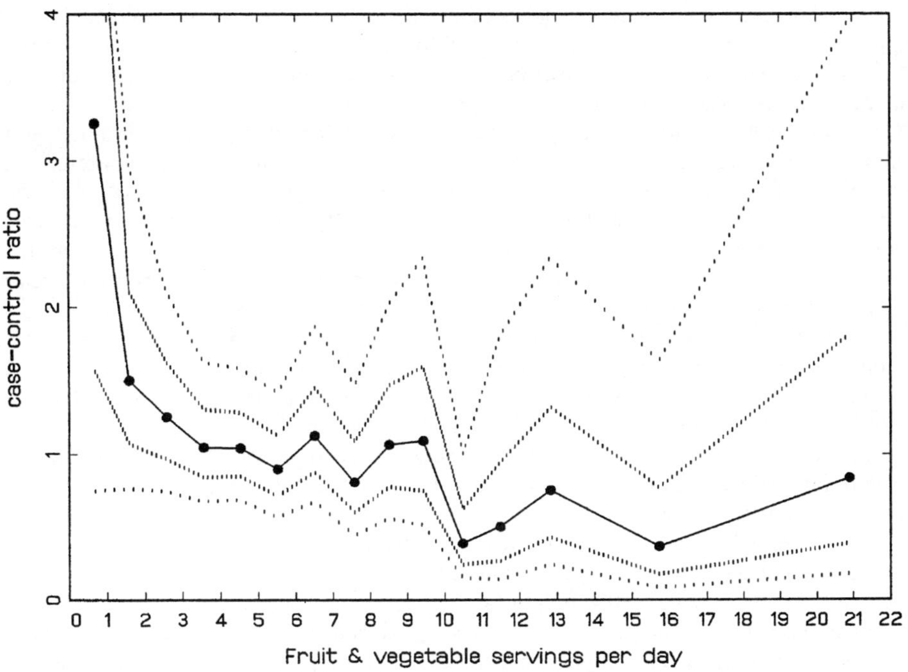

FIGURE 17–1 • Plot of case-control ratios and 80% and 99% confidence limits from data in Table 17–4, using arithmetic scale.

a plot of estimates versus exposure level was monotone. The term "dose–response," however, can refer to any pattern whatsoever, and here we use it in this general sense. That is, *dose–response* will here mean the pattern relating the outcome or effect measure to exposure, whatever it may be. The term "trend" is often used as a synonym for "dose–response," though it is more general still, as in "the trend in risk was upward but fluctuations occurred in later years." In particular, a trend may be observed over time, age, weight, or other variables for which the concept of "dose" is meaningless.

Figure 17–1 presents the case-control ratios A_j/B_j computed from Table 17–4, plotted against the category means, and connected by straight line segments. The inner dotted lines are approximate 80% confidence limits, and the fainter outer dotted lines are 99% limits. These limits are computed using the variance estimate

$$\hat{V} = \widehat{\text{Var}}[\ln(A_j/B_j)] = 1/A_j + 1/B_j$$

in the formula

$$\exp[\ln(A_j/B_j) + Z_\gamma \hat{V}^{1/2}]$$

where Z_γ is the 100γ percentile of the standard normal distribution ($Z_{0.80} = 1.282$, $Z_{0.99} = 2.576$). The figure gives an impression of a steeper trend in the ratios at low consumption levels (less than three servings per day) than at higher levels. If no important bias or error is present, the trends in Figure 17–1 should reflect those in the underlying source-population rates.

A common approach to graphing risk or rate ratios uses a single reference level; for example, with X_0 as the reference level in rate ratios, one would plot $I_1/I_0, \ldots, I_J/I_0$ or their logarithms against the nonreference exposure levels $X_1, \ldots, X_J$. With this approach, the resulting curve is proportional to the curve obtained by plotting the rates, but it appears to be less precisely estimated (Easton et al., 1991).

PLOTTING CONFIDENCE LIMITS

Although it is helpful to plot confidence limits along with point estimates, care must be taken to prevent the graph from visually overemphasizing imprecise points. The conventional approach of placing error bars around the points produces such overemphasis. Thus, we recommend instead that the upper and lower limits receive their own graph line, as in Figure 17–1, rather than connecting the limits to their point estimate by error bars. The resulting graphs of the lower and upper limits together form a *confidence band* for the curve being estimated.

Two serious problems arise in plotting estimated associations or effects that are derived using a shared reference level. One is that the widths of the confidence intervals at nonreference levels depend on the size of the counts in the chosen reference category; the other is that no confidence interval is generated for the curve at the reference category. If the counts in the reference category are smaller than those in other categories, the confidence limits around the estimates at the nonreference levels will be far apart and will thus make the shape of the dose–response curve appear much more imprecisely estimated than it actually is. Graphs of confidence limits for rates, risks, and case-control ratios do not suffer from these problems but are sometimes not an option (as in matched case-control studies). A more general solution, known as *floating absolute risk* (Easton et al., 1991; Greenland et al., 1999c), circumvents the problems but is designed for regression analyses and so will not be described here. To address the problems in tabular analyses of cohort or unmatched case-control data, we again recommend plotting rates, risks, case-control ratios, or their transforms, rather than rate ratios, risk ratios, or odds ratios. For matched case-control analyses, we suggest taking as the reference category the one that yields the narrowest confidence intervals, although a narrower confidence band can be obtained using the floating absolute risk method.

The limits obtained using the methods presented earlier in this book are known as pointwise limits. If no bias is present, a 90% pointwise confidence band has at least a 90% chance (over study repetitions) of containing the true rate, risk, or effect at any single observed exposure level. Nonetheless, there is a much lower chance that a conventional pointwise confidence band contains the entire true dose–response curve. That is, there will be *less* than a 90% chance that the true curve runs inside the pointwise band at every point along the graph. Construction of confidence bands that have a 90% chance of containing the true curve everywhere is best accomplished using regression methods; see Hastie and Tibshirani (1990, sec. 3.8).

As a final caution, note that neither the pointwise limits nor the corresponding graphical confidence band provide an appropriate test of the overall null hypothesis of no exposure–outcome association. For example, it is possible (and not unusual) for all the 99% confidence limits for the exposure-specific associations to contain the null value, and yet the trend statistic may yield a P-value of less than 0.01 for the association between exposure and disease.

VERTICAL SCALING

Rates, risks, and ratio measures are often plotted on a semilogarithmic graph, in which the vertical scale is logarithmic. Semilogarithmic plotting is equivalent to plotting the log rates, log risks, or log ratios against exposure, and is useful as a preliminary to log-linear (exponential) and logistic regression. Such regressions assume linear models for the log rates, log risks, or log odds, and departures from the models are easiest to detect visually when using a logarithmic vertical scale. Figure 17–2 is a plot of the case-control ratios and confidence limits from Figure 17–1, using a logarithmic vertical scale. In this scale, the difference in trend at high and low doses appears less than in Figure 17–1.

There are various arguments for examining semilogarithmic plots (Gladen and Rogan, 1983), but there can be subject-matter reasons for also examining plots with other scales for the vertical or horizontal axis (Morgenstern and Greenland, 1990; Devesa et al., 1995). In particular, the untransformed scale (that is, direct plotting of the measures) is important to examine when one wishes to convey information about absolute effects and health impacts. For example, suppose the average risks at levels X_0, X_1, X_2 of a potentially modifiable exposure follow the pattern $R_0 = 0.001$, $R_1 = 0.010$, $R_2 = 0.050$. A plot of the risk ratios $R_0/R_0 = 1$, $R_1/R_0 = 10$, $R_2/R_0 = 50$ against X_0, X_1, X_2 will indicate that the proportionate risk reduction produced by moving from level X_2 to level X_1 is $(50 - 10)/50 = 0.80$. This reduction is over 80% of the maximum potential reduction of $(50 - 1)/50 = 0.98$ produced by moving from X_2 to X_0. In other words, reducing exposure from X_2 to X_1 may yield most of the total potential risk reduction. A plot of the log risk ratios at X_0, X_1, X_2 (which are 0, 2.3, 3.9) will not make clear the preceding point and may convey

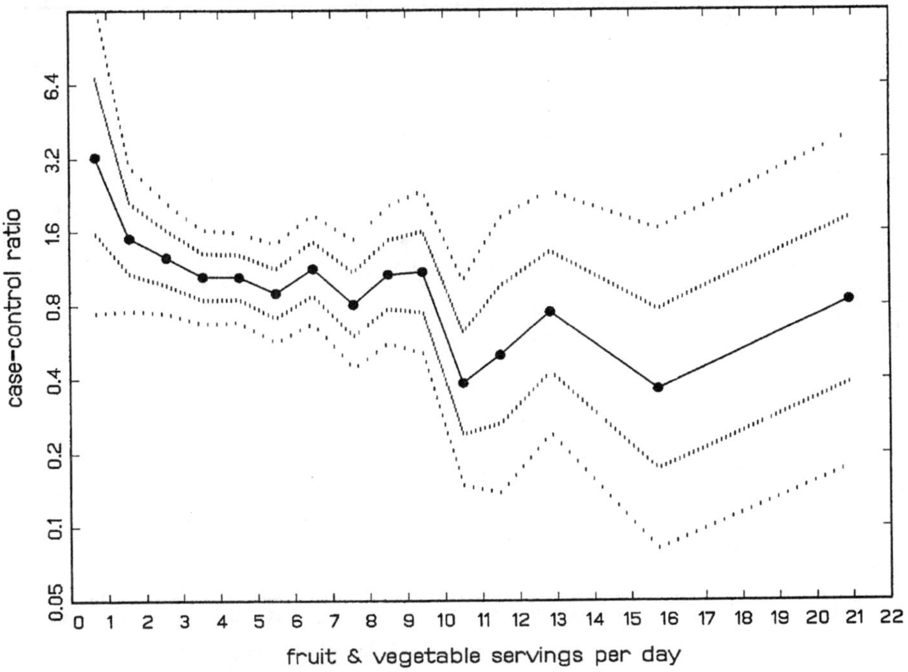

FIGURE 17–2 • Plot of case-control ratios and 80% and 99% confidence limits from data in Table 17–4, using logarithmic vertical scale.

the mistaken impression that moving from X_2 to X_1 does not achieve most of the possible benefit from exposure modification.

Another approach to graphical analysis is to plot attributable and prevented fractions (relative to a common reference level) against exposure levels. Attributable fractions are plotted above the horizontal axis for exposure levels with risks higher than the reference level risk, and preventable fractions are plotted below the horizontal axis for levels with risks lower than the reference level (Morgenstern and Greenland, 1990).

INCREMENTAL (SLOPE) PLOTS

The slope (direction) of a curve may be assessed directly by plotting incremental (adjacent) differences, such as $I_1 - I_0$, $I_2 - I_1, \ldots, I_J - I_{J-1}$, or incremental ratios, such as I_1/I_0, $I_2/I_1, \ldots, I_J/I_{J-1}$, against the category boundaries (Maclure and Greenland, 1992). Incremental differences will be greater than 0 and incremental ratios will be greater than 1 wherever the trend is upward; the differences will be less than 0 and the ratios less than 1 wherever the trend is downward. Figure 17–3 displays the incremental odds ratios and their 80% and 99% confidence limits from the data in Table 17–4 plotted on a logarithmic vertical scale against the category boundaries. This graph supplements Figure 17–2 by showing that the data are fairly consistent with an unchanging slope in the logarithmic trend across consumption, which corresponds to an exponential trend on the original scale.

Because incremental ratios are based on division by a shifting reference quantity, their pattern does not follow that of underlying rates or risks, and so they are not well suited for evaluating health impacts. They need logarithmic transformation to avoid distorted impressions produced by the shifting reference level. Suppose, for example, that average risks at X_0, X_1, X_2 are $R_0 = 0.02$, $R_1 = 0.01$, $R_2 = 0.02$, such as might occur if exposure was a nutrient for which both deficiency and excess are harmful. On the untransformed scale the change in risk from X_0 to X_1 is exactly opposite the change in risk from X_1 to X_2. As a result, in going from X_0 to X_2 the exposure effects cancel out to yield identical risks at X_0 and X_2. Yet the incremental risk ratios are $R_1/R_0 = 1/2$ and

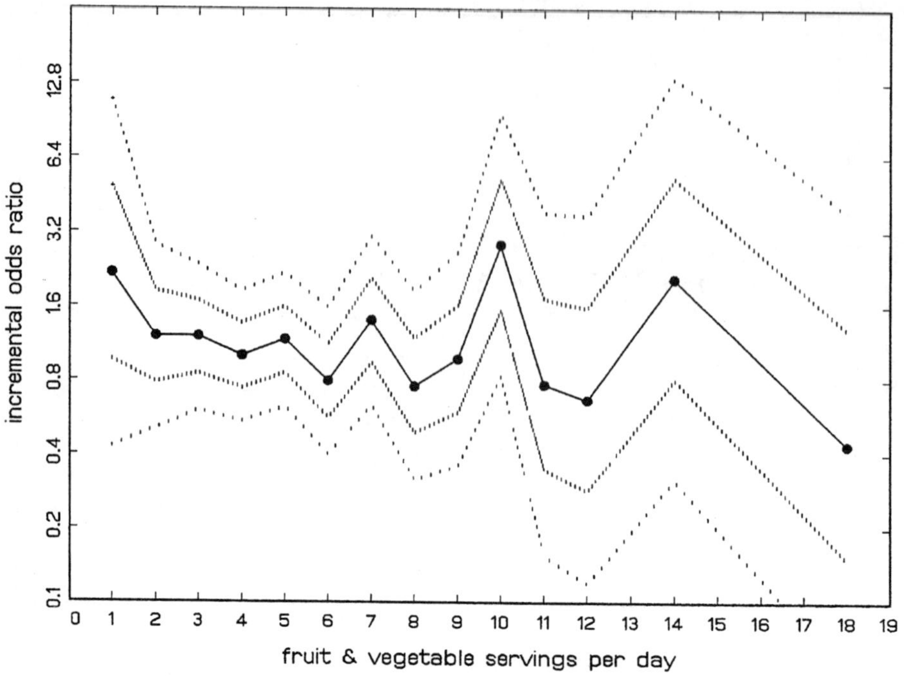

FIGURE 17–3 • Plot of incremental odds ratios and 80% and 99% confidence limits from data in Table 17–4, using logarithmic vertical scale.

$R_2/R_1 = 2$, so that the second exposure increment will appear visually to have a larger effect than the first if the ratios are plotted on the arithmetic scale. In contrast, on a logarithmic scale R_1/R_0 will be the same distance below zero as R_2/R_1 is above zero. This equidistance shows that the effects of the two increments cancel exactly.

HORIZONTAL SCALING AND CATEGORY SCORES

One must also choose a horizontal (exposure) scale for a plot. When each exposure level X_0, $X_1, \ldots, X_J$ represents a unique exposure value, an obvious choice is to use this unique value. For example, if X_j corresponds to "j previous pregnancies," one may simply use number of previous pregnancies as the horizontal axis. If, however, the exposure levels represent internally heterogeneous categories, such as 5-year groupings of exposure time, a numeric value or score must be assigned to each category to form the horizontal scale.

Category midpoints are perhaps the simplest choice that will often yield reasonable scores. For example, this scheme would assign scores of $s_0 = 0$, $s_1 = 2.5$, $s_2 = 7$, and $s_3 = 12$ years for exposure categories of 0, 1 to 4, 5 to 9, and 10 to 14 years. Midpoints do not, however, provide scores for open-ended categories such as 15+ years.

Two slightly more involved choices that do provide scores for open-ended categories are category means and medians. Category means have an advantage that they will on average produce a straight line if there is no bias and the true dose–response curve is a line. If, however, there are categories within which exposure has large nonlinear effects (such as an exponential trend and a fivefold risk increase from the lower to the upper end of a category), no simple scoring method will provide an undistorted dose–response curve (Greenland, 1995b). Thus, avoidance of very broad categories is advisable when strong effects may be present within such categories.

One automatic, common, and poor method of scoring categories is to assign them ordinal numbers (that is, $s_j = j$, so that $0, 1, \ldots, J$ is assigned to category $X_0, X_1, \ldots, X_J$). If any category is internally heterogeneous, it will only be accidental that such ordinal scores yield a biologically meaningful horizontal axis. If the categories span unequal intervals, as in

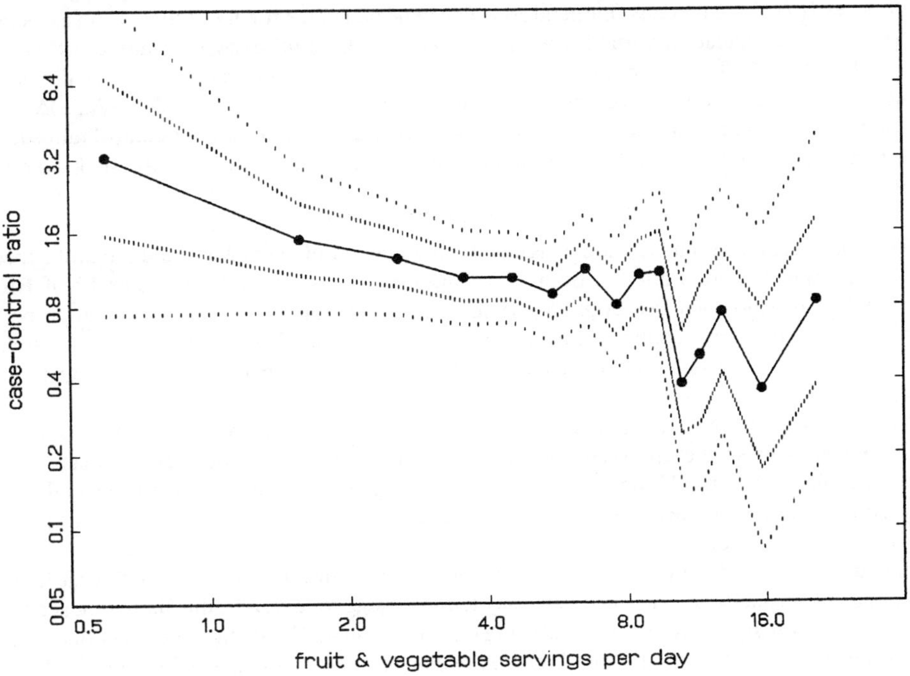

FIGURE 17–4 • Plot of case-control ratios and 80% and 99% confidence limits from data in Table 17–4, using logarithmic horizontal and vertical scales.

Tables 17–3 and 17–4, ordinal scores can easily yield quantitatively meaningless dose–response curves and harm the power of trend tests (Lagakos, 1988; Greenland, 1995a, 1995b). These shortcomings arise because the distance between the ordinal scores is always 1, and this distance will not in general correspond to any difference in average exposure or effect across the categories.

In choosing the horizontal scale, it is possible to transform exposure in any fashion that is of scientific interest. Suppose, for example, one has a carcinogenesis model that predicts the logarithm of lung cancer rates will increase linearly with the logarithm of exposure. To check the prediction, one may plot the logarithms of the rates against the category-specific means of log exposure. Equivalently, one may plot the rates against the geometric means of the exposure categories, using logarithmic scales for both axes. (Recall that the geometric mean exposure is the antilog of the mean of the logarithms of the individual exposures.) Under the theory, the resulting plot should on average follow a line if no bias is present. Figure 17–4 presents the same results as in Figure 17–2, but plotted with logarithmic horizontal and vertical scales. With this scaling, the entire curve appears not too far from a straight line, considering the statistical uncertainty in the results.

In the preceding example, a different (and nonlinear) curve would result if one used the arithmetic means (the second column of Table 17–4) as scores for the exposure categories. The difference between the geometric and arithmetic means will tend to be small if the categories are narrow, but it may be large for broad categories. This potential for discrepancy is yet another reason we recommend keeping categories as narrow as practical. When examining a logarithmic exposure scale, geometric means will provide a more meaningful analysis than will arithmetic means, because the logarithm of the geometric mean is the average of the logarithms of the potentially unique individual exposure measurements, whereas the logarithm of the arithmetic mean is not.

SMOOTHING THE GRAPH

Small counts may produce graphs with highly implausible fluctuations. As mentioned earlier, a common approach to this problem is to add $1/2$ to each table cell. A superior approach is to average the observed counts with expected counts (Chapter 12 of Bishop et al., 1975; Greenland, 2006b). A simple way to do so is as follows. Suppose there are $J + 1$ exposure levels and I strata, for a total of $K = I(J + 1)$ case cells (numerators). The expected value for A_{ji} if there is no association of exposure *or* stratification variables with the outcome (the null expected number of cases) is $E_{ji} = (M_{1+}/T_{++})T_{ji}$ for person-time data, which is just the overall crude rate times the person-time at exposure j, stratum i. For count data, this expected value is $E_{ji} = (M_{1+}/N_{++})N_{ji}$. The smoothed case count that replaces A_{ji} in graphing rates or proportions or case-control ratios is then a weighted average of the observed cases and null expected number of cases. One such average is

$$S_{ji} = [M_{1+}A_{ji} + (K/2)E_{ji}]/(M_{1+} + K/2)$$

in which the observed counts A_{ji} are weighted by the number of cases M_{1+}, and the null expected number of cases E_{ji} are weighted by half the number of case cells K (Chapter 12 of Bishop et al., 1975). The smoothed case count S_{ji} yields a smoothed rate S_{ji}/T_{ji} or smoothed proportion S_{ji}/N_{ji} or smoothed case-control ratio $S_{ji}/(N_{ji} - S_{ji})$. The numbers in Table 17–4 are so large that this smoothing approach produces a barely perceptible difference in the graphs in Figures 17–1 through 17–4.

There are other simple averaging schemes, each of which can greatly improve accuracy of rate or risk estimates when the observed counts A_{ji} are small. More complex schemes can do even better (Greenland, 2006b). All operate as in the preceding equation by putting more weight on the observed value as the sample size grows and putting more weight on the expected value as the cases are spread over more cells.

The curves obtained using null expectations in the averaging formula are somewhat flattened toward the null. Because unsmoothed data may tend to exaggerate trends, this flattening is not necessarily a bad property. If desired, the flattening can be eliminated by using expected values derived from a logistic regression model that includes exposure and confounder effects rather than null expected values. If, however, one goes so far as to use a regression model for the graphical analysis, one can instead use model extensions such as splines (Chapter 20) to generate smoothed graphs.

Two cautions should be observed in using the above weighted-averaging approach. First, the smoothed counts are designed to take care of only sporadic small counts (especially zeros and ones). If the data are consistently sparse (such as pair-matched data), only summary sparse-data measures (such as Mantel-Haenszel estimates) should be graphed. Second, one need not and should not compute sparse-data summaries or trend statistics from the smoothed counts. The purpose of the smoothed counts is only to stabilize estimates that depend directly on cell sizes, such as stratum-specific and standardized rates, proportions, and case-control ratios.

If the exposure measurement is continuous (or nearly so), one may instead use more sophisticated smoothing techniques. One such method (kernel smoothing) is discussed below, and others are described in Chapters 20 and 21.

TREND STATISTICS

In examining tables and trend graphs, a natural question to ask is whether the outcome measure tends to increase or decrease in value as the exposure score increases. If the outcome measure is a rate, for example, we could ask whether the true rates tend to increase with the scores. We can suggest an answer to this question based on visual inspection of the graph, but one usually wants some formal statistical assessment as well.

The standard approach to statistical assessment of trend is to perform a regression analysis of the variation in the outcome measure with the scores. Because this approach typically involves many subtleties and computer-based calculations, we defer discussion of such analysis until the chapters on regression. The basic qualitative question—"Does the outcome measure tend to go up or down with the exposure scores?"—can, however, be addressed by a relatively simple and popular trend test developed by Mantel (1963). Unfortunately, its simplicity and popularity have led to extensive misinterpretation of the P-value derived from the test (Maclure and Greenland, 1992). Therefore, before we present the statistic, we explain its meaning.

Consider two hypotheses about the true outcome measures. Under the *null hypothesis,* these measures are not associated with the exposure scores. Under the *linear hypothesis,* the true measures will fall along a line when plotted against the scores. (The hypothesis is sometimes said to be *log-linear* if the outcome measures are logarithms of more basic measures such as rates or rate ratios.) The null hypothesis is a special case of the linear hypothesis, the one in which the line is horizontal. The Mantel trend P-value is often misinterpreted as a P-value for the linear hypothesis; it is not, however. Rather, it is a P-value for testing the *null* hypothesis. If no bias is present, it provides a valid test of that hypothesis, in that the P-value will tend toward small values *only* if the null hypothesis is false.

In addition to validity, we would like a statistic to have the highest power possible, so that *if* the null hypothesis is false, the P-value will tend toward small values. The Mantel test will be powerful when the linear hypothesis holds for the rate, risk, log rate, or log odds. That is, if any of these outcome measures has a linear relation to the scores, the Mantel test will have good power relative to the best power achievable from the study. If, however, the relation of the outcomes to the scores is nonlinear to the point of being nonmonotonic, the Mantel test may have poor power relative to the best achievable. In some extreme situations involving U-shaped relations between outcome measures and scores, the Mantel test may have little chance of detecting even a strong association.

The basic cautions in using the Mantel test may be summarized as follows: As always, a large P-value means only that the test did not detect an association; it does *not* mean that the null hypothesis is true or probably true, nor does it mean that further analyses will not reveal some violation of the null. A small P-value means only that some association was detected by the test; it does *not* mean that the association of the outcome with exposure is linear or even that it is monotone. The test is related to the linear hypothesis only in that it is much more capable of detecting linear and log-linear associations than nonmonotone associations.

With these cautions in mind, we now describe the test. The Mantel trend statistic is a type of score statistic, and it is a direct generalization of the Mantel-Haenszel statistic for binary exposures. It has the form

$$\chi_{\text{trend}} = \frac{S - E}{V^{1/2}} \qquad [17\text{–}4]$$

where S is the sum of the case scores when every person is assigned the score in his or her category, and E and V are the expected value and variance of S under the null hypothesis. S and E may be computed from $S = \sum_i \sum_j A_{ji} s_j$ and $E = \sum_i M_{1i} E_i$, where s_j is the score assigned to category j and E_i is the expected case score in stratum i under the null hypothesis; $E_i = \sum_j T_{ji} s_j / T_{+i}$ for person-time data and $E_i = \sum_j N_{ji} s_j / N_{+i}$ for pure count data. For person-time data,

$$V = E_i M_{1i} V_i \qquad \text{where} \qquad V_i = \sum_j T_{ji} s_j^2 / T_{+i} - E_i^2$$

whereas for pure count data,

$$V = \sum_i \frac{M_{1i} M_{0i}}{N_{+i} - 1} V_i \qquad \text{where} \qquad V_i = \sum_i N_{ji} s_j^2 / N_{+i} - E_i^2$$

In either case, V_i is the variance of the scores in stratum i under the null hypothesis. If there are only two exposure categories ($J = 1$), χ_{trend} simplifies to the usual Mantel-Haenszel statistic described in Chapter 15.

If no bias is present and the null hypothesis is correct, χ_{trend} will have a standard normal distribution. Thus, its observed value can be found in a standard normal table to obtain a P-value for the null hypothesis. Special care is needed in interpreting the sign of χ_{trend} and the P-values based on it, however. A negative value for χ_{trend} may only indicate a trend that is predominantly but not consistently decreasing; similarly, a positive value may only indicate a trend that is predominantly but not consistently increasing. We emphasize again that a small P-value from this statistic means only that an association was detected, *not* that this association is linear or even monotone.

The data in Table 17–4 have only one stratum. Using the arithmetic category means as the scores, the formulas simplify to

$$S = \sum_j A_j s_j = 13(0.68) + \cdots + 5(20.91) = 2694.3$$

$$E = M_1 \sum_j N_j s_j / N_+ = 488[17(0.68) + \cdots + 11(20.91)]/976 = 2870.8$$

$$V = \frac{M_1 M_0}{N_+ - 1}\left(\sum_j N_j s_j^2 / N_+ - E^2/M_1^2\right)$$

$$= \frac{488^2}{975}[17(0.68^2)/976 + \cdots + 11(20.91^2)/976 - 5.8828^2] = 2814.6$$

and so $\chi_{\text{trend}} = (2694.3 - 5.8828)/2814.6^{1/2} = -3.33$, which has a two-sided P-value of 0.0009. If we use the mean log servings as the scores, we instead get $\chi_{\text{trend}} = -3.69$ and $P = 0.0002$. This larger χ_{trend} and smaller P reflect the fact that the log case-control ratios appear to follow a line more closely when plotted against log servings (Fig. 17–4) than when plotted against servings (Fig. 17–2).

The Mantel statistic is well suited for sparse stratifications, in that it remains valid even if all the counts A_{ji} are only zeros or ones, and even if there is never more than two subjects per stratum. Thus, it may be applied directly to matched data. It is, however, a large-sample statistic, in that it requires (among other things) at least two of the exposure-specific case totals A_{j+} be large and (for pure count data) at least two of the exposure-specific noncase totals B_{j+} be large. When there is doubt about the adequacy of sample size for the test, one may instead use a stratified permutation (exact) test, which, like the Mantel test, is available in several computer packages, including Egret and StatXact (Cytel, 2006).

One positive consequence of their sparse-data validity is that neither the Mantel test nor its permutation counterparts require that one collapse subjects into heterogeneous exposure categories. In particular, the Mantel statistic can be applied directly to continuous exposure data, in which each subject may have a unique exposure value. By avoiding degradation of exposure into broad categories, the power of the test can be improved (Lagakos, 1988; Greenland, 1995a). This improvement is reflected in the preceding example, in that χ_{trend} obtained from the broad categories in Table 17–3 using mean log servings is -2.95, two-sided $P = 0.003$, whereas the χ_{trend} obtained using the individual data in Table 17–4 on log servings is -3.77, two-sided $P = 0.0002$. To compute χ_{trend} from subject-specific data, note that the formula for S, E, and V can use "categories" that contain only a single person. For example, in the data in Table 17–4, there was one person (a case) who reported eating only 1 serving every other week, which is $^1/_{14}$ serving per day. Using subject-specific data, this person is the sole member of the first ($j = 1$) serving category, which has $A_l = 1$, $B_1 = 0$, $N_1 = 1$, and $s_1 = \ln(^1/_{14})$. This category contributes to the sums in S, E, and V the amounts $A_1 s_1 = \ln(^1/_{14})$, $M_1 N_1 s_1/N_+ = 488[\ln(^1/_{14})]/976$, and $N_1 s_1^2/N_+ = \ln(^1/_{14})^2/976$. By applying the above formulas to each case and control separately and summing the results over all subjects, we obtain a χ_{trend} of -3.77, which yields a smaller P-value than any of the categorical (grouped) analyses.

The Mantel statistic takes on an exceptionally simple and well-known form in matched-pair case-control studies. For such studies, $M_{1i} = M_{0i} = 1$ and $N_i = 2$ in all strata. Let s_{1i} and s_{0i} be the case and control scores or exposures in pair (stratum) i. We then have S = sum of case exposures $= \sum_i s_{1i}$, $E_i = (s_{1i} + s_{0i})/2$, and

$$V_i = \left(s_{1i}^2 + s_{0i}^2\right)/2 - (s_{1i} + s_{0i})^2/2^2 = (s_{1i} - s_{0i})^2/4$$

so that

$$S - E = \sum_i s_{1i} - \sum_i (s_{1i} + s_{0i})/2 = \sum_i (s_{1i} - s_{0i})/2 = \sum_i d_i/2$$

and

$$V^{1/2} = \left(\sum_i d_i^2\right)^{1/2} / 2$$

where $d_i = s_{1i} - s_{0i}$ = case-control exposure difference. Thus

$$\chi_{\text{trend}} = \sum_i d_i \Big/ \left(\sum_i d_i^2\right)^{1/2}$$

This may be recognized as the classical t-statistic for testing pairwise differences (Dixon and Massey, 1969). When exposure is dichotomous, χ_{trend} simplifies further, to the McNemar matched-pairs statistic (Chapter 16).

SPECIAL HANDLING OF THE ZERO LEVEL

When exposure is a non-negative physical or temporal quantity (such as grams, years, rads, or pack-years of exposure), some authors recommend routine deletion of the zero level (unexposed) before computation of trend estimates or statistics. Such deletion cannot be justified in all situations, however. In any given situation, a number of context-specific factors must be evaluated to develop a rationale for retaining or deleting the unexposed (Greenland and Poole, 1995).

One valid rationale for deleting the unexposed arises if there is good evidence that such subjects differ to an important extent from exposed subjects on uncontrolled confounders or selection factors. This hypothesis is plausible when considering, for example, alcohol use: Abstainers may differ in many health-related ways from drinkers. If such differences are present, the estimated outcome measure among the unexposed may be biased to a different extent than the estimates from other categories. This differential bias can distort the shape of the dose–response curve and bias the entire sequence of estimates. Suppose, for example, that j = years exposed, and the corresponding true risks R_j fall on a straight line with a slope of 0.010/year, with $R_0 = 0.010$, $R_1 = 0.020$, $R_2 = 0.030$, $R_3 = 0.040$. The sequence of risks relative to the unexposed risk will then also be linear: $R_1/R_0 = 2$, $R_2/R_0 = 3$, $R_3/R_0 = 4$. Suppose next that the net bias in the estimated risks is 0% (none) among the unexposed but is −30% among the four exposed levels. The expected estimates for the R_j will then be 0.010, 0.014, 0.021, 0.028. The resulting risk curve will no longer be a straight line (which has a constant slope throughout); instead, the slope will increase from $0.014 - 0.010 = 0.004$/year to $0.021 - 0.014 = 0.007$/year after the first year, whereas the resulting risk ratios will be 1.4, 2.1, and 2.8, all downward biased.

On the other hand, if the unexposed group is not subject to bias different from the exposed, there is no sound reason to discard them from the analysis. In such situations, deleting the unexposed will simply harm the power and precision of the study, severely if many or most subjects are unexposed. In real data analyses, one may be unsure of the best approach. If so, it is not difficult to perform analyses both with and without the unexposed group to see if the results depend on its inclusion. If such dependence is found, this fact should be reported as part of the results.

Another problem that arises in handling the zero exposure level is that one cannot take the logarithm of zero. Thus, if one retains the zero exposed in a dose–response analysis, one cannot use the log transform $\ln(x)$ of exposure, or plot exposure on a logarithmic scale. A common solution to this problem is to add a small positive number c to the exposure before taking the logarithm; the resulting transform is then $\ln(c + x)$. For example, one could use $\ln(1 + x)$, in which case subjects with zero exposure have a value of $\ln(1 + 0) = \ln(1) = 0$ on the new scale. This solution has a drawback of being arbitrary, as the transform $\ln(1 + x)$ depends entirely on the units used to measure exposure. For example, if exposure is measured in servings per day, persons who eat 0, 1, and 5 servings per day will have $\ln(1 + x)$ equal to $\ln(1) = 0$, $\ln(2) = 0.7$, and $\ln(6) = 1.8$, so that the first two people are closer together than the second two. If we instead use servings per week, the same people will have $\ln(1 + x)$ equal to 0, $\ln(1 + 7) = 2.1$, and $\ln[1 + 7(5)] = 3.6$, so that the second two people will be closer together than the first two. Likewise, use of a different added number, such as $\ln(0.1 + x)$ instead of $\ln(1 + x)$, can make a large difference in the results. There is no general solution for this arbitrariness except to be aware that $\ln(c + x)$ represents a broad variety of transforms, depending on both c and the units of exposure measurement. The smaller c is, the more closely the transform produces a logarithmic shape, which is extremely steep near $x = 0$ and which levels off rapidly as x increases; as c is increased, the transform moves gradually toward a linear shape.

MOVING AVERAGES

Categorical analysis of trends is apparently simple, but it involves the complexities of choosing the number of categories, the category boundaries, and the category scores. A simpler alternative with potentially better statistical properties is to plot a *moving average* or *running mean* of the outcome variable across exposure levels. This approach may be viewed as a smoothing technique suitable for exposures measured on a fine quantitative scale. It involves moving a window (interval) across the range of exposure; one computes a rate, risk, or relative-risk estimate within the window each time one moves the window.

The width of the window may be fixed, or it may be varied as the window is moved; often this variation is done to keep the same number of subjects in each window. The window radius is half its width and so is also known as its half-width. The main choice to be made is that of this radius. Once the radius is selected, one plots the average outcome for each window against the exposure value at the center of the window. The number and spacing of window moves depends on how much detail one wants in the final graph; with a computer graphing algorithm, the number of windows used can be made as large as desired. For example, in plotting rates against pack-years of smoking, one could have the window center move from 0 to 20 in increments of 0.5 pack-years, with a radius of 4 pack-years.

To improve statistical performance, it is customary to employ weighted averaging within a window, such that any subject at the center of the window is given maximum weight, with weight smoothly declining to zero for subjects at the ends of the window. There are a number of standard weighting functions in use, all of which tend to yield similar-looking curves in typical epidemiologic data. These weight functions are also known as *kernels;* hence, the weighted averaging process is often called *kernel smoothing,* and algorithms for carrying out the process are called *kernel smoothers* (Hastie and Tibshirani, 1990; Hastie et al., 2001).

To describe the weighted-averaging process, let x be a given exposure value, and let h be the radius of the window centered at x. The weight (kernel) function we will use is defined by

$$\begin{aligned} w_u(x) &= \text{weight to give to a person whose exposure level is } u \\ &\quad\ \text{when estimating the average outcome at exposure level } x \\ &= 1 - (u-x)^2/h^2 \qquad \text{when } |x-u| < h \\ &= 0 \text{ otherwise} \end{aligned}$$

This function reaches a maximum of 1 when $u = x$, drops toward 0 as u moves away from x, and is 0 when u is more than h units from x (for then u is outside the window centered at x). For example, consider a window centered at $x = 9$ pack-years with radius $h = 4$. The weight given a person with 9 pack-years is $w_9(9) = 1 - (9-9)^2/4^2 = 1$, whereas the weights given persons with 7, 11, 5, and 13 pack-years are

$$w_7(9) = 1 - (7-9)^2/4^2 = 0.75 = 1 - (11-9)^2/4^2 = w_{11}(9)$$

and

$$w_5(9) = 1 - (5-9)^2/4^2 = 0 = 1 - (13-9)^2/4^2 = w_{13}(9)$$

Thus, persons whose exposure level is near x are given more weight for estimating the average outcome at x than persons whose exposure level is further from x. Persons whose exposure level is outside the window centered at x are given zero weight.

When averaging rates or proportions, the statistical properties of the smoothed estimate may be further improved by multiplying the kernel weight $w_u(x)$ by the denominator (person-time or number of persons) observed at u. When this is done, the formula for the moving weighted-average rate at x becomes

$$\hat{I}_x = \frac{\sum_u T_u w_u(x) A_u / T_u}{\sum_u T_u w_u(x)} = \frac{\sum_u w_u(x) A_u}{\sum_u w_u(x) T_u} = \frac{\sum_u w_u(x) A_u \big/ \sum_u w_u(x)}{\sum_u w_u(x) T_u \big/ \sum_u w_u(x)} = \frac{\overline{A}(x)}{\overline{T}(x)}$$

where A_u is the number of cases and T_u is the amount of person-time observed at exposure level u. Note that A_u/T_u is the rate observed at exposure level u. The rate estimate $\hat{I}_x$ is just the ratio of two weighted averages with weights $w_u(x)$: the weighted average number of cases observed, $\overline{A}(x)$, and the weighted average amount of person-time observed, $\overline{T}(x)$. To estimate the average risk at x, we would instead use the number of persons observed at u, N_u, in place of the person-time T_u in the preceding formula.

For case-control data, we could plot the moving weighted-average case-control ratio by using control counts B_u in place of T_u. To adjust for confounders, the smoothed rate or risk estimates or case-control ratios may be computed within strata (using the same window weights in each stratum), and then standardized (averaged) across strata, to obtain moving standardized averages.

Weighted averaging can be applied directly to uncategorized data and so does *not* require any choice of category boundaries or category scores. It is much simpler to illustrate for categorical data, however, and so we construct an example from the data in Table 17–4. To do so, we must consider choice of the exposure scale on which we wish to construct the weights $w_u(x)$. This choice is a different issue from the choice of plotting scale considered earlier, because once we construct the moving averages, we can plot them on any axis scales we wish.

The kernel weights $w_u(x)$ depend on the distance from u to x, and so their relative magnitude as u varies will depend strongly on whether and how one transforms exposure before computing the weights. For example, one could measure distances between different numbers of servings per day on an arithmetic (untransformed) scale, in which case u and x represent servings per day. A common alternative is to measure distances on a geometric (log-transformed) scale, in which case u and x represent the logarithms of servings per day. The moving weighted averages described here tend to work better when the outcome being averaged (such as a rate or risk) varies linearly across the exposure scale used to construct the weights. Comparing Figures 17–2 and 17–4 shows that a log transform of servings per day yields a more linear plot than does an untransformed scale, and so we use weights based on log servings for our illustration.

The radius h based on log exposure has a simple interpretation on the original (untransformed) scale. If x represents a log exposure level, then only persons whose log exposure level u is between $x - h$ and $x + h$ will have nonzero weight for the average computed at x. Taking antilogs, we see that only persons whose exposure level e^u is between $e^{x-h} = e^x e^{-h}$ and $e^{x+h} = e^x e^h$ will have nonzero weight in the average computed at the exposure level e^x. For example, if we use a radius of $h = \ln(2)$ to construct the weights at 8 servings per day, only persons whose daily number of servings is between $\exp[\ln(8) - \ln(2)] = 4$ and $\exp[\ln(8) + \ln(2)] = 16$ servings will have nonzero weight in the average case-control ratio.

As one example, we compute the average case-control ratio for the third category in Table 17–4, using a radius on the log-servings scale of $h = \ln(2) = 0.69$. Only the logarithmic means of categories 2, 3, 4, and 5 are within a distance of 0.69 from 0.94, the logarithmic mean of category 3, so only the case-control ratios of categories 2, 3, 4, and 5 will have nonzero weights. The weights for these categories are

$$w_{0.45}(0.94) = 1 - (0.45 - 0.94)^2/0.69^2 = 0.50$$

$$w_{0.94}(0.94) = 1 - (0.94 - 0.94)^2/0.69^2 = 1.00$$

$$w_{1.26}(0.94) = 1 - (1.26 - 0.94)^2/0.69^2 = 0.78$$

$$w_{1.51}(0.94) = 1 - (1.51 - 0.94)^2/0.69^2 = 0.32$$

The weighted average case-control ratio for $e^{0.94} = 2.56$ servings per day is thus

$$\frac{\overline{A}(0.94)}{\overline{B}(0.94)} = \frac{0.50(36) + 1.00(55) + 0.78(70) + 0.32(77)}{0.50(24) + 1.00(44) + 0.78(67) + 0.32(74)} = \frac{152.2}{131.9} = 1.15$$

We repeat this averaging process for each category in Table 17–4, and obtain 15 smoothed case-control ratios. The solid line in Figure 17–5 provides a log-log plot of these ratios, with dotted lines for the 80% and 99% confidence bands. Because of their complexity, we omit the variance formulas used to obtain the bands; for a discussion of confidence bands for smoothed curves, see Hastie and Tibshirani (1990). Comparing this curve to the unsmoothed curve in Figure 17–4, we see that the averaging has provided a much more stable and smooth curve. The smoothed curve is also much more in accord with what we would expect from a true dose–response curve, or even one that is biased in some simple fashion.

As the final step in our graphical analysis, we replot the curve in Figure 17–5 using the original (arithmetic) scales for the coordinate axes. Figure 17–6 shows the result: The slightly nonlinear log-log curve in Figure 17–5 becomes a profoundly nonlinear curve in the original scale. Figure 17–6 suggests that most of the apparent risk reduction from fruit and vegetable consumption occurs in going from less than 1 serving per day to 2 servings per day, above which only a very gradual (but consistent) decline in risk occurs. Although the initial large reduction is also apparent in the original categorical plot in Figure 17–1, the gradual decline is more clearly imaged by the smoothed curve in Figure 17–6.

We have used both the transformed (Fig. 17–5) and untransformed (Fig. 17–6) scales in our smoothing analysis. As mentioned earlier, moving averages tend to work best (in the sense of having the least bias) when the curve being smoothed is not too far from linear; in our example, this led us to use logarithmic exposure and outcome scales for computing the moving averages.

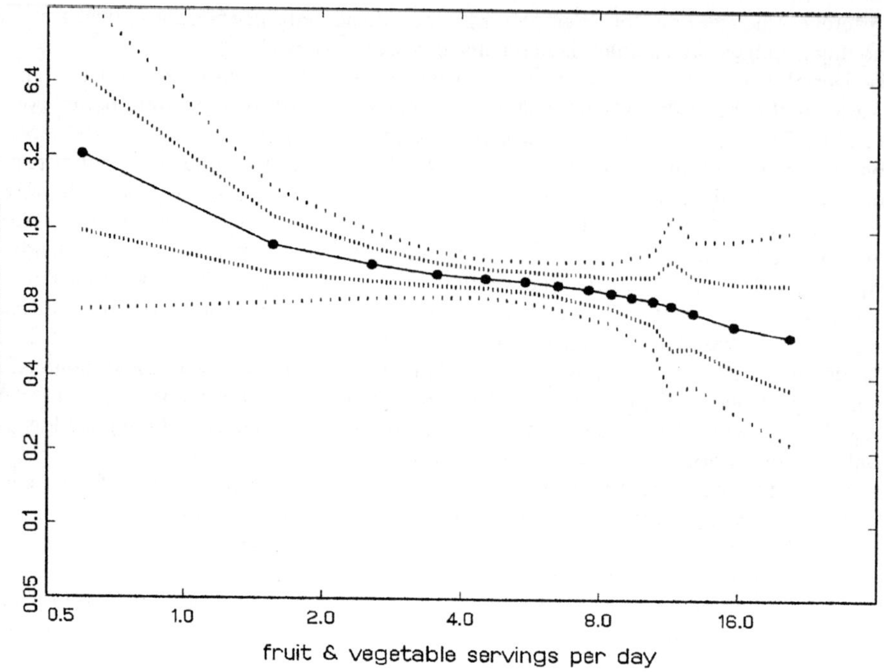

FIGURE 17–5 • Plot of running weighted-average (kernel-smoothed) case-control ratios from data in Table 17–4, using logarithmic horizontal and vertical scales and logarithmic weight (kernel) function.

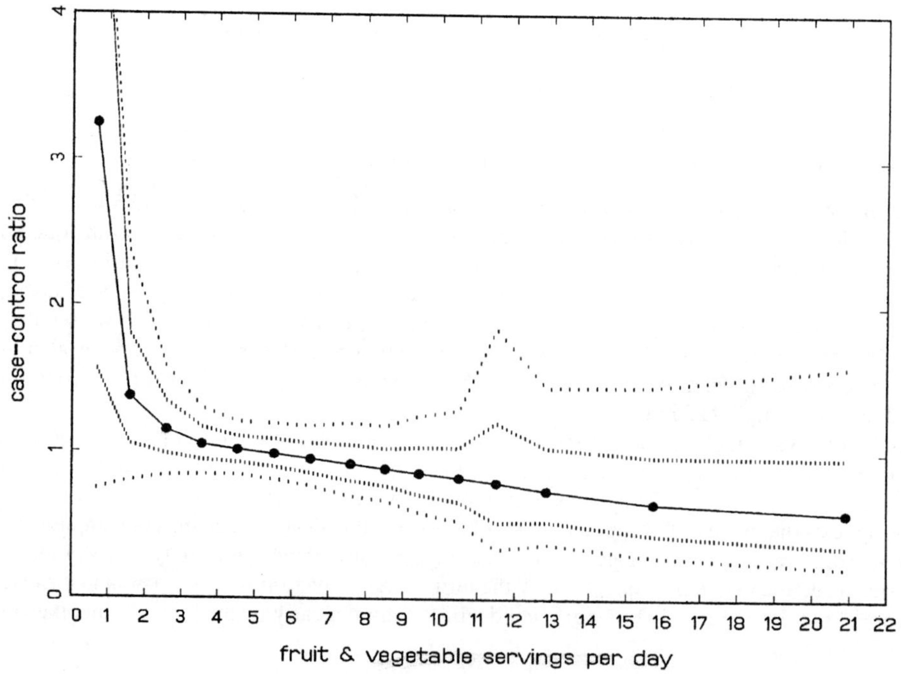

FIGURE 17–6 • Plot of running weighted-average case-control ratios from data in Table 17–4, using arithmetic scale and logarithmic weight function.

Nevertheless, transforming the results back to the original scale can be important for interpretation; in our example, this transformation makes clear that, even after smoothing, the association under study is concentrated largely at the lowest intake levels.

VARIABLE-SPAN SMOOTHERS

Instead of being constant, the window width $2h$ can be allowed to vary with x so that there are either a fixed number of subjects or (equivalently) a fixed percentage of subjects in each window. For example, the width may be chosen so each window has as close to 100 subjects as possible. (It may not be possible to have exactly 100 subjects in some windows, because there may be subjects with identical exposure values that have to be all in or all out of any window.) The width may instead be chosen so that each window has as close to 50% of all subjects as possible. These types of windows are called (asymmetric) *nearest-neighbor* windows. The proportion of subjects in each window is called the *span* of the window.

In a person-time rate analysis or in an analysis in which the number of cases is far less than the number of noncases, the window widths can be chosen to include a fixed percentage of cases instead of subjects. There are many more sophisticated methods for choosing window widths, but the basic nearest-neighbor approaches just described are adequate for exploratory analyses. The larger the span is, the smoother the curve that will be generated. With a computer program, it is a simple matter to graph a moving average for several different spans. Such a process can provide a feel for the stability of patterns observed in the graphs.

CATEGORICAL ESTIMATES AS MOVING AVERAGES

The curves obtained from moving weighted averages tend to be biased toward flatness, especially when wide windows are used or the curve is highly nonlinear in the scales used for averaging. The latter problem is one of the reasons we used the log scale rather than the original scale when smoothing the curve in the example. Nonetheless, moving averages are less biased than the curves obtained using fixed categories of width that are less than the window width of the moving weighted average. The curves obtained by plotting rates or risks from fixed categories are special cases of moving averages in which only a few (usually four to six) nonoverlapping windows are used. Curves from fixed categories correspond to using a weight function $w_u(x)$ that equals 1 for all exposure levels u in the category of x and equals 0 for all u outside the category. In other words, the fixed-category curves in Figures 17–1 through 17–4 may be viewed as just very crude versions of moving-average graphs.

MORE GENERAL SMOOTHERS

One way to avoid flattening of the smoothed curve is to use a running-weighted regression curve (such as *a running weighted line*) rather than a running weighted average. Moving averages and running curves are examples of *scatterplot smoothers* (Hastie and Tibshirani, 1990). Such techniques can be extended to include covariate adjustment and other refinements; see the discussion of nonparametric regression in Chapter 21. Software that produces and graphs the results from such smoothers is becoming more widely available. We strongly recommend use of smoothers whenever one must study trends or dose–response with a continuous exposure variable, and a substantial number of subjects are spread across the range of exposure. The smoothed curves produced by these techniques can help alert one to violations of assumptions that underlie common regression models, can make more efficient use of the data than categorical methods, and can be used as presentation graphics.

BASIC ANALYSIS OF MULTIPLE OUTCOMES

Several special points should be considered in analyses of data in which the individual outcomes are classified beyond a simple dichotomy of "diseased/nondiseased" or "case/control." Such data arise when disease is subclassified by subtype, or competing causes of death are studied, or multiple case or control groups are selected in a case-control study. For example, studies of cancer usually subdivide cases by cancer site; a study of cancer at a given site may subdivide cases by stage at diagnosis or by histology; and in hospital-based case-control studies, controls may be subdivided according to diagnosis.

The simplest approach to multiple-outcome analysis is to perform repeated dichotomous-outcome analyses, one for each disease rate or risk in a cohort study, or one for each case-control group combination in a case-control study. Such repeated analyses are rarely sufficient, however; for example, in case-control studies with multiple control groups, one should also conduct a comparison of the control groups. It can also be important to examine simultaneous estimates of all effects of interest (Thomas et al., 1985). The most statistically efficient way to perform simultaneous comparisons involves methods such as polytomous logistic regression, described in Chapter 20. These methods also lend themselves directly to sensible multiple-comparison procedures based on hierarchical regression (Greenland, 1992a, 1997b; see Chapter 21).

We recommend that one begin with tabular analyses, cross-classifying all outcomes (including the noncases or denominators) against the exposure variable. Table 17–5 presents results on the association of male genital implants with cancers diagnosed a year or more following the implant (Greenland and Finkle, 1996). The estimates in the table were adjusted using 5-year age categories and 1-year categories for year of diagnosis. The first panel of the table compares the five different diagnoses chosen as control diseases, using the largest group (colon polyps) as referent. The differences observed here were judged small enough to warrant combination of the controls into one group for the main analysis in the second panel of the table. This analysis suggests an association of the implants with liver cancer and possibly bone and connective-tissue cancer as well.

TABLE 17–5

Case-Control Data on Male Genital Implants (Penile and Testicular) and Cancers Diagnosed >1 Year after Implant

	Implant				
	Yes	No	Odds Ratio	(95% Limits)	*P*-Value
I. Comparisons of Control Diseases					
Benign stomach tumors[a]	6	1,718	1.24	(0.48, 2.59)	0.63
Deviated septum	17	7,874	1.04	(0.61, 1.76)	0.88
Viral pneumonia	10	3,616	1.22	(0.63, 2.38)	0.55
Gallstones	49	20,986	0.91	(0.64, 1.29)	0.60
Colon polyps	94	32,707	1.00	(reference group)	
II. Comparison of Cancers against Combined Controls					
Liver[a]	10	1,700	2.47	(1.22, 4.44)	0.02
Bone[a]	19	4,979	1.70	(1.02, 2.65)	0.04
Connective tissue[a]	8	2,119	1.54	(0.69, 2.92)	0.27
Brain	26	10,296	1.14	(0.75, 1.73)	0.53
Lymphomas	10	4,068	1.02	(0.54, 1.93)	0.95
Myelomas[a]	3	1,455	0.84	(0.20, 2.21)	0.76
Leukemias[a]	5	2,401	0.89	(0.31, 1.94)	0.79
All control diseases	176	66,901	1.00	(reference group)	

[a] Median-unbiased estimates and mid-*P* statistics; remainder are Mantel-Haenszel statistics. Statistics were derived with stratification on age in 5-year intervals from 30 to 89 years of age and year of diagnosis in 1-year intervals from 1989 to 1994. *P*-values are two-sided.

From Greenland S, Finkle WD. A case-control study of prosthetic implants and selected chronic diseases. *Ann Epidemiol.* 1996;6:530–540.

As with an analysis of a polytomous exposure, analysis of multiple diseases should include examination of a simultaneous statistic that tests for all exposure–disease associations. For unstratified data, one can use the Pearson χ^2 statistic, which when applied to the numbers in the second panel of Table 17–5 has a value of 10.23 with seven degrees of freedom (the number of cancers). This statistic yields $P = 0.18$ for the joint hypothesis of no exposure–cancer association, indicating that the spread of estimates and P-values seen in the table is fairly consistent with purely random variation. This fact would not be apparent from examining only the pairwise comparisons in the table. We further discuss simultaneous analysis of multiple outcome data in the next section.

SIMULTANEOUS STATISTICS FOR TABULAR DATA

Earlier we mentioned the multiple-comparisons problem inherent in separate pairwise comparisons of multiple exposure levels. This problem is ordinarily addressed by presenting a *simultaneous* or *joint* analysis of the exposure levels. In the remainder of this chapter, we describe the principles of simultaneous analysis in more detail.

To understand better the distinction between separate and joint analyses of multiple exposure levels, consider the following $J(J + 1)/2$ questions regarding an exposure with $J + 1$ levels (one question for each pair i, j of exposure levels):

Question ij: Do exposure levels X_i and X_j have different rates of disease?

For an exposure with three levels ($J = 2$), this represents $2(3)/2 = 3$ different questions. Each of these questions could be addressed by conducting a Mantel-Haenszel comparison of the corresponding pair of exposure levels. We would then get three different Mantel-Haenszel statistics, χ_{MH10}, χ_{MH20}, χ_{MH21}, which compare exposure levels X_1 to X_0, X_2 to X_0, and X_2 to X_1. In the absence of biases, χ_{MHij} would have a standard normal distribution under the single null hypothesis:

H_{0ij}: Exposure levels X_i and X_j have the same disease rate, regardless of the rates at other levels.

Thus, in Table 17–3, the first P-value of 0.005 refers to the hypothesis that the ≤ 2 category has the same polyp rate as the >6 category, regardless of the rate in any other exposure category.

Contrast the above set of questions and hypotheses, which consider only two exposures at a time, with the following question that considers all exposure levels simultaneously:

Joint Question: Are there *any* differences among the rates of disease at different exposure levels?

This question is a compound of all the separate (pairwise) questions, in that it is equivalent to asking whether there is a difference in the rates between *any* pair of exposure levels. To address this joint question statistically, we need to use a test statistic (such as the Pearson statistic χ^2_{P} or the Mantel trend statistic χ_{trend}) that specifically tests the joint null hypothesis:

H_{Joint}: There is no difference among the disease rates at different exposure levels.

This hypothesis asserts that the answer to the joint question is "no."

We may extend the Pearson statistic to test joint hypotheses other than the joint null. To do so, we must be able to generate expected values under non-null hypotheses. For example, if exposure has three levels indexed by $j = 0, 1, 2$ ($J = 2$), we must be able to generate expected values under the hypothesis that the rate ratios IR_1 and IR_2 comparing level 1 and 2 to level 0 are 2 and 3 (H_{Joint}:$IR_1 = 2$, $IR_2 = 3$), as well as under other hypotheses. Consider the person-time data in Table 17–1. Under the hypothesis that the true rate ratios for $X_1, \ldots, X_J$ versus X_0 are $IR_1, \ldots, IR_J$, the expectation of A_j is

$$E_j = \frac{IR_j T_j}{\sum\limits_k IR_k T_k}. \qquad [17\text{–}5]$$

The summation index k in the denominator ranges from 0 to J; IR_0 (the rate ratio for X_0 versus X_0) is equal to 1 by definition. To obtain a test statistic for the hypothesis that the true rate ratios are $IR_1, \ldots, IR_J$, we need only substitute these expected values into the Pearson χ^2 formula (equation 17–1 or 17–2). If there is no bias and the hypothesis is correct, the resulting χ^2_{P} will have approximately a χ^2 distribution with J degrees of freedom. Again, the accuracy of the approximation depends on the size of the expected values E_j.

Although the non-null Pearson statistic can be extended to stratified data, this extension requires the expected numbers to be large in all strata, and so methods based on regression models are preferable (Chapter 21).

JOINT CONFIDENCE REGIONS

Rarely is a particular non-null hypothesis of special interest. The Pearson statistic based on non-null expected values (formula 17–5) can, however, be used to find *joint* (or simultaneous) *confidence regions*. Such a region is the generalization of a confidence interval to encompass several measures at once. To understand the concept, suppose that exposure has three levels, X_0, X_1, X_2, and that we are interested in the log rate ratios $\ln(IR_1)$ and $\ln(IR_2)$ comparing levels X_1 and X_2 to X_0. Figure 17–7 shows an elliptical region in the plane of possible values for $\ln(IR_2)$ and $\ln(IR_1)$. Such a region is called a *C% confidence region* for $\ln(IR_1)$ and $\ln(IR_2)$ if it is constructed by a method that produces regions containing the pair of true values for $\ln(IR_1)$, $\ln(IR_2)$ with at least $C\%$ frequency.

Suppose we have an approximate statistic for testing that the pair of true values equals a particular pair of numbers, such as the simultaneous Pearson statistic χ^2_P described earlier. Then we can construct an approximate $C\%$ confidence region for the pair of true values by taking it to be the set of all points that have a P-value greater than $1 - C/100$. For example, to get an approximate 90% confidence region for IR_1, IR_2 in the preceding examples, we could take the region to be the set of all points that have $P \geq 0.10$ by the Pearson χ^2 test. We could also obtain a 90% confidence region for $\ln(IR_1)$, $\ln(IR_2)$ just by plotting these points for IR_1, IR_2, using logarithmic axes.

The notion of joint confidence region extends to any number of measures. For example, in studying a four-level exposure with three rate ratios, IR_1, IR_2, IR_3, we could use the Pearson statistic to obtain a three-dimensional confidence region. Given large enough numbers, the corresponding region for $\ln(IR_1)$, $\ln(IR_2)$, $\ln(IR_3)$ would resemble an ellipsoid.

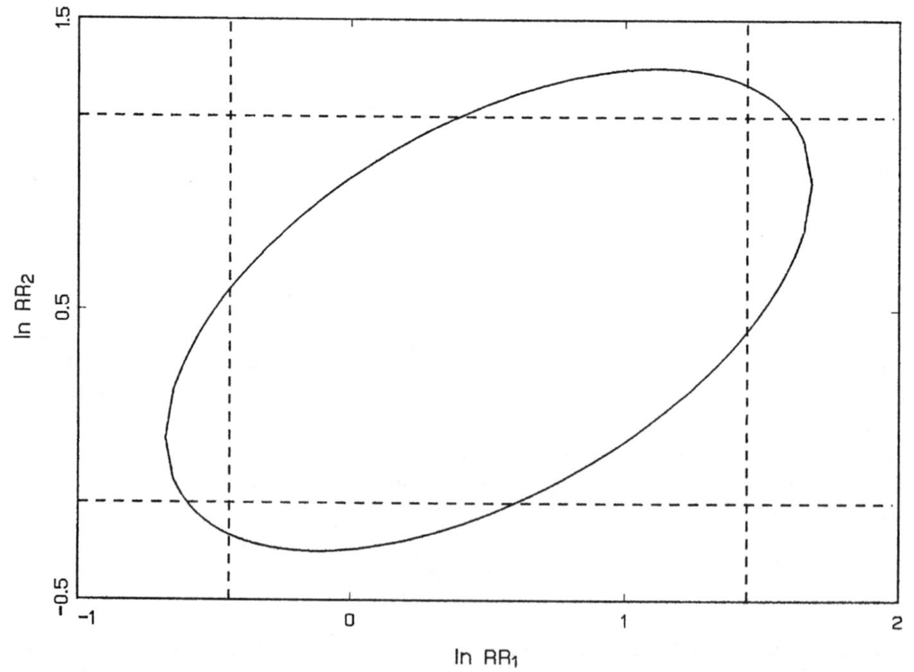

FIGURE 17–7 • Graphical comparison of single 95% confidence intervals (dashed lines) and a joint 95% confidence region (ellipse).

TABLE 17–6

General Data Layout for Simultaneous Analysis of Three Diseases in a Person-Time Follow-up Study

	Exposure Level			
	X_J	...	X_0	Totals
Disease		...		
D_3	A_{3J}	...	A_{20}	M_3
D_2	A_{2J}	...	A_{20}	M_2
D_1	A_{1J}	...	A_{10}	M_1
All diseases D	A_J	...	A_0	M
Person-time	T_J	...	T_0	T

SIMULTANEOUS ANALYSIS OF MULTIPLE OUTCOMES

Table 17–6 illustrates a general data layout for simultaneous analysis of three diseases in a person-time follow-up study. There are several parameters that can be studied with these data, among them:

1. The association of the combined-disease outcome D ("All diseases") with exposure
2. The association of each disease D_h ($h = 1, 2, 3$) with exposure
3. The differences among the separate exposure–disease associations

For example, we could have D = colon cancer with D_1 = ascending, D_2 = transverse, and D_3 = descending colon cancer. The associations of exposure with the combined site D and separate sites D_I could be examined one at a time, using any of the methods described earlier for analyzing a single-disease outcome. We also have the option of analyzing the separate sites simultaneously.

To understand the distinction between separate and joint analyses, consider the following questions (one each for $h = 1, 2, 3$):

Question h: Is exposure associated with disease D_h?

For the colon cancer example, this represents three different questions, one for each of the ascending ($h = 1$), transverse ($h = 2$), and descending ($h = 3$) sites. Each of these questions could be examined separately by repeatedly applying the unordered Pearson statistic or the Mantel trend statistic described earlier in this chapter, each time using a different row for the number of cases but keeping the same denominators T_j. The unordered analyses would yield three Pearson statistics χ^2_{P1}, χ^2_{P2}, χ^2_{P3}, one for each disease site D_h, and we might also obtain three corresponding trend statistics χ_{T1}, χ_{T2}, χ_{T3}. In the absence of biases, the statistic χ^2_{Ph} would have approximately a χ^2 distribution with J degrees of freedom if the following null hypothesis (a "no" answer to Question h) was true:

H_{0h}: Exposure is unassociated with disease D_h, regardless of the exposure association with any other disease site.

Similarly, in the absence of biases, the statistic χ_{Th} would have approximately a standard normal distribution if H_{0h} were true.

Contrast the three questions that consider one disease site at a time with the following question that considers all sites simultaneously:

Joint Question: Is exposure associated with *any* of the sites D_1, D_2, D_3?

Logically, the answer to this question is "no" if and only if the answer is "no" to all of the three preceding questions. That is, the joint null hypothesis,

H_{Joint}: Exposure is not associated with any site.

is equivalent to stating that H_{0h} is true for every site D_h. A test statistic for H_{Joint} that does not require or make use of any ordering of exposure is the joint Pearson statistic,

$$\chi^2_{P+} = \sum_h E_j(A_{hj} - E_{hj})^2/E_{hj} \qquad [17\text{–}6]$$

where $E_{hj} = M_h T_j/T_+$ is the expectation of A_{hj} under the joint null hypothesis H_{Joint}. With I diseases, this statistic has approximately a χ^2 distribution with IJ degrees of freedom if there is no bias and H_{Joint} is true. Note that $\chi^2_{P+} = \sum_h \chi^2_{Ph}$. For pure count data, χ^2_{P+} is equal to $N_+/(N_+ - 1)$ times the generalized Mantel-Haenszel statistic for pure count data. The latter statistic generalizes to stratified data without an increase in degrees of freedom, but requires matrix inversion (Somes, 1986). Alternatively, one may test H_{Joint} using a deviance statistic computed using a polytomous logistic regression program (Chapters 20 and 21).

A test statistic for H_{Joint} that makes use of ordered exposure scores $s_0, s_1, \ldots, s_J$ is the joint trend statistic

$$\chi^2_{T+} = \sum_h (S_h - E_h)^2/V_h \qquad [17\text{–}7]$$

where

$$S_h = \sum_j A_{hj}s_j, \quad E_h = M_h \sum_j T_j s_j/T$$

and

$$V_h = M_h\left(\sum_j T_j s_j/T - E_h^2\right)$$

χ^2_{T+} has approximately a χ^2 distribution with the number of diseases as its degrees of freedom if there are no biases and the joint null is true. For person-time data, $\chi^2_{T+} = \sum_h \chi^2_{Th}$. Like the Mantel-Haenszel statistic, the stratified version of χ^2_{T+} requires matrix inversion, but it is also easily computed using a polytomous logistic regression program. If both the disease and exposure have ordered scores, a one-degree-of-freedom statistic can be constructed for testing H_{Joint} that will usually be more powerful than χ^2_{T+} (Mantel, 1963).

RELATION BETWEEN SIMULTANEOUS AND SINGLE COMPARISONS

It is an important and apparently paradoxical fact that the simple logical relations between simultaneous and single-comparison hypotheses do *not* carry over to simultaneous and single-comparison statistics. For example, the joint null hypothesis that there is no difference in disease rates across exposure levels can be false if and only if at least one of the single null hypotheses is false. Nonetheless, it is possible to have the P-value from the multiple-disease statistic χ^2_P be much smaller than every one of the P-values from the single-disease statistics χ^2_{Ph}. For example, suppose we had rates at three disease sites and four exposure levels ($J = 3$ with three nonreference levels), with $\chi^2_{P1} = \chi^2_{P2} = \chi^2_{P3} = 6.3$ with $J = 3$ degrees of freedom for each disease separately. These statistics each yield $P = 0.10$, but the joint statistic is then $\chi^2_{P+} = 6.3 + 6.3 + 6.3 = 18.9$ on $3 + 3 + 3 = 9$ degrees of freedom, which yields $P = 0.03$.

Conversely, a joint null hypothesis can be true if and only if all the single null hypotheses are true. Yet it is possible for the P-value from one or more (but not all) of the single statistics to be much smaller than the P-value from the joint statistic, χ^2_P. For example, with rates at two disease sites and four exposure levels, we could get $\chi^2_{P1} = 0$ and $\chi^2_{P2} = 8.4$ with three degrees of freedom for the two sites, which yield P-values of 1.0 and 0.04. But then $\chi^2_{P+} = 0 + 8.4 = 8.4$ with six degrees of freedom, which has a P-value of 0.2. The results in the second panel of Table 17–5 illustrate a similar phenomenon for pure count data: The liver and bone cancer associations have $P = 0.02$ and $P = 0.04$, yet the joint P-value for all seven diseases is 0.18.

Similar examples can be found using other statistics, such as the simultaneous trend statistic χ^2_{T+}. In general, simultaneous (joint hypothesis) P-values do not have a simple logical relation to the single-hypothesis P-values. This counterintuitive lack of relation also applies to confidence intervals. For example, a simultaneous 95% confidence region for two rate ratios need not contain a point contained in the two one-at-a-time 95% confidence intervals; conversely, a point in the simultaneous 95% confidence region may not be in all of the one-at-a-time confidence intervals.

A resolution of the apparent paradox may be obtained by overlaying a simultaneous 95% confidence region for two log rate ratios with two single 95% confidence intervals, as in Figure 17–7. The single 95% confidence intervals are simply a vertical band for $\ln(RR_1)$ and a horizontal band for $\ln(RR_2)$. For a valid study design, the vertical band contains $\ln(RR_1)$ with at least 95% probability (over study repetitions) and the horizontal band contains $\ln(RR_2)$ with at least 95% probability; nonetheless, the overlap of these bands (which is the dashed square) contains the true pair ($\ln(RR_1)$, $\ln(RR_2)$) with as little as $0.95(0.95) \doteq 0.90$ or 90% probability. In contrast, the joint 95% confidence region is the ellipse, which contains the true pair ($\ln(RR_1)$ $\ln(RR_2)$) with at least 95% probability over study repetitions. Note that two of the square's corners are outside the ellipse; points inside these corners are inside the overlap of the single confidence intervals, but outside the joint confidence region. Conversely, there are sections inside the ellipse that are outside the square; points inside these sections are inside the joint confidence region but outside one or the other single confidence interval.

Figure 17–7 may help one visualize why a joint confidence region and the single confidence intervals have very different objectives: Simultaneous methods use a single region to try to capture *all* the true associations at once at a given minimum frequency, while keeping the area (or volume) of the region as small as possible. In contrast, single methods use a single interval to capture just one true association at a given minimum frequency, while keeping this one interval as narrow as possible. Overlapping the regions produced by the single intervals will not produce joint confidence regions that are valid at the confidence level of the single intervals.

CHAPTER 18

Introduction to Bayesian Statistics

Sander Greenland

Frequentism versus Subjective Bayesianism 329
- Subjective Probabilities Should Not Be Arbitrary 330
- The Posterior Distribution 330
- Frequentist–Bayesian Parallels 331
- Empirical Priors 331
- Frequentist–Bayesian Divergences 332
- Frequentist Fantasy versus Observational Reality 332
- Summary 333

Simple Approximate Bayesian Methods 333

Information-Weighted Averaging 334
- A Single Two-Way Table 334
- Bayesian Interpretation of Frequentist Results 335
- Adjustment 336
- Varying the Prior 336
- Bayes versus Semi-Bayes 337

Prior Data: Frequentist Interpretation of Priors 337
- Reverse-Bayes Analysis 338
- Priors with Non-Null Center 339
- Choosing the Sizes of the Prior Denominators 339
- Non-Normal Priors 340
- Further Extensions 340

Checking the Prior 340

Discussion 341
- Data Alone Say Nothing at All 341
- Data Priors as a General Diagnostic Device 341
- The Role of Markov-Chain Monte Carlo 342
- Connections to Sensitivity Analysis 342
- Some Cautions on Use of Priors 342

Conclusions 343

Chapters 10 and 13 briefly introduced the central concepts of Bayesian statistics. Beginning with Laplace in the 18th century, these methods were used freely alongside other methods. In the 1920s, however, several influential statisticians (R. A. Fisher, J. Neyman, and E. Pearson) developed bodies of frequentist techniques intended to supplant entirely all others, based on notions of objective probability represented by relative frequencies in hypothetical infinite sequences of randomized experiments or random samplings. For the rest of the 20th century these methods dominated statistical research and became the sole body of methods taught to most students. Chapters 14 through 17 describe the fundamentals of these frequentist methods for epidemiologic studies.

In the context of randomized trials and random-sample surveys in which they were developed, these frequentist techniques appear to be highly effective tools. As the use of the methods spread from designed surveys and experiments to observational studies, however, an increasing number of statisticians questioned the objectivity and realism of the hypothetical infinite sequences invoked by frequentist methods (e.g., Lindley, 1965; DeFinetti, 1974; Cornfield, 1976; Leamer, 1978; Good, 1983; Berger and Berry, 1988; Berk et al., 1995; Greenland, 1998a). They argued that a subjective

Bayesian approach better represented situations in which the mechanisms generating study samples and exposure status were heavily nonrandom and poorly understood. In those settings, which typify most epidemiologic research, the personal judgments of the investigators play an unavoidable and crucial role in making inferences and often override technical considerations that dominate statistical analyses (as perhaps they should; cf. Susser, 1977).

In the wake of such arguments, Bayesian methods have become common in advanced training and research in statistics (e.g., Leonard and Hsu, 1999; Carlin and Louis, 2000; Gelman et al., 2003; Efron, 2005), even in the randomized-trial literature for which frequentist methods were developed (e.g., Spiegelhalter et al., 1994, 2004). Elementary training appears to have lagged, however, despite arguments for reform (Berry, 1997). The present chapter illustrates how the conventional frequentist methods introduced in Chapter 15 can be used to generate Bayesian analyses. In particular, it shows how basic epidemiologic analyses can be conducted with a hand calculator or ordinary software packages for stratified analysis (Greenland, 2006a). The same computational devices can also be used to conduct Bayesian regression analyses with ordinary regression software (Greenland, 2007a; Chapter 21). Thus, as far as computation is concerned, it is a small matter to extend current training and practice to encompass Bayesian methods.

The chapter begins with a philosophical section that criticizes standard objections to Bayesian approaches, and that delineates key parallels and differences between frequentist and Bayesian methods. It does not address distinctions within frequentist and Bayesian traditions. See Chapter 10 and Goodman (1993) for reviews of the profound divergence between Fisherian and Neyman-Pearsonian frequentism. The present chapter argues that observational researchers (not just statisticians) need training in subjective Bayesianism (Lindley, 1965; DeFinetti, 1974; Goldstein, 2006) to serve as a counterweight to the alleged objectivity of frequentist methods. For this purpose, neither "objective" Bayesian methods (Berger, 2004) nor "pure likelihood" methods (Royall, 1997) will do, because they largely replicate the pretense of objectivity that renders frequentist methods so misleading in observational research.

Much of the modern Bayesian literature focuses on a level of precision in specifying a prior and analytic computation that is far beyond anything required of frequentist methods or by the messy problems of observational data analysis. Many of these computing methods obscure important parallels between traditional frequentist methods and Bayesian methods. High precision is unnecessary given the imprecision of the data and the goals of everyday epidemiology. Furthermore, subjective Bayesian methods are distinguished by their use of informative prior distributions; hence their proper use requires a sound understanding of the meaning and limitations of those distributions, not a false sense of precision. In observational studies, neither Bayesian nor other methods require extremely precise computation, especially in light of the huge uncertainties about the processes generating observational data (represented by the likelihood function), as well as uncertainty about prior information.

After an introduction to the philosophy of Bayesian methods, the chapter focuses on basic Bayesian approaches that display prior distributions as prior estimates or prior data, and that employ the same approximate formulas used by frequentist methods (Lindley, 1964; Good, 1965, 1983; Bedrick et al., 1996; Greenland 2001b, 2003b, 2006a, 2007a, 2007b; Greenland and Christensen, 2001). Even for those who prefer other computing methods, the representation of prior distributions as prior data is helpful in understanding the strength of the prior judgments.

FREQUENTISM VERSUS SUBJECTIVE BAYESIANISM

There are several objections that frequentists have raised against Bayesian methods. Some of these are legitimate but apply in parallel to frequentist methods (and indeed to all of statistics) in observational studies. Most important, perhaps, is that the assumptions or models employed are at best subjective judgments. Others are propaganda—e.g., that adopting a Bayesian approach introduces arbitrariness that is not already present. In reality, the Bayesian approach makes explicit those subjective and arbitrary elements that are shared by all statistical inferences. Because these elements are hidden by frequentist conventions, Bayesian methods are left open to criticisms that make it appear only they are using those elements.

SUBJECTIVE PROBABILITIES SHOULD NOT BE ARBITRARY

In subjective (personalist) Bayesian theory, a prior for a parameter is a probability distribution Pr(parameters) that shows how a particular person would bet about parameters if she disregarded the data under analysis. This prior need not originate from evidence preceding the study; rather, it represents information apart from the data being analyzed. When the only parameter is a risk ratio, RR, the 50th percentile (median) of her prior Pr(RR) is a number RR_{median} for which she would give even odds that $RR < RR_{median}$ versus $RR > RR_{median}$, i.e., she would assign $Pr(RR < RR_{median}) = Pr(RR > RR_{median})$ if she disregarded the analysis data. Similarly, her 95% prior limits are a pair of numbers RR_{lower} and RR_{upper} such that she would give 95:5 = 19:1 odds that the true risk ratio is between these numbers, i.e., $Pr(RR_{lower} < RR < RR_{upper}) = .95$ if she disregarded the analysis data.

Prior limits may vary considerably across individuals; mine may be very different from yours. This variability does not mean, however, that the limits are arbitrary. When betting on a race with the goal of minimizing losses, no one would regard it reasonable to bet everything on a randomly drawn contestant; rather, a person would place different bets on different contestants, based on their previous performance (but taking account of differences in the past conditions from the present). Similarly, in order for a Bayesian analysis to seem reasonable or credible to others, a prior should reflect results from previous studies or reviews. This reflection should allow for possible biases and lack of generalizability among studies, so that prior limits might be farther apart than frequentist meta-analytic confidence limits (even if the latter incorporated random effects).

The prior Pr(parameters) is one of two major inputs to a Bayesian analysis. The other input is a function Pr(data|parameters) that shows the probability the analyst would assign the observed data for any given set of parameter values (usually called the *likelihood function*; see Chapter 13). In subjective-Bayesian analysis this function is another set of bets: The model for Pr(data|parameters) summarizes how one would bet on the study outcome (the data) if one knew the parameters (e.g., the exposure-covariate specific risks). Any such model should meet the same credibility requirements as the prior. This requirement parallels the frequentist concern that the model should be able to approximate reality. In fact, any competent Bayesian has the same concern, albeit perhaps with more explicit doubts about whether that can be achieved with standard models.

The same need for credibility motivates authors to discuss other literature when writing their research reports. Credible authors pay attention to past literature in their analyses, e.g., by adjusting for known or suspected confounders, by not adjusting for factors affected by exposure, and by using a dose–response model that can capture previously observed patterns (e.g., the J-shaped relation of alcohol use to cardiovascular mortality). They may even vary their models to accommodate different views on what adjustments should be done. In a similar manner, Bayesian analyses need not be limited to using a single prior or likelihood function. Acceptability of an analysis is often enhanced by presenting results from different priors to reflect different opinions about the parameter, by presenting results using a prior that is broad enough to assign relatively high probability to each discussant's opinion (a "consensus" prior), and by presenting results from different degrees of regression adjustment (which involves varying the likelihood function).

THE POSTERIOR DISTRIBUTION

Upon seeing the outcome of a race on which a person had bet, she would want to update her bets regarding the outcome of another race involving the same contestants. In this spirit, Bayesian analysis produces a model for the posterior distribution Pr(parameters|data), a probability distribution that shows how she should bet about the parameters *after* examining the analysis data.

As a minimal criterion of reasonable betting, suppose she would never want to place her bets in a manner that allows an opponent betting against her to guarantee a loss. This criterion implies that her bets should obey the laws of probability, including Bayes's theorem,

$$\text{Pr(parameters|data)} = \text{Pr(data|parameters)Pr(parameters)/Pr(data)}$$

where the portion Pr(data) is computed from the likelihood function and the prior (for a review of these arguments, see Greenland, 1998a). The 50th percentile (median) of her posterior about a risk ratio RR is a number RR_{median} for which $Pr(RR < RR_{median}|data) = Pr(RR > RR_{median}|data)$, where "|data" indicates that this bet is formulated in light of the analysis data. Similarly, her 95% posterior limits are a pair of numbers RR_{lower} and RR_{upper} such that after analyzing the data she would give 95:5 = 19:1 odds that the true relative risk is between these numbers, i.e., $Pr(RR_{lower} < RR < RR_{upper}|data) = 0.95$.

As with priors, posterior distributions may vary considerably across individuals, not only because they may use different priors Pr(parameters), but also because they may use different models for the data probabilities Pr(data|parameters). This variation is only to be expected given disagreement among observers about the implications of past study results and the present study's design. Bayesian analyses can help pinpoint sources of disagreement, especially in that they distinguish sources in the priors from sources in the data models.

FREQUENTIST–BAYESIAN PARALLELS

It is often said (incorrectly) that "parameters are treated as fixed by the frequentist but as random by the Bayesian." For frequentists and Bayesians alike, the value of a parameter may have been fixed from the start, or it may have been generated from a physically random mechanism. In either case, both suppose that it has taken on some fixed value that we would like to know. The Bayesian uses probability models to express personal uncertainty about that value. In other words, the "randomness" in these models represents personal uncertainty; it is *not* a property of the parameter, although it should accurately reflect properties of the mechanisms that produced the parameter.

A crucial parallel between frequentist and Bayesian methods is their dependence on the model chosen for the data probability Pr(data|parameters). Statistical results are as sensitive to this choice as they are to choice of priors. The choice should thus ideally reflect the best available knowledge about forces that influence the data, including effects of unmeasured variables, biased selection, and measurement errors (such as misclassification). Instead, the choice is almost always a default built into statistical software, based on assumptions of random sampling or random treatment assignment (which are rarely credible in observational epidemiology), plus additivity assumptions. Worse, the data models are often selected by mechanical algorithms that are oblivious to background information and, as a result, often conflict with contextual information. These problems afflict the majority of epidemiologic analyses today, in the form of models (such as the logistic, Poisson, and proportional-hazards models) that make interaction and dose–response assumptions that are rarely if ever justified. These models are never known to be correct and in fact cannot hold exactly, especially when one considers possible study biases (Greenland, 1990, 2005b).

Acceptance of results derived from these models (whether the results are frequentist or Bayesian) thus requires the doubtful assumption that existing violations have no important effect on results. The model for Pr(data|parameters) is thus a weak link in the chain of reasoning leading from data to inference, shared by both frequentist and Bayesian methods. In practice, the two approaches often use the same model for Pr(data|parameters), whence divergent outputs from the methods must arise elsewhere. A major source of divergence is the explicit prior Pr(parameters) used in Bayesian reasoning. The methods described in this chapter will show the mechanics of this divergence and provide a sense of when it will be important.

EMPIRICAL PRIORS

The addition of the prior Pr(parameter) raises the point that the validity of the Bayesian answer will depend on the validity of the prior model as well as the validity of the data model. If the prior should not just be some arbitrary opinion, however, what should it be?

One answer arises from frequentist shrinkage-estimation methods (also known as Stein estimation, empirical-Bayes, penalized estimation, and random-coefficient or ridge regression) to improve repeated-sampling accuracy of estimates. These methods use numerical devices that translate directly into priors (Leamer, 1978; Good, 1983; Titterington, 1985) and thus leave unanswered the same question asked of subjective Bayesians: Where should these devices come from? Empirical-Bayes and random-coefficient methods assume explicitly that the parameters as well as the data would vary randomly across repetitions according to an actual frequency distribution Pr(parameters) that can be estimated from available data. As in Bayesian analyses, these methods compute posterior coefficient distributions using Bayes's theorem. Given the randomness of the coefficients, however, the resulting posterior intervals are also frequentist confidence intervals in the sense of containing the true (if varying) parameter values in the stated percentage of repetitions (Carlin and Louis, 2000).

Those who wish to extend Bayes–frequentist parallels into practice are thus led to the following empirical principle: When true frequency distributions exist and are known for the data or the parameter distribution (as in multilevel random sampling; Goldstein, 2003), they should be used as the distributions in Bayesian analysis. This principle reflects the idea of placing odds on race contestants based on their past frequencies of winning and corresponds to common notions of induction (Greenland, 1998b). Such frequency-based priors are more accurately termed "empirical" rather than "subjective," although the decision to accept the empirical evidence remains a subjective judgment (and subject to error). Empirical priors are mandated in much of Bayesian philosophy, such as the "principal principle" of Lewis (1981), which states that when frequency probabilities exist and are known (as in games of chance and in quantum physics), one should use them as personal probabilities. More generally, an often-obeyed (if implicit) inductive principle is that the prior should be found by fitting to available empirical frequencies, as is often done in frequentist hierarchical regression (Good, 1965, 1983, 1987; Greenland, 2000d; Chapter 21). The fitted prior is thus no more arbitrary than (and may even be functionally identical to) a fitted second-stage frequentist model. With empirical priors, the resulting frequentist and Bayesian interval estimates may be numerically identical.

FREQUENTIST–BAYESIAN DIVERGENCES

Even when a frequentist and a Bayesian arrive at the same interval estimate for a parameter, the interpretations remain quite different. Frequentist methods pretend that the models are laws of chance in the real world (indeed, much of the theoretical literature encourages this illusion by calling distributions "laws"). In contrast, subjective-Bayesian methods interpret the models as nothing more than summaries of tentative personal bets about how the data and the parameters would appear, rather than as models of a real random mechanism. The prior model *should* be based on observed frequencies when those are available, but the resulting model for the posterior Pr(parameters|model) is a summary of personal bets after seeing the data, not a frequency distribution (although if the parameters are physically random, it will also represent a personal estimate of their distribution).

It is important to recognize that the subjective-Bayesian interpretation is much less ambitious (and less confident) than the frequentist interpretation, insofar as it treats the models and the analysis results as systems of personal judgments, possibly poor ones, rather than as some sort of objective reality. Probabilities are nothing more than expressions of opinions, as in common phrasings such as "It will probably rain tomorrow." Reasonable opinions are based heavily on frequencies in past experience, but they are never as precise as results from statistical computations.

FREQUENTIST FANTASY VERSUS OBSERVATIONAL REALITY

For Bayesian methods, there seems no dispute that the results should be presented with reference to the priors as well as to the data models and the data. For example, a posterior interval should be presented as "*Given these priors, models, and data*, we would be 95% certain that the parameter is in this interval."

A parallel directive should be applied to frequentist presentations. For example, 95% confidence intervals are usually presented as if they account for random error, without regard for what that random error is supposed to represent. For observational research, one of many problems with frequentist ("repeated-sampling") interpretations is that it is not clear what is "random" when no random sampling or randomization has been done. Although "random variation" may be present even when it has not been introduced by the investigator, in observational studies there is seldom a sound rationale for claiming it follows the distributions that frequentist methods assume, or any known distribution (Greenland, 1990). At best, those distributions refer only to thought experiments in which one asks, "*If* data were repeatedly produced by the *assumed* random-sampling process, the statistics would have their stated properties (e.g., 95% coverage) across those repetitions." They do not refer to what happens under the distributions actually operating, for the latter are unknown.

Thus, what they do say is extremely hypothetical, so much so that to understand them fully is to doubt their relevance for observational research (Leamer, 1978).

Frequentist results are hypothetical whenever one cannot be certain that the assumed data model holds, as when uncontrolled sources of bias (such as confounding, selection bias, and measurement error) are present. In light of such problems, claims that frequentist methods are "objective" in an observational setting seem like propaganda or self-delusion (Leamer, 1978; Good, 1983; Berger and Berry, 1988; Greenland, 1998a, 2005b). At best, frequentist methods in epidemiology represent a dubious social convention that mandates treating observational data as if they arose from a fantasy of a tightly designed and controlled randomized experiment on a random sample (that is, as if a thought experiment were reality). Like many entrenched conventions, they provoke defenses that claim utility (e.g., Zeger, 1991; Efron, 2005) without any *comparative* empirical evidence that the conventions serve observational research better than would alternatives. Other defenses treat the frequentist thought experiments as if they were real—an example of what has been called the mind-projection fallacy (Jaynes and Bretthorst, 2003).

Were we to apply the same truth-in-packaging standard to frequentists as to Bayesians, a "statistically significant" frequentist result would be riddled with caveats such as "*If* these data had been generated from a randomized trial with no drop-out or measurement error, these results would be very improbable were the null true; but because they were not so generated we can say little of their actual statistical significance." Such brutal honesty is of course rare in presentations of observational epidemiologic results because emphasizing frequentist premises undermines the force of the presentation.

SUMMARY

A criticism of Bayesian methods is that the priors must be arbitrary, or subjective in a pernicious or special way. In observational studies, however, the prior need be no more arbitrary than the largely arbitrary data models that are routinely applied to data, and can often be given a scientific foundation as or more firm than that of frequentist data models. Like any analysis element, prior models should be scrutinized critically (and rejected as warranted), just as should frequentist models. When relevant and valid external frequency data are available, they should be used to build the prior model (which may lead to inclusion of those data as part of the likelihood function, so that the external and current data become pooled).

When prior frequency data are absent or invalid, however, other sources of priors will enter, and must be judged critically. Later sections will show how simple log relative-risk priors can be translated into "informationally equivalent" prior frequency data, which aids in this judgment, and which also allows easy extension of Bayesian methods to regression analysis and non-normal priors (Greenland, 2007ab).

SIMPLE APPROXIMATE BAYESIAN METHODS

Exact Bayesian analysis proceeds by computing the posterior distribution via Bayes's theorem, which requires Pr(data). The latter can be difficult to evaluate (usually requiring multiple integration over the parameters), which seems to have fostered the misimpression that practical Bayesian analyses are inherently more complex computationally than frequentist analyses. But this impression is based on an unfair comparison of *exact* Bayesian methods to *approximate* frequentist methods.

Frequentist teaching evolved during an era of limited computing, so they focused on simple, large-sample approximate methods for categorical data. In contrast, the Bayesian resurgence occurred during the introduction of powerful personal computers and advanced Monte Carlo algorithms, hence much Bayesian teaching focuses on exact methods, often presented as if simple approximations are inadequate. But Bayesian approximations suitable for categorical data have a long history (Lindley 1964; Good 1965), are as accurate as frequentist approximations, and are accurate enough for epidemiologic studies. The approximations also provide insights into the meaning of both Bayesian and frequentist methods and hence are the focus of the remainder of this chapter.

In the examples that follow, the outcome is very rare, so we may ignore distinctions among risk, rate, and odds ratios, which will be generically described as "relative risks" (RR). Because a normal distribution has equal mode, median, and mean, we may also ignore distinctions among these measures of location when discussing a normal ln(RR). When we take the antilog $e^{\ln(RR)} = RR$, however, we obtain a log-normal distribution, for which mode < median and geometric mean < arithmetic mean. Only the median transforms directly: median $RR = e^{\text{median}\ln(RR)}$.

INFORMATION-WEIGHTED AVERAGING

Information (or precision) is here defined as the inverse of the variance (Leonard and Hsu, 1999, sec. 3.4). Weighting by information shows how simple Bayesian methods parallel frequentist summary estimation based on inverse-variance weighting (Chapters 15 and 33). It assumes that both the prior model and the data model are adequately approximated by normal distributions. This assumption requires that the sample sizes (both actual and prior) are large enough for the approximation to be adequate. As with the approximate frequentist methods on which they are based, there is no hard-and-fast rule on what size is adequate, in part because of disagreement about how much inaccuracy is tolerable (which depends on context). As mentioned in earlier chapters, however, the same approximations in frequentist categorical statistics are arguably adequate down to cell sizes of 4 or 5 (Agresti, 2002).

A SINGLE TWO-WAY TABLE

Table 18–1 shows case-control data from Savitz et al. (1988), the first widely publicized study to report a positive association between residential magnetic fields and childhood leukemia. Although previous studies had reported positive associations between household wiring and leukemia, strong field effects seemed unlikely at the time, and very strong effects seemed very unlikely. Suppose we model these *a priori* ideas by placing 2:1 odds on a relative risk (RR) between ½ and 2 and 95% probability on RR between ¼ and 4 when comparing children above and below a 3 milligauss (mG) cutpoint for fields. These bets would follow from a normal prior for the log relative risk ln(RR) that satisfies

$$\exp(\text{prior mean} - 1.96 \cdot \text{prior standard deviation}) = 1/4$$

$$\exp(\text{prior mean} + 1.96 \cdot \text{prior standard deviation}) = 4$$

Solving this pair of equations, we get

$$\text{Prior mean of } \ln(RR) = \text{average of the limits} = \frac{\ln(1/4) + \ln(4)}{2} = 0$$

$$\text{Prior standard deviation of } \ln(RR) = \frac{\text{width of interval in } \ln(RR) \text{ units}}{\text{width of interval in standard deviation units}}$$

$$= \frac{\ln(4) - \ln(1/4)}{2(1.96)} = 0.707$$

$$\text{Prior variance of } \ln(RR) = 0.707^2 = 0.500 = 1/2$$

TABLE 18–1

Case-Control Data on Residential Magnetic Fields ($X = 1$ is >3 mG average exposure, $X = 0$ is ≤3 mG) and Childhood Leukemia (Savitz et al., 1988) and Frequentist Results

	$X = 1$	$X = 0$	
Cases	3	33	Table odds ratio = RR estimate = 3.51
Controls	5	193	95% confidence limits = 0.80, 15.4

ln(OR) = ln(RR) estimate = ln(3.51), estimated variance = 0.569

Thus, the normal prior distribution that would produce the stated bets has mean zero and variance $1/2$.

Three of 36 cases and five of 198 controls had estimated average fields above 3 milligauss (mG). These data yield the following frequentist RR estimates:

$$\text{Estimated RR} = \text{sample odds ratio} = 3(193)/5(33) = 3.51$$

$$\text{Estimated variance of log odds ratio} = 1/3 + 1/33 + 1/5 + 1/193 = 0.569$$

$$95\% \text{ confidence limits} = \exp[\ln(3.51) \pm 1.96 \cdot 0.569^{1/2}] = 0.80, 15.4$$

Assuming there is no prior information about the prevalence of exposure, an approximate posterior mean for ln(RR) is just the average of the prior mean ln(RR) of 0 and the data estimate ln(3.51), weighted by the information (inverse variance) of $1/(1/2)$ and $1/0.569$, respectively:

$$\text{Posterior mean for } \ln(\text{RR}) = \text{expected } \ln(\text{RR}) \text{ given data}$$
$$\approx [0/(1/2) + \ln(3.51)/0.569]/[1/(1/2) + 1/0.569] = 0.587$$

The approximate posterior variance of ln(RR) is the inverse of the total information:

$$\text{Posterior variance for } \ln(\text{RR}) \approx 1/[1/(1/2) + 1/0.569] = 0.266$$

Together, this mean and variance produce

$$\text{Posterior median for RR} \approx \exp(0.587) = 1.80$$

$$95\% \text{ posterior limits for RR} \approx \exp(0.587 \pm 1.96 \cdot 0.266^{1/2}) = 0.65, 4.94$$

The posterior RR of 1.80 is close to a simple geometric averaging of the prior RR (of 1) with the frequentist estimate (of 3.51), because the data information is $1/0.569 = 1.76$ whereas the prior information is $1/(1/2) = 2$, giving almost equal weight to the two. This equal weighting arises because both the study (with only three exposed cases and five exposed controls) and the prior are weak. Note too that the posterior RR of 1.80 is much closer to the frequentist odds ratios from other studies, which average around 1.7 (Greenland, 2005b).

BAYESIAN INTERPRETATION OF FREQUENTIST RESULTS

The weighted-averaging formula shows that the frequentist results arise from the Bayesian calculation when the prior information is made negligibly small relative to the data information . In this sense, frequentist results are just extreme Bayesian results, ones in which the prior information is zero, asserting that absolutely nothing is known about the RR outside of the study. Some promote such priors as "letting the data speak for themselves." In reality, the data say nothing by themselves: The frequentist results are computed using probability models that assume complete absence of bias, and so filter the data through false assumptions.

A Bayesian analysis that uses these frequentist data models is subject to the same criticism. Even with no bias, however, assuming absence of prior information is empirically absurd. Prior information of zero implies that a relative risk of (say) 10^{100} is as plausible as a value of 1 or 2. Suppose the relative risk were truly 10^{100}; then every child exposed above 3 mG would have contracted leukemia, making exposure a sufficient cause. The resulting epidemic would have come to everyone's attention long before the above study was done because the leukemia rate would have reflected the prevalence of high exposure, which is about 5% in the United States. The actual rate of leukemia is 4 cases per 100,000 person-years, which implies that the relative risk cannot be extremely high. Thus there are ample background data to rule out such extreme relative risks.

So-called objective-Bayes methods (Berger, 2006) differ from frequentist methods only in that they make these unrealistic "noninformative" priors explicit. The resulting posterior intervals represent inferences that no thoughtful person could make, because they reflect nothing of the subject under study or even the meaning of the variable names. Genuine prior bets are more precise. Even exceptionally "strong" relations in noninfectious-disease epidemiology (such as smoking and lung cancer) involve RR of the order of 10 or 1/10, and few noninfectious study exposures are even that far from the null. This situation reflects the fact that, for a factor to reach the level of formal epidemiologic study, its effects must be small enough to have gone undetected by clinical practice or by surveillance systems. There is almost always some surveillance (if only informal, through the health care system) that implies limits on the effect size. If these limits are huge, frequentist results serve as a rough approximation to a Bayesian analysis that uses an empirically based prior for the RR; otherwise the frequentist results may be very misleading.

ADJUSTMENT

To adjust for measured confounders without using explicit priors for their confounding effects, one need only set a prior for the adjusted RR and then combine the prior ln(RR) with the adjusted frequentist estimate by inverse-variance averaging. For example, in a pooled analysis of 14 studies of magnetic fields (>3 mG vs. less) and childhood leukemia (Greenland, 2005b, Table 18–1), the only important measured confounder was the source of the data (i.e., the variable coding "study"), and thus stratification by study was crucial. The maximum-likelihood odds-ratio estimate of the common odds ratio across the studies was 1.69, with 95% confidence limits of 1.28, 2.23; thus the log odds ratio was $\ln(1.69) = 0.525$ with variance estimate $[\ln(2.23/1.28)/3.92]^2 = 0.0201$. Combining this study-adjusted frequentist result with a normal(0,½) prior yields

$$\text{Posterior mean for } \ln(\text{RR}) \approx [0/(^1\!/_2) + \ln(1.69)/0.0201]/[1/(^1\!/_2) + 1/0.0201] = 0.504$$

$$\text{Posterior variance for } \ln(\text{RR}) \approx 1/[1/(^1\!/_2) + 1/.0201] = 0.0193$$

$$\text{Posterior median for RR} \approx \exp(0.504) = 1.66$$

$$95\% \text{ posterior limits for RR} \approx \exp(0.504 \pm 1.96 \cdot 0.0193^{1/2}) = 1.26, 2.17$$

This posterior hardly differs from the frequentist results, reflecting that the data information is $1/0.0201 = 50$, or 25 times the prior information of $1/(^1\!/_2) = 2$. In other words, the data information dominates the prior information.

One can also make adjustments based on priors for confounding, which may include effects of unmeasured variables (Leamer, 1974; Graham, 2000; Greenland, 2003c, 2005b).

VARYING THE PRIOR

Many authors have expressed skepticism over the existence of an actual magnetic field effect, so much so that they have misinterpreted positive findings as null because they were not "statistically significant" (e.g., UKCCS, 1999). The Bayesian framework allows this sort of prejudice to be displayed explicitly in the prior, rather than forcing it into misinterpretation of the data (Higgins and Spiegelhalter, 2002). Suppose that the extreme skepticism about the effect is expressed as a normal prior for ln(RR) with mean zero and 95% prior limits for RR of 0.91 and 1.1 (cf. Taubes, 1994). The prior standard deviation is then $[\ln(1.1) - \ln(0.91)]/3.92 = 0.0484$. Averaging this prior with the frequentist summary of ln(1.69) yields 95% posterior RR limits of 0.97, 1.16. Here, the prior weight is $1/0.0484^2 = 427$, more than 8 times the data information of 50, and so the prior dominates the final result.

It can be instructive to examine how the results change as the prior changes (Leamer, 1978; Spiegelhalter et al., 1994, 2004; Greenland, 2005b). Using a normal(0, v) prior, a simple approach examines the outputs as the variance v ranges over values that different researchers hold. For example, when examining a relative risk (RR), prior variances of ⅛, ½, 2, 4 for ln(RR) correspond to 95% prior intervals for RR of (½, 2), (¼, 4), (1/16, 16), (1/50, 50). The frequentist results represent another (gullible) extreme prior based on two false assumptions: first, that the likelihood (data) model is correct (which is falsified by biases); and second, that nothing is known about any explicit parameter, corresponding to infinite v and hence no prior upper limit on RR (which is falsified by surveillance data). At the other extreme, assertions of skeptics often correspond to priors with $v < ^1\!/_8$ and hence a 95% prior interval within (½, 2).

BAYES VERSUS SEMI-BAYES

The preceding example analyses are *semi*-Bayes in that they do not introduce an explicit prior for all the free parameters in the problem. For example, they do not use a prior for the population exposure prevalence $\Pr(X = 1)$ or for the relation of adjustment factors to exposure or the outcome. Semi-Bayes analyses are equivalent to Bayesian analyses in which those parameters are given noninformative priors and correspond to frequentist mixed models (in which some but not all coefficients are random). As with frequentist analyses, the cost of using no prior for a parameter is that the results fall short of the accuracy that could be achieved if a realistic prior were used. The benefit is largely one of simplicity in not having to specify priors for many parameters. Good (1983) provides a general discussion of cost–benefit trade-offs of analysis complexity, under the heading of "Type-II rationality." Good (1983) and Greenland (2000d) also describe how multilevel (hierarchical) modeling subsumes frequentist, semi-Bayes, and Bayes methods, as well as shrinkage (empirical-Bayes) methods.

PRIOR DATA: FREQUENTIST INTERPRETATION OF PRIORS

Having expressed one's prior bets as intervals about the target parameter, it is valuable to ask what sort of data would have generated those bets as confidence intervals. In the previous examples, we could ask: What would constitute data "equivalent" to the prior? That is, what experiment would convey the same information as the normal (0, ½) prior for ln(RR)? Answers to such Bayesian questions can be found by frequentist thought experiments (Higgins and Spiegelhalter, 2002, app. 2), which show how Bayesian methods parallel frequentist methods for pooled analysis of multiple studies.

Suppose we were given the results of a trial with N_1 children randomized to exposure $(X = 1)$ and N_0 to no exposure (a trial that would be infeasible and unethical in reality but, as yet, allowed in the mind), as in Table 18–2. With equal allocation, $N_1 = N_0 = N$. The frequentist RR estimate then equals the ratio of the number of treated cases A_1 to the number of untreated cases A_0:

$$\text{Estimated RR} = (A_1/N)/(A_0/N) = A_1/A_0$$

Given the rarity of leukemia, N would be very large relative to A_1 and A_0. Hence $1/N \approx 0$, and

$$\text{Estimated variance for ln(RR)} = 1/A_1 + 1/A_0 - 1/N - 1/N \approx 1/A_1 + 1/A_0$$

(Chapter 14). To yield our prior for RR, these estimates must satisfy

$$\text{Estimated RR} = A_1/A_0 = 1$$

so $A_1 = A_0 = A$, and

$$\text{Estimated variance of ln(RR) estimate} \approx 1/A_1 + 1/A_0 = 1/A + 1/A = 2/A = 1/2$$

so $A_1 = A_0 = A = 4$. Thus, data roughly equivalent to a normal(0, ½) prior would comprise 4 cases in each of the treated and the untreated groups in a very large randomized trial with equal allocation, yielding a prior estimate RR_{prior} of 1 and a ln(RR) variance of ½. The value of N would not matter provided it was large enough so that $1/N$ was negligible relative to $1/A$. Table 18–3 shows an example.

TABLE 18–2

General Notation for 2 × 2 Prior-Data Layout

	$X = 1$	$X = 0$	
Cases	A_1	A_0	Table RR $= RR_{prior} = (A_1/N_1)/(A_0/N_0)$
Total	N_1	N_0	$= (A_1/A_0)/(N_1/N_0)$

TABLE 18–3

Example of Bayesian Analysis via Frequentist Methods: Data Approximating a Log-Normal Prior, Reflecting 2:1 Certainty That RR Is Between 1/2 and 2, 95% Certainty That RR Is between 1/4 and 4, and Result of Combination with Data from Table 18–1. ($X = 1$ is >3 mG average exposure, $X = 0$ is ≤3 mG)

	$X = 1$	$X = 0$	
Cases	4	4	Table RR = RR_{prior} = 1
Total	100,000	100,000	Approximate 95% prior limits = 0.25, 4.00

$\ln(RR_{prior}) = 0$, approximate variance $= 1/4 + 1/4 = 1/2$

Approximate posterior median and 95% limits from stratified analyses combining prior with Table 18–1:

From information (inverse-variance) weighting of RR estimates: 1.80, 95% limits 0.65, 4.94

From maximum-likelihood (ML) estimation: 1.76, 95% limits 0.59, 5.23

Expressing the prior as equivalent data leads to a general method for doing Bayesian and semi-Bayes analyses with frequentist software:

1. Construct data equivalent to the prior, then
2. Add those prior data to the actual study data as a distinct (prior) stratum.

The resulting point estimate and C% confidence limits from the frequentist analysis of the augmented (actual + prior) data provide an approximate posterior median and C% posterior interval for the parameter.

In the example, this method leads to a frequentist analysis of two strata: one stratum for the actual study data (Table 18–1) and one stratum for the prior-equivalent data (Table 18–3). Using information weighting (which assumes both the prior and the likelihood are approximately normal), these strata produce a point estimate of 1.80 and 95% limits of 0.65, 4.94, as above. A better approximation is supplied by using maximum likelihood (ML) to combine the strata, which here yields a point estimate of 1.76 and 95% limits of 0.59, 5.23. This approximation assumes only that the posterior distribution is approximately normal.

With other stratification factors in the analysis, the prior remains just an extra stratum, as above. For example, in the pooled analysis there were 14 strata, one for each study (Greenland, 2005b, Table 18–1). Adding the prior data used above with $A = 4$ and $N = 100{,}000$ as if it were a 15th study, and applying ML, the approximate posterior median RR and 95% limits are 1.66 and 1.26, 2.17, the same as from information weighting.

After translating the prior to equivalent data, one might see the size of the hypothetical study and decide that the original prior was overconfident, implying a prior trial larger than seemed justified. For a childhood leukemia incidence of $4/10^5$ years, 8 cases would require 200,000 child-years of follow-up, which is quite a bit larger than any real randomized trial of childhood leukemia. If one were not prepared to defend the amount of one's prior information as being this ample, one should make the trial smaller. In other settings one might decide that the prior trial should be larger.

REVERSE-BAYES ANALYSIS

Several authors describe how to apply Bayes's theorem in reverse (inverse-Bayes analysis) by starting with hypothetical posterior results and asking what sort of prior would have led to those results, given the actual data and data models used (Good, 1983; Matthews, 2001). One hypothetical posterior result of interest has the null as one of the 95% limits. In the above pooled analysis, this posterior leads to the question: How many prior cases per group (A) would be needed to make the lower end of the 95% posterior interval equal 1?

Repeating the ordinary Bayes analysis with different A and N until the lower posterior limit equals 1, we find that $A = 275$ prior leukemia cases per group (550 total) forces the lower end of the 95% posterior interval to 1.00. That number is more than twice the number of exposed cases seen in all epidemiologic studies to date. At a rate of about 4 cases/10^5 person-years, a randomized trial capable of producing $2A = 550$ leukemia cases under the null would require roughly $550/(4/10^5)$ >13 million child-years of follow-up. The corresponding prior variance is $2/275 = 0.00727$, for a 95% prior interval of

$$\exp(0 \pm 1.96 \cdot 0.00727^{1/2}) = 0.85, 1.18$$

Although this is an extremely skeptical prior, it is not as skeptical as many of the opinions written about the relation (Taubes, 1994). Upon seeing this calculation, we might fairly ask of skeptics, "Do you actually have evidence for the null that is equivalent to such an impossibly large, perfect randomized trial?" Without such evidence, the calculation shows that any reasonable posterior skepticism about the association must arise from methodologic shortcomings of the studies. These shortcomings correspond to shortcomings of standard frequentist data models; see Greenland (2005b) and Chapter 19.

PRIORS WITH NON-NULL CENTER

Suppose we shift the prior estimate RR_{prior} for RR to 2, with 95% prior limits of ½ and 8. This shift corresponds to $\ln(RR_{prior}) = \ln(2)$ with a prior variance of ½. Combining this prior with the Savitz data by information weighting yields

$$\text{Posterior variance} \approx 1/[1/(1/2) + 1/0.569] = 0.266 \qquad \text{(as before)}$$

$$\text{Posterior ln(RR) median} \approx [\ln(2)/(1/2) + \ln(3.51)/0.569]/[1/(1/2) + 1/0.569] = 0.956$$

$$\text{Posterior RR median} \approx \exp(0.956) = 2.60$$

$$\text{95\% posterior RR limits} \approx \exp(0.956 \pm 1.96 \cdot 0.266^{1/2}) = 0.95, 7.15$$

One can accomplish the same by augmenting the observed data set with a stratum of prior data. To preserve approximate normality, we keep $A_1 = A_0$ (so $A_1/A_0 = 1$) and adjust the denominator quotient N_1/N_0 to obtain the desired $RR_{prior} = (A_1/A_0)/(N_1/N_0) = 1/(N_1/N_0) = N_0/N_1$. In the preceding example this change means keeping $A_1 = A_0 = 4$ and $N_1 = 100{,}000$, but making $N_0 = 200{,}000$, so that

$$RR_{prior} = (4/100{,}000)/(4/200{,}000) = 200{,}000/100{,}000 = 2$$

The approximate prior variance of ln(RR) remains ¼ + ¼ = ½. Thus, data equivalent to the upshifted prior would be the observation of 4 cases in each of the treated and the untreated groups in a randomized trial with a 1:2 allocation to $X = 1$ and $X = 0$.

CHOOSING THE SIZES OF THE PRIOR DENOMINATORS

The absolute size of N_1 and N_0 used will matter little, provided both $N_1 > 100 \cdot A_1$ and $N_0 > 100 \cdot A_0$. Thus, if we enlarge A_1 and A_0, we enlarge N_1 and N_0 proportionally to maintain disease rarity in the prior data. Although it may seem paradoxical, this rarity is simply a numerical device that can be used even with common diseases. This procedure works because standard frequentist RR estimators do not combine baseline risks across strata. By placing the prior data in a separate stratum, the baseline risk in the prior data may take on any small value, without affecting either the baseline risk estimates for the actual data or the posterior RR estimates. N_1 and N_0 are used only to move the prior estimate RR_{prior} to the desired value: When they are very large, they cease to influence the prior variance and only their ratio, N_1/N_0, matters in setting the prior.

For the thought experiment used to set N_1 and N_0, one envisions an experimental group that responds to treatment (X) with the relative risk one expects, but in which the baseline risk is so low that the distinctions among odds, risk, and rate ratios become unimportant. The estimator applied to the total (augmented) data will determine what is estimated. An odds-ratio estimator will produce an odds-ratio estimate, a risk-ratio estimator will produce a risk-ratio estimate, and a rate-ratio estimator will produce a rate-ratio estimate. For rate-ratio analyses, N_1 and N_0 represent person-time rather than persons.

NON-NORMAL PRIORS

The addition of prior data shown above (with very large N_1, N_0) corresponds to using an F distribution with $2A_1$, $2A_0$ degrees of freedom as the RR prior (Jones, 2004; Greenland, 2007b). With $A_1 = A_0 = A$, the above log-normal approximation to this prior appears adequate down to about $A = 4$; for example, at $A = 4$, the approximate 95% RR interval of ($^1\!/\!_4$, 4) has 93.3% exact prior probability from an $F(8, 8)$ distribution; at $A = 3$ the approximate 95% interval is (1/5, 5) and has 92.8% exact probability from an $F(6, 6)$. These are minor discrepancies compared to other sources of error, and the resulting discrepancies for the posterior percentiles are smaller still. As with the accuracy of maximum likelihood, the accuracy of the posterior approximation depends on the total information across strata (prior + data). Nonetheless, if we want to introduce prior data that represent even less information or that represent non-normal ln(RR) priors, we can employ prior data with $A_1 \neq A_0$ to induce ln(RR)-skewness, and with A_1, $A_0 < 3$ to induce heavier tails than the normal distribution. Generalizations beyond the F distribution are also available (Greenland, 2003b, 2007b).

FURTHER EXTENSIONS

Prior-data methods extend easily to multivariable modeling and to settings in which some or all variables (including the outcome) have multiple levels. For example, one may add a prior stratum for each regression coefficient in a model; coefficients for continuous variables can be represented as trials comparing two levels of the variable (e.g., 800 vs. 0 mcg/day folic acid supplementation); and prior correlations can be induced using a hierarchical prior-data structure (Greenland, 2003c, 2007a).

CHECKING THE PRIOR

A standard recommendation is to check homogeneity of measures before summarizing them across strata. An analogous recommendation is to check the compatibility of the data and the prior (Box, 1980), which is subsumed under the more general topic of Bayesian model checking (Geweke, 1998; Gelman et al., 2003; Spiegelhalter et al., 2004). For normal priors, one simple approximate check examines the P-value from the "standardized" difference,

$$(\text{Frequentist estimate} - \text{prior estimate})/(\text{frequentist variance} + \text{prior variance})^{1/2},$$

which is the analog of the frequentist two-stratum homogeneity statistic (Chapter 15). Like frequentist homogeneity tests, this check is neither sensitive nor specific, and it assumes that the prior is normal and the observed counts are "large" (>4). A small P-value does indicate, however, that the prior and the frequentist results are too incompatible to average by information weighting.

For the pooled magnetic field data with a normal(0, ½) prior ($A_1 = A_0 = 4 << N_1 = N_0$), the check is $[\ln(1.69) - 0]/(0.0201 + ½)^{1/2} = 0.72$, $P = 0.47$. Thus, by this check the prior and the frequentist result appear to be compatible, largely because the prior is compatible with such a broad range of results. Despite this compatibility, their average may still be misleading (e.g., as a result of study biases). In contrast, with the skeptical normal $(0, 0.0484^2)$ prior ($A_1 = A_0 = 427 << N_1 = N_0$), the check is $[\ln(1.69) - 0]/(0.0201 + 0.0484^2)^{1/2} = 3.50$, $P = 0.0005$, which indicates extreme incompatibility of the prior and the frequentist result, and which suggests that the average would be misleading because at least one of the prior and the frequentist result is misleading (and perhaps both are).

The P-value for the exposure–disease (X-Y) association in the actual data equals the homogeneity P-value from comparing the frequentist result to a dogmatic normal (0, 0) prior concentrated entirely at the null with zero variance (equivalent to overwhelming prior data, e.g., $A = 10^{100}$ and $N = 10^{100,000}$). For the pooled-data example this P-value is 0.0002, corresponding to the usual interpretation that a small P-value is indicative of a conflict between the null and the data. The P-value comparing the prior mean to the frequentist estimate can be viewed as a generalization of the usual P-value to allow testing of nondogmatic ("fuzzy") hypotheses in which the true parameter is specified only up to a distribution, rather than asserted to equal a single number.

DISCUSSION

DATA ALONE SAY NOTHING AT ALL

It is sometimes recommended that the prior should be given up if it appears to be in conflict with the "actual data" (e.g., Robins and Greenland, 1986). The conflict, however, is between the prior and the frequentist result from the data *model*; without a model for the data-generating mechanism, the data alone can conflict with nothing (Robins, 2001).

If we truly believed the frequentist results were from perfect data from a randomized trial conducted on a random sample from the target population, we would no doubt afford them precedence over a prior composed from mere impressions of other evidence. Indeed, a key inferential property of randomized studies is that, if they are precise enough, they force agreement among those who believe that the randomization was carried out properly and not undermined by subsequent events. Observational studies stray from this ideal, however, and do so to an unknown extent. A conflict between a prior and a frequentist result can arise from an invalid data model (resulting from study biases or an incorrect analytic method), as opposed to an incorrect prior. Thus, an apparent conflict only calls attention to a discrepancy in need of explanation. This situation is starkly illustrated by the magnetic-field controversy, in which many scientists still postulate that the frequentist result (rather than their skeptical prior) is in error.

Although (as is often said) frequentist statistics better reflect the data than do Bayesian statistics, those data should not be regarded as sacrosanct when making inferences beyond the observations. Even rough but contextually well-informed priors can provide information as reliable as or more reliable than current observations. To put it negatively, one may be justifiably afraid of the unreliability of subjective priors, but this fear does not license exclusive reliance on unreliable data. Frequentist statistics and their "objective" Bayesian analogs indeed stay closer to the observations, but this closeness will harm inference when those observations are riddled with error and better external information is available. Conversely, for the goal of data description (as opposed to inference), neither Bayesian nor frequentist modeling results are an adequate substitute for tabular and graphical data summaries.

DATA PRIORS AS A GENERAL DIAGNOSTIC DEVICE

The data representation of priors is far more important and general than is realized by most of the statistics community today. For teaching, data priors provide both a Bayesian interpretation of frequentist statistics (as Bayesian statistics with no prior data) and a frequentist interpretation of Bayesian statistics (as frequentist statistics based in part on external data). For analysis, data priors provide a critical perspective on a proposed prior and can lead to refinements to better match the level of prior information one wishes to assume. Other prior representations are also conceptually helpful; for example, the penalized-likelihood approach illustrates how Bayesian statistics can be viewed as frequentist statistics with probabilistic constraints on parameters (Greenland, 2000c, 2001b). These interpretations show that entering and deleting variables in a regression are extremes along a continuum in which the variable may enter partially, to the extent allowed by the constraint (Leamer, 1978; Greenland, 1999b, 2000a).

Data representations are not limited to conjugate priors (priors that have the same functional form as the likelihood function). Any prior that can be viewed as a product of likelihood functions can be translated into data, namely, the data arising from the statistical studies represented by the functions. These functions may be of varying forms, and those forms may differ from that of the actual-data likelihood (i.e., they may be nonconjugate). The translation clarifies the evidential claims that the prior is making. Conversely, to say that a given prior cannot be viewed as augmenting data means that one could not envision a series of studies that would lead to the prior (let alone point to actual studies that produce the prior). Such a prior is arguably nonempirical in principle and hence scientifically meaningless (in the same sense that a theory that is empirically untestable in principle is scientifically meaningless). Translation between forms for a prior is thus a scientific (as opposed to statistical) diagnostic for priors.

THE ROLE OF MARKOV-CHAIN MONTE CARLO

Translation of the prior into various forms does not dictate the manner of posterior computation. One could, for example, translate for diagnostic purposes and then sample from the posterior distribution using a Markov-chain Monte Carlo (MCMC) program such as WinBUGS (www.mrc-bsu.cam.ac.uk/bugs/welcome.shtml). Nonetheless, MCMC is subject to technical problems that are not always easily detected; indeed, as of this writing (2007) the WinBUGS website carries the warning: "MCMC is inherently less robust than analytic statistical methods." MCMC also does not display the parallels between frequentist and Bayesian analyses. Hence it is arguably inadequate alone or as a starting point for Bayesian instruction, and analytic methods are valuable for starting and checking MCMC analyses.

One can question, however, whether MCMC analyses are necessary once approximate results are in hand. Given perfectly correct models, and if allowed to run long enough, MCMC can produce more accurate results than the methods described above. Nonetheless, upon considering all the poorly understood sources of bias that plague observational research, our models are always highly inaccurate, and MCMC refinements may only add a false sense of precision to inaccurate results.

CONNECTIONS TO SENSITIVITY ANALYSIS

There is a close and complementary connection between Bayesian methods and sensitivity analyses (Chapter 19), in which parameters fixed at defaults by frequentist methods are varied to see their effect on statistics. Simple sensitivity analyses will reveal unlimited sensitivities to certain variations and hence convey no information unless coupled with contextual information to determine what variations are meaningful (Greenland, 1998c). That contextual information is none other than prior information, which can be formalized in a prior distribution for use in Bayesian or analogous prior-sampling methods for risk and decision analysis (Eddy et al., 1992; Greenland, 2001c, 2003c, 2005b; Chapter 19). In this format, one can also conduct Bayesian sensitivity analysis by seeing how results vary as the prior is varied. For this process, data representations can help one judge which priors are credible enough to examine.

SOME CAUTIONS ON USE OF PRIORS

Many have argued for integrating the Bayesian perspective into the teaching of basic methods (e.g., see Berry, 1997, and the ensuing discussion). The prior-data approach facilitates this goal because it requires no new statistical formulas or software. Standard frequentist methods for stratified and regression analysis become Bayesian by adding just a few data records and covariates.

With this new capacity, however, comes risk of abuse. Although Bayesian methods are now widely accepted as a way to improve inferences using prior information (e.g., Carlin and Louis, 2000; Gelman et al., 2003), one cannot expect improvement over ordinary methods using just any prior. Worsening could occur from using a badly misinformed prior (a prior that assigns relatively low probability to values near the truth), which suggests being generous in setting the spread of the prior. If the resulting prior remains highly influential, subject-matter justification will be especially important, as will statistical checks of the compatibility of priors with the likelihood. Among basic diagnostics are visual comparisons of prior and likelihood summaries or graphs, e.g., comparing the prior mode and limits to the maximum-likelihood (ML) estimate and confidence limits, or comparing entire graphs. Another simple check is the P-value for comparing the actual and prior data as if the latter were an actual data stratum, as described above. Although a large P-value means only that the check detected no problem, a small P-value indicates incompatibility of the prior with the model for the actual data, which could arise from faulty prior information, faulty actual data (resulting from, e.g., study defects), a faulty model for the data (i.e., a faulty likelihood model), or some combination.

Concerns about background information argue for retaining frequentist results to compare with Bayesian results whenever the former are sensible to apply, and for using vaguely informative and relatively simple priors. "Vaguely informative" is a context-dependent notion, however, in which the percentiles of the prior distribution would be viewed as at least reasonable if not liberally inclusive by all those working in the research topic. With 95% limits of $1/4$, 4 and 2:1 (67%) limits of $1/2$, 2, the normal(0, 0.5) prior for ln(RR) may often seem reasonable when the RR is expected to be in the "weak" ($1/2$, 2) range and there is no strong directional information. But in some contexts (e.g., environmental and occupational research), only adverse health effects are of serious concern, and the use of more directional priors may then be justifiable.

Vaguely informative should not be construed as noninformative. Noninformative priors correspond to using values of A_1 and A_0 of zero, which give back the ML estimate and confidence interval as the posterior mode and interval. So-called reference priors (Berger, 2006) correspond to using very small values and thus give similar results. Such "objective Bayesian" methods confer none of the predictive benefits obtainable from well-informed priors, rarely make sense on subject-matter grounds (Greenland, 1998b, 2006a), and (like frequentist methods) break down in the face of nonidentification (Greenland, 2005b). In essence, they discard prior information, the key source of Bayesian strengths as well as weaknesses. Thus, like frequentism, objective Bayesianism leads to mechanical procedures that software or a robot could apply to data. Such decontextualized algorithmic statistics form the bulk of current statistical training. Epidemiologic inference requires contextual input, however, and prior specification is one crucial aspect that should not be automatic.

CONCLUSIONS

Bayesian and frequentist methods address different questions. Bayesian methods address questions of the form: "Having seen the data, what betting odds should I place on this hypothesis versus another?" and seek to use contextual information to improve the bet. The methods focus on the observed data, rather than on counterfactual data as might arise under a hypothetical long run. In contrast, frequentist methods address questions of the form: "If I applied this method to a hypothetical long run of studies like this one, how would it behave over that long run?" and seek methods with desirable long-run properties (properties such as correct confidence-interval coverage rates; see Chapters 10 and 13). Frequentist methods do not provide odds of hypotheses, nor do they address whether the particular inference they produce from the observed data is better than other inferences one could make from those data, without reference to a long run.

Despite their focus on actual data, Bayesian methods exhibit desirable frequentist (long-run) properties when both they and the evaluation are well-informed by the scientific context (Gustafson and Greenland, 2006b). Thus, even for a frequentist, Bayesian thinking is necessary as part of a broad and well-rounded approach. Bayesian and related methods become particularly worthwhile when conventional frequentist statistics become questionable and priors matter, as when confronting sparse data, multiple comparisons, collinearity, or nonidentification (Greenland, 1993a, 2000c, 2000d, 2000e, 2001b, 2003c, 2005b, 2007a; Greenland et al., 2000; Gustafson and Greenland, 2006b). Frequentist interval estimates inevitably get interpreted as if they were Bayesian, without appreciating that the priors implicit in those interpretations are rarely if ever contextually plausible. Because this appreciation seems essential for proper interpretation of frequentist as well as Bayesian methods in observational settings (e.g., see Leamer, 1978; Rubin, 1991; Greenland, 2003c, 2005b, 2006a), the inclusion of Bayesian perspectives in teaching would be helpful even if frequentist results remained the norm for presentation.

A major flaw shared by conventional statistical methods (be they frequentist, likelihoodist, or Bayesian), however, is that they pretend the data came from an ideal study in which all important influences on the data (including those of the investigators and the subjects) can be approximated by a known model. In observational epidemiology, this assumption can be drastically flawed, resulting in far too much certainty placed on statistical results. Chapter 19 discusses how statistics can approach this problem in a contextually informed manner by using bias models with explicit priors for unknown bias parameters.

In summary, Bayesian analysis can be performed easily by information weighting of prior estimates with frequentist estimates (as if doing a meta-analysis of prior studies and the current study). More generally, it can be done by representing prior information as hypothetical study data to be added to the analysis as new strata (as if doing a pooled analysis of prior studies and the current study). This data-prior approach provides a diagnostic for contextual strength and relevance of the prior, and also facilitates Bayesian regression analysis (Greenland, 2007a, 2007b). Both approaches allow one to produce Bayesian analyses from formulas and software for frequentist analyses, and both facilitate introduction of Bayesian ideas into introductory statistics training alongside the corresponding frequentist approaches.

CHAPTER 19

Bias Analysis

Sander Greenland and Timothy L. Lash

Introduction 345
The Need for Bias Analyses 346
Caveats about Bias Analysis 347
Analysis of Unmeasured Confounders 348
External Adjustment 348
Relation of Unadjusted to Adjusted Odds Ratios 351
Combination with Adjustment for Measured Confounders 352
Analysis of Misclassification 352
Exposure Misclassification 353
Nondifferentiality 355
Application to the Resins-Lung Cancer Example 356
Relation of Predictive Values to Sensitivity and Specificity 357
Disease Misclassification 358
Confounder Misclassification 359
Misclassification of Multiple Variables 360
A Matrix Adjustment Method 360
Use of Validation Data 361
Selection Bias 362
Multiple-Bias Analyses 363
Probabilistic Bias Analysis 364
Probabilistic Sensitivity Analysis 364
Analysis of Uncontrolled Confounding 365
Some Easily Generated Distributions 370
Trapezoidal Distributions 371
Generating Dependent Variables 371
Analysis of Misclassification 372
Analysis of Selection Bias 375
Comparative and Combined Analyses 376
Bayesian and Semi-Bayesian Analysis 378
Conclusion 380

INTRODUCTION

This chapter provides an introduction to quantitative methods for evaluating potential biases (systematic errors) in individual studies. The first half of this chapter covers basic methods to assess sensitivity of results to confounding by an unmeasured variable, misclassification, and selection bias. These methods quantify systematic errors by means of *bias parameters,* which in a sensitivity analysis are first fixed at hypothetical values and then varied to see how the results vary with the parameters.

The second half of this chapter extends basic bias-sensitivity analysis by assigning a prior probability distribution to the bias parameters (probabilistic bias modeling) to produce *distributions* of results as output. The methods are typically implemented via simulation, and their outputs have a natural interpretation as semi-Bayesian posterior distributions (Chapter 18) for exposure effects. They are "semi-" Bayesian because they use prior distributions for the bias parameters but not for the effect under study. We focus on the special case in which the observed data can be represented in a 2×2 table of an exposure indicator X (coded $1 = $ present, $0 = $ absent) and a disease indicator D. Many of the basic principles and difficulties of bias analysis can be illustrated with this simple case, because the 2×2 table can be thought of as a stratum from a larger data set.

Most statistical methods also assume specific models for the form of effects (of exposure, modifiers, and confounders) and of random errors. Use of erroneous model forms is sometimes called *specification error* and can lead to systematic errors known as *specification biases*. *Model-sensitivity analysis* addresses these biases by seeing how the results change as the model form is changed (Leamer, 1985; Draper, 1995; Saltelli et al., 2000). We do not cover model-sensitivity analysis, because it involves technical issues of model selection beyond the scope of this chapter; see Chapter 21 for further discussion.

We also do not address general *missing-data bias* (bias due to nonrandomly incomplete data); see Robins et al. (1994) and Little and Rubin (2002) for discussions, especially under the heading of *informatively* or *nonignorably missing data* (Lyles and Allen, 2002). All the problems we discuss can be viewed as extreme cases of missing-data bias: Uncontrolled confounding is due to missing data on a confounder; misclassification is due to missing data on the true variables; and selection bias is due to nonrandomly missing members of the source population.

All methods, whether conventional methods or those described here, consider the data as given; that is, they assume that we have the data and that the data have not been corrupted by miscodings, programming errors, forged responses, etc. Thus, the methods assume that there is no misclassification due to data processing errors or investigator fraud. Such problems arise from isolated events that may affect many records, and their correction depends entirely on detection (e.g., via logic checks, data examination, and comparison of data sources). Thus, we do not see such problems as falling within the sphere of sensitivity analysis.

THE NEED FOR BIAS ANALYSES

Our discussion of statistical methods has so far focused on accounting for measured confounders and random errors in the data-generating process. Randomization of exposure assignment is the conventional assumption of statistical methods for causal inference within a study cohort, for it makes confounding a chance phenomenon. Random sampling forms the analogous conventional assumption of statistical methods for inference from the sample to a larger population (e.g., from a case-control study to a source population), for it makes sampling error a chance phenomenon. Most methods assume that measurement error is absent, but those that account for errors assume that the errors are random (Carroll et al., 2006). Upon stratification, these assumptions (that confounding, sampling errors, and measurement errors are random) are made within levels of the stratifying variables. We will call methods based on these randomness assumptions *conventional methods*.

By assuming that all errors are random and that any modeling assumptions (such as homogeneity) are correct, all uncertainty about the effect of errors on estimates is subsumed within conventional standard deviations for the estimates (standard errors), such as those given in earlier chapters (which assume no measurement error), and any discrepancy between an observed association and the target effect may be attributed to chance alone. When the assumptions are incorrect, however, the logical foundation for conventional statistical methods is absent, and those methods may yield highly misleading inferences. Epidemiologists recognize the possibility of incorrect assumptions in conventional analyses when they talk of residual confounding (from nonrandom exposure assignment), selection bias (from nonrandom subject selection), and information bias (from imperfect measurement). These biases rarely receive quantitative analysis, a situation that is understandable given that the analysis requires specifying values (such as amount of selection bias) for which little or no data may be available. An unfortunate consequence of this lack of quantification is the switch in focus to those aspects of error that are more readily quantified, namely, the random components.

Systematic errors can be and often are larger than random errors, and failure to appreciate their impact is potentially disastrous. The problem is magnified in large studies and pooling projects, because in those studies the large size reduces the amount of random error, and as a result the random error may be only a small component of total error. In such studies, a focus on "statistical significance" or even on confidence limits may amount to nothing more than a decision to focus on artifacts of systematic error as if they reflect a real causal effect.

Addressing concerns about systematic errors in a constructive fashion is not easy, but is nonetheless essential if the results of a study are to be used to inform decisions in a rational fashion. The process of addressing bias quantitatively we shall call *bias analysis*. As described in a number of books (e.g., Eddy et al., 1992; National Research Council, 1994; Vose, 2000), the basic ideas have existed for decades under the topic of sensitivity analysis and the more general topics of *uncertainty analysis, risk assessment,* and *risk analysis.* These topics address more sources of uncertainty than we shall address, such as model misspecification and informatively missing data. Here we focus only on the effects of basic validity problems.

A discomforting aspect of these analyses is that they reveal the highly tentative and subjective nature of inference from observational data, a problem that is concealed by conventional statistical analysis. Bias analysis requires educated guesses about the likely sizes of systematic errors, guesses that are likely to vary considerably across observers. The conventional approach is to make the guess qualitatively by describing the study's limitations. An assessment of the extent of bias, compared with the extent of exposure effects, therefore becomes an exercise in intuitive reasoning under uncertainty.

The ability to reason under uncertainty has been studied by cognitive psychologists and sociologists, who have found it susceptible to many predictable patterns of mistakes (Kahneman et al., 1982; Gilovich, 1993; Gilovich et al., 2002). This literature, where it deals with situations analogous to epidemiologic inference, indicates that the qualitative approach tends to favor exposure effects over systematic errors as an explanation for observed associations (Lash, 2007). Quantitative methods such as those described in this chapter offer a potential safeguard against these failures, by providing insight into the importance of various sources of error and by helping to assess the uncertainty of study results. For example, such assessments may argue persuasively that certain sources of bias cannot by themselves plausibly explain a study result, or that a bias explanation cannot be ruled out. As discussed in Chapters 2 and 18, and later in this section, the primary caution is that what appears "plausible" may vary considerably across persons and time.

There are several reasons why quantitative methods that take account of uncontrolled biases have traditionally seen much less development than methods for addressing random error. First, until recently, randomized experiments supplied much of the impetus for statistical developments. These experiments were concentrated in agriculture, manufacturing, and clinical medicine and often could be designed so that systematic errors played little role in the final results. A second reason is that most uncontrolled biases cannot be analyzed by conventional methods (i.e., without explicit priors for bias parameters) unless additional "validation" data are available. Such data are usually absent or very limited. Furthermore, validation studies may themselves be subject to systematic errors beyond those present in the main study, such as potentially biased selection for validation (e.g., if validation requires further subject consent and participation). As a result, investigators must resort to less satisfactory partial analyses, or quantify only the uncertainty due to random error.

Editors and reviewers in the health sciences seldom call on authors to provide a quantitative assessment of systematic errors. Because of the labor and expertise required for a bias analysis, and the limited importance of single studies for policy issues, it makes little sense to require such an analysis of every study. For example, studies whose conventional 95% confidence limits exclude no reasonable possibility will be viewed as inconclusive regardless of any further analysis. It can be argued that the best use of effort and journal space for single-study reports is to focus on a thorough description of the study design, methods, and data, to facilitate later use of the study data in reviews, meta-analyses, and pooling projects (Greenland et al., 2004).

On the other hand, any report with policy implications may damage public health if the claimed implications are wrong. Thus it is justifiable to demand quantitative bias analysis in such studies. Going further, it is arguably an ethical duty of granting agencies and editors to require a thorough quantitative assessment of relevant literature and of systematic errors to support claimed implications for public policy or medical practice. Without the endorsement of these gatekeepers of funding and publication, there is little motivation to collect validation data or to undertake quantitative assessments of bias.

CAVEATS ABOUT BIAS ANALYSIS

As noted above, results of a bias analysis are derived from inputs specified by the analyst, a point that should be emphasized in any presentation of the methods or their results. These inputs are constructed from judgments, opinions, or inferences about the likely magnitude of bias sources or parameters. Consequently, bias analyses do not establish the existence or absence of causal effects any more than do conventional analyses. Rather, they show how the analysts developed their output judgments (inferences) from their input judgments.

An advantage of bias analysis over a qualitative discussion of study limitations is that it allows mathematics to replace unsound intuitions and heuristics at many points in judgment formation. Nonetheless, the mathematics should not entice researchers to phrase judgments in objective terms that mask their subjective origin. For example, a claim that "our analysis indicates the conventional results are biased away from the null" would be misleading. A better description would say that "our analysis indicates that, *under the values we chose for the bias parameters,* the conventional results *would be* biased away from the null." The latter description acknowledges the fact that the results are sensitive to judgmental inputs, some of which may be speculative. The description, by its nature, should also encourage the analyst to present evidence that the values chosen for the bias parameters cover the range of reasonable combinations of those parameters.

The more advanced methods of this chapter require input distributions (rather than sets of values) for bias parameters, but the same caveat holds: The results of the bias analysis apply only under those chosen distributions. The analysis will be more convincing if the analyst provides evidence that the chosen distributions assign high probability to reasonable combinations of the parameters.

To some extent, similar criticisms apply to conventional frequentist and Bayesian analyses (Chapters 13–18 and 20–21), insofar as those analyses require many choices and judgments from the investigators. Examples include choice of methods used to handle missing data (Chapter 13), choice of category boundaries for quantitative variables (Chapter 13 and 17), choice of methods for variable selection (Chapter 21), and choice of priors assigned to effects under study (Chapter 18). As the term "conventional" connotes, many choices have default answers (e.g., a binomial model for the distribution of a dichotomous outcomes). Although the scientific basis for these defaults is often doubtful or lacking (*e.g.*,missing-data indicators; percentile boundaries for continuous variables; stepwise variable selection; noninformative priors for effects), deviations from the defaults may prompt requests for explanations from referees and readers.

Bias analysis requires more input specifications than do conventional analyses, and as yet there is no accepted convention regarding these specifications. As a result, input judgments are left entirely to the analyst, opening avenues for manipulation to produce desired output. Thus, when examining a bias analysis, a reader must bear in mind that other reasonable inputs might produce quite different results. This input sensitivity is why we emphasize that bias analysis is a collection of methods for explaining and refining subjective judgments in light of data (like the subjective Bayesian methods of Chapter 18), rather than a method for detecting nonrandom data patterns. In fact, a bias analysis can be made to produce virtually any estimate for the study effect without altering the data or imposing an objectionable prior on that effect. Such outcome-driven analyses, however, may require assignment of values or distributions to bias parameters that have doubtful credibility. Therefore, it is crucial that the inputs used for a bias analysis be described in detail so that those inputs can be examined critically by the reader.

ANALYSIS OF UNMEASURED CONFOUNDERS

Sensitivity analysis and external adjustment for confounding by dichotomous variables appeared in Cornfield et al. (1959) and were further elaborated by Bross (1966, 1967), Yanagawa (1984), Axelson and Steenland (1988), and Gail et al. (1988). Extensions of these approaches to multiple-level confounders are available (Schlesselman, 1978, correction by Simon, 1980b; Flanders and Khoury, 1990; Rosenbaum, 2002); see Chapter 33 for an example. Although most of these methods assume that the odds ratios or risk ratios are constant across strata, it is possible to base external adjustment on other assumptions (Yanagawa, 1984; Gail et al., 1988). Practical extensions to multiple regression analyses typically involve modeling the unmeasured confounders as latent (unobserved) variables (e.g., Lin et al., 1998; Robins et al., 1999a; Greenland, 2005b; McCandless et al., 2007)).

EXTERNAL ADJUSTMENT

Suppose that we have conducted an analysis of an exposure X and a disease D, adjusting for the recorded confounders, but we know of an unmeasured potential confounder and want to assess the possible effect of failing to adjust for this confounder. For example, in a case-control study of occupational exposure to resin systems (resins) and lung cancer mortality among male workers at a transformer assembly plant, Greenland et al. (1994) could adjust for age and year of death, but

TABLE 19–1

Crude Data for Case-Control Study of Occupational Resins Exposure (X) and Lung Cancer Mortality (Greenland et al., 1994); Controls Are Selected Noncancer Causes of Death

	$X = 1$	$X = 0$	Total
Cases ($D = 1$)	$A_{1+} = 45$	$A_{0+} = 94$	$M_{1+} = 139$
Controls ($D = 0$)	$B_{1+} = 257$	$B_{0+} = 945$	$M_{0+} = 1202$

Odds ratio after adjustment for age and death year: 1.77.
Age-year adjusted conventional 95% confidence limits for OR_{DX}: 1.18, 2.64.

they had no data on smoking. Upon adjustment for age and year at death, a positive association was observed for resins exposure and lung cancer mortality ($OR = 1.77$, 95% confidence limits = 1.18, 2.64). To what extent did confounding by smoking affect this observation?

For simplicity, suppose that resins exposure and smoking are treated as dichotomous: $X = 1$ for resin-exposed, 0 otherwise; $Z = 1$ for smoker, 0 otherwise. We might wish to know how large the resins/smoking association has to be so that adjustment for smoking removes the resins-lung cancer association. The answer to this question depends on a number of parameters, among them (a) the resins-specific associations (i.e., the associations within levels of resins exposure) of smoking with lung cancer, (b) the resins-specific prevalences of smoking among the controls, and (c) the prevalence of resins exposure among the controls. Resins prevalence is observed, but we can only speculate about the first two quantities.

It is this speculation, or educated guessing, that forms the basis for sensitivity analysis. We will assume various plausible combinations of values for the smoking/lung cancer association and resins-specific smoking prevalences, then see what values we get for the smoking-adjusted resins-lung cancer association. If all the latter values are substantially elevated, we have a basis for doubting that the unadjusted resins-lung cancer association is due entirely to confounding by smoking. Otherwise, confounding by smoking is a plausible explanation for the observed resins-lung cancer association.

We will use the crude data in Table 19–1 for illustration. There is no evidence of important confounding by age or year in these data, probably because the controls were selected from other chronic-disease deaths. For example, the crude odds ratio is 1.76 versus an age-year adjusted odds ratio of 1.77, and the crude 95% confidence limits are 1.20 and 2.58 versus 1.18 and 2.64 after age-year adjustment. If it is necessary to stratify on age, year or both, we could repeat the computations given below for each stratum and then summarize the results across strata, or we could use regression-based adjustments (Greenland, 2005b).

Consider the general notation for the expected stratified data given in Table 19–2. We will use hypothesized values for the stratum-specific prevalences to fill in this table and solve for an assumed

TABLE 19–2

General Layout (Expected Data) for Sensitivity Analysis and External Adjustment for a Dichotomous Confounder Z

	$Z = 1$			$Z = 0$		
	$X = 1$	$X = 0$	Total	$X = 1$	$X = 0$	Total
Cases	A_{11}	A_{01}	M_{11}	$A_{1+} - A_{11}$	$A_{0+} - A_{01}$	$M_{1+} - M_{11}$
Controls	B_{11}	B_{01}	M_{01}	$B_{1+} - B_{11}$	$B_{0+} - B_{01}$	$M_{0+} - M_{01}$

common odds ratio relating exposure to disease within levels of Z,

$$OR_{DX} = \frac{A_{11}B_{01}}{A_{01}B_{11}} = \frac{(A_{1+} - A_{11})(B_{0+} - B_{01})}{(A_{0+} - A_{01})(B_{1+} - B_{11})}$$

Suppose that the smoking prevalences among the exposed and unexposed populations are estimated or assumed to be P_{Z1} and P_{Z0}, and the odds ratio relating the confounder and disease within levels of exposure is OR_{DZ} (i.e., we assume odds-ratio homogeneity). Assuming that the control group is representative of the source population, we set $B_{11} = P_{Z1}B_{1+}$ and $B_{01} = P_{Z0}B_{0+}$. Next, to find A_{11} and A_{01}, we solve the pair of equations

$$OR_{DZ} = \frac{A_{11}(B_{1+} - B_{11})}{(A_{1+} - A_{11})B_{11}}$$

and

$$OR_{DZ} = \frac{A_{01}(B_{0+} - B_{01})}{(A_{0+} - A_{01})B_{01}}$$

These have solutions

$$A_{11} = OR_{DZ}A_{1+}B_{11}/(OR_{DZ}B_{11} + B_{1+} - B_{11}) \qquad [19\text{–}1]$$

and

$$A_{01} = OR_{DZ}A_{0+}B_{01}/(OR_{DZ}B_{01} + B_{0+} - B_{01}) \qquad [19\text{–}2]$$

Having obtained data counts corresponding to A_{11}, A_{01}, B_{11}, and B_{01}, we can put these numbers into Table 19–2 and compute directly a Z-adjusted estimate of the exposure-disease odds ratios OR_{DX}. The answers from each smoking stratum should agree.

The preceding estimate of OR_{DX} is sometimes said to be "indirectly adjusted" for Z, because it is the estimate of OR_{DX} that one would obtain if one had data on the confounder Z and disease D that displayed the assumed prevalences and confounder odds ratio OR_{DZ}. A more precise term for the resulting estimate of OR_{DX} is "externally adjusted," because the estimate makes use of an estimate of OR_{DZ} obtained from sources external to the study data. The smoking prevalences must also be obtained externally; occasionally (and preferably), they may be obtained from a survey of the underlying source population from which the subjects were selected. (Because we assumed the odds ratios are constant across strata, the result does not depend on the exposure prevalence.)

To illustrate external adjustment with the data in Table 19–1, suppose that the smoking prevalences among the resins exposed and unexposed are 70% and 50%. Then

$$B_{11} = P_{Z1}B_{1+} = 0.70(257) = 179.9$$

and

$$B_{01} = P_{Z0}B_{0+} = 0.50(945) = 472.5$$

Taking $OR_{DZ} = 5$ for the resins-specific smoking/lung cancer odds ratio, equations 19–1 and 19–2 yield

$$A_{11} = 5(45)179.9/[5(179.9) + 257 - 179.9] = 41.45$$

and

$$A_{01} = 5(94)472.5/[5(472.5) + 945 - 472.5] = 78.33$$

Putting these results into Table 19–2, we obtain the stratum-specific resins-lung cancer odds ratios

$$OR_{DX} = \frac{41.45(472.5)}{179.9(78.33)} = 1.39$$

TABLE 19–3

Sensitivity of Externally Adjusted Resins–Cancer Odds Ratio OR_{DX} to Choice of P_{Z1} and P_{Z0} (Smoking Prevalences among Exposed and Unexposed), and OR_{DZ} (Resins-Specific Smoking–Cancer Odds Ratio)

			OR_{DZ}		
P_{Z1}	P_{Z0}	OR_{XZ}	5	10	15
0.40	0.30	1.56	$OR_{DX} = 1.49$	$OR_{DX} = 1.42$	$OR_{DX} = 1.39$
0.55	0.45	1.49	1.54	1.49	1.48
0.70	0.60	1.56	1.57	1.54	1.53
0.45	0.25	2.45	1.26	1.13	1.09
0.60	0.40	2.25	1.35	1.27	1.24
0.75	0.55	2.45	1.41	1.35	1.33

and

$$OR_{DX} = \frac{(45 - 41.45)(945 - 472.5)}{(257 - 179.9)(94 - 78.33)} = 1.39$$

which agree (as they should). We see that confounding by smoking could account for much of the crude resins odds ratio if there were a much higher smoking prevalence among the resin exposed relative to the unexposed.

In a sensitivity analysis, we repeat the above external adjustment process using other plausible values for the prevalences and the confounder effect (see Sundararajan et al., 2002; Marshall et al., 2003; and Maldonado et al., 2003 for examples). Table 19–3 presents a summary of results using other values for the resins-specific smoking prevalences and the smoking odds ratio. The table also gives the smoking-resins odds ratio

$$OR_{XZ} = O_{Z1}/O_{Z0} = P_{Z1}(1 - P_{Z0})/(1 - P_{Z1})P_{Z0}$$

where $O_{Zj} = P_{Zj}/(1 - P_{Zj})$ is the odds of $Z = 1$ versus $Z = 0$ when $X = j$. There must be a substantial exposure-smoking association to remove most of the exposure-cancer association. Because there was no reason to expect an exposure-smoking association at all, Table 19–3 supports the notion that the observed resins-cancer association is probably not due entirely to confounding by the dichotomous smoking variable used here. We would have to consider a polytomous smoking variable to further address confounding by smoking.

RELATION OF UNADJUSTED TO ADJUSTED ODDS RATIOS

An equivalent approach to that just given uses the following formulas for the ratio of the unadjusted to Z-adjusted odds ratios (Yanagawa, 1984):

$$\begin{aligned}\frac{OR_{DX\text{-unadjusted}}}{OR_{DX\text{-adjusted}}} &= \frac{(OR_{DZ}O_{Z1} + 1)(O_{Z0} + 1)}{(OR_{DZ}O_{Z0} + 1)(O_{Z1} + 1)} \\ &= \frac{(OR_{DZ}OR_{XZ}O_{Z0} + 1)(O_{Z0} + 1)}{(OR_{DZ}O_{Z0} + 1)(OR_{XZ}O_{Z0} + 1)} \\ &= \frac{OR_{DZ}OR_{XZ}P_{Z0} + 1 - P_{Z0}}{(OR_{DZ}P_{Z0} + 1 - P_{Z0})(OR_{XZ}P_{Z0} + 1 - P_{Z0})} \\ &= \frac{OR_{DZ}P_{Z1} + 1 - P_{Z1}}{OR_{DZ}P_{Z0} + 1 - P_{Z0}}\end{aligned} \qquad [19\text{–}3]$$

Assuming that Z is the sole uncontrolled confounder, this ratio can be interpreted as the degree of bias due to failure to adjust for Z. This series of equations shows that when Z is not associated with the disease ($OR_{DZ} = 1$) or is not associated with exposure ($OR_{XZ} = 1$), the ratio of the unadjusted and adjusted odds ratios is 1, and there is no confounding by Z. In other words, a confounder must be associated with the exposure and the disease in the source population (Chapter 9). Recall, however, that these associations are not sufficient for Z to be a confounder, because a confounder must also satisfy certain causal relations (e.g., it must not be affected by exposure or disease; see Chapters 4, 9, and 12). The equations in 19–3 also show that the ratio of unadjusted to adjusted odds ratios depends on the prevalence of $Z = 1$; i.e., the degree of confounding depends not only on the magnitude of the associations but also on the confounder distribution.

In many circumstances, we may have information about only one or two of the three parameters that determine the unadjusted/adjusted ratio. Nonetheless, it can be seen from 19–3 that the ratio cannot be further from 1 than are $OR_{DZ}/(OR_{DZ}P_{Z0} + 1 - P_{Z0})$, $OR_{XZ}/(OR_{XZ}P_{Z0} + 1 - P_{Z0})$, $1/(OR_{DZ}P_{Z0} + 1 - P_{Z0})$, or $1/(OR_{XZ}P_{Z0} + 1 - P_{Z0})$; the ratio is thus bounded by these quantities. Furthermore, because the bound $OR_{DZ}/(OR_{DZ}P_{Z0} + 1 - P_{Z0})$ cannot be further from 1 than OR_{DZ}, the ratio cannot be further from 1 than OR_{DZ}, and similarly cannot be further from 1 than OR_{XZ} (Cornfield et al., 1959; Bross, 1967). Thus, the odds-ratio bias from failure to adjust Z cannot exceed the odds ratio relating Z to D or to X.

These methods readily extend to cohort studies. For data with person-time denominators T_{ji}, we use the T_{ji} in place of the control counts B_{ji} in the previous formulas to obtain an externally adjusted rate ratio. For data with count denominators N_{ji}, we use the N_{ji} in place of the B_{ji} to obtain an externally adjusted risk ratio (Flanders and Khoury, 1990). Bounds analogous to those above can be derived for risk differences (Kitagawa, 1955). Improved bounds can also be derived under deterministic causal models relating X to D in the presence of uncontrolled confounding (e.g., Maclehose et al., 2005). There is also a large literature on bounding causal risk differences from randomized trials when uncontrolled confounding due to noncompliance may be present; see Chapter 8 of Pearl, 2000 for references.

COMBINATION WITH ADJUSTMENT FOR MEASURED CONFOUNDERS

The preceding equations relate the unadjusted odds ratio to the odds ratio adjusted only for the unmeasured confounder (Z) and thus ignore the control of any other confounders. If adjustment for measured confounders has an important effect, the equations must be applied using bias parameters conditioned on those measured confounders. To illustrate, suppose that age adjustment was essential in the previous example. We should then have adjusted for confounding by smoking in the age-adjusted or age-specific odds ratios. Application of the previous equations to these odds ratios will require age-specific parameters, e.g., P_{Z0} will be the age-specific smoking prevalence among unexposed noncases, OR_{DZ} will be the age-specific association of smoking with lung cancer among the unexposed, and OR_{XZ} will be the age-specific association of smoking with resins exposure among noncases.

Although most estimates of confounder–disease associations are adjusted for major risk factors such as age, information adjusted for other parameters is often unavailable. Use of unadjusted parameters in the preceding equations may be misleading if they are not close to the adjusted parameters (e.g., if the unadjusted and age-adjusted odds ratios associating smoking with exposure are far apart). For example, if age is associated with smoking and exposure, adjustment for age could partially adjust for confounding by smoking, and the association of smoking with exposure will change upon age adjustment. Use of the age-unadjusted smoking–exposure odds ratio (OR_{XZ}) in the preceding equations will then give a biased estimate of the residual confounding by smoking after age adjustment. More generally, proper external adjustment in combination with adjustments for measured confounders requires information about the unmeasured variables that is conditional on the measured confounders.

ANALYSIS OF MISCLASSIFICATION

Nearly all epidemiologic studies suffer from some degree of measurement error, which is usually referred to as classification error or *misclassification* when the variables are discrete. The effect of even modest amounts of error can be profound, yet rarely is the error quantified (Jurek et al., 2007). Simple situations can be analyzed, however, using basic algebra (Copeland et al., 1977; Greenland, 1982a; Kleinbaum et al., 1984), and more extensive analyses can be done using software that performs matrix algebra (e.g., SAS, GAUSS, MATLAB, R, S-Plus) (Barron, 1977; Greenland and Kleinbaum, 1983; Greenland, 1988b). We will focus on basic methods for dichotomous variables. We will then briefly discuss methods that allow use of validation study data, in which classification rates are themselves estimated from a sample of study subjects.

EXPOSURE MISCLASSIFICATION

Consider first the estimation of exposure prevalence from a single observed category of subjects, such as the control group in a case-control study. Define the following quantities in this category:

X = 1 if exposed, 0 if not
X^* = 1 if *classified* as exposed, 0 if not
PVP = probability that someone classified as exposed is truly exposed
= predictive value of an exposure "positive" = $\Pr(X = 1|X^* = 1)$
PVN = probability that someone classified as unexposed is truly unexposed
= predictive value of an exposure "negative" = $\Pr(X = 0|X^* = 0)$
${B_1}^*$ = number classified as exposed (with $X^* = 1$)
${B_0}^*$ = number classified as unexposed (with $X^* = 0$)
B_1 = expected number truly exposed (with $X = 1$)
B_0 = expected number truly unexposed (with $X = 0$)

If they are known, the predictive values can be used directly to estimate the numbers truly exposed (B_1) and truly unexposed (B_0) from the misclassified counts ${B_1}^*$ and ${B_0}^*$ via the expected relations

$$\begin{aligned} B_1 &= PVP \cdot {B_1}^* + (1 - PVN){B_0}^* \\ B_0 &= PVN \cdot {B_0}^* + (1 - PVP){B_1}^* \end{aligned} \qquad [19\text{–}4]$$

Note that the total M_0 is not changed by exposure misclassification:

$$\begin{aligned} M_0 &= B_1 + B_0 \\ &= PVN \cdot {B_0}^* + (1 - PVP){B_1}^* + PVP \cdot {B_1}^* + (1 - PVN){B_0}^* \\ &= (PVP + 1 - PVP){B_1}^* + (PVN + 1 - PVN){B_0}^* \\ &= {B_1}^* + {B_0}^* \end{aligned}$$

Thus, once we have estimated B_1, we can estimate B_0 from $B_0 = M_0 - B_1$. From the preceding equations we can estimate the true exposure prevalence as $P_{e0} = B_1/M_0$. Parallel formulas for cases or person-time follow by substituting A_1, A_0, ${A_1}^*$, and ${A_0}^*$ or T_1, T_0, ${T_1}^*$, and ${T_0}^*$ for B_1, B_0, ${B_1}^*$, and ${B_0}^*$ in equations 19–4. The adjusted counts obtained by applying the formula to actual data are only estimates derived under the assumption that the true predictive values are PVP and PVN and there is no other error in the observed counts (e.g., no random error). To make this clear, one should denote the solutions in equations 19–4 by $\hat{B}_1$ and $\hat{B}_0$ instead of B_1 and B_0; for notational simplicity, we have not done so.

Unfortunately, predictive values are seldom available, and when they are, their applicability is highly suspect, in part because they depend directly on exposure prevalence, which varies across populations (see formulas 19–9 and 19–10). For example, those study participants who agree to participate in a much more extensive validation substudy of food intake or medication usage (highly cooperative subjects) may have different patterns of intake and usage than other study participants. Owing to variations in exposure prevalence across populations and time, predictive values from a different study are even less likely to apply to a second study. Even when one can reliably estimate predictive values for a study, these estimates must be allowed to vary with disease and confounder levels, because exposure prevalence will vary across these levels.

These problems in applying predictive values lead to alternative adjustment methods, which use classification parameters that do not depend on true exposure prevalence. The following four probabilities are common examples of such parameters:

$$\begin{aligned}
\text{Se} &= \text{probability that someone exposed is classified as exposed}\\
&= \text{sensitivity} = \Pr(X^* = 1|X = 1)\\
\text{Fn} &= \text{probability that someone exposed is classified as unexposed}\\
&= \text{false-negative probability} = \Pr(X^* = 0|X = 1) = 1 - \text{Se}\\
\text{Sp} &= \text{probability that someone unexposed is classified as unexposed}\\
&= \text{specificity} = \Pr(X^* = 0|X = 0)\\
\text{Fp} &= \text{probability that someone unexposed is classified as exposed}\\
&= \text{false-positive probability} = \Pr(X^* = 1|X = 0) = 1 - \text{Sp}
\end{aligned}$$

The following equations then relate the expected misclassified counts to the true counts:

$$\begin{aligned}
B_1{}^* &= \text{expected number of subjects classified as exposed}\\
&= \text{Se}\,B_1 + \text{Fp}\,B_0
\end{aligned} \qquad [19\text{–}5]$$

and

$$\begin{aligned}
B_0{}^* &= \text{expected number of subjects classified as unexposed}\\
&= \text{Fn}\,B_1 + \text{Sp}\,B_0
\end{aligned} \qquad [19\text{–}6]$$

Note that Se + Fn = Sp + Fp = 1, showing again that the total is unchanged by the exposure misclassification:

$$\begin{aligned}
M_0 &= B_1 + B_0 = (\text{Se} + \text{Fn})B_1 + (\text{Sp} + \text{Fp})B_0\\
&= \text{Se}\,B_1 + \text{Fp}\,B_0 + \text{Fn}\,B_1 + \text{Sp}\,B_0 = B_1{}^* + B_0{}^*
\end{aligned}$$

In most studies, one observes only the misclassified counts $B_1{}^*$ and $B_0{}^*$. If we assume that the sensitivity and specificity are equal to Se and Sp (with Fn = 1 − Se and Fp = 1 − Sp), we can estimate B_1 and B_0 by solving equations 19–5 and 19–6. From equation 19–6, we get

$$B_0 = (B_0{}^* - \text{Fn}\,B_1)/\text{Sp}$$

We can substitute the right side of this equation for B_0 in equation 19–5, which yields

$$B_1{}^* = \text{Se}\,B_1 + \text{Fp}(B_0{}^* - \text{Fn}\,B_1)/\text{Sp}$$

We then solve for B_1 to get

$$\begin{aligned}
B_1 &= (\text{Sp}\,B_1{}^* - \text{Fp}\,B_0{}^*)/(\text{Se Sp} - \text{Fn Fp})\\
&= (B_1{}^* - \text{Fp}\,M_0)/(\text{Se} + \text{Sp} - 1) \qquad [19\text{–}7]\\
B_0 &= M_0 - B_1 = (B_0{}^* - \text{Fn}\,M_0)/(\text{Se} + \text{Sp} - 1).
\end{aligned}$$

From these equations we can also estimate the true exposure prevalence as $P_{e0} = B_1/M_0$. Again, the B_1 and B_0 obtained by applying equation 19–7 to actual data are only estimates derived under the assumption that the true sensitivity and specificity are Se and Sp.

Sensitivity analysis for exposure classification proceeds by applying equation 19–7 for various pairs of classification probabilities (Se, Sp) to the observed noncase counts $B_1{}^*$ and $B_0{}^*$. To construct a corrected measure of association, we must also apply analogous equations to estimate A_1 and A_0 from the observed (misclassified) case counts $A_1{}^*$ and $A_0{}^*$:

$$A_1 = (A_1{}^* - \text{Fp}\,M_1)/(\text{Se} + \text{Sp} - 1) \qquad [19\text{–}8]$$

from which we get $A_0 = M_1 - A_1$, where M_1 is the observed case total. These formulas may be applied to case-control, closed-cohort, or prevalence-survey data. For person-time follow-up data, equation 19–7 can be modified by substituting T_1, T_0, $T_1{}^*$, and $T_0{}^*$ for B_1, B_0, $B_1{}^*$, and $B_0{}^*$.

The formulas may be applied within strata of confounders as well. After application of the formulas, we may compute "adjusted" stratum-specific and summary effect estimates from the estimated true counts. Finally, we tabulate the adjusted estimates obtained by using different pairs (Se, Sp), and thus obtain a picture of how sensitive the results are to various degrees of misclassification.

Formulas 19–7 and 19–8 can yield negative adjusted counts, which are impossible values for the true counts. One way this can arise is if Se + Sp <1, which implies that the classification is assigning values worse than randomly, in the following sense: Imagine that we conduct a coin toss with a probability p of heads to decide whether someone was exposed or not, setting $X^* = 1$ when the coin toss yielded heads (p may be any number between 0 and 1). The sensitivity and specificity of this completely random classification are then p and $1 - p$, respectively, and Se + Sp = 1. We will henceforth assume that our actual classification method is better than a coin toss, in the sense that Se + Sp > 1.

Even with this assumption, the solution B_1 to equation 19–7 will be negative if Fp > $B_1{}^*/M_0$, i.e., if the assumed false-positive probability exceeds the observed prevalence of exposure in the noncases, or, equivalently, if Sp < $B_0{}^*/M_0$. In parallel, B_0 will be negative if Fn > $B_0{}^*/M_0$ (equivalently, Se < $B_1{}^*/M_0$), A_1 will be negative if Fp > $A_1{}^*/M_1$, and A_0 will be negative if Fn > $A_0{}^*/M_1$. A negative solution indicates that either other errors (e.g., random errors) have distorted the observed counts, the value chosen for Se or for Sp is wrong, or some combination of these problems.

Although sensitivity and specificity do not depend on the true exposure prevalence, they are influenced by other characteristics. Because predictive values are functions of sensitivity and specificity (see formulas 19–9 and 19–10, later), they too will be affected by these characteristics, as well as by any characteristic that affects prevalence. For example, covariates that affect exposure recall (such as age and comorbidities) will alter the classification probabilities for self-reported exposure history and may vary considerably across populations. In such situations, sensitivity and specificity may not generalize well from one population to another (Begg, 1987). This lack of generalizability is one reason why varying classification probabilities in the formulas (sensitivity analysis) is crucial even when estimates are available from the literature.

Valid variances for adjusted estimates cannot be calculated from the adjusted counts using conventional formulas (such as those in Chapters 14–18), even if we assume that sensitivity and specificity are known or are unbiased estimates from a validation study. This problem arises because conventional formulas do not take account of the data transformations and random errors in the adjustments. Formulas that do so are available (Selén, 1986; Espeland and Hui, 1987; Greenland, 1988b, 2007c; Gustafson, 2003; Greenland and Gustafson, 2006). Probabilistic sensitivity analysis (discussed later) can also account for these technical issues, and for other sources of bias as well.

NONDIFFERENTIALITY

In the preceding description, we assumed nondifferential exposure misclassification, that is, the same values of Se and Sp applied to both the cases (equation 19–8) and the noncases (equation 19–7). To say that a classification method is nondifferential with respect to disease means that it has identical operating characteristics among cases and noncases, so that sensitivity and specificity do not vary with disease status. We expect this property to hold when the mechanisms that determine the classification are identical among cases and noncases. In particular, we expect nondifferentiality when the disease is unrelated to exposure measurement. This expectation is reasonable when the mechanisms that determine exposure classification precede the disease occurrence and are not affected by uncontrolled risk factors, as in many cohort studies, although even then it is not guaranteed to hold (Chapter 9). Thus, to say that there is nondifferential misclassification (such as when exposure data are collected from records that predate the outcome) means that neither disease nor uncontrolled risk factors result in different accuracy of response for cases compared to noncases.

Put more abstractly, nondifferentiality means that the classification X^* is independent of the outcome D (i.e., the outcome conveys no information about X) conditional on the true exposure X and adjustment variables. Although this condition may seldom be met exactly, it can be examined on the basis of qualitative mechanistic considerations. Intuition and judgment about the role of the outcome in exposure classification errors are the basis for priors about measurement behavior. Such judgments provide another reason to express such priors in terms of sensitivity and specificity, as we will do later, rather than predictive values.

As discussed in Chapter 9, differentiality should be expected when exposure assessment can be affected by the outcome. For example, in interview-based case-control studies, cases may be more likely to recall exposure (correctly or falsely) than controls, leading to higher sensitivity or lower specificity among cases relative to controls (*recall bias*). When differential misclassification is a reasonable possibility, we can extend the sensitivity analysis by using different sensitivities and specificities for cases and noncases. Letting Fp_1, Fp_0 be the case and noncase false-positive probabilities, and Fn_1, Fn_0 the case and noncase false-negative probabilities, the corrected odds ratio for a single 2-by-2 table simplifies to

$$\frac{(A_1{}^* - Fp_1M_1)(B_0{}^* - Fn_0M_0)}{(A_0{}^* - Fn_1M_1)(B_1{}^* - Fp_0M_0)}$$

This formula is sensible, however, only if all four parenthetical terms in the ratio are positive.

APPLICATION TO THE RESINS-LUNG CANCER EXAMPLE

As a numerical example, we adjust the resins-lung cancer data in Table 19–1 under the assumption that the case sensitivity and specificity are 0.9 and 0.8, and the control sensitivity and specificity are 0.8 and 0.8. This assumption means that exposure detection is somewhat better for cases. (Because this study is record-based with deaths from other diseases as controls, it seems unlikely that the actual study would have had such differential misclassification.) From equations 19–7 and 19–8, we obtain

$$B_1 = [257 - 0.2(1{,}202)]/[0.8 + 0.8 - 1] = 27.67$$

$$B_0 = 1{,}202 - 27.67 = 1{,}174.33$$

$$A_1 = [45 - 0.2(139)]/[0.8 + 0.9 - 1] = 24.57$$

$$A_0 = 139 - 24.57 = 114.43$$

These yield an adjusted odds ratio of 24.57(1,174.33)/114.43(27.67) = 9.1. This value is much higher than the unadjusted odds ratio of 1.8, despite the fact that exposure detection is better for cases.

By repeating the preceding calculation, we obtain a resins-misclassification sensitivity analysis for the data in Table 19–1. Table 19–4 provides a summary of the results of this analysis. As can be seen, under the nondifferential misclassification scenarios along the descending diagonal, the adjusted odds-ratio estimates (2.34, 2.42, 10.7, 11.0) are always further from the null than

TABLE 19–4

Adjusted Resins-Lung Cancer Mortality Odds Ratios under Various Assumptions about the Resins Exposure Sensitivity (Se) and Specificity (Sp) among Cases and Controls

Cases		Controls			
		Se: 0.90	0.80	0.90	0.80
Se	Sp	Sp: 0.90	0.90	0.80	0.80
0.90	0.90	2.34[a]	2.00	19.3	16.5
0.80	0.90	2.83	2.42[a]	23.3	19.9
0.90	0.80	1.29	1.11	10.7[a]	9.1
0.80	0.80	1.57	1.34	12.9	11.0[a]

[a] Nondifferential misclassification.

the unadjusted estimate computed directly from the data (1.76, which corresponds to the adjusted estimate assuming Se = Sp = 1, no misclassification). This result reflects the fact that, if the exposure is dichotomous and the misclassification is better than random, nondifferential, and independent of all other errors (whether systematic or random), the bias produced by the exposure misclassification is toward the null. We caution, however, that this rule does not extend automatically to other situations, such as those involving a polytomous exposure (see Chapter 9).

In one form of recall bias, cases remember true exposure more than do controls, i.e., there is higher sensitivity among cases (Chapter 9). Table 19–4 shows that, even if we assume that this form of recall bias is present, adjustment may move the estimate away from the null; in fact, three adjusted estimates (2.00, 16.5, 9.1) are further from the null than the unadjusted estimate (1.76). These results show that the association can be considerably diminished by misclassification, even in the presence of recall bias. To understand this apparently counterintuitive phenomenon, one may think of the classification procedure as having two components: a nondifferential component shared by both cases and controls, and a differential component reflecting the recall bias. In many plausible scenarios, the bias toward the null produced by the nondifferential component overwhelms the bias away from the null produced by the differential component (Drews and Greenland, 1990).

Table 19–4 also shows that the specificity is a much more powerful determinant of the observed odds ratio than is the sensitivity in this example (e.g., with Se = 0.8 and Sp = 0.9, the adjusted estimate is 2.42, whereas with Se = 0.9 and Sp = 0.8, the adjusted estimate is 10.7), because the exposure prevalence is low. In general, when exposure prevalence is low, the odds-ratio estimate is more sensitive to false-positive error than to false-negative error, because false positives arise from a larger group and thus can easily overwhelm true positives.

Finally, the example shows that the uncertainty in results due to the uncertainty about the classification probabilities can be much greater than the uncertainty conveyed by conventional confidence intervals. The unadjusted 95% confidence interval in the example extends from 1.2 to 2.6, whereas the misclassification-adjusted odds ratios range above 10 if we allow specificities of 0.8, even if we assume that the misclassification is nondifferential, and to as low as 1.1 if we allow differential misclassification. Note that this range of uncertainty does not incorporate random error, which is the only source of error reflected in the conventional confidence interval.

RELATION OF PREDICTIVE VALUES TO SENSITIVITY AND SPECIFICITY

Arguments are often made that the sensitivity and specificity of an instrument will be roughly stable across similar populations, at least within levels of disease and covariates such as age, sex, and socioeconomic status. Nonetheless, as mentioned earlier, variations in sensitivity and specificity can occur under many conditions—for example, when the measure is an interview response and responses are interviewer-dependent (Begg, 1987). These variations in sensitivity and specificity will also produce variations in predictive values, which can be seen from formulas that relate the predictive values to sensitivity and specificity. To illustrate the relations, again consider exposure classification among noncases, where $M_0 = B_1 + B_0 = B_1{}^* + B_0{}^*$ is the noncase total, and let $P_{e0} = B_1/M_0$ be the true exposure prevalence among noncases. Then, in expectation, the predictive value positive among noncases is

$$\begin{aligned} PVP_0 &= (\text{number of correctly classified subjects in } B_1{}^*)/B_1{}^* \\ &= \text{Se } B_1/(\text{Se } B_1 + \text{Fp } B_0) \\ &= \text{Se}(B_1/M_0)/[\text{Se}(B_1/M_0) + \text{Fp}(B_0/M_0)] \\ &= \text{Se}P_{e0}/[\text{Se}P_{e0} + \text{Fp}(1 - P_{e0})] \end{aligned} \quad [19\text{–}9]$$

Similarly, in expectation, the predictive value negative among noncases is

$$PVN_0 = \text{Sp}(1 - P_{e0})/[\text{Fn}P_{e0} + \text{Sp}(1 - P_{e0})] \quad [19\text{–}10]$$

Equations 19–9 and 19–10 show that predictive values are a function of the sensitivity, specificity *and* the unknown true exposure prevalence in the population to which they apply. When adjustments are based on internal validation data and those data are a random sample of the entire study, there is no issue of generalization across populations. In such situations the predictive-value approach is simple and efficient (Marshall, 1990; Brenner and Gefeller, 1993). We again emphasize, however, that validation studies may be afflicted by selection bias, thus violating the randomness assumption used by this approach.

DISEASE MISCLASSIFICATION

Most formulas and concerns for exposure misclassification also apply to disease misclassification. For example, Equation 19–4 and 19–7 can be modified to adjust for disease misclassification. For disease misclassification in a closed-cohort study or a prevalence survey, *PVP* and *PVN* will refer to the predictive values for disease, and A, B, and N will replace B_1, B_0, and M_0. For the adjustments using sensitivity and specificity, consider first the estimation of the incidence proportion from a closed cohort or of prevalence from a cross-sectional sample. The preceding formulas can then be adapted directly by redefining Se, Fn, Sp, and Fp to refer to disease. Let

$D = 1$ if diseased, 0 if not
$D^* = 1$ if classified as diseased, 0 if not
Se = Probability someone diseased is classified as diseased
= Disease sensitivity = $\Pr(D^* = 1|D = 1)$
Fn = False-negative probability = 1 − Se
Sp = Probability someone nondiseased is classified as nondiseased
= disease specificity = $\Pr(D^* = 0|D = 0)$
Fp = False-positive probability = 1 − Sp

Suppose that A and B are the true number of diseased and nondiseased subjects, and A^* and B^* are the numbers classified as diseased and nondiseased. Then equations 19–5 through 19–7 give the expected relations between A, B and A^*, B^*, with A, B replacing B_1, B_0; A^*, B^* replacing $B_1{}^*$, $B_0{}^*$; and $N = A + B = A^* + B^*$ replacing M_0. With these changes, equation 19–7 becomes

$$A = (A^* - \text{Fp}\,N)/(\text{Se} + \text{Sp} - 1) \qquad [19\text{–}11]$$

and $B = N - A$. These equations can be applied separately to different exposure groups and within strata, and "adjusted" summary estimates can then be computed from the adjusted counts. Results of repeated application of this process for different pairs of Se, Sp can be tabulated to provide a sensitivity analysis. Also, the pair Se, Sp can either be kept the same across exposure groups (nondifferential disease misclassification) or allowed to vary across groups (differential misclassification). As noted earlier, however, special variance formulas are required (Selén, 1986; Espeland and Hui, 1987; Greenland, 1988b; Greenland, 2007c; Gustafson, 2003).

The situation differs slightly for person-time follow-up data. Here, one must replace the specificity Sp and false-positive probability Fp with a different concept, that of the *false-positive rate,* Fr:

Fr = number of false-positive diagnoses (noncases diagnosed as cases) per unit person-time.

We then have

$$A^* = \text{Se}\,A + \text{Fr}\,T \qquad [19\text{–}12]$$

where T is the true person-time at risk. Also, false-negatives (of which there are Fn A) will inflate the observed person-time T^*; how much depends on how long the false-negatives are followed. Unless the disease is very common, however, the false negatives will add relatively little person-time and we can take T to be approximately T^*. Upon doing so, we need only solve equation 19–12 for A:

$$A = (A^* - \text{Fr}\,T^*)/\text{Se} \qquad [19\text{–}13]$$

and get an adjusted rate A/T^*. Sensitivity analysis then proceeds (similarly to before) by applying equation 19–13 to the different exposure groups, computing adjusted summary measures, and repeating this process for various combinations of Se and Fr (which may vary across subcohorts).

The preceding analysis of follow-up data is simplistic, in that it does not account for possible effects if exposure lengthens or shortens the time from incidence to diagnosis. These effects have generally not been correctly analyzed in the medical literature (Greenland, 1991a, Greenland, 1999a; see the discussion of standardization in Chapter 4). In these cases, one should treat time of disease onset as the outcome variable and adjust for errors in measuring this outcome using methods for continuous variables (Carroll et al., 2006).

Often studies make special efforts to verify case diagnoses, so that the number of false positives within the study will be negligible. If such verification is successful, we can assume that $\mathrm{Fp} = 0$, $\mathrm{Sp} = 1$, and equations 19–11 and 19–13 then simplify to $A = A^*/\mathrm{Se}$. If we examine a risk ratio RR under these conditions, then, assuming nondifferential misclassification, the observed RR^* will be

$$RR^* = \frac{A_1{}^*/N_1}{A_0{}^*/N_0} = \frac{\mathrm{Se}\, A_1/N_1}{\mathrm{Se}\, A_0/N_0} = \frac{A_1/N_1}{A_0/N_0} = RR$$

In other words, with perfect specificity, nondifferential sensitivity of disease misclassification will not bias the risk ratio. Assuming that the misclassification negligibly alters person-time, the same will be true for the rate ratio (Poole, 1985) and will also be true for the odds ratio when the disease is uncommon. The preceding fact allows extension of the result to case-control studies in which cases are carefully screened to remove false positives (Brenner and Savitz, 1990).

Suppose now that the cases cannot be screened, so that in a case-control study there may be many false cases (false positives). It would be a severe mistake to apply the disease-misclassification adjustment equation 19–11 to case-control data if (as is almost always true) Se and Sp are determined from other than the study data themselves (Greenland and Kleinbaum, 1983), because the use of different sampling probabilities for cases and controls alters the sensitivity and specificity within the study relative to the source population. To see the problem, suppose that all apparent cases $A_1{}^*$, $A_0{}^*$ but only a fraction f of apparent noncases $B_1{}^*$, $B_0{}^*$ are randomly sampled from a closed cohort in which disease has been classified with sensitivity Se and specificity Sp. The expected numbers of apparent cases and controls selected at exposure level j is then

$$A_j{}^* = \mathrm{Se}\, A_j + \mathrm{Fp}\, B_j$$

and

$$f \cdot B_j{}^* = f(\mathrm{Fn}\, A_j + \mathrm{Sp}\, B_j)$$

The numbers of true cases and noncases at exposure level j in the case-control study are

$$\mathrm{Se}\, A_j + f \cdot \mathrm{Fn}\, A_j = (\mathrm{Se}\, + f \cdot \mathrm{Fn})A_j$$

and

$$\mathrm{Fp}\, B_j + f \cdot \mathrm{Sp}\, B_j = (\mathrm{Fp}\, + f \cdot \mathrm{Sp})B_j$$

whereas the numbers of correctly classified cases and noncases in the study are $\mathrm{Se}\, A_j$ and $f \cdot \mathrm{Sp}B_j$. The sensitivity and specificity in the study are thus

$$\mathrm{Se}\, A_j/(\mathrm{Se} + f \cdot \mathrm{Fn})A_j = \mathrm{Se}/(\mathrm{Se} + f \cdot \mathrm{Fn})$$

and

$$f \cdot \mathrm{Sp}\, B_j/(\mathrm{Fp} + f \cdot \mathrm{Sp})B_j = f \cdot \mathrm{Sp}/(\mathrm{Fp} + f \cdot \mathrm{Sp})$$

The study specificity can be far from the population specificity. For example, if $\mathrm{Se} = \mathrm{Sp} = 0.90$, all apparent cases are selected, and controls are 1% of the population at risk, the study specificity will be $0.01(0.90)/[0.1 + 0.01(0.90)] = 0.08$. Use of the population specificity 0.90 instead of the study specificity 0.08 in a sensitivity analysis could produce extremely distorted results.

CONFOUNDER MISCLASSIFICATION

The effects of dichotomous confounder misclassification lead to residual and possibly differential residual confounding (Greenland, 1980; Chapter 9). These effects can be explored using the methods discussed previously for dichotomous exposure misclassification (Savitz and Baron, 1989; Marshall and Hastrup, 1996; Marshall et al., 1999). One may apply equations 19–7 and 19–8 to the confounder within strata of the exposure (rather than to the exposure within strata of the confounder) and then compute a summary exposure–disease association from the adjusted data. The utility of this approach is limited, however, because most confounder adjustments involve more than two strata. We discuss a more general (matrix) approach below.

MISCLASSIFICATION OF MULTIPLE VARIABLES

So far, our analyses have assumed that only one variable requires adjustment. In many situations, age and sex (which tend to have negligible error) are the only important confounders, the cases are carefully screened, and only exposure remains seriously misclassified. There are, however, many other situations in which not only exposure but also major confounders (such as smoking level) are misclassified. Disease misclassification may also coexist with these other problems, especially when studying disease subtypes.

In examining misclassification of multiple variables, it is commonly assumed that the classification errors for each variable are independent of *errors* in other variables. This assumption is different from that of nondifferentiality, which asserts that errors for each variable are independent of the *true values* of the other variables. Neither, either one, or both assumptions may hold, and both have different implications for bias. As mentioned in Chapter 9, the generalization that "nondifferential misclassification of exposure always produces bias toward the null" is false if the errors are dependent or if exposure has multiple levels.

If all the classification errors are independent across variables, we can apply the adjustment formulas in sequence for each misclassified variable, one at a time. For example, in a prevalence survey we may first obtain counts adjusted for exposure misclassification from equations 19–7 and 19–8, then further adjust these counts for disease misclassification using equation 19–11. If, however, the classification errors are dependent across variables, we must turn to more complex adjustment methods such as those based on matrix adjustment of counts (Greenland and Kleinbaum, 1983; Selén, 1986; Espeland and Hui, 1987; Greenland, 1988b). Dependent errors most easily arise when a common method, such as an interview or medical record review, is used to ascertain more than one variable involved in the analysis (Lash and Fink, 2003b). Matrix methods are also useful for adjustments of polytomous (multilevel) variables.

A MATRIX ADJUSTMENT METHOD

We now briefly outline one simple matrix approach that is the natural generalization of the formulas given earlier (Barron, 1977; Greenland and Kleinbaum, 1983; Kleinbaum et al., 1984; Greenland, 1988b), and can be applied under any misclassification setting, including dependent and differential misclassification of polytomous variables. Imagine that we have a multiway table of data classified by disease, one or more exposures, and one or more stratification variables (all of which may have multiple levels). Suppose that this table has K cells. We can list these cells in any order and index them by a subscript $k = 1, \ldots\ldots, K$. Suppose that $C_k{}^*$ subjects are classified into cell k, whereas C_k subjects truly belong in that cell. Next, define

p_{mk} = probability of being classified into cell m when the true cell is k.

Then, in expectation,

$$C_m{}^* = \sum_{k=1}^{K} p_{mk} C_k \qquad [19\text{–}14]$$

This equation is a generalization of equations 19–5 and 19–6.

If we write C^* and C for the vectors of $C_m{}^*$ and C_k, and P for the matrix of p_{mk}, then equation 19–14 reduces to $C^* = PC$. The adjusted counts, assuming that P contains the true classification probabilities, can then be found from the observed (misclassified) counts C^* by inverting P, to get $C = P^{-1}C^*$. The practical utility of this formula in a given application will of course depend on the information available to specify plausible values for the p_{mk}.

USE OF VALIDATION DATA

In the previous sensitivity formulas we assumed that Se and Sp were educated guesses, perhaps suggested by or estimated from external literature. Suppose instead that classification probabilities can be estimated directly from an internal validation subsample of the study subjects, and the latter subsample is itself free of bias. In particular, suppose that the sampling is random within levels of exposure, disease, and any adjustment covariates. A number of statistically efficient ways of using these data are then available, beginning with the predictive-value approaches described earlier, but also including two-stage and missing-data analysis methods. From such methods, correctly classified counts may be estimated using maximum-likelihood or related techniques, and full statistics (including confidence intervals) can be obtained for the resulting effect estimates (e.g., Tennenbein, 1970; Selén, 1986; Espeland and Hui, 1987; Greenland, 1988b; Marshall, 1990; Lyles, 2002; Greenland, 2007c). Regression methods may also be used to adjust for errors in continuous measurements (e.g., Rosner et al., 1989; Speigelman et al., 2000, 2001, 2005; Carroll et al., 2006; Freedman et al., 2004). Robins et al. (1994) and Carroll et al. (2006) review and compare a number of methods and their relation to missing-data techniques, and discuss general methods for continuous as well as discrete variables.

A general adjustment formula for the predictive-value approach follows if we have estimates of

q_{km} = probability of truly belonging to cell k when classified into cell m

We can then obtain estimates of the true counts from the formula

$$C_k = \sum_{m=1}^{M} q_{km} C_m{}^*, \qquad [19\text{–}15]$$

which is a generalization of equation 19–4. In the matrix algebra formulation, we can write this equation as $C = QC^*$, where Q is the matrix of q_{km}. Adjustment methods more efficient and more general than the preceding approach can be obtained using likelihood-based techniques; see Carroll et al. (2006) for a model-based treatment.

An important caution in interpreting the results from formal adjustment methods is that most methods assume the validation standard is measured without error. If, however, the validation measurement taken as the truth is itself subject to error, then the adjusted estimate will also be biased, possibly severely so (Wacholder et al., 1993). Many studies labeled as validation studies actually substitute one imperfect measure of a variable for another. They are thus measures of agreement, not validity. For binary exposures, the bias in the adjusted estimate can be kept below that of the unadjusted estimate if the validation measurement has higher sensitivity and specificity than the regular measurement, and the adjustment method does not assume nondifferentiality (Brenner, 1996). More generally, by introducing assumptions (models) for the joint relation of the available measurements to each other and to the true values, as well as assumptions about randomness of validation sampling, further adjustments can be made to account for errors in the validation measurements (Spiegelman et al., 1997ab, 2000, 2001, 2005). These assumptions may then be subjected to sensitivity analyses of the impact of assumption violations.

We have underscored the random-sampling assumptions in validation methods because of the high potential for selection bias in many validation studies. Validation studies often require an additional respondent burden (e.g., to complete a diet diary in addition to a food frequency questionnaire), leading to questions about the representativeness of those who volunteer to participate. Even when no burden is imposed, selection bias may occur. For example, studies that validate self-reported history by record review sometimes treat those who refuse permission to review their records as if they were no different from those who permit review. Nonetheless, one reason to refuse permission may be to avoid detection of an inaccurate self-report. If this type of refusal is common enough, extrapolation of the results from those who permit review to the larger study group will exaggerate the validity of self-reported history. Sensitivity analysis of selection bias (discussed next) can be used to assess such problems.

In summary, when the validation study is itself subject to systematic error and bias, sensitivity analysis remains an important adjunct to more formal adjustment methods.

SELECTION BIAS

Selection bias (including response and follow-up bias) is perhaps the simplest to deal with mathematically and yet is often the hardest to address convincingly, although attempts have been made (e.g., Tang et al., 2000; Greenland, 2003c; Lash and Fink, 2004). The chief obstacle is lack of sufficient information to perform a quantitative analysis. It is thus unsurprising that many subject-matter controversies (such as those once surrounding exogenous estrogens and endometrial cancer; see Chapter 9) can be reduced to disputes about selection bias in case-control studies.

Some early writings mistakenly implied that selection bias, like confounding, can always be controlled if one obtains data on factors affecting selection . Although some forms of selection bias ("selection confounding") can be controlled like confounding, other forms can be impossible to control without external information; see Chapter 12. An example of controllable selection bias is that induced by matching in case-control studies. As discussed in Chapter 11, one need only control the matching factors to remove the bias. Other examples include two-stage studies, which employ biased selection with known selection probabilities and then use those probabilities to adjust for the selection bias (Walker, 1982a; White, 1982b; Breslow and Cain, 1988; Flanders and Greenland, 1991; Weinberg and Wacholder, 1990; Chapter 15). Examples of ordinarily uncontrollable bias occur when controls are matched to cases on factors affected by exposure or disease and for which the population distribution is unknown, such as intermediate causal factors or disease symptoms (Greenland and Neutra, 1981; Chapter 12).

Selection bias is controllable when the factors that affect selection are measured on all study subjects, and either (a) these factors are antecedents of both exposure and disease, and so can be controlled like confounders (Chapter 12), or (b) one knows the joint distribution of these factors (including exposure and disease, if they jointly affect selection) in the entire source population, and so can adjust for the bias using methods such as shown in equation 19–3 or the one given below. A condition equivalent to (b) is that one knows the selection probabilities for each level of the factors affecting selection. Unfortunately, this situation is rare. It usually occurs only when the study incorporates features of a population survey, as in two-stage designs (Walker, 1982a; White, 1982b) and randomized recruitment (Weinberg and Sandler, 1991). In most studies, one can usually only control as appropriate and hope that no other factors (such as intermediates or disease symptoms) have influenced selection.

There is a well-known decomposition for the odds ratio that can be used for sensitivity analysis of selection bias. Suppose that S_{Aj} and S_{Bj} are the probabilities of case and noncase selection at exposure level j. (For a dichotomous exposure, $j = 1$ for the exposed and 0 for the unexposed.) Alternatively, in a density-sampled case-control study, let S_{Bj} be the person-time rate of control selection at exposure level j. Then the population case counts can be estimated by A_j/S_{Aj} and the population noncase counts (or person-times) can be estimated by B_j/S_{Bj}. Therefore, the adjusted odds ratio or rate-ratio estimate comparing exposure level j to level 0 is

$$\frac{(A_j/S_{Aj})(B_0/S_{B0})}{(A_0/S_{A0})(B_j/S_{Bj})} = \frac{A_jB_0}{A_0B_j}\left(\frac{S_{Aj}S_{B0}}{S_{A0}S_{Bj}}\right)^{-1} \qquad [19\text{–}16]$$

for example, see Walker (1982a) and Kleinbaum et al. (1984). In words, an adjusted estimate can be obtained by dividing the sample odds ratio by a selection bias factor $S_{Aj}S_{B0}/S_{A0}S_{Bj}$. Equation 19–16 can be applied within strata of confounders, and the selection bias factor can vary across the strata. Generalizations of this formula to regression settings are also available (Scharfstein et al., 1999; Greenland, 2003c). It can also be applied repeatedly to account for independent sources of selection bias. We will illustrate its application in the section on probabilistic sensitivity analysis.

The obstacle to any application is determining or even getting a vague idea of the selection probabilities S_{Aj} and S_{Bj}. Again, these usually can be estimated only if the study in question incorporates survey elements to determine the true population frequencies. Otherwise, a sensitivity analysis based on equation 19–16 may have to encompass a broad range of possibilities. Equation 19–16 does provide one minor insight: No bias occurs if the selection bias factor is 1. One way the latter will occur is if disease and exposure affect selection independently, in the sense that $S_{Aj} = t_A u_j$ and $S_{Bj} = t_B u_j$, where t_A and t_B are the marginal selection probabilities for cases and noncases, and u_j is the marginal selection probability at exposure level j (in density studies, t_B will be the marginal rate of control selection). Occasionally one may reason that such independence will hold, or independence can be forced to hold through careful sampling. Nonetheless, when refusal is common and subjects know their own exposure and disease status, there may be good reasons to doubt the assumption (Criqui et al., 1979).

Now suppose that the selection bias is a consequence of having a covariate Z affected by exposure X that influenced selection (e.g., as when Z is an intermediate, or is affected by exposure X and the study disease D). Recall that equation 19–3 gives the ratio of the unadjusted OR_{DX} to the Z-adjusted OR_{DXZ} in terms of the prevalence P_{Z0} of $Z = 1$ among unexposed noncases, the odds ratio OR_{DZ} relating Z to D given X, and the odds ratio OR_{XZ} relating Z to X given D. Our present situation is the reverse of that when Z is an unmeasured confounder: we now have the Z-stratified OR_{DX} but want the unadjusted OR_{DX}. The inverses of the expressions in 19–3 are equal to the ratio of the adjusted and unadjusted DX odds ratios and thus equal the selection bias produced by stratifying on Z, assuming that the Z-specific DX odds ratio (OR_{DX}) is constant across Z levels (Greenland, 2003a). If the odds ratio for the association of Z with selection does not vary with D or X, we can estimate OR_{DX}, OR_{DZ}, and OR_{XZ} from the data and then do a sensitivity analysis of selection bias as a function of O_{Z0}, which equals the product of the true (population) odds of $Z = 1$ versus $Z = 0$ and the ratio of selection probabilities when $Z = 1$ versus $Z = 0$ (the degree of Z-related selection bias).

MULTIPLE-BIAS ANALYSES

Sensitivity analyses for different biases may be combined into a multiple-bias analysis. This combination, however, requires proper ordering of the adjustments, because order can make a difference. As a general rule, adjustments should be made in the *reverse* of the order in which the problems occurred during the data-generation process, much as one undoes package wrappings in the reverse of the order of the wrappings (Greenland, 1996c, 2005b). In particular, because differential misclassification bias as a function of sensitivity and specificity does not reduce to a simple multiplicative bias factor in the odds ratio, the result of the combined adjustment will depend on the order in which misclassification adjustment is made.

Confounding originates in population causal relations (Chapters 4, 9, and 12) and so is usually the first problem to occur, but selection from the source population may occur before or after classification. As an example, suppose that we wish to make adjustments for uncontrolled smoking confounding and exposure misclassification, and we have external data indicating a likely joint distribution for smoking and exposure. Suppose also that these external data are themselves based on exposure measurements misclassified in a manner similar to the study data (as would be the case if the data came from the same cohort as the study data). The external adjustment for smoking will then yield a hypothetical smoking-stratified table of *misclassified* exposure by disease, which then must be adjusted for misclassification. In other words, the smoking stratification should precede the misclassification adjustment. On the other hand, if the joint distribution of smoking and exposure used for external adjustment was a purely hypothetical one referring to the *true* exposure, the misclassification adjustment should precede the construction of the hypothetical smoking-stratified table.

To complicate matters further, the ordering of classification may differ for different variables; e.g., in a case-control study, exposure classification typically occurs after selection, but disease classification typically occurs before. Sometimes even the ordering of classification steps for a single variable is mixed; e.g., in the resins example, job information came from records that preceded the study, but exposure classification based on the jobs came from hygienist evaluations made after selection. An ideal analysis would make separate adjustments for each source of exposure misclassification, with misclassification adjustments occurring both before and after selection-bias adjustments.

Another problem in multiple-bias analysis is the complexity of examining and presenting results from multiple adjustments. The minimum number of parameters for a realistic analysis of an effect is arguably three confounding parameters, four classification probabilities, and four selection probabilities. Yet if we assigned only five values to each of these $3 + 4 + 4 = 11$ bias parameters, and eliminated half the combinations from each of the three parameter groups based on symmetry considerations, we would still have $5^{11}/2^3 > 6$ million combinations to consider. This problem has led to development of probabilistic methods for summarizing over these combinations, which we address next.

PROBABILISTIC BIAS ANALYSIS

The methods in the preceding sections describe simple sensitivity analyses that provide a quantitative assessment of one bias at a time, or as ordered adjustments. The bias parameters (e.g., associations of an unmeasured confounder with the exposure and outcome; false-positive and false-negative classification probabilities; selection probabilities) are assigned one value or a limited number of values. Although these methods yield an estimate of the direction and magnitude of bias, they treat the bias parameters as if they were perfectly measured themselves (one assigned value) or as if they can only take on a limited combination of values (as in Tables 19–3 and 19–4). Neither treatment is likely correct. In addition, when a set of adjustments arises from different combinations of bias parameters, these simple methods provide no sense of which adjustment is most plausible and which adjustment is least plausible. All combinations are treated as if they are equally likely, and presentation of multiple combinations is both cumbersome and difficult to interpret (Greenland, 1998c).

The simple methods we have presented do not combine the adjustment for systematic error with the random error reflected in the conventional confidence interval. The effect of adjustments on the P-value and confidence interval can be nonintuitive. For example, although an adjustment for nondifferential misclassification of a binary exposure can easily move a small unadjusted association far from the null (see Table 19–4), the same adjustment will either have no effect on the P-value or, through an overwhelming increase in variance, will make the P-value larger than it was before adjustment. Therefore, the adjustment does not yield stronger evidence against the null hypothesis, even though it yields an estimate of association that is farther from the null (Greenland and Gustafson, 2006).

As we have mentioned, a major problem with conventional statistical analysis is its exclusive focus on random error as the only source of uncertainty. Early attempts to integrate bias analysis with random-error analysis applied sensitivity analyses to P-values and confidence limits (Greenland and Robins, 1985a; Rosenbaum, 2002), for example by repeatedly applying conventional formulas to the adjusted data obtained from multiple scenarios. Such approaches, however, may convey an unduly pessimistic or conservative picture of the uncertainty surrounding results. For example, the lowest lower 95% limit and highest upper 95% limit from a broad-ranging analysis will contain a very wide interval that could have a coverage rate much greater than 95%. This problem occurs in part because sensitivity analyses treat all scenarios equally, regardless of plausibility. Probabilistic bias analysis provides a more coherent approach by integrating the results using explicit prior distributions for the bias parameters. This approach is the focus of the remainder of the chapter.

We will illustrate probabilistic bias analysis in perhaps its simplest and most common form, Monte-Carlo sensitivity analysis (MCSA), also known as Monte-Carlo risk assessment. After outlining this approach, we apply it to adjustments for an unmeasured confounder, misclassification, and selection bias, following the outline and example used above for simple sensitivity analysis. We conclude with a brief description of Bayesian bias analysis, which provides a more general approach to probabilistic bias analysis based on the same models and distributions. Both approaches can be thought of as supplying a posterior distribution for the target parameter (e.g., an effect measure), in the sense described in Chapter 18. The chief limitation of MCSA (which it shares with conventional frequentist methods) is that it implicitly assumes we have no prior information about the target parameter and certain other parameters. In contrast, the Bayesian approach can use prior information on any and all the parameters of the models.

PROBABILISTIC SENSITIVITY ANALYSIS

Probabilistic sensitivity analysis extends simple sensitivity analysis by assigning probability distributions to the bias parameters (Hoffman and Hammonds, 1994; Lash and Silliman, 2000; Greenland, 2001c, 2003c, 2005b; Lash and Fink, 2003a; Phillips, 2003), rather than using a few fixed values for the parameters. Assuming that the data under analysis provide no information about the bias parameters, these distributions must be developed based on information outside the data, such as experiences in other studies. The distributions for the bias parameters are then Bayesian prior distributions, as described in Chapter 18.

At each iteration of a Monte-Carlo sensitivity analysis, values for the bias parameters are randomly selected from their assigned probability distributions and then used in the sensitivity-analysis formulas given earlier to produce an adjusted estimate. There may be adjustments for multiple biases as well as for random error. Repeating this random selection-and-adjustment process, we generate a frequency distribution of adjusted estimates of the target parameter. This distribution can be summarized using percentiles, such as the median (the 50th percentile), and using intervals between percentiles. For example, the 2.5th and 97.5th percentiles of the distribution are the limits of an interval that contains 95% of the simulated estimates.

Percentiles and intervals from the MCSA distribution depict in a compact and accessible way the frequency of estimates obtained from repeated adjustment for systematic errors (or both systematic and random errors) based on the priors. To distinguish them from confidence intervals, we will call them *simulation intervals* or *MCSA intervals*. Conventional confidence intervals implicitly assume absence of uncontrolled systematic error, and they usually cover the true value with much less than their stated frequency when this assumption is not approximately correct. In the latter case, if the priors used in MCSA assign high relative probability to the actual values of the bias parameters, the resulting simulation interval typically has better coverage of the true value than the corresponding conventional confidence interval (e.g., Gustafson and Greenland, 2006b).

Suppose that our overall model of bias and random error is a good approximation to the actual data-generating process, that we have negligible background information about the target parameter, and that our distributions for the bias parameters fairly reflect our best information about the biases. The MCSA summaries then provide a reasonable sense of where the target parameter is "most likely" to be, where "most likely" is meant in a Bayesian (betting) sense as described in Chapter 18. The final MCSA distribution incorporates biases judged potentially important and random error. It provides a sense of the total uncertainty about the target parameter that is warranted under the assumed models and distributions, given the data. This more complete sense of uncertainty stems from using a model that makes fewer assumptions than are used by conventional statistical methods, which neglect unmeasured sources of bias.

ANALYSIS OF UNCONTROLLED CONFOUNDING

We will illustrate a Monte-Carlo analysis of confounding by smoking, an unmeasured potential confounder, in the study of the association between occupational resins exposure and lung cancer mortality (Table 19–1). Multiple combinations of the bias parameters yielded the 18 adjusted estimates in Table 19–3. Our probabilistic sensitivity analysis begins by assigning prior probability distributions to each of the bias parameters, which are the prevalence of smoking in those exposed to resins (P_{Z1}), the prevalence of smoking in those unexposed to resins (P_{Z0}), and the odds ratio associating smoking with lung cancer mortality (OR_{DZ}).

As an initial simple illustration, we give P_{Z0} and P_{Z1} independent prior distributions that are uniform between 0.40 and 0.70. These bounds reflect that we know smoking prevalence among men in the United States was high (over 50%) during the time under study (Centers for Disease Control, 2006), but we do not know how the study population differed from the general population, nor do we know how smoking was associated with exposure, if at all. To draw a uniform random number p between 0.40, 0.70, one can use a uniform random-number generator (available in most statistical software) to get a number u between 0 and 1, and then transform u to $p = 0.40 + (0.70 - 0.40)u = 0.4 + 0.3u$.

We emphasize that our use of independent uniform distributions is unrealistic. One problem is that the uniform distribution imposes sharp boundaries on supported (allowed) values, where in fact no sharp boundary exists, and makes the probabilities jump from 0 to a maximum value at those boundaries. Another problem is that the uniform distribution makes all supported values equally probable, when in fact there will be differences in plausibility among these values. We will describe later how to obtain more realistic distributions for proportions, and how to deal with dependencies.

Our prior distribution for OR_{DZ} is log-normal with 95% limits of 5 and 15. To simulate from this distribution, at iteration i we draw $\ln(OR_{DZ,i})$ from a normal distribution with 95% limits of ln(5) and ln(15), reflecting our high certainty that the odds ratio OR_{DZ} for the smoking indicator Z

is between 5 and 15. The solid curve in Figure 19–1a shows the density of this distribution. The limits imply that the mean of this symmetrical distribution is $[\ln(15) + \ln(5)]/2 = 2.159$. Because the number of standard deviations between the upper and lower 95% limits is $2(1.96) = 3.92$, the standard deviation (SD) of this distribution is $[\ln(15) - \ln(5)]/3.92 = 0.280$. To draw a normal random number w with mean = 2.159 and SD = 0.280, one can use a standard (mean = 0, SD = 1) normal random-number generator (available in most software) to get a number z, and then transform z to w = mean + $z \cdot$ SD $= 2.159 + z(0.280)$. Finally, we use w as our draw of $\ln(OR_{DZ})$ and hence e^w as our draw of OR_{DZ}.

To generate a large number (K) of adjusted estimates based on the chosen distributions, we proceed as follows. At iteration i (where i goes from 1 to K) we execute the following steps:

1. For each bias parameter, draw a random value from its prior distribution: $P_{Z0,\text{i}}$ from a uniform(0.40, 0.70), $P_{Z1,i}$ from a uniform (0.40, 0.70), and $\ln(OR_{DZ,\text{i}})$ from a normal with mean = 2.159 and SD = 0.280.
2. Using the bias parameter values drawn in step 1, solve equation 19–1 or 19–3 to obtain the corresponding $OR_{DX,\text{i}}$ adjusted for smoking. Record this value.

Repeating steps 1 and 2 K times generates a frequency distribution of K externally adjusted $OR_{DX,i}$. Ideally, K is chosen so that the simulated percentiles of most interest (such as the median OR_{DX}) are accurate to the number of digits used for presentation (e.g., three digits). This criterion may require far more iterations than needed to obtain sufficient accuracy for practical purposes, however.

In this example, after one simulation run of K = 20,000 iterations, the median $OR_{DX,i}$ equaled 1.77 with 95% simulation limits of 1.25 and 2.50, which have a ratio of $2.50/1.25 = 2.00$. We use the ratio of limits to measure the width of the interval because the measure of association being simulated is itself a ratio measure. Note that this ratio of limits will vary with the chosen interval percentage. The limits and their ratio reflect only our uncertainty about the bias parameters, as modeled by their prior distributions. They should be contrasted with the conventional 95% confidence limits for OR_{DX} of 1.18 and 2.64, which have a ratio of $2.64/1.18 = 2.24$. The similar ratios of limits reflect the fact that our priors induce uncertainty about confounding that is comparable with our uncertainty about random error.

Incorporating Adjustment for Random Error

We next generate a distribution for OR_{DX} that incorporates both sources of uncertainty (confounding and random error). We take each adjusted $\ln(OR_{DX,i})$ and subtract from it a random error generated from a normal distribution with a standard deviation equal to the conventional standard deviation estimate for the log odds ratio. From the formula in Chapter 14, that estimated standard deviation is $\hat{SD} = (1/45 + 1/94 + 1/257 + 1/945)^{1/2} = 0.1944$. Thus, to incorporate independent random error into our simulation, we add a third step to each iteration:

3. Draw a number z_i from a standard normal distribution. Then construct a smoking and random-error-adjusted odds ratio

$$OR_{DX,i}{}^* = \exp[\ln(OR_{DX,i}) - \text{z}_i\, \hat{SD}] \qquad [19\text{–}17]$$

If we apply step 3 without steps 1 and 2, the resulting frequency distribution will adjust for random error only and its 2.5th and 97.5th percentiles will approach the conventional confidence limits (Fig. 19–2a) as K grows large. As described above, repeating steps 1 and 2 without step 3 generates a distribution of $OR_{DX,i}$ that is adjusted for smoking only. Repeating all three steps together generates a distribution of $OR_{DX,i}{}^*$ that are adjusted for smoking and for random error. After one simulation run of K = 20,000 iterations, the median $OR_{DX,i}{}^*$ equals 1.77 with 95% simulation limits 1.04 and 3.03, which have a ratio of $3.03/1.04 = 2.91$. In contrast, the conventional 95% confidence limits for OR_{DX} have a ratio of 2.24, which is only $2.24/2.91 \approx 77\%$ that of the new ratio.

The larger ratio of upper to lower limits from the simulation results reflects the fact that our priors allow for some uncertainty about a source of uncontrolled confounding. The simulation returns the conventional interval if in step 1 of our simulation we make $P_{Z1,i} = P_{Z0,i}$, for then smoking and exposure are unassociated in every iteration, and there is no confounding by smoking. In other

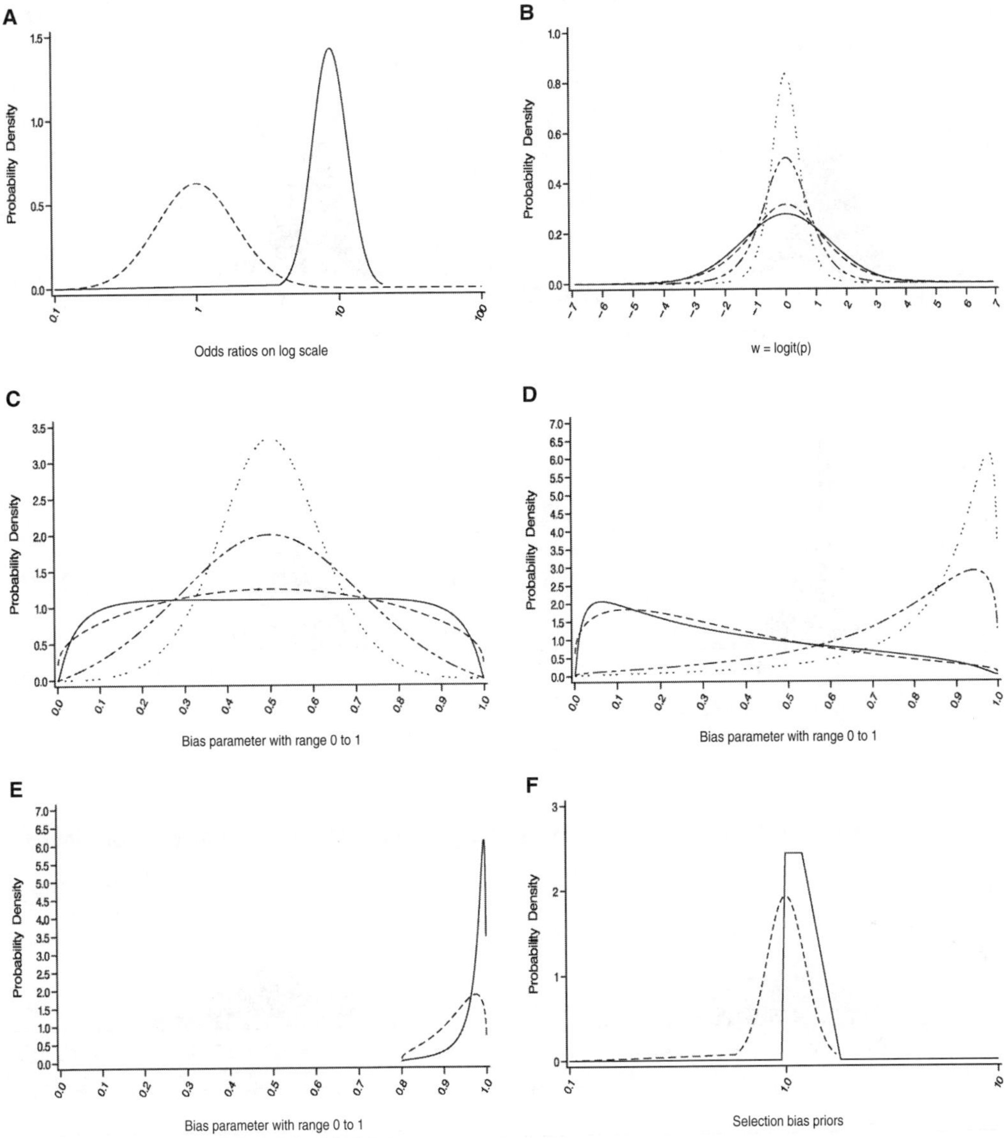

FIGURE 19–1 • Probability densities for distributions discussed in text. **(a)** Densities for unmeasured-confounding example: solid curve (——), normal prior for $\ln(OR_{DZ})$ with mean ln(10) and standard deviation 0.280; dashed curve (— —), normal prior for $\ln(OR_{XZ})$ with mean 0 and standard deviation 0.639. **(b)** Densities for unbounded w with location m and scale factor s: solid curve (——), normal density $m = 0$ and standard deviation $= \sigma = s = 1.45$; dashed curve (— —), logistic density with $m = 0$, $s = 0.8$, $\sigma = 0.8\pi/3^{1/2} = 1.45$; mixed dashed curve (— - - —), logistic density with $m = 0$ and $s = 0.5$; dotted curve (··· ···), logistic density with $m = 0$ and $s = 0.3$. **(c)** Densities for a proportion p, where $w = \text{logit}(p)$ has location m and scale factor s: solid curve (——), logit-normal density with $m = 0$ and $\sigma = s = 1.45$; dashed curve (— —), logit-logistic density with $m = 0$ and $s = 0.8$; mixed dashed curve (— - - —), logit-logistic density with $m = 0$ and $s = 0.5$; dotted curve (··· ···), logit-logistic density with $m = 0$ and $s = 0.3$. **(d)** Densities for a proportion p, where $w = \text{logit}(p)$ has location m and scale factor s: solid curve (——), normal density with $m = \text{logit}(0.5) = 0$ and $\sigma = s = 1.45$; dashed curve (— —), logit-logistic density with $m = \text{logit}(0.3)$ and $s = 0.8$; mixed dashed curve (— - - —), logit-logistic density with $m = \text{logit}(0.8)$ and $s = 0.8$; dotted curve (··· ···), logit-logistic density with $m = \text{logit}(0.9)$ and $s = 0.8$. **(e)** Densities for misclassification example: solid curve (——), prior for sensitivity Se_i of resin exposure classification, where $Se_i = 0.8 + 0.2\ \text{expit}(w)$ and w has a logistic distribution with $m = \text{logit}(0.8)$ and $s = 0.8$; dashed curve (— —), prior for specificity Sp_i of resin exposure classification, where $Sp_i = 0.8 + 0.2\ \text{expit}(w)$ and w has a logistic distribution with $m = \text{logit}(0.7)$ and $s = 0.8$. **(f)** Densities for selection-bias example (semilogarithmic plot): solid curve (——), normal prior for log selection-bias factor with mean $\ln(1) = 0$ and standard deviation 0.207; dashed curve (— —), trapezoidal prior density for log selection-bias factor with $b_l = -\ln(0.95)$, $b_u = -\ln(1.8)$, $m_l = -\ln(1) = 0$, $m_u = -\ln(1.2)$.

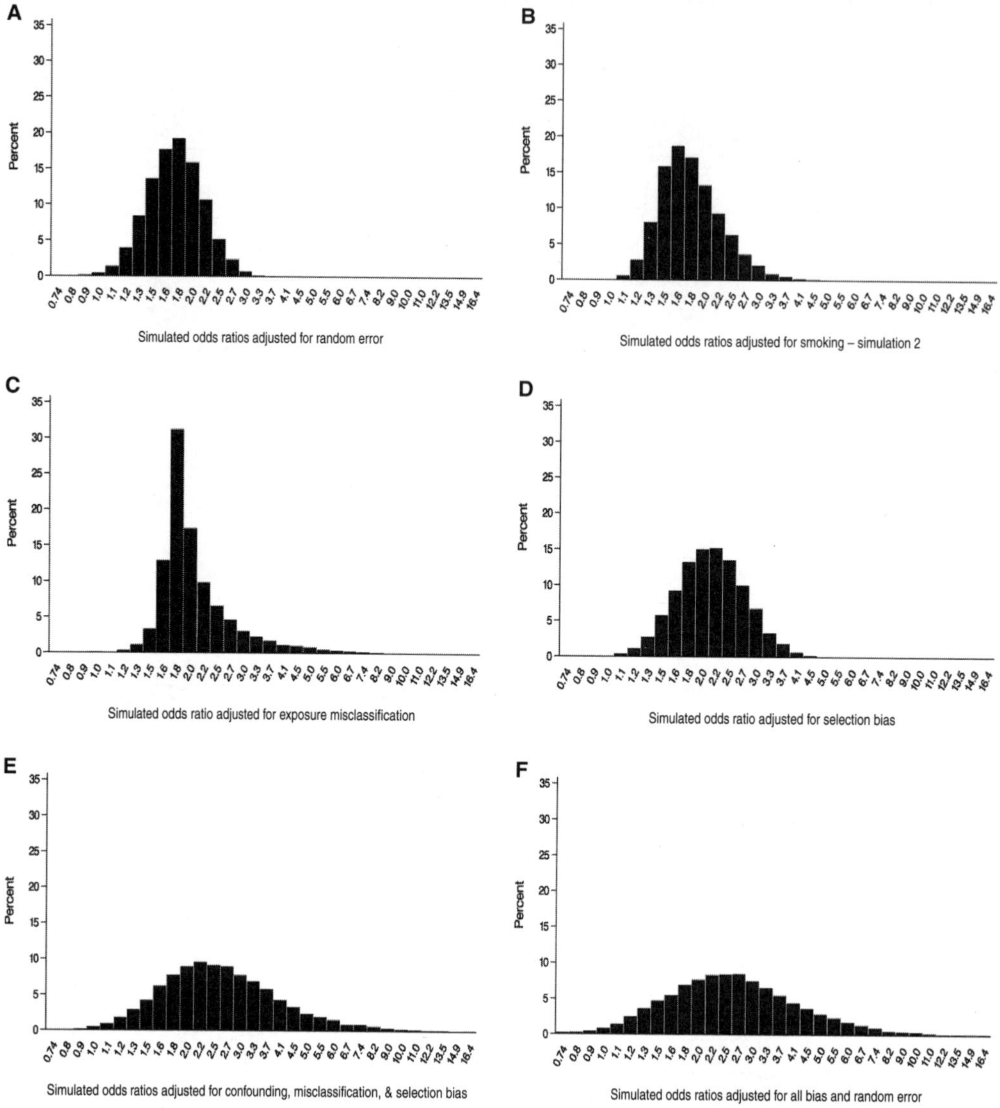

FIGURE 19–2 • Histograms of simulation results ($K = 20{,}000$) from Monte-Carlo sensitivity analysis of bias in the resins-lung cancer example. **(a)** Adjustment for random error only: median = 1.77, 95% simulation limits = 1.18, 2.64 (equal to the conventional 95% confidence limits), ratio of limits = 2.24. **(b)** Adjustment for unmeasured confounding by smoking, without random error: median = 1.77, 95% simulation limits = 1.26, 3.06, ratio of limits = 2.43. **(c)** Adjustment for misclassification of resin exposure, without random errror: median = 1.92, 95% simulation limits = 1.46, 4.90, ratio of limits = 3.36. **(d)** Adjustment for selection biases, without random error: median = 2.14, 95% simulation limits = 1.32, 3.57, ratio of limits = 2.70. **(e)** Adjustment for uncontrolled confounding by smoking, misclassification of resin exposure, and selection biases, without random error: median = 2.52, 95% simulation limits = 1.21, 7.54, ratio of limits = 6.23. **(f)** Adjustment for uncontrolled confounding by smoking, misclassification of resin exposure, and selection biases, with random error: median = 2.54, 95% simulation limits = 1.10, 7.82, ratio of limits = 7.11.

words, the conventional interval is equivalent to a simulation interval that assumes that there is no uncontrolled confounding.

Step 3 as given above uses the same normal approximation to random error on the log odds ratio scale as used in conventional statistics (e.g., Chapters 14 through 16). An alternative that is sometimes easier to employ (particularly with the record-level adjustments described later) is *resampling*. At each iteration, before making the bias adjustment in step 2, a new data set of the same size as the old is sampled with replacement from the original data set (separately for cases and controls in a case-control study, to maintain the original case and control numbers). The distribution of estimates obtained with this added step adjusts simultaneously for random error and the unmeasured confounder, whereas the distribution of estimates from the original data adjusts only for the unmeasured confounder. Rather than using the resampled data directly, more sophisticated *bootstrap* approaches use the resampled data to make adjustments for statistical biases as well as for random error (Efron and Tibshirani, 1994; Davison and Hinkley, 1997; Carpenter and Bithell, 2000).

Building More Realistic Prior Distributions

The uniform distributions assigned to the prevalences P_{Z1} and P_{Z0} of smoking in exposed and unexposed assign the same probability to every possible pair of values for these prevalences. Thus a 70% smoking prevalence in the exposed and 40% prevalence in the unexposed is assigned the same probability as a 50% prevalence for both. But we have no basis for expecting that any difference actually occurred, and we think that small differences are more likely than large ones. Furthermore, if we knew the smoking prevalence in one group, it would lead us to expect a similar prevalence in the other. As a result of placing overly high probabilities on large differences, the preceding simulation may exaggerate the uncertainty due to confounding. It may also understate uncertainty by excluding improbable—but possible—large values for the differences. One way to give higher probabilities to pairs with smaller differences, and thus more accurately reflect our uncertainty, is to generate the pairs so that the two prevalences are correlated. We will discuss generation of correlated pairs under misclassification.

Another way to better represent our uncertainty is to switch to a bias formula in which it is reasonable to treat the bias parameters as independent (Greenland, 2001c). Formula 19–3 is an example. Using this formula, instead of sampling from a distribution for P_{Z1} we may instead sample from a distribution for OR_{XZ}, the exposure-confounder odds ratio. Unlike with P_{Z1}, knowing OR_{XZ} will have little if any influence on our expectation for P_{Z0}, so giving OR_{XZ} and P_{Z0} independent priors is not unreasonable.

Another feature of the uniform prior distributions for P_{Z1} and P_{Z0} is that they impose sharp bounds on OR_{XZ}, excluding as impossible values that are less than $(1-0.7)0.4/0.7(1-0.4) = 2/7$ or more than $0.7(1-0.4)/(1-0.7)0.4 = 7/2 = 3.5$. Because we do not know for certain that OR_{XZ} is within these bounds, we can better reflect our uncertainty by using a distribution that allows some chance of falling outside these bounds. For illustration, suppose that we assign $\ln(OR_{XZ})$ a normal distribution with 95% prior limits at the extreme values from the uniform distributions for P_{Z1} and P_{Z0}, which are $\pm\ln[0.7(1-0.4)/(1-0.7)0.4] = \pm\ln(3.5)$. The mean of this normal distribution is 0, and the width of the 95% prior interval is $2\cdot\ln(3.5)$, so the SD is $2\cdot\ln(3.5)/3.92 = 0.639$. The dashed curve in Figure 19–1a shows the density of this distribution. We then replace step 1 above with

1.′ For each bias parameter, draw a random value from its prior distribution: $P_{Z0,i}$ from a uniform distribution (0.40, 0.70), $\ln(OR_{XZ,i})$ from a normal distribution with mean = 0 and SD = 0.639, and $\ln(OR_{DZ,i})$ from a normal distribution with mean = 2.16 and SD = 0.280.

Repeating steps 1′ through 3 K times generates a new frequency distribution of K externally adjusted $OR_{DX,i}$ (Fig. 19–2b) and also a frequency distribution of K externally adjusted $OR_{DX,i}{}^*$ that are adjusted for random error as well. After one simulation run of $K = 20{,}000$ iterations, the median $OR_{DX,i}{}^*$ equaled 1.77 with 95% simulation limits 1.05 and 3.47, which have a ratio of $3.47/1.05 = 3.30$. The conventional 95% confidence limits for OR_{DX} have a ratio of $2.64/1.18 = 2.24$, which is only $2.24/3.30 \approx 2/3$ that of the new ratio. The earlier simulation limits based on unrealistic independent priors have a ratio of $3.03/1.04 = 2.91$, which is only $2.91/3.30 = 88\%$ that of the new ratio.

Analysis of Uncontrolled Confounding via Direct Bias Simulation

Confounding analyses are sometimes conducted by placing a prior directly on the amount of confounding in the conventional estimate (Robins et al., 1999b; Bodnar et al., 2006). For example, if earlier studies of the same association measured the confounder in question and reported both the unadjusted and adjusted estimates, the adjusted could be divided into the unadjusted to provide an estimate of the bias due to failing to adjust for the confounder; one can also construct confidence intervals for this ratio (Greenland and Mickey, 1988). These results and other considerations can be used as a basis for a prior on the size of the bias factor in a study that fails to adjust for the confounder.

SOME EASILY GENERATED DISTRIBUTIONS

As mentioned earlier, the uniform is a rigid and unrealistic distribution. Although prior distributions are usually little more than educated guesses or bets about the parameters (hopefully reflecting relevant external data), flexible alternatives are needed to capture the rough distinctions that can be made (e.g., among "likely," "probable," "reasonable," and "implausible" values). One alternative we have illustrated for log odds ratios is the normal distribution. This choice can be adequate as long as our uncertainty about the parameter can be approximated by a symmetric, unbounded, and peaked distribution. Often, however, our uncertainty is better represented by a distribution with asymmetries, boundaries, or broad areas of equally probable values. Although normal random numbers can be transformed to capture these properties, other distributions better suited for this purpose can be derived from uniform random numbers.

Logistic Distributions

Consider a number u generated from the uniform distribution between 0 and 1. Let m and s be any fixed numbers with $s > 0$, and let

$$w = m + s \cdot \text{logit}(u) \quad \text{where logit}(u) = \ln(u) - \ln(1 - u) \qquad [19\text{–}18]$$

The new random number w has what is known as a *logistic distribution* recentered at m and rescaled by s. It has mean, median, and mode at m, and scale s. Like a normal distribution, it is symmetric with an unbounded range, but it has heavier tails, reflected in the fact that the standard deviation of a logistic distribution is $\sigma = (\pi/3^{1/2})s \approx 1.81s$, or 81% larger than the scale factor s. In contrast, for a normal distribution, the standard deviation σ and the scale factor s are equal ($\sigma = s$), which is why elementary statistics books rarely distinguish the scale factor from the standard deviation. Figure 19–1b shows densities of logistic distributions for various choices of s, along with the density of a normal distribution with $\sigma = 1.81(0.8) \approx 1.45$ for comparison (solid curve). Relative to the normal, the logistic spreads mass from the center hump into the tails. Thus a logistic prior can be used as an alternative to a normal prior when extreme values are not considered as highly improbable as a normal prior makes them appear.

The logistic prior can be generalized further into recentered and rescaled log-F distributions (also known as generalized-conjugate distributions). These distributions can generate a large variety of shapes, including skew distributions, and can be extended further to encompass multiple correlated parameters (Greenland, 2003b, 2007b; Jones, 2004). These distributions can also be translated into "prior data," along the lines described in Chapter 18 (Greenland, 2007b).

Transformation to Proportions and Bounded Variables

Now let $p = \text{expit}(w) = e^w/(1 + e^w)$ where w has an unbounded distribution with median m, such as a normal, logistic, or log-F distribution. The new random number p has a distribution from 0 to 1 with median expit(m). Consider first the special case in which w has a logistic distribution with $m = 0$. The distribution of p is then symmetric about 0.5 and is uniform if, in addition, $s = 1$. If $s < 1$, however, the distribution of p will give more probability to the middle values (near 0.5) than to extreme values (near 0 and 1), and if $s > 1$ it will give more probability to the extremes (near 0 and 1) than to the middle. For $s = 0.9$, the distribution of p is largely flat from 0.1 to 0.9, then falls off, and for $s = 0.8$, the distribution of p is a rounded hill or semicircle between 0 and 1. As s gets smaller, the hill becomes less rounded and more peaked; for $s = 0.3$ the density of p becomes a bell curve between 0 and 1. Figure 19–1c shows the density of p for various choices of s when w is logistic and $m = 0$, and also for p when w is normal with $\sigma = 1.45$ and $m = 0$. We caution that for logistic distributions with $s > 1$ or normal distributions with $\sigma > 1.6$, the resulting density for p is bimodal.

With nonzero m, the distribution of p becomes skewed even if the starting distribution of $w = \text{logit}(p)$ is symmetric. Suppose that we start with a symmetric distribution for w that is determined by its median m and scale factor s, such as a normal or a logistic distribution. To skew the distribution of p to a median of, say, 0.3, we shift w by $m = \text{logit}(0.3)$, so that $w = m + s \cdot \text{logit}(u)$, where u is again uniform. Thus, starting from a uniform u, we get

$$p = \text{expit}(w) = \text{expit}[m + s \cdot \text{logit}(u)]$$

Figure 19–1d shows the density of the distribution of p for various choices of m when $s = 0.8$. If we take the logit of p, we get back the logistic or normal distribution that we started with. Therefore, by analogy with the term "log-normal" for a variable whose log has a normal distribution, we say that the distribution of $p = \text{expit}(w)$ is *logit-logistic* if w is logistic, and is *logit-normal* if w is normal (Lesaffre et al., 2006).

We can also shift and rescale the range of p to get yet another random number q that falls between a desired minimum (lower boundary) b_l and maximum (upper boundary) b_u, by setting $q = b_l + (b_u - b_l)p$. If $w = \text{logit}(p)$ has a distribution determined by its median m and scale factor s, four parameters specify the distribution of q: m, s, and the boundaries b_l and b_u. The median of $q$is then $b_l + (b_u - b_l)\text{expit(m)}$.

TRAPEZOIDAL DISTRIBUTIONS

A *trapezoidal distribution* has as parameters a minimum (lower boundary) b_l, a maximum (upper boundary) b_u, a lower mode m_l, and an upper mode m_u. The minimum and maximum set the range of values allowed (supported) by the distribution, and the lower and upper modes set a zone of indifference in which all values are considered equally probable. The density of the distribution has a lower triangular "tail" sloping upward between b_l and m_l, a flat "table" between m_l and m_u, and an upper triangular "tail" sloping downward between m_u and b_u. The density is symmetric if $b_u - m_u = m_l - b_l$, and becomes more peaked as m_u and m_l become closer. In the extreme case with $m_l = m_u$, the density becomes triangular with a sharp peak at the modes. At the other extreme, at which the lower mode equals the minimum ($m_l = b_l$) and the upper mode equals the maximum ($m_u = b_u$), the density becomes uniform.

A trapezoidal random number t can be obtained from a random uniform (0, 1) number u as follows:

Let $v = [b_l + m_l + u \cdot (b_u + m_u - b_l - m_l)]/2$. Then

(i) If $m_l \le v \le m_u$, then $t = v$.

(ii) If $v < m_l$, then $t = b_l + [(m_l - b_l)(2v - m_l - b_l)]^{1/2}$. [19–19]

(iii) If $v > m_u$, then $t = b_u - [2(b_u - m_u)(v - m_u)]^{1/2}$.

The trapezoidal distribution is a useful candidate prior for logically bounded quantities such as proportions, and for other quantities when one is comfortable with placing sharp lower and upper bounds on the possible values. Uncertainty about the bounds to use can be accommodated by setting those bounds very wide to accommodate all remotely reasonable possibilities, thus making the tails long (i.e., making $m_l - b_l$ and $b_u - m_u$ large relative to $m_u - m_l$).

GENERATING DEPENDENT VARIABLES

So far we have discussed only use of independent distributions for the different bias parameters. For realism, however, it is sometimes essential to build dependence into these distributions. Earlier we noted that the prevalence of smoking in those exposed to resins (P_{Z1}) and in those unexposed to resins (P_{Z0}) were likely similar, although both may have been in a wide range (we used 0.4 to 0.7). More generally, when considering analogous classification or selection probabilities across different subgroups (e.g., cases and controls, men and women), it is often unrealistic to consider the probabilities equal (nondifferential) across the subgroups, but it is usually even more unrealistic to pretend that they are completely unrelated, for we often expect these probabilities to be similar across the subgroups. Even if we think that they are not necessarily close together, finding evidence that a probability of misclassification (or of refusal) is high in one subgroup will lead us to think it high in other subgroups. In other words, we usually expect analogous bias parameters to be positively associated across subgroups.

If we can translate the degree of association we expect between two unknown parameters π and τ into a correlation coefficient r, there is a simple way to generate pairs of random draws of π and τ that have that correlation. At each iteration, we first generate three (instead of two) independent random numbers, labeled h_1, h_2, h_3. These three numbers need not come from the same distribution; all that matters is that they are drawn independently and have the same variance. Then the pair of random numbers

$$g_1 = r^{1/2}h_1 + (1-r)^{1/2}h_2 \qquad g_2 = r^{1/2}h_1 + (1-r)^{1/2}h_3 \qquad [19\text{–}20]$$

will have correlation r across the iterations. Now g_1 and g_2 may not have the location, spread, or shape desired for the π and the τ distributions (i.e., they might not have the desired mean and standard deviation, or the desired bounds, or desired modes). If, however, the h_k are all drawn from distributions with mean 0 and variance 1, then g_1 and g_2 will also have mean 0 and variance 1; in that case, to get different means μ_1, μ_2 and variances σ_1^2, σ_2^2 for the pair members, we use instead $\mu_1 + \sigma_1 g_1$, $\mu_2 + \sigma_2 g_2$, which will still have correlation r. For this reason it is often easiest to start with distributions for h_k that have means of 0 and variances of 1, and then transform the output pair to have the desired means and variances. This approach can be generalized to create multiple correlated parameters via hierarchical modeling (Greenland, 2003c, 2005b).

Use of equation 19–20 will be illustrated in application to differential misclassification adjustment. If the inputs h_k are normal, the output pair g_1 and g_2 will also be normal. If the inputs h_k have the same distribution (e.g., all logistic or all trapezoidal), the distributions of the outputs g_1 and g_2 will tend to have a more normal shape than the inputs. When using equation 19–20 with non-normal inputs, one should create histograms of the final generated variables to check that they have acceptable distributions. If we require non-normality of one or both of the final pair members, we can transform g_1 or g_2 or both in a nonlinear fashion. For example, starting with normal g_1 and g_2, we could use $\exp(g_1)$ and $\text{expit}(g_2)$ to obtain a final pair with $\exp(g_1)$ a positive log-normal number and $\text{expit}(g_2)$ a logit-normal number between 0 and 1. Nonlinear transforms sometimes have little effect on the final pair correlation if r is positive, but they can be changed dramatically by certain transformations (Greenland, 1996e). Hence if nonlinear transforms are used, one should check the actual correlation as well as means and variances of the final pairs generated.

ANALYSIS OF MISCLASSIFICATION

Consider again Table 19–4, which shows the results of our initial sensitivity analysis of misclassification. The four bias parameters that govern these results are the sensitivities and specificities of exposure classification among cases and controls. For a Monte-Carlo sensitivity analysis of misclassification paralleling Table 19–4, one needs to assign prior distributions to the four bias parameters. A simple way to use the simulation draws from these distributions is as follows. At each iteration, the misclassification-adjusted counts B_{1i}, B_{0i}, A_{1i}, and A_{0i} are derived from Se_i and Sp_i using equations 19–7 and 19–8. The misclassification-adjusted odds-ratio estimate from iteration i is then $OR_{DX,i} = A_{1i}B_{0i}/A_{0i}B_{1i}$. Finally, formulas 19–7 and 19–8 are applied iteratively using draws from these distributions.

Nondifferential Misclassification

To continue the resins-lung cancer example assuming nondifferential misclassification, at each iteration we draw two independent uniform random numbers u_1, u_2 and transform them to logistic draws $g_1 = \text{logit}(0.9) + 0.8 \cdot \text{logit}(u_1)$ and $g_2 = \text{logit}(0.7) + 0.8 \cdot \text{logit}(u_2)$. We then set

$$\text{Se}_i = 0.8 + 0.2 \cdot \text{expit}(g_1) \qquad \text{and} \qquad \text{Sp}_i = 0.8 + 0.2 \cdot \text{expit}(g_2)$$

which force Se_i and Sp_i to lie between 0.8 and 1, with a median of $0.8 + 0.2(0.9) = 0.98$ for Se_i and a median of $0.8 + 0.2(0.7) = 0.94$ for Sp_i. Figure 19–1e shows the resulting densities for Se_i and Sp_i. After one simulation run of $K = 20{,}000$ iterations, the median $OR_{DX,i}$ adjusted for nondifferential misclassification is 2.01, and the 95% simulation limits are 1.78 and 4.71, which have a ratio of 2.65. This ratio is 18% greater than the ratio of the conventional confidence limits. As in the confounding examples, one can also account for random error by applying formula 19–17 (step 3) to generate $OR_{DX,i}{}^*$ from the $OR_{DX,i}$. With random error added, the median $OR_{DX,i}{}^*$ is 2.10 and the 95% simulation limits are 1.32 and 4.99, which have a ratio of 3.78. These limits are shifted upward relative to the conventional limits of 1.18 and 2.64, and have a ratio about 70% greater than that of the conventional limits. This shift arises because the assumed exposure misclassification is nondifferential, and other, downward sources of bias are not included in the adjustment model.

Treatment of Negative Adjustments

To avoid negative adjusted counts, the prior distributions for sensitivity and specificity must be bounded by $Se \geq B_1{}^*/M_0$ and $Sp \geq B_0{}^*/M_0$ among noncases, and by $Se \geq A_1{}^*/M_1$ and $Sp \geq A_0{}^*/M_1$ among cases. If a distribution is used that extends into the region of negative adjustment (i.e., if it allows draws that violate any of these inequalities), there are several options. If one regards the region as a reasonable possibility and regards the prior distribution as fair, one may set the negative counts to 0 and then tally the resulting 0 or infinite odds ratios in the final simulation percentiles. On the other hand, if one does not regard the region as realistic, one can either revise the prior distribution to fall above the region, or let the simulation do this revision automatically by having it discard draws that fall in the region.

If draws are discarded, the result is the same as using a distribution that is truncated at the point where the region of negative adjustments begins. One should thus check whether the resulting truncated distribution still appears satisfactory. As an example, Fox et al. (2005) used trapezoidal prior distributions for the parameters in the resins-lung cancer example. For nondifferential misclassification scenarios, at Monte-Carlo iteration i, Fox et al. independently drew a sensitivity Se_i and a specificity Sp_i from a trapezoidal distribution with $b_l = 75\%$, $b_u = 100\%$, $m_l = 85\%$, and $m_u = 95\%$. This distribution results in negative adjusted counts when $Sp_i \leq B_0{}^*/M_0 = 945/1{,}202 = 0.786$. Discarding these draws (as Fox et al. did) truncates the distribution at 0.786, so that the actual simulation distribution is no longer trapezoidal. Instead, the probability of $Sp < 0.786$ is 0. The resulting prior density jumps from 0 to about $(0.786 - 0.75)/(0.85 - 0.75) \approx 40\%$ of its maximum at 0.786, and continues upward, paralleling the original trapezoidal density.

Using this truncated prior, the median adjusted odds ratio obtained by Fox et al. was 2.5, with 95% simulation limits of 1.7 and 14 before accounting for random error, and limits of 1.4 and 15 (ratio $15/1.7 \approx 9$) after accounting for random error. The distribution assigned to sensitivity and specificity was meant to parallel the fixed values used in Table 19–4, rather than to reflect actual prior beliefs about the values; as a consequence, all of the adjusted odds ratios from the earlier sensitivity analysis that assumed nondifferential misclassification (the descending diagonal of Table 19–4) fall within the 95% simulation limits.

Record-Level Adjustment

To obtain their results, Fox et al. (2005) actually used a simulation procedure more complex but approximately equivalent to the one based on equations 19–7 and 19–8. At each iteration, the adjusted counts $A_{1,i}$ and $B_{1,i}$ derived from Se_i and Sp_i are used to compute the prevalences among cases and controls, then predictive values are estimated from equations 19–9 and 19–10. For each data record, these predictive values are used to impute the "true" values of exposure from the observed misclassified values. The resulting adjusted data set at iteration i is then used to compute an adjusted odds ratio. The advantage of this procedure is that it retains the same form even if further adjustments are needed (e.g., for age, sex, and other confounders recorded in the data). It also parallels multiple imputation for measurement-error adjustment based on validation data (Cole et al., 2006), and so is easily combined with imputations for missing data. The disadvantage is that it can be computationally demanding, because it requires construction of a new data set at each iteration.

Differential Misclassification

To allow for differential misclassification, we must generate separate sensitivities $Se_{1,i}$, $Se_{0,i}$ and separate specificities $Sp_{1,i}$, $Sp_{0,i}$ for cases and controls. In doing so, however, we must note that case sensitivities are not *a priori* independent of the control sensitivities, nor are the case specificities *a priori* independent of the control specificities, and take these facts into account in the simulations. For example, if we found out the sensitivity and specificity for the controls, the information would definitely influence the distributions we would assign to the case sensitivity and specificity. One way to address this dependence in the resins-lung cancer example is as follows. At each iteration i, we:

1. Draw three independent uniform random numbers u_1, u_2, u_3, transform them to logistic numbers $h_k = \text{logit}(0.9) + 0.8 \cdot \text{logit}(u_k)$, and use formula 19–20 to generate pairs of numbers g_1 and g_2 from the h_k, with correlation $r = 0.8$. We then set

$$\text{Se}_{1,i} = 0.8 + 0.2 \cdot \text{expit}(g_1) \qquad \text{and} \qquad \text{Se}_{0,i} = 0.8 + 0.2 \cdot \text{expit}(g_2)$$

2. Draw three more independent uniform random numbers u_4, u_5, u_6, transform them to logistic numbers $h_k = \text{logit}(0.7) + 0.8 \cdot \text{logit}(u_k)$, and use formula 19–20 to generate pairs of numbers g_3 and g_4 from the h_k, with correlation $r = 0.8$. We then set

$$\text{Sp}_{1,i} = 0.8 + 0.2 \cdot \text{expit}(g_3), \text{Sp}_{0,i} = 0.8 + 0.2 \cdot \text{expit}(g_4)$$

$\text{Se}_{1,i}$, $\text{Sp}_{1,i}$ are then used to adjust the case counts via formula 19–8, and $\text{Se}_{0,i}$, $\text{Sp}_{0,i}$ are used to adjust the control counts via formula 19–7.

After one simulation run of $K = 20{,}000$ iterations, the correlation of $\text{Se}_{1,i}$ and $\text{Se}_{0,i}$ was 0.76 and the correlation of $\text{Sp}_{1,i}$ and $\text{Sp}_{0,i}$ was 0.78. The median $OR_{DX,i}$ was 1.92 and the 95% simulation limits were 1.46 and 4.90, which have a ratio of 3.36 (Fig. 19–2c). This ratio is $3.36/2.24 \approx 1.5$ times larger than the ratio of the conventional limits, and is $3.36/2.65 \approx 1.27$ times larger than the ratio of the limits from the nondifferential simulations. Upon adding random error using formula 19–17, the median $OR_{DX,i}{}^*$ is 2.01 and the 95% simulation limits are 1.20 and 5.13, which have a ratio of 4.28 (Fig. 19–2d). This ratio is $4.28/3.36 \approx 1.27$ times larger than that without random error.

We use the same classification priors for cases and controls, because in this study we have no basis for presuming that any difference exists. By generating separately the parameters for cases and controls with a correlation less than 1, however, we produce a limited and random degree of differentiality at each draw. The distribution of differentiality is partially controlled by the correlation parameter r, with less differentiality expected as r approaches 1. With the same priors for cases and controls, a correlation of 1 corresponds to nondifferentiality, because it would make $g_1 = g_2$ and $g_3 = g_4$ and thus create the same sensitivity and specificity for cases and controls at every iteration. The distribution of differentiality is also controlled by the final transformation to sensitivity and specificity, with less differentiality expected as the bounds become narrower. Equality of the distributions for cases and controls simply reflects our ignorance about how differentiality might have occurred, if it occurred.

Had the exposure histories been based on subject recall rather than on records, we would have made the case sensitivity distribution higher and the case specificity distribution lower relative to the control distributions, to build some recall bias into our priors. A more-detailed model for the underlying continuous exposure measurement could also lead to a difference in the case and control distributions for sensitivity and specificity, even if the continuous error distribution was the same for both cases and controls (Flegal et al., 1991).

The sensitivity distribution is set higher than the specificity distribution because the dichotomy into exposed versus unexposed corresponds to positive exposure versus no exposure in the original quantitative exposure evaluation. It thus favors sensitivity over specificity. If a very high cutpoint is used, the sensitivity distribution might be set lower than the specificity distribution.

Both the differential and nondifferential results are more compatible with larger odds ratios than the conventional result. One should bear in mind that disagreements are due entirely to the different priors underlying the analyses. The conventional result assumes perfect classification and gives a result equivalent to a simulation in which the prior probability that $\text{Se} = \text{Sp} = 1$ is 100%. In contrast, our simulations allow for the possibility that both false-positive and false-negative exposure misclassification might be common. One's preferences should depend on which priors better reflect one's own judgment about the exposure classification that generated Table 19–1.

In all the preceding simulations, sensitivities were generated independently of specificities. An independence judgment might be justified if there were forces that move the correlation of sensitivity with specificity in the positive direction, other forces that moved the correlation in the negative direction, and we do not know the relative strength of these forces (Greenland, 2005b). As an upward force on the correlation, the association of the original quantitative exposure assessment with true exposure level is unknown: If it is high, then both sensitivity and specificity will be high; and if it is low, then both sensitivity and specificity will be low. As a downward force, sensitivity will decline and specificity will increase as the cutpoint chosen for dichotomization is increased. An ideal analysis would attempt to model the relative contribution of these forces to the final correlation. In the present example, however, the cutpoint is known and at its minimum, hence arguably the downward force is eliminated and sensitivity and specificity should have been given a positive correlation.

ANALYSIS OF SELECTION BIAS

As noted earlier, when the factors affecting selection are measured on all study subjects and are not affected by exposure or disease, the selection bias produced by the factors can be controlled by adjusting for the factors. Thus, if such a factor Z is unmeasured but we can assign prior distributions to its prevalence and its associations with exposure and disease, we can conduct a Monte-Carlo sensitivity analysis of selection bias using the formulas presented earlier for analysis of confounding. When selection bias arises because exposure X affects Z and Z influences selection, the inverse of formula 19–3 gives the selection bias produced by stratifying on Z. If Z is measured, the quantities OR_{DZ} and OR_{XZ} can be estimated from the data, and the simulation requires only a prior on the prevalence of $Z = 1$ within one of the exposure–disease combinations, e.g., prevalence odds O_{Z0} among the unexposed noncases. If Z is unmeasured however, priors on OR_{DZ} and OR_{XZ} will be needed as well.

If data are available that indicate the size of the selection bias factor $S_{Aj}S_{B0}/S_{A0}S_{Bj}$ in equation 19–16, they can be used to create a prior directly for this factor. Draws from this prior are then divided into the odds-ratio estimate to provide a selection-bias adjusted estimate from that iteration. This approach generalizes easily to regression-model coefficients (Greenland, 2003c).

Consider again the resins-lung cancer example. In this study, 71 of 210 (34%) lung cancer cases and 787 of 1,989 (40%) control deaths were omitted from the analysis because of lack of adequate job records for exposure reconstruction, due mostly to routine record disposal during the history of the facility under study (Greenland et al., 1994). If lack of records were strongly related to both resin exposure and cause of death, considerable selection bias could result. The magnitude could be bounded by the (absurd) extremes in which either all 71 missing cases were exposed and all 787 missing controls were unexposed, which yields a bias factor of $(45 + 71)(945 + 787)/45(945) = 4.7$, or all 71 missing cases were unexposed and all 787 missing controls were exposed, which yields a bias factor of $94(257)/(94 + 71)(257 + 787) = 0.14$.

Because we see only a small association between lack of records and cause of death, we expect the bias (if any) from lack of records to be small; hence these bounds are of no help. Instead, we assign a normal prior to the component of bias in the log odds ratio due to missing records with mean 0 (no bias) and standard deviation 0.207 (Fig. 19–1f, solid curve), which yields 95% prior probability of the bias factor falling between $\exp(\pm 1.96 \cdot 0.207) = 0.67$ and 1.5, and 2:1 odds of the factor falling between $\exp(\pm 0.97 \cdot 0.207) = 0.82$ and 1.22. Draws z from a standard normal distribution are thus used to adjust the resin-lung cancer odds ratio by dividing $\exp(0.207z)$ into the odds ratio. A more thorough analysis would attempt to relate lack of records to dates of employment, trends in resin use, and trends in mortality from lung cancer and the control diseases (lack of records was far more frequent among earlier employees than later employees, and was modestly associated with cause of death).

Other sources of selection bias include use of lung cancer deaths as a substitute for incident cases, and use of other deaths as controls. To build a prior distribution for these sources, assume for the moment that lack of records is not a source of bias. Given the relative socioeconomic homogeneity of the underlying occupational cohort, we expect similar survival rates among the exposed and unexposed, making it plausible that the use of deaths for cases produced little bias. Thus we neglect case-selection bias, i.e., we assume that $S_{A1} \approx S_{A0}$. On the other hand, use of other deaths as controls is suspect. For example, if resins exposure is positively associated with death from these control causes of deaths, controls will exhibit too much exposure relative to the source population (i.e., $S_{B1} > S_{B0}$), leading to $S_{B0}/S_{B1} \approx S_{A1}S_{B0}/S_{A0}S_{B1} < 1$ if $S_{A1} \approx S_{A0}$. Furthermore, if resin association with control deaths were the sole source of selection bias, the inverse of this bias factor, S_{B1}/S_{B0}, would equal the rate ratio for that association (for related discussion, see "Number of Control Groups" in Chapter 8). Thus a prior for the control selection bias in this example is approximated by a prior for the inverse of the odds ratio relating resin exposure to the control causes of death. Equivalently, a prior for the log selection-bias factor is approximated by the negative of the prior for the log odds ratio relating exposure to control deaths.

The control deaths were primarily from cardiovascular causes, which were chosen based on a prior that assigned low probability to an association with the study exposures. Even if there were an association, occupational factors for cardiovascular deaths usually have small ratios (less than smoking–cardiovascular disease rate ratios, which are typically on the order of 2), as one would expect owing to the high frequency and heterogeneity of cardiovascular deaths. To roughly capture these ideas, we assign a trapezoidal prior to the log selection-bias factor for control selection bias, with $b_l = -\ln(.95)$, $b_u = -\ln(1.8)$, $m_l = -\ln(1) = 0$, and $m_u = -\ln(1.2)$ (Fig. 19–1f, dashed). Draws w from this distribution are then used to adjust the resin-lung cancer odds ratio by dividing e^w into the odds ratio.

Combining the two selection-bias adjustments under the assumption of independence of the sources, at each iteration we draw a standard normal z and a trapezoidal w, then divide the resin–lung cancer odds ratio by $\exp(0.207z + w)$. After one simulation run with $K = 20{,}000$ iterations, the median $OR_{DX,i}$ is 2.14 and the 95% simulation limits are 1.32 and 3.57, which have a ratio of 2.70 (Fig. 19–2d). This ratio is $2.70/2.24 \approx 1.21$ times larger than the ratio of the conventional limits. After accounting for random error using formula 19–17, the median $OR_{DX,i}{}^*$ is 2.15 and the 95% simulation limits are 1.14 and 4.14, which have a ratio 3.63, $3.63/2.24 \approx 1.62$ times larger than the ratio of the conventional limits. The conventional limits are obtained from a simulation in which the priors for both selection-bias factors assign 100% probability to 1 (no bias).

Another form of selection bias arises in meta-analyses, in which studies may be selectively excluded because of inclusion criteria or publication bias. A number of methods for dealing with publication bias have been developed, including sensitivity analyses; see Chapter 33 for citations.

COMPARATIVE AND COMBINED ANALYSES

Table 19–5 summarizes the results of the Monte-Carlo analyses given here. With the example prior distributions, it appears that random error, confounding, and selection bias make similar contributions to uncertainty about the resins-lung cancer odds ratio, whereas exposure classification errors are a somewhat larger source of uncertainty.

Extension of these methods to multiple probabilistic bias analysis is straightforward if the parameters from each source of bias (confounding, exposure misclassification, disease misclassification, confounder misclassification, selection bias) can be treated as if they are independent. An important caution is that, even if the parameters from each source are independent, the order of adjustment can still matter if misclassification adjustment is made. As discussed earlier, adjustments should be made in reverse order of their occurrence. Thus, some misclassification adjustments may come before selection-bias adjustments, whereas others may come after.

If all the tabular data counts are large and random error is independent of the bias parameters, the order in which random error is added will usually not matter much, especially when (as in the present example) random error turns out to be small compared with potential biases. Nonetheless, the sensitivity of random-error adjustment to order can be investigated by comparing results from resampling the data first, versus adding random error last as in formula 19–17. No ordering is universally justified, however, because random variation can occur at any stage of the data-generating process. Exposure and disease occurrence have random components (which lead to random components in confounding), and selection and classification errors have random components. An ideal analysis would also model these sources separately, although again, given large enough data counts, their combination into one step may have little effect.

TABLE 19–5

Summary of Results from Monte-Carlo Sensitivity Analyses of Biases in Study of Occupational Resins Exposure (X) and Lung Cancer Mortality (Table 19–1)

Bias Model	Without Incorporating Random Error			With Random Error Incorporated		
	Median	2.5th & 97.5th Percentiles	Ratio of Limits	Median	2.5th & 97.5th Percentiles	Ratio of Limits
1. None (conventional)	1.77	1.77, 1.77	1.00	1.77	1.18, 2.64	2.24
2. P_{Z0} & $P_{Z1} \sim$ uniform (0.4, 0.7); $\ln(OR_{DZ}) \sim$ normal (2.159, 0.280)	1.77	1.25, 2.50	2.00	1.77	1.04, 3.03	2.91
3. $P_{Z0} \sim$ uniform (0.4, 0.7); $\ln(OR_{XZ}) \sim$ normal (0, 0.639); $\ln(OR_{DZ}) \sim$ normal (2.159, 0.280)	1.77	1.26, 3.06	2.43	1.80	1.05, 3.47	3.30
4. $Se = 0.8 + 0.2 \cdot \text{expit}(g_1)$ & $Sp = 0.8 + 0.2 \cdot \text{expit}(g_2)$, where $g_1 = \text{logit}(0.9) + 0.8 \cdot \text{logit}(u_1)$ & $g_2 = \text{logit}(0.7) + 0.8 \cdot \text{logit}(u_2)$ and u_1 & $u_2 \sim$ uniform (0, 1)	2.01	1.78, 4.71	2.65	2.10	1.32, 4.99	3.78
5. $Se_1 = 0.8 + 0.2 \cdot \text{expit}(g_1)$ & $Se_0 = 0.8 + 0.2 \cdot \text{expit}(g_2)$, where g_1 & $g_2 = \text{logit}(0.9) + 0.8 \cdot \text{logit}(u_k)$ with $r = 0.8$; $Sp_1 = 0.8 + 0.2 \cdot \text{expit}(g_3)$ & $Sp_0 = 0.8 + 0.2 \cdot \text{expit}(g_4)$, where g_3 & $g_4 = \text{logit}(0.7) + 0.8 \cdot \text{logit}(u_k)$ with $r = 0.8$, and $u_k \sim$ uniform (0, 1)	1.92	1.46, 4.90	3.36	2.01	1.20, 5.13	4.28
6. $\ln(S_{A0}S_{B0}/S_{A0}S_{B1}) \sim 0.207z +$ trapezoidal with $b_1 = -\ln(0.95)$, $b_u = -\ln(1.8)$, $m_1 = -\ln(1)$ & $m_u = -\ln(1.2)$	2.14	1.32, 3.57	2.70	2.15	1.14, 4.14	3.63
7. Combined in order 5, then 6, then 3	2.52	1.21, 7.54	6.23	2.54	1.10, 7.82	7.11

In the resins-lung cancer example, we assume that the study problems occurred in the order of confounding, selection bias, and misclassification. Thus, at each iteration of our multiple-bias analysis, we

1. Draw sensitivities and specificities to adjust the odds ratio for misclassification.
2. Draw the selection-bias factors to divide into this misclassification-adjusted odds ratio.
3. Draw the independent confounding parameters P_{Z0}, OR_{DZ}, OR_{XZ}, to create a confounding factor to divide into the odds ratio adjusted for misclassification and selection.

We use the priors illustrated earlier, allowing differential misclassification. After one simulation run of $K = 20{,}000$ iterations, the resulting median $OR_{DX,i}$ is 2.52 and the 95% simulation limits are 1.21 and 7.54, which have a ratio of 6.23 (Fig. 19–2e). This ratio is $6.23/2.24 \approx 2.8$ times larger than the ratio of conventional limits, demonstrating that random error is of far less importance than total bias uncertainty under our priors. Adding random error using formula 19–17 gives a median $OR_{DX,i}{}^*$ of 2.54 and 95% simulation limits of 1.10 and 7.82, which have a ratio of 7.11 (Fig. 19–2f). This ratio is $7.11/2.24 \approx 3.2$ times larger than the ratio of conventional limits, demonstrating that the conventional limits grossly understate the uncertainty one should have if one accepts our priors.

Figures 19–2a through 19–2d display the separate sources of uncertainty that contributed to the final risk assessment in Figure 19–2f. Other sets of priors could give very different results. Nonetheless, we expect that any set of priors that is reasonably consistent with the limited study design (a record-based mortality case-control study in an occupational cohort) will also yield a combined simulation interval that is much wider than the conventional confidence interval, because the simulation interval will incorporate uncertainty about biases as well as random error.

The priors we chose did lead to a point of agreement with the conventional analysis: Both analyses suggest that workplace exposure to resins is associated with lung cancer in the underlying cohort. In our final combined assessment, the proportion of simulations in which the adjusted *OR* estimate fell below 1 was 0.014; the analogous conventional statistic is the upper-tailed *P*-value for testing $OR_{DX} \leq 1$, which from Table 19–1 is 0.002. We emphasize, however, that this degree of agreement with the conventional result might not arise from bias analyses with other defensible sets of priors.

Our assessment assumed independence among the different sources of uncertainty (random error, confounding, misclassification, selection bias). Parameter dependencies within and between the different steps (1 to 3) can be accommodated by inducing correlations using formula 19–20. Our ability to specify such correlations knowledgeably is often limited. Nonetheless, information about the mechanisms responsible for the correlations is often available; for example, vitamin intakes estimated from food-intake data have substantially correlated errors owing to the errors in capturing food and supplement consumption. Hierarchical models (Chapter 21) can be used to capture available information about such correlations (Greenland, 2003c, 2005b).

BAYESIAN AND SEMI-BAYESIAN ANALYSIS

Bayesian approaches to bias analysis begin with a bias model as used in a sensitivity analysis, then add prior distributions for the bias parameters. Thus they involve the same initial work, inputs, and assumptions as probabilistic sensitivity analysis (PSA). They may also employ prior distributions for other parameters in the problem, such as one for the effect under study. As discussed in Chapter 18, if all parameters are given an explicit prior, the analysis is fully Bayesian; otherwise it is semi-Bayesian. To describe these methods, we will use the term *distribution* to refer to what is technically known as a probability density or mass function.

If only the bias parameters are given explicit priors, the only difference between semi-Bayesian analysis and PSA is in the ensuing computations. To outline the differences, suppose that:

- Y represents the observed data under analysis; above, Y is the four counts in Table 19–1.
- β represents all the bias parameters; above, β would contain the parameters involving an unmeasured confounder, sensitivities and specificities, and selection-bias factors.
- α represents all other parameters in the problem; above, α would contain the effect of interest (the log odds ratio adjusted for all bias and random error) and the true exposure prevalence.

- $P(\beta)$ represents the joint prior distribution of the bias parameters; if, as above, parameters for different bias sources are given independent priors, $P(\beta)$ is just the product of all the bias-prior distributions.
- $P(\varepsilon)$ represents the assumed distribution of random errors; above, $P(\varepsilon)$ was approximated by a normal distribution on the log odds-ratio scale.

For a Monte-Carlo (simulation) analysis, PSA iterates through draws of the bias parameters β from their prior $P(\beta)$, along with draws of random errors ε from $P(\varepsilon)$, then plots or tabulates the adjusted results, as in Table 19–5. It is thus a simple extension of classical sensitivity analysis using priors to choose the possible bias-parameter values, and adding random-error adjustment.

In contrast, a Monte-Carlo Bayesian analysis iterates through draws of all parameters from the joint *posterior distribution* $P(\alpha, \beta|Y)$ for both α and β. From Bayes's theorem (Chapter 18), the posterior $P(\alpha, \beta|\text{Y})$ is proportional to $P(Y|\alpha, \beta)P(\alpha, \beta)$, where $P(\alpha,\beta)$ is the joint prior distribution for α and β and $P(Y|\alpha,\beta)$ is the probability of seeing the data Y given the parameters α and β. The latter data probability is a function of α, β, and the random-error distribution $P(\varepsilon)$. In a semi-Bayesian bias analysis, all values of α are taken to have equal prior probability, in that $P(\alpha, \beta)$ is assumed to equal $P(\beta)$; i.e., a "noninformative" prior for α is assumed. The semi-Bayesian posterior distribution is thus proportional to $P(Y|\alpha, \beta)P(\beta)$.

Posterior sampling can be computationally demanding and technically subtle, especially when the data contain no direct information about certain parameters, as in the bias models used earlier (e.g., see Carlin and Louis, 2000, Gelman et al., 2003, Gustafson, 2003, 2005). Computational details can be largely handled by free Internet software such as WinBUGS (MRC, 2004), however. As a result, bias analyses using Monte-Carlo Bayesian methods have begun to appear in the epidemiologic literature (Gustafson, 2003; Steenland and Greenland, 2004; Chu et al., 2006; McCandless et al., 2007). There are also analytic approximations to Bayesian analyses that are easy to implement using ordinary commercial software, such as the prior-data approach in Chapter 18 (Greenland, 2006a, 2007a, 2007b), and that can be adapted to bias analysis and combined with Monte-Carlo methods (Greenland and Kheifets, 2006).

Under the models for bias discussed earlier in this chapter, PSA with random error included tends to give results similar to semi-Bayesian bias analysis, provided the priors do not lead to impossible outputs (e.g., negative adjusted counts) in the sensitivity analysis (Greenland, 2005b). For example, in an analysis of smoking as an unmeasured confounder in an occupational cohort study of silica exposure and lung cancer, Steenland and Greenland (2004) obtained conventional 95% confidence limits of 1.31 and 1.93. In contrast, the 95% MCSA simulation limits (including random error) were 1.15 and 1.78, while the Bayesian posterior simulation limits using the same confounding prior and a noninformative prior for the silica effect were 1.13 and 1.84. In general, we expect the PSA and semi-Bayesian results to be similar when, under the assumed model and prior, the data provide no information about the bias parameters, i.e., when the posterior distribution $P(\beta|Y)$ equals the prior $P(\beta)$ (Greenland, 2005b). The confounding and selection models used earlier are examples. Gustafson (2005) provides a general discussion of conditions for the latter equality.

Although they are less transparent computationally than PSA, Bayesian approaches have advantages in interpretation and flexibility. First, unlike with PSA, the Bayesian output distribution is guaranteed to be a genuine posterior probability distribution. This guarantee means, for example, that the 95% Bayesian interval is a fair betting interval under the assumed prior and data model (Chapter 18). Second, Bayesian analysis has no difficulty accommodating priors that would sometimes yield impossible outputs in sensitivity analysis. Recall that an impossible sensitivity-analysis output might reflect a problem with the data (e.g., large random error) rather than the prior; hence such an output is not a sufficient reason to reject or modify the prior. Third, Bayesian analyses can reveal counterintuitive phenomena in uncertainty assessments that are not apparent in PSA (Gustafson and Greenland, 2006a).

Fourth and perhaps most important, the Bayesian formulation facilitates use of prior information about any parameter in the analysis, not just those in the sensitivity models. For example, in addition to bias priors, one can use priors for effects of measured confounders (Greenland, 2000c; Gustafson and Greenland, 2006b) or for the effect under study (Greenland, 2001c; Greenland and Kheifets, 2006). As explained in Chapter 18, the "noninformative" effect priors implicit in conventional methods, in PSA, and in semi-Bayesian analysis are always contextually absurd, in that they treat effects that are enormous and effects that are small as if they were equally probable. The consequence of this treatment is unnecessary imprecision and greater susceptibility to false-positive results. Nonetheless, PSA provides an easily implemented bridge between ordinary sensitivity analysis and Bayesian analysis, and will often be sufficient for bias analysis, especially when random error is a small component of total uncertainty.

CONCLUSION

Bias analysis is a quantitative extension of the qualitative speculations that characterize good discussions of study results. In this regard, it can be viewed as an attempt to move beyond conventional statistics, which are based on implausible randomization and random-error assumptions (Greenland, 1990; Greenland, 2005b), and the more informed but informal inferences that recognize the importance of biases, but do not attempt to estimate their magnitude.

No analysis should be expected to address every conceivable source of uncertainty. There will be many sources that will be of minor importance in a given context, and preliminary considerations will often identify just a few sources of concern. At one extreme, conventional results may show that the random error in a study is potentially so large that no important inference could be drawn under any reasonable scenario (as in studies with few exposed cases). In that case, bias analysis will be a superfluous exercise. Bias analysis may also be justifiably avoided if the author is content with a descriptive approach to the study report, and can refrain from making inferences or recommendations (Greenland et al., 2004).

Nonetheless, bias analysis will often be essential to obtain an accurate picture of the net uncertainty one should have in light of study data and a given set of prior judgments. The results quantify the degree to which a study should seem informative under those priors, rather than classifying the study into crude and often misleading categories of "valid" versus "invalid" or "high quality" versus "low quality" based on qualitative assessments. This quantification can be most important for large studies, pooled analyses, and meta-analyses claiming to have clear findings. It can even become essential to the public interest when results are likely to be used for public policy or medical practice recommendations. In these settings, conventional results can become an impediment to sound recommendations if they appear to provide conclusive inferences and are not tempered by formal bias analysis.

As mentioned in the introduction, a danger of quantitative bias analyses is the potential for analysts to exaggerate or obscure reported associations by manipulating bias parameters or priors. As various controversies have revealed, however, there is ample opportunity for investigators to inject their own biases (or those of their sponsors) by manipulating study protocols, study data, and conventional analyses (e.g., see Curfman et al., 2006, regarding Vioxx and coronary events). Thus, as with all methods, the potential for abuse is not an argument against honest use, nor does it argue for the superiority of conventional approaches.

Honest use of sensitivity and Bayesian analyses involves attempts to base priors and models on empirical evidence, uninfluenced by the consequences (both analytically and politically). As emphasized in the introduction, however, it also requires presentation of results as judgments based on the chosen models and priors, rather than as data analyses or as objective study findings. Because conventional results are themselves based on doubtful models and implicit priors of no bias, they would be presented as nothing more than ill-founded judgments if they were subject to the same truth-in-packaging requirement (Greenland, 2005b).

An advantage of formal bias analyses over narrative evaluations of conventional results is that opinions and prejudices about parameter values are made explicit in the priors, thus opening the assumptions underpinning any inferences to public scrutiny and criticism. Readers can evaluate the reasonableness of the analysis in light of their own priors and background information. When controversy arises, alternative analyses will be needed. Once a bias analysis is programmed, however, alternative bias models and priors can be examined with little extra effort. Comparisons of alternative formulations can be viewed as a sensitivity analysis of the bias analysis (Greenland, 1998c). Such comparisons allow observers to isolate more easily sources of disagreement and identify formulations that best reflect their own judgment, thereby helping move debates beyond qualitative assertions and counterassertions.

CHAPTER 20

Introduction to Regression Models

Sander Greenland

Why Model? 381
Regression Functions 382
Frequentist Regression 382
Other Concepts of Population 383
Regression and Causation 383
Binary Regression 383
Multiple Regression 384
Regression Measures of Effect 385
Regression Standardization 386
Multivariate Regression 388
Frequentist versus Bayesian Regression 388
Basic Regression Models 389
Model Specification and Model Fitting 389
Background Example 390
Vacuous Models 390
Constant Models 391
Linear Risk Models 392
Recentering 392
Rescaling 392
Exponential Risk Models 393
Logistic Models 394
Other Risk and Odds Models 395
Rate Models 395
Incidence-Time and Hazard Models 396
Trend Models: Univariate Exposure Transforms 398
Interpreting Models after Transformation 399
Outcome Transformations 400
Multiple Regression Models 400
Relations among Multiple-Regression Models 401
Product Terms (Statistical Interactions) 402
Trends and Product Terms 404
Interpreting Product-Term Models 405
Regression Models and Biologic Interactions 406
Categorical Regressors 407
Trend Models in Multiple Regression 408
Categorical Trends 409
Regression with Category Scores 410
Power Models 410
Regression Splines 410
Models for Trend Variation 412
Extensions of Logistic Models 413
Polytomous Logistic Models 413
Ordinal Logistic Models 414
Generalized Linear Models 416

WHY MODEL?

Basic tabular and graphical methods (Chapters 13 through 18) are an essential component of epidemiologic analysis and are often sufficient, especially when one need consider only a few variables at a time. They are, however, limited in the number of variables that they can examine simultaneously. Even sparse-strata methods (such as Mantel-Haenszel) require that some strata have two or more subjects; yet, as more and more variables or categories are added to a stratification, the number of subjects in each stratum may eventually fall to 0 or 1.

Regression analysis encompasses a vast array of techniques designed to overcome the numerical limitations of simpler methods. This advantage is purchased at a cost of stronger assumptions, which are compactly represented by a *regression model*. Such models (and hence the assumptions they represent) have the advantage of being explicit; a disadvantage is that the models may not be well understood by the intended audience or even the user.

Regression models can and should be tailored by the analyst to suit the topic at hand; the latter process is sometimes called *model specification.* This process is part of the broader task of *regression modeling,* which will be discussed in the next chapter. To ensure that the assumptions underlying the regression analysis are realistic, it is essential that the modeling process be actively guided by the scientists involved in the research, rather than be left solely to mechanical algorithms. Such active guidance requires familiarity with the variety and interpretation of models, as well as familiarity with the scientific context and subject matter. This chapter thus focuses primarily on forms of models and their interpretation, rather than on the more technical issues of model fitting and testing.

A crucial point is that a regression *function* is distinct from a model for that function. A regression *model* is another, simpler function used to approximate or estimate the true regression function. This distinction is often obscured and even unrecognized in elementary treatments of regression, which in turn has generated much misunderstanding of regression modeling. Therefore, this chapter provides separate discussions of regression functions and regression models.

This chapter provides only outlines of key topics. It begins with the general theory needed to understand regression analysis, and then provides details of various model forms. Although the focus is on models for risks, rates, and survival times, the general theory applies to any outcome, and several of the model forms described (transformed-outcome, ordinal-logistic, and generalized-linear models) apply to continuous outcomes. More detailed treatments of regression analysis can be found in many books, including Mosteller and Tukey (1977), Leamer (1978), Breslow and Day (1980, 1987), McCullagh and Nelder (1989), Clayton and Hills (1993), Hosmer and Lemeshow (2000), Agresti (2002), Dobson (2001), Hardin and Hilbe (2001), McCulloch and Searle (2001), Hoffman (2003), and Berk (2004). Leamer (1978) and Berk (2004) are particularly recommended for their attention to deficiencies of regression analysis in scientific applications. Berk gives special attention to causal analysis via regression, whereas Mosteller and Tukey (1977) provide detailed connections of regression analysis to descriptive analysis.

REGRESSION FUNCTIONS

There are two primary interpretations of regression functions, frequentist and Bayesian, which correspond to two different interpretations of probability (see Chapter 18). We focus primarily on the frequentist interpretation, but we briefly discuss the Bayesian interpretation at the end of this section. In both interpretations, the term *regression* is often used to refer to the regression function.

FREQUENTIST REGRESSION

In the frequentist view, the *regression* of a variable Y on another variable X is the function that describes how the average (mean) value of Y changes across population subgroups defined by values of X. This function is often written as $E(Y|X = x)$, which should be read as "the average of Y when the variable X takes on the specific value x." The "E" part of the notation stands for "expectation," which here is just another word for "population mean."

As an example, suppose that Y stands for "height" to the nearest centimeter at some time t, X stands for "weight" to the nearest kilogram at time t, and the population of interest is that of Denmark at time t. If we subclassify the Danish population at t into categories of weight X, compute the average height in each category, and tabulate or graph these average heights against the weight categories, the result displays the regression, $E(Y|X = x)$, of height Y on weight X in Denmark at time t. Several important points should be emphasized:

1. The *concept* of regression involves no modeling. Some describe this fact by saying that the concept of regression is essentially "nonparametric." The regression of Y on X is just a graphical property of the physical world, like the orbital path of Earth around the Sun.
2. There is nothing mathematically sophisticated about the regression function. Each point on a regression curve could be computed by taking the average of Y within a subpopulation defined as having a particular value of X. In the example, the value of the regression function at $X = 50$ kg, $E(Y|X = 50)$, is just average height at time t among Danes who weigh 50 kg at time t.

3. A regression function cannot be unambiguously computed until we carefully define X, Y, *and* the population over which the averages are to be taken. We will call the latter population the *target population* of the regression. This population is all too often left out of regression definitions, often resulting in confusion.

Some ambiguity is unavoidable in practice. In our example, is time t measured to the nearest year, day, minute, or millisecond? Is the Danish population all citizens, all residents, or all persons present in Denmark at t? We may decide that leaving these questions unanswered is tolerable, because varying the definitions over a modest range will not change the result to an important extent. But if we left time completely out of the definition, the regression would become hopelessly ambiguous, for now we would not have a good idea of who to include or exclude from our average: Should we include people living in Denmark in prehistoric times, or in the time of King Canute (the 11th century A.D.), or in the distant future (a thousand years from now)? The choice could strongly influence our answer, because of the large changes in height-to-weight relations that have occurred over time.

OTHER CONCEPTS OF POPULATION

It is important to distinguish between our usage of "target population" and our usage of "source population." The target population of regression is defined without regard to our observations; for example, the regression of diastolic blood pressure on cigarette usage in China is defined whether or not we conduct a study in China (the target for this regression). A source population is a source of subjects for a particular study and is defined by the selection methods of the study; for example, a random-sample survey of all residents of Beijing would have Beijing as its source population. The concepts of target and source populations connect only insofar as inferences about a regression function drawn from a study are most easily justified when the source population of the study is identical to the target population of the regression. Otherwise, issues of generalization from the source to the target have to be addressed (see Chapter 9).

In some literature, regression functions (and many other concepts) are defined in terms of averages within a "superpopulation" or "hypothetical universe." A superpopulation is an abstraction of a target population, sometimes said to represent the distribution (with respect to all variables of interest) of all possible persons that ever were or ever could be targets of inference for the analysis at hand. Because the superpopulation approach focuses on purely hypothetical distributions, we believe it has encouraged substitution of mathematical theory for the more prosaic task of connecting study results to populations of immediate public health concern. Thus, in this chapter we define a regression function in terms of averages within a real (target) population.

REGRESSION AND CAUSATION

When considering a regression function $E(Y|X = x)$, the variable Y is termed the dependent variable, outcome variable, or *regressand,* and the variable X is termed the independent variable, predictor, covariate, or *regressor.* The "dependent/independent" terminology is most common but also problematic, because it invites confusion with unrelated probabilistic and causal concepts of dependence and independence. For example, if Y is age and X is blood pressure, $E(Y|X = x)$ represents the average age of persons given blood pressure, X. But it is blood pressure X that causally depends on age Y, not the other way around.

More generally, for any pair of variables X and Y, we can consider either the regression of Y on X, $E(Y|X = x)$, or the regression of X on Y, $E(X|Y = y)$. Thus, the concept of regression does not imply any causal or even temporal relation between the regressor and the regressand. For example, Y could be blood pressure at the start of follow-up of a cohort, and X could be blood pressure after 1 year of follow-up. Then, $E(Y|X = x)$ represents the average initial blood pressure among cohort members whose blood pressure after 1 year of follow-up is x. Below we will introduce a notation that distinguishes causation from association in regression.

BINARY REGRESSION

The concept of regression applies to variables measured on any scale: The regressand and the regressor may be continuous or discrete, or even binary. For example, Y could be an indicator of diabetes ($Y = 1$ for present, $Y = 0$ for absent), and X could be an indicator for sex ($X = 1$ for female, $X = 0$ for male). Then $E(Y|X = 1)$ represents the average of the diabetes indicator Y among women, and $E(Y|X = 0)$ represents the average of Y among men.

When the regressand Y is a binary indicator (0, 1) variable, $E(Y|X = x)$ is called a *binary regression,* and this regression simplifies in a very useful manner. Specifically, when Y can be only 0 or 1, the average $E(Y|X = x)$ equals the proportion of population members who have $Y = 1$ among those who have $X = x$. For example, if Y is the diabetes indicator, $E(Y|X = x)$ is the proportion with diabetes (i.e., with $Y = 1$) among those with $X = x$. To see this, let N_{yx} denote the number of population members who have $Y = y$ and $X = x$. Then the number of population members with $X = x$ is $N_{1x} + N_{0x} = N_{+x}$, and the average of Y among these members, $E(Y|X = x)$, is

$$\frac{N_{1x} \cdot 1 + N_{0x} \cdot 0}{N_{1x} + N_{0x}} = \frac{N_{1x}}{N_{+x}}$$

which is just the proportion with $Y = 1$ among those with $X = x$.

The epidemiologic ramifications of the preceding relation are important. Let $\Pr(Y = y|X = x)$ stand for "the proportion (of population members) with $Y = y$ among those with $X = x$" (which is often interpreted as the probability of $Y = y$ in the subpopulation with $X = x$). If Y is a binary indicator, we have just seen that

$$E(Y|X = x) = \Pr(Y = 1|X = x)$$

that is, the average of Y when $X = x$ equals the proportion with $Y = 1$ when $X = x$. Thus, if Y is an indicator of *disease presence* at a given time, the regression of Y on X, $E(Y|X = x)$, provides the proportion *with* the disease at that time, or prevalence proportion, given $X = x$. For example, if $Y = 1$ indicates diabetes presence on January 1, 2010, and X is weight on that day, $E(Y|X = x)$ provides diabetes prevalence as a function of weight on that day. If Y is instead an indicator of *disease incidence* over a time interval, the regression of Y on X provides the proportion getting disease over that interval, or incidence proportion, given $X = x$. For example, if $Y = 1$ indicates stroke occurrence in 2010 and X is weight at the start of the year, $E(Y|X = x)$ provides the 2010 stroke incidence (proportion) as a function of initial weight.

MULTIPLE REGRESSION

The concept of multiple regression (or multivariable regression) is a simple extension of the ideas discussed above to situations in which there are multiple (two or more) regressors. To illustrate, suppose that Y is a diabetes indicator, X_1 stands for "sex" (coded 1 for females, 0 for males), and X_2 stands for "weight" (in kilograms). Then the regression of Y on X_1 and X_2, written $E(Y|X_1 = x_1, X_2 = x_2)$, provides the average of Y among population members of a given sex X_1 and weight X_2. For example, $E(Y|X_1 = 1, X_2 = 70)$ is the average diabetes indicator (and, hence, the diabetes prevalence) among women who weigh 70 kg.

We can add as many regressors as we want. For example, we could add age (in years) to the last regression. Let X_3 stand for "age." Then $E(Y|X_1 = x_1, X_2 = x_2, X_3 = x_3)$ provides the diabetes prevalence among population members of a given sex, weight, and age. Continuing to add regressors produces a very clumsy notation, however, and so we adopt a simple convention: We will let $\mathbf{X}$ without a subscript represent the ordered list of all the regressors we want to consider. Thus, in our diabetes example, $\mathbf{X}$ will stand for the horizontal list (X_1, X_2, X_3) of "sex," "weight," and "age." Similarly, we will let $\mathbf{x}$ without a subscript stand for the horizontal ordered list of values (x_1, x_2, x_3) for $\mathbf{X} = (X_1, X_2, X_3)$. Thus, if we write $E(Y|\mathbf{X} = \mathbf{x})$, it is a shorthand for

$$E(Y|X_1 = x_1, X_2 = x_2, X_3 = x_3)$$

when there are three regressors under consideration.

More generally, if there are n regressors $X_1, \ldots, X_n$, we will write $\mathbf{X}$ for the ordered list $(X_1, \ldots, X_n)$ and $\mathbf{x}$ for the ordered list of values $(x_1, \ldots, x_n)$. The horizontal ordered list of variables $\mathbf{X}$ is called a *row vector* of regressors, and the horizontal ordered list of values $\mathbf{x}$ is called a *row vector* of values. Above, the vector $\mathbf{X}$ is composed of the $n = 3$ items "sex," "weight," and "age," and the list $\mathbf{x}$ is composed of specific values for sex (0 or 1), weight (kilograms), and age (years). The number of items n in $\mathbf{X}$ is called the length or dimension of $\mathbf{X}$.

REGRESSION MEASURES OF EFFECT

As discussed earlier, regression functions do not involve any assumptions of time order or causal relations. Thus, regression coefficients and quantities derived from them represent measures of association, not measures of effect. To interpret the exposure coefficients as measures of effect, the exposure variables **X** must be interpretable as potential intervention variables (Chapter 4) and the regression function must be modeled to provide an unconfounded representation of the effects of interest. Issues of selection bias and measurement error do not arise at this point because here and throughout this chapter the models are assumed to refer to population relations, before selection and measurement.

To make this unconfounded representation more precise, suppose that **X** is the vector containing the exposures of interest, **Z** is another vector containing the other regressors, and that the regressors in **Z** are proper confounder candidates, i.e., they are unaffected by **X** or Y (see Chapters 9 and 12). We may then write

$$E(Y|\text{Set}[\mathbf{X}=\mathbf{x}], \mathbf{Z}=\mathbf{z})$$

for the average value Y would have *if* everyone in the target population with $\mathbf{Z}=\mathbf{z}$ had their **X** value set to **x**. This *potential average outcome* can be very different from the actual average $E(Y|\,\mathbf{X}=\mathbf{x}, \mathbf{Z}=\mathbf{z})$. The latter refers only to those population members with $\mathbf{X}=\mathbf{x}$ and $\mathbf{Z}=\mathbf{z}$, whereas the former refers to *all* population members with $\mathbf{Z}=\mathbf{z}$, including those who actually had **X** equal to values other than **x**. Thus the potential average outcome generalizes the potential-outcome concept from Chapter 4 to regressions. In terms of causal diagrams (Chapter 12), the potential average $E(Y|\,\text{Set}[\mathbf{X}=\mathbf{x}], \mathbf{Z}=\mathbf{z})$ refers to a graph that has no arrow into any member of **X** for the subpopulation with $\mathbf{Z}=\mathbf{z}$.

As an example, suppose the target population is all persons born between 1901 and 1950 and surviving to age 50 years, Y is an indicator of death by age 80, **X** contains only X_1 = pack-years of cigarettes smoked by age 50, and $\mathbf{Z}=(Z_1, Z_2)$ where $Z_1=1$ if female, 0 if male and Z_2 = year of birth. Then

$$E\{Y|X_1=20, \mathbf{Z}=(1, 1940)\}$$

is the average risk of dying by age 80 years (mortality proportion) among women born in 1940 and surviving to age 50 who smoked 20 pack-years by age 50. In contrast,

$$E\{Y|\text{Set}[X_1=20], \mathbf{Z}=(1, 1940)\}$$

is the average risk of dying by age 80 among all women born in 1940 and surviving to age 50 *if* all such women had smoked 20 pack-years by age 50.

In Chapter 4 we defined effect measures as contrasts (such as differences and ratios) of occurrence in the *same* population under different conditions. In regression analysis, we may define effect measures as contrasts of averages in the same population under different conditions. Because occurrence measures are averages, this definition subsumes the preceding definition. As an example, consider the average of Y in the subpopulation with $\mathbf{Z}=\mathbf{z}$ when **X** is set to $\mathbf{x}^*$ versus that average when **X** is set to **x**. The ratio effect measure is

$$\frac{E\{Y|\text{Set}[\mathbf{X}=\mathbf{x}^*], \mathbf{Z}=\mathbf{z}\}}{E\{Y|\text{Set}[\mathbf{X}=\mathbf{x}], \mathbf{Z}=\mathbf{z}\}}$$

the difference effect measure is

$$E\{Y|\text{Set}[\mathbf{X}=\mathbf{x}^*], \mathbf{Z}=\mathbf{z}\} - E\{Y|\text{Set}[\mathbf{X}=\mathbf{x}], \mathbf{Z}=\mathbf{z}\}$$

and the attributable fraction is

$$\frac{E\{Y|\text{Set}[\mathbf{X}=\mathbf{x}^*], \mathbf{Z}=\mathbf{z}\} - E\{Y|\text{Set}[\mathbf{X}=\mathbf{x}], \mathbf{Z}=\mathbf{z}\}}{E\{Y|\text{Set}[\mathbf{X}=\mathbf{x}^*], \mathbf{Z}=\mathbf{z}\}}$$

In the example, the ratio

$$\frac{E\{Y|\text{Set}[X_1=20], \mathbf{Z}=(1, 1940)\}}{E\{Y|\text{Set}[X_1=0], \mathbf{Z}=(1, 1940)\}}$$

measures the *effect* of smoking 20 pack-years by age 50 versus no smoking on the risk of dying by age 80 among women born in 1940. On the other hand, the ratio

$$\frac{E\{Y|X_1 = 20, \mathbf{Z} = (1, 1940)\}}{E\{Y|X_1 = 0, \mathbf{Z} = (1, 1940)\}}$$

represents only the *association* of smoking 20 pack-years by age 50 versus no smoking with the risk among women born in 1940, because it contrasts two different subpopulations (one with $X_1 = 20$, the other with $X_1 = 0$).

To infer that all associational measures estimated from our analysis equal their corresponding effect measures, we have to make the following assumption of no confounding given $\mathbf{Z}$ (which is sometimes expressed by stating that there is no residual confounding):

$$E(Y|\mathbf{X} = \mathbf{x}, \mathbf{Z} = \mathbf{z}) = E(Y|\text{Set}[\mathbf{X} = \mathbf{x}], \mathbf{Z} = \mathbf{z})$$

This assumption states that the average we observe or estimate in the subpopulation with both $\mathbf{X} = \mathbf{x}$ and $\mathbf{Z} = \mathbf{z}$ is equal to what the average in the larger subpopulation with $\mathbf{Z} = \mathbf{z}$ would have been if everyone had $\mathbf{X}$ set to $\mathbf{x}$. It is important to appreciate the strength of the assumption. In the above example, the no-confounding assumption entails

$$E\{Y|X_1 = 20, \mathbf{Z} = (1, 1940)\} = E\{Y|\text{Set}[X_1 = 20], \mathbf{Z} = (1, 1940)\}$$

which states that the risk we will observe among women born in 1940 who smoked 20 pack-years by age 50 equals the risk we would have observed in *all* women born in 1940 if they all had smoked 20 pack-years by age 50. The social variables associated with both smoking and death should lead us to doubt that the two quantities are even approximately equal.

The dubiousness of no-confounding assumptions is often the chief limitation in using epidemiologic data for causal inference. This limitation applies to both tabular and regression methods. Randomization of persons to values of $\mathbf{X}$ can largely overcome this limitation because it ensures that effect estimates follow an identifiable probability distribution centered around the true effect. The remaining strategy is to ensure there are enough well-measured confounders in $\mathbf{Z}$ so that the no-confounding assumption is at least plausible. This strategy often leads to few subjects at each value $\mathbf{x}$ of $\mathbf{X}$ and $\mathbf{z}$ of $\mathbf{Z}$, which in turn leads to the sparse-data problems that regression modeling attempts to address (Robins and Greenland, 1986).

REGRESSION STANDARDIZATION

Regression modeling alone is often insufficient to address sparse-data problems. For example, when the number of observed values of $\mathbf{X}$ or $\mathbf{Z}$ is comparable to the number of observations, it may be impossible to estimate reliably any regressor-specific outcome or effect. It may still be possible to estimate averages over the regressors, however. It then becomes important to define relevant averages.

Standardization is weighted averaging of an outcome measure over a distribution (Chapter 3). A *standard distribution* W for the vector of regressors $\mathbf{Z} = (Z_1, \ldots, Z_K)$ is a set of weights $w(\mathbf{z})$, one for each value $\mathbf{z}$ of $\mathbf{Z}$, that sum or integrate to 1: $\sum_{\mathbf{z}} w(\mathbf{z}) = 1$. The regression of Y on $\mathbf{X}$ *standardized* to W is then the average of $E(Y|\mathbf{X} = \mathbf{x}, \mathbf{Z} = \mathbf{z})$ weighted by the $w(\mathbf{z})$ (Lane and Nelder, 1982),

$$E_W(Y|\mathbf{X} = \mathbf{x}) = \sum_{\mathbf{z}} w(\mathbf{z}) E(Y|\mathbf{X} = \mathbf{x}, \mathbf{Z} = \mathbf{z})$$

If Y and $\mathbf{Z}$ are independent given $\mathbf{X}$, $E_W(Y|\mathbf{X} = \mathrm{x}) = E(Y|\mathbf{X} = \mathbf{x})$, the unstandardized (crude) expectation when $\mathbf{X} = \mathbf{x}$, but otherwise the two will not be equal for most weighting schemes. Ideally, the standardizing weights $w(\mathbf{z})$ will reflect the distribution of the covariates $\mathbf{Z}$ in a target population of subject-matter relevance.

For the rest of this section, suppose that $\mathbf{X}$ is a single intervention variable, which we will denote X. Then, if the regression is generalizable to the target, the distribution of $\mathbf{Z}$ is unaffected by X, and $\mathbf{Z}$ is sufficient for confounding control (Chapter 12), $E_W(Y|X = x)$ will represent the expectation of Y under the intervention $X = x$ in that population, i.e.,

$$E_W(Y|X = x) = E(Y|\text{Set}[X = x]) \text{ for that population.}$$

A caution, however, is that if X and $\mathbf{Z}$ affect Y, then even if X does not affect $\mathbf{Z}$ directly, X will likely affect the person-time distribution of $\mathbf{Z}$, leading to failure of this equation if W is a person-time distribution (Chapter 4; Greenland, 1996a).

Often, the standard weights are by default taken to be $w(\mathbf{z}) = \Pr(\mathbf{Z} = \mathbf{z})$, the proportion with $\mathbf{Z} = \mathbf{z}$ in the study cohort or source population. The resulting averages are then said to be *marginal* or *population-averaged* or *standardized to the total*. This standard is appropriate when X is a treatment variable and one wants to compare the effect of different treatment choices for the entire population, as in field trials. In that case, if $\mathbf{Z}$ is sufficient for confounding control, the standardized mean equals the marginal potential outcome of the total population under treatment $X = x$:

$$E_W(Y = y|X = x) = E(Y = y|\text{Set}[X = x])$$

(Chapter 4; Pearl, 1995, 2000). In many settings, however, concern is with effects in a particular subpopulation. A more relevant weighting then uses the proportion with $\mathbf{Z} = \mathbf{z}$ among those in that subpopulation. For example, suppose that $X = 0$ represents those unexposed and $X > 0$ those exposed. If interest is in effects among the exposed, $w(\mathbf{z}) = \Pr(\mathbf{Z} = \mathbf{z}|X > 0)$ will be the relevant standard, whereas if interest is in effects among the unexposed, $w(\mathbf{z}) = \Pr(\mathbf{Z} = \mathbf{z}|X = 0)$ will be the relevant standard. If X and $\mathbf{Z}$ are independent, however, all these standards are identical, for then

$$w(\mathbf{z}) = \Pr(\mathbf{Z} = \mathbf{z}|X > 0) = \Pr(\mathbf{Z} = \mathbf{z}|X = x) = \Pr(\mathbf{Z} = \mathbf{z})$$

for any value x of X.

Standardized outcome measures at different levels of exposure X can be contrasted to form standardized measures of association or effect. For example, standardized ratios, differences, and attributable fractions contrasting $X = x_1$ with $X = x_0$ have the form

$$E_W(Y|X = x_1)/E_W(Y|X = x_0),$$

$$E_W(Y|X = x_1) - E_W(Y|X = x_0),$$

and

$$[E_W(Y|X = x_1) - E_W(Y|X = x_0)]/E_W(Y|X = x_1)$$

More generally, one can compare outcomes under different distributions for X (Chapter 4; Morgenstern and Bursic, 1982; Bruzzi et al., 1985; Greenland and Drescher, 1993; Greenland, 2004d). Suppose that X would have a distribution $\Pr_1(X = x)$ after an intervention and a distribution $\Pr_0(X = x)$ without the intervention. Suppose also that the standardizing covariates are sufficient for confounding control and are unaffected by the intervention. Then the standardized ratios, differences, and attributable fractions contrasting the outcome with and without the intervention have the above forms but with

$$\sum_x E_W(Y|X = x)\Pr_1(X = x) \quad \text{and} \quad \sum_x E_W(Y|X = x)\Pr_0(X = x)$$

in place of

$$E_W(Y|X = x_1) \quad \text{and} \quad E_W(Y|X = x_0).$$

Comparison of $X = x_1$ with $X = x_0$ is just the extreme special case of these general measures when $\Pr_1(X = x_1) = 1$ and $\Pr_0(X = x_0) = 1$, as, for example, when an intervention shifts everyone from $X = 1$ (exposed) to $X = 0$ (unexposed). These standardized measures become measures of the effect of shifting the X distribution when the $\mathbf{Z}$ distribution is given by the standard W, assuming that the regressors $\mathbf{Z}$ are sufficient for confounding control and are unaffected by X, and the relations are generalizable (stable) under the interventions.

If only a single measure of effect is desired, the regressor-specific no-confounding assumption can be replaced by a less restrictive assumption tailored to that measure. To illustrate, suppose that X is pack-years of smoking we are interested only in what the effect of smoking 20 versus 0 pack-years would be on *everyone* in the target, regardless of sex or birth year, as measured by the causal risk ratio

$$E[Y|\text{Set}(X = 20)]/E[Y|\text{Set}(X = 0)]$$

The corresponding measure of association is the risk ratio for 20 versus 0 pack-years, standardized to the total population, $E_W(Y|X = 20)/E_W(Y|X = 0)$, where $w(\mathbf{z}) = \Pr(\mathbf{Z} = \mathbf{z})$. The no-confounding assumption is now that this standardized ratio equals the causal ratio. This summary assumption may hold even if there is confounding within levels of sex and birth year or there is confounding when using other standards (although it would still be implausible in this example).

MULTIVARIATE REGRESSION

Multiple regression concerns averages within levels of multiple regressors. Sometimes this process is called "multivariate analysis." In advanced statistics, however, the term *multivariate regression* is usually reserved for regressions in which there are multiple *regressands*. To illustrate, suppose that Y_1 is an indicator of the presence of diabetes, Y_2 is diastolic blood pressure, and $\mathbf{Y}$ is the list (Y_1, Y_2) composed of these two variables. Also, let $\mathbf{X}$ be the list (X_1, X_2, X_3) composed of the sex indicator, weight, and age. Then the multivariate regression of diabetes and blood pressure on sex, weight, and age provides the average diabetes indicator *and* average blood pressure for each specific combination of sex, weight, and age:

$$E(Y_1, Y_2|X_1 = x_1, X_2 = x_2, X_3 = X_3) = E(\mathbf{Y}|\mathbf{X} = \mathbf{x})$$

There may be any number of regressands in the list $\mathbf{Y}$ and regressors in the list $\mathbf{X}$ of a multivariate regression. Multivariate regression notation allows one to express the separate regressions for each regressand in one equation.

FREQUENTIST VERSUS BAYESIAN REGRESSION

In frequentist theory, an expectation is interpreted as an average in a specific subgroup of a specific population. The regression $E(Y|\mathbf{X} = \mathbf{x})$ thus represents an objective functional relation among theoretically measurable variables (the average of Y as a function of the variables listed in $\mathbf{X}$). It may be that this relation has not been observed, perhaps because it exists but we are unable to measure it, or because it does not yet exist. Examples of the former and latter are the regressions of blood pressure on weight in Spain 10 years ago and 10 years from now. In either situation, the regression is an external relation that one tries to estimate, perhaps by projecting (extrapolating) from current knowledge about presumably similar relations. For example, one might use whatever survey data one can find on blood pressure and weight to estimate what the regression of blood pressure on weight would look like in Spain 10 years ago or 10 years from now. In this approach, one tries to produce an *estimate* $\hat{E}(Y|\mathbf{X} = \mathbf{x})$ of the true regression $E(Y|\mathbf{X} = \mathbf{x})$.

In subjective Bayesian theory (Chapter 18), an expectation is what we would or should expect to see in a given target population. This notion of expectation corresponds roughly to a prediction of what we would see if we could observe the target in question. The regression $E(Y|\mathbf{X} = \mathbf{x})$ does not represent an objective relation to be estimated, but instead represents a subjective (personal) expectation about how the average of Y varies across levels of $\mathbf{X}$ in the target population. Like the frequentist regression estimate, however, it is something one constructs from whatever data one may find that seems to be informative about this variation.

Both frequentist and Bayesian authors have noted that the two approaches often yield similar interval estimates (Cox and Hinkley, 1974; Good, 1983). It is increasingly recognized that divergences are usually due to differences in the criteria for a "good" point estimate: Frequentists traditionally prefer criteria of unbiased prediction (e.g., having an average error of 0), whereas Bayesians more often prefer criteria of closeness (e.g., having the smallest average squared error possible). When analogous criteria are adopted in both approaches, Bayesian and frequentist methods can yield similar numeric results in standard epidemiologic applications.

Nonetheless, Bayesians and frequentists interpret their results differently. The Bayesian presents a prediction, denoted by $E(Y|\mathbf{X} = \mathbf{x})$, as his or her "best bet" about the average of Y when $\mathbf{X} = \mathbf{x}$, according to some criteria for "best bet." The frequentist presents a prediction, denoted by $\hat{E}(Y|\mathbf{X} = \mathbf{x})$ (or, more commonly, $\hat{Y}_{\mathbf{X}=\mathbf{x}}$), as "the" best estimate of the average of Y when $\mathbf{X} = \mathbf{x}$, according to some criteria for "best estimate" (such as minimum variance among statistically unbiased estimators). Too often, the latter criteria are presumed to be universally shared but are not really shared or even properly understood by epidemiologists; one could and would reach different conclusions using other defensible criteria (such as minimum mean squared error). For these reasons, it can be valuable to consider both frequentist and Bayesian interpretations of the models, methods, and results.

BASIC REGRESSION MODELS

In any given instance, the true regression of Y on $\mathbf{X}$, $E(Y|\mathbf{X} = \mathbf{x})$, can be an extremely complicated function of the regressors $\mathbf{X}$. Thus, even if we observe this function without error, we may wish to formulate simplified pictures of reality that yield *models* for this regression. These models, though inevitably incorrect, can be very useful. A classic example is the representation of the distance from the earth to the sun, Y, as a function of day of the year T. To the nearest kilometer, this distance is a complex function of T because of the gravitational effects of the moon and of the other planets in the solar system. If we represent the orbit of the earth around the sun as a circle with the sun at the center, our regression model will predict the distance $E(Y|T = t)$ by a single number (about 150 million kilometers) that does not change with t. This model is adequate if we can tolerate a few percent error in our predictions. If we represent the orbit of the earth as an ellipse, our regression model will predict the earth–sun distance as smoothly and cyclically varying over the course of a year (within a range of about 147 to 153 million kilometers). Although it is not perfectly accurate, this model is adequate if we can tolerate a few tenths of a percent error in our predictions.

MODEL SPECIFICATION AND MODEL FITTING

Our description of the preceding models must be refined by distinguishing between the *form* of a model and a *fitted* model. "Circle" and "ellipse" refer to forms, that is, general classes of shapes. The circular model form corresponds to assuming a constant earth–sun distance over time; the elliptical model form allows this distance to vary over a temporal cycle. The process of deciding between these two forms is a simple example of *model specification.*

If we decide to use the circular form, we must also select a value for the radius (which is the earth–sun distance in the model). This radius specifies which circle (out of the many possible circles) to use as a representation of the earth's orbit and is an example of a model *parameter.* The process of selecting the "best" estimate of the radius is an example of *model fitting,* and the circle that results is sometimes called the *fitted model* (although the latter term is sometimes used instead to refer to the model form).

There are two important relations between a set of data and a model fit to those data. First, there is "distance" from the fitted model to the data; second, there is "resistance" or "stability" of the fitted model, which is the degree to which the model predictions or parameter estimates change when the data themselves are changed. Chapter 21 describes a few approaches to evaluating distance and stability, including *delta-beta* analysis.

Depending on our accuracy requirements, we may have on hand several simplified pictures of reality and hence several candidate models. At best, our choice may require a trade-off between simplicity and accuracy, as in the preceding example. There is an old dictum (often referred to as *Occam's razor*) that one should not introduce needless complexity for purposes of prediction or explanation. Following this dictum, if we need only 2% accuracy in predicting the earth's distance from the sun, then we should not bother with the ellipse model and instead use the constant distance derived from the circle model.

There is a more subtle benefit from this advice than avoiding needless mental exertion. Suppose that we are given two models, one (the more complex) containing the other (the more simple) as a special case, and some data with which to fit the two models. Then the more complex model will be able to fit the available data more closely than the simpler model, in the sense that the predictions from the more complex model will (on average) be closer to what is seen in the data than will the predictions from the simpler model. This is so in the preceding example because the ellipse contains the circle as a special case. Nonetheless, there is a penalty for this closeness to the data: The predictions obtained from the more complex model tend to be less stable than those obtained from the simpler model.

Consider now the use of the two different model forms to predict events outside of the data set to which the models were fitted. One example is forecasting the earth's distance from the sun; another is predicting the incidence of AIDS at a time 5 years in the future. Intuitively, we might expect that if one model is both closer to the data and more stable than the other, that model will give more accurate predictions. The choice among models is rarely so clear-cut, however. Usually, one model will be closer to the data, while the other will be more stable, and it will be difficult to tell which will be more accurate. We often face this dilemma in a choice between a more complex and simpler model.

To summarize, model specification is the process of selecting a model form, whereas model fitting is the process of using data to estimate the parameters in a model form. There are many methods of model fitting, and the topic is so vast and technical that we will only superficially outline a few key elements. Nearly all commercial computer programs are based on one of just a few fitting methods, so that nearly all users (statisticians as well as epidemiologists) are forced to base their analyses on the assumptions of these few methods. We will discuss specification and fitting methods in Chapter 21.

BACKGROUND EXAMPLE

The following epidemiologic example will be used at various points to illustrate specific models. In the 1990s a controversy arose over whether women with no history of breast cancer but thought to be of high risk (because of family history and perhaps other factors) should be given the drug tamoxifen as a prophylactic regimen. Evidence suggested that tamoxifen might prevent breast cancer (Fisher et al., 1998) but also cause or promote endometrial and liver cancer.

One measure of the net effect of tamoxifen prophylaxis up to a given age is the change in risk of death by that age. Suppose that the regress and Y is an indicator of death by age 70 years ($Y = 1$ for dead, 0 for alive). The regressors $\mathbf{X}$ include

X_1 = years of tamoxifen therapy
X_2 = age (in years) at start of tamoxifen therapy
X_3 = age at menarche
X_4 = age at menopause
X_5 = parity

Suppose that the target population is American women born between 1925 and 1950 who survived to age 50 years and did not use tamoxifen before that age. If tamoxifen was not taken during follow-up, we set age at tamoxifen start (X_2) to 70, because women who started at age 70 or later and women who never took tamoxifen have the same exposure history during the age interval under study.

In this example, the regression $E(Y|\mathbf{X} = \mathbf{x})$ is just the average risk, or incidence proportion, of death by age 70 among women in the target population who have $\mathbf{X} = \mathbf{x}$. Therefore, we will write $R(\mathbf{x})$ as a shorthand for $E(Y|\mathbf{X} = \mathbf{x})$. We will also write R for the crude (overall) average risk $E(Y)$, $R(x_1)$ for the average risk $E(Y|X_1 = x_1)$ in the subpopulation defined by having $X_1 = x_1$ (without regard to the other variables), and so on.

VACUOUS MODELS

A model so general that it implies nothing at all, but simply re-expresses the overall average risk in a different notation, is

$$E(Y) = R = \alpha \qquad [20\text{–}1]$$

There is only one regression parameter (or coefficient) α in this model, and it corresponds to the average risk in the target population. A model such as model 20–1 that has no implication (i.e., that imposes no restriction or constraint) is said to be *vacuous*.

Two models are said to be *equivalent* if they have identical implications for the regression. Given that $R > 0$, a model that is equivalent to model 20–1 is

$$E(Y) = R = \exp(\alpha) \qquad [20\text{–}2]$$

Model 20–2 has no implication beyond forcing R to be positive. In this model, α is the natural logarithm of the overall average risk:

$$\alpha = \ln(R)$$

Given that $R > 0$ and $R < 1$, a model that is equivalent to models 20–1 and 20–2 is

$$E(Y) = R = \text{expit}(\alpha) \qquad [20\text{–}3]$$

where expit(α) is the *logistic* transform of α, defined as

$$\text{expit}(\alpha) = e^{\alpha}/(1 + e^{\alpha})$$

Model 20–3 has no implication beyond forcing R to fall between 0 and 1. Now, however, the parameter α in model 20–3 is the logit (log odds) of the overall average risk:

$$\alpha = \ln\left(\frac{R}{1-R}\right) = \text{logit}(R)$$

CONSTANT MODELS

In comparing the complexity and implications of two models A and B, we say that model A is more general, more flexible, or more complex than model B, or that A contains B, if all the implications of model A are also implications of model B, but not vice versa (that is, if B imposes some restrictions beyond those imposed by A). Other ways of stating this relation are that B is simpler, stronger, or stricter than A, B is contained or nested within A, or B is a special case of A.

The following model is superficially similar to model 20–1 but is in fact much more strict:

$$E(Y|X_1 = x_1) = R(x_1) = \alpha \qquad [20\text{–}4]$$

This model implies that the average risks of the subpopulations defined by years of tamoxifen use are identical. The parameter α represents the common value of these risks. This model is called a *constant* regression because it allows no variation in average risks across levels of the regressor. To see that it is a special case of model 20–1, note that $E(Y)$, the overall average, is just an average of all the X_1-specific averages $E(Y|X_1 = x_1)$. Hence, if all the X_1-specific averages equal α, as in model 20–4, then the overall average must equal α as well, as in model 20–1.

Given that $R(x_1) > 0$ and $R(x_1) < 1$, the following two models are equivalent to model 20–4:

$$R(x_1) = \exp(\alpha) \qquad [20\text{–}5]$$

which can be rewritten as

$$\ln[R(x_1)] = \alpha$$

and

$$R(x_1) = \text{expit}(\alpha) = e^{\alpha}/(1 + e^{\alpha}) \qquad [20\text{–}6]$$

which can be rewritten as

$$\text{logit}[R(x_1)] = \alpha$$

In model 20–5, α is the common value of the log risks $\ln[R(x_1)]$, whereas in model 20–6, α is the common value of the logits, logit$[R(x_1)]$. Each of the models (models 20–4 through 20–6) is a special case of the more general models (models 20–1 through 20–3). In other words, models 20–4 through 20–6 are simpler, stronger, or stricter than models 20–1 through 20–3, and are contained or nested within models 20–1 through 20–3.

A constant regression is of course implausible in most situations. For example, age is related to most health outcomes. In the above example, we expect the average death risk to vary across the subgroups defined by age at start (X_2). There are infinite ways to model these variations. Chapter 21 discusses the problem of selecting a useful model from among the many choices. The present chapter describes some of the more common choices, focusing on models for average risks (incidence proportions), incidence odds, and person-time incidence rates. The models for risks and odds can also be used to model prevalence proportions and prevalence odds.

LINEAR RISK MODELS

Consider the model

$$R(x_1) = \alpha + \beta_1 x_1 \quad [20\text{–}7]$$

This model allows the average risk to vary across subpopulations with different values for X_1, but only in a linear fashion. The model implies that subtracting the average risk in the subpopulation with $X_1 = x_1$ from that in the subpopulation with $X_1 = x_1 + 1$ will always yield β_1, *regardless* of what x_1 is. Under model 20–7,

$$R(x_1 + 1) = \alpha + \beta_1(x_1 + 1)$$

and

$$R(x_1) = \alpha + \beta_1 x_1$$

so

$$R(x_1 + 1) - R(x_1) = \beta_1$$

β_1 thus represents the difference in risk between the subpopulation defined by having $X_1 = x_1 + 1$ and that defined by having $X_1 = x_1$. The model implies that this difference does not depend on the reference level x_1 for X_1 used for the comparison.

Model 20–7 is an example of a *linear* risk model. It is a special case of model 20–1; it also contains model 20–4 as a special case: Model 20–4 is the special case of model 20–7 in which $\beta_1 = 0$ and so average risks do not vary across levels of X_1. Linear risk models (such as model 20–7) are easy to understand, but they have a severe technical problem that makes them difficult to fit in practice: There are combinations of α and β_1 that will produce impossible values (less than 0 or greater than 1) for one or more of the risks $R(x_1)$. Several models partially or wholly address this problem by transforming the linear term $\alpha + \beta_1 x_1$ before equating it to the risk. We will study two of these models.

RECENTERING

Under model 20–7,

$$R(0) = \alpha + \beta_1 \cdot 0 = \alpha$$

so α represents the average risk for the subpopulation with $X_1 = 0$. In the present example, 0 is a possible value for X_1 (tamoxifen) and so this interpretation of α presents no problem. Suppose, however, that we model X_3 (age at menarche) instead of X_1:

$$R(X_3) = \alpha + \beta_3 X_3$$

Because age at menarche cannot equal 0, α has no meaningful interpretation in this model. To avoid such interpretational problems, it is useful to recenter a variable for which 0 is impossible (such as X_3), by subtracting some frequently observed value from it before putting it in the model. For example, age 13 is a frequently observed value for age at menarche. We can redefine X_3 to be "age at menarche minus 13 years." With this redefinition, $R(X_3) = \alpha + \beta_3 X_3$ refers to a different model, one in which $R(0) = \alpha$ represents the average risk for women who were age 13 at menarche. We will see later that such recentering is advisable when using any model, and it is especially important when product terms ("interactions") are used in a model.

RESCALING

A simple way of describing β_1 in model 20–7 is that it is the difference in risk per unit increase in X_1. Often the units used to measure X_1 are small relative to exposure increases of substantive interest. Suppose, for example, that X_1 is diastolic blood pressure (DBP) measured in mm Hg; β_1 is then the risk difference per millimeter increase in DBP. A 1-mm Hg increase, however, will be of no clinical interest; instead, we will want to consider increases of at least 5 and possibly 10 or 20 mm Hg. Under model 20–7, the difference in risk per 10 mm Hg increase is 10 β_1. If we want to have β_1 represent the difference in risk per 10 mm Hg, we need only redefine X_1 as DBP divided by 10; X_1 will then be DBP in cm Hg.

Division of a variable by a constant, as just described, is sometimes called *rescaling* of the variable. Such rescaling is advisable whenever it changes the measurement unit to a more meaningful value. Unfortunately, rescaling is often done in a way that makes the measurement unit *less* meaningful, by dividing the variable by its sample standard deviation (SD). The sample SD is an irregular unit that is unique to the study data and that depends heavily on how subjects were selected into the analysis. For example, the SD of DBP might be 12.7 mm Hg in one study and 15.3 mm Hg in another study. Suppose that each study divides DBP by its SD before entering it in model 20–7. In the first study, β_1 refers to the change in risk per 12.7 mm Hg increase in DBP, whereas in the second study β_1 refers to the change in risk per 15.3 mm Hg. Rescaling by the SD thus renders the coefficients interpretable only in peculiar and different units, so that they cannot be compared directly with one another or to coefficients from other studies.

We will see later that rescaling is even more important when product terms are used in a model. We thus recommend that rescaling be done using simple and easily interpreted constants for the divisions. Methods that involve division by sample SDs (such as transformations of variables to Z-scores), however, should be avoided (Greenland et al., 1986, 1991).

EXPONENTIAL RISK MODELS

Consider the following model:

$$R(x_1) = \exp(\alpha + \beta_1 x_1) \qquad [20\text{–}8]$$

The exponential function (exp) is always positive, so model 20–8 will produce positive $R(x_1)$ for any combination of α and β_1. Model 20–8 is sometimes called an *exponential* risk model. It is a special case of the vacuous model 20–2; it also contains the constant model 20–5 as the special case in which $\beta_1 = 0$.

To understand the implications of the exponential risk model, we can recast it in an equivalent form by taking the natural logarithm of both sides:

$$\ln[R(x_1)] = \ln[\exp(\alpha + \beta_1 x_1)] = \alpha + \beta_1 x_1 \qquad [20\text{–}9]$$

Model 20–9 is often called a *log-linear* risk model. The exponential/log-linear model allows risk to vary across subpopulations defined by X_1, but only in an exponential fashion. To interpret the coefficients, we may compare the log risks under model 20–9 for the two subpopulations defined by $X_1 = x_1 + 1$ and $X_1 = x_1$:

$$\ln[R(x_1 + 1)] = \alpha + \beta_1(x_1 + 1)$$

and

$$\ln[R(x_1)] = \alpha + \beta_1 x_1$$

so

$$\ln[R(x_1 + 1)] - \ln[R(x_1)] = \ln[R(x_1 + 1)/R(x_1)] = \beta_1$$

Thus, under models 20–8 and 20–9, β_1 represents the log risk ratio comparing the subpopulation defined by having $X_1 = x_1 + 1$ and that defined by $X_1 = x_1$, regardless of the chosen reference level x_1. Also, $\ln[R(0)] = \alpha + \beta_1 \cdot 0 = \alpha$ if $X_1 = 0$; thus, α represents the log risk for the subpopulation with $X_1 = 0$ (and so is meaningful only if X_1 can be zero).

We can derive another equivalent interpretation of the parameters in the exponential risk model by noting that

$$R(x_1 + 1) = \exp[\alpha + \beta_1(x_1 + 1)]$$

and

$$R(x_1) = \exp(\alpha + \beta_1 x_1)$$

so

$$R(x_1 + 1)/R(x_1) = \exp[\alpha + \beta_1(x_1 + 1) - (\alpha + \beta_1 x_1)] = \exp(\beta_1)$$

Thus, under models 20–8 and 20–9, $\exp(\beta_1)$ represents the *ratio* of risks between the subpopulations defined by $X_1 = x_1 + 1$ and $X_1 = x_1$, and this ratio does not depend on the reference level x_1 (because x_1 does not appear in the final expression for the risk ratio). Also, $R(0) = \exp(\alpha + \beta_1 \cdot 0) = e^{\alpha}$, so e^{α} represents the average risk for the subpopulation with $X_1 = 0$.

As with linear risk models, exponential risk models have the technical problem that some combinations of α and β_1 will yield risk values greater than 1, which are impossible. This problem will not be a practical concern, however, if all the fitted risks and their confidence limits fall well below 1.

LOGISTIC MODELS

As will be discussed in Chapter 21, neither linear nor exponential risk models can be used to analyze case-control data if no external information is available to allow estimation of risks in the source population, whereas the following model can be used without such information:

$$\begin{aligned} R(x_1) &= \text{expit}(\alpha + \beta_1 x_1) \\ &= \frac{\exp(\alpha + \beta_1 x_1)}{1 + \exp(\alpha + \beta_1 x_1)} \end{aligned} \qquad [20\text{–}10]$$

This model is called a *logistic* risk model, after the logistic function (expit) in the core of its definition. Because the range of the logistic function is between 0 and 1, the model will only produce risks between 0 and 1, regardless of the values for α, β_1, and x_1. The logistic model is perhaps the most commonly used model in epidemiology, so we examine it in some detail. Model 20–10 is a special case of model 20–3, but unlike model 20–3, it is not vacuous because it constrains the X_1-specific risks to follow a particular (logistic) pattern. The constant model 20–6 is the special case of the logistic model in which $\beta_1 = 0$.

To understand the implications of the logistic model, it is helpful to recast it as a model for the odds. First, note that, under the logistic model (equation 20–10),

$$\begin{aligned} 1 - R(x_1) &= 1 - \frac{\exp(\alpha + \beta_1 x_1)}{1 + \exp(\alpha + \beta_1 x_1)} \\ &= \frac{1}{1 + \exp(\alpha + \beta_1 x_1)} \end{aligned}$$

Because $R(x_1)/[1 - R(x_1)]$ is the odds, we divide each side of equation 20–10 by the preceding expression and find that, under the logistic model, the odds of disease $O(x_1)$ when $X_1 = x_1$ is

$$\begin{aligned} O(x_1) = \frac{R(x_1)}{1 - R(x_1)} &= \frac{\dfrac{\exp(\alpha + \beta_1 x_1)}{1 + \exp(\alpha + \beta_1 x_1)}}{\dfrac{1}{1 + \exp(\alpha + \beta_1 x_1)}} \\ &= \exp(\alpha + \beta_1 x_1) \end{aligned} \qquad [20\text{–}11]$$

This model form (equation 20–11) shows that the logistic risk model is equivalent to an exponential *odds* model.

Taking logarithms of both sides of equation 20–11, we see that the logistic model is also equivalent to the log-linear odds model

$$\ln[O(x_1)] = \alpha + \beta_1 x_1 \qquad [20\text{–}12]$$

Recall that the logit of risk is defined as the log odds:

$$\text{logit}[R(x_1)] = \ln\{R(x_1)/[(1 - R(x_1)]\} = \ln[O(x_1)]$$

Hence, from equation 20–12, the logistic model can be rewritten in one more equivalent form,

$$\text{logit}[R(x_1)] = \alpha + \beta_1 x_1 \qquad [20\text{–}13]$$

This equivalent of the logistic model is often called the logit-linear risk model, or *logit model*.

As a general caution regarding terms, note that "log-linear model" can refer to any one of several different models, depending on the context: In addition to log-linear *risk* models (equation 20–9) and log-linear *odds* models (equation 20–12) given earlier, there are also the log-linear *rate* models and log-linear *incidence-time* models described below, as well as log-linear *count* models (Chapter 21).

We can derive two equivalent interpretations of the logistic model parameters. First,

$$\ln[O(x_1 + 1)] = \alpha + \beta_1(x_1 + 1)$$

$$\ln[O(x_1)] = \alpha + \beta_1 x_1$$

so

$$\ln[O(x_1 + 1)] - \ln[O(x_1)] = \ln[O(x_1 + 1)/O(x_1)] = \beta_1$$

Thus, under the logistic model (equation 20–10), β_1 represents the log odds ratio comparing the subpopulations with $X_1 = x_1 + 1$ and $X_1 = x_1$. Also, $\ln[O(0)] = \alpha + \beta_1 \cdot 0 = \alpha$; thus, α is the log odds (logit) for the subpopulation with $X_1 = 0$ (and so is meaningful only if X_1 can be 0). Equivalently, we have

$$O(x_1 + 1)/O(x_1) = \exp(\beta_1)$$

and

$$O(0) = \exp(\alpha)$$

so that $\exp(\beta_1)$ is the odds ratio comparing the subpopulations with $X_1 = x_1 + 1$ and $X_1 = x_1$, and $\exp(\alpha)$ is the odds for the subpopulation with $X_1 = 0$.

OTHER RISK AND ODDS MODELS

In addition to those given so far, several other risk models are occasionally mentioned but rarely used in epidemiology. The linear odds model is obtained by replacing the average risk by the odds in the linear risk model:

$$O(x_1) = \alpha + \beta_1 x_1 \qquad [20\text{–}14]$$

Here, β_1 is the *odds* difference between subpopulations with $X_1 = x_1 + 1$ and $X_1 = x_1$, and α is the odds for the subpopulation with $X_1 = 0$. Like risk, the odds cannot be negative; unfortunately, some combinations of α and β_1 in model 20–14 will produce negative odds. As a result, this model (like the linear risk model) may be difficult to fit and gives unsatisfactory results in many settings.

Another model replaces the logistic transform (expit) in the logistic model (equation 20–10) by the inverse of the standard normal distribution, which also has a range between 0 and 1. The resulting model, called a *probit* model, has seen much use in bioassay. Its absence from epidemiologic use may stem from the fact that (unlike the logistic model) its parameters have no simple epidemiologic interpretation, and the model appears to have no advantage over the logistic in epidemiologic applications.

Several attempts have been made to use models that are mixtures of different basic models. These mixtures have various drawbacks, including difficulties in fitting the models and interpreting the parameters (Moolgavkar and Venzon, 1987). We thus do not describe them here.

RATE MODELS

Instead of modeling average risks, we may model person-time incidence rates. If we let Y denote the *rate* observed in a study subpopulation (so that Y is the observed number of cases per unit of observed person-time), the regression $E(Y|\mathbf{X} = \mathbf{x})$ represents the average number of cases per unit of person-time in the target subpopulation defined by $\mathbf{X} = \mathbf{x}$. We will denote this expected rate or "average rate" by $I(\mathbf{x})$.

Most rate models are analogs of risk and odds models. For example, the model

$$I(x_1) = E(Y|X_1 = x_1) = \alpha + \beta_1 x_1 \quad [20\text{–}15]$$

is a linear *rate* model, analogous to (but different from) the linear risk and odds models (equations 20–7, 20–14). This rate model implies that the difference in average rates between subpopulations with $X_1 = x_1 + 1$ and $X_1 = x_1$ is β_1, regardless of x_1. Also, α is the average rate for the subpopulation with $X_1 = 0$. This model can be problematic, because some combinations of α and β_1 in model 20–15 can produce negative rate values, which are impossible.

To prevent the latter problem, most rate modeling begins with an exponential *rate* model such as

$$I(x_1) = \exp(\alpha + \beta_1 x_1) \quad [20\text{–}16]$$

Because the exponential (exp) can never be negative, this model will not produce negative rates, regardless of α, β_1, or x_1. The model is equivalent to the log-linear *rate* model

$$\ln[I(x_1)] = \alpha + \beta_1 x_1 \quad [20\text{–}17]$$

The parameter β_1 in models 20–16 and 20–17 is the log of the rate ratio comparing the subpopulation with $X_1 = x_1 + 1$ to the subpopulation with $X_1 = x_1$, regardless of x_1; hence, $\exp(\beta_1)$ is the corresponding rate ratio $I(x_1 + 1)/I(x_1)$. Also, α is the log of the rate for the subpopulation with $X_1 = 0$; hence, $\exp(\alpha)$ is the average rate $I(0)$ when $X_1 = 0$. The exponential rate model (model 20–16) is analogous to, but different from, the exponential risk model (equation 20–8) and the exponential odds model (equation 20–11).

INCIDENCE-TIME AND HAZARD MODELS

We can also model the average time to occurrence of an event, starting from some designated zero time such as birth (in which case, "time" is age), start of treatment, or some calendar date (Cox and Oakes, 1984; Hosmer and Lemeshow, 1999; Kalbfleisch and Prentice, 2002). These are called incidence-time, waiting-time, failure-time, or survival-time models. Let T stand for time of the event measured from zero. One approach to incidence time regression is to use a linear model for log incidence time, such as

$$E[\ln(T)|X_1 = x_1] = \alpha - \beta_1 x_1 \quad [20\text{–}18]$$

Because T is always positive, $\ln(T)$ is always defined. In this model, α is the average log incidence time in the subpopulation with $X_1 = 0$, and $-\beta_1$ is the difference in average log incidence times when comparing the subpopulation with $X_1 = x_1 + 1$ to the subpopulation with $X_1 = x_1$ (regardless of the value x_1). Model 20–18 is an example of an *accelerated-life model* (Cox and Oakes, 1984), which is a building block for the method of *g-estimation* (see Chapter 21).

Note that the sign of β_1 in the model is reversed from its sign in earlier models. This reversal is done so that, if the outcome event at T is undesirable, then, as in earlier models, positive values of β_1 will correspond to harmful effects from increasing X_1, and negative values will correspond to beneficial effects. For example, under the model, if T is death time and β_1 is positive, an increase in X_1 will be associated with earlier death.

Another generalization of the basic accelerated-life model, similar but not identical to model 20–18, is the log-linear model for expected incidence time,

$$\ln[E(T|X_1 = x_1)] = \alpha - \beta_1 x_1 \quad [20\text{–}19]$$

Model 20–19 differs from model 20–18 because the log of an average is greater than the average of the logs (unless T does not vary). Model 20–19 can be rewritten as

$$\begin{aligned} E(T|X_1 = x_1) &= \exp(\alpha - \beta_1 x_1) = \exp(-\beta_1 x_1)e^{\alpha} \\ &= \exp(-\beta_1 x_1)T_0 \end{aligned}$$

where $T_0 = E(T|X_1 = 0) = e^{\alpha}$. Under model 20–19, e^{α} is the average incidence time in the subpopulation with $X_1 = 0$, and $e^{-\beta_1}$ is the ratio of average incidence times in the subpopulation with $X_1 = x_1 + 1$ and the subpopulation with $X_1 = x_1$. As with model 20–18, the sign of β_1 is negative so that positive values of β_1 will correspond to harmful effects.

More common approaches to modeling incidence times impose a model for the risk of the event up to each point in time, or for the rate of the event "at" each point in time. The most common such model is the *Cox model,* also known as the *proportional-hazards model.* We can give an approximate description of this model as follows: Suppose that we specify a time span Δt that is small enough so that the risk of having the event in any interval t to $t + \Delta t$ among those who survive to t without the event is very small. The Cox model then implies that the rates in any such short interval will follow an exponential model like equation 20–16, with α but not β_1 allowed to vary with time t.

If we write $I(t; x_1)$ for the average rate in the interval t to $t + \Delta t$ among persons who survive to t and have $X_1 = x_1$, the Cox model implies that

$$I(t; x_1) \approx \exp(\alpha_t + \beta_1 x_1) \qquad [20\text{–}20]$$

Under the model, the approximation ($\approx$) improves as Δt gets smaller. Note that the intercept α_t may vary with time, but in this simple Cox model the coefficient β_1 of X_1 is assumed to remain constant. This constancy means that, at any time t, the rate ratio comparing subpopulations with $X_1 = x_1 + 1$ and $X_1 = x_1$ will be

$$I(t; x_1 + 1)/I(t; x_1) \approx \exp[\alpha_t + \beta_1(x_1 + 1)]/\exp(\alpha_t + \beta_1 x_1) = \exp(\beta_1)$$

so that β_1 is the log rate ratio per unit of X_1, regardless of either the reference level x_1 *or* the time t at which it is computed. As a consequence, when plotted over time, the rate curves at $X_1 = x_1 + 1$ and at $X_1 = x_1$ will be proportional, having the constant ratio $\exp(\beta_1)$.

Under the Cox model (equation 20–20), the rate at time t for the subpopulation with $X_1 = 0$ is given by $I(t; 0) \approx \exp(\alpha_t)$. If we denote this "baseline" rate by $h_0(t)$ instead of $\exp(\alpha_t)$, we have

$$I(t; x_1) \approx \exp(\alpha_t + \beta_1 x_1) = \exp(\alpha_t)\exp(\beta_1 x_1) = h_0(t)\exp(\beta_1 x_1) = \exp(\beta_1 x_1)h_0(t)$$

The last expression is the standard form of the model given in most textbooks. The term "Cox model" has become fairly standard, although a special case of the model was proposed by Sheehe (1962).

The approximate form of the Cox model (equation 20–20) may be seen as an extension of the exponential rate model (equation 20–16) in which the rates may vary over time. In statistical theory, the assumption is made that, at each time t, the rate $I(t; x_1)$ approaches a limit $h(t; x_1)$ as Δt goes to zero. This limit is usually called the *hazard* or *intensity* of the outcome at time t. The Cox model is then defined as a model for these hazards,

$$h(t; x_1) = \exp(\beta_1 x_1)h_0(t)$$

In epidemiologic studies, these hazards are purely theoretical quantities; thus, it is important to understand the approximate forms of the model given above and what those forms imply about observable rates.

The Cox model may be extended to allow X_1 to vary over time. Let us write $X_1(t)$ as an abbreviation for "the exposure as of time t" and $x_1(t)$ for the actual numerical value of $X_1(t)$ at time t. Then the *Cox model with time-dependent covariates* implies that the incidence rate at time t in the subpopulation that has exposure level $x_1(t)$ at time t is

$$I[t; x_1(t)] \approx h[t; x_1(t)] = \exp[\beta_1 x_1(t)]h_0(t) \qquad [20\text{–}21]$$

This model may be the most widely used model for time-dependent exposures. Usually, a time-dependent exposure $X_1(t)$ is not defined as the actual amount at time t, but instead is some cumulative and lagged index of exposure up to t (see Chapter 16). For example, if time is measured in months and exposure is cumulative tamoxifen lagged 3 months, $X_1(t)$ will mean "cumulative amount of tamoxifen taken up to month $t - 3$" and $x_1(t)$ will be a value for this variable.

Even if $X_1(t)$ is a summarized history, it refers to a person's history as of time t, not to his or her time at risk, and may even be calculated using data that precede start of follow-up. Thus no issue of immortal person-time (Chapter 7) arises in defining or computing $X_1(t)$. In particular, if exposure can begin before start of follow-up, this historical $X_1(t)$ will depend on exposure that precedes that start. If, however, data on exposure before follow-up are unavailable, then $X_1(t)$ will be censored at start of follow-up.

There are biases that can arise in use of Cox models to estimate effects of time-dependent exposures (Robins et al., 1992a; Robins and Greenland, 1994). See the section of Chapter 21 on modeling longitudinal data for further discussion and references.

TREND MODELS: UNIVARIATE EXPOSURE TRANSFORMS

Consider again the linear risk model (equation 20–7). If this model is correct, a plot of average risk across the subpopulations defined by X_1 (that is, a plot of risk against X_1) will yield a line. Ordinarily, however, there is no compelling reason to think that the model is correct, and we may wish to entertain other possible models for the trend in risk across exposure levels. We can generate an unlimited variety of such models by *transforming* exposure, that is, by replacing X_1 in the model by some function of X_1.

To illustrate, we can replace years exposed in model 20–7 by its logarithm, to get

$$R(x_1) = \alpha + \beta_1 \ln(x_1) \qquad [20\text{–}22]$$

This equation still defines a linear risk model, because a plot of average risk against the new regressor $\ln(X_1)$ will yield a line. But it is a very different model from model 20–7, because if model 20–22 is correct, a plot of average risk against years exposed (X_1) will yield a *logarithmic curve* rather than a line. Such a curve starts off very steep for $X_1 < 1$, but it levels off rapidly beyond $X_1 > 1$.

As discussed in Chapter 17, a technical problem can arise in using the logarithmic transform: It is not defined if X_1 is negative or zero. If the original exposure measurement can be negative or zero, it is common practice to add a number c to X_1 that is big enough to ensure that $X_1 + c$ is always positive. The resulting model is

$$R(x_1) = \alpha + \beta_1 \ln(x_1 + c) \qquad [20\text{–}23]$$

The shape of the curve represented by this model (and hence results derived using the model) can be very sensitive to the value chosen for c, especially when the values of X_1 may be less than 1. Frequently, c is set equal to 1, although there is usually no compelling reason for this choice.

Among other possibilities for exposure transforms are simple power curves of the form

$$R(x_1) = \alpha + \beta_1 x_1^p \qquad [20\text{–}24]$$

where p is some number (typically $1/2$ or 2) chosen in advance according to some desired property. For example, with X_1 as years exposed, use of $p = 1/2$ yields the *square-root* model

$$R(x_1) = \alpha + \beta_1 x_1^{1/2}$$

which produces a trend curve that levels off as X_1 increases above zero. In contrast, use of $p = 2$ yields the simple *quadratic* model

$$R(x_1) = \alpha + \beta_1 x_1^2$$

which produces a trend that rises more and more steeply as X_1 increases above zero.

One technical problem can arise when using the power model (equation 20–24): It is not defined if p is fractional and X_1 can be negative. To get around this limitation, we may add some number c to X_1 that is big enough to ensure that $X_1 + c$ is never negative, and then use $(x_1 + c)^p$ in the model; nonetheless, the result may again be sensitive to the choice of c.

The trend implications of linear and exponential models are vastly different, and hence the implications of exposure transforms are also different. Consider again the exponential risk model (equation 20–8). If this model is correct, a plot of average risk against X_1 will yield an exponential curve rather than a line. If β_1 is positive, this curve starts out slowly but rises more and more rapidly as X_1 increases; it eventually rises more rapidly than does any power curve (equation 20–24). Such rapid increase is often implausible, and we may wish to use a slower-rising curve to model risk.

One means of moderating the trend implied by an exponential model is to replace x_1 by a fixed power x_1^p with $0 < p < 1$, for example,

$$R(x_1) = \exp(\alpha + \beta_1 x_1^{1/2})$$

Another approach is to take the logarithm of exposure. This transform produces a new model:

$$\begin{aligned} R(x_1) &= \exp[\alpha + \beta_1 \ln(x_1)] \\ &= \exp(\alpha)\exp[\beta_1 \ln(x_1)] \\ &= e^{\alpha} \exp[\ln(x_1)]^{\beta_1} = e^{\alpha} x_1^{\beta_1} \end{aligned} \qquad [20\text{–}25]$$

A graph of risk against exposure under this model produces a power curve, but now (unlike model 20–24) the power is the unspecified (unknown) coefficient β_1 instead of a prespecified value p, and the multiplier of the exposure power is e^{α} (which must be positive) instead of β_1. Model 20–25 may thus appear to be more appropriate than model 20–24 when we want the power of X_1 to appear as an unknown coefficient β_1 in the model, rather than as a prespecified value p. As earlier, however, X_1 must always be positive in order to use model 20–25; otherwise, we must add a constant c to it such that $X_1 + c$ is always positive.

When β_1 is negative in model 20–25, risk declines more and more gradually across increasingly exposed subpopulations. For example, if $\beta_1 = -1$, then under model 20–25, $R(x_1) = e^{\alpha} x_1^{-1} = e^{\alpha}/x_1$, which implies that risk declines 50% (from $e^{\alpha}/1$ to $e^{\alpha}/2$) when going from $X_1 = 1$ to $X_1 = 2$, but declines less than 10% (from $e^{\alpha}/10$ to $e^{\alpha}/11$) when going from $X_1 = 10$ to $X_1 = 11$.

The exposure transforms and implications just discussed carry over to the analogous models for odds and rates. For example, we can modify the logistic model (which is an exponential odds model) by substituting the odds $O(x_1)$ for the risk $R(x_1)$ in models 20–22 through 20–25. Similarly, we can modify the rate models by substituting the rate $I(x_1)$ for $R(x_1)$. Each model will have implications for the odds or rates analogous to those described earlier for the risk; because the risks, odds, and rates are functions of one another (Chapter 3), each model will have implications for other measures as well.

Any trend in the odds will appear more gradual when transformed into a risk trend. To see this, note that

$$R(x_1) = O(x_1)/[1 + O(x_1)] < O(x_1)$$

and hence

$$O(x_1)/R(x_1) = 1 + O(x_1)$$

This ratio of odds to risk grows as the odds (and the risks) get larger. Thus, the logistic risk model, which is an exponential odds model, implies a less than exponential trend in the risk. Conversely, any trend in the risks will appear steeper when transformed into an odds trend. Thus, the exponential risk model implies a greater than exponential trend in the odds. Of course, when all the risks are low (less than 10% for all possible X_1 values), the risks and odds will be similar and so there will be little difference between the shape of the curves produced by analogous risk and odds models.

The relation of risk and odds trends to rate trends is more complex in general, but in typical applications follows the simple rule that rate trends tend to fall between the less steep risk and more steep odds trends. For example, an exponential rate model typically implies a less than exponential risk trend but more than exponential odds trend. To see why these relations can be reasonable to expect, recall that, if incidence is measured over a span of time Δt in a closed population, then $R(x_1) < I(x_1)\Delta t < O(x_1)$. When the risks are uniformly low, we obtain $R(x_1) \approx I(x_1)\Delta t \approx O(x_1)$ (Chapter 3), and so there will be little difference in the curves produced by analogous risk, rate, and odds models.

INTERPRETING MODELS AFTER TRANSFORMATION

One drawback of models with transformed regressors is that the interpretation of the coefficients depends on the transformation. As an example, consider the model 20–25, which has $\ln(x_1)$ in place of x_1. Under this model, the risk ratio for a one-unit increase in X_1 is

$$\begin{aligned} R(x_1+1)/R(x_1) &= e^{\alpha}(x_1+1)^{\beta_1}/e^{\alpha}x_1^{\beta_1} \\ &= [(x_1+1)/x_1]^{\beta_1} \end{aligned}$$

which will depend on the value x_1 used as the reference level: If $\beta_1 = 1$ and x_1 is 1, the risk ratio is 2, but if $\beta_1 = 1$ and x_1 is 2, the ratio is 1.5. Here, β_1 is the power to which x_1 is raised, and so it determines the shape of the trend. The interpretation of the intercept α is also altered by the transformation. Under model 20–25, $R(1) = e^{\alpha} 1^{\beta_1} = e^{\alpha}$; thus, α is the log risk when $X_1 = 1$, rather than when $X_1 = 0$, and so is meaningful only if 1 is a possible value for X_1.

As a contrast, consider again the model $R(x_1) = \exp(\alpha + \beta_1 x_1^{1/2})$. Use of $x_1^{1/2}$ rather than x_1 moderates the rapid increase in the slope of the exponential dose–response curve, but it also leads to difficulties in coefficient interpretation. Under the model, the risk ratio for a 1-unit increase in X_1 is

$$\exp\left[\alpha + \beta_1(x_1 + 1)^{1/2}\right] / \exp(\alpha + \beta_1 x_1^{1/2}) = \exp\left\{\beta_1\left[(x_1 + 1)^{1/2} - x_1^{1/2}\right]\right\}$$

Here, β_1 is the log risk ratio per unit increase in the *square root* of X_1, which is rather obscure in meaning. Interpretation may proceed better by considering the shape of the curve implied by the model, for example, by plotting $\exp(\alpha + \beta_1 x_1^{1/2})$ against possible values of X_1 for several values of β_1. (The intercept α is less important in this model, because it determines only the vertical scale of the curve rather than its shape.) Such plotting is often needed to understand and compare different transforms.

OUTCOME TRANSFORMATIONS

Suppose now that Y is quantitative (e.g., CD4 count, diastolic blood pressure) and $h(y)$ is a transform (function) defined for all possible values y of Y. We may then model the regression of $h(Y)$ instead of Y. This transformation of the outcome is often done to ensure that the model does not allow impossible values for Y, such as a negative value for a count. One example is model 20–18 for log incidence time $\ln(T)$. The general form is

$$E[h(Y)|X_1 = x_1)] = \alpha + \beta_1 x_1$$

Interpretation of coefficients with a transformed outcome $h(Y)$ depends on the outcome transformation h, for with the transform β_1 will be the change in the expected $h(Y)$ per unit increase in X_1. If the regressor X_1 is also replaced by a transform, interpretation of the model coefficient can become very obscure. For example, suppose that Y is birth weight, $h(y)$ is the natural log $\ln(y)$, X_1 is previous number of pregnancies, and the model is

$$E[\ln(Y)|X_1 = x_1)] = \alpha + \beta_1 x_1^{1/2}$$

Then β_1 will be the change in the expected log birth weight $E[\ln(Y)|X_1 = x_1]$ per unit increase in the square root of previous number of pregnancies X_1. Graphing this regression function against X_1 (rather than against $X_1^{1/2}$) can aid in interpretation by showing the expected log birth weight as a function of previous number of pregnancies, but it is still not straightforward because the regression is for log birth weight, not birth weight.

An alternative to transforming the outcome is to transform the regression itself. Model 20–19 provides an example of this approach with incidence time T as the outcome. As was shown there (using T in place of Y), transforming the regression $E(Y|X_1 = x_1)$ leads to a model different from that obtained by transforming the outcome Y, and leaves the interpretation of the final model in terms of the expectation of the original Y. Transformation of the regression is covered later, under the topic of *generalized linear models*.

MULTIPLE REGRESSION MODELS

Suppose now that we wish to model the full multiple regression $E(Y|\mathbf{X} = \mathbf{x})$. Each of the previous models for the single regression $E(Y|X_1 = x_1)$ can be extended to handle this more general situation by using the following device: In any model for the single regression, replace $\beta_1 x_1$ by

$$\beta_1 x_1 + \beta_2 x_2 + \ldots + \beta_n x_n \qquad [20\text{–}26]$$

To illustrate the idea, suppose that we wish to model average risk of death by age 70 years across female subpopulations defined by

X_1 = years of tamoxifen therapy
X_2 = age at start of tamoxifen use
X_3 = age at menarche

with $\mathbf{X} = (X_1, X_2, X_3)$. Then the multiple linear risk model for $R(\mathbf{x})$ is

$$R(\mathbf{x}) = \alpha + \beta_1 x_1 + \beta_2 x_2 + \beta_3 x_3$$

whereas the multiple logistic risk model is

$$R(\mathbf{x}) = \text{expit}(\alpha + \beta_1 x_1 + \beta_2 x_2 + \beta_3 x_3)$$

If instead we wished to model the death rate, we could use the multiple linear rate model

$$I(\mathbf{x}) = \alpha + \beta_1 x_1 + \beta_2 x_2 + \beta_3 x_3$$

or a multiple exponential rate model,

$$I(\mathbf{x}) = \exp(\alpha + \beta_1 x_1 + \beta_2 x_2 + \beta_3 x_3)$$

Because formula 20–26 can be clumsy to write out when there are three or more regressors ($n \geq 3$), several shorthand notations are in use. Let $\boldsymbol{\beta}$ represent the vertical list (column vector) of coefficients $\beta_1, \ldots, \beta_n$. Recall that $\mathbf{x}$ stands for the horizontal list (row vector) of values $x_1, \ldots, x_n$. If we let $\mathbf{x}\boldsymbol{\beta}$ stand for $\beta_1 x_1 + \ldots + \beta_n x_n$, we can represent the multiple linear risk model by

$$R(\mathbf{x}) = \alpha + \mathbf{x}\boldsymbol{\beta} = \alpha + \beta_1 x_1 + \ldots + \beta_n x_n \qquad [20\text{–}27]$$

the multiple logistic model by

$$R(\mathbf{x}) = \text{expit}(\alpha + \mathbf{x}\boldsymbol{\beta}) \qquad [20\text{–}28]$$

the multiple exponential rate model by

$$I(\mathbf{x}) = \exp(\alpha + \mathbf{x}\boldsymbol{\beta}) \qquad [20\text{–}29]$$

and so on for all the models discussed earlier.

RELATIONS AMONG MULTIPLE-REGRESSION MODELS

The multiple-regression models 20–27 through 20–29 are not more general than the single-regression models 20–7, 20–10, and 20–16, nor do they contain those models as special cases, because they refer to entirely different subclassifications of the target population. The single-regression models refer to variations in averages across subpopulations defined by levels of just one variable; the multiple-regression models, in contrast, refer to variations across the much finer subdivisions defined by the levels of several variables. For example, it is at least logically possible for $R(x_1)$ to follow the single-logistic model (equation 20–10) without $R(\mathbf{x})$ following the multiple-logistic model (equation 20–28); conversely, it is possible for $R(\mathbf{x})$ to follow the multiple-logistic model without $R(x_1)$ following the single-logistic model.

The preceding point is often overlooked because the single-regression models are often confused with multiple-regression models in which all regressor coefficients except one are 0. The difference, however, is analogous to the differences discussed earlier between the vacuous models 20–1 through 20–3 (which are so general as to imply nothing) and the constant regression models 20–4 through 20–6 (which are so restrictive as to be unbelievable in typical situations). To see this analogy, consider the multiple-logistic model

$$R(\mathbf{x}) = \text{expit}(\alpha + \beta_1 x_1) \qquad [20\text{–}30]$$

The right side of this equation is the same as in the single-logistic model (equation 20–10), but the left side is crucially different: It is the multiple-risk regression $R(\mathbf{x})$, instead of the single-regression $R(x_1)$. Unlike model 20–10, model 20–30 *is* a special case of the multiple-logistic model (equation 20–28), the one in which $\beta_2 = \beta_3 = \ldots = \beta_n = 0$. Unlike model 20–10, model 20–30 asserts that risk does not vary across subpopulations defined by $X_1, X_2, \ldots, X_n$ *except* to the extent that X_1 varies. This model is far more strict than model 20–28, which allows risk to vary with $X_2, \ldots, X_n$ as well as X_1 (albeit only in a logistic fashion). It is also far more strict than model 20–10, which says absolutely nothing about whether or how risk varies across subpopulations defined by $X_2, \ldots, X_n$, within specific levels of X_1.

We must be careful to distinguish between models that refer to different multiple regressions. For example, compare the two exponential rate models

$$I(x_1, x_2) = \exp(\alpha + \beta_1 x_1 + \beta_2 x_2) \qquad [20\text{–}31]$$

and

$$I(x_1, x_2, x_3) = \exp(\alpha + \beta_1 x_1 + \beta_2 x_2) \qquad [20\text{–}32]$$

These are different models. The first is a model for the regression of rates on X_1 and X_2 only, whereas the second is a model for the regression of rates on X_1, X_2, and X_3. The first model in no way refers to X_3, whereas the second asserts that rates do not vary across levels of X_3 if one looks within levels of X_1 and X_2. Model 20–32 is the special case of

$$I(x_1, x_2, x_3) = \exp(\alpha + \beta_1 x_1 + \beta_2 x_2 + \beta_3 x_3)$$

in which $\beta_3 = 0$, whereas model 20–31 is not.

Many textbooks and software manuals fail to distinguish between models such as 20–31 and 20–32, and instead focus only on the appearance of the right-hand side of the models. Most software fits the less restrictive model that ignores other covariates (equation 20–31 in the preceding example) rather than the more restrictive model (equation 20–32) when requested to fit a model with only X_1 and X_2 as regressors. Note that if the less restrictive model is inadequate, then the more restrictive model must also be inadequate.

Unfortunately, if the less restrictive model appears adequate, it does *not* follow that the more restrictive model is also adequate. For example, it is possible for the model form $\exp(\alpha + \beta_1 x_1 + \beta_2 x_2)$ to describe adequately the double regression $I(x_1, x_2)$ (which means it describes adequately the rate variation across X_1 and X_2 when X_3 is ignored), and yet at the same time describe poorly the triple regression $I(x_1, x_2, x_3)$ (which means that it describes inadequately the rate variation across X_1, X_2, and X_3). That is, a model may describe poorly the rate variation across X_1, X_2, and X_3 even if it describes adequately the rate variation across X_1 and X_2 when X_3 is ignored. The decision as to whether the model is acceptable should depend on whether the rate variation across X_3 is relevant to the analysis objectives. For example, if the objective is to estimate the effect of changes in X_1 on the death rate, and X_2 and X_3 are both potential confounders (as in the tamoxifen example), we want the model to describe adequately the rate variation across all three variables. But if X_3 is instead affected by the study exposure X_1 (such as when X_1 is past estrogen exposure and X_3 is an indicator of current uterine bleeding), we usually will not want to include X_3 in the regression model (because we will not want to adjust our exposure-effect estimate for X_3).

PRODUCT TERMS (STATISTICAL INTERACTIONS)

Each model form we have described has differing implications for measures of association derived from the models. Consider again the linear risk model with three regressors X_1, X_2, and X_3 , and let x_1^* and x_1 be any two values for X_1. Under the model, the risks at $X_1 = x_1^*$ and $X_1 = x_1$ and their difference, *RD*, when $X_2 = x_2$ and $X_3 = x_3$ are

$$R(x_1^*, x_2, x_3) = \alpha + \beta_1 x_1^* + \beta_2 x_2 + \beta_3 x_3$$

$$R(x_1, x_2, x_3) = \alpha + \beta_1 x_1 + \beta_2 x_2 + \beta_3 x_3$$

$$RD = \beta_1(x_1^* - x_1)$$

Thus, the model implies that the risk difference between two subpopulations with the same X_2 and X_3 levels depends only on the difference in their X_1 levels. In other words, the model implies that the risk differences for X_1 within levels of X_2 and X_3 will not vary across levels of X_2 and X_3. Such an implication may be unacceptable, in which case we can either modify the linear model or switch to another model. A simple way to modify a model is to add *product terms*. For example, suppose we want to allow the risk differences for X_1 to vary across levels of X_2. We can add the product of X_1 and X_2 to the model as a fourth variable. The risks and their differences will then be

$$R(x_1^*, x_2, x_3) = \alpha + \beta_1 x_1^* + \beta_2 x_2 + \beta_3 x_3 + \gamma_{12} x_1^* x_2$$

$$R(x_1, x_2, x_3) = \alpha + \beta_1 x_1 + \beta_2 x_2 + \beta_3 x_3 + \gamma_{12} x_1 x_2 \quad [20\text{–}33]$$

$$RD = \beta_1(x_1^* - x_1) + \gamma_{12}(x_1^* - x_1)x_2 = (\beta_1 + \gamma_{12}x_2)(x_1^* - x_1) \quad [20\text{–}34]$$

Under model 20–33, the risk difference for $X_1 = x_1^*$ versus $X_1 = x_1$ is given by formula 20–34, which depends on X_2.

A model (e.g., equation 20–33) that allows variation of the risk difference for X_1 across levels of X_2 will also allow variation in the risk difference for X_2 across levels of X_1. As an example, let x_2^* and x_2 be any two possible values for X_2. Under model 20–33, the risks at $X_2 = x_2^*$ and $X_2 = x_2$ and their difference RD when $X_1 = x_1$, $X_3 = x_3$ are

$$R(x_1, x_2^*, x_3) = \alpha + \beta_1 x_1 + \beta_2 x_2^* + \beta_3 x_3 + \gamma_{12} x_1 x_2^*$$

$$R(x_1, x_2, x_3) = \alpha + \beta_1 x_1 + \beta_2 x_2 + \beta_3 x_3 + \gamma_{12} x_1 x_2$$

$$RD = \beta_2(x_2^* - x_2) + \gamma_{12}x_1(x_2^* - x_2) = (\beta_2 + \gamma_{12}x_1)(x_2^* - x_2) \quad [20\text{–}35]$$

Thus, under the model, the risk difference for $X_2 = x_2^*$ versus $X_2 = x_2$ is given by formula 20–35, which depends on X_1. Formulas 20–34 and 20–35 illustrate how product terms modify a model in a symmetric way. The term $\gamma_{12}x_1x_2$ allows the risk differences for X_1 to vary with X_2 and the risk differences for X_2 to vary with X_1.

If we have three regressors in a model, we have three unique two-way regressor products (x_1x_2, x_1x_3, x_2x_3) that we can put in the model. More generally, with n regressors, there are $\binom{n}{2}$ pairs and hence $\binom{n}{2}$ two-way products we can use. It is also possible to add triple products (e.g., $x_1x_2x_3$) or other complex combinations to the model, but such additions are rare in practice (notable exceptions are body mass indices, such as weight/height^2 [Michels et al., 1998]). A model without product terms is sometimes called a "main-effects only" model, and can be viewed as the special case of a model with product terms (the special case in which all the product coefficients γ_{ij} are 0).

Consider next an exponential risk model with the above three variables. Under this model, the risks at $X_1 = x_1^*$ and $X_1 = x_1$ and their ratio RR when $X_2 = x_2$, $X_3 = x_3$ are

$$R(x_1^*, x_2, x_3) = \exp(\alpha + \beta_1 x_1^* + \beta_2 x_2 + \beta_3 x_3)$$

$$R(x_1, x_2, x_3) = \exp(\alpha + \beta_1 x_1 + \beta_2 x_2 + \beta_3 x_3)$$

$$RR = \exp[\beta_1(x_1^* - x_1)] \quad [20\text{–}36]$$

Thus, the model implies that the risk ratio comparing two subpopulations with the same X_2 and X_3 levels depends only on the difference in their X_1 levels. In other words, the model implies that the risk ratios for X_1 will be constant across levels of X_2 and X_3. If this implication is unacceptable, product terms can be inserted, as with the linear model. These terms allow the risk ratios to vary in a limited fashion across levels of other variables.

The preceding discussion of product terms can be applied to linear and exponential models in which the odds or rate replace the risk. For example, without product terms, the logistic model implies that the odds ratios for each regressor are constant across levels of the other regressors (because the logistic model is an exponential odds model); we can add product terms to allow the odds ratios to vary. Likewise, without product terms, the exponential rate model implies that the rate ratios for each regressor are constant across levels of the other regressors; we can add product terms to allow the rate ratios to vary.

Although product terms can greatly increase the flexibility of a model, the type of variation allowed by product terms can be very limited. For example, model 20–33 implies that raising X_2 by 1 unit (i.e., comparing subpopulations that have $X_2 = x_2 + 1$ instead of $X_2 = x_2$) will yield a risk difference for X_1 of

$$[\beta_1 + \gamma_{12}(x_2 + 1)](x_1^* - x_1) = (\beta_1 + \gamma_{12}x_2)(x_1^* - x_1) + \gamma_{12}(x_1^* - x_1)$$

In other words, the model implies that shifting our comparison to subpopulations that are 1 unit higher in X_2 will change the risk difference for X_1 in a linear fashion, by an amount $\gamma_{12}(x_1^* - x_1)$, regardless of the reference values x_1, x_2, x_3 of X_1, X_2, X_3.

TRENDS AND PRODUCT TERMS

Each of the preceding models forces or assumes a particular shape for the graph obtained when average outcome (regression) is plotted against the regressors. Consider again the tamoxifen example. Suppose we wished to plot how the risk varies across subpopulations with different number of years exposure but with the same age at start of exposure and the same age at menarche. Under the linear risk model, this involves plotting the average risk

$$R(x_1, x_2, x_3) = \alpha + \beta_1 x_1 + \beta_2 x_2 + \beta_3 x_3$$

against X_1, while keeping X_2 and X_3 fixed at some values x_2 and x_3. By doing so, we obtain a line with an intercept equal to $\alpha + \beta_2 x_2 + \beta_3 x_3$ and a slope equal to β_1. Whenever we change X_2 and X_3 and replot $R(x)$ against X_1, the intercept will change (unless $\beta_2 = \beta_3 = 0$), but the slope will remain β_1. Because lines with the same slope are parallel, we can say that the linear risk model given above implies *parallel linear* trends in risk with increasing tamoxifen (X_1) as one moves across subpopulations of different starting age (X_2) and menarche age (X_3). Each change in X_2 and X_3 adds some constant (possibly negative) amount to the X_1 curve. For this reason, the linear risk model is sometimes called an *additive* risk model.

If we plot risks against X_2, we will get analogous results: The linear risk model given above implies parallel linear relations between average risk and X_2 as one moves across levels of X_1 and X_3. Likewise, the model implies parallel linear relations between average risk and X_3 across levels of X_1 and X_2. Thus, the linear model implies additive (parallel) relations among all the variables.

If we are not satisfied with the linearity assumption but we wish to retain the additivity (parallel-trend) assumption, we can transform the regressors. If we are not satisfied with the parallel-trend assumption, we can allow the trends to vary across levels of other regressors by adding product terms to the model. For example, adding the product of X_1 and X_2 to the model yields model 20–33, which can be rewritten as

$$R(x_1, x_2, x_3) = \alpha + (\beta_1 + \gamma_{12} x_2) x_1 + \beta_2 x_2 + \beta_3 x_3$$

From this reformulation, we see that the slope for the line obtained by plotting average risk against X_1 while keeping X_2, X_3 fixed at x_2, x_3 will be $\beta_1 + \gamma_{12} x_2$. Thus, the slope of the trend in risk across X_1 will vary across levels of X_2 (if $\gamma_{12} \neq 0$), and so the trend lines for X_1 will not be parallel. We also see that γ_{12} is the difference in the X_1-trend slopes between subpopulations with the same X_3 value but 1 unit apart in their X_2 value.

An entirely different approach to producing nonparallel trends begins with an exponential model. For example, under the exponential risk model (equation 20–36), a plot of average risk against X_1 while keeping X_2 and X_3 fixed at x_2 and x_3 will produce an *exponential* curve rather than a line. This exponential curve will have intercept $\exp(\alpha + \beta_2 x_2 + \beta_3 x_3)$. If, however, we change the value of X_2 or X_3 and replot risk against X_1, we will *not* obtain a parallel risk curve. Instead, the new curve will be *proportional* to the old one: A change in X_2 or X_3 *multiplies* the entire X_1 curve by some amount. For this reason, the exponential model is sometimes called a *multiplicative risk* model. If we are not satisfied with this proportionality-of-trends assumption, we can insert product terms into the model, which will allow for certain types of nonproportional trends. Proportional trends in risk appear parallel when plotted on a logarithmic vertical scale; when product terms with nonzero coefficients are present, logarithmic trends appear nonparallel.

Analogous comments and definitions apply if we substitute odds or rates for risks in the preceding arguments. For example, consider the multiple logistic model in the exponential odds form:

$$O(\mathbf{x}) = \exp(\alpha + \beta_1 x_1 + \beta_2 x_2 + \beta_3 x_3)$$

A plot of the disease odds $O(\mathbf{x})$ against X_1 while keeping X_2 and X_3 fixed will produce an exponential curve; a plot of the log odds (logit) against X_1 while keeping X_2 and X_3 fixed will produce a line. If we change the value of X_2 or X_3 and replot the odds against X_1, we will obtain a new curve that is proportional to the old; that is, the new odds curve will equal the old curve multiplied by some constant amount. Thus, the logistic model is sometimes called a multiplicative odds model. For analogous reasons, the exponential rate model is sometimes called a multiplicative rate model. In both these models, inserting product terms into the model allows certain types of departures from proportional trends.

INTERPRETING PRODUCT-TERM MODELS

Several important cautions should be highlighted when attempting to build models with product terms and interpret coefficients in models with product terms. First, the "main-effect" coefficient β_j will be meaningless when considered alone if its regressor X_j appears in a product with another variable X_k that cannot be 0. In the tamoxifen example, X_1 is years of exposure, which can be 0, while X_3 is age at menarche (in years), which is always greater than 0. Consider the model

$$\begin{aligned} R(x_1, x_2, x_3) &= \alpha + \beta_1 x_1 + \beta_2 x_2 + \beta_3 x_3 + \gamma_{13} x_1 x_3 \\ &= \alpha + \beta_1 x_1 + \beta_2 x_2 + (\beta_3 + \gamma_{13} x_1) x_3 \\ &= \alpha + (\beta_1 + \gamma_{13} x_3) x_1 + \beta_2 x_2 + \beta_3 x_3 \end{aligned} \quad [20\text{–}37]$$

Under this model, $\beta_1 + \gamma_{13}x_3$ is the slope for the trend in risks across X_1 given $X_2 = x_2$ and $X_3 = x_3$. Thus, if X_3 is 0, this slope will be $\beta_1 + \gamma_{13}0 = \beta_1$, and so β_1 could be interpreted as the slope for X_1 in subpopulations of a given X_2 and with $X_3 = 0$. But X_3 is age at menarche and so it cannot be 0; thus β_1 has no simple epidemiologic interpretation. In contrast, because X_1 is years of exposure and so can be 0, β_3 does have a simple interpretation: Under model 20–37, $\beta_3 + \gamma_{13}x_1$ is the slope for X_3 given $X_1 = x_1$; hence $\beta_3 + \gamma_{13} \cdot 0 = \beta_3$ is the slope for X_3 in subpopulations with no tamoxifen exposure ($X_1 = 0$).

As mentioned earlier, if a regressor X_j cannot be zero, one can ensure a simple interpretation of the intercept a by recentering the regressor, that is, by subtracting a reference value from the regressor before entering it in the model. Such recentering also helps provide a simple interpretation for the coefficients of variables that appear with X_3 in product terms. In the example, we can recenter by redefining X_3 to be age at menarche minus 13 years. With this change, β_1 in model 20–37 will now be the slope for X_1 (years of tamoxifen) in subpopulations of a given X_2 (age at start of tamoxifen) in which this new X_3 is 0 (that is, in which the age at menarche was 13).

Rescaling can also be important for interpretation of product-term coefficients. As an example, suppose that X_1 is serum cholesterol in mg/dL and X_2 is diastolic blood pressure (DBP) in mm Hg, and that the product of X_1 and X_2 is entered into the model without rescaling—say, as $\gamma_{12}x_1x_2$ in an exponential rate model. Then γ_{12} represents the difference in the log rate ratio for a 1-mg/dL increase in cholesterol when comparing subpopulations 1 mm Hg apart in DBP. Even if this term is important, it will appear to be very small in magnitude because of the small units used to measure cholesterol and DBP. To avoid such deceptive appearances, we can rescale X_1 and X_2 so that their units represent important increases in cholesterol and DBP. For example, we can redefine X_1 as cholesterol divided by 20 and X_2 as DBP divided by 10. With this rescaling, γ_{12} represents the difference in the log rate ratio for a 20-mg/dL increase in cholesterol when comparing subpopulations that are 10 mm Hg apart in DBP.

Another caution is that, in most situations, a product term in a model should be accompanied by terms for all variables and products contained within that product. For example, if one enters $\gamma_{12}x_1x_2$ in a model, β_1x_1 and β_2x_2 should also be included in that model; and if one enters $\delta_{123}x_1x_2x_3$ in a model, all of β_1x_1, β_2x_2, β_3x_3, $\gamma_{12}x_1x_2$, $\gamma_{13}x_1x_3$, and $\gamma_{23}x_2x_3$ should be included in that model. This rule, sometimes called the *hierarchy principle* (Bishop et al., 1975), is useful in avoiding models with bizarre implications. As an example, suppose that X_1 is serum lead concentration and X_2 is age minus 50 years. If $\gamma_{12} > 0$, the 1-year mortality-risk model

$$R(x_1, x_2) = \exp(\alpha + \beta_2 x_2 + \gamma_{12} x_1 x_2)$$

implies that serum lead is positively related to risk among persons older than age 50 ($X_2 > 0$), is unrelated to risk among persons of age 50 ($X_2 = 0$), and is negatively related to risk among persons younger than age 50 ($X_2 < 0$); if $\gamma_{12} < 0$, it implies a negative relation over 50 and a positive relation below 50. Rarely (if ever) will we have grounds for assuming that such unusual relations hold. To prevent use of absurd models, many regression programs automatically enter all terms contained within a product when the user instructs the program to enter the product into the model.

Models that violate the hierarchy principle often arise when one variable is not defined for all subjects. As an example, suppose in a study of breast cancer in women that X_1 is age at first birth (AFB) and X_2 is parity. Because X_1 is undefined for nulliparous women ($X_2 = 0$), one sometimes sees the breast cancer rate modeled by a function in which age at first birth appears only in a product term with parity, such as $\exp(\alpha + \beta_2 x_2 + \gamma_1 x_1 x_2)$. The rationale for this model is that the rate will remain defined even when age at first birth (X_1) is undefined, because $x_1 x_2$ will be 0 when parity (X_2) is 0. But this type of model assumes that the coefficient relating X_1 to the outcome is always a multiple of X_2, which is rarely plausible; e.g., here it says that the multiplier $\gamma_1 x_2$ of age at first birth is 6 times higher for a woman with six births than for a woman with one birth.

One can sometimes avoid violating the hierarchy principle if there is a reasonable way to extend variable definitions to all subjects. Thus, in the tamoxifen example, age at start of tamoxifen was extended to the untreated by setting it to age 70 years (end of follow-up) for those subjects, and for those subjects who started at age 70 or later. The rationale for this extension is that, within the age interval under study, untreated subjects and subjects starting tamoxifen at age 70 or later will have identical exposures.

Another caution is that product terms are commonly labeled "interaction terms" or "statistical interactions." We avoid these labels because they may inappropriately suggest the presence of biologic (mechanical) interactions between the variables in a product term. In practice, regression models are applied in many situations in which there is no effect of the regressors on the regressand (outcome). Even in causal analyses, the connections between product terms and biologic interactions can be very indirect and can depend on many biologic assumptions. In the next section, we will briefly describe the simplest of these connections.

REGRESSION MODELS AND BIOLOGIC INTERACTIONS

In Chapter 5 we defined interaction response types for binary factors and showed that absence of such interactions implies additivity of causal risk differences. In the absence of confounding, the latter additivity condition is equivalent to a multiple-linear risk model. To see this equivalence, consider two binary risk factors X_1 and X_2. Additivity of risk differences corresponds to

$$R(1,1) - R(0,0) = [R(1,0) - R(0,0)] + [R(0,1) - R(0,0)]$$

which yields

$$R(1,1) = R(0,0) + [R(1,0) - R(0,0)] + [R(0,1) - R(0,0)]$$

Define $\alpha = R(0,0)$, $\beta_1 = R(1,0) - R(0,0)$, and $\beta_2 = R(0,1) - R(0,0)$. The equation for $R(1,1)$ can then be rewritten

$$R(1,1) = \alpha + \beta_1 + \beta_2$$

The definitions of α, β_1, β_2 also yield

$$R(0,0) = \alpha, \quad R(1,0) = \alpha + \beta_1, \quad R(0,1) = \alpha + \beta_2$$

The last four risk equations can be represented by the single formula

$$R(x_1, x_2) = \alpha + \beta_1 x_1 + \beta_2 x_2$$

where x_1 and x_2 can be either 0 or 1. This formula is a special case of the multiple-linear risk model (equation 20–27). Thus, in the absence of confounding, departure of risks from the multiple-linear risk model implies a departure from risk-difference additivity, which in turn implies that interaction response types are present. As discussed in Chapter 5, however, risk-difference additivity is a population phenomenon that may arise from a balance between synergistic and antagonistic responses, rather than absence of interactions. Hence, neither risk-difference additivity nor the linear-risk model implies absence of biologic interactions between X_1 and X_2.

Consider next the extension of the linear-risk model with a product term,

$$R(x_1, x_2) = \alpha + \beta_1 x_1 + \beta_2 x_2 + \beta_3 x_1 x_2$$

One occasionally sees the product ("interaction") coefficient β_3 used as a measure of the population frequency of interactions between X_1 and X_2. Such usage is incorrect, insofar as the magnitude of β_3 reflects only the net balance among the different response types listed in Chapter 5. For example, $\beta_3 > 0$ implies only that synergistic response types are more frequent than antagonistic and competitive response types, not that antagonistic and competitive response types are absent; $\beta_3 < 0$ implies only that antagonistic and competitive responses are more frequent than synergistic responses, not that synergistic responses are absent; and $\beta_3 = 0$ implies only that synergistic responses are balanced by antagonistic and competitive responses, not that interactions are absent.

The preceding concepts and observations extend to situations involving polytomous or continuous regressors (Greenland, 1993b).

CATEGORICAL REGRESSORS

Consider a regressor whose possible values are discrete and few, and perhaps purely nominal (that is, with no natural ordering or quantitative meaning). An example is marital status (never married, currently married, formerly married). Such regressors may be entered into a multiple-regression model using *category indicator variables*. To use this approach, we first choose one level of the regressor as the *reference level* against which we want to compare risks or rates. For each of the remaining levels (the *index* levels), we create a binary variable to indicate whether a person is at that level (1 if at the level, 0 if not). We then enter these indicators into the regression model.

The entire set of indicators is called the *coding* of the original regressor. To code marital status, we can take "currently married" as the reference level and define

$X_1 = 1$ if formerly married, 0 if currently or never married
$X_2 = 1$ if never married, 0 if currently or formerly married (i.e., ever married)

There are $2 \cdot 2 = 4$ possible numerical combinations of values for X_1 and X_2, but only three of them are logically possible. The impossible combination is $X_1 = 1$ (formerly married) and $X_2 = 1$ (never married). Note, however, that we need two indicators to distinguish the three levels of marital status, because one indicator can only distinguish two levels.

In general, we need $J - 1$ indicators to code a variable with J levels. Although these indicators will have 2^{J-1} possible numerical combinations, only J of these combinations will be logically possible. For example, we need four indicators to code a variable with five levels. These indicators have $2^4 = 16$ numerical combinations, but only 5 of the 16 combinations will be logically possible.

Interpretation of the indicator coefficients depends on the model form and the chosen coding. For example, in the logistic model

$$R(x_1, x_2) = \text{expit}(\alpha + \beta_1 x_1 + \beta_2 x_2) \qquad [20\text{–}38]$$

$\exp(\beta_2)$ is the odds ratio comparing $X_2 = 1$ persons (never married) to $X_2 = 0$ persons (ever married) within levels of X_1. Because one cannot have $X_2 = 1$ (never married) and $X_1 = 1$ (formerly married), the only level of X_1 within which we can compare $X_2 = 1$ to $X_2 = 0$ is the zero level (never or currently married). Thus, $\exp(\beta_2)$ is the odds ratio comparing never married ($X_2 = 1$) to currently married ($X_2 = 0$) people among those never or currently married ($X_1 = 0$). In a similar fashion, $\exp(\beta_1)$ compares those formerly married to those currently married among those ever married.

In general, the type of indicator coding just described, called *disjoint category coding,* results in coefficients that compare each index category to the reference category. With this coding, for a given person, no more than one indicator in the set can equal 1; all the indicators are 0 for persons in the reference category. A different kind of coding is *nested indicator coding*. In this type of coding, levels of the regressor are grouped, and then codes are created to facilitate comparisons both within and across groups. For example, suppose we wish to compare those not currently married (never or formerly married) to those currently married, and also compare those never married to those formerly married. We can then use the indicators

$Z_1 = 1$ if never or formerly married (i.e., not currently married), 0 otherwise (currently married)
$Z_2 = 1$ if never married, 0 if ever married

Z_2 is the same as the X_2 used above, but Z_1 is different from X_1. The combination $Z_1 = 0$ (currently married), $Z_2 = 1$ (never married) is impossible; $Z_1 = Z_2 = 1$ for people who never married. In the logistic model

$$R(z_1, z_2) = \text{expit}(\alpha + \beta_1 z_1 + \beta_2 z_2) \qquad [20\text{–}39]$$

$\exp(\beta_2)$ is now the odds ratio comparing those never married ($Z_2 = 1$) to those ever married ($Z_2 = 0$) among those not currently married ($Z_1 = 1$). Similarly, $\exp(\beta_1)$ is now the odds ratio comparing those formerly married ($Z_1 = 1$) to those currently married ($Z_1 = 0$) among those ever married ($Z_2 = 0$).

There can be many options for coding category indicators. The choice among these options may be dictated by which comparisons are of most interest. As long as each level of the regressor can be uniquely represented by the indicator coding, the choice of coding will not alter the assumptions represented by the model. There is, however, one technical point to consider in choosing codes. The precision of the estimated coefficient for an indicator depends directly on the numbers of subjects at each indicator level. For example, suppose that in the data there are 1,000 currently married subjects, 200 formerly married subjects, and only 10 never married subjects. Then an indicator that has "never married" as one of its levels (0 or 1) has a much less precise coefficient estimate than other indicators. If "never married" is chosen as the reference level for a disjoint coding scheme, all the indicators will have that level as their zero level, and so all will have very imprecise coefficient estimates. To maximize precision, many analysts prefer to use disjoint coding in which the largest category (currently married in the preceding example) is taken as the reference level.

In choosing a coding scheme, one need not let precision concerns prevent one from making interesting comparisons. Coding schemes that distinguish among the same categories produce equivalent models. Therefore, one may fit a model repeatedly using different but equivalent coding schemes, in order to easily examine all comparisons of interest. For example, one could fit model 20–38 to compare those never or formerly married with those currently married, then fit model 20–39 to compare the never with formerly married.

Although indicator coding is essential for purely nominal regressors, it can also be used to study quantitative regressors, especially when one expects qualitative differences between persons at different levels. Consider number of marriages as a regressor. We might suspect that people of a given age who have had one marriage tend to be qualitatively distinct from people of the same age who have had no marriage or two marriages, and that people who have had several marriages are even more distinctive. We thus might want to code number of marriages in a manner that allows qualitative distinctions among its levels. If "one marriage" is the most common level, we might use it as the reference level and use

$X_1 = 1$ if never married, 0 otherwise
$X_2 = 1$ if two marriages, 0 otherwise
$X_3 = 1$ if three or more marriages, 0 otherwise

We use one variable to represent "three or more" because there might be too few subjects with three or more marriages to produce acceptably precise coefficients for a finer division of levels. The coding just given will provide comparisons of those never married, twice married, and more-than-twice married to those once married. Other codings could be used to make other comparisons.

TREND MODELS IN MULTIPLE REGRESSION

Multiple regression models can be extended to produce much more flexible trend models than those provided by simple transformations. The latter restrict trends to follow basic shapes, such as quadratic or logarithmic curves. The use of multiple terms for each exposure and confounder allows more detailed assessment of trends and more complete control of confounding than is possible with simple transformations.

CATEGORICAL TRENDS

One way to extend trend models is to categorize the regressor and then use a category-indicator coding such as discussed earlier. The resulting analysis may then parallel the categorical (tabular) trend methods discussed in Chapter 17. Much of the advice given there also applies here. To the extent allowed by the data numbers and background information, the categories should represent scientifically meaningful constructs within which risk is not expected to change dramatically. Purely mathematical categorization methods such as percentiles (quantiles) can do very poorly in this regard and so are best avoided when prior risk information is available (Greenland, 1995a, 1995c). On the other hand, the choices of categories should *not* be dictated by the results produced; for example, manipulation of category boundaries to maximize the effect estimate will produce an estimate that is biased away from the null, whereas manipulation of boundaries to minimize a P-value will produce a downwardly biased P-value. Similarly, manipulation to minimize the estimate or maximize the P-value will produce a null-biased estimate or an upwardly biased P-value.

Two common types of category codes are used in trend models. *Disjoint coding* produces estimates that compare each index category (level) to the reference level. Consider coding weekly servings of fruits and vegetables with

$X_1 = 1$ for <15, 0 otherwise
$X_2 = 1$ for 36 to 42, 0 otherwise
$X_3 = 1$ for >42, 0 otherwise

In the rate model

$$\ln[I(x_1, x_2, x_3)] = \alpha + \beta_1 x_1 + \beta_2 x_2 + \beta_3 x_3 \qquad [20\text{–}40]$$

$\exp(\beta_1)$ is the rate ratio comparing the "<15" category with the "15 to 35" category (which is the referent), and so on, whereas $\exp(\alpha)$ is the rate in the "15 to 35" category (the category for which all the X_j are 0). When model 20–40 is fitted, we can plot the fitted rates on a graph as a step function, as was done in Chapter 17 for category-specific rates. This plot provides a crude impression of the trends across (but not within) categories.

Confounders may be added to the model in order to control confounding, and these too may be coded using multiple indicators or any of the methods described later. We may plot the model-adjusted trends by fixing each confounder at a reference level and allowing the exposure level to vary.

Incremental coding (nested coding) can be useful when one wishes to compare each category against its immediate predecessor (Maclure and Greenland, 1992). For "number of servings per week," we could use

$Z_1 = 1$ for >14, 0 otherwise
$Z_2 = 1$ for >35, 0 otherwise
$Z_3 = 1$ for >42, 0 otherwise

Note that if $Z_2 = 1$, then $Z_1 = 1$, and if $Z_3 = 1$, then $Z_1 = Z_2 = 1$. In the model

$$\ln[I(z_l, z_2, z_3)] = \alpha + \beta_1 z_1 + \beta_2 z_2 + \beta_3 z_3 \qquad [20\text{–}41]$$

$\exp(\beta_1)$ is the rate ratio comparing the "15 to 35" category ($Z_1 = 1$ and $Z_2 = Z_3 = 0$) to the <15 category ($Z_1 = Z_2 = Z_3 = 0$). Similarly, $\exp(\beta_2)$ is the rate ratio comparing the "36 to 42" category ($Z_1 = Z_2 = 1$ and $Z_3 = 0$) to the "15 to 35" category ($Z_1 = 1$ and $Z_2 = Z_3 = 0$). Finally, $\exp(\beta_3)$ compares the >42 category ($Z_1 = Z_2 = Z_3 = 1$) to the "36 to 42" category ($Z_1 = Z_2 = 1$

and $Z_3 = 0$). Thus, $\exp(\beta_1)$, $\exp(\beta_2)$, and $\exp(\beta_3)$ are the incremental rate ratios across adjacent categories. Again, we may add confounders to the model and plot adjusted trends.

REGRESSION WITH CATEGORY SCORES

A common practice in epidemiology is to divide each covariate into categories, assign a score to each category, and enter scores into the model instead of the original variable values. The issues involved in assigning such scores were discussed in Chapter 17 under the heading, "Horizontal Scaling and Category Scores" in the "Dose–Response and Trend Analysis" section. Briefly, ordinal scores or codes (e.g., 1, 2, 3, 4, 5 for a series of five categories) should be avoided, as they can yield quantitatively meaningless dose–response curves and harm the power and precision of the results (Lagakos, 1988; Greenland, 1995b, 1995c). Category midpoints can be much less distortive but are not defined for open-ended categories; category means or medians can be even less distortive and are defined for open-ended categories. Unfortunately, if there are important nonlinear effects within categories, no simple scoring method will yield an undistorted dose–response curve, nor will it achieve the power and precision obtainable by entering the uncategorized covariates into the model (Greenland, 1995b, 1995c). We thus recommend that categories be kept narrow and that scores be derived from category means or medians, rather than from midpoints or ordinal scores. We further recommend that one also examine models using the covariates in their uncategorized (continuous) form whenever associations are clearly present.

POWER MODELS

Another approach to trend analysis and confounder control is to use multiple power terms for each regressor. Such an approach does not require categorization, but it does require care in selection of terms. Traditionally, the powers used are positive integers (e.g., x_1, x_1^2, x_1^3), but fractional powers may also be used (Royston and Altman, 1994). As an illustration, suppose that X_1 represents the actual number of servings per week (instead of an indicator). We can model trends across this regressor by using X_1 in the model along with the following powers of X_1:

$X_2 = X_1^{1/2}$ = square root of X_1
$X_3 = X_1^2$ = square of X_1

The multiple-regression model

$$\ln[I(x_1, x_2, x_3)] = \alpha + \beta_1 x_1 + \beta_2 x_2 + \beta_3 x_3$$

is now just another way of writing the *fractional polynomial* model

$$\ln[I(x_1)] = \alpha + \beta_1 x_1 + \beta_2 x_1^{1/2} + \beta_3 x_1^2 \qquad [20\text{–}42]$$

We can plot fitted rates from this model using very narrow spacing to produce *a smooth curve* as an estimate of rate trends across X_1. As always, we may also include confounders in the model and plot model-adjusted trends.

Power models have several advantages over categorical models. Most important, they make use of information about differences within categories, which is ignored by categorical models and categorical analyses (Greenland, 1995a, 1995b, 1995c). Thus, they can provide a more complete picture of trends across exposure and more thorough control of confounders. They also provide a smoother picture of trends. One disadvantage of power models is a potentially greater sensitivity of estimates to *outliers,* that is, persons with unusual values or unusual *combinations* of values for the regressors. This problem can be addressed by performing influence analysis (Chapters 13 and 21).

REGRESSION SPLINES

Often it is possible to combine the advantages of categorical and power models through the use of *spline models.* Such models can be defined in a number of equivalent ways, and we present only the simplest. In all approaches, one first categorizes the regressor, as in categorical analysis (although fewer, broader categories may be sufficient in a spline model). The boundaries between these categories are called the *knots* or *join points* of the spline. Next, one chooses the *power* (or order) of the spline, according to the flexibility one desires within the categories (higher powers allow more flexibility).

Use of category indicators corresponds to a zero-power spline, in which the trend is flat within categories but may jump suddenly at the knots; thus, category-indicator models are just special and unrealistic types of spline models. In a first-power or *linear* spline, the trend is modeled by a series of connected line segments. The trend within each category corresponds to a line segment; the slope of the trend may change only at the knots, and no sudden jump in risk (discontinuity in trend) can occur.

To illustrate how a linear spline may be represented, let X_1 again be "number of servings per week" but now define

$X_2 = X_1 - 14$ if $X_1 > 14$, 0 otherwise
$X_3 = X_1 - 35$ if $X_1 > 35$, 0 otherwise

Then the log-linear rate model

$$\ln[I(x_1, x_2, x_3)] = \alpha + \beta_1 x_1 + \beta_2 x_2 + \beta_3 x_3 \qquad [20\text{–}43]$$

produces a log-rate trend that is a series of three line segments that are connected at the knots (category boundaries) of 14 and 35. To see this, note that when X_1 is less than 14, X_2 and X_3 are 0, so the model simplifies to a line with slope β_1:

$$\ln[I(x_1, x_2, x_3)] = \alpha + \beta_1 x_1$$

in this range. When X_1 is greater than 14 but less than 35, the model simplifies to a line with slope $\beta_1 + \beta_2$:

$$\begin{aligned}\ln[I(x_1, x_2, x_3)] &= \alpha + \beta_1 x_1 + \beta_2 x_2 \\ &= \alpha + \beta_1 x_1 + \beta_2(x_1 - 14) \\ &= \alpha - 14\beta_2 + (\beta_1 + \beta_2)x_1\end{aligned}$$

Finally, when X_1 is greater than 35, the model becomes a line with slope $\beta_1 + \beta_2 + \beta_3$:

$$\begin{aligned}\ln[I(x_1, x_2, x_3)] &= \alpha + \beta_1 x_1 + \beta_2 x_2 + \beta_3 x_3 \\ &= \alpha + \beta_1 x_1 + \beta_2(x_1 - 14) + \beta_3(x_1 - 35) \\ &= \alpha - 14\beta_2 - 35\beta_3 + (\beta_1 + \beta_2 + \beta_3)x_1\end{aligned}$$

Thus, β_1 is the slope of the spline in the first category, β_2 is the change in slope in going from the first to the second category, and β_3 is the change in slope in going from the second to the third category.

The pattern produced by a linear spline appears to be more realistic than a categorical trend, but it can suddenly change its slope at the knots. To smooth out such sudden changes, we may increase the order of the spline. Increasing the power to 2 produces a second-power or *quadratic* spline, which comprises a series of parabolic curve segments smoothly joined together at the knots. To illustrate how such a trend may be represented, let X_1, X_2, and X_3 be as just defined. Then the model

$$\ln[I(x_1, x_2, x_3)] = \alpha + \beta_1 x_1 + \gamma_1 x_1^2 + \gamma_2 x_2^2 + \gamma_3 x_3^2 \qquad [20\text{–}44]$$

will produce a log-rate trend that is a series of three parabolic segments smoothly connected at the knots of 14 and 35. The coefficient γ_1 corresponds to the curvature of the trend in the first category, while γ_2 and γ_3 correspond to the changes in curvature when going from the first to the second category and from the second to the third category. A still smoother curve could be fit by using a third-power or *cubic* spline, but for epidemiologic purposes the quadratic spline is often smooth and flexible enough.

One disadvantage of quadratic and cubic splines is that the curves in the end categories (tails) may become very unstable, especially if the category is open-ended. This instability may be reduced by *restricting* one or both of the end categories to be a line segment rather than a curve. To restrict the lower category to be linear in a quadratic spline, we need only remove the *first* quadratic term $\gamma_i x_1^2$ from the model. To restrict the upper category, we must subtract the *last* quadratic term from all the quadratic terms; in doing so, we must remove the last term from the model because it will be 0 after the subtraction.

To illustrate an upper category restriction, suppose we wish to restrict the above quadratic spline model for log rates (20–44) so that it is linear in the upper category only. Define

$Z_1 = X_1 =$ number of servings per week
$Z_2 = X_1^2 - X_3^2$
$Z_3 = X_2^2 - X_3^2$

Then the model

$$\ln[I(z_l, z_2, z_3)] = \alpha + \beta_1 z_1 + \beta_2 z_2 + \beta_3 z_3 \qquad [20\text{–}45]$$

will produce a log-rate trend that comprises smoothly connected parabolic segments in the first two categories ("<14" and "15 to 35"), and a line segment in the last category (">35") that is smoothly connected to the parabolic segment in the second category. (If we also wanted to force the log-rate curve in the first category to follow a line, we would remove Z_2 from the model.)

To plot or tabulate the curve from a spline model, we select a set of X_1 values spaced across the range of interest, compute the set of spline terms for each X_1 value, combine these terms with the coefficients in the model to get the model-predicted outcomes, and plot these predictions. To illustrate, suppose that X_1 is servings per week and we wish to plot model 20–45 with $\alpha = -6.00$, $\beta_1 = -0.010$, $\beta_2 = -0.001$, and $\beta_3 = 0.001$ over the range 0 to 50 servings per week in 5-serving increments. We then compute Z_1, Z_2, Z_3 at 0, 5, 10, ..., 50 servings per week, then compute the predicted rate

$$\exp(-6.00 - 0.010z_1 - 0.001z_2 + 0.001z_3)$$

at each set of Z_1, Z_2, Z_3 values and plot these predictions against the corresponding X_1 values 0, 5, 10, ..., 50. For example, at $X_1 = 40$ we get $Z_1 = 40$, $Z_2 = 40^2 - (40 - 35)^2 = 1{,}575$, and $Z_3 = (40 - 14)^2 - (40 - 35)^2 = 651$, for a predicted rate of

$$\exp[-6.00 - 0.010(40) - 0.001(1{,}575) + 0.001(651)] = 6.6/10{,}000 \text{ years}$$

As with other trend models, we may obtain model-adjusted trends by adding confounder terms to our spline models. The confounder terms may be splines or any other form we prefer; spline plotting will be simplified, however, if the confounders are centered before they are entered into the analysis, for then the above plotting method may be used without modification. Further discussions of splines and their application are given by Hastie and Tibshirani (1990), Wahba (1990), de Boor (2001), and Hastie et al. (2001).

MODELS FOR TREND VARIATION

We may allow trends to vary across regressor levels by entering products among regressor terms. For example, suppose that X_1, X_2, X_3 are power terms for fruit and vegetable intake, while W_1, W_2, W_3, W_4 are spline terms for age. To allow the fruit-vegetable trend in log rates to vary with age, we could enter into the model all $3 \cdot 4 = 12$ products of the X_j and W_k, along with the X_j and W_k. If in addition there is an indicator $Z_1 = 1$ for female, 0 for male, the resulting model is

$$\begin{aligned} &\ln[R(x_1, x_2, x_3, w_1, w_2, w_3, w_4, z_1)] \\ &\quad = \alpha + \beta_1 x_1 + \beta_2 x_2 + \beta_3 x_3 + \beta_4 w_1 + \beta_5 w_2 + \beta_6 w_3 + \beta_7 w_4 + \beta_8 z_1 \\ &\quad\quad + \gamma_{11} x_1 w_1 + \gamma_{12} x_1 w_2 + \cdots + \gamma_{33} x_3 w_3 + \gamma_{34} x_3 w_4 \end{aligned}$$

The same model form may be used if X_1, X_2, X_3 and W_1, W_2, W_3, W_4 represent category indicators or other terms for fruit-vegetable intake and age.

Models with products among multiple trend terms can be difficult to fit and may yield quite unstable results unless large numbers of cases are observed. Given enough data, however, such models can provide more realistic pictures of dose–response relations than can simpler models. Results from such models may be easily interpreted by plotting or tabulating the fitted trends for the key exposures of interest at various levels of the "modifying" regressors. In the preceding example, this process would involve plotting the model-fitted rates against fruit and vegetable intake for each of several ages (e.g., for ages evenly spaced within the range of case ages).

The results may also be summarized using standardization over the confounders and modifiers, which will be discussed in the next chapter.

EXTENSIONS OF LOGISTIC MODELS

Polytomous and continuous outcomes are often analyzed by reducing them to just two categories and applying a logistic model. For example, CD4 counts might be reduced to the dichotomy ≤ 200, >200; cancer outcomes might be reduced to cancer and no cancer. Alternatively, multiple categories may be created with one designated as a referent, and the other categories compared one at a time to the referent using separate logistic models for each comparison. Although they are not necessarily invalid, these approaches disregard the information contained in differences within categories, in differences between nonreference categories, and in ordering among the categories. As a result, models designed specifically for polytomous or continuous outcomes can yield far more precision and power than simple dichotomous-outcome analyses.

This section briefly describes several extensions of the multiple logistic model (equation 20–28) to polytomous and ordinal outcomes. Analogous extensions of other models are possible.

POLYTOMOUS LOGISTIC MODELS

Suppose that an outcome variable Y has $I+1$ mutually exclusive outcome categories or levels $y_0, \ldots, y_1$, where category y_0 is considered the reference category. The second part of Table 17–5 provides an example in which Y is a disease outcome variable, with $y_0 =$ all control diseases as the reference category, and $I = 7$ other categories $y_1, \ldots, y_7$ corresponding to the cancer outcomes listed in the table. Let $R_i(\mathbf{x})$ denote the average risk of falling in outcome category $y_i (i = 1, \ldots, I)$ given that the regressors $\mathbf{X}$ equal $\mathbf{x}$; that is, let

$$R_i(\mathbf{x}) = \Pr(Y = y_i|\mathbf{X} = \mathbf{x})$$

The *polytomous logistic model* for this risk is then

$$R_i(\mathbf{x}) = \frac{\exp(\alpha_i + \mathbf{x}\boldsymbol{\beta}_i)}{1 + \sum_{j=1}^{I} \exp(\alpha_j + \mathbf{x}\boldsymbol{\beta}_j)} \quad [20\text{–}46]$$

For the example in the second part of Table 17–5, this is a model for the risk of falling in cancer category y_i $(i = 1, \ldots, 7)$. When Y has only two levels, I equals 1, and so formula 20–46 simplifies to the multiple logistic model (equation 20–28).

Model 20–46 represents I separate risk equations, one for each nonreference outcome level $y_1, \ldots, y_I$. Each equation has its own intercept α_i and vector of coefficients $\boldsymbol{\beta}_i = (\beta_{i1}, \ldots, \beta_{in})$, with a distinct coefficient β_{ik} corresponding to every combination of a regressor X_k and nonreference outcome level y_i $(i = 1, \ldots, I)$. Thus, with n regressors in $\mathbf{X}$, the polytomous logistic model involves I intercepts and $I \cdot n$ regressor coefficients. For example, with seven nonreference outcome levels and three regressors, the model would involve seven intercepts and $7 \cdot 3 = 21$ regressor coefficients, for a total of 28 model parameters.

The polytomous logistic model can be written more simply as a model for the odds. To see this, note that the risk of falling in the reference category must equal 1 minus the sum of the risks of falling in the nonreference categories:

$$R_0(\mathbf{x}) = \Pr(Y = y_0|\mathbf{X} = \mathbf{x})$$

$$= 1 - \sum_{i=1}^{I} \exp(\alpha_i + \mathbf{x}\boldsymbol{\beta}_i)/[1 + \sum_{j=1}^{I} \exp(\alpha_j + \mathbf{x}\boldsymbol{\beta}_j)]$$

$$= 1/[1 + \sum_{j=1}^{I} \exp(\alpha_j + \mathbf{x}\boldsymbol{\beta}_j)] \qquad [20\text{–}47]$$

Dividing equation 20–47 into 20–46, we get a model for $O_i(\mathbf{x}) = R_i(\mathbf{x})/R_0(\mathbf{x})$ = the odds of falling in outcome category y_i versus category y_0:

$$O_i(x) = \frac{\exp(\alpha_i + \mathbf{x}\boldsymbol{\beta}_i)/[1 + \sum_j \exp(\alpha_j + \mathbf{x}\boldsymbol{\beta}_j)]}{1/[1 + \sum_j \exp(\alpha_j + \mathbf{x}\boldsymbol{\beta}_j)]}$$

$$= \exp(\alpha_i + \mathbf{x}\boldsymbol{\beta}_i) \qquad [20\text{–}48]$$

This form of the model provides a familiar interpretation for the coefficients. Suppose $\mathbf{x_1}$ and $\mathbf{x_0}$ are two different vectors of values for the regressors $\mathbf{X}$. Then the ratio of the odds of falling in category y_i versus y_0 when $\mathbf{X} = \mathbf{x}^*$ versus $\mathbf{X} = \mathbf{x}$ is

$$\frac{O_i(\mathbf{x}^*)}{O_i(\mathbf{x})} = \frac{\exp(\alpha_i + \mathbf{x}^*\boldsymbol{\beta}_i)}{\exp(\alpha_i + \mathbf{x}\boldsymbol{\beta}_i)} = \exp[(\mathbf{x}^* - \mathbf{x})\boldsymbol{\beta}_i]$$

From this equation, we see that the antilog $\exp(\beta_{ik})$ of a coefficient β_{ik} corresponds to the proportionate change in the odds of outcome y_i versus y_0 when the regressor X_k increases by 1 unit.

The polytomous logistic model is most useful when the levels of Y have no meaningful order, as with the cancer types in Table 17–5. For further reading about the model, see McCullagh and Nelder (1989) and Hosmer and Lemeshow (2000).

ORDINAL LOGISTIC MODELS

Suppose that the levels $y_0, \ldots, y_I$ of Y follow a natural order. Order arises, for example, when Y is a clinical scale, such as y_0 = normal, y_1 = dysplasia, y_2 = neoplasia, rather than just a cancer indicator; Y is a count, such as number of malformations found in an individual; or the Y levels represent categories of a physical quantity, such as CD4 count (e.g., >500, 200 to 500, <200). There are at least four different ways to extend the logistic model to such outcomes.

Recall that the logistic model is equivalent to an exponential odds model. One extension uses an exponential model to represent the odds of falling in outcome category y_i versus falling in category y_{i-1} (the next lowest category):

$$\frac{R_i(\mathbf{x})}{R_{i-1}(\mathbf{x})} = \frac{\Pr(Y = y_i|\mathbf{X} = \mathbf{x})}{\Pr(Y = y_{i-1}|\mathbf{X} = \mathbf{x})} = \exp(\alpha_i^* + \mathbf{x}\boldsymbol{\beta}^*) \qquad [20\text{–}49]$$

for $i = 1, \ldots, I$. This may be called the *adjacent-category logistic model,* because taking logarithms of both sides yields the equivalent *adjacent-category logit* model (Agresti, 2002). It may be seen as a special case of the polytomous logistic model: From formula 20–48, the polytomous logistic model implies that

$$\frac{R_i(\mathbf{x})}{R_{i-1}(\mathbf{x})} = \frac{R_i(\mathbf{x})/R_0(\mathbf{x})}{R_{i-1}(\mathbf{x})/R_0(\mathbf{x})} = \frac{\exp(\alpha_i + \mathbf{x}\boldsymbol{\beta}_i)}{\exp(\alpha_{i-1} + \mathbf{x}\boldsymbol{\beta}_{i-1})}$$

$$= \exp[(\alpha_i - \alpha_{i-1}) + \mathbf{x}(\boldsymbol{\beta}_i - \boldsymbol{\beta}_{i-1})]$$

The adjacent-category logistic model sets $\alpha_i^* = \alpha_i - \alpha_{i-1}$, and forces the I coefficient differences $\boldsymbol{\beta}_i - \boldsymbol{\beta}_{i-1}$ ($i = 1, \ldots, I$) to equal a common value $\boldsymbol{\beta}^*$. If there is a natural distance d_i between adjacent outcome categories y_i and y_{i-1} (such as the difference between the category means), the model can be modified to use these distances as follows:

$$R_i(\mathbf{x})/R_{i-1}(\mathbf{x}) = \exp(\alpha_i^* + \mathbf{x}\boldsymbol{\beta}^* d_i) \qquad [20\text{–}50]$$

for $i = 1, \ldots, I$. This model allows the coefficient differences $\boldsymbol{\beta}_i - \boldsymbol{\beta}_{i-1}$ to vary with the distances d_i between categories. For further discussion of adjacent-category models, see Agresti (2002) and Greenland (1994a).

A different extension uses an exponential model to represent the odds of falling *above* category y_i versus falling *in or below* category y_i:

$$\frac{\Pr(Y > y_i|\mathbf{X} = \mathbf{x})}{\Pr(Y \leq y_i|\mathbf{X} = \mathbf{x})} = \exp(\alpha_i^* + \mathbf{x}\boldsymbol{\beta}^*) \qquad [20\text{–}51]$$

where $i = 0, \ldots,$ I. This is called the *cumulative-odds* or *proportional-odds* model. It can be derived by assuming that Y was obtained by categorizing a special type of continuous variable (McCullagh and Nelder, 1989). Yet another extension uses an exponential model to represent the odds of falling *above* outcome category y_i versus *in* category y_i:

$$\frac{\Pr(Y > y_i|\mathbf{X} = \mathbf{x})}{\Pr(Y = y_i|\mathbf{X} = \mathbf{x})} = \exp(\alpha_i^* + \mathbf{x}\boldsymbol{\beta}^*) \qquad [20\text{–}52]$$

where $i = 0, \ldots, I$. This is called the *continuation-ratio model.* A similar extension uses an exponential model to represent the odds of falling *in* category y_i versus falling *below* y_i:

$$\frac{\Pr(Y = y_i|\mathbf{X} = \mathbf{x})}{\Pr(Y < y_i|\mathbf{X} = \mathbf{x})} = \exp(\alpha_i^* + \mathbf{x}\boldsymbol{\beta}^*) \qquad [20\text{–}53]$$

where $i = 1, \ldots, I$. This model may be called the *reverse continuation-ratio model.* It can be derived by reversing the order of the Y levels in model 20–52, but in any given application it is not equivalent to model 20–52 (Greenland, 1994a).

Certain guidelines may be of use for choosing among ordinal models, although none is absolute. First, the adjacent-category and cumulative-odds models are *reversible,* in that only the signs of the coefficients change if the order of the Y levels is reversed. In contrast, the two continuation-ratio models are not reversible. This observation suggests that the continuation-ratio models may be more appropriate for modeling irreversible disease stages (e.g., osteoarthritic severity), whereas the adjacent-category and cumulative-odds models may be more appropriate for potentially reversible outcomes (such as cell counts) (Greenland, 1994a). Second, because the coefficients of adjacent-category models contrast pairs of categories, the model appears best suited for discrete outcomes with few levels (e.g., cell types along a normal–dysplastic–neoplastic scale). Third, because the cumulative-odds model can be derived from categorizing certain special types of continuous outcomes, it is often considered most appropriate when the outcome under study is derived by categorizing a single underlying continuum (e.g., blood pressure) (McCullagh and Nelder, 1989). For a more detailed comparative discussion of ordinal logistic models and guidelines for their use, see Greenland (1994a).

All the preceding ordinal models simplify to the ordinary logistic model when there are only two outcome categories ($I = 2$). They can also be applied to continuous Y, although most software requires categorizing Y for this purpose. Categorization may be a problem insofar as results from all the preceding models (including the cumulative-odds model) can be sensitive to the choice of the Y categories (Greenland, 1994a; Strömberg, 1996). One advantage of the continuation-ratio models (20–52 and 20–53) over their competitors is that they can be fitted with ordinary software without categorization of Y, even if Y is continuous (Greenland, 1994a). The primary caution is that conditional maximum likelihood (see Chapters 15 and 21) must be used for model fitting if the observed outcomes are sparsely scattered across the levels of Y (as will be inevitable if Y is continuous). If Y is continuous (e.g., BMI, blood pressure, etc.), this requirement can be met by using a Cox (proportional-hazards) regression program to fit the models, as follows: Let $y_{\min}$ and $y_{\max}$ be the minimum and maximum values of Y in the data. Then model 20–52 can be fitted by using $T = Y - y_{\min} + 1$ as the survival-time variable in the program, whereas model 20–53 can be fitted by using $T = y_{\max} - Y + 1$ as the survival-time variable.

Finally, all the above models can be generalized to allow variation in the coefficients $\boldsymbol{\beta}$ across levels of Y, as in the polytomous logistic model (Peterson and Harrell, 1990; Greenland, 1994a; Ananth and Kleinbaum, 1997; Cole and Ananth, 2001; Kuss, 2006). When this variation is modeled, the adjacent-category model is known as the *stereotype* model.

GENERALIZED LINEAR MODELS

Consider again the exponential risk and rate models,

$$R(\mathbf{x}) = \exp(\alpha + \mathbf{x}\boldsymbol{\beta}) \qquad \text{and} \qquad I(\mathbf{x}) = \exp(\alpha + \mathbf{x}\boldsymbol{\beta})$$

and the logistic risk model,

$$R(\mathbf{x}) = \text{expit}(\alpha + \mathbf{x}\boldsymbol{\beta})$$

We can replace the "exp" in the exponential models and the "expit" in the logistic model by other reasonable functions. In fact, each of these models is of the general form

$$E(Y|\mathbf{X} = \mathbf{x}) = f(\alpha + \mathbf{x}\boldsymbol{\beta}) \qquad [20\text{–}54]$$

where $f(u)$ is a function that is smooth and strictly increasing as u increases. That is, as $\alpha + \mathbf{x}\boldsymbol{\beta}$ gets larger, $f(\alpha + \mathbf{x}\boldsymbol{\beta})$ gets larger, but it never jumps or bends suddenly.

For any such function $f(u)$, there is always an inverse function $g(v)$ that "undoes" $f(u)$, in the sense that $g[f(u)] = u$ whenever $f(u)$ is defined. Hence, a general form equivalent to 20–54 is

$$g[E(Y|\mathbf{X} = \mathbf{x})] = \alpha + \mathbf{x}\boldsymbol{\beta} \qquad [20\text{–}55]$$

A model of the form 20–55 is called *a generalized linear model*. The function $g(v)$ is called the *link function* for the model; thus, the link function is $\ln(v)$ for the log-linear model and logit(v) for the logit-linear model. The term $\alpha + \mathbf{x}\boldsymbol{\beta}$ is called the *linear predictor* for the model and is often abbreviated η (Greek letter eta); that is, $\eta = \alpha + \mathbf{x}\boldsymbol{\beta}$ by definition.

Almost all the models in the chapter are generalized linear models. Ordinary linear models (such as the linear risk model) are the simplest examples, in which $f(u)$ and $g(v)$ are both the identity function, i.e., $f(u) = u$ and $g(v) = v$, so that

$$E(Y|\mathbf{X} = \mathbf{x}) = \alpha + \mathbf{x}\boldsymbol{\beta}$$

The inverse of the exponential function $\exp(u)$ is the natural log function $\ln(v)$. Hence the generalized-linear forms of the exponential risk and rate models are the log-linear risk and rate models

$$\ln[R(\mathbf{x})] = \alpha + \mathbf{x}\boldsymbol{\beta} \quad \text{and} \quad \ln[I(\mathbf{x})] = \alpha + \mathbf{x}\boldsymbol{\beta}$$

Thus the exponential risk and rate models correspond to a natural-log link function, because $\ln[\exp(u)] = u$. Similarly, the inverse of the logistic function expit(u) is the logit function logit(v). Hence the generalized-linear form of the logistic-risk model is the logit-linear risk model

$$\text{logit}[R(\mathbf{x})] = \alpha + \mathbf{x}\boldsymbol{\beta}$$

Thus the logistic model corresponds to the logit link function, because logit[expit(u)] $= u$.

The choices for f and g are virtually unlimited. In epidemiology, however, only the logit link $g(v) = \text{logit}(v)$ is in common use for risks, and only the log link $g(v) = \ln(v)$ is in common use for rates. These link functions are almost always the software default, and are sometimes the only options in software for risk and rate modeling. Some packages, however, allow selection of linear risk, rate, or odds models, and some allow users to define their own link function.

The choice of link function can have a profound effect on the shape of the trend or dose–response surface allowed by the model, especially if exposure is represented by only one or two terms. For example, if exposure is represented by a single term $\beta_1 x_1$ in a risk model, use of the identity link results in a linear risk model and a linear trend for risk; use of the log link results in an exponential (log-linear) risk model and an exponential trend for risk; and use of a logit link results in a logistic model and an exponential trend for the odds.

Generalized linear models differ from transformed-outcome models in that they transform the regression (conditional expectation) of Y by a link function g before imposing linearity assumptions, rather than by transforming Y itself. The generalized linear forms (20–54 and 20–55) may thus be applied to any type of outcome, including a discrete or continuous Y. They may even be combined with a transformation $h(Y)$ of Y to create a generalized linear model for the transformed outcome,

$$g\{E[h(Y)|\mathbf{X} = \mathbf{x}]\} = \alpha + \mathbf{x}\boldsymbol{\beta}$$

and (as always) the variables in **X** may be transforms of the original regressors. Because of their great flexibility, generalized linear models encompass a much broader range of forms for risks and rates than the linear, log-linear, and logistic models. One example is the complementary log-log risk model,

$$R(\mathbf{x}) = 1 - \exp[-\exp(\alpha + \mathbf{x}\boldsymbol{\beta})]$$

which translates to the generalized linear form

$$\ln\{-\ln[1 - R(\mathbf{x})]\} = \alpha + \mathbf{x}\boldsymbol{\beta}$$

This model corresponds to the link function $\ln[-\ln(1 - v)]$ and arises naturally in certain biology experiments. For further reading on generalized linear models, see McCullagh and Nelder (1989), Dobson (2001), Hardin and Hilbe (2001), McCulloch and Searle (2001), and Hoffman (2003).

CHAPTER 21

Introduction to Regression Modeling

Sander Greenland

Model Searching 419
Role of Prior Information 419
Selection Strategies 420
Model Fitting 421
Residual Distributions 421
Overdispersion 422
Sample-Size Considerations 422
Data Grouping and Count Data 423
Model Checking 423
Tabular Checks 423
Tests of Regression and R^2 424
Tests of Fit 425
Global Tests of Fit 427
Model Diagnostics 427
Delta-Beta Analysis 428
Resampling Analysis and Bootstrapping 428
Model Sensitivity Analysis 429
Modeling in Unmatched Case-Control Studies and Related Designs 429
Multiplicative-Intercept Models for Density Studies 430
Multiplicative-Intercept Models for Cumulative and Prevalence Studies 431
Other Models for Case-Control Studies 431
Case-Cohort and Two-Stage Studies 432
Stratified Models 432
Modeling Matched Data 434
Hierarchical (Multilevel) Regression 435
Why Add a Second Stage? 436
Specifying the Prior Standard Deviation 437
Hierarchical Regression and Model Selection 437
Smoothing with Hierarchical Regression 438
Summary 439
Model-Based Estimates of Incidence and Prevalence 439
Nonparametric Regression 440
Model-Based Standardization 442
Standardization Using Outcome Models 443
Standardized Measures versus Coefficients 443
Standardization Using Full-Data Models 444
Standardization Using Exposure Models: Inverse-Probability Weighting 444
Standardization in Case-Control Studies 445
Marginal-Outcome Modeling 446
Scoring Methods 446
Confounder Scores and Balancing Scores 446
Outcome Scores 447
Exposure Scores 447
Outcome versus Exposure Modeling 449
Model Combination and Doubly Robust Estimation 450
Scoring in Case-Control Studies 451
Modeling Longitudinal Data 451
Time-Dependent Exposures and Covariates 452
Recurrent Outcomes 452
Structural Models and g-Estimation 453

Chapter 20 provided an introduction to regression concepts and basic model forms. The present chapter provides brief introductions to the following topics: model selection; model fitting; model checking; modeling of case-control, stratified, and matched data; and the more general techniques of hierarchical and nonparametric regression, which address certain limitations of conventional modeling approaches. It then discusses model-based estimation of incidence, prevalence, and standardized (marginal) measures of effect, including inverse-probability-weighting and confounder-scoring methods. It closes with a brief overview of longitudinal data analysis.

MODEL SEARCHING

How do we find a model or set of models that will be acceptable for our purposes? There are far too many model forms to allow us to examine most or even much of the total realm of possibilities. There are several systematic, mechanical, and traditional algorithms for finding models (such as stepwise and best-subset regression) that lack logical or statistical justification and that perform poorly in theory, simulations, and case studies; see Sclove et al. (1972), Bancroft and Han (1977), Draper et al. (1979), Freedman (1983), Flack and Chang (1987), Freedman et al. (1988), Hurvich and Tsai (1990), Faraway (1992), Weiss (1995), Greenland (1993b, 2000c, 2001b), Harrell (2001), and Viallefont et al. (2001).

One serious problem is that the P-values and standard errors (SE) obtained from the final model after variables are selected using significance-testing criteria (such as "F-to-enter" and "F-to-remove") will be downwardly biased, usually to a large degree. In particular, the SE estimates obtained from the selected model ignore the variability induced by model selection, thus underestimating the standard deviations (SDs) of the point estimates obtained by applying the algorithms across different random samples. As a result, the final models selected by the algorithms will tend to yield P-values that are much too small and confidence intervals that are much too narrow (and hence fail to cover the true coefficient values with the stated frequency); see the citations in the preceding paragraph. Unfortunately, significance-testing with no accounting for selection is the basis for most variable-selection procedures in standard packaged software.

Other criteria for selecting variables, such as "change-in-point-estimate" criteria, do not necessarily perform better than significance testing; for example, see Maldonado and Greenland (1993a). Viable alternatives to significance testing in model selection have emerged only gradually with advances in computing and with deeper insights into the problem of model selection. We outline the conventional approaches after first reinforcing one of the most essential and neglected starting points for good modeling: laying out existing information in a manner that can help avoid models that are in conflict with established facts. In a later section, we describe an alternative to model selection provided by hierarchical regression.

ROLE OF PRIOR INFORMATION

The dependence of regression results on the chosen model can be either an advantage or a drawback. When simple tabular analyses (Chapters 14 through 17) require severe simplification of the analysis variables, use of a model structure that is capable of reasonably approximating reality can improve the accuracy of the estimates by avoiding such reduction. On the other hand, use of a model that is incapable of even approximating reality can decrease accuracy to less than that of tabular analysis.

This trade-off underscores the desirability of using flexible (and possibly complex) models. One should take care to avoid models that are entirely unsupported by background knowledge. For example, in a cohort study of lung cancer, it is reasonable to restrict rates to increase with age, because there is enormous background literature documenting that this trend is found in all human populations. In contrast, one would want to avoid restricting cardiovascular disease (CVD) rates to increase strictly with alcohol consumption, because there is evidence suggesting that the alcohol–CVD relation is not strictly increasing (Maclure, 1993).

Prior knowledge about most epidemiologic relations is usually too limited to provide much guidance in model selection. A natural response might be to use models that are as flexible as possible (a flexible model can reproduce a wide variety of curves and surfaces). Unfortunately, flexible models have limitations. The more flexible the model, the larger is the sample needed for the usual estimation methods (such as maximum likelihood) to provide approximately unbiased coefficient estimates. Also, after a certain point, increasing flexibility may increase variability of estimates so much that the accuracy of the estimates is decreased relative to estimates from simpler models, despite the greater faithfulness of the flexible model to reality. As a result, it is usual practice to employ models that are severely restrictive in arbitrary ways, such as logistic models (Robins and Greenland, 1986).

Fortunately, estimates obtained from the most common epidemiologic regression models, exponential (log-linear) and logistic models, retain some interpretability even when the underlying (true) regression function is not particularly close to those forms (Maldonado and Greenland, 1993b, 1994). For example, under common conditions, rate- or risk-ratio estimates obtained from those models can be interpreted as approximate estimates of standardized rate or risk ratios, using the total source population as the standard (Greenland and Maldonado, 1994). To ensure that such interpretations are reasonable, the model used should at least be able to replicate qualitative features of the underlying regression function. For example, if the underlying regression may have a reversal in the slope of the exposure–response curve, we should use a model that is capable of exhibiting such reversal (even if it cannot replicate the exact shape of the true curve).

SELECTION STRATEGIES

Even with ample prior information, there will always be an overwhelming number of model choices, and so model search strategies are needed. Many strategies have been proposed, although none has been fully justified.

Some strategies begin by specifying a minimal model form that is among the most simple credible forms. Here "credible" means "compatible with available information." Thus, we start with a model of minimal computational or conceptual complexity that does not conflict with background information. There may be many such models; in order to help ensure that our analysis is credible to the intended audience, however, the starting model form should be one that most researchers will view as a reasonable possibility.

To specify a simple yet credible model form, one needs some knowledge of the background scientific literature on the relations under study. This knowledge includes information about relations of potential confounders to the study exposures and study diseases, as well as relations of study exposures to the study diseases. Thus, specification of a simple yet credible model can demand much more initial effort than is routinely used in model specification.

Once we have specified a minimal starting model, we can add complexities that seem necessary (by some criteria) in light of the data. Such a search process is an *expanding* search (Leamer, 1978). Its chief drawback is that often there are too many possible expansions to consider within a reasonable length of time. If, however, one neglects to consider any possible expansion, one risks missing an important shortcoming of the initial model. As a general example, if our minimal model involves only first-order (linear) terms for 12 variables, we have $\binom{12}{2} = 66$ possible two-way products among these variables to consider, as well as 12 quadratic terms, for a total of 78 possible expansions with just one second-order term. An analyst may not have the time, patience, or resources to examine all the possibilities in detail; this predicament usually leads to use of automatic significance-testing procedures to select additional terms, which (as mentioned above) can lead to distorted statistics.

Some strategies begin by specifying an initial model form that is flexible enough to approximate any credible model form. A flexible starting point can be less demanding than a simple one in terms of the need for background information. For example, rather than concern ourselves with what the literature suggests about the shape of a dose–response curve, we can employ a starting model form that can approximate a wide range of curves. Similarly, rather than concern ourselves with what the literature suggests about joint effects, we can employ a form that can approximate a wide range of joint effects. We can then search for a simpler but adequate model by removing from the flexible model any complexities that appear to be unnecessary in light of the data. Such a search process, based on simplifying a complex model, is a *contracting* or simplifying search (Leamer, 1978).

The chief drawback of a purely contracting search is that a sufficiently flexible prior model may be too complex to fit to the available data. This drawback arises because more complex models generally involve more parameters; with more parameters in a model, more data are needed to produce trustworthy point and interval estimates. Conventional model-fitting methods may yield biased estimates or may completely fail to yield any estimates (e.g., not converge) if the fitted model is too complex. For example, if our flexible model for 12 variables contains all first- and second-order terms, there will be 12 first-order plus 12 quadratic plus 66 product terms, for a total of 90 coefficients. Fitting this model by conventional methods may be well beyond what our data can support.

Because of potential fitting problems, contracting searches begin with something much less than a fully flexible model. Some begin with a model as flexible as can be fitted, or maximal model. As with minimal models, maximal models are not unique. In order to produce a model that can be fitted with conventional methods, one may have to limit flexibility of dose–response, flexibility of joint effects, or both. It is also possible to start a model search anywhere in between the extremes of minimal and maximal models, and proceed by expanding as seems necessary and contracting as seems reasonable based on the data (although, again, resource limitations often lead to mechanical use of significance tests for this process). Unsurprisingly, such *stepwise* searches share some advantages and disadvantages with purely expanding and purely contracting searches. Like other searches, care should be taken to ensure that the starting and ending points do not conflict with prior information.

The results obtained following a model search can be very sensitive to the choice of starting model. One can check for this problem by conducting several searches, starting at different models. Nonetheless, there are always far too many possible models to search through them all, and with many variables to consider, model search strategies always risk producing a misleading model form. Modern methods to address this problem and other modeling issues can be found in the literature on statistical learning, for example, under topics such as cross-validation, model averaging, nonparametric regression, smoothing, and boosting (Hastie et al., 2001). There is also a large Bayesian literature on the topic (e.g., Brown et al., 2002). Some of these methods reduce the selection problem by merging models or their results, for example, by averaging over competing models (Draper, 1995; Raftery, 1995; Carlin and Louis, 2000; Hastie et al., 2001; Viallefont et al., 2001), by using inferential methods that account for the selection process (Ye, 1998; Hastie et al., 2001; Harrell, 2001; Efron, 2004; Shen et al., 2004), or by embedding the models in a hierarchical model that contains them all as special cases (Greenland, 1999).

The literature on model selection and averaging has focused largely on prediction problems, but it has begun to influence causal-inference methodology (Hill and McCulloch, 2008) and has close connections to several topics that we discuss later. As discussed in later sections, hierarchical modeling can be used for model averaging and smoothing, and any prediction method can be used as part of standardized effect estimation. Penalized fitting and other shrinkage methods also allow fitting of much larger models than feasible with conventional methods, often eliminating the need for variable selection in confounding control (Greenland, 2008).

MODEL FITTING

RESIDUAL DISTRIBUTIONS

Conventional model-fitting methods correspond to the estimation methods for categorical analyses, as described in Chapters 13 through 16. Different fitting methods lead to different estimates, and so in presenting results one should specify the method used to derive the estimates. The vast majority of programs use *maximum-likelihood* (ML) estimation, which is based on very specific assumptions about how the observed values of Y tend to distribute (vary) when the vector of regressors $\mathbf{X}$ is fixed at a given value x. This distribution is called the (random) error distribution or *residual distribution* of Y.

If Y is the person-time rate observed at a given value $\mathbf{x}$ of $\mathbf{X}$, and T is the corresponding observed person-time, it is conventionally assumed that the number of cases observed, $A = YT$, will tend to vary according to a Poisson distribution if the person-time is fixed at its observed value (see Chapter 14). Hence, conventional ML regression analysis of person-time rates is usually called *Poisson regression*. If, on the other hand, Y is the proportion of cases observed at a given value $\mathbf{x}$ of $\mathbf{X}$ out of a person-count total N, it is conventionally assumed that the number of cases observed, $A = YN$, will tend to vary according to a *binomial distribution* if the number of persons (person count) N is fixed at its observed value. Hence, conventional ML regression analysis of prevalence or incidence proportions (average risks) is sometimes called *binomial regression*. Note that if $N = 1$, the proportion diseased Y can be only 0 or 1; in this situation, $A = YN$ can be only 0 or 1 and is said to have a Bernoulli distribution (which is just a binomial distribution with $N = 1$).

The binomial distribution can be deduced from the homogeneity and independence assumptions discussed in Chapter 14. As noted there, its use is inadvisable if there are important violations of either assumption, e.g., if the disease is contagious over the study period.

If Y is the number of exposed cases in a 2×2 table, the conventionally assumed distribution for Y is the *hypergeometric*. As discussed in Chapter 14, ML fitting in this situation is usually referred to as *conditional maximum likelihood* (CML). CML fitting is closely related to partial-likelihood methods, which are used for fitting Cox models in survival analysis. More details on maximum-likelihood model fitting can be found in textbooks on nonlinear regression, such as McCullagh and Nelder (1989), Clayton and Hills (1993), Hosmer and Lemeshow (2000), Agresti (2002), Dobson (2001), Hardin and Hilbe (2001), McCulloch and Searle (2001), and Hoffman (2003).

OVERDISPERSION

What if the residual distribution of the observed Y does *not* follow the conventionally assumed residual distribution? Under a broad range of conditions, it can be shown that the resulting ML-fitted values (ML estimates) will remain approximately unbiased if no other source of bias is present (White, 1982a, 1993; Royall, 1986). Nonetheless, the estimated SDs obtained from the program will be biased. In particular, if the actual variance of Y given $\mathbf{X} = \mathbf{x}$ (the *residual variance*) is greater than that implied by the conventional distribution, Y is said to suffer from *overdispersion* or *extravariation*, and the estimated SDs and P-values obtained from an ordinary maximum-likelihood regression program will be too small.

In Poisson regression, overdispersion is sometimes called "extra-Poisson variation"; in binomial regression, overdispersion is sometimes called "extra-binomial variation." Typically, such overdispersion arises when there is dependence among the recorded outcomes, as when the outcome Y is the number infected in a group, or Y is the number of times a person gets a disease. As an example, suppose that Y is the number of eyes affected by glaucoma in an individual. In a natural population, $Y = 0$ for most people and $Y = 2$ for most of the remainder, with $Y = 1$ very infrequently. In other words, the Y values will be largely limited to the extremes of 0 and 2. In contrast, a binomially distributed variable with the same possible values (0, 1, or 2) and the same mean as Y will have a higher probability of 1 than 2, and hence a smaller variance than Y (these facts may be deduced from the binomial formula in Chapter 13).

Two major approaches have been developed to cope with potential overdispersion, both of which are based on modeling the residual distribution. One approach is to use maximum likelihood, but with a residual distribution that allows a broader range of variation for Y, such as the negative binomial in place of the Poisson or the beta-binomial in place of the binomial (McCullagh and Nelder, 1989). Such approaches can be computationally intensive, but they have been implemented in some software. The second and simpler approach is to model only the residual variance of Y, rather than specify the residual distribution completely. Fitting methods that employ this approach are discussed by various authors under the topics of quasi-likelihood, pseudo-likelihood, and estimating-equation methods; see McCullagh and Nelder (1989), McCullagh (1991), and Diggle et al. (2002) for descriptions of these methods. Interestingly, Mantel-Haenszel methods can be viewed as special cases of such methods applied to categorical data (Liang, 1987; Schouten et al., 1993).

SAMPLE-SIZE CONSIDERATIONS

One drawback of all the fitting methods discussed so far is that they depend on some sort of "large-sample" (asymptotic) approximations, which usually require that the number of parameters in the model be much less than (roughly, not more than 10% of) the number of cases observed (Pike et al., 1980; Peduzzi et al., 1996), although in some examples even a 10:1 case:parameter ratio is insufficient (Greenland et al., 2000a). When the sample size is insufficient, highly distorted estimates (i.e., sparse-data bias) may occur without warning.

Methods that do not use large-sample approximations (exact methods) can be used to fit certain models. These methods require the same residual-distribution assumptions as maximum-likelihood methods, however. An example is exact logistic regression (Hirji, 2006). Unfortunately, exact fitting methods for incidence and prevalence models are so computationally demanding that they cannot fit models as complex as can be fit with other methods, and they incur methodologic objections based on their failure to constrain the size of the estimated relative risks when such constraints are most needed (see Chapter 18). Alternative approaches are available that meet these objections and permit fitting of incidence and prevalence models while retaining approximately valid small-sample results. These alternatives include *penalized-likelihood estimation* and related "shrinkage" methods of Stein estimation, random-coefficient regression, ridge regression, and Bayesian regression (Efron and Morris, 1975; Copas, 1983; Titterington, 1985; Carlin and Louis, 2000; Gelman et al., 2003; Greenland 2000c, 2001b, 2007a). Penalized likelihood can also be used for fitting hierarchical models, and can in fact be viewed as a form of hierarchical modeling, which will be discussed later.

DATA GROUPING AND COUNT DATA

The usual input to regression programs is in the form of an observed numerator of case counts and a corresponding denominator of counts or person-time, one pair for each observed value **x** of the vector of regressors **X**. It is commonly thought that rate models such as equation 20-17 require the regressors to be grouped into categories. This is not so: Most rate-regression programs can make use of ungrouped regressor data, in which an individual record contains an indicator of whether the individual got disease, which serves as the case count (1 if the individual got disease, 0 if not) and also contains the person-time at risk observed for the person. The only issue is then whether there are sufficient data overall to allow the fitting methods to work properly (Greenland et al., 2000a).

Conversely, suppose that each component of **X** is a categorical (discrete) variable, such as marital status, parity, sex, and age category. The multiway contingency table formed by cross-classifying all subjects on each **X** component then has a cell for each value **x** of **X**. Such tables are often analyzed using a log-linear model for the number of observations (subject count) $A_{\mathbf{x}}$ expected in cell **x** of the table, $\ln(A_{\mathbf{x}}) = \alpha + \mathbf{x}\boldsymbol{\beta}$. Although software for log-linear count modeling is available in some packages, count data can be easily analyzed using any program for Poisson (rate) regression, by entering $A_{\mathbf{x}}$ as the rate numerator at regressor value **x**, and giving each count a person-time denominator of 1. This approach eliminates the need for special software and provides greater modeling flexibility than is available in many tabular-analysis packages.

MODEL CHECKING

It is important to check a fitted model against the data. The extent of these checks may depend on what purpose we want the model to serve. At one extreme, we may only want the fitted model to provide approximately valid *summary* estimates or trends for a few key relationships. For example, we may want only to estimate the average increment in risk produced by a unit increase in exposure. At the other extreme, we may want the model to provide approximately valid *regressor-specific* predictions of outcomes, such as exposure-specific risks by age, sex, and ethnicity. The latter goal is more demanding and requires more detailed scrutiny of results, sometimes on a subject-by-subject basis.

Model diagnostics can detect discrepancies between data and a model only within the range of the data, and then only when there are enough observations to provide adequate diagnostic power. For example, there has been much controversy concerning the health effects of "low-dose" radiation exposure (exposures that are only modestly in excess of natural background levels). This controversy arose because the natural incidence of key outcomes (such as leukemia) is low, and few cases had been observed in "low-dose" cohorts. As a result, several proposed dose–response models "fitted the data adequately" in the low-dose region, in that each model passed the conventional battery of diagnostic checks. Nonetheless, the health effects predicted by these models conflicted to an important extent.

More generally, one should bear in mind that a good-fitting model is not the same as a correct model. In particular, a model may appear to be correct in the central range of the data but produce grossly misleading predictions for combinations of covariate values that are poorly represented or absent in the data.

TABULAR CHECKS

Both tabular methods (such as Mantel-Haenszel) and regression methods produce estimates by merging assumptions about population structure (such as that of a common odds ratio or of an explicit regression model) with observed data. When an estimate is derived using a regression model, especially one with many regressors, it may become difficult to judge how much the estimate reflects the data and how much it reflects the model.

To investigate the source of results, we recommend that one compare model-based results to the corresponding tabular (categorical-analysis) results. As an illustration, suppose we wish to check a logistic model in which X_1 is the exposure under study, and four other regressors, X_2, X_3, X_4, and X_5, appear in the model, with X_1, X_2, X_3 continuous, X_4, X_5 binary, and products among X_1, X_2, and X_4 in the model. Any regressor in a model must appear in the corresponding tabular analysis. Because X_2 and X_4 appear in products with X_1 and the model is logistic, they should be treated as modifiers of the X_1 odds ratio in the corresponding tabular analysis. X_3 and X_5 do not appear in products with X_1 and so should be treated as pure confounders (adjustment variables) in the corresponding tabular analysis. Because X_1, X_2, X_3 are continuous in the model, they must have at least three levels in the tabular analysis, so that the results can at least crudely reflect trends seen with the model. If all three of these regressors are categorized into four levels, the resulting table of disease (two levels) by all regressors will have $2 \cdot 4^3 \cdot 2^2 = 512$ cells, and perhaps many zero cells.

From this table, we can attempt to compute three (for exposure strata 1, 2, and 3 versus 0) adjusted odds ratios (e.g., using the Mantel-Haenszel summary) for each of the $4 \times 2 = 8$ combinations of X_2 and X_4, adjusting all $3 \times 8 = 24$ odds ratios for the $4 \times 2 = 8$ pure-confounder levels. Some of these 24 adjusted odds ratios may be infinite or undefined as a result of small numbers, which will indicate that the corresponding regression estimates are largely model projections. Similarly, the tabular estimates may not exhibit a pattern seen in the regression estimates, which will suggest that the pattern was induced by the regression model rather than the data. For example, the regression estimates might exhibit a monotone trend with increasing exposure even if the tabular estimates did not. Interpretation of such a conflict will depend on the context: If we are certain that dose–response is monotone (e.g., smoking and esophageal cancer), the monotonicity of the regression estimates will favor their use over the tabular results; in contrast, doubts about monotonicity (e.g., as with alcohol and coronary heart disease) will lead us to use the tabular results or switch to a model that does not impose monotonicity.

TESTS OF REGRESSION AND R^2

Most programs supply a "test of regression" or "test of model," which is a test of the hypothesis that all the regression coefficients (except the intercept α) are zero. For instance, in the exponential rate model

$$I(\mathbf{x}) = \exp(\alpha + \mathbf{x}\boldsymbol{\beta})$$

the "test of regression" provides a P-value for the null hypothesis that all the components of $\boldsymbol{\beta}$ are 0, that is, that $\beta_1 = \cdots = \beta_n = 0$. Similarly, the "test of R^2" provided by linear regression programs is just a test that all the regressor coefficients are 0. A small P-value from these tests suggests that the variation in outcomes observed across regressor values appears improbably large under the hypothesis that the regressors are unrelated to the outcome. Such a result suggests that at least one of the regressors is related to the outcome. It does *not,* however, imply that the model fits well or is adequate in any way.

To understand the latter point, suppose that $\mathbf{X}$ comprises the single indicator $X_1 = 1$ for smokers, 0 for nonsmokers, and the outcome Y is average 20-year risk of lung cancer. In most any study of reasonable size and validity, "the test of regression" (which here is just a test of $\beta_1 = 0$) will yield a small P-value. Nonetheless, the model is inadequate to describe variation in risk, because it neglects amount smoked, age at start, and sex. More generally, a small P-value from the test of regression tells us only that at least one of the regressors in the model should be included in some form or another; it does not tell us which regressor or what form to use, nor does it tell us anything about what has been left out of the model. Conversely, a large P-value from the "test of regression" does not imply that all the regressors in the model are unimportant or that the model fits well. It is always possible that transformation of those regressors will result in a small P-value, or that their importance cannot be discerned given the random error in the data.

A closely related mistake is interpreting the squared multiple-correlation coefficient R^2 for a regression as a goodness-of-fit measure. R^2 indicates only the proportion of Y variance that is attributable to variation in the fitted mean of Y. Although $R^2 = 1$ (the largest possible value) does

TABLE 21–1

Hypothetical Cohort Data Illustrating Inappropriateness of R^2 for Binary Outcomes (See Text)

	$X_1 = 1$	$X_1 = 0$
$Y = 1$	1,900	100
Total	100,000	100,000

Risk ratio = 19, $R^2 = 0.008$.

correspond to a perfect fit, R^2 can also be close to 0 under a correct model if the residual variance of Y (i.e., the variance of Y around the true regression curve) is always close to the total variance of Y.

The preceding limitations of R^2 apply in general. Correlational measures such as R^2 can become patently absurd measures of fit or association when the regressors and regressand are discrete or bounded (Rosenthal and Rubin, 1979; Greenland et al., 1986; Cox and Wermuth, 1992; Greenland, 1996e). As an example, consider Table 21–1, which shows a large association of a factor with a rare disease. The logistic model $R(x) = \text{expit}(\alpha + \beta_1 x_1)$ fits these data perfectly because it uses two parameters to describe only two proportions; thus, it is a saturated model. Furthermore, $X_1 = 1$ is associated with a 19-fold increase in risk, yet the correlation coefficient for X_1 and Y (derived using standard formulas) is only 0.09, and the R^2 for the regression is only 0.008.

Correlation coefficients and R^2 can give even more distorted impressions when multiple regressors are present (Greenland et al., 1986, 1991). For this reason, we strongly recommend against their use as measures of association or effect when modeling incidence or prevalence.

TESTS OF FIT

Tests of model fit check for nonrandom incompatibilities between the fitted regression model and the data. To do so, however, these tests must assume that the fitting method used was appropriate; in particular, test validity may be sensitive to assumptions about the residual distribution that were used in fitting. Conversely, it is possible to test assumptions about the residual distribution, but these tests usually have little power to detect violations unless a parametric regression model is assumed. Thus, useful model tests cannot be performed without making some assumptions.

Many tests of regression models are *relative,* in that they test the fit of an index model by assuming the validity of a more elaborate *reference* model that contains it. A test that assumes a relatively simple reference model (i.e., one that has only a few more coefficients than the index model) can have much better power than a test that assumes a more complex reference model if the simpler reference model is a good approximation to the true regression. The cost is that the test may have much worse power if the simpler model is a poor approximation.

When models are fitted by maximum likelihood, a standard method for testing the fit of a simpler model against a more complex model is the *deviance test,* also known as the log-likelihood ratio test. Suppose that X_1 represents cumulative dose of an exposure, and that the index model we want to test is

$$R(x_1) = \text{expit}(\alpha + \beta_1 x_1)$$

a simple linear-logistic model. When we fit this model, a ML program should supply either a "residual deviance statistic" $D(\tilde{\alpha}, \tilde{\beta}_1)$, or a "model log-likelihood" $L(\tilde{\alpha}, \tilde{\beta}_1)$, where $\tilde{\alpha}, \tilde{\beta}_1$ are the ML estimates for this simple model, $D(\tilde{\alpha}, \tilde{\beta}_1) = -2L(\tilde{\alpha}, \tilde{\beta}_1)$, and $L(\tilde{\alpha}, \tilde{\beta}_1)$ is the maximum of the likelihood function (Chapter 13) for the model. Suppose we want to test the fit of the index model taking as the reference the fractional-polynomial logistic model

$$R(x_1) = \text{expit}(\alpha + \beta_1 x_1 + \beta_2 x_1^{1/2} + \beta_3 x_1^2)$$

of which the index model is the special case with $\beta_2 = \beta_3 = 0$. We then fit this model and get either the residual deviance $D(\hat{\alpha}, \hat{\beta}_1, \hat{\beta}_2, \hat{\beta}_3)$ or the log-likelihood $L(\hat{\alpha}, \hat{\beta}_1, \hat{\beta}_2, \hat{\beta}_3)$ for the model, where $\hat{\alpha}, \hat{\beta}_1, \hat{\beta}_2, \hat{\beta}_3)$ are the ML estimates for this power model. The deviance statistic for testing the linear-logistic model against the power-logistic model (that is, for testing $\beta_2 = \beta_3 = 0$) is then

$$\Delta D(\beta_2, \beta_3) = D(\hat{\alpha}, \hat{\beta}_1) - D(\hat{\alpha}, \hat{\beta}_1, \hat{\beta}_2, \hat{\beta}_3)$$

This statistic is related to the model log-likelihoods by the equation

$$\Delta D(\beta_2, \beta_3) = -2[L(\hat{\alpha}, \hat{\beta}_1) - \hat{\alpha}, \hat{\beta}_1, \hat{\beta}_2, \hat{\beta}_3)]$$

If the linear-logistic model is correct (so that $\beta_2 = \beta_3 = 0$) and the sample is large enough, this statistic has an approximately χ^2 distribution with 2 degrees of freedom, which is the difference in the number of parameters in the two models.

A small P-value from this statistic suggests that the linear-logistic model is inadequate or fits poorly; that is, either or both the terms $\beta_2 x_1^{1/2}$ and $\beta_3 x_1^2$ capture deviations of the true regression from the linear-logistic model. A large P-value does *not,* however, imply that the linear-logistic model is adequate or fits well; it means only that no need for the terms $\beta_2 x_1^{1/2}$ and $\beta_3 x_1^2$ was detected by the test. In particular, a large P-value from this test leaves open the possibility that $\beta_2 x_1^{1/2}$ and $\beta_3 x_1^2$ are important for describing the true regression function, but the test failed to detect this condition; it also leaves open the possibility that some other terms that are not present in the reference model may be important. These unexamined terms may involve X_1 or other regressors.

Now consider a more general description. Suppose that we want to test an index model against a reference model in which it is nested (contained) and that this reference model contains p more unknown parameters (coefficients) than the index model. We fit both models and obtain either residual deviances of D_i and D_r for the index and reference models, or log-likelihoods L_i and L_r. If the sample is large enough and the index model is correct, the deviance statistic

$$\Delta D = D_i - D_r = -2(L_i - L_r) \qquad [21-1]$$

will have an approximately χ^2 distribution with p degrees of freedom. Again, a small P-value suggests that the index model does not fit well, but a large P-value does *not* mean that the index model fits well, except in the very narrow sense that the test did not detect a need for the extra terms in the reference model.

Whatever the size of the deviance P-value, its validity depends on three assumptions (in addition to absence of study biases). First, it assumes that ML fitting of the models is appropriate; in particular, there must be enough subjects to justify use of ML to fit the reference model, and the assumed residual distribution must be correct. Second, it assumes that the reference regression model is approximately correct. Third, it assumes that the index model being tested is nested within the reference model. The third is the only assumption that is easy to check: In the previous example, we can see that the linear-logistic model is just the special case of the power-logistic model in which $\beta_2 = \beta_3 = 0$. In contrast, if we used the linear-logistic model as the index model (as above) but used the power-linear model

$$R(x_1) = \alpha + \beta_1 x_1 + \beta_2 x_1^{1/2} + \beta_3 x_1^2$$

as the reference model, the resulting deviance difference would be meaningless, because the latter model does *not* contain the linear-logistic model as a special case.

Comparison of nonnested models is a more difficult task. If the compared models have the same number of parameters, it has been suggested that (absent other considerations) one should choose the model with the highest log-likelihood (Walker and Rothman, 1982). In the general case, other strategies include basing comparisons on measures of fit that adjust for the number of model parameters. Examples include the *Akaike information criterion* (AIC), often defined as the model deviance plus $2p$, where p is the number of model parameters; the *Schwarz information criterion* or *Bayesian information criterion* (BIC), often defined as the model deviance plus $p \cdot \ln(N)$, where N is the number of observations; and criteria based on *cross-validation* (Hastie et al., 2001). Larger values of these criteria suggest poorer out-of-sample predictive performance of the model. The definitions of these criteria vary considerably across textbooks (e.g., cf. Leonard and Hsu, 1999, p. 8); fortunately, the differences do not affect the ranking of models by each criterion.

As mentioned earlier, a major problem induced by model-selection strategies is that they invalidate the conventional confidence intervals and P-values. Nonetheless, advances in computing have led to strategies that address these selection effects via bootstrapping or related methods (Hastie et al., 2001), or that finesse the selection problem by averaging over the competing models (Draper, 1995; Raftery, 1995; Greenland, 1999; Carlin and Louis, 2000; Hastie et al., 2001; Viallefont et al., 2001).

GLOBAL TESTS OF FIT

One special type of deviance test of fit can be performed when Y is a proportion or rate. Suppose that, for every distinct regressor value $\mathbf{x}$, at least four cases can be expected if the index model is correct; also, if Y is a proportion, suppose that at least four noncases can be expected if the index model is correct. (This criterion, though somewhat arbitrary, originated because it ensures that the chance of a particular cell count being 0 is less than 2% if the cell variation is Poisson.) We can then test our index model against the *saturated* regression model

$$E(Y|\mathbf{X} = \mathbf{x}) = \alpha_{\mathbf{x}} \qquad [21-2]$$

where $\alpha_{\mathbf{x}}$ is a distinct parameter for every distinct observed value $\mathbf{x}$ of $\mathbf{X}$; that is, $\alpha_{\mathbf{x}}$ may represent a different number for every value $\mathbf{x}$ of $\mathbf{X}$ and may vary in any fashion as $\mathbf{X}$ varies. This model is so general that it contains all other regression models as special cases.

The degrees of freedom for the test of the index model against the saturated model (equation 21–2) is the number of distinct $\mathbf{X}$-values (which is the number of parameters in the saturated model) minus the number of parameters in the index model, and is often called the *residual degrees of freedom* for the model. This *residual* deviance test is sometimes called a "global test of fit" because it has some power to detect any systematic incompatibility between the index model and the data. Another well-known global test of fit is the *Pearson* χ^2 *test,* which has the same degrees-of-freedom and sample-size requirements as the saturated-model deviance test.

Suppose that we observe K distinct regressor values and we list them in some order $\mathbf{x}_1, \ldots, \mathbf{x}_K$. The statistic used for the Pearson test has the form of a residual sum of squares:

$$\text{RSS}_{\text{Pearson}} = \sum_k (Y_k - \hat{Y}_k)^2 / \hat{V}_k = \Sigma_k [(Y_k - \hat{Y}_k) / \hat{S}_k]^2 \qquad [21-3]$$

where the sum is over all observed values $1, \ldots, K$, Y_k is the rate or risk observed at value $\mathbf{x}_k$, $\hat{Y}_k$ is the rate or risk predicted (fitted) at $\mathbf{x}_k$ by the model, $\hat{V}_k$ is the estimated variance of Y_k when $\mathbf{X} = \mathbf{x}_k$, and $\hat{S}_k = \hat{V}_k^{1/2}$ is the estimated SD of Y_k under the model. In Poisson regression, $Y_k = \exp(\hat{\alpha} + \mathbf{x}_k\hat{\beta})$ and $\hat{V}_k = \hat{Y}_k / T_k$, where T_k is the person-time observed at $\mathbf{x}_k$; in binomial regression, $Y_k = \text{expit}(\hat{\alpha} + \mathbf{x}_k\hat{\beta})$ and $\hat{V}_k = \hat{Y}_k(1 - \hat{Y}_k)/N_k$, where N_k is the number of persons observed at $\mathbf{x}_k$. The quantity $(Y_k - \hat{Y}_k)/\hat{S}_k$ is sometimes called the *standardized residual* at value $\mathbf{x}_k$; it is the distance between Y_k and $\hat{Y}_k$ expressed in units of the estimated SD of Y_k under the model.

Other global tests have been proposed that have fewer degrees of freedom and less restrictive sample-size requirements than the deviance and Pearson tests (Hosmer and Lemeshow, 2000). A major drawback of all global tests of fit, however, is their low power to detect model problems (Hosmer et al., 1997). If any of the tests yields a low P-value, we can be confident that the tested (index) model is unsatisfactory and needs modification or replacement (albeit the tests provide no clue as to how to proceed). If, however, they all yield a high P-value, it does not mean that the model is satisfactory. In fact, the tests are unlikely to detect any but the most gross conflicts between the fitted model and the data. Therefore, global tests should be regarded as crude preliminary screening tests only, to allow quick rejection of grossly unsatisfactory models.

The deviance and Pearson statistics are sometimes used directly as measures of distance between the data and the model. Such use is most easily seen for the Pearson statistic. The second form of the Pearson statistic shows that it is the sum of squared standardized residuals; in other words, it is a sum of squared distances between data values and model-fitted values of Y, measured in standard-deviation units. The deviance and Pearson global test statistics can also be transformed into measures of prediction error under the model (McCullagh and Nelder, 1989; Hosmer and Lemeshow, 2000).

MODEL DIAGNOSTICS

Suppose now we have found a model that has passed preliminary checks such as tests for additional terms and global tests of fit. Before adopting this model as a source of estimates, it is wise to check the model further against the basic data, and assess the trustworthiness of any model-based inferences we wish to draw. Such activity is subsumed under the topic of *model diagnostics* and its subsidiary topics of residual analysis, influence analysis, and model-sensitivity analysis (Belsley et al., 2004). These topics are vast, and we can only mention a few approaches here. In particular, residual analysis is not discussed here, largely because its proper use involves a number of technical complexities when dealing with the censored data and nonlinear models predominant in epidemiology (McCullagh and Nelder, 1989).

DELTA-BETA ANALYSIS

One important form of influence analysis available in some packaged software is *delta-beta* ($\Delta\beta$) *analysis*. For a data set with N subjects total, estimated model coefficients (or approximations to them) are recomputed N times over, each time deleting exactly one of the subjects from the model fitting. Alternatively, the data set may be simplified to N groups of subjects, each group containing subjects with a unique regressor pattern (e.g., a particular exposure–age–sex–education combination), and the regression then recomputed deleting one group at a time. For individually matched data comprising N matched sets, the delta-beta analysis may be done deleting one matched set at a time. In all these approaches, the output is N different sets of coefficient estimates. These sets are then examined to see if any one subject, group, or matched set influences the resulting estimates to an unusual extent.

To illustrate, suppose our objective is to estimate the rate-ratio per unit increase in an exposure X_1, to be measured by $\exp(\hat{\beta}_1)$, where $\hat{\beta}_1$ is the estimated exposure coefficient in an exponential-rate model. For each subject, the entire model (confounders included) is refitted without that subject. Let $\hat{\beta}_{1(-i)}$ be the estimate of β_1 obtained when subject i is excluded from the data. The difference $\hat{\beta}_{1(-i)} - \hat{\beta}_1 \equiv \Delta\hat{\beta}_{1(-i)}$ is called the *delta-beta* for β_1 for subject i. The influence of subject i on the results can be assessed in several ways. One way is to examine the effect on the rate-ratio estimate. The proportionate change in the estimate from dropping subject i is

$$\exp(\hat{\beta}_{1(-i)})/\exp(\hat{\beta}_1) = \exp(\hat{\beta}_{1(-i)} - \hat{\beta}_1) = \exp(\Delta\hat{\beta}_{1(-i)})$$

for which a value of 1.30 indicates that dropping subject i increases the estimate by 30%, and a value of 0.90 indicates that dropping subject i decreases the estimate by 10%. One can also assess the effect of dropping the subject on confidence limits, P-values, or any other quantity of interest.

Some packages compute "standardized" delta-betas of the form $\Delta\hat{\beta}_{1(-i)}/\hat{s}_1$, where $\hat{s}_1$ is the estimated standard error for $\hat{\beta}_1$. By analogy with Z-statistics, any standardized delta-beta below -1.96 or above 1.96 is often interpreted as being unusual. This interpretation can be misleading, however, because $\hat{s}_1$ is not the standard deviation of the delta-beta $\Delta\hat{\beta}_{1(-i)}$, and so this type of standardized delta-beta does not have a standard normal distribution.

It is possible that one or a few subjects or matched sets are so influential that deleting them alters the conclusions of the study, even when N is in the hundreds (Pregibon, 1981). In such situations, comparison of the records of those subjects to others may reveal unusual combinations of regressor values among those subjects. Such unusual combinations may arise from previously undetected data errors, and should at least lead to enhanced caution in interpretation. For instance, it may be only mildly unusual to see a woman who reports having had a child at age 45 or a woman who reports natural menopause at age 45. The combination in one subject, however, may arouse suspicion of a data error in one or both regressors, a suspicion worth the labor of further data scrutiny if that woman or her matched set disproportionately influences the results.

Delta-beta analysis must be replaced by a more complex analysis if the exposure of interest appears in multiple model terms, such as indicator terms, power terms, product terms, or spline terms. In that situation, one must focus on changes in estimates of specific effects or summaries, for example, changes in estimated risk ratios.

RESAMPLING ANALYSIS AND BOOTSTRAPPING

Variability in results due to "random" vagaries of subject selection and outcome occurrence are supposedly addressed by the confidence limits supplied by statistical programs for associational measures and regression coefficients. Unfortunately, these limits are usually based on distributional assumptions or approximations whose validity may be uncertain in a given application. A less formal but more visually immediate assessment of random variability can be obtained through elementary *resampling analysis* (Simon and Burstein, 1985), in which the entire data set of N subjects (or matched sets) is repeatedly random-sampled as if it were itself a source population. Specifically, we may take K random samples of size N (the size of the study sample) each from the data set by sampling *with* replacement (if we sampled without replacement, we would always end up with our original sample). For each sample, we may repeat our analysis, to obtain K estimated exposure coefficients or K estimated dose–response curves. These K results can be plotted in a single histogram or graph. The plot provides a visual impression of the extent to which random variability might have influenced the results.

The resampling analysis just described is the first step in *nonparametric bootstrapping*. Bootstrapping employs resampling to produce better estimates, P-values, and diagnostics than are available using standard methods. It has become a vast topic area (Hall, 1992; Efron and Tibshirani, 1994; Davison and Hinkley, 1997), although the numerous subtleties involved in proper (as opposed to naïve) bootstrapping blunted initial hopes for widespread use (Young, 1994; Carpenter and Bithell, 2000). For example, direct use of bootstrap percentiles as confidence limits is easy and popular, but can perform poorly. Problems include instability of the estimated percentiles if K is not huge (on the order of 10,000 or more; e.g., see Hill and Reiter, 2006), as well as finite-sample biases. One can address these problems by estimating the variance and finite-sample bias of the effect estimate from the bootstrap samples, then constructing the confidence interval from these estimates. More sophisticated bootstrap procedures can address the problems thoroughly, but can be complicated compared with naïve percentile methods (Hall, 1992; Efron and Tibshirani, 1994; Davison and Hinkley, 1997; Carpenter and Bithell, 2000). Furthermore, complexities in the sampling design (such as nearest-neighbor matching) can invalidate bootstrap estimates based on simple random resampling of individual records (Abadie and Imbens, 2006).

MODEL SENSITIVITY ANALYSIS

A valuable diagnostic procedure, which is often a by-product of the model-selection approaches described in the following, is model sensitivity analysis (Leamer, 1985; Draper, 1995; Saltelli et al., 2000). Given the variety of models available for fitting, it is inevitable that quite a few can be found that fit reasonably well by all standard tests and diagnostics. Model sensitivity analysis seeks to identify a spectrum of such acceptable models, and asks whether various estimates and tests are sensitive to the choice of model used for inference. Those results that are consistent (stable) across acceptable model-based and stratified analyses can be presented using any one of the analyses. On the other hand, results that vary across analyses need to be reported with much more uncertainty than is indicated by their (unstable) confidence intervals; in particular, one should report the fact that the estimates were unstable.

The credibility, value, and results of a sensitivity analysis are themselves sensitive to the spectrum of models investigated for acceptability. Most such analyses cover limited territory, in part because most software has a restricted range of model forms that can be examined easily. Typically, only exponential-Poisson and Cox models for rates and binomial-logistic models for risks are available, although some packages supply linear rate and linear odds models. The similar restrictions imposed by these models results in severe limitations on the range of analysis. Nonetheless, within these limits there are vast possibilities for the terms representing the effects of exposures, confounders, and modifiers.

MODELING IN UNMATCHED CASE-CONTROL STUDIES AND RELATED DESIGNS

So far, we have assumed that the regressand (outcome variable) is some sort of occurrence measure (risk, prevalence rate, incidence time) observed in a cohort or population of interest. In case-control studies, however, we observe two disproportionate samples, one taken from cases of the study disease and the other from the underlying population at risk. This sampling distorts the frequency of disease in the study away from that in the source population. Nonetheless, the reasoning that shows we can estimate incidence ratios from case-control data (Chapter 8) also shows that, for a broad class of models, we can validly model case-control data *as if* it were cohort data. The one caution is that only the incidence ratios and attributable fractions estimated from the models are valid; to estimate risks, rates, and their differences, some external data must be used.

MULTIPLICATIVE-INTERCEPT MODELS FOR DENSITY STUDIES

Consider an unmatched case-control study that uses density (risk-set) sampling of controls (Chapter 8). For simplicity, let us assume that the source and target populations are identical. Suppose that rates across subpopulations of the underlying source population follow a *multiplicative-intercept* model

$$I(\mathbf{x}) = \exp(\alpha)r(\mathbf{x}\boldsymbol{\beta}) \qquad [21\text{–}4]$$

where $r(\mathbf{x}\boldsymbol{\beta})$ is a rate-ratio ("relative risk") function that equals 1 when $\mathbf{x}\boldsymbol{\beta} = 0$ (Greenland, 1981; Thomas, 1981b; Weinberg and Wacholder, 1993). The most common form uses $r(\mathbf{x}\boldsymbol{\beta}) = \exp(\mathbf{x}\boldsymbol{\beta})$, which yields the exponential-rate model

$$I(\mathbf{x}) = \exp(\alpha + \mathbf{x}\boldsymbol{\beta})$$

Taking $r(\mathbf{x}\boldsymbol{\beta}) = 1 + \mathbf{x}\boldsymbol{\beta}$ instead yields the linear rate-ratio model

$$I(\mathbf{x}) = \exp(\alpha)(1 + \mathbf{x}\boldsymbol{\beta})$$

Let $T(\mathbf{x})$ be the person-time at risk in the source population at value $\mathbf{X} = \mathbf{x}$ over the study period. Suppose that a fraction f of the cases is randomly sampled over the period, and controls are randomly sampled over the period at a rate of h controls per unit person-time. Then expected numbers of cases (A) and controls (B) observed at value $\mathbf{X} = \mathbf{x}$ is

$$A(\mathbf{x}) = f \cdot \exp(\alpha)r(\mathbf{x}\boldsymbol{\beta})T(\mathbf{x})$$

and

$$B(\mathbf{x}) = h \cdot T(\mathbf{x})$$

so that

$$A(\mathbf{x})/B(\mathbf{x}) = (f/h)\exp(\alpha)r(\mathbf{x}\boldsymbol{\beta})$$

If we let $\alpha^* = \ln(f/h) + \alpha$, we see that

$$\begin{aligned} A(\mathbf{x})/B(\mathbf{x}) &= \exp[\ln(f/h) + \alpha]r(\mathbf{x}\boldsymbol{\beta}) \\ &= \exp(\alpha^*)r(\mathbf{x}\boldsymbol{\beta}) \end{aligned}$$

Thus, $A(\mathbf{x})/B(\mathbf{x})$ follows a multiplicative-intercept model with covariate coefficients identical to those of the population rate model. The only difference is that the intercept α^* is shifted away from α by a factor $\ln(f/h)$.

Now suppose we take $r(\mathbf{x}\boldsymbol{\beta}) = \exp(\mathbf{x}\boldsymbol{\beta})$. Let $N(\mathbf{x}) = A(\mathbf{x}) + B(\mathbf{x})$ be the total number of study subjects (cases and controls) expected at value $\mathbf{X} = \mathbf{x}$. The proportion of this total expected to be cases is then

$$\begin{aligned} A(\mathbf{x})/N(\mathbf{x}) &= A(\mathbf{x})/[A(\mathbf{x}) + B(\mathbf{x})] \\ &= [A(\mathbf{x})/B(\mathbf{x})]/[1 + A(\mathbf{x})/B(\mathbf{x})] \\ &= \exp(\alpha^*)r(\mathbf{x}\boldsymbol{\beta})/[1 + \exp(\alpha^*)r(\mathbf{x}\boldsymbol{\beta})] \\ &= \exp(\alpha^* + \mathbf{x}\boldsymbol{\beta})/[1 + \exp(\alpha^* + \mathbf{x}\boldsymbol{\beta})] \\ &= \text{expit}(\alpha^* + \mathbf{x}\boldsymbol{\beta}) \end{aligned}$$

Thus, the ratio $A(\mathbf{x})/N(\mathbf{x})$ follows a logistic model with covariate coefficients $\boldsymbol{\beta}$ identical to those of the population rate model. As a consequence, to estimate the population coefficients $\boldsymbol{\beta}$ from density-sampled case-control data under an exponential-rate model, we need only model the case-control data using logistic regression. In particular, the estimate $\hat{\beta}_1$ of a particular coefficient obtained from the logistic model fitting is interpretable as an estimate of the change in the log rate ratio per unit increase in X_k.

The preceding remarkable observation appeared in various forms beginning with Sheehe (1962). More generally, valid SE estimates for the estimate of $\boldsymbol{\beta}$ can be obtained by modeling the case-control data as if it were cohort data; only the estimates of the intercept term α and its standard error are biased by the case-control sampling (Prentice and Breslow, 1978). Note that a "rare-disease" assumption is *not* needed for any of these results.

Because the population rate ratios are functions of the $\boldsymbol{\beta}$ only, the intercept term α is not needed for most purposes. If α is desired, however, and the case-control sampling ratio f/h is known or can be estimated, then α can be estimated by subtracting $\ln(f/h)$ from the estimate of α^* (Prentice and Breslow, 1978); see below. Given estimates of α and $\boldsymbol{\beta}$, one may use the fitted model to estimate and plot the population rates (Greenland, 1981; Benichou and Wacholder, 1994). Given estimates of only α^* and $\boldsymbol{\beta}$, one can still use the estimates of the case-control ratios $\exp(\alpha^*)r(\mathbf{x}\boldsymbol{\beta})$ as proportional substitutes for rates in tables and plots (Greenland et al., 1999).

If we know or can estimate f/h, we can estimate α in the preceding models by substituting our estimates of α^* and $\ln(f/h)$ into the equation $\alpha = \alpha^* - \ln(f/h)$ (Prentice and Breslow, 1978; Greenland, 1981). We can in turn estimate f/h from the overall (crude) disease rate in the source population. To see this, let A_c be the total number of cases, let T_c be the total person-time at risk in the source population during the study period, and let $I_c = A_c/T_c$. Also, let A_+ and B_+ be the total number of cases and controls. We then have the expected relation

$$\frac{A_+}{B_+} = \frac{fA_c}{hT_c} = \left(\frac{f}{h}\right)I_c$$

so that $f/h = A_+/(B_+I_c)$, the observed case-control ratio by the overall disease rate in the source population (Greenland, 1981).

MULTIPLICATIVE-INTERCEPT MODELS FOR CUMULATIVE AND PREVALENCE STUDIES

Suppose we have a cumulative or prevalence case-control study with random sampling of fractions f of cases and h of noncases. If the odds in the source follows a multiplicative-intercept model $O(\mathbf{x}) = \exp(\alpha)r(\mathbf{x}\boldsymbol{\beta})$, the expected case-control ratio will follow the model

$$A(\mathbf{x})/B(\mathbf{x}) = \exp(\alpha^*)r(\mathbf{x}\boldsymbol{\beta})$$

where $\alpha^* = \alpha + \ln(f/h)$. If we know or can estimate f/h, then we may obtain an estimate of α from the equation $\alpha = \alpha^* - \ln(f/h)$ (Anderson, 1972; Greenland, 1981). Given the overall (crude) odds O_c in the source population, we can in turn estimate f/h from the equation $f/h = A_+/(B_+O_c)$, the observed case-control ratio divided by the overall odds in the source population.

Because the logistic model $R(\mathbf{x}) = \text{expit}(\alpha + \mathbf{x}\boldsymbol{\beta})$ is identical to the exponential odds model $O(\mathbf{x}) = \exp(\alpha + \mathbf{x}\boldsymbol{\beta})$, an argument parallel to that given for density studies shows that the proportions expected to be cases in the study will follow the logistic model

$$A(\mathbf{x})/N(\mathbf{x}) = \text{expit}(\alpha^* + \mathbf{x}\boldsymbol{\beta})$$

(Anderson, 1972; Mantel, 1973; Prentice and Pyke, 1979). Thus, to estimate the population logistic coefficients $\boldsymbol{\beta}$, we need only model the case-control data using logistic regression as if it were a cohort or survey. Similarly, a linear odds-ratio model $O(\mathbf{x}) = \exp(\alpha)(1 + \mathbf{x}\boldsymbol{\beta})$ induces the additive case-control ratio model $A(\mathbf{x})/B(\mathbf{x}) = \exp(\alpha^*)(1 + \mathbf{x}\boldsymbol{\beta})$. A few software packages allow fitting these linear odds-ratio models (some call them "additive logistic models") to data.

OTHER MODELS FOR CASE-CONTROL STUDIES

Estimation of the selection ratio f/h allows fitting of other models to case-control data (Greenland, 1981). As an example, suppose the source population follows a linear rate model

$$I(\mathbf{x}) = \alpha + \mathbf{x}\boldsymbol{\beta}$$

In a density case-control study, the expected numbers of cases and controls will be

$$A(\mathbf{x}) = f \cdot (\alpha + \mathbf{x}\boldsymbol{\beta})T(\mathbf{x})$$

and

$$B(\mathbf{x}) = hT(\mathbf{x})$$

and the ratio will be

$$A(\mathbf{x})/B(\mathbf{x}) = (f/h)(\alpha + \mathbf{x}\boldsymbol{\beta}) = \alpha^* + \mathbf{x}\boldsymbol{\beta}^*$$

where $\alpha^* = (f/h)\alpha$ and $\boldsymbol{\beta}^* = (f/h)\boldsymbol{\beta}$. Thus, $\boldsymbol{\beta}$ will be distorted by the factor f/h in the case-control data, and we will not be able to estimate $\boldsymbol{\beta}$ validly unless we know or can estimate f/h. If we have an estimate of f/h, however, we can divide our case-control estimates of α^* and $\boldsymbol{\beta}^*$ by our estimate of f/h to obtain estimates of α and $\boldsymbol{\beta}$. Parallel arguments show that, under linear and exponential risk models, we can estimate the covariate coefficients from cumulative or prevalence case-control data if we know or can estimate f/h.

CASE-COHORT AND TWO-STAGE STUDIES

Suppose that a cohort is studied using a case-cohort design, with random sampling of fractions f of cases and h of the total cohort at start of follow-up. As with a cumulative case-control study, if the underlying cohort follows a multiplicative-intercept odds model, the ratios of expected case and noncase numbers will also follow a multiplicative-intercept model. The bias in the intercept will be different, however. In addition to the fraction f of all cases that composes the case sample, a fraction h of all cases is expected to appear in the total-cohort sample. Furthermore, we expect a fraction f of the latter cases also to appear in the case sample, so that we expect a fraction fh of all cases to appear in both samples. Thus, the fraction of all cases with $\mathbf{X} = \mathbf{x}$ who will appear in the case-cohort study will be $f + h - fh$, and

$$\alpha^* = \alpha + \ln[(f + h - fh)/h] = \alpha + \ln(f/h + 1 - f)$$

In case-cohort studies, f and h are usually chosen by the investigator, so once α^* is estimated, this equation can be solved for α. If f/h is unknown, it can be estimated directly from case-cohort data as the ratio of the numbers of cases in the case sample and the cohort sample, although this estimate may be very unstable. Standard regression programs can be used to fit a broad range of risk models to case-cohort data (Prentice, 1986; Schouten et al., 1993), provided the data are entered with special formats or weights. The chief obstacle to these approaches is that they may require extra programming to obtain correct standard-deviation estimates.

A variety of methods exist for analyzing two-stage data (Breslow and Cain, 1988; Cain and Breslow, 1988; Flanders and Greenland, 1991; Robins et al., 1994; Breslow and Holubkov, 1997a, 1997b), but each requires special programming. Perhaps the conceptually simplest approach is to adopt a missing-data viewpoint, in which subjects in the second-stage sample are complete subjects, while subjects who are only in the first-stage sample are those with data missing on the second-stage covariates (Robins et al., 1994). This approach allows analysis of two-stage data with missing-data software. The same approach can be used to analyze case-cohort and nested case-control data when full-cohort data are available (Wacholder, 1996).

STRATIFIED MODELS

Suppose we have data that are divided into K strata indexed by $k = 1, \ldots, K$, with the strata defined by potential confounders in the list $\mathbf{Z} = (z_1, \ldots, z_m)$. For example, suppose we have data stratified on $Z_1 = 1$ if female, 0 if male and $Z_2 = 1$ if age is 50 to 54 years, 2 if age is 55 to 59 years, 3 if age is 60 to 64 years, and 4 if age is 64 to 69 years. Here, $\mathbf{Z} = (Z_1, Z_2)$ comprises a sex indicator and one four-level age-category variable. Together, Z_1 and Z_2 define $2 \times 4 = 8$ sex–age strata. Suppose also we have another list of variables $\mathbf{X}$, including the study exposures and potential confounders other than those in **Z**. A *stratified model* is a model for the stratum-specific regressions. As discussed below, such models are central to modeling of matched data.

To illustrate this concept, suppose we index the strata by $k = 1, \ldots, 8$ with the above eight sex-age strata and that $\mathbf{X} = (X_1, X_2)$. One possible stratified logistic risk model is then

$$R_k(\mathbf{x}) = \text{expit}(\alpha_k + \beta_1 x_1 + \beta_2 x_2) \qquad [21\text{–}5]$$

This model asserts that, within each stratum, risk varies with X_1 and X_2 according to a simple logistic model, and only the intercept of the model changes across strata. More general models allow other parameters to change across strata. For example, the model

$$\begin{aligned} R_k(\mathbf{x}) &= \text{expit}(\alpha_k + \beta_1 x_1 + \beta_2 x_2 + \gamma_1 x_1 z_1 + \gamma_2 x_2 z_1) \\ &= \text{expit}[\alpha_k + (\beta_1 + \gamma_1 z_1)x_1 + (\beta_2 + \gamma_2 z_1)x_2] \end{aligned}$$

allows the X_1 and X_2 coefficients to vary with sex: For men, $Z_1 = 0$ and so in male strata,

$$R_k(\mathbf{x}) = \text{expit}(\alpha_k + \beta_1 x_1 + \beta_2 x_2)$$

For women, $Z_1 = 1$ and so in female strata,

$$R_k(\mathbf{x}) = \text{expit}[\alpha_k + (\beta_1 + \gamma_1)x_1 + (\beta_2 + \gamma_2)x_2]$$

We could also build models in which the coefficients varied with the age group (Z_2 level) of the strata, by including product terms with Z_2 or with indicators of different levels of Z_2.

Stratum-specific models can be defined for any outcome measure and model form. For example, we could use a stratum-specific linear-odds model

$$O_k(\mathbf{x}) = \alpha_k + \beta_1 x_1 + \beta_2 x_2 \qquad [21\text{–}6]$$

One special consideration in using stratum-specific models arises if the strata are sparse, in that there are too few subjects per stratum to allow estimation of the intercepts α_k. In those situations, special fitting methods (known as *sparse-data* methods) must be used. Such methods do not provide estimates of the intercepts α_k, and they are available only for multiplicative-intercept models of the form $\exp(\alpha_k)r(\mathbf{x}\boldsymbol{\beta})$; equation 21–5 is an example, whereas equation 21–6 is not. Because sparse stratifications are common, these methods correspond to an important application of stratified models. Nonetheless, although these methods can reduce sparse-data problems, they are not immune to those problems (Greenland, 2000e, Greenland et al., 2000a).

Conditional maximum-likelihood (CML) is the most common sparse-data fitting method for stratified logistic models. CML fitting of stratified logistic models is usually called "conditional logistic regression" (Breslow and Day, 1980; McCullagh and Nelder, 1989; Clayton and Hills, 1993; Hosmer and Lemeshow, 2000). CML can also be used to fit the stratified linear odds-ratio model

$$O_k(\mathbf{x}) = \exp(\alpha_k)(1 + \mathbf{x}\boldsymbol{\beta}^*) \qquad [21\text{–}7]$$

Note, however, that this model is *not* equivalent to the stratified linear-odds model (model 21–6), because model 21–7 implies that

$$O_k(\mathbf{x}) = \exp(\alpha_k) + \exp(\alpha_k)\mathbf{x}\boldsymbol{\beta}^* = \exp(\alpha_k) + \mathbf{x}\boldsymbol{\beta}_k^* \qquad [21\text{–}8]$$

where $\boldsymbol{\beta}_k^* = \exp(\alpha_k)\boldsymbol{\beta}^*$ varies across strata. Parallel observations apply to linear risk and rate models. As a consequence, neither risk nor rate additivity corresponds to a stratified linear relative-risk model (Greenland, 1993d).

CML is limited to multiplicative-intercept models for the rate or odds; it is not appropriate for a multiplicative-intercept model for risks, such as model 21–5. Confidence intervals obtained from standard conditional logistic programs also assume that subject outcomes are independent within strata. To overcome these restrictions, other sparse-data fitting methods have been developed that are generalizations of the Mantel-Haenszel methods discussed in earlier chapters. Examples include methods for fitting logistic models to sparse data with dependent outcomes (Liang, 1987) and methods for fitting exponential and linear risk models to sparse cohort data (Stijnen and van Houwelingen, 1993; Greenland, 1994b).

MODELING MATCHED DATA

The general principles for modeling in matched studies are the same as those for stratified analysis of matched studies (see Chapter 16). Most importantly, all matching factors should be treated as potential confounders, in that one should assess whether failure to control them will affect interval estimates. Any matching factor for which control affects these estimates to an important degree should be controlled. What is an "important degree" depends on the subject matter, however.

A crucial point is that complete control of the matching in matched-data modeling requires use of a stratified model with each unique matching category defining its own stratum (which often results in a sparse stratification). In such a model, each matching stratum (that is, each unique combination of matching factors) is given its own unique intercept term. Consider a cumulative case-control study of the relation of smoking X_1 and alcohol use X_2 to risk of laryngeal cancer, matched on sex Z_1 ($Z_1 = 1$ female, 0 male) and age Z_2 in six 5-year categories from 45–49 to 70–74, coded by $Z_2 = 1, \ldots, 6$. There are then $2 \times 6 = 12$ unique matching strata, which we may index by 1–12. A model that treats smoking and alcohol as having linear logistic relations to disease risk within matching strata, and that also allows adjustment for any selection bias produced by the matching, is

$$R_k(x_1, x_2) = \text{expit}(\alpha_k + \beta_1 x_1 + \beta_2 x_2) \qquad [21\text{–}9]$$

where $k = 1, \ldots, 12$, according to the age–sex stratum.

To be more precise, suppose that the source cohort follows model 21–9 and that cases and controls are randomly sampled within matching strata. Using arguments similar to those for unmatched data, it can be shown that the ratios of expected case numbers $A_k(x_1, x_2)$ to expected totals $N_k(x_1, x_2)$ from the matched case-control data will follow the logistic model

$$A_k(x_1, x_2)/N_k(x_1, x_2) = \text{expit}(\alpha_k^* + \beta_1 x_1 + \beta_2 x_2)$$

where $\alpha_k^* = \alpha_k + \ln(f_k/h_k)$ and f_k and h_k are the sampling fractions for cases and controls in matching stratum k. If instead we conduct a density case-control study of the rate of laryngeal cancer and the source population follows the stratified exponential rate model

$$I(x_1, x_2) = \exp(\alpha_k + \beta_1 x_1 + \beta_2 x_2)$$

the expected data will follow the previous logistic model with $\alpha_k^* = \alpha_k + \ln(f_k/h_k)$, where h_k is the control sampling rate in stratum k.

Suppose that X_4 is the actual age (in years) of a subject and $X_3 = Z_1 = 1$ female, 0 male. A model that does *not* allow full adjustment for the matching is

$$R(\mathbf{x}) = \text{expit}(\alpha + \beta_1 x_1 + \beta_2 x_2 + \beta_3 x_3 + \beta_4 x_4), \qquad [21\text{–}10]$$

where $\mathbf{x} = (x_1, x_2, x_3, x_4)$. Unlike the first model, this model implies that the age variable has a linear logistic relation to risk, and that the age and sex effects on the odds are multiplicative. Even if the underlying source population follows this model, the case-control matching on age can alter the age trend in the expected matched data away from the linear logistic form to a highly nonlinear form (Greenland, 1986a, 1997b). Use of a linear logistic trend for age can only be rationalized if the model (equation 21–10) gives confidence limits for the smoking and alcohol effect estimates that are not substantially different from those obtained using the stratified model (equation 21–9).

Sometimes a variable is not matched closely enough to prevent important confounding by the variable within matching strata. We can address this problem in a stratified analysis by using finer strata for the variable. For example, if age is matched in only 10-year intervals, we can split each of these intervals into two 5-year or even five 2-year strata. We can accomplish this split with a model that has separate intercepts for each of the finer strata. If, as a result, there are few subjects per stratum, sparse-data fitting methods will be needed.

Modeling permits an alternative to finer stratification, however: One can model the effects of within-stratum variation of the matching variable. For example, if the subjects are matched on sex and on age using two 10-year strata of 55 to 64 years and 65 to 74 years, we can make a model-based adjustment for age variation within the four matching strata by adding a term to the model for the effect of age variation within strata. For example, define X_5 to be the deviation of a person's age from the mean age of the controls in the person's matching category. If the mean ages of women 55 to 64, men 55 to 64, women 65 to 74, and men 65 to 74 are 60, 59, 70, and 68, respectively, then X_5 equals age minus 60, age minus 59, age minus 70, or age minus 68, depending on which matching category a person is in. We then add X_5 directly to the stratified case-control model as $\beta_3 x_5$, which yields

$$\text{expit}(\alpha_k^* + \beta_1 x_1 + \beta_2 x_2 + \beta_3 x_5)$$

(there is no term for sex or age alone, because the latter are matching variables and thus their stratum-specific effects are included in the intercepts α_k^*). This process is just one of many ways to model the within-stratum age effects.

Other models beside the logistic can be used for matched data, such as the linear odds-ratio model (equation 21–5). We again caution, however, that the linear odds-ratio model does not correspond to the linear odds model 21–4 (Greenland, 1993d) and therefore does not approximate the linear risk or rate model even if the outcome is uncommon. As with unmatched data, external information is required to fit linear rate or linear or exponential risk models to matched case-control data. The information required is more detailed, however. In density studies we must know or estimate the selection ratios f_k/h_k. These ratios can be estimated by dividing the matching-stratum-specific rates or odds into the matching-stratum-specific case-control ratios (Greenland, 1981).

HIERARCHICAL (MULTILEVEL) REGRESSION

Often there is information about the regressors that will be valuable if not essential to incorporate into the analysis. For example, in a study of vitamin intakes and disease, we would know that some vitamins are water-soluble whereas others are fat-soluble; and in a study of chlorinated hydrocarbon levels in tissues, we would know the degree of chlorination of the measured compounds. One way to use such information is to create a model for the original regression coefficients as a function of this information. Thus the vitamin coefficients could be regressed on an indicator of whether they were for a water-soluble or fat-soluble vitamin; and chlorinated hydrocarbon coefficients could be regressed on a measure of their degree of chlorination. This process is called *hierarchical* or *multilevel* modeling, to reflect that more than one level of modeling is done (Greenland, 2000d).

Consider a case-control study of foods $\mathbf{X}$ and their relations to breast cancer in women (Witte et al., 1994, 2000; Greenland, 2000c), with confounders $\mathbf{W}$, and an indicator $Y = 1$ for cases, 0 for controls. An ordinary regression analysis would use maximum likelihood to estimate $\boldsymbol{\beta}$ in the logistic model

$$R(\mathbf{x}, \mathbf{w}) = \text{expit}(\alpha + \mathbf{x}\boldsymbol{\beta} + \mathbf{w}\boldsymbol{\gamma}) \qquad [21\text{–}11]$$

The coefficients $\boldsymbol{\beta}$ in model 21–11 represent food-item effects; with density-sampled controls, each coefficient represents the unit change in the log rate of breast cancer per unit increase in food item.

Hierarchical regression goes beyond the ordinary model (equation 21–11) to add a model for some or all of the coefficients in $\boldsymbol{\beta}$ or $\boldsymbol{\gamma}$. In the example, a natural choice is to model the food-item effects in $\boldsymbol{\beta}$ as a function of nutrient content. Suppose that for each food item X_j we have a list (row vector) $\mathbf{z}_j = (z_{1j}, z_{2j}, \ldots, z_{pj})$ of p elements giving the vitamin, mineral, fat, protein, carbohydrate, and fiber content of each unit of the food item. For instance, if X_6 is skim milk measured in units of 250 mL (one serving), z_{16}, z_{26}, z_{36}, etc. could be the thiamine, riboflavin, niacin, etc., content of 250 mL of skim milk; such information could be obtained from nutrient tables. We may then model the food effects β_j in $\boldsymbol{\beta}$ in model 21–11 as a function of the nutrient contents of the foods, for example, using linear regression:

$$\beta_j = \pi_1 z_{1j} + \pi_2 z_{2j} + \cdots + \pi_p z_{pj} + \delta_j = \mathbf{z}_j\boldsymbol{\pi} + \delta_j \qquad [21\text{–}12]$$

where $\boldsymbol{\pi}$ is the column vector containing $\pi_1, \ldots, \pi_p$, and δ_j is the deviation of the effect of food item j from the sum $\pi_1 z_{1j} + \cdots + \pi_p z_{pj} = \mathbf{z}_j\boldsymbol{\pi}$. A term $\pi_k z_{kj}$ in model 21–12 represents the *linear* portion of the contribution of nutrient k to the effect β_j of food item j. The deviation δ_j is called the *residual effect* of item j; it represents effects of food item j that are not captured by the sum $\mathbf{z}_j\boldsymbol{\pi}$. Such residual effects can arise from interactions among the modeled nutrients, as well as from unmeasured nutrients. These residual effects δ_j are usually assumed to be independent random quantities having means of 0 and standard deviations τ_j.

The linear model (equation 21–12) for the food-item effects in model 21–11 is called a *second-stage model* or *prior model,* with nutrient contents **Z** as the second-stage regressors or prior regressors. The original model 21–11 is called a *first-stage model,* and **X** and **W** are the *first-stage regressors*. Taken together, the two models 21–11 and 21–12 constitute a two-stage *hierarchical regression model*. The τ_j are called *second-stage standard deviations* or *prior standard deviations*; they may be fixed in advance using background information (Greenland, 1992a, 1993b, 1994c, 2000c, 2000d; Witte et al., 1994, 2000) or estimated using a variance model (Breslow and Clayton, 1993; Goldstein, 2003; Gelman et al., 2003; Skrondal and Raabe-Hesketh, 2004). For simplicity, in this section we assume that the τ_j are all equal to a single known value τ.

The two-stage formulation in 21–11 and 21–12 arises naturally in many epidemiologic contexts besides food-nutrient studies. One common example is in occupational studies, in which the first-stage exposures in **X** are job histories (e.g., years spent as a welder) and second-stage regressors in **Z** are exposures associated with each unit of job experience (e.g., level of metal dust exposure in the job) (Greenland, 1992a; Steenland et al., 2000; De Roos et al., 2001). Hierarchical models may have as many stages as one desires (Good, 1983, 1987; Goldstein, 2003). For example, we could add a third-stage model in which the nutrient effects in $\boldsymbol{\pi}$ depend on the chemical properties of the nutrients (e.g., antioxidant activity, fat solubility, etc.).

In multilevel modeling terminology, model stages are called model levels (Greenland, 2000d; Goldstein, 2003). For example, model 21–11 is a level-1 model with level-1 regressors **X** and **W**, whereas model 21–12 is a level-2 model with level-2 regressors **Z**. Hierarchical models are also known as empirical-Bayes models (Deely and Lindley, 1981; Morris, 1983; Good, 1987; Yanagimoto and Kashiwagi, 1990; Carlin and Louis, 2000), in which case model 21–12 is sometimes called a *prior model* with prior covariates **Z**. These models provide a logical foundation for deriving ridge regression and other "shrinkage" estimation methods (Leamer, 1978).

Hierarchical models can be reformulated as *random-coefficient models* or *mixed models* (Robinson, 1991; Breslow and Clayton, 1993; McCulloch and Searle, 2001; Goldstein, 2003); in the preceding hierarchical model, the δ_j are the random coefficients. In the mixed-model formulation, the higher-stage models are substituted into the lower-stage models to obtain a single model that combines elements from all stages. To illustrate, note that the second-stage model as in model 21–12 represents J equations, one for each β_j. The equations may be combined into a single matrix equation, $\boldsymbol{\beta} = \mathbf{Z}\boldsymbol{\pi} + \boldsymbol{\delta}$, where **Z** is the matrix with rows $\mathbf{z_j}$ and $\boldsymbol{\delta}$ is the vector of the δ_j. We may then substitute this form of the second-stage model into model 21–11 to obtain

$$R(\mathbf{x}, \mathbf{w}) = \text{expit}[\alpha + \mathbf{x}(\mathbf{Z}\boldsymbol{\pi} + \boldsymbol{\delta}) + \mathbf{w}\boldsymbol{\gamma}] = \text{expit}(\alpha + \mathbf{x}\mathbf{Z}\boldsymbol{\pi} + \mathbf{x}\boldsymbol{\delta} + \mathbf{w}\boldsymbol{\gamma})$$

In this formulation, the random δ_j become coefficients of x_j. The model is "mixed" because it contains both the "fixed" coefficients π_j in $\boldsymbol{\pi}$ and the random δ_j coefficients in $\boldsymbol{\delta}$. Note, however, that "fixed" means only that the coefficients in $\boldsymbol{\pi}$ have not been given explicit prior distributions in the model. Treating the coefficients in $\boldsymbol{\pi}$ as fixed gives results equivalent to assigning the coefficient a "noniformative" prior distribution, which is equivalent to assigning overly high probabilities to contextually absurd values of $\boldsymbol{\pi}$ (see Chapter 18).

There are numerous methods for fitting a hierarchical model such as model 21–11 plus 21–12. These include Monte-Carlo techniques (Gelman et al., 2003), which require special software, and approximations such as penalized likelihood, penalized quasi-likelihood (PQL) (Breslow and Clayton, 1993; Greenland, 1997b) and related methods, which can be carried out with procedures in software such as SAS (Witte et al. 2000). When the τ_j are fixed in advance, data augmentation can be used to fit the models with any logistic regression program (Greenland, 2001b, 2007a).

WHY ADD A SECOND STAGE?

It is natural to ask what is gained by adding model 21–12 to model 21–11, or, in general, what is gained by elaborating our ordinary models with more stages. Statistical theory, simulation studies, and several decades of applications all yield the same answer: Addition of a second-stage model can yield tremendous gains in the accuracy of predictions and effect estimates; for example, see Efron and Morris (1975, 1977), Morris (1983), Brandwein and Strawderman (1990), Greenland (1993a, 1997b, 2000c, 2000d), and Witte and Greenland (1996). The chief proviso is that the second-stage model, like the first-stage model, should be carefully formulated so that it makes efficient use of the available data and is scientifically reasonable. For example, the strength of model 21–12 is that it allows us to make use of existing nutrient-content information about foods in our estimation of food effects.

If one is interested in effects of the second-stage covariates, hierarchical models can offer more realistic representations of effects than conventional models. Consider, for example, the conventional model used to study nutrient effects,

$$R(\mathbf{z}, \mathbf{w}) = \text{expit}(\alpha + \mathbf{c}\boldsymbol{\pi} + \mathbf{w}\boldsymbol{\gamma}) \qquad [21\text{–}13]$$

where $\mathbf{c} = (c_1, \ldots, c_p)$ represents the list of nutrient contents of an individual's diet. The contents c_k are obtained from the food history by multiplying each food quantity x_j by its content z_{kj} of nutrient k, and then summing these products across food items; that is, $c_k = \sum_j x_j z_{kj}$. The latter equations can be combined into the single equation $\mathbf{c} = \sum_j x_j z_j = \mathbf{xZ}$.

The conventional model makes no allowance for the possibilities that nutrients that are not in $\mathbf{z}$ may affect risk, or that there may be important nonlogistic effects of nutrients. In contrast, the more general hierarchical model (model 21–11 plus 21–12) allows for the possibility that there are food effects beyond $\mathbf{c}\boldsymbol{\pi}$ by adding to the model the random coefficients δ_j. The greater generality of the hierarchical model over the conventional model can be seen in the mixed model formulation of the hierarchical model by noting that $\mathbf{c}\boldsymbol{\pi} = \mathbf{xZ}\boldsymbol{\pi}$:

$$\begin{aligned} R(\mathbf{x}, \mathbf{z}, \mathbf{w}) &= \text{expit}(\alpha + \mathbf{xZ}\boldsymbol{\pi} + \mathbf{x}\boldsymbol{\delta} + \boldsymbol{\gamma}\mathbf{w}) \\ &= \text{expit}(\alpha + \mathbf{c}\boldsymbol{\pi} + \mathbf{x}\boldsymbol{\delta} + \boldsymbol{\gamma}\mathbf{w}) \end{aligned} \qquad [21\text{–}14]$$

Here, $\mathbf{x}\boldsymbol{\delta} = x_1\delta_1 + \cdots + x_n\delta_n$ represents food-item effects that are not captured by the term $\mathbf{c}\boldsymbol{\pi}$ for the measured nutrients. The conventional model for $R(\mathbf{z}, \mathbf{w})$ is thus a special case of the hierarchical model for $R(\mathbf{x}, \mathbf{z}, \mathbf{w})$ in which all the δ_j are (dubiously) assumed to be zero.

SPECIFYING THE PRIOR STANDARD DEVIATION

Assuming that all the residual effects δ_j are 0 corresponds to assuming that their common standard deviation τ is 0. A credible analysis will employ a more reasonable (positive) value for τ. Doing so requires careful consideration of the scientific application. In the food-nutrient example, δ_j is only one component of the log rate ratio for the effect of one unit of food item j. We expect little effect on breast cancer from one unit of a food item (a unit such as "100 g of celery per day"); thus we expect δ_j to be rather small. For example, if we are 95% certain that the rate ratio per unit of food item j is between ½ and 2, we should be at least 95% certain that δ_j is within the interval ln(½) = −0.7 and ln(2) = 0.7. In fact, δ_j represents the log rate ratio per unit of food item j *after* adjusting out all the linear-logistic effects of measured nutrients. Therefore, we should be 95% certain that δ_j is in a much smaller interval, say, ln(2/3) = −0.4 to ln(3/2) = 0.4. If the δ_j are normally distributed with SD τ, saying that we are 95% certain that δ_j is between −0.4 and 0.4 is equivalent to saying that $1.96\tau = 0.4$, or that $\tau = 0.2$.

When τ is fixed in advance using background scientific information, the resulting penalized-likelihood estimates are sometimes called generalized ridge-regression or semi-Bayes estimates (Titterington, 1985; Greenland, 1992a, 2000c). Specifying τ in advance can yield better small-sample estimates than estimating τ, but this specification must be done carefully to avoid harming confidence-interval coverage (Greenland, 1993b). Further discussions of specifying τ can be found in Greenland (1992a, 1993b, 1994c, 2000d, 2001b) and Witte et al. (1994, 2000).

It is also possible to assign a prior distribution to τ instead of a single value (sometimes called Bayes empirical-Bayes modeling; Deely and Lindley, 1981), in which case the τ is influenced by the data, but interpretation and specification of this prior can be difficult. As a result, some authors have used "noninformative" or "objective" priors for τ. Again, use of "noninformative" priors has the drawback of assigning overly high probabilities to contextually absurd values of τ.

HIERARCHICAL REGRESSION AND MODEL SELECTION

Hierarchical regression and its variants (such as shrinkage estimation) can provide a solution to much of the arbitrariness and inconsistency inherent in conventional variable selection and model selection procedures (Greenland, 2000c, 2008). Recall that backward elimination (contracting search) procedures ideally begin with a maximal model that is flexible enough to approximate any reasonably possible regression function. Forward selection (expanding search) procedures begin with a minimal model that has only those terms considered essential (e.g., confounder effects), along with one or a few simple exposure terms. Both procedures use somewhat arbitrary criteria to search for a final model. This final model is then incorrectly treated as if it had been specified *a priori,* which in turn leads to invalidly narrow confidence intervals and invalidly small P-values (Sclove et al., 1972; Freedman, 1983; Freedman et al., 1988; Hurvich and Tsai, 1990; Greenland, 1993b; Viallefont et al., 2001).

One hierarchical approach takes a maximal model as the first-stage model, and then specifies a second-stage model such that, when $\tau = 0$ (so that all $\delta_j = 0$), a minimal model holds. By fixing τ at a scientifically reasonable positive value or by estimating it from the data, the resulting fitted hierarchical model will represent a justifiable compromise between the maximal and minimal models. Consider the problem of selecting product terms to include in a model. Backward elimination begins with a maximal model that contains all the product terms among all the regressors and proceeds to delete terms according to some criterion. Forward selection begins with a minimal model that contains no product term and proceeds to add terms according to some criterion. With either procedure, those product terms in the final model may be similar to what they would be in the maximal model, whereas those product terms that are not in the final model have their coefficients set to 0. Thus, these procedures may be viewed as making an "all-or-nothing" choice for each product term.

As an alternative, one can use a hierarchical approach to move ("shrink") each product-term coefficient part way to 0, and so compromise (average) between the extremes of putting each coefficient completely in or completely out of the model. For example, one can use the maximal model as the first-stage model, and then penalize the product-term coefficients for their distance from 0. Suppose there are six binary regressors in the analysis; these yield $\binom{6}{2} = 15$ possible product terms. If the 15 product terms have coefficients $\boldsymbol{\theta} = (\theta_1, \theta_2, \ldots, \theta_{15})$ in the maximal model, one can shrink the estimates of these coefficients toward 0 using a very simple second-stage model in which the θ_j are independent identically distributed random variables with mean 0 and standard deviation τ. In the notation of model 21–12, this model corresponds to making $\theta_j = \delta_j$; there is no second-stage covariate.

SMOOTHING WITH HIERARCHICAL REGRESSION

Consider next the problems of trend modeling. A maximal model allows the regressand (outcome) to depend on the regressor in an arbitrary fashion by having as many coefficients as there are values of the regressor. A minimal model might allow only a linear dependence of the regressand on exposure, and so have only one coefficient for the regressor. Alternatively, the minimal model might allow a more general relation, such as a quadratic dependence (which involves two coefficients for the regressor). In either case, a hierarchical approach uses the maximal model as the first-stage model and then penalizes the regressor coefficients for their distance from the values predicted by the minimal model (Greenland, 1996d).

As an example, suppose the regressor in question is age measured in 11 five-year categories from 35–39 to 85–89, and the regressand is the logarithm of the lung cancer rate. One maximal model for the age trend would include an intercept plus 10 indicator variables for age, e.g., one for each category from 40–44 to 85–89 (there may also be additional terms for other regressors, such as study exposures, smoking, sex, occupation). Let $\boldsymbol{\gamma} = (\gamma_1, \ldots, \gamma_{10})$ be the vector of coefficients of these indicators.

One minimal model for the age trend would include an intercept α plus a single age variable, e.g., the midpoints 37, 42, 47, ..., 87 of the 11 age categories (along with the terms for the other regressors). Let θ be the coefficient of age in this model. The minimal model predicts that the categorical coefficients from the maximal model should follow a simple linear trend,

$$\gamma_j = \theta \cdot 5j \qquad [21\text{–}15]$$

The product $5j$ is the number of years from age 37 (the midpoint of the reference age category, which is category 0) to the midpoint of category j.

The hierarchical approach allows random deviations of the category-specific age terms γ_j from the simple linear model (model 21–15), so that the second-stage model is

$$\gamma_j = \theta \cdot 5j + \delta_j \qquad [21\text{–}16]$$

where the δ_j are independent identically distributed random variables with a mean of 0. Under this approach, the estimates of age-category specific rates will be pulled toward (averaged with) the line predicted by the minimal model (21–15), and so when they are graphed they will exhibit a much smoother trend than that produced by fitting the maximal model (which allows the γ_j to fluctuate in an arbitrary fashion). The smoothness of the curve generated from the hierarchical modeling depends on the size of the prior standard deviation τ for the δ_j. When τ is very large (>2 in exponential and logistic regression), the second-stage model is virtually ignored, and the results are close to those from fitting the maximal model only. When τ is very small, the $\hat{\delta}_j$ will be forced to be near 0 and the fitted curve will be nearly the same as the curve from the minimal (log-linear) model. By allowing use of τ of moderate size, the hierarchical approach enables fitting of models between these extremes of roughness and oversimplification.

SUMMARY

The methods of hierarchical regression can be derived from a number of superficially disparate approaches, among them empirical-Bayes and semi-Bayesian regression; random-coefficient regression; multilevel analysis; penalized-likelihood analysis; ridge regression; and Stein estimation (shrinkage). In addition, all the methods described in this chapter so far—including ordinary regression, overdispersed regression, correlated-outcome regression, and smoothing—can be derived as special cases of hierarchical regression. Hierarchical regression can thus be viewed as a general approach to regression analysis to improve flexibility and accuracy of models and estimates.

MODEL-BASED ESTIMATES OF INCIDENCE AND PREVALENCE

In Chapter 20 we focused primarily on interpreting the model coefficients as differences or log ratios of risks, rates, odds, or prevalences. These interpretations are not very useful when the exposure of interest is represented by more than one continuous model term. To illustrate, suppose we analyze the association of average ounces of alcohol per day X_1 with the 1-year death rate in a cohort of women, adjusting for age X_2, and we use the exponential model

$$I(\mathbf{x}) = \exp(\alpha + \beta_1 x_1 + \gamma_1 x_1^2 + \beta_2 x_2)$$

This is equivalent to the log-linear rate model

$$\log[I(\mathbf{x})] = \alpha + \beta_1 x_1 + \gamma_1 x_1^2 + \beta_2 x_2$$

The coefficient β_1 does not have any straightforward interpretation. It is sometimes called the "linear component of the alcohol effect." It does *not,* however, represent the change in the log rate per unit increase in average daily alcohol consumption, because this change also depends on the coefficient γ_1 of x_1^2 and so depends on the reference level for X_1. For example, under the model, the change in log rate when moving from the $X_1 = 0$ (nondrinker) subpopulation to the $X_1 = 1$ subpopulation is

$$\alpha + \beta_1 1 + \gamma_1 1^2 + \beta_2 x_2 - (\alpha + \beta_1 0 + \gamma_1 0^2 + \beta_2 x_2) = \beta_1 + \gamma_1$$

whereas the change from $X_1 = 2$ to $X_1 = 3$ is

$$\alpha + \beta_1 3 + \gamma_1 3^2 + \beta_2 x_2 - (\alpha + \beta_1 2 + \gamma_1 2^2 + \beta_2 x_2) = \beta_1 + 5\gamma_1$$

The larger the quadratic coefficient γ_1 relative to β_1, the greater will be the disparity between these two changes.

Transforming model results into a table or graph of model-based estimates can provide an easily interpreted summary of results when exposure appears in multiple terms. As an example, consider first a model (such as the preceding one) in which there is no product term containing both exposure and other regressors. In this situation, one may summarize the modeling results by selecting a series of exposure levels and presenting model-based estimates for each selected level. Suppose in the preceding example that alcohol use ranged from 0 to 7 oz/day in the data set. One could then present the model-fitted rates at 0, 1, 2, 3, 5, and 7 oz/day, keeping age X_2 fixed at a reference level x_2. To compute these quantities, we simply exponentiate the fitted log rates at $X_1 = 0, 1, 2, 3, 5, 7$. These fitted rates have the general form

$$\hat{I}(x_1, x_2) = \exp(\hat{\alpha} + \hat{\beta}_1 x_1 + \hat{\gamma}_1 x_1^2 + \hat{\beta}_2 x_2)$$

The levels of the study exposure used in a presentation can be selected based on simplicity and interest, but they are best kept within the range of observed exposure values. One could also select the exposure means in the categories used in tabular (categorical) analyses; this choice allows meaningful comparisons between the model-based and tabular estimates, and ensures that the exposure levels are within the observed range. As rough guidelines to minimize statistical variability of the fitted estimates, we recommend that the reference value for a continuous variable (such as age) be close to its sample mean, while the reference value for a discrete variable (such as ethnicity) be a value frequently observed in both cases and persons still at risk.

Suppose now that there are product terms between the focal exposure and other regressors, as in the model

$$I(\mathbf{x}) = \exp(\alpha + \beta_1 x_1 + \gamma_1 x_1^2 + \beta_2 x_2 + \gamma_2 x_1 x_2 + \gamma_3 x_1^2 x_2)$$

Here, the rate ratios relating alcohol use (X_1) to death change with age (X_2), and hence the curves relating alcohol use to the death rate are not proportional across levels of age. To display this phenomenon, one can tabulate or graph the model-fitted rates at several different age levels in the study age range. These fitted rates have the form

$$\hat{I}(x_1, x_2) = \exp(\hat{\alpha} + \hat{\beta}_1 x_1 + \hat{\gamma}_1 x_1^2 + \hat{\beta}_2 x_2 + \hat{\gamma}_2 x_1 x_2 + \hat{\gamma}_3 x_1^2 x_2)$$

As will be discussed later, it is also straightforward to construct model-based summary effect estimates, such as model-based standardized risk and rate ratios, and attributable-fraction estimates (Lane and Nelder, 1982; Bruzzi et al., 1985; Flanders and Rhodes, 1987; Greenland, 1991c, 2001e, 2004a, 2004b; Greenland and Holland, 1991; Greenland and Drescher, 1993; Joffe and Greenland, 1995).

Confidence limits to accompany model-based estimates can be obtained by setting limits for the term $\alpha + \mathbf{x\beta}$ in the model and then transforming the limits as necessary, or by simulation or bootstrap methods. Some packaged programs will supply a variance estimate $\hat{V}$ or a standard-deviation estimate $\hat{V}^{1/2}$ for a linear combination of model parameters. Such programs will thus supply a variance $\hat{V}$ estimate for $\hat{\alpha} + \mathbf{x}\hat{\boldsymbol{\beta}}$ because $\alpha + \mathbf{x\beta}$ is the linear combination of α and $\beta_1, \ldots, \beta_n$, with coefficients $1, x_1, \ldots, x_n$. We may then set 95% confidence limits for $\hat{\alpha} + \mathbf{x}\hat{\boldsymbol{\beta}}$ using the formula

$$\hat{\alpha} + \mathbf{x}\hat{\boldsymbol{\beta}} \pm 1.96\,\hat{V}^{1/2}$$

(other confidence levels use another multiplier in place of 1.96). If $\alpha + \mathbf{x\beta}$ is the log rate when $\mathbf{X} = \mathbf{x}$, we simply take the antilog of its limits to obtain limits for the rate; if $\alpha + \mathbf{x\beta}$ is a logit (log odds), we take the logistic transform (expit) of its limits to obtain limits for the risk when $\mathbf{X} = \mathbf{x}$. For further descriptions of model-based confidence limits for risk ratios, rate ratios, attributable fractions, and other measures, see Flanders and Rhodes (1987), Greenland (1991c, 2001e, 2004a, 2004b), Benichou and Gail (1990b), Greenland and Drescher (1993), and Joffe and Greenland (1995).

NONPARAMETRIC REGRESSION

So far the discussion has concerned only parametric trend models, in part because all can be fitted using conventional regression software by creating the appropriate regressors (e.g., splines) from the original data. There are, however, several methods that can provide greater model flexibility. Among these methods are *kernel regression,* which generalizes the moving-weighted-average approach described in Chapter 17; *smoothing splines,* which generalize the regression splines described in Chapter 20 (Hastie and Tibshirani, 1990; Simonoff,1996); and *penalized splines,* which are a transitional form between regression splines and smoothing splines that use a hierarchical-regression structure for smoothing, as described earlier (Wahba et al., 1995). Hastie et al. (2001) provide an extensive overview of these topics and related approaches, while Wasserman (2006) provides an introduction. Related hierarchical methods can be used to smooth multiway contingency tables (see Chapter 12 of Bishop et al., 1975, and Greenland, 2006b).

A key characteristic of these techniques is that their primary output is a graph or table of trends, rather than a summary estimate of association or effect. Nonetheless, as discussed later, it is possible to summarize over these outputs using standardization. Kernel regression and smoothing splines are often classified as *nonparametric regression,* because they do not even yield an explicit model or formula for the regression function. Instead, they yield only a list or plot of fitted (estimated) values for the true regression function at specific values for the regressors. This property is a strength, in that assumptions about the shape of the regression are kept to a minimum, but it is a limitation in that a table or graph is needed to describe fully the results from these methods.

For the latter reason, many analysts regard nonparametric regression as a useful exploratory procedure to suggest which parametric model forms to use for trend analyses. As with variable selection, such use of the data to select the model can invalidate P-values and confidence intervals from the final model. Nonetheless, we believe that this exploration is valuable whenever there is a possibility that simpler trend analyses may not be adequate. The chief obstacle to such exploration is sample size: Nonparametric regression requires a fairly large number of subjects across the exposure range of interest to realize its potential flexibility. Even within these limits, however, nonparametric regression can be used for standardized estimation, as described below.

A common type of nonparametric regression is *locally linear kernel regression* (Fan and Gijbels, 1996; Hastie et al., 2001). Suppose that we wish to estimate the regression of Y on $\mathbf{X}$, and we assume that the graph of this function is smooth. Then, over short distances along the regressor axes, the regression can be approximated by a linear function. (This follows from the fact that smooth functions are differentiable.) Just how short these distances are depends on how good an approximation we want. Also, better performance of the method is usually obtained by transforming the regression first. For example, when examining rates, it is usually better to approximate linearly the logarithm of the regression, $\ln[I(\mathbf{x})]$; and when examining risks or proportions, it is usually better to approximate linearly the logit of the regression, $\text{logit}[R(\mathbf{x})]$, because these transforms ensure that the approximation does not go outside logical bounds (0 for rates, 0 and 1 for risks).

Suppose that $h(\mathbf{x})$ is the true value of the transformed regression function. Local linear kernel regression produces a fitted (estimated) value $\hat{h}(\mathbf{x})$ for each distinct regressor value $\mathbf{x}$ by fitting a different *weighted* linear regression model for each $\mathbf{x}$. In the regression at a given value $\mathbf{x}$ for $\mathbf{X}$, the weights vary from 0 to 1, depending on the distance of each data point from $\mathbf{x}$. Any observation with $\mathbf{X} = \mathbf{x}$ receives weight 1 because it has 0 distance from $\mathbf{x}$; the weights decline smoothly as one moves across data points whose $\mathbf{X}$ values are farther and farther from $\mathbf{x}$. Eventually, for data points with $\mathbf{X}$ values very far from $\mathbf{x}$, the weights may be 0 or very close to 0. The weights may also vary inversely with the estimated variances of the outcomes.

To graph or estimate the regression (or its log or logit) in the manner just described can be computationally intensive, because an entire regression model must be fitted for every distinct value of $\mathbf{X}$ that one wishes to plot. Suppose, for example, that $\mathbf{X}$ contains just one regressor, $X_1 =$ years smoked, and that we want our plot to show the fitted rate at 1-year intervals from 0 to 40. Then we have to fit a different log-linear regression with different weights for every one of the 41 years from 0 to 40. To estimate $h(0)$, persons with $X_1 = 0$ have weight 1, and the weights tend to drop off toward 0 as X_1 increases; to estimate $h(20)$, persons with $X_1 = 20$ have weight 1, and the weights tend to drop off toward 0 as X_1 moves away from 20; and so on for all the X_1 values. The regressors $\mathbf{X}$ may include confounders as well as exposures of interest, so that the fitted curves can be confounder-adjusted (in a locally linear fashion). The fitted regression may be local (nonparametric) in one, several, or all the regressors in $\mathbf{X}$. When the fitted estimates are based on a mix of local and fully specified (parametric) elements, this approach is sometimes called "semiparametric."

In locally linear regression, the analyst can control the "waviness" or complexity of the fitted curves (or surface) by varying the rapidity with which the weights fall off as one moves away from the regressor value $\mathbf{x}$ being fitted. In most software, this rapidity is controlled by a *smoothing parameter* that gives a simpler, smoother-looking curve when set high and a more complex, wavy curve when set low. Typically, this parameter can be varied from 0 to 1 or from 0 to infinity. When this parameter is 0, the fitted curve gives weight 0 to everything but observations exactly at **x** and simply "connects the dots" (the observed Y values), producing a jagged, unstable graph. At the other extreme, with a very large smoothing parameter, the resulting curve is practically the same as that from generalized-linear regression analysis (in which the same $\boldsymbol{\beta}$ applies to all **x**).

Some software allows the analyst to experiment with the smoothing parameter to find the most plausible-looking curve; other software estimates a "best" value for this parameter according to some statistical criterion, such as cross-validation sum-of-squares (Hastie and Tibshirani, 1990; Hastie et al., 2001) and plots the results. Also, the smoothing procedure may allow the smoothing parameter to vary with **X**; procedures that do so are called *variable-span* smoothers. Usually, the decline is made more rapid if there are many observations near x, less rapid if there are few. Examples of variable-span smoothers are the LOWESS and LOESS procedures (Hastie and Tibshirani, 1990; Fan and Gijbels, 1996). Because smoothing procedures encounter difficulties when **X** contains more than a few regressors, most software will impose further assumptions beyond smoothness. The most common assumption is that contributions of the separate regressors to the transformed regression are additive; in that case the resulting model is called a *generalized-additive model* (Hastie and Tibshirani, 1990; Hastie et al., 2001).

MODEL-BASED STANDARDIZATION

Suppose that the main objective of modeling is to control confounding by a vector of covariates $\mathbf{Z} = (Z_1, \ldots, Z_K)$ while examining the association of an exposure variable X with an outcome variable Y. A direct approach to this problem is to fit a model for the regression of Y on X and **Z**, which has been the focus of discussion so far. For example, if Y is binary, the most common direct approach fits the group-specific logistic risk model

$$\Pr(Y = 1|X = x, \mathbf{Z} = \mathbf{z}) = \text{expit}(\alpha + x\beta + \mathbf{z}\boldsymbol{\gamma}) \qquad [21\text{–}17]$$

then uses the odds-ratio estimate $\exp(\hat{\beta})$ as the **Z**-adjusted estimate of the association of X with Y.

In the outcome model, the association $\exp(\beta)$ is a **Z**-*conditional* measure, which is supposed to represent the effect of X on Y within strata defined by values of **Z**, provided that **Z** is sufficient for confounding control. As described in Chapter 20, if the conditional effect varies with some component Z_k in the vector **Z** (i.e., if Z_k modifies the effect measure β), the model will at the least need product terms between X and Z_k to capture the variation, and there will be a separate effect measure for every level of Z_k. More sophisticated approaches use a hierarchical or nonparametric regression to estimate $E(Y|X, \mathbf{Z})$. These approaches can lead to a unique effect estimate for every value of **Z**, perhaps with no simple systematic pattern in the estimates.

To address the complexity and potential instability of results when homogeneity is not assumed, one can instead focus on using a model to estimate a standardized measure from the regression. It turns out that several modern statistical methods such as marginal modeling and inverse-probability weighting can be viewed as forms of standardized-effect estimation, and this view connects standardization to confounder scoring (below). To describe the general ideas, as in Chapter 20 let W be a standard distribution for the vector of potential confounders and modifiers **Z**. W is a set of weights $w(\mathbf{z})$, one for each value **z** of **Z**, that sum or integrate to 1, that is, $\sum_{\mathbf{z}} w(\mathbf{z}) = 1$, and the regression of Y on X *standardized* to W is the average of $E(Y|X = x, \mathbf{Z} = \mathbf{z})$ weighted by the $w(\mathbf{z})$,

$$E_W(Y|X = x) = \sum_{\mathbf{z}} w(\mathbf{z})E(Y|X = x, \mathbf{Z} = \mathbf{z}) \qquad [21\text{–}18]$$

As explained in Chapter 20, risk and prevalence parameters are expected proportions, and rates are expected counts per unit of person-time. They can thus be substituted into the standardization formula. For example, a standardized incidence rate is $I_W(x) = \sum_{\mathbf{z}} w(\mathbf{z})I(x, \mathbf{z})$, and a standardized risk is $R_W(x) = \sum_{\mathbf{z}} w(\mathbf{z})R(x, \mathbf{z})$. The latter is an example of a standardized probability, which has the general form

$$\Pr_W(Y = y|X = x) = \sum_{\mathbf{z}} w(\mathbf{z})\Pr(Y = y|X = x, \mathbf{Z} = \mathbf{z}) \qquad [21\text{–}19]$$

The standardization methods discussed next apply with all these forms, although most of the illustrations will be in the probability form.

STANDARDIZATION USING OUTCOME MODELS

Suppose that we know or can validly estimate the weights $w(\mathbf{z})$ for a standard. There are then several approaches to model-based (or smoothed) standardization, depending on the type of model employed. The most straightforward is to model the conditional (X, **Z**-specific) outcomes $E(Y|X = x, \mathbf{Z} = \mathbf{z})$ or $I(x, \mathbf{z})$ or $\Pr(Y = y|X = x, \mathbf{Z} = \mathbf{z})$ and then use the model-fitted (predicted) outcomes in the preceding formulas (Lane and Nelder, 1982). For example, if we fit a model for the X, **Z**-specific incidence rates $I(x, \mathbf{z})$ to a cohort and obtain fitted rates $\hat{I}(x, \mathbf{z})$, the estimated standardized rate is $\hat{I}_W(x) = \sum_{\mathbf{z}} w(\mathbf{z})\hat{I}(x, \mathbf{z})$. The model may be anything we choose, and in particular may contain products between X and components of **Z**, and may have a hierarchical (multilevel) structure. The specific estimates $\hat{I}(x, \mathbf{z})$ may even be from a fitted nonparametric regression, such as those produced by data-driven prediction algorithms (Hastie et al., 2001).

Details of standardization of risks, rates, ratios, and attributable-fractions using parametric models are given by Lane and Nelder, 1982, Bruzzi et al., 1985, Flanders and Rhodes, 1987, Greenland, 1991c, 2001e, 2004a, 2004b; Greenland and Holland, 1991, Greenland and Drescher, 1993, and Joffe and Greenland, 1995, among others. Most of these articles also supply variance formulas; these formulas can be unwieldy, however, and one can instead obtain confidence limits via simulation or bootstrapping (Greenland, 2004c). As always, the interpretation of these standardized estimates as effect estimates assumes that no uncontrolled bias is present, and in particular that **Z** is sufficient for confounding control and has a distribution unaffected by X. Again, the latter assumption is likely to be violated when the standard W is a person-time distribution and X and **Z** affect Y (Chapter 4; Greenland, 1996a)

STANDARDIZED MEASURES VERSUS COEFFICIENTS

To see the relation of standardization to the simpler approach of using a single exposure coefficient as the summary, suppose that the outcome model is of the additive form

$$E(Y|X = x, \mathbf{Z} = \mathbf{z}) = \alpha + x\beta + g(\mathbf{z}) \qquad [21\text{–}20]$$

where $g(\mathbf{z})$ is any function of **Z** [most commonly, $g(\mathbf{z}) = \mathbf{z}\boldsymbol{\gamma}$]. Substitution of 21–20 into the standardization formula (21–18) yields

$$\begin{aligned} E_W(Y|X = x+1) &= \sum_{\mathbf{z}} w(\mathbf{z})[\alpha + (x+1)\beta + g(\mathbf{z})] \\ &= \sum_{\mathbf{z}} w(\mathbf{z})[\alpha + \beta + x\beta + g(\mathbf{z})] \\ &= \sum_{\mathbf{z}} w(\mathbf{z})\beta + \sum_{\mathbf{z}} w(\mathbf{z})[\alpha + x\beta + g(\mathbf{z})] \\ &= \beta \sum_{\mathbf{z}} w(\mathbf{z}) + E_W(Y|X = x) \end{aligned}$$

Because $\sum_{\mathbf{z}} w(\mathbf{z}) = 1$, we get $E_W(Y|X = x+1) = \beta + E_W(Y|X = x)$ and so $E_W(Y|X = x+1) - E_W(Y|X = x) = \beta$. In other words, under an additive model for the X contribution to the conditional outcome $E(Y|X = x, \mathbf{Z} = \mathbf{z})$, the standardized difference for a unit increase in X is equal to the X coefficient, regardless of the weighting W.

Next, suppose that the outcome model is of the log-additive (multiplicative) form

$$E(Y = y|X = x, \mathbf{Z} = \mathbf{z}) = \exp[\alpha + x\beta + g(\mathbf{z})] \qquad [21\text{–}21]$$

Substitution of 21–21 into the standardization formula 21–18 yields

$$\begin{aligned} E_W(Y|X = x+1) &= \sum_{\mathbf{z}} w(\mathbf{z}) \exp[\alpha + (x+1)\beta + g(\mathbf{z})] \\ &= \sum_{\mathbf{z}} w(\mathbf{z}) \exp(\beta) \exp[\alpha + x\beta + g(\mathbf{z})] \\ &= \exp(\beta) \sum_{\mathbf{z}} w(\mathbf{z}) \exp[\alpha + x\beta + g(\mathbf{z})] \\ &= \exp(\beta)\, E_W(Y|X = x) \end{aligned}$$

and so $E_W(Y|X = x+1)/E_W(Y|X = x) = \exp(\beta)$. In other words, under a multiplicative model for the X contribution to $E(Y|X = x, \mathbf{Z} = \mathbf{z})$, the log-standardized ratio for a unit increase in X is equal to the X coefficient, regardless of the weighting W.

The preceding results show that if we are willing to make strong assumptions about homogeneity of the X association with Y across values of $\mathbf{Z}$, we can bypass weighted averaging and use model coefficients as standardized measures. The problem with this usage is its strong dependence on the homogeneity assumptions. With weighted averaging, we can use products of X and $\mathbf{Z}$ components or even more complex regression models, and thus we need not depend on homogeneity assumptions. Nonetheless, if we use an additive model and nonadditivity (modification of the differences by $\mathbf{Z}$) is present, the resulting X-coefficient β can be a good approximation of the population-averaged difference with weights $w(\mathbf{z}) = \Pr(\mathbf{Z} = \mathbf{z})$, provided the $\mathbf{Z}$ contribution $g(\mathbf{Z})$ is well modeled. In a similar fashion, if we use a multiplicative model when modification of the ratios by $\mathbf{Z}$ is present, the resulting $\exp(\beta)$ can be a good approximation of the population-averaged ratio, again provided the $\mathbf{Z}$ contribution $g(\mathbf{Z})$ is well modeled (Greenland and Maldonado, 1994).

Unfortunately, unless risk is low at all $X, \mathbf{Z}$ combinations, the results just described do not carry over to logistic or linear odds models, reflecting the problem of noncollapsibility of odds ratios discussed in Chapter 4. In particular, when $\beta \neq 0$ and $\boldsymbol{\gamma} \neq 0$ in the regression model 21–17, the conditional odds ratio $\exp(\beta)$ will be farther from 1 than the odds ratio obtained by first standardizing the risks from the model and then combining them in an odds ratio (Greenland et al., 1999b). For similar reasons, the results do not carry over to exponential and linear rate models unless X has negligible effect on person-time (Greenland, 1996a).

STANDARDIZATION USING FULL-DATA MODELS

From basic probability,

$$\Pr(Y = y|X = x, \mathbf{Z} = \mathbf{z}) = \Pr(Y = y, X = x, \mathbf{Z} = \mathbf{z})/\Pr(X = x, \mathbf{Z} = \mathbf{z})$$

and

$$\Pr(X = x, \mathbf{Z} = \mathbf{z}) = \sum_{y} \Pr(Y = y, X = x, \mathbf{Z} = \mathbf{z})$$

Substitution into the standardization formula 21–19 yields

$$\Pr_W(Y = y|X = x) = \sum_{\mathbf{z}}[w(\mathbf{z})\Pr(\mathbf{Y} = \mathbf{y}, \mathbf{X} = \mathbf{x}, \mathbf{Z} = \mathbf{z})/\sum_{\mathbf{y}} \Pr(\mathbf{Y} = \mathbf{y}, \mathbf{X} = \mathbf{x}, \mathbf{Z} = \mathbf{z})] \qquad [21\text{–}22]$$

We can thus model the full (joint) distribution $\Pr(Y = y, X = x, \mathbf{Z} = \mathbf{z})$ of Y, X, and $\mathbf{Z}$, and then substitute the fitted values into this alternate standardization formula. When $w(\mathbf{z}) = \Pr(\mathbf{Z} = \mathbf{z})$ or $w(\mathbf{z})$ is the $\mathbf{Z}$ distribution in a special group, such as $w(\mathbf{z}) = \Pr(\mathbf{Z} = \mathbf{z}|X > 0)$, the same model can be used to estimate the weights as well, and thus can provide an integrated modeling approach to standardization (see Chapter 4 of Bishop et al., 1975). In particular, one may use a log-linear count model for the number of subjects expected at each combination of Y, X, and $\mathbf{Z} = \mathbf{z}$.

When $\mathbf{Z}$ is continuous or has many components, full modeling of $\Pr(Y = y, X = x, \mathbf{Z} = \mathbf{z})$ may become impractical or require use of unrealistically strong assumptions. In these situations, modeling only the outcome probability $\Pr(Y = y|X = x, \mathbf{Z} = \mathbf{z})$ can be far more robust than modeling the entire joint distribution $\Pr(Y = y, X = x, \mathbf{Z} = \mathbf{z})$. Other robust approaches can be based on exposure modeling.

STANDARDIZATION USING EXPOSURE MODELS: INVERSE-PROBABILITY WEIGHTING

Consider the probability formula

$$\Pr(Y = y|X = x, \mathbf{Z} = \mathbf{z}) = \Pr(Y = y, X = x, \mathbf{Z} = \mathbf{z})/\Pr(\mathbf{Z} = \mathbf{z})\Pr(X = x|\mathbf{Z} = \mathbf{z})$$

Substitution into the standardization formula 21–19 yields

$$\Pr_W(Y = y|X = x) = \sum_{\mathbf{z}} w(\mathbf{z})\Pr(Y = y, X = x, \mathbf{Z} = \mathbf{z})/\Pr(\mathbf{Z} = \mathbf{z})\Pr(X = x|\mathbf{Z} = \mathbf{z}) \qquad [21\text{–}23]$$

A standardized proportion can thus be viewed as a weighted sum of the proportions $\Pr(Y = y, X = x, \mathbf{Z} = \mathbf{z})$ with weights $w(\mathbf{z})/\Pr(\mathbf{Z} = \mathbf{z})\Pr(X = x|\mathbf{Z} = \mathbf{z})$. The weights are the product of two factors: the standardizing weight $w(\mathbf{z})$ and the inverse-probability weight $1/\Pr(\mathbf{Z} = \mathbf{z})\Pr(X = x|\mathbf{Z} = \mathbf{z})$. Thus, standardization can be viewed as a modified *inverse-probability weighted* procedure (IPW, also known as *Horvitz-Thompson* estimation) (Horvitz and Thompson, 1952; Rosenbaum, 1987; Sato and Matsuyama, 2003).

Because the term $\Pr(\mathbf{Z} = \mathbf{z})$ can be difficult to estimate if $\mathbf{Z}$ is continuous or has many components, the general IPW reformulation is not often used. With the total-population weighting $w(\mathbf{z}) = \Pr(\mathbf{Z} = \mathbf{z})$, however, the IPW formulation simplifies to

$$\Pr_W(Y = y|X = x) = \sum_{\mathbf{z}} \Pr(Y = y, X = x, \mathbf{Z} = \mathbf{z})/\Pr(X = x|\mathbf{Z} = \mathbf{z}) \qquad [21\text{–}24]$$

(Robins et al., 2000). $\Pr_W(Y = y|X = x)$ can thus be estimated by first fitting a model for $\Pr(X = x|\mathbf{Z} = \mathbf{z})$, the probability of exposure $X = x$ given covariates $\mathbf{Z} = \mathbf{z}$, then substituting the fitted values for $\Pr(X = x|\mathbf{Z} = \mathbf{z})$ into 21–24, to create a weighted summation over $\mathbf{Z}$ of the observed proportions with $Y = y, X = x, \mathbf{Z} = \mathbf{z}$. The same fitted exposure model can be used to standardize to a particular exposure group instead of the total. For example, to standardize to those with $X > 0$, $w(\mathbf{z}) = \Pr(\mathbf{Z} = \mathbf{z}|X > 0)$ and formula 21–23 becomes

$$\Pr_W(Y = y|X = x) = \sum_{\mathbf{z}} \Pr(Y = y, X = x, \mathbf{Z} = \mathbf{z})\Pr(X > 0|\mathbf{Z} = \mathbf{z})/\Pr(X = x|\mathbf{Z} = \mathbf{z})$$

(Sato and Matsuyama, 2003). This formula is just a modification of formula 21–24 with the summation weight multiplied by $\Pr(X > 0|\mathbf{Z} = \mathbf{z}) = \sum_{x>0} \Pr(X = x|\mathbf{Z} = \mathbf{z})$.

Because pure IPW estimation models only $\Pr(X = x|\mathbf{Z} = \mathbf{z})$ rather than the entire joint distribution $\Pr(Y = y, X = x, \mathbf{Z} = \mathbf{z})$, it can be more robust than full modeling when $\mathbf{Z}$ has many values. The price, however, is that IPW estimation can be more unstable when some values of X are uncommon, for then the weight denominator $\Pr(X = x|\mathbf{Z} = \mathbf{z})$ can get quite small, making the estimated weight highly unstable. As discussed below, some stabilization of IPW estimation can be achieved by fitting a marginal model to the total-population standardized outcomes, using modified weights.

Although IPW applies to any exposure variable, when X is binary $\Pr(X = 1|\mathbf{Z} = \mathbf{z})$ is often called the exposure *propensity score* (Rosenbaum and Rubin, 1983). Note, however, that IPW uses $\Pr(X = 0|\mathbf{Z} = \mathbf{z})$ for those with $X = 0$, rather than using $\Pr(X = 1|\mathbf{Z} = \mathbf{z})$ for everyone, as is done in propensity scoring (see below).

STANDARDIZATION IN CASE-CONTROL STUDIES

Suppose now that we have case-control data and sufficient external information to estimate the selection ratio f/h for cases and controls. As discussed earlier, one can fit incidence models to the data by modifying the coefficient estimates to reflect the selection ratios. The resulting incidence estimates can be used in outcome-model based standardization.

Suppose next that only ratios or attributable fractions are of interest and the data are unmatched. A simple approach treats the fitted case-control ratios as if they were incidence estimates and enters them directly into the outcome-model formula (21–19). This approach is valid because both the numerator and denominator will be distorted by the same factor (f/h), which will cancel out of the formula. Extensions to matched data are also possible (Greenland, 1987b). For cumulative or prevalence case-control studies, these techniques assume that $\Pr(Y = 1|X = x, \mathbf{Z} = \mathbf{z})$ is uniformly small.

An alternative approach multiplies the weight of each subject by the inverse of its relative probability of selection. This method can be used with any sampling design in which these relative probabilities are known, such as two-stage designs (Flanders and Greenland, 1991; Chapter 15). This approach can become unstable and inefficient (Scott and Wild, 2002), however, and modification of the weights is needed to deal with these problems (Robins et al., 1994, 2000). Approaches based on exposure modeling encounter further problems, as will be discussed under scoring for case-control studies.

MARGINAL-OUTCOME MODELING

An important refinement of IPW estimation adds an explicit model for the standardized outcomes and fits this model with stabilized weights. For example, if Y is binary and $w(\mathbf{z}) = \Pr(\mathbf{Z} = \mathbf{z})$, the standardized outcomes can be given a marginal logistic model such as

$$\Pr_W(Y = 1|X = x) = \text{expit}(\alpha + x\beta) \qquad [21\text{–}25]$$

When $\mathbf{Z}$ is sufficient for confounding control, $\Pr_W(Y = 1|X = x) = \Pr(Y = 1|\text{Set}[X = x])$ and so formula 21–25 becomes the marginal causal model

$$\Pr(Y = 1|\text{Set}[X = x]) = \text{expit}(\alpha + x\beta)$$

which is commonly called a *marginal structural model* (MSM). This marginal model can be fitted using IPW by using estimates of $1/\Pr(X = x|\mathbf{Z} = \mathbf{z})$ as the individual weights in a regression program (Robins et al., 2000). Better performance, however, is obtained by using estimates of $\Pr(X = x)/\Pr(X = x|\mathbf{Z} = \mathbf{z})$ as the weights. These "stabilized" weights are estimated by modeling $\Pr(X = x)$ as well as $\Pr(X = x|\mathbf{Z} = \mathbf{z})$ and then taking the ratio of the fitted values. As before, the approach extends easily to other weightings, e.g., with $w(\mathbf{z}) = \Pr(\mathbf{Z} = \mathbf{z}|X > 0)$, marginal modeling uses the regression weight

$$\Pr(X = x)\Pr(X > 0|\mathbf{Z} = \mathbf{z})/\Pr(X = x|\mathbf{Z} = \mathbf{z})$$

The stabilized marginal modeling approach requires fitting three distinct models, so it is more work than pure IPW modeling. It also can be less robust if the marginal model is restrictive. Nonetheless, if $\mathbf{Z}$ is complicated, it can remain more robust than full modeling of the joint distribution $\Pr(Y = y, X = x, \mathbf{Z} = \mathbf{z})$. General issues comparing IPW methods and modeling of $\Pr(Y = y|X = x, \mathbf{Z} = \mathbf{z})$ are discussed in the next section. Marginal structural modeling tends to produce less stable results than does modeling outcome probabilities, but has the advantage of extending straightforwardly to longitudinal causal modeling (Robins et al., 2000; Hernán et al., 2000).

SCORING METHODS

CONFOUNDER SCORES AND BALANCING SCORES

There has been much work on defining and estimating a function $g(\mathbf{Z})$ of measured confounders $\mathbf{Z}$, called a *confounder score*, that can be treated as a single confounder in subsequent analyses. The target parameter in older work was not always clearly defined. In more precise work, the goal has been to estimate an X effect on Y standardized to the total or exposed source population.

Standardization without modeling is equivalent to taking $g(\mathbf{Z})$ to be a categorical compound variable with a distinct level for every possible value of $\mathbf{Z}$. For example, if $\mathbf{Z}$ = (sex, age), then $g(\mathbf{Z}) = g(\text{sex, age})$ is the compound "sex–age." This two-dimensional $g(\mathbf{Z})$ has as possible values every sex–age combination $g(\mathbf{z})$, such as $g(\text{male}, 60)$ = "male age 60 years," and the effect measure of interest might be a sex–age standardized risk ratio. This two-dimensional score will control all confounding by sex and age if the latter is measured with enough accuracy.

Unfortunately, the strata of a compound variable rapidly become too sparse for analysis as the number of possible values for $\mathbf{Z}$ increases. For example, if $\mathbf{Z}$ is composed of 8 levels for age, 4 levels for housing density, 6 levels for income, 5 levels for education, and 2 levels for sex, it will have 1920 possible levels, far too many strata to use directly in most studies. Thus, attention has focused on model-based construction of a simpler composite score that would control all confounding by $\mathbf{Z}$.

Consider first a score $g(\mathbf{Z})$ with the property that Y and $\mathbf{Z}$ are independent given the exposure and the score. In other words, suppose that when X is at a particular value x and $g(\mathbf{Z})$ is at a particular value c, Y does not depend on the value of $\mathbf{Z}$:

$$\Pr\{Y = y|X = x, \mathbf{Z} = \mathbf{z}, g(\mathbf{Z}) = c\} = \Pr\{Y = y|X = x, g(\mathbf{Z}) = c\}$$

If a score $g(\mathbf{Z})$ satisfies this equation, Y will have a "balanced" (equal) distribution across the values of $\mathbf{Z}$ within strata defined by X and $g(\mathbf{Z})$; hence $g(\mathbf{Z})$ may be called an *outcome-balancing* score.

Consider next a score $g(\mathbf{Z})$ with the property that Y and X are independent given the score. In other words, suppose that $\mathbf{Z}$ does not depend on the value of X when $g(\mathbf{Z})$ is at a particular value c:

$$\Pr\{\mathbf{Z} = \mathbf{z}|X = x, g(\mathbf{Z}) = c\} = \Pr\{\mathbf{Z} = \mathbf{z}|g(\mathbf{Z}) = c\}$$

Such a $g(\mathbf{Z})$ will on average "balance" the distribution of $\mathbf{Z}$ across the levels of X. An equivalent condition is that X does not depend on the value of $\mathbf{Z}$ when $g(\mathbf{Z})$ is at a particular value c:

$$\Pr\{X = x|\mathbf{Z} = \mathbf{z}, g(\mathbf{Z}) = c\} = \Pr\{X = x|g(\mathbf{Z}) = c\}$$

If a score $g(\mathbf{Z})$ satisfies this condition, X will have a "balanced" (equal) distribution across the levels of $\mathbf{Z}$ within strata defined by $g(\mathbf{Z})$; hence, $g(\mathbf{Z})$ may be called an *exposure-balancing* score.

Because of the balance they create, stratification on outcome-balancing or exposure-balancing scores will be sufficient for control of confounding by $\mathbf{Z}$ when estimating marginal (average) effects. Analyses that employ balancing scores may be unnecessarily complicated and inefficient, however. For example, if there is no confounding by any component of $\mathbf{Z}$, no score involving $\mathbf{Z}$ will be necessary and use of such a score will unnecessarily increase variances (and possibly introduce bias if some component of $\mathbf{Z}$ should not be controlled). The key issue is how to construct a score that is at once simple and sufficient. Many regression approaches have been proposed for this purpose, and the following subsections review several that have been have been used in epidemiologic research.

OUTCOME SCORES

Scores that are constructed to predict the outcome are called *outcome scores*. Early outcome-scoring methods were based on fitting a model for the regression of the outcome Y on $\mathbf{Z}$ alone (e.g., Bunker et al., 1969). For a disease indicator Y, one could fit a logistic model

$$\Pr(Y = 1|\mathbf{Z} = \mathbf{z}) = \text{expit}(\alpha^* + \mathbf{z}\boldsymbol{\gamma}^*)$$

then use the fitted probability expit $(\hat{\alpha} + \mathbf{z}\hat{\boldsymbol{\gamma}}^*)$ for each subject as the values $g(\mathbf{z})$ of the confounder score. This fitted probability is also known as a *risk score* or *prognostic score*. Because the fitted probability is just a one-to-one function of the fitted linear combination $\mathbf{z}\hat{\boldsymbol{\gamma}}^*$, one can equivalently take $g(\mathbf{z}) = \mathbf{z}\hat{\boldsymbol{\gamma}}^*$ as the confounder score.

Analyses using risk scores obtained by regressing Y on $\mathbf{Z}$ alone (without X) appeared in various forms through the 1970s. Such scores are *not* outcome-balancing, and adjusting for them results in null-biased estimates of the $\mathbf{Z}$-adjusted association of X on Y. This bias arises because the term $\mathbf{z}\boldsymbol{\gamma}^*$ incorporates any effect of X that is confounding the $\mathbf{Z}$ effect, and hence adjustment for $\mathbf{z}\boldsymbol{\gamma}^*$ adjusts away part of the X effect (Miettinen, 1976b; Greenland, 1984b). If the model is correct, however, the adjustment can give correct null P-values (Pike et al., 1979; Cook and Goldman, 1989).

To remove the bias, one may use as the confounder score the fitted value of the linear term at $X = 0$ from a model with both X and $\mathbf{Z}$, such as $g(\mathbf{z}) = \mathbf{z}\hat{\boldsymbol{\gamma}}$ from fitting the risk model 21–17 (Miettinen, 1976b; Pike et al., 1979). This score will be outcome balancing on average if the model is correct. Nonetheless, because the score is estimated, the resulting standard errors may be downwardly biased, leading to downwardly biased P-values and overly narrow confidence intervals. Thus, on theoretical grounds as well as labor, none of these basic outcome-score approaches is clearly better than just using $\exp(\hat{\beta})$ from the outcome model (21–17) as the effect estimate, nor are they better than model-based standardization.

EXPOSURE SCORES

Scores that are constructed to predict the exposure are called *exposure scores*. Miettinen (1976b) suggested creating an exposure score by regressing X on Y and $\mathbf{Z}$, and then (by analogy with risk scoring) setting $Y = 0$. In the context of cohort studies, Rosenbaum and Rubin (1983) argued instead that one should model the probability of X as a function of $\mathbf{Z}$ only, which for a binary X could be

$$\Pr(X = 1|\mathbf{Z} = \mathbf{z}) = e_1(\mathbf{z}) = \text{expit}(\nu + \mathbf{z}\boldsymbol{\theta})$$

They called this probability of $X = 1$ the *propensity score* for X, and showed that, if the fitted model is correct, $e_1(\mathbf{z})$ is the coarsest exposure-balancing score, in that no further simplification of the score preserves its property of balancing $\mathbf{Z}$ across levels of X. Note, however, that simpler scores than $e_1(\mathbf{z})$ may be sufficient for control of confounding by $\mathbf{Z}$. For example, if Z_1 is not confounding given the remaining covariates in $\mathbf{Z}$ then there is no need to balance Z_1, and a score without Z_1 would be sufficient and simpler.

Subsequent work showed (rather paradoxically) that if one knows the correct model for the propensity score, using the score from fitting that model has better statistical properties than using the true score $e_1(\mathbf{z})$ (Rosenbaum, 1987; Robins et al., 1992b). Thus, if the preceding model were correct, using fitted score $\hat{e}_1(\mathbf{z}) = \text{expit}(\hat{\nu} + \mathbf{z}\hat{\boldsymbol{\theta}})$ would be better than using $e_1(\mathbf{z}) = \text{expit}(\nu + \mathbf{z}\boldsymbol{\theta})$ with the true ν and $\boldsymbol{\theta}$. Although this theory shows that the propensity-score approach, taking $g(\mathbf{z}) = \hat{e}_1(\mathbf{z})$, is a viable competitor to direct modeling of the regression of Y on X and $\mathbf{Z}$, the propensity model is unknown in observational studies and the theory leaves open how the exposure model should be built. Studies suggest that the criteria for selection of variables for adjustment (inclusion in $\mathbf{Z}$) should be the same as those used for outcome regression (e.g., Brookhart et al., 2006). These criteria can be roughly summarized by the common-sense rule that important confounders should be forced into the model. Because the strength of confounding by a covariate Z_k is determined by its association with both X and Y, selection based on either association alone can easily select nonconfounders over confounders.

As with analyses based on modeling Y, selection based on conventional variable-selection criteria (e.g., coefficient $P < 0.05$) can be especially harmful. For example, stepwise propensity modeling will retain a variable that is unassociated with Y if it is "significantly" associated with X, resulting in adjustment for a nonconfounder; yet it will remove a confounder whose association with X is "nonsignificant," resulting in uncontrolled confounding. On the other hand, it will retain variables that discriminate strongly between exposed and unexposed even if they have no relation to Y other than through X and so are not confounders, thus harming the efficiency of propensity-score stratification by reducing overlap between the exposed and unexposed groups. For similar reasons, ability of the propensity model to discriminate between the exposed and unexposed should not be a criterion for determining a good model; e.g., a model that discriminates perfectly will leave no exposed and unexposed subjects in the same stratum of the fitted score.

As with any modeling procedure, once the exposure model has been fitted, checks of its adequacy are advisable. A simple diagnostic is to check that the exposure and the covariates $\mathbf{Z}$ are independent given the exposure score, as they should be if the score is adequate. This check is often done by examining the covariate-exposure associations after stratifying the data on the fitted scores.

Given that the score appears adequate, the question is how it should be used for adjustment. Scores have been used for stratification, matching, or as a covariate in regressions of Y on exposure (Rosenbaum, 2002; Rubin, 2006). As noted earlier, the fitted propensity score $\hat{e}_1(\mathbf{z})$ can also be used to construct inverse-probability weights for marginal modeling of the dependence of Y on X (Robins et al., 2000; Hirano et al., 2003; Lunceford and Davidian, 2004). For example, those with $X = 1$ could receive weight $w = 1/\hat{e}_1(\mathbf{z})$; those with $X = 0$ would then receive weight $\hat{w} = 1/\hat{e}_0(\mathbf{z})$; where $\hat{e}_0(\mathbf{z}) = 1 - \hat{e}_1(\mathbf{z})$ is the fitted value of $\Pr(X = 0|\mathbf{Z} = \mathbf{z})$. In other words, a model for the regression of Y on X is fitted in which each subject receives a weight $1/\hat{e}_x(\mathbf{z})$, the inverse of the probability of getting the exposure the subject actually had.

One objection to stratification and matching on a fitted score is that they involve score categorization, which may introduce residual confounding (Robins et al., 1992b; Lunceford and Davidian, 2004). Similarly, direct use of the score as a regressor in an outcome model may introduce further model misspecification, although this problem may be minimized by modeling the association between the score and the outcome flexibly (e.g., using polynomial regression or splines). Matching on the score can avoid these problems but can invalidate conventional interval estimates for the effect (Hill and Reiter, 2006; Abadie and Imbens, 2006).

In contrast, weighting requires neither categorization nor specification of the score effect on Y. It also generalizes easily to an exposure variable X with more than two levels, including time-varying exposures (Hernán et al., 2000, 2001). Its chief drawback is that it can lead to instabilities due to fitted probabilities near 0 (Robins et al., 2000). A related approach that does not require categorization uses a special transform of $\hat{e}_x(z)$ in a conditional-outcome model and then averages over that model (Bang and Robins, 2005).

Because of differences in implicit weightings, different approaches may be estimating different parameters if there is modification of the X effect measure across levels of $\mathbf{Z}$ (Stürmer et al., 2005, 2006; Kurth et al., 2006). For example, standardization over propensity-score strata corresponds to standardization by $w(\mathbf{z}) = \Pr(\mathbf{Z} = \mathbf{z})$, and use of other summaries over the strata often approximates this standardization (Greenland and Maldonado, 1994). But propensity-score matching will alter the cohort distribution of $\mathbf{Z}$ and thus lead to a different standard than simply using everyone in the propensity-score analysis. If matching is based on taking all those with $X = 1$ and using their score to select n matches with $X = 0$, the resulting cohort will in expectation have the $\mathbf{Z}$ distribution $\Pr(\mathbf{Z} = \mathbf{z}|X = 1)$ of the exposed, and so that distribution will now be the standard.

In a similar fashion, weighting by $1/\hat{e}_1(\mathbf{z})$ and $1/\hat{e}_0(\mathbf{z})$ is equivalent to standardization to the distribution in the total cohort, $\Pr(\mathbf{Z} = \mathbf{z})$ (Robins et al., 2000). To standardize to the distribution in the exposed, $\Pr(\mathbf{Z} = \mathbf{z}|X = 1)$, the weights $w(\mathbf{z})$ must be modified to $\hat{e}_1(\mathbf{z})/\hat{e}_1(\mathbf{z}) = 1$ for the exposed and $\hat{e}_1(\mathbf{z})/\hat{e}_0(\mathbf{z})$ for the unexposed (Sato and Matsuyama, 2003). This standard is appropriate if the goal is to estimate net effect that exposure had on the exposed. To standardize to the distribution in the unexposed, $\Pr(\mathbf{Z} = \mathbf{z}|X = 0)$, the weights $w(\mathbf{z})$ must be modified to $\hat{e}_0(\mathbf{z})/\hat{e}_1(\mathbf{z})$ for the exposed and $\hat{e}_0(\mathbf{z})/\hat{e}_0(\mathbf{z}) = 1$ for the unexposed. This standard is appropriate if the goal is to estimate the net effect that exposure would have on the unexposed.

Propensity-score and IPW methods are based on modeling the full probability $\Pr(X = x|\mathbf{Z} = \mathbf{z})$ of X given $\mathbf{Z}$. When X is continuous, this task can be more difficult to do accurately than modeling only the regression of X on $\mathbf{Z}$, $E(X = x|\mathbf{Z} = \mathbf{z})$, which is the $\mathbf{Z}$-conditional mean of exposure X. *E-estimation* and *intensity scoring* are based on adjustment using a fitted model for the exposure regression $E(X = x|\mathbf{Z} = \mathbf{z})$, subject to constraints on the conditional regression $E(Y|X = x, \mathbf{Z} = \mathbf{z})$ (Robins et al., 1992b; Brumback et al., 2003). Like IPW, these methods generalize to time-varying exposures and confounders, where they are known as *g-estimation* (see below).

OUTCOME VERSUS EXPOSURE MODELING

There has been some controversy over the relative merits of outcome modeling and exposure modeling approaches, especially with regard to their model dependence. A few facts should be noted at the outset. First, confounding that is not captured by the measured $\mathbf{Z}$ (e.g., because of measurement error in $\mathbf{Z}$ or failure to include some confounders in $\mathbf{Z}$) cannot be accounted for by either approach. Thus neither approach addresses a truly intrinsic problem of observational studies—residual confounding by mismeasured or unmeasured confounders (Rubin, 1997; Joffe and Rosenbaum, 1999). In a similar fashion, adjustment for inappropriate covariates, such as those affected by X or Y (e.g., intermediates) will produce bias, regardless of the approach.

If $\mathbf{Z}$ is a confounder, mismodeling of either $E(Y|X = x, \mathbf{Z} = \mathbf{z})$ or $\Pr(X = x|\mathbf{Z} = \mathbf{z})$ can leave residual confounding by $\mathbf{Z}$. It thus is always possible that results from neither, only one, or each approach suffers bias from mismodeling. The relative bias of the approaches may depend heavily on the modeling strategy. As a simple example, suppose that just one covariate Z_k in $\mathbf{Z}$ is the only confounder in a study, and that both the outcome models will be built by selecting only those covariates in $\mathbf{Z}$ with $P < 0.05$ in the fitted model. If Z_k has $P < 0.05$ in the outcome model but $P > 0.05$ in the exposure model, it will be selected into the outcome model and there will be no confounding of results from that model, but it will be left out of the exposure model, resulting in confounding of results from that model. Conversely, if Z_k has $P > 0.05$ in the outcome model but $P < 0.05$ in the exposure model, it will be left out of the outcome model, resulting in confounding of results from that model, but it will be selected into the exposure model and there will be no confounding of results from that model.

The specification issue is often framed as a question of how accurately we can model the dependence of Y on X and $\mathbf{Z}$ versus how accurately we can model the dependence of X on $\mathbf{Z}$. In both approaches the final step may be to average (standardize) over the modeling results. In each approach, this averaging can reduce sensitivity to mismodeling. For example, when one standardizes model-based estimates of $E(Y|X = x, \mathbf{Z} = \mathbf{z})$ over a $\mathbf{Z}$-distribution similar to that in the data, the resulting summary estimates will be far more stable and less sensitive to misspecification than the $E(Y|X = x, \mathbf{Z} = \mathbf{z})$ estimates. This robustness arises from the averaging of residual errors to 0 over the data distribution of the regressors. Although this average need not be 0 within levels of X, one can check the X-specific averages: Large values indicate that X was mismodeled.

Early simulation studies reported higher specification robustness for propensity scoring (Drake, 1993; Drake and Fisher, 1995), but with only one confounder, no provision for model modification or expansion (and thus no adaptivity to context), and no explicit justification of parameter settings chosen for simulation. Use of modern modeling strategies in simulation (e.g., hierarchical or nonparametric modeling) can change comparisons dramatically, sometimes in favor of outcome modeling (e.g., Hill and McCulloch, 2008).

The potential accuracy and difficulty of each approach also depends heavily on context as well as modeling strategy. For example, in a study of nutrient intakes and lung cancer, it is doubtful that modeling of intakes (the exposures) will be any simpler or more accurate than modeling of lung cancer risk. Exposure modeling would also be more laborious insofar as a new exposure model would have to be be created for every nutrient we wish to examine. As an opposite example, in a focused study of a medical procedure or prescription drug and survival, we may have far more ability to model accurately who will receive the procedure or drug than who will survive the study period. Thus, one cannot judge whether outcome or exposure modeling is preferable without knowledge about the topic under study.

On the latter issue, it is frequently overlooked that adjustment via exposure modeling requires at least two models: the exposure model for X given $\mathbf{Z}$, and a model for adjustment of the X, Y association by the fitted exposure model. The latter model may involve only Y, X, and the fitted score, and may be far simpler than the model for $E(Y|X = x, \mathbf{Z} = \mathbf{z})$ if $\mathbf{Z}$ is complicated or contains many variables. Nonetheless, that simplicity reflects only transference of complexity to modeling $\Pr(X = x|\mathbf{Z} = \mathbf{z})$.

A parallel statistical issue is the amount of sample information available for each model. In this regard the exposure model often has an advantage in practice (Cepeda et al., 2003). To illustrate, suppose that Y is binary and X and $\mathbf{Z}$ are purely categorical. If, as often happens in cohort studies, the sample numbers with $Y = 1$ at each level of X, $\mathbf{Z}$ tend to be very small, estimates of conditional risk $\Pr(Y = 1|X = x, \mathbf{Z} = \mathbf{z})$ may require a restrictive model, or may become unstable and suffer small-sample biases (Greenland et al., 2000a). If at the same time the numbers at each level of X, $\mathbf{Z}$ are large, stable estimates of the exposure probabilities $\Pr(X = x|\ \mathbf{Z} = \mathbf{z})$ can still be obtained. Note, however, that this small-sample bias advantage of exposure modeling does not lead to greater efficiency, because the final precision of any estimate remains limited by the small numbers at $Y = 1$. Note also that the advantage will switch to outcome modeling if the outcome ($Y = 1$) is common but the exposure ($X = 1$) is rare.

The relative precision of summary estimates from outcome and exposure modeling is difficult to evaluate because of the noncomparable models used by the two approaches. Theoretical results that assume homogeneous exposure effects and correct specification of both models (e.g., Robins et al., 1992b) find precision or power advantages for outcome modeling, as observed in examples and simulations (e.g., Drake and Fisher, 1995). This advantage is purchased by risk of downwardly biased standard errors if effects are heterogeneous. This risk can be reduced by use of X–$\mathbf{Z}$ product terms or more flexible outcome models, which in turn reduces the efficiency of outcome modeling. The same theory confirms empirical reports that inclusion of nonconfounders is less harmful to precision in exposure modeling than in outcome modeling (assuming, of course, that the nonconfounders are unaffected by exposure; see Chapters 9 and 12), although this difference may not be enough to compensate for the lower precision of exposure modeling relative to outcome modeling (Robins et al., 1992b; Lunceford and Davidian, 2004).

Again, different approaches may be estimating different parameters, which can lead to disparate results even when all the models are correct (Stürmer et al., 2005, 2006; Kurth et al., 2006; Austin et al., 2007). As mentioned above, coefficients from outcome models and marginal models reflect an approximate total-population weighting (Greenland and Maldonado, 1994), but propensity-score matching can greatly alter the population and hence the weighting. Meaningful comparisons require modification of the weights to give the methods the same standard, as described earlier.

MODEL COMBINATION AND DOUBLY ROBUST ESTIMATION

A straightforward resolution of the choice between outcome modeling and exposure modeling is to do both, and if disagreement appears, to attempt to discern the reason. Another resolution is to combine the two approaches, for example, by entering the score directly in a model for Y along with

X and $\mathbf{Z}$, or by using the propensity score for matching and then regressing Y on X and $\mathbf{Z}$ in the matched sample (Rubin and Thomas, 2000; Rubin, 2006). Alternatively, one may use the inverse-probability weights estimated from modeling $\Pr(X = x|\mathbf{Z} = \mathbf{z})$ to fit the model for $E(Y|X = x, \mathbf{Z} = \mathbf{z})$, then standardize over the fitted expected outcomes (Kang and Schafer, 2007). Intuitively, the idea is that if propensity scoring or IPW fails to adjust fully for $\mathbf{Z}$, the regression adjustment for $\mathbf{Z}$ may compensate, and vice versa.

This idea is formalized in the theory of *doubly robust estimation,* which shows how to combine outcome and exposure modeling in a fashion that gives a valid estimate if either model is correct (Scharfstein et al., 1999; Van der Laan and Robins, 2003; Kang and Schafer, 2007). The theory justifies the IPW regression approach and leads to new approaches to marginal modeling (Bang and Robins, 2005). The term *doubly robust* reflects the fact that these methods have two ways to get the right answer, although this property does not necessarily improve performance when neither model is correct (Kang and Schafer, 2007).

SCORING IN CASE-CONTROL STUDIES

In most case-control studies, selection probabilities are intentionally set much higher for cases than for potential controls, and they may also vary with covariates $\mathbf{Z}$ as a result of matching. One consequence is that models for Y and for X fitted to the data will be distorted relative to the population. As discussed earlier, however, in most studies one can fit outcome models as if the data were from a cohort study, and the distortions will cancel out of incidence-ratio and attributable-fraction estimates from the models. If one has population data, these data can be used to remove the distortions in the outcome models to obtain incidence estimates as well (Greenland 1981, 2004d).

Unlike outcome modeling, at present no published exposure-scoring proposal for case-control data has strong theoretical or empirical support. The situation is complicated because the distortion of the relation of X to $\mathbf{Z}$ produced by case-control sampling does not cancel out of estimation formulas, even when there is no matching. As a result, simply fitting the propensity score to the data without regard to outcome status or sampling will result in a biased score estimate and thus can lead to residual confounding (Mansson et al., 2007). One naïve solution to this problem is to assume the controls are representative of the population and fit an exposure model to the controls only (Miettinen, 1976b). Unfortunately, this practice can lead to distorted score-specific estimates because the resulting scores will fit the controls far better than the cases. One consequence of this distortion is the spurious appearance of variation in effect measures across levels of the propensity score (effect-measure modification) even when there is none (Mansson et al., 2007).

One could instead fit a model for $\Pr(X = 1|Y = y, \mathbf{Z} = \mathbf{z})$ to both the cases and controls, and then use the fitted value of $\Pr(X = 1|Y = 0, \mathbf{Z} = \mathbf{z})$ as the exposure score (Miettinen, 1976b). The effectiveness of this strategy in eliminating the aforementioned distortions depends in part on the number of product terms between Y and $\mathbf{Z}$ components in the model: With many outcome-covariate products, the fitted values of $\Pr(X = 1|Y = 0, \mathbf{Z} = \mathbf{z})$ will approach those obtained by fitting the controls alone, leading back to the original distortions. Performance of this and any scoring strategy will also depend on the method used to adjust for the estimated score.

MODELING LONGITUDINAL DATA

This section provides a brief description of certain issues that can arise in studies involving time-dependent exposures and confounders (such as smoking, alcohol use, drug use, treatment compliance, occupational exposures, diet, exercise, stress, weight, blood pressure, serum cholesterol, cancer screening, and health insurance status) or recurrent outcomes (such as angina, back pain, allergy attacks, asthma attacks, seizures, and depression). It focuses primarily on the problem that a time-dependent covariate may both affect and be affected by the study exposure, and thus act as both a confounder and an intermediate. Similarly, a recurrent outcome may both affect and be affected by a time-dependent exposure and thus act as a confounder as well as an outcome.

Data that contain multiple measurements over time on each subject are often called *repeated-measures* or *longitudinal data*. Although there is a voluminous literature on the analysis of such data, most of it does not give methods that adjust properly for confounding by intermediate or outcome variables. In particular, standard methods of time-dependent Cox modeling (Cox and Oakes, 1984;

Kalbfleish and Prentice, 2002), random-effects regression (Stiratelli et al., 1984), and correlated logistic regression ("GEE" analysis) (Liang and Zeger, 1986; Zeger and Liang, 1992; Diggle et al., 2002) give biased effect estimates when exposure affects a confounder or is affected by the study outcome (Robins et al., 1992a; Robins and Greenland, 1994; Robins et al., 1999b).

TIME-DEPENDENT EXPOSURES AND COVARIATES

All the methods for effect estimation we have considered up to now, and those considered in most textbooks, implicitly assume that the study exposure does not affect any covariate used to create strata or used as a regressor. As discussed in earlier chapters, they also assume that there is no confounding within strata or within levels of other covariates in the analysis model. These two assumptions are often incompatible when the exposure and covariates vary over time.

To illustrate, suppose that we wish to study the overall long-term effect of coffee use on myocardial infarction (MI) risk. Serum cholesterol is a reasonable candidate as a confounder, because coffee drinkers may have more unmeasured factors associated with elevated cholesterol (such as personality traits) and because serum cholesterol is positively associated with MI risk. On the other hand, serum cholesterol is also a reasonable candidate as an intermediate, because coffee use may elevate serum cholesterol levels (Chapter 33).

The net effect of both the preceding scenarios will be a positive association of coffee use and serum cholesterol. Given that serum cholesterol is also positively associated with MI, adjustment for serum cholesterol will most likely decrease the estimated effect of coffee use on MI (indeed, this decrease has been observed in some studies). Because coffee use and elevated serum cholesterol may be associated through common causes, some of this decrease could be attributed to removal of confounding by cholesterol, in which case the unadjusted estimate will be biased. Nonetheless, because part of the coffee–cholesterol association may be due to a coffee effect on cholesterol, part of the decrease in the estimated coffee effect may reflect adjustment for a variable (again, cholesterol) affected by coffee use, and so will not reflect removal of confounding. This reasoning implies that the adjusted estimate is also biased.

As one might expect, resolution of this dilemma requires that one have longitudinal data on the exposure (here, coffee use) and every covariate that plays a dual role of confounder and intermediate (here, serum cholesterol). It also requires use of an estimation method that adjusts for the confounding effect of the covariate *and no more*. In particular, we do not want to adjust for the effect of exposure on the confounder. Unfortunately, conventional methods, such as time-dependent Cox regression and Poisson regression, cannot fulfill this requirement (Robins et al., 1992a). Robins has developed a number of approaches that can properly adjust the estimated effect of a time-varying exposure for a time-varying covariate if longitudinal data are available (Robins, 1987, 1989, 1993, 1997, 1999; Robins et al., 1992a). These methods may be necessary even if exposure and the covariate affected by exposure have no effect on risk; such situations arise when the covariate is a proxy for unmeasured confounders.

Suppose now that we are interested only in the direct effect of coffee use on MI, apart from any effect it has on cholesterol. That is, we may wish to estimate the part of the coffee effect on MI that is *not* attributable to any increase in cholesterol it produces. Here again, conventional adjustment methods may be biased for this direct effect (Robins and Greenland, 1992, 1994; see Chapter 12). Fortunately, the same methods developed by Robins for adjusting for confounding by an intermediate variable can be extended to the problem of estimating direct effects (Robins and Greenland, 1994; Petersen et al., 2006).

The problems described above are examples of the more general problem of determining what variables must be measured (e.g., full coffee use and cholesterol histories, versus summaries such as average levels) and how these variables must be accounted for in the analysis, given that a particular effect is of interest. As discussed in Chapter 12, graphical approaches to this problem have been developed, along with explicit algorithms for making such determinations.

RECURRENT OUTCOMES

Consider next a situation in which the outcome may recur. Examples commonly arise in studies of respiratory disease, neurologic disorders, and psychiatric conditions. For example, the outcome may be asthma attack (yes or no) recorded for each day of the study period, along with fixed covariates (such as sex) and time-varying covariates (such as activity, medication, air pollution, and weather variables). In some situations, the outcome may affect (as well as be affected by) the exposure and other covariates. For example, having an asthma attack one day may influence a person's activity level the next day; furthermore, it may directly affect the risk of an asthma attack the next day. Thus, earlier outcomes may act as confounders when estimating effects of exposures on later outcomes.

Unfortunately, conventional methods for analyzing recurrent outcomes, such as generalized estimating equation or GEE regression (Zeger and Liang, 1992; Diggle et al., 2002) and random-effects logistic regression (Stiratelli et al., 1984), do not adjust for the effects of outcomes on exposures or covariates, nor do they properly adjust for the effects of earlier outcomes on later outcomes (Robins et al., 1999b). These methods assume implicitly that the outcome does not affect the exposure and other covariates, and they impose symmetric relations between outcomes at different times (note that causal relations are inherently asymmetric; in particular, earlier outcomes can affect later outcomes, but not vice versa). The methods of Robins do not require such assumptions, and they can be applied to the analysis of recurrent outcomes (Robins et al., 1999b).

STRUCTURAL MODELS AND G-ESTIMATION

Variables in a model are sometimes classified as *endogenous* or internal if they can be affected by other variables in the model, *exogenous* or external if not (see Chapter 12). For example, in a longitudinal study of asthma attacks, physical activity and medication variables will be endogenous variables, whereas air pollution and weather variables will be exogenous variables. With this terminology, the message of the present section can be summarized thus: Methods such as classical standardization, correlated-outcome (random-effects and GEE) regression, and Cox regression can give biased answers when some of the confounders are endogenous. To avoid this bias, methods based on multiple model equations (such as those of Robins) are needed.

The topic of modeling multiple causal relations with multiple equations is known in social sciences as *structural-equations modeling*. This topic is so vast that we cannot review it here. A classic introduction to linear structural equations is Duncan (1975), while Pearl (2000) provides a modern nonparametric perspective that is equivalent to the approach of Robins (1997). Several issues in structural-equation modeling arise when estimating effects of time-dependent exposures. One strong objection to the social science literature on structural equations is that the methods often involve implausibly strong assumptions, such as linear relations among all variables (Freedman, 1985, 1987). To avoid such difficulties, Robins developed semiparametric methods that attempt to minimize assumptions about the functional forms of the causal relations and error distributions, and that have some robustness to violations of the assumptions that are made (Robins et al., 1992a, 1992b; Robins, 1993, 1997, 1998a, 1998b, 1999; Mark and Robins, 1993a; Robins and Greenland, 1994; Witteman et al., 1998).

Most of these methods are based on *structural nested failure-time* (SNFT) and *structural nested mean* (SNM) models, which generalize the potential-outcome models described in Chapters 4 and 20 to longitudinal treatments (i.e., time-dependent exposures that may influence and be influenced by other time-dependent variables). The robustness of structural nested modeling arises from the fact that it makes no assumption about the causal relations among the covariates beyond that required by the time ordering (causes must precede effects). The only causal dependence it models is that of the outcome on the exposure. Along with the latter causal model, it employs another model for the regression of the study exposure at each point in time on the exposure, covariate, and disease history of each subject up to that point in time.

Mathematically, structural nested failure-time models are a generalization of the strong accelerated-life model described in Chapter 20. To describe the model, suppose that a person is actually given fixed treatment $X = x_a$ and "fails" (e.g., dies) at time Y_a, where Y_a is the potential outcome of the person under $X = x_a$. Assuming zero is a meaningful reference value for X, the basic causal accelerated-life model assumes the survival time of the person when given $X = 0$ instead would have been $Y_0 = \exp(x_a\beta)Y_a$, where Y_0 is the potential outcome of the person under $X = 0$, and the factor $\exp(x_a\beta)$ is the amount by which setting $X = 0$ would have expanded (if $x_a\beta > 0$) or contracted (if $x_a\beta < 0$) survival time relative to setting $X = x_a$.

Suppose next that X can vary over time, and that the actual survival interval $S = (0, Y_a)$ is partitioned into K successive intervals of length $\Delta t_1, \ldots, \Delta t_K$, such that $X = x_k$ in interval k. A basic structural-nested model for the survival time of the person had X been held at 0 over time is then

$$Y_0 = \sum_k \exp(x_k \beta) \, \Delta t_k$$

The distribution of Y_0 across persons may be further modeled as a function of baseline covariates.

Structural nested models are most easily fitted using a two-step procedure called *g-estimation* (Robins et al., 1992; Robins and Greenland, 1994; Robins, 1998a). To illustrate the basic idea, assume no censoring of Y, no measurement error, and let X_k and $\mathbf{Z}_k$ be the treatment and covariates at interval k. Then, under the model, a hypothesized value β_h for β produces for each person a computable value $Y_0(\beta_h) = \sum_k \exp(x_k \beta_h) \Delta t_k$ for Y_0. Next, suppose that for all k, Y_0 and X_k are independent given the treatment history $X_1, \ldots, X_{k-1}$ and covariate history $\mathbf{Z}_1, \ldots, \mathbf{Z}_k$ up to time k (as will occur if treatment is sequentially randomized given these histories). If $\beta = \beta_h$, then $Y_0(\beta_h) = Y_0$ and so must be independent of X_k given the histories. One can test this conditional independence of $Y_0(\beta_h)$ and the X_k with any standard method. For example, one could use a permutation test or some approximation to one, such as the log-rank test (Chapter 16) stratified on the treatment and covariate histories.

Subject to further modeling assumptions, one could instead use a test that the coefficient of $Y_0(\beta_h)$ is zero in a model for the regression of X_k on $Y_0(\beta_h)$ and the histories. In either case, the set of all β_h that have a P-value greater than α by this test form a $1 - \alpha$ confidence interval for β, and the value of β_h with $P = 1$ (the value b for β that makes $Y_0(b)$ and the X_k conditionally independent) is a valid estimator of β (Robins, 1998a). G-estimation can be implemented in any package that allows preprocessing and creation of the new covariates $Y_0(\beta_h)$ for regression analysis (Witteman et al., 1998; Sterne et al., 2002; Tilling et al., 2002).

If (as usual) censoring is present, g-estimation becomes more complex (Robins, 1998a). As a simpler though more restrictive approach to censored longitudinal data with time-varying treatments, one can fit a marginal structural model (MSM) for the potential outcomes using a generalization of inverse-probability weighting (Robins, 1998b, 1999; Robins et al., 2000; Hernán et al., 2000, 2001). Unlike standard time-dependent Cox models, both SNFT and marginal-structural model fitting require special attention to the censoring process, but they make weaker assumptions about that process. Their greater complexity is the price one must pay for the generality of the procedures: Both structural nested and marginal structural models can yield unconfounded effect estimates in situations in which standard models appear to fit well but yield very biased results (Robins et al., 1992a, 1999b, 2000; Robins and Greenland, 1994).

One important application of g-estimation is in adjusting for noncompliance (nonadherence) when estimating treatment effects from randomized trials (Robins and Tsiatis, 1991; Mark and Robins, 1993ab). Typical analysis of randomized trials use the "intent-to-treat" rule, in which subjects are compared based on their assigned treatment, regardless of compliance. Estimates of biologic treatment effects based on this rule tend to be biased because noncompliance causes assigned treatment to become a misclassified version of received treatment. On the other hand, noncompliers tend to differ from compliers with respect to risk, and hence conventional analyses of received treatment tend to be confounded. Thus, we face the dilemma (analogous to that with confounding intermediates) of bias in either conventional analysis.

Subject to certain assumptions that are usually more plausible than those required for the validity of conventional analyses, it is possible to escape the dilemma by using assigned treatment as a fixed exogenous covariate and received treatment as an endogenous time-dependent exposure whose effect is represented in a structural nested model. See Mark and Robins (1993b), White et al. (2002), Cole and Chu (2005), and Greenland et al. (2008) for more details.

As with all statistical methods, inferences from g-estimation and marginal structural modeling are conditional on the model being correct, and the model is not likely to be exactly correct even if its fit appears good. Nonetheless, the validity of the P-value for the null hypothesis $\beta = 0$ from g-estimation will be fairly insensitive to misspecification of the form of the model for Y_0, although the power of the corresponding test may be severely impaired by the misspecification

(Robins, 1998a). Of course, in observational studies g-estimation and marginal structural modeling share all the usual limitations of conventional methods, including the assumption that all errors are random as described by the model (no uncontrolled confounding, selection bias, or measurement error). In particular, inferences from the methods are only conditional on an uncertain assumption of "no sequential confounding," that Y_0 and the X_k are independent given the treatment and covariate histories used for stratification or modeling of Y_0 and the X_k. When this assumption is in doubt, one will need to turn to sensitivity analysis to assess the effect of its violation (Brumback et al., 2004).

Section IV

Special Topics

CHAPTER 22

Surveillance

James W. Buehler

History of Surveillance 460
Objectives of Surveillance 462
Descriptive Epidemiology of Health Problems 462
Links to Services 464
Links to Research 464
Evaluation of Interventions 465
Planning and Projections 466
Education and Policy 467
Summary 467
Elements of a Surveillance System 467
Case Definition 467
Population under Surveillance 469
Cycle of Surveillance 470
Confidentiality 470
Incentives to Participation 470
Surveillance Ethics 471
Summary 471
Approaches to Surveillance 472
Active versus Passive Surveillance 472
Notifiable Disease Reporting 472
Laboratory-Based Surveillance 472
Volunteer Providers 473
Registries 473
Surveys 473
Information Systems 474
Sentinel Events 475
Record Linkages 475
Combinations of Surveillance Methods 475
Summary 476
Analysis, Interpretation, and Presentation of Surveillance Data 476
Analysis and Interpretation 476
Presentation 478
Attributes of Surveillance 479
Conclusion 479

People who manage programs to prevent or control specific diseases need reliable information about the status of those diseases or their antecedents in the populations they serve. The process that is used to collect, manage, analyze, interpret, and report this information is called *surveillance*. Surveillance systems are networks of people and activities that maintain this process and may function at local to international levels. Because surveillance systems are typically operated by public health agencies, the term "public health surveillance" is often used (Thacker and Berkelman, 1988). Locally, surveillance may provide the basis for identifying people who need treatment, prophylaxis, or education. More broadly, surveillance can inform the management of public health programs and the direction of public health policy (Sussman et al., 2002).

When new public health problems emerge, the rapid implementation of surveillance is critical to an effective early response. Likewise, as public health agencies expand their domain to include a broader spectrum of health problems, establishing surveillance is often a first step to inform priority setting for new programs. Over time, surveillance is used to identify changes in the nature or extent of health problems and the effectiveness of public health interventions. As a result, surveillance systems may grow from simple *ad hoc* arrangements into more elaborate structures.

The modern concept of surveillance was shaped by programs to combat infectious diseases, which depended heavily on legally mandated reporting of "notifiable" diseases (Langmuir, 1963). Health problems now monitored by surveillance reflect the diversity of epidemiologic inquiry and public health responsibilities, including acute and chronic diseases, reproductive health, injuries, disabilities, environmental and occupational health hazards, and health risk behaviors (Thacker and Berkelman, 1988). An equally diverse array of methods is used to obtain information for surveillance, ranging from traditional case reporting to adapting data collected primarily for other purposes, such as computerized medical care records.

Surveillance systems are generally called on to provide descriptive information regarding when and where health problems are occurring and who is affected—the basic epidemiologic parameters of time, place, and person. The primary objective of surveillance is most commonly to monitor the occurrence of disease over time within specific populations. When surveillance systems seek to identify all, or a representative sample of, occurrences of a health event in a defined population, data from surveillance can be used to calculate incidence rates and prevalence. Surveillance can characterize persons or groups who are affected by health problems and identify groups at highest risk. Surveillance is often used to describe health problems themselves, including their manifestations and severity, the nature of etiologic agents (e.g., antibiotic resistance of microorganisms), or the use and effect of treatments.

Populations under surveillance are defined by the information needs of prevention or control programs. For example, as part of a hospital's program to monitor and prevent hospital-acquired infections, the target population would be patients receiving care at that hospital. At the other extreme, the population under surveillance may be defined as the global population, as is the case for a global network of laboratories that collaborate with the World Health Organization in tracking the emergence and spread of influenza strains (Kitler et al., 2002). For public health agencies, the population under surveillance usually represents residents within their political jurisdiction, which may be a city, region, or nation.

All forms of epidemiologic investigation require a balance between information needs and the limits of feasibility in data collection. For surveillance, this balance is often the primary methodologic challenge. As an ongoing process, surveillance depends on long-term cooperation among persons at different levels in the health delivery system and coordinating agencies. Asking too much of these participants or failing to demonstrate the usefulness of their participation threatens the operation of any surveillance system and wastes resources. Another dimension of this balance lies in the interpretation of surveillance data, regardless of whether surveillance depends on primary data collection or adaptation of data collected for other purposes. Compared with data from targeted research studies, the advantage of surveillance data is often their timeliness and their breadth in time, geographic coverage, or number of people represented. To be effective, surveillance must be as streamlined as possible. As a result, surveillance data may be less detailed or precise compared with those from research studies. Thus, analyses and interpretation of surveillance data must exploit their unique strengths while avoiding overstatement.

HISTORY OF SURVEILLANCE

The modern concept of surveillance has been shaped by an evolution in the way health information has been gathered and used to guide public health practice (Table 22–1) (Thacker and Berkelman, 1992; Eylenbosch and Noah, 1988). Beginning in the late 1600s and 1700s, death reports were first used as a measure of the health of populations, a use that continues today. In the 1800s, Shattuck used morbidity and mortality reports to relate health status to living conditions, following on the earlier work of Chadwick, who had demonstrated the link between poverty and disease. Farr combined data analysis and interpretation with dissemination to policy makers and the public, moving beyond the role of an archivist to that of a public health advocate.

In the late 1800s and early 1900s, health authorities in multiple countries began to require that physicians report specific communicable diseases to enable local prevention and control activities, such as quarantine of exposed persons or isolation of affected persons. Eventually, local reporting systems coalesced into national systems for tracking certain endemic and epidemic infectious diseases, and the term *surveillance* evolved to describe a population-wide approach to monitoring health and disease.

TABLE 22–1

Key Events in the History of Public Health Surveillance

Date	Events
Late 1600s	von Leibnitz calls for analysis of mortality reports in health planning.
	Graunt publishes *Natural and Political Observations Made upon the Bills of Mortality,* which defines disease-specific death counts and rates.
1700s	Vital statistics are used in describing health increases in Europe.
1840–1850	Chadwick demonstrates relationship between poverty, environmental conditions, and disease.
	Shattuck, in report from Massachussets Sanitary Commission, relates death rates, infant and maternal mortality, and communicable diseases to living conditions.
1839–1879	Farr collects, analyzes, and disseminates to authorities and the public data from vital statistics for England and Wales.
Late 1800s	Physicians are increasingly required to report selected communicable diseases (e.g., smallpox, tuberculosis, cholera, plague, yellow fever) to local health authorities in European countries and the United States.
1925	All states in the United States begin participating in national morbidity reporting.
1935	First national health survey is conducted in the United States.
1943	Cancer registry is established in Denmark.
Late 1940s	Implementation of specific case definition demonstrates that malaria is no longer endemic in the southern United States.
1955	Active surveillance for cases of poliomyelitis demonstrates that vaccine-associated cases are limited to recipients of vaccine from one manufacturer, allowing continuation of national immunization program.
1963	Langmuir formulates modern concept of surveillance in public health, emphasizing role in describing health of populations.
1960s	Networks of "sentinel" general practitioners are established in the United Kingdom and The Netherlands.
	Surveillance is used to target smallpox vaccination campaigns, leading to global eradication.
	WHO broadens its concept of surveillance to include a full range of public health problems (beyond communicable diseases).
1980s	The introduction of microcomputers allows more effective decentralization of data analysis and electronic linkage of participants in surveillance networks.
1990s and 2000s	The Internet is used increasingly to transmit and report data. Public concerns about privacy and confidentiality increase in parallel with the growth in information technology.
2001	Cases of anthrax associated with exposure to intentionally contaminated mail in the United States lead to growth in "syndromic surveillance" aimed at early detection of epidemics.

Adapted from Thacker SB, Berkelman RL. History of public health surveillance. In: Halperin W, Baker EL, Monson RR. *Public Health Surveillance.* New York: Van Nostrand Reinhold, 1992:1–15; and Eylenbosch WJ, Noah ND. Historical aspects. In: Eylenbosch WJ, Noah ND, eds. *Surveillance in Health and Disease.* Oxford: Oxford University Press, 1988:1–8.

Important refinements in the methods of notifiable disease reporting occurred in response to specific information needs. In the late 1940s, concern that cases of malaria were being overreported in the southern United States led to a requirement that case reports be documented. This change in surveillance procedures revealed that malaria was no longer endemic, permitting a shift in public health resources and demonstrating the utility of specific case definitions. In the 1960s, the usefulness of outreach to physicians and laboratories by public health officials to identify cases of disease and solicit reports (active surveillance) was demonstrated by poliomyelitis surveillance during the implementation of a national poliomyelitis immunization program in the United States. As a result of these efforts, cases of vaccine-associated poliomyelitis were shown to be limited to recipients of vaccine from one manufacturer, enabling a targeted vaccine recall, calming of public fears, and continuation of the program. The usefulness of active surveillance was further demonstrated during the smallpox-eradication campaign, when surveillance led to a redirection of vaccination efforts away from mass vaccinations to highly targeted vaccination programs.

Throughout the 1900s, alternatives to disease reporting were developed to monitor diseases and a growing spectrum of public health problems, leading to an expansion in methods used to conduct surveillance, including health surveys, disease registries, networks of "sentinel" physicians, and use of health databases. In 1988, the Institute of Medicine in the United States defined three essential functions of public health: assessment of the health of communities, policy development based on a "community diagnosis," and assurance that necessary services are provided, each of which depends on or can be informed by surveillance (Institute of Medicine, 1988).

In the 1980s, the advent of microcomputers revolutionized surveillance practice, enabling decentralized data management and analysis, automated data transmission via telephone lines, and electronic linkage of participants in surveillance networks, as pioneered in France (Valleron et al., 1986). This automation of surveillance was accelerated in the 1990s and early 2000s by advances in the science of informatics and growth in the use of the Internet (Yasnoff et al., 2000). In the early 2000s, the increasing threat of bioterrorism provided an impetus for the growth of systems that emphasized the earliest possible detection of epidemics, enabling a timely and maximally effective public health response. These systems involve automation of nearly the entire process of surveillance, including harvesting health indicators from electronic records, data management, statistical analysis to detect aberrant trends, and Internet-based display of results. Despite this emphasis on informatics, the interpretation of results and the decision to act on surveillance still requires human judgment (Buehler et al., 2003).

While the balance between privacy rights and governments' access to personal information for disease monitoring has been debated for over a century, the increasing automation of health information, both for medical care and public health uses, has led to heightened public concerns about potential misuse (Bayer and Fairchild, 2000; Hodges et al., 1999). This concern is exemplified in the United States by the implementation in 2003 of the privacy rules of the Health Insurance Portability and Accountability Act of 1996, which aim to protect privacy by strictly regulating the use of electronic health data yet allowing for legitimate access for public health surveillance (Centers for Disease Control and Prevention, 2003a). In the United Kingdom, the Data Protection Act of 1998, prompted by similar concerns, has called into question the authority of public health agencies to act on information obtained from surveillance (Lyons et al., 1999). As the power of information technologies grow, such controversies regarding the balance between public health objectives and individual privacy are likely to increase in parallel with the capacity to automate public health surveillance.

OBJECTIVES OF SURVEILLANCE

DESCRIPTIVE EPIDEMIOLOGY OF HEALTH PROBLEMS

Monitoring trends, most often trends in the rate of disease occurrence, is the cornerstone objective of most surveillance systems. The detection of an increase in adverse health events can alert health agencies to the need for further investigation. When outbreaks or disease clusters are suspected, surveillance can provide a historical perspective in assessing the importance of perceived or documented changes in incidence. Alternatively, trends identified through surveillance can provide an indication of the success of interventions, even though more detailed studies may be required to evaluate programs formally.

For example, the effectiveness of the national program to immunize children against measles in the United States has been gauged by trends in measles incidence. Following the widespread use of measles vaccine, measles cases declined dramatically during the 1960s. In 1989–1990, however, a then-relatively large increase in measles cases identified vulnerabilities in prevention programs, and subsequent declines demonstrated the success of redoubled vaccination efforts (Centers for Disease Control and Prevention, 1996) (Fig. 22–1).

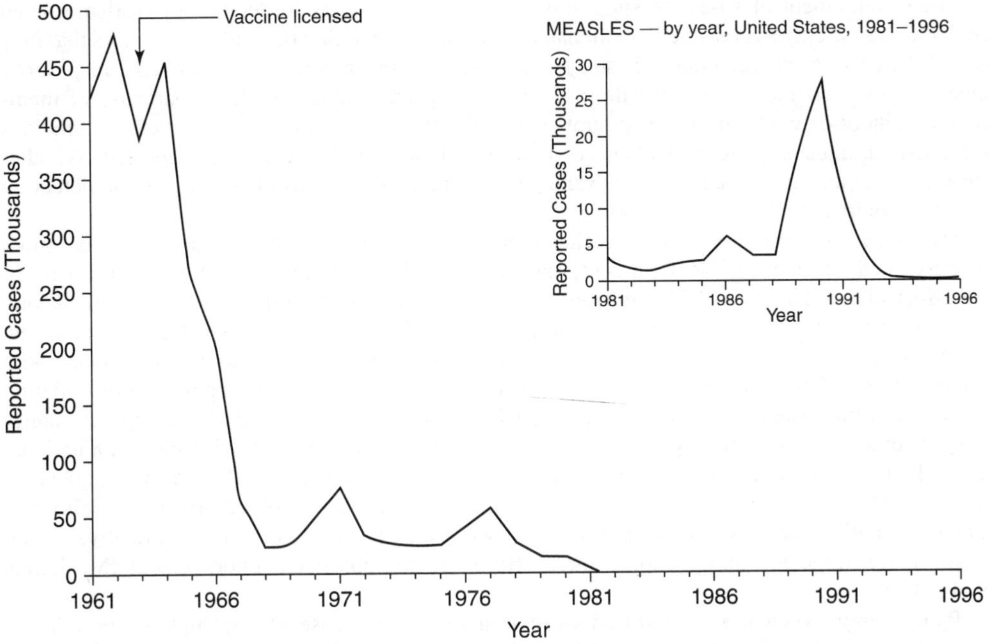

FIGURE 22–1 • Measles, by year of report, 1961–1996, United States. (Reproduced from Centers for Disease Control and Prevention. Summary of notifiable diseases, United States, 1996. *Morb Mortal Wkly Rep.* 1996;45:43.)

Information on the common characteristics of people with health problems permits identification of groups at highest risk of disease, while information on specific exposures or behaviors provides insight into etiologies or modes of spread. In this regard, surveillance can guide prevention activities before the etiology of a disease is defined. This role was demonstrated in the early 1980s, when surveillance of the acquired immunodeficiency syndrome (AIDS) provided information on the sexual, drug using, and medical histories of people with this newly recognized syndrome. Surveillance data combined with initial epidemiologic investigations defined the modes of human immunodeficiency virus (HIV) transmission before HIV was discovered, permitting early prevention recommendations (Jaffe et al., 1983). Equally important, the observation that nearly all persons with AIDS had an identified sexual, drug-related, or transfusion exposure was effective in calming public fears about the ways in which the disease was *not* transmitted, i.e., that the presumed infectious agent was not transmissible via casual contact or mosquito bites.

Detection of outbreaks is an often-cited use of surveillance. In practice, astute clinicians commonly detect outbreaks before public health agencies receive and analyze information on case reports. This pattern has been often been the case for clusters of new diseases, including toxic shock syndrome, legionnaires disease, and AIDS. Contacts between health departments and clinicians engendered by surveillance, however, can increase the likelihood that clinicians will inform health departments when they suspect that outbreaks are occurring. Some outbreaks may not be recognized if individual clinicians are unlikely to encounter a sufficient number of affected persons to perceive an increase in incidence. In such instances, surveillance systems that operate on a broad geographic basis may detect outbreaks. Such detection occurred in 1983 in Minnesota, where laboratory-based surveillance of salmonella infections detected an increase in isolates of a particular serotype, *Salmonella newport*. Subsequent investigation of these cases documented a specific pattern of antibiotic resistance in these isolates and a link to meat from cattle that had been fed subtherapeutic doses of antibiotics to promote growth (Holmberg, 1984). The results of this investigation, which was triggered by findings from routine surveillance in one state, contributed to a national reassessment of policies in the United States regarding the use of antibiotics in animals raised for human consumption.

The development of so-called syndromic surveillance systems to detect bioterrorism-related epidemics as quickly as possible has emphasized automated tracking of disease indicators that may herald the onset of an epidemic. These systems monitor nonspecific syndromes (e.g., respiratory illness, gastrointestinal illness, febrile rash illness) and other measures (e.g., purchase of medications, school or work absenteeism, ambulance dispatches) that may increase before clinicians recognize an unusual pattern of illness or before illnesses are diagnosed and reported. Whether these approaches offer a substantial advantage over traditional approaches to epidemic detection has been controversial (Reingold, 2003).

Data may also be collected on the characteristics of the disease itself, such as the duration, severity, method of diagnosis, treatment, and outcome. This information provides a measure of the effect of the disease and identification of groups in whom the illness may be more severe. For example, surveillance of tetanus cases in the United States in 1989–1990 documented that deaths were limited to persons >40 years of age and that the risk of death among persons with tetanus increased with increasing age. This observation emphasized the importance of updating the immunization status of adults as part of basic health services, particularly among the elderly (Prevots et al., 1992). Among patients with end-stage kidney disease receiving care in a national network of dialysis centers in the United States, surveillance of a simple indicator that predicts the risk of morbidity and reflects the sufficiency of dialysis (reduction in blood urea levels following dialysis) identified centers with subpar performance levels. For those centers with relatively poor performance, targeted quality improvement efforts led to subsequent improvement (McClellan et al., 2003).

By describing where most cases of a disease occur or where disease rates are highest, surveillance provides another means for targeting public health interventions. Depicting surveillance data using maps has long been a standard approach to illustrate geographic clustering, highlight regional differences in prevalence or incidence, and generate or support hypotheses regarding etiology. A classic example is the use of maps by John Snow to support his observations that cholera cases in London in 1854 were associated with consumption of drinking water from a particular well, the Broad Street pump (Brody et al., 2000). In the United States, men of African descent have higher rates of prostate cancer compared with other men, and death rates for prostate cancer are highest in the Southeast (Fig. 22–2). This observation, coupled with observations that farmers are at increased risk for prostate cancer and that farming is a common occupation in affected states, prompted calls for further investigation of agricultural exposures that may be linked to prostate cancer (Dosemeci et al., 1994).

LINKS TO SERVICES

At the community level, surveillance is often an integral part of the delivery of preventive and therapeutic services by health departments. This role is particularly true for infectious diseases for which interventions are based on known modes of disease transmission, therapeutic or prophylactic interventions are available, and receipt of a case report triggers a specific public health response. For example, notification of a case of tuberculosis should trigger a public health effort to assure that the patient completes the full course of therapy, not only to cure the disease but also to minimize the risk of further transmission and prevent recurrence or emergence of a drug-resistant strain of *Mycobacterium tuberculosis*. In countries with sufficient public health resources, such a report also prompts efforts to identify potential contacts in the home, workplace, or school who would benefit from screening for latent tuberculosis infection and prophylactic therapy. Likewise for certain sexually transmitted infections, case reports trigger investigations to identify, test, counsel, and treat sex partners. Thus, at the local level, surveillance not only provides aggregate data for health planners, it also serves to initiate individual preventive or therapeutic actions.

LINKS TO RESEARCH

Although surveillance data can be valuable in characterizing the basic epidemiology of health problems, they seldom provide sufficient detail for probing more in-depth epidemiologic hypotheses. Among persons reported with a disease, surveillance may permit comparisons among different groups defined by age, gender, date of report, etc. Surveillance data alone, however, do not often

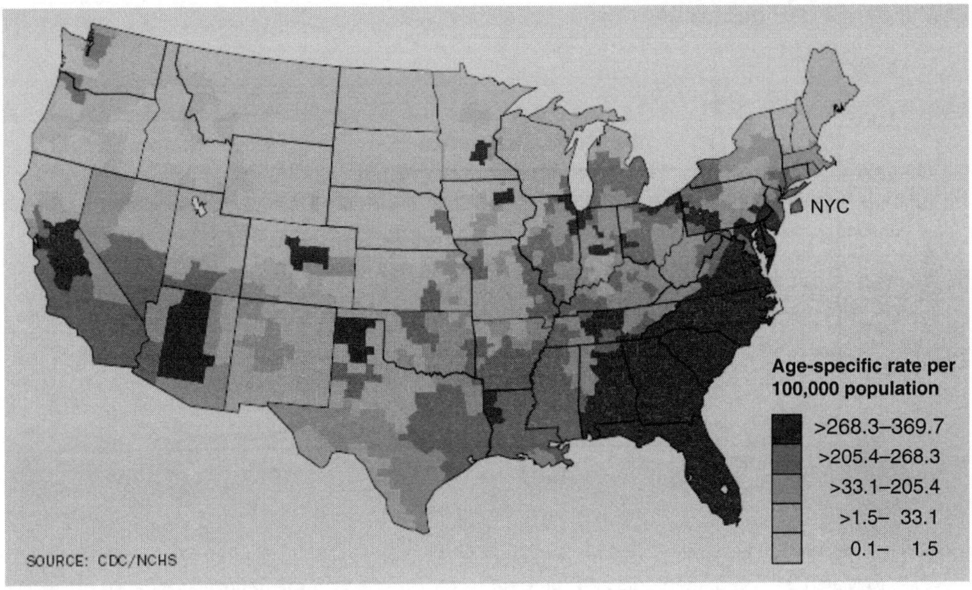

FIGURE 22–2 • Prostate cancer death rates, by place of residence, black males, age 70 years, 1988–1992. United States. (Reproduced from Pickle LW, Mungiole M, Jones GK, White AA. *Atlas of United States Mortality*. Hyattsville, MD: National Center for Health Statistics; 1996. DHHS Publication No. (PHS) 97-1015, p. 67.)

provide a comparison group of people without the health problem in question. Nonetheless, surveillance can provide an important bridge to researchers by providing clues for further investigation and by identifying people who may participate in research studies. This sequence of events occurred shortly after the detection of an epidemic of toxic shock syndrome in 1979. Rapidly initiated surveillance illustrated that the outbreak was occurring predominantly among women and that disease onset was typically during menstruation (Davis et al., 1980). This finding led to case-control studies that examined exposures associated with menstruation. These studies initially found an association with tampon use and subsequently with use of a particular tampon brand. This information led to the recall of that tampon brand and recommendations concerning tampon manufacture (Centers for Disease Control, 1990d).

EVALUATION OF INTERVENTIONS

Evaluation of the effect of public health interventions is complex. Health planners need information about the effectiveness of interventions, yet full-scale evaluation may not be feasible. By charting trends in the numbers or rates of events or the characteristics of affected persons, surveillance may provide a comparatively inexpensive and sufficient assessment of the effect of intervention efforts. In some instances, the temporal association of changes in disease trends and interventions are so dramatic that surveillance alone can provide simple and convincing documentation of the effect of an intervention. Such was the case in the outbreak of toxic shock syndrome, when cases fell sharply following removal from the market of the tampon brand associated with the disease (Fig. 22–3).

In other instances, the role of surveillance in assessing the effect of interventions is less direct. For example, the linkage of information from birth and death certificates is an important tool in the surveillance of infant mortality and permits monitoring of birth-weight-specific infant death rates. This surveillance has demonstrated that in the United States, declines in infant mortality during the latter part of the 20th century were due primarily to a reduction in deaths among small, prematurely born infants. Indirectly, this decline is a testament to the effect of advances in specialized obstetric and newborn care services for preterm newborns. In contrast, relatively little progress has been made in reducing the proportion of infants who are born prematurely (Buehler et al., 2000).

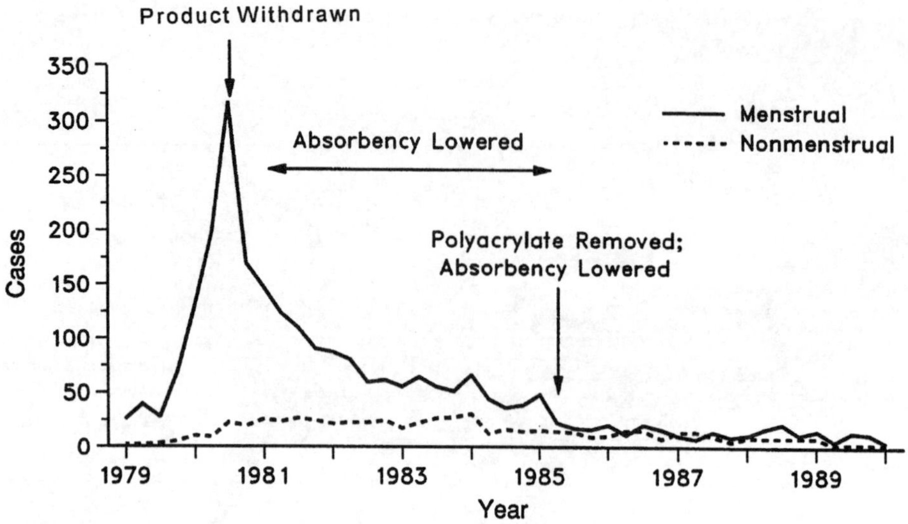

FIGURE 22–3 • Reported cases of toxic shock syndrome, by quarter: United States, January 1, 1979, to March 31, 1990. (Reproduced from Centers for Disease Control. Reduced incidence of menstrual toxic-shock syndrome—United States, 1980–1990. *Morb Mortal Wkly Rep.* 1990;39:421–424.)

Following recognition of widespread HIV transmission during the late 1980s and early 1990s in Thailand, the Thai government instituted a multifaceted national HIV prevention program. Surveillance data demonstrated that one element of this program—aggressive promotion of condom use for commercial sex encounters—was associated with an increase in condom use and parallel declines in HIV and other sexually transmitted infections among military conscripts, one of several sentinel populations among whom HIV trends had been monitored. Although this observation provides compelling support for the effectiveness of the condom promotion strategy, it is impossible to definitively parse attribution among various program elements and other influences on HIV risk behaviors (Celentano et al., 1998).

PLANNING AND PROJECTIONS

Planners need to anticipate future demands for health services. Observed trends in disease incidence, combined with other information about the population at risk or the natural history of a disease, can be used to anticipate the effect of a disease or the need for care.

During earlier years of the global HIV epidemic, widespread transmission was not manifest because of the long interval between the asymptomatic phase of HIV infection and the occurrence of severe disease. In Thailand, HIV prevention programs noted earlier were prompted by findings from a comprehensive system of HIV serologic surveys during a period when the full effect of HIV infection on morbidity and mortality was yet to be seen. These surveys, established to monitor HIV prevalence trends, revealed a dramatic increase in HIV infections among illicit drug users in 1988, followed by subsequent increases among female sex workers, young men entering military service (most of whom were presumably infected through sexual contact with prostitutes), women infected through sexual contact with their boyfriends or husbands, and newborn infants infected through perinatal mother-to-infant transmission (Weninger et al., 1991). The implications of these data, both for the number of future AIDS cases and the potential for extension of HIV transmission, prompted the prevention program.

Techniques for predicting disease trends using surveillance data can range from the application of complex epidemiologic models to relatively simple strategies, such as applying current disease rates to future population estimates. The World Health Organization used this latter strategy to predict global trends in diabetes through 2025, applying the most recently available age- and country-specific diabetes prevalence estimates obtained from surveillance and other sources to population projections. Despite the limitations of the data used to make these calculations and of the assumptions underlying this approach, the resulting prediction that increases in diabetes will be greater among developing than developed countries provides a starting point for diabetes prevention and care planners (King et al., 1998).

EDUCATION AND POLICY

The educational value of surveillance data extends from their use in alerting clinicians to community health problems to informing policy makers about the need for prevention or care resources. Influenza surveillance illustrates this spectrum. Local surveillance based on reporting and specimen collection by "sentinel" physician practices can identify the onset of the influenza season and prevalent influenza strains (Brammer et al., 2002; Fleming et al., 2003). Public health departments can use this information to alert clinicians to the appearance of influenza, provide timely guidance on the evaluation of patients with respiratory illness, and inform the use of antiviral or other medications. Globally, surveillance of influenza through an international network of laboratories is used to predict which strains are likely to be most prevalent in an upcoming season and guide vaccine composition and manufacture (Kitler et al., 2002). Documentation of the extent of influenza-related morbidity and mortality, combined with assessments of vaccine use and effectiveness, can shape public debates about policies for vaccine manufacture, distribution, purchase, and administration, as happened during the 2003–2004 influenza season in the United States, when illness peaked earlier than usual and demand for vaccine exceeded supply (Meadows, 2004).

Surveillance and other epidemiologic or scientific evidence provide an essential perspective in shaping public health policy and must be effectively integrated with other perspectives that are often brought to bear in political decision making. The complexity of this process is heightened when conflicting values about priorities or optimal interventions clash, as is evident in the development of HIV-prevention policy. Surveillance data illustrate the extent of transmission attributable to illicit drug use or sexual intercourse, and other studies shed light on the effectiveness of intervention strategies such as needle–syringe exchange and drug treatment programs and promotion of condom use and sexual abstinence (Valdiserri et al., 2003). How prevention resources are allocated among these and other strategies is shaped not only by epidemiologic and cost-effectiveness data but also by the values of those contributing to policy development.

SUMMARY

The primary objective of surveillance is to monitor the incidence or prevalence of specific health problems, to document their effect in defined populations, and to characterize affected people and those at greatest risk. At the community level, surveillance can guide health departments in providing services to people; in the aggregate, surveillance data can be used to inform and evaluate public health programs. Trends detected through surveillance can be used to anticipate future trends, assisting health planners. In addition to providing basic information on the epidemiology of health problems, surveillance can lead to hypotheses or identify participants for more detailed epidemiologic investigations. To be effective, surveillance data must be appropriately communicated to the full range of constituents who can use the data, ranging from health care providers to policy makers.

ELEMENTS OF A SURVEILLANCE SYSTEM

CASE DEFINITION

Defining a case is fundamental and requires an assessment of the objectives and logistics of a surveillance system. Surveillance definitions must balance competing needs for sensitivity, specificity, and feasibility. For diseases, requiring documentation through evidence of diagnostic tests may be important. Equally important are the availability of tests, how they are used, and the ability of surveillance personnel to obtain and interpret results. Because of the need for simplicity, surveillance case definitions are typically brief.

For some diseases, definitions may be stratified by the level of confirmation, e.g., probable versus confirmed cases, depending on available information (Centers for Disease Control and

Prevention, 1997). For surveillance of health-related behaviors or exposures, surveillance definitions may depend on self-reports, observation, or biologic specimen collection and measurement. For an individual disease or health problem, no single definition is ideal. Rather, appropriate definitions vary widely in different settings, depending on information needs, methods of reporting or data collection, staff training, and resources. For example, successful surveillance definitions for hepatitis A, an infection that results in short-term liver dysfunction, range from "yellow eyes"—a hallmark clinical sign of jaundice that accompanies the disease—to a definition that requires laboratory-based documentation of infection with hepatitis A virus combined with signs of acute illness and clinical or laboratory evidence of liver dysfunction (Buehler and Berkelman, 1991). The first definition is very simple and could be used by field staff with minimal training, e.g., in a refugee camp, where the occurrence of epidemic hepatitis A has been documented, where laboratory testing is not readily available, and where the inclusion of some people with jaundice caused by other diseases will not substantially affect the usefulness of the data. The second definition is appropriate in a developed country where diagnostic testing is done routinely to distinguish various types of viral hepatitis and where the clinical and public health response depends on a specific diagnosis. Requiring all elements of this definition, however, would exclude some people who indeed have acute hepatitis A infection, such as those with asymptomatic infection, which is common in children, or those in whom diagnostic testing was deemed unnecessary, e.g., those with characteristic illness and a clear history of exposure to others with documented infection. In such instances, case definitions may be expanded to include epidemiologically linked cases. While expanding a definition in this way increases its sensitivity and relevance to real-world situations, it may also make it more complex and difficult to implement.

For diseases with long latency or a chronic course, developing a case definition depends on decisions regarding which phase to monitor: asymptomatic, early disease, late disease, or death. For example, in establishing a system to monitor ischemic heart disease, potential definitions may be based on symptoms of angina, diagnostic tests for coronary artery occlusion, functional impairment arising from the disease, hospital admission for myocardial infarction, or death due to myocardial infarction. Each of these definitions would measure different segments of the population with coronary artery disease, each would have strengths and limitations, and each would require a unique approach and data source to implement. If death were chosen as the outcome to measure, one approach might be to monitor death certificates that specify coronary artery disease as the underlying cause of death. This approach has the advantage of being relatively simple and inexpensive, assuming a satisfactory vital registration system is already well established, but it is limited by variations in physicians' diligence in establishing diagnoses and completing death certificates. In addition, trends in deaths may be affected not only by trends in incidence but also by advances in care that would avert deaths. Depending on the objectives of the proposed surveillance system and the needs of the information users, using death certificates to monitor coronary artery disease trends may be sufficient or completely unsatisfactory.

Ideally, surveillance case definitions should both inform and reflect clinical practice. This objective may be difficult to achieve when surveillance definitions are less inclusive than the more intuitive criteria that clinicians often apply in diagnosing individual patients or when surveillance taps an information source with limited detail. This dilemma arises from the role of surveillance in monitoring diseases at the population level, the need for simplicity in order to facilitate widespread use, and variations in the importance of specificity. Surveillance definitions employ a limited set of "yes/no" criteria that can be quickly applied in a variety of settings, while clinicians add to such criteria additional medical knowledge and their subjective understanding of individual patients. This difference in perspective can sometimes be perplexing to public health personnel and clinicians alike. Similarly, confusion may arise when definitions established for surveillance are used for purposes beyond their original intent. For example, much of the public debate that preceded the 1993 revision of the surveillance definition for AIDS in the United States was prompted by the Social Security Administration's use of the surveillance definition as a criterion for disability benefits (United States Congress Office of Technology Assessment, 1992). That many with disabling illness failed to meet AIDS surveillance criteria illustrated both the limits of the definition as a criterion for program eligibility and the need to revise the definition to meet surveillance objectives amidst growing awareness of the spectrum of severe HIV-related morbidity.

Often, monitoring disease is insufficient, and there is a need to monitor exposures or behaviors that predispose to disease, especially when public health resources are invested in preventing these exposures or altering behaviors. The trade-offs inherent in defining diseases extend to surveillance definitions for environmental exposures and behaviors. For example, smoking is the leading cause of preventable death in the United States, and thus there is a strong interest in monitoring tobacco use. To this end, the Behavioral Risk Factor Surveillance System in the United States monitors smoking and other health behaviors (Centers for Disease Control and Prevention, 2002). The case definition for "current cigarette smoking" requires a "yes" response to the question, "Have you smoked at least 100 cigarettes in your entire life?" combined with reporting smoking "every day" or "some days" in response to the question, "Do you now smoke cigarettes every day, some days, or not at all?" Observed trends in smoking prevalence using this definition will be affected by the cutoff criteria built into the questions, by telephone ownership, and by participants' ability or willingness to respond accurately, which may reflect trends in the perceived social desirability of smoking. In contrast, the Health Survey for England involves visits to households to conduct interviews and collect blood specimens. The Survey has monitored levels of self-reported smoking and plasma cotinine (a nicotine metabolite) among participants. This approach allows a more precise definition of exposure to tobacco smoke, both among smokers and household contacts, and permits more detailed evaluation of the effects of tobacco exposure (Jarvis et al., 2001), but it is more costly than a telephone survey and necessarily involves many fewer participants. This example reveals an essential polarity in surveillance: For a given cost, more detailed information can be collected from a smaller number of people, permitting the use of more precise definitions and more detailed analyses, or less detailed and precise information can be obtained from a larger number of people, permitting more widespread monitoring.

POPULATION UNDER SURVEILLANCE

All surveillance systems target specific populations, which may range from people at specific institutions (e.g., hospitals, clinics, schools, factories, prisons), to residents of local, regional, or national jurisdictions, to persons living in multiple nations. In some instances, surveillance may seek to identify all occurrences, or a representative sample, of specific health events within the population of a defined geographic area (population-based systems). In other instances, target sites may be selected for conducting surveillance, based on an *a priori* assessment of their representativeness, a willingness of people at the sites to participate in a surveillance system, and the feasibility of incorporating them into a surveillance network (convenience sampling).

Population-based surveillance systems include notifiable disease reporting systems, which require health care providers to report cases of specific diseases to health departments, and systems based on the use of vital statistics. Other population-based surveillance systems depend on surveys designed to sample a representative group of people or facilities, such as those conducted by the National Center for Health Statistics in the United States, including surveys of outpatient care providers, hospitals, and the population (National Center for Health Statistics, accessed 2007). Information from these surveys can be used for national-level surveillance of a wide variety of illnesses, provided they occur with sufficient frequency and geographic dispersion to be reliably included in the survey data. National surveys, however, may be limited in their ability to provide information for specific geographic subdivisions.

Despite the desirability of surveillance systems that seek to include all or a statistically representative sample of events, in many situations such an approach is not feasible. Because of the need to identify a group of participants with sufficient interest, willingness, and capability, some surveillance systems are focused on groups of nonrandomly selected sites, often with intent to include a mix of participants that represents different segments of the target population. In these situations, the actual population under surveillance may be the group of people who receive medical care from certain clinics, people who live in selected cities, people who work in selected factories, etc. Examples of this approach include (a) the Centers for Disease Control and Prevention's (CDC) network of 122 cities that report weekly numbers of deaths attributed to pneumonia and influenza in order to detect influenza epidemics through the recognition of excess influenza-related mortality (Brammer et al., 2002), and (b) HIV seroprevalence surveys in the United Kingdom that sample persons receiving treatment for sexually transmitted infections, drug users, and pregnant women at sentinel clinics in London and elsewhere (Nicoll et al., 2000).

CYCLE OF SURVEILLANCE

Surveillance systems can be described as information loops or cycles, with information coming into the collecting organization and information being returned to those who need it. A typical surveillance loop begins with the recognition of a health event, notification of a health agency (with successive transfer of information from local to central agencies), analysis and interpretation of aggregated data, and dissemination of the results. This process can involve varying levels of technical sophistication ranging from manual systems to record data and transport reports by courier to systems involving telecommunications, radio or satellite technology, or the Internet. An early example of the use of telecommunications to support this cycle is a French network, established in 1984, that enabled participating general practitioners to report communicable diseases to national health authorities, send messages, obtain summaries of surveillance data, and receive health bulletins (Valleron et al., 1986). Regardless of the level of technology employed in a surveillance system, the critical measure of success is whether information gets to the right people in time to be useful.

CONFIDENTIALITY

Personal identifying information is necessary to identify duplicate reports, obtain follow-up information when necessary, provide services to individuals, and use surveillance as the basis for more detailed investigations. Protecting the physical security and confidentiality of surveillance records is both an ethical responsibility and a requirement for maintaining the trust of participants. Laws that mandate disease reporting to health departments generally provide concomitant protections and sanctions to prevent inappropriate release of identifying information. Procedures to protect security include limiting access of personnel to sensitive data, adequate locks for rooms and files where data are stored, and use of passwords, encryption, and other security measures in computer and Internet systems. Agencies that maintain surveillance data should articulate policies that specify the terms and conditions of access to data not only for agency staff but also for guest researchers who may have an interest in analyzing surveillance information (Centers for Disease Control and Prevention, 2003b). Assuring adherence to confidentiality policies and security procedures should be an essential part of staff training and ongoing performance assessment.

As a further safeguard against violations of confidentiality, personal identifying information should not be collected or kept when it is not needed. Surveillance data may be stored electronically in different versions, with and without identifiers, with only the latter made accessible to users who do not need identifiers, as is often the case for most analyses. Although personal identifying information may be needed locally, it is generally not necessary for that information to be forwarded to more central agencies. For example, because of the links of HIV infection to certain sexual behaviors and intravenous drug use and because of concerns about discrimination against HIV-infected people, the HIV/AIDS epidemic generated unprecedented attention to the protection of confidentiality in surveillance. In the United States, cases of HIV infection and AIDS are first reported to local or state health departments, which in turn forward reports to the CDC. Names are obtained by state health departments to facilitate follow-back investigations when indicated, update case reports when relevant additional information becomes available (e.g., a person with HIV infection develops AIDS or a person with AIDS dies), and cull duplicate reports. States do not forward names to the CDC, where monitoring national AIDS trends does not require names (Centers for Disease Control and Prevention, 1999b).

INCENTIVES TO PARTICIPATION

Successful surveillance systems depend on effective collaborative relationships and on the usefulness of the information they generate. Providing information back to those who contribute to the system is the best incentive to participation. This feedback may be in the form of reports, seminars, or data that participants can analyze themselves. Often, individual physicians, clinics, or hospitals are interested in knowing how they compare with others, and special reports distributed confidentially to individual participants may be welcomed. Documenting how surveillance data are used to improve services or shape policy emphasizes to participants the importance of their cooperation.

Other incentives may be more immediate, such as payment for case reports. From the perspective of agencies conducting surveillance, payment of health care providers for case reports is undesirable because of the cost and because it lacks the spirit of voluntary collaboration based on mutual interests in public health. In some situations, however, payments may be appropriate and effective. For example, during the smallpox-eradication campaign, progressively higher rewards were offered for case reports as smallpox became increasingly rare and as the goal of eradication was approached (Foster et al., 1980). For people who participate in surveys, respondents may be paid or provided other incentives for their time and willingness to complete interviews or provide specimens.

Last, there may be legal incentives to participation. Requirements for reporting certain conditions can be incorporated into licensure or certification requirements for physicians, hospitals, or laboratories. Enforcing such laws, however, may create an adversarial relationship between health agencies and those with whom long-term cooperation is desired. Alternatively, health care providers may be liable for the adverse consequences of failing to report, e.g., permitting continued transmission of a communicable disease.

SURVEILLANCE ETHICS

Assuring the ethical practice of public health surveillance requires an ongoing effort to achieve a responsible balance among competing interests and risks and benefits (Bayer and Fairchild, 2000). These competing interests include the legitimate desire of people to protect their privacy against unwarranted government intrusion and the responsibilities of governments to protect the health of their constituents and to obtain the information needed to direct public health interventions. The risks of surveillance may act at the individual or group levels. People may suffer embarrassment or discrimination if information about their health is released inappropriately. Many surveillance systems will not publish frequencies when the total is below a critical number, such as fewer than five, because persons contributing to so low a total might be readily identified. Conversely, groups with high rates of disease may be stigmatized by publicity surrounding the dissemination of surveillance data that illustrate health disparities, especially when the adverse effects of health disparities fall on groups that suffer economic or social deprivation (Mann et al., 1999).

Reducing these individual risks requires that surveillance data be collected judiciously and managed responsibly. Reducing the risk of stigmatization among groups with high disease rates often depends on emphasizing that surveillance data alone do not explain the underlying reasons for health disparities. Both individual and group risks will be countered by constructive actions to address the problems that surveillance brings to light (Public Health Leadership Society, 2002).

Surveillance systems may or may not be subject to formal oversight by ethical review boards. For example, in the United States, public health surveillance systems are generally managed under the authority of public health laws. As a result, they are subject to oversight through the process of governance that shapes those laws and are deemed to be outside the purview of regulations that govern research, although the boundary between public health practice and research remains controversial (MacQueen and Buehler, 2004; Fairchild and Bayer, 2004). The protocols of researchers who seek to use surveillance data, for example, to identify cases for a case-control study, are ordinarily subject to review by a human-subject research board because such research seeks to develop information that can be generalized to other situations and because the scope of information collected is beyond what is needed for immediate prevention or disease control.

SUMMARY

Surveillance systems require an operational definition of the disease or condition under surveillance and of the target population. Events within the target population may be usefully monitored by attempting to identify all occurrences, occurrences within a statistically defined sample, or occurrences within a convenience sample. Surveillance systems encompass not only data collection but also analysis and dissemination. The "cycle" of information flow in surveillance may depend on manual or technologically advanced methods, including the Internet. The protection of confidentiality is essential and requires protecting the physical security of data as well as policies against inappropriate release. The best incentive to maintaining participation in surveillance systems is demonstration of the usefulness of the information collected. The ethical conduct of public health surveillance requires an appreciation of both the benefits and risks of obtaining population health information.

APPROACHES TO SURVEILLANCE

ACTIVE VERSUS PASSIVE SURVEILLANCE

The terms *active* and *passive* surveillance are used to describe two alternative approaches to surveillance. An active approach means that the organization conducting surveillance initiates procedures to obtain reports, such as regular telephone calls or visits to physicians or hospitals. A passive approach to surveillance means that the organization conducting surveillance does not contact potential reporters and leaves the initiative for reporting to others.

Although the terms *active* and *passive* are conceptually useful, they are insufficient for describing a surveillance method. Instead, it is important to describe how surveillance is conducted, who is contacted, how often the contacts are made, and what, if any, backup procedures are in place to identify cases that are not originally reported. For example, it may not be feasible to contact all potential reporters. Thus, in taking an active approach to surveillance, a health agency may elect to contact routinely only large medical centers, and special investigations may be done periodically to identify cases that had not been reported through routine procedures.

NOTIFIABLE DISEASE REPORTING

Under public health laws, certain diseases are deemed "notifiable," meaning that physicians or laboratories must report cases to public health officials. Traditionally, this approach has been used mainly for infectious diseases and mortality. More recently, notifiable diseases have often included cancers. Regulations that mandate disease reporting have varying time requirements and designate varying levels of responsibility for reporting. For example, some diseases are of such urgency that reporting to the local health department is required immediately or within 24 hours to allow an effective public health response; others with less urgency can be reported less rapidly. In addition, persons or organizations responsible for reporting vary and may include the individual physician, the laboratory where the diagnosis is established, or the facility (clinic or hospital) where the patient is treated.

In the United States, each state has the authority to designate which conditions are reportable by law. The Council of State and Territorial Epidemiologists agrees on a set of conditions that are deemed nationally reportable, and state health departments voluntarily report information on cases of these diseases to the CDC. Tabulations of these reports are published by the CDC in the *Morbidity and Mortality Weekly Report* and in an annual summary (Centers for Disease Control and Prevention, 2004a).

LABORATORY-BASED SURVEILLANCE

Using diagnostic laboratories as the basis for surveillance can be highly effective for some diseases. The advantages of this approach include the ability to identify patients seen by many different physicians, especially when diagnostic testing for a particular condition is centralized; the availability of detailed information about the results of the diagnostic test, e.g., the serum level of a toxin or the antibiotic sensitivity of a bacterial pathogen; and the promotion of complete reporting through use of laboratory licensing procedures. The disadvantages are that laboratory records alone may not provide information on epidemiologically important patient characteristics and that patients having laboratory tests may not be representative of all persons with the disease.

An example of the utility of laboratory-based surveillance is a 10-state project for selected bacterial pathogens in the United States. Surveillance personnel routinely contact all hospital laboratories within the target areas and thus have obtained population-based estimates of the occurrence of a variety of severe infections. Data from this system have been used to monitor the effect of vaccinations against *Streptococcus pneumoniae,* inform the development of guidelines for preventing mother-to-newborn transmission of Group B streptococcal disease, and monitor trends in food-borne illness caused by selected bacterial pathogens (Pinner et al., 2003).

VOLUNTEER PROVIDERS

Special surveillance networks are sometimes developed to meet information needs that exceed the capabilities of routine approaches. This situation may occur because more detailed or timely information is required, because there is need to obtain information on a condition that is not legally deemed to be reportable, or because there is a logical reason to focus surveillance efforts on practitioners of a certain medical specialty.

For example, in 1976–1977, an outbreak of Guillain-Barré syndrome, a severe neurologic disorder, occurred in association with the swine influenza vaccination campaign in the United States. National surveillance for Guillain-Barré syndrome was initiated in anticipation of the 1978–1979 influenza season because of continuing concerns about the safety of influenza vaccines in following years. Persons with this syndrome are likely to be treated by neurologists, so the CDC and state epidemiologists enlisted the assistance of members of the American Academy of Neurology. Data from this surveillance system enabled health authorities to determine that the 1978–1979 influenza vaccine was not associated with an elevated risk of Guillain-Barré syndrome (Hurwitz et al., 1981).

The participation of a physician, clinic, or hospital in such a surveillance network requires commitment of resources and time. While obtaining a random sample of sites or providers is desirable, the participation rate may be low and limited to those with the greatest interest or capability. In that situation, it would be more expedient to identify volunteer participants and to enlist a representative group of participants based on geography or the characteristics of their patient populations.

In a number of countries, physicians have organized surveillance networks to monitor illnesses that are common in their practices and to assess their approach to diagnosis and care, complementing investigations done in academic research centers. For example, the Pediatric Research in Office Settings project, a network of over 500 pediatricians across the United States, monitored the characteristics, evaluation, treatment, and outcomes of febrile infants and observed that physicians' judgments led to departures from established care guidelines that were both cost-saving and beneficial to patient outcomes (Pantell et al., 2004). Physician networks may collaborate with public health agencies, as in the case of influenza surveillance in Europe (Aymard et al., 1999).

REGISTRIES

Registries are listings of all occurrences of a disease, or category of disease (e.g., cancer, birth defects), within a defined area. Registries collect relatively detailed information and may identify patients for long-term follow-up or for specific laboratory or epidemiologic investigation.

The Surveillance, Epidemiology, and End Result project of the National Cancer Institute in the United States began in 1973 in five states and has grown into a wide-ranging network of statewide, metropolitan, and rural registries that together represent approximately one fourth of the nation's population, including areas selected to assure inclusion of major racial and ethnic groups (National Cancer Institute, accessed 2007). Through contacts with hospitals and pathologists, the occurrence of incident cases of cancer is monitored, and ascertainment is estimated to be nearly complete. Data collected on cancer patients include demographic characteristics, exposures such as smoking and occupational histories, characteristics of the cancer (site, morphology, and stage), treatment, and outcomes. In addition to providing a comprehensive approach to monitoring the occurrence of specific cancers, patients identified through these centers have been enrolled in a variety of further studies. One of these was the Cancer and Steroid Hormone Study, which examined the relation between estrogen use and breast, ovarian, and endometrial cancer (Wingo et al., 1988).

SURVEYS

Periodic or ongoing surveys provide a method for monitoring behaviors associated with disease, personal attributes that affect disease risk, knowledge or attitudes that influence health behaviors, use of health services, and self-reported disease occurrence. For example, the Behavioral Risk

Factor Surveillance System is an ongoing telephone survey that is conducted by all state health departments in the United States and monitors behaviors associated with leading causes of morbidity and mortality, including smoking, exercise, seat-belt use, and the use of preventive health services (Indu et al., 2003). The survey includes a standard core of questions; over time, additional questions have been included, with individual states adding questions of local interest. Surveys based on in-person interviews, such as the National Health and Nutrition Examination Survey in the United States or the Health Survey for England, include physical examinations and specimen collection and can be used to monitor the prevalence of physiologic determinants of health risk, such as blood pressure, cholesterol levels, and hematocrit (National Center for Health Statistics, 2007; Jarvis et al., 2001).

In countries where vital registration systems are underdeveloped, surveys have long been used to estimate basic population health measures, such as birth and fertility rates and infant, maternal, and overall mortality rates, as well as trends in illnesses that are major causes of death, such as respiratory and gastrointestinal illness (White et al., 2000). In several sub-Saharan African countries, national health surveys have been expanded to measure HIV prevalence and to validate prevalence estimates based on sentinel antenatal clinic surveys (World Health Organization and UNAIDS, 2003).

INFORMATION SYSTEMS

Information systems are large databases collected for general rather than disease-specific purposes, which can be applied to surveillance. In some instances, their use for monitoring health may be secondary to other objectives. Vital records are primarily legal documents that provide official certification of birth and death, yet the information they provide on the characteristics of newborns or the causes of death have long been used to monitor health. Records from hospital discharges are computerized to monitor the use and costs of hospital services. Data on discharge diagnoses, however, are a convenient source of information on morbidity. Insurance billing records, both private and government-sponsored, provide information on inpatient and outpatient diagnoses and treatments.

For example, Workers' Compensation is a legally mandated system in the United States that provides insurance coverage for work-related injuries and illnesses. Examination of claims in Massachusetts for work-related cases of carpal tunnel syndrome, a musculoskeletal problem aggravated by repetitive hand-wrist movements, has been used to monitor trends of this condition and complement data from physician reports (Davis et al., 2001). In Ohio, claims data were used for surveillance of occupational lead poisoning and identified worksites that required more intensive supervision by regulatory investigators (Seligman et al., 1986).

Because these information systems serve multiple objectives, their use for surveillance (or research) requires care. These massive systems may not be collected with stringent data quality procedures for those items of greatest interest to epidemiologists. Furthermore, they are subject to variability among contributing sites, and they are susceptible to systematic variations that can artificially influence trends. For example, in many health data systems, diagnoses are classified and coded using the International Classification of Diseases (ICD). Approximately once a decade, the ICD is revised to reflect advancing medical knowledge, and interim codes may be introduced between revisions when new diseases emerge. Changes in coding procedures can affect assessment of trends. In 1987, special codes for HIV infection (categories 042.0–044.9) were implemented in the United States. That year, analysis of vital records indicated that the number of deaths attributed to *Pneumocystis carinii* pneumonia (code 136.3), a major complication of HIV infection, dropped precipitously. This drop did not reflect an advance in the prevention or treatment of *Pneumocystis* infection; rather it reflected a shift from the use of code 136.3 to 042.0 (the new code for HIV infection with specified infections, including *Pneumocystis*) (Buehler et al., 1990).

In addition, methods for assigning diagnoses and ICD codes may vary among areas. Under the 9th revision of the ICD, which has been updated to the 10th revision for mortality coding, for a person who died from an overdose of cocaine, the cause of death may have been assigned ICD code 304.2 (cocaine dependence), code 305.6 (cocaine abuse), code 986.5 (poisoning by surface and infiltration anesthetics, including cocaine), or code E855.2 (unintentional poisoning by local anesthetics, including cocaine). If postmortem toxicology studies were pending when coding was done (or if the results of toxicology tests are noted on death certificates after the preparation of computerized records), code 799.9 (unknown or unspecified cause) may have been assigned. Thus, use of computerized death certificates to compare the incidence of fatal cocaine intoxication over time or among areas may yield spurious results if coding variations are not considered (Pollock et al., 1991).

The user of these large data sets must be careful. They may be available in "public access" formats, but their accessibility should not blind the potential user to their intricacies.

SENTINEL EVENTS

The occurrence of a rare disease known to be associated with a specific exposure can alert health officials to situations where others may have been exposed to a potential hazard. Such occurrences have been termed *sentinel events* because they are harbingers of broader public health problems. Surveillance for sentinel events can be used to identify situations where public health investigation or intervention is required.

For example, in 1983, Rutstein et al. proposed a list of sentinel occupational health events to serve as a framework for national surveillance of work-related diseases and as a guide to clinicians in caring for persons with occupational diseases. The detection of diseases on this list should trigger health and safety investigations of the workplace, identify settings where worker protection should be improved, or identify workers needing medical screening or treatment. The list included the diseases, etiologic agents, and industries or occupations where the exposure was likely (e.g., bone cancer due to radium exposure in radium processors) (Rutstein et al., 1983).

RECORD LINKAGES

Records from different sources may be linked to extend their usefulness for surveillance by providing information that one source alone may lack. For example, in order to monitor birth-weight-specific infant death rates, it is necessary to link information from corresponding birth and death certificates for individual infants. The former provides information on birth weight and other infant and maternal characteristics (e.g., gestational age at delivery, number and timing of prenatal visits, mother's age and marital status, hospital where birth occurred), and the latter provides information on the age at death (e.g., neonatal versus postneonatal) and causes of death. By combining information based on individual-level linked birth and death records, a variety of maternal, infant, and hospital attributes can be used to make inferences about the effectiveness of maternal and infant health programs or to identify potential gaps in services (Buehler et al., 2000).

In addition, linkage of surveillance records to an independent data source can be used to identify previously undetected cases and thus measure and improve the completeness of surveillance. For example, a number of state health departments in the United States have linked computerized hospital discharge records to AIDS case reports to evaluate the completeness of AIDS surveillance. Hospital discharges in persons likely to have AIDS are identified using a "net" of diagnostic codes that specify HIV infection or associated conditions. For persons identified from hospital records who do not match to the list of reported cases, investigations are conducted to confirm whether the people indeed have AIDS (representing previously unreported cases), whether they have signs of HIV infection but have not yet developed AIDS, or whether they have no evidence of HIV infection (Lafferty et al., 1988).

COMBINATIONS OF SURVEILLANCE METHODS

For many conditions, a single data source or surveillance method may be insufficient to meet information needs, and multiple approaches are used that complement one another. For example, as already noted, influenza surveillance in the United States is based on a mix of approaches, including monitoring of trends in deaths attributed to "pneumonia and influenza" in 122 cities, networks of sentinel primary care physicians to monitor outpatient visits for "influenza-like illness," targeted collection of respiratory samples to identify prevalent influenza strains, reports from state epidemiologists to track levels of "influenza activity," and participation in the World Health Organization's international network of laboratories to track the global emergence of new influenza strains (Brammer et al., 2002).

National diabetes surveillance in the United States tracks prevalence and incidence of diabetes, death rates, hospitalizations, diabetes-related disabilities, the use of outpatient and emergency services for diabetes care, the use of services for end-stage renal disease (a major complication of diabetes), and the use of diabetes preventive services. This multifaceted surveillance system draws on a mosaic of data sources, including four different surveys conducted by the National Center for Health Statistics (National Health Interview Survey, National Hospital Discharge Survey, National Ambulatory Care Survey, National Hospital Ambulatory Medical Care Survey), death certificates, the United States Renal Data System—a surveillance system for end-stage renal disease funded by the National Institutes of Health, the Behavioral Risk Factor Surveillance System, and the census (Centers for Disease Control and Prevention, 1999a).

SUMMARY

A wide array of methods can be employed to conduct surveillance, with the selection of a method depending on information needs and resources. These include notifiable disease reporting, which is based on legally mandated reporting by health care providers; reporting from laboratories for conditions diagnosed using laboratory tests; reporting from networks of volunteer health care providers; the use of registries, which provide comprehensive population-based data for specific health events; population surveys; information from vital records and other health data systems; and monitoring of "sentinel" health events to detect unrecognized health hazards. The terms *active* and *passive* surveillance describe the role that agencies conducting surveillance take in obtaining surveillance information from reporting sources. Linkage of surveillance records to other information sources may be used to expand the scope of surveillance data, or combinations of multiple sources may be used to provide complementary perspectives.

ANALYSIS, INTERPRETATION, AND PRESENTATION OF SURVEILLANCE DATA

ANALYSIS AND INTERPRETATION

The analysis of surveillance data is generally descriptive and straightforward, using standard epidemiologic techniques. Analysis strategies used in other forms of epidemiologic investigation are applicable to surveillance, including standardizing rates for age or other population attributes that may vary over time or among locations, controlling for confounding when making comparisons, taking into account sampling strategies used in surveys, and addressing problems related to missing data or unknown values. In addition to these concerns, there are special situations or considerations that may arise in the analysis and interpretation of surveillance data, including the following.

Attribution of Date

In analyzing trends, a decision must often be made whether to examine trends by the date events occurred (or were diagnosed) or the date they were reported. Using the date of report is easier but subject to irregularities in reporting. Using the date of diagnosis provides a better measure of disease occurrence. Analysis by date of diagnosis, however, will underestimate incidence in the most recent intervals if there is a relatively long delay between diagnosis and report. Thus, it may be necessary to adjust recent counts for reporting delays, based on previous reporting experience (Karon et al., 1989).

Attribution of Place

It is often necessary to decide whether analyses will be based on where events or exposures occurred, where people live, or where health care is provided, which may all differ. For example, if people cross geographic boundaries to receive medical care, the places where care is provided may differ from where people reside. The former may be more important in a surveillance system that monitors the quality of health care, whereas the latter would be important if surveillance were used to track the need for preventive services among people who live in different areas. Census data, the primary source for denominators in rate calculations, are based on place of residence, and thus place of residence is commonly used. For notifiable disease reporting systems, this requires cross-jurisdiction (e.g., state-to-state) reporting among health departments when an illness in a resident of one area is diagnosed and reported in another.

Use of Geographic Information Systems (GIS)

Geographic coordinates (latitude and longitude) for the location of health events or place of residence can be entered into computerized records, allowing automated generation of maps using GIS computer software. By combining geographic data on health events with the location of hazards, environmental exposures, or preventive or therapeutic services, GIS can facilitate the study of spatial associations between exposures or services and health outcomes (Cromley, 2003). Given the importance of maps for presenting surveillance data, it is not surprising that the use of GIS has grown rapidly in surveillance practice.

Detection of a Change in Trends

Surveillance uses a wide array of statistical measures to detect increases (or decreases) in the numbers or rates of events beyond expected levels. The selection of a statistical method depends on the underlying nature of disease trends (e.g., seasonal variations, gradual long-term declines), the length of time for which historical reference data are available, the urgency of detecting an aberrant trend (e.g., detecting a one-day increase versus assessing weekly, monthly, or yearly variations), and whether the objective is to detect temporal aberrations or both temporal and geographic clustering (Janes et al., 2000; Waller et al., 2004). For example, to identify unusually severe influenza seasons, the CDC uses time-series methods to define expected seasonal norms for deaths attributed to "pneumonia and influenza" and to determine when observed numbers of deaths exceed threshold values (Fig. 22–4). Automated systems aimed at detecting the early onset of bioterrorism-related epidemics have drawn on statistical techniques developed for industrial quality control monitoring, such as the CUSUM method employed in the CDC's Early Aberration Reporting System (Hutwagner et al., 2003).

In assessing a change detected by surveillance, the first question to ask is, "Is it real?" There are multiple artifacts that can affect trends, other than actual changes in incidence or prevalence, including changes in staffing among those who report cases or manage surveillance systems, changes in the use of health care services or reporting because of holidays or other events, changes in the interest in a disease, changes in surveillance procedures, changes in screening or diagnostic criteria, and changes in the availability of screening, diagnostic, or care services. The second question to ask is, "Is it meaningful?" If an increase in disease is recognized informally or because a statistical

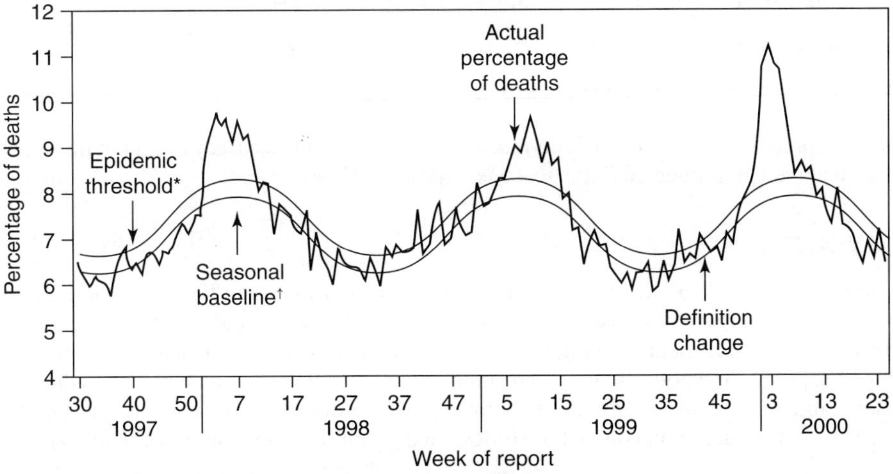

FIGURE 22–4 • Percentage of deaths attributed to pneumonia or influenza, 122 cities in the United States, 1997–2003 influenza seasons. (Reproduced from Brammer TL, Murray EL, Fukuda K, et al. Surveillance for influenza—United States, 1997–98, 1988–99, and 1999–2000 seasons. In *Surveillance Summaries*, October 25, 2002. *Morb Mortal Wkly Rep.* 2002:51(No. SS-7):6.)

threshold was surpassed, judgment is required to determine whether the observation reflects a potential public health problem and the extent and aggressiveness of the next-step investigations, which may range from re-examining surveillance data to launching a full-scale epidemiologic investigation. This judgment is particularly important for systems that monitor nonspecific syndromes that may reflect illness with minimal public health importance or the earliest stage of potentially severe disease. "False alarms" may be common if statistical thresholds are set too low, increasing the likelihood that alarms are triggered by random variations. Such foibles emphasize the importance of being familiar with how data are collected and analyzed and with the local context of health care services.

Assessing Completeness of Surveillance

If two independent surveillance or data systems are available for a particular condition and if records for individuals represented in these systems can be linked to one another, then it is possible to determine the number represented by both and the number included in one but not the other. Using capture-recapture analysis, the number missed by both can be estimated, in turn allowing an estimate of the total number of cases in the population and calculation of the proportion identified by each (see Chapter 23). The accuracy of this approach depends on the likelihood of detection by one system being independent of detection by the other, an assumption that is rarely met in practice. Violations of this assumption may lead to an underestimate of the total number of cases in a population (Hook and Regal, 2000) and thus to an overestimation of the completeness of surveillance. This approach also depends on the accuracy of record linkages, which in turn depends on the accuracy and specificity of the identifying information used to make linkages. If names are not available, proxy markers for identity, such as date of birth combined with sex, may be used. Even if names are available, they can change, be misspelled, or be listed under an alias. Software that converts names to codes, such as Soundex, can aid in avoiding linkage errors from spelling and punctuation. Nonetheless, other errors in recording or coding data can lead to false matches or non-matches. In addition to matches based on complete alignment of matching criteria, standards should be set and validated for accepting or rejecting near matches. Although computer algorithms can accomplish most matches and provide measures of the probability that matches are correct, manual validation of at least a sample of matched and nonmatched is advisable.

Smoothing

Graphic plots of disease numbers or rates by time or small geographic area may yield an erratic or irregular picture owing to statistical variability, obscuring visualization of underlying trends or geographic patterns. To solve this problem, a variety of temporal or geographic "smoothing" techniques may be used to clarify trends or patterns (Devine, 2004).

Protection of Confidentiality

In addition to suppressing data when reporting a small number of cases or events that could enable recognition of an individual, statistical techniques may be used to introduce perturbations into data in a way that prevents recognition of individuals but retains overall accuracy in aggregate tabulations or maps (Federal Committee on Statistical Methodology, 1994).

PRESENTATION

Because surveillance data have multiple uses, it is essential that they be widely and effectively disseminated, not only to those who participate in their collection, but also to the full constituency of persons who can use them, ranging from public health epidemiologists and program managers to the media, public, and policy makers. The mode of presentation should be geared to the intended audience. Tabular presentation provides a comprehensive resource to those with the time and interest to review the data in detail. In contrast, well-designed graphs or maps can immediately convey key points.

In addition to issuing published surveillance reports, public health agencies are increasingly using the Internet to post reports, allowing for more frequent updates and widespread access. In addition, interactive Internet-based utilities can allow users to obtain customized surveillance reports, based on their interest in specific tabulations.

Depending on the nature of surveillance findings and the disease or condition in question, the release of surveillance reports may attract media and public interest. This eventuality should be anticipated, if possible in collaboration with a media communications expert, to plan for media inquiries, identify and clarify key public health messages that arise from the data (respecting both the strengths and limits of data), and to draw attention to related steps that program managers, policy makers, or members of the public can take to promote health.

ATTRIBUTES OF SURVEILLANCE

Surveillance systems have multiple attributes that can be used to evaluate existing systems or to conceptualize proposed systems (Centers for Disease Control and Prevention, 2001). Because enhancements in some attributes are likely to be offset by degradations in others, the utility and cost of surveillance depends on how well the mix of attributes is balanced to meet information needs. These attributes are

Sensitivity. To what extent does the system identify all targeted events? For purposes of monitoring trends, low sensitivity may be acceptable if sensitivity is consistent over time and detected events are representative. For purposes of assessing the impact of a health problem, high sensitivity (or an ability to correct for under-ascertainment) is required.

Timeliness. How promptly does information flow through the cycle of surveillance, from information collection to dissemination? The need for timeliness depends on the public health urgency of a problem and the types of interventions that are available.

Predictive value. To what extent are reported cases really cases? Does surveillance measure what it aims to measure?

Representativeness. To what extent do events detected through the surveillance represent persons with the condition of interest in the target population? A lack of representativeness may lead to misdirection of health resources.

Data quality. How accurate and complete are descriptive data in case reports, surveys, or information systems?

Simplicity. Are surveillance procedures and processes simple or complicated? Are forms easy to complete? Is data collection kept to a necessary minimum? Is software "user-friendly"? Are Internet Web pages easy to navigate? Are reports presented in a straightforward manner?

Flexibility. Can the system readily adapt to new circumstances or changing information needs?

Acceptability. To what extent are participants in a surveillance system enthusiastic about the system? Does their effort yield information that is useful to them? Does the public support allowing public health agencies access to personal health information for surveillance purposes?

Certain attributes are likely to be closely related and mutually reinforcing. For example, simplicity is likely to enhance acceptability. Others are likely to be competing. Efforts to promote timeliness may require sacrifices in completeness or data quality. Efforts to assure complete reporting may be compromised by inclusion of some who do not have the disease in question. This balance of attributes is also relevant to evaluating automated surveillance systems aimed at early epidemic detection. For example, lowering statistical thresholds to assure timely and complete detection of possible epidemics is likely to result in more frequent "false alarms" (Centers for Disease Control and Prevention, 2004b).

CONCLUSION

Surveillance is a process for monitoring and reporting on trends in specific health problems among defined populations. In conducting surveillance, there are multiple options for virtually every component of a surveillance system, from the selection of a data source to the application of statistical analysis methods to the dissemination of results. Selecting among these options requires consideration of the objectives of a particular system, the information needs of the intended users, and the optimal mix of surveillance attributes, such as timeliness and completeness. Ultimately, the test of a surveillance system depends on its success or failure in contributing to the prevention and control of disease, injury, disability, or death.

An example of such success is provided by the role of surveillance in national and international efforts to stop the spread of severe acute respiratory syndrome (SARS) in 2003. In February 2003, the world learned about an epidemic of severe respiratory illness in southern China that had begun in November of the preceding year. The full threat of SARS was recognized when news reports about the outbreak in China came to the attention of the World Health Organization, as cases appeared in Hong Kong and Vietnam among travelers from China, and eventually as international travelers or their contacts became ill on multiple continents. The objectives of SARS surveillance were multiple: first, to characterize the illness, its risk of transmission, and duration of infectiousness; second, to obtain specimens from affected persons, enabling the identification of the etiologic agent, description of the human immune response, and development of diagnostic tests; and, third, to inform prevention and control activities, such as the development of public education, the identification of ill and exposed persons, and the implementation of isolation or quarantine measures commensurate with the extent of transmission in local areas. Developing a case definition for this new disease of unknown cause was challenging because its signs and symptoms were similar to those of other respiratory illnesses. Sensitivity was achieved by including relatively general indicators of respiratory illness. Specificity was achieved by requiring evidence of exposure based on travel or contact history, by limiting the definition to relatively severe disease (even though, as with other newly discovered diseases, there may have been an unrecognized spectrum of milder illness), and by excluding persons with other known diagnoses. Surveillance had to be flexible as the etiologic agent was identified, as tests were developed that allowed the diagnosis of SARS to be established or excluded, and as the list of affected countries expanded and contracted. The World Health Organization promoted international consistency by promulgating a standard case definition that was widely used, with limited modifications by individual countries as indicated by the local epidemiologic situations. The public health response to SARS also raised profound ethical questions about the balance between individual rights and the protection of public health, ranging from familiar questions about reporting the names of affected persons to health departments to less familiar questions in modern times about the use of quarantine. The complexity of these questions was heightened because SARS affected countries with widely varying traditions regarding civil liberties, the use of police powers, and governance. Altogether, surveillance and the broader spectrum of prevention and control measure contributed to the interruption of recognized transmission by July 2003, just months after the disease was first recognized by the international community, averting what could have been a much more extensive and deadly international epidemic. Based on the experience of 2003, the World Health Organization and individual nations refined surveillance and prevention strategies in anticipation of subsequent respiratory illness seasons and a possible re-emergence of the disease (Heyman and Rodier, 2004; Schrag et al., 2004; Gostin et al., 2003; Weinstein, 2004).

CHAPTER 23

Using Secondary Data

Jørn Olsen

Epidemiology in Ideal Circumstances 482
Analysis of Secondary Data from Complete Populations 482
Use of Secondary Data and Validity 483
Epidemiologic Studies Based Fully on Existing Registers 483
Examples of the Use of Secondary Data 484
Multigeneration Registers 484
Sibs and Half-Sibs 484
Stress and Pregnancy 485
Vaccines and Autism 485
Linkage of Data 486
Validation of Data 487
Data Quality 487
Quantification of Bias Related to Misclassification 488
Monitoring 488
Ethics of Secondary Data Access 490
Conclusion 491

In this chapter we define *secondary data* as data generated for a purpose different from the research activity for which they are used. This is not a very precise definition—data may be generated for different purposes that may overlap with the objective of the study. The important issue for research is not so much whether data are primary or secondary, but whether the data are adequate to shed light on the research question to be studied and to assure that data with an unfilled research potential are not destroyed.

It is never possible to design a perfect study, ensure perfect compliance with the protocol, get error-free data, and analyze those data with appropriate statistical models. Because epidemiologists conduct their research in the real world, we often have to settle for less than the ideal, and weigh the pros and cons of different design options. In this decision process we sometimes have to choose between using already existing data and generating new data. Using existing data may sometimes be the best option available, or even the only option. For example, it has been suggested that an influenza infection during pregnancy can increase the risk of schizophrenia in the offspring decades later. To explore this hypothesis we could generate primary data and wait for 20 to 30 years to explore this idea, or we could look for existing data that were generated back in time. These secondary data could be used to scrutinize the hypothesis.

If we decide to use secondary data, we must be confident of the validity of those data or at least have a good idea of their limitations. The same is true for primary data, but for primary data we can build quality control into the design, whereas secondary data often must be taken as is. Secondary data may on occasion be the best source for study data. For example, nonresponse might bias the collection of primary data and secondary data could be available for all. More often, secondary data might be the best source given the available resources.

Those who are charged with collecting and maintaining secondary data can enhance their utility by ensuring that data with an unused research potential are archived in a way that makes it possible to find and use the data. Making data available for research is an important part of the research structure, and some countries have a system for archiving data for research following standardized norms for data documentation (research data archives). Furthermore, adequate meta-analyses often require access to raw data from the studies to be included.

Keeping large stores of data, especially personally identifiable data, requires a high degree of data security to reduce the risk of unwanted disclosure. Most countries have laws on data protection, but it is advisable to add good practice rules to the daily work routines.

EPIDEMIOLOGY IN IDEAL CIRCUMSTANCES

Imagine a country where all citizens are given a personal identification number at birth, which they keep for the rest of their lives, and where most written information generated by public authorities is stored in computers and is identifiable through this identification number. Imagine that this information includes an electronic medical file, all contacts to the health care system, all diagnoses made, all prescribed medicines, all social benefits, all birth defects, all immunizations, and more. Imagine that a similar registration system is used for income, work history, education, social grouping, and residence, and then envision a register system that can link family members together and link the members of society to huge biobanks that include everyone in the population. Imagine that all this information is stored and kept over time. In this vision, the entire country is a cohort. Although this scenario may provoke privacy concerns, with some justification, it also describes an ideal world for epidemiologists, demographers, and social scientists, if the information being collected is available for scientific use. If the health care system, as well as the social system, is furthermore organized in the same way for the entire country, then we have a country-cohort that allows efficient evaluation of preventives and therapies after they are introduced. In fact, some countries have some of the resources that allow for research on complete national populations.

ANALYSIS OF SECONDARY DATA FROM COMPLETE POPULATIONS

As discussed in Parts I and II of this book, etiologic inference must face numerous validity problems such as confounding, selection bias, and measurement error. In a study on the entire population, selection bias due to nonresponse is avoided. What remains are problems of evaluating accuracy of data on exposures, diseases, confounders, adjusting for confounding as well as possible with the data available, and potential problems with loss to follow-up. Most studies based on registers have limited data for confounder control, measurement inaccuracy is frequently a problem, and loss to follow-up is a concern only with substantial migration out of the population.

On the other hand, the alternative to the analysis of secondary data may well be expensive data collection with attendant low response rates. It is not unusual that almost 50% refuse to take part in a case-control study and more may decline to be enrolled in a long-term and time-consuming follow-up study. Even simple cross-sectional surveys may suffer from low participation rates. Loss to follow-up among study participants is usually much more extensive than emigration from a population.

Retrospective case-control studies are especially vulnerable to selection bias related to nonresponse, because the decision to participate in a study may be a function of the case status and the exposure experience, especially if the hypothesis is known to the subjects. Use of secondary data in a case-control study may avoid this problem if the case-control analysis can be based entirely on existing secondary data. Such a design may also solve problems of differential recall if the secondary data were collected before disease onset.

In prospective studies, participants cannot base their decision to participate on an event that may happen in the future, but nonresponse may still be related to the endpoints under study through factors present at the time of invitation, such as social conditions, age, type of education, number of working hours, altruistic attitudes towards research, etc. If these factors can be fully adjusted for in the analysis, the association with nonresponse and the endpoint should disappear. Unfortunately, the available data (whether primary or secondary) may not be complete and accurate enough to enable such full adjustment, and so substantial bias due to nonresponse as well as self-selection for exposure may remain. Although people in a follow-up study cannot base their decision to participate or the length of their participation in a study on an event that will happen in the future, they are able to base their decisions on their perceived risk of getting the disease under study. If this perceived risk predicts the event and their participation in the study correlates with both the risk and the exposure under study, bias may result in a number of different scenarios. How one should classify this type of bias is a matter of choice. It may be considered a self-selection bias, or (following Chapters 10 and 12) the self-selection may be said to create confounding that may be impossible to remove, e.g., confounding by unknown genetic factors. Following Hernan et al. (2004), such a bias can be classified as confounding, if based on common causes, or selection bias if based on common effects. Using a process-oriented terminology focuses on the selection and emphasizes the need to make this selection as small as possible and to "blind" its conditions as much as possible. Biases such as this may be found in studies of familial diseases, or in a study of reproductive failures in multiparous women, who use their previous pregnancy experience to estimate their risk.

Although we want as good data as possible for our research, there may be a trade-off between data quality and bias. It is possible that too much attention on data collection may introduce bias. For example, if data on cardiovascular diseases are collected within a study on the use of hormones and their cardiovascular effects, clinicians may be influenced by the hormonal hypothesis when making the diagnosis, unless they are blinded to the exposure data. This problem may not exist in routine clinical work, because clinicians rarely take environmental exposures into consideration when making diagnoses (although there are exceptions, such as smoking and bronchitis, use of oral contraceptive methods and venous diseases, high blood pressure and stroke, etc.). Data quality with emphasis on precision may be a poorer alternative to data quality with emphasis on unbiasedness. For example, gestational age may be determined with greater precision by using ultrasound measures compared with gestational age data based on the last menstrual period. Ultrasound measures, however, are based on comparing fetal size with standards of fetal growth, and in a study of exposures that interfere with fetal growth at an early stage (before the ultrasound measure), the estimate may be biased by the exposure. Although the error may be small and have no clinical relevance, it may be significant for the comparisons on which the research questions rest.

USE OF SECONDARY DATA AND VALIDITY

Most epidemiologic studies rest on some use of secondary data. A follow-up study often identifies the cohorts from existing data sources such as medical files, membership lists, occupational records, prescription data, etc. A case-control study usually departs from an existing register of some sort for the disease in question. For example, a case-control study of use of cellular phones and brain cancers will usually be based on an existing register of brain cancer or based on repeated search for new cancer cases in clinical records from relevant hospital departments. Controls may be selected from the source population by direct sampling if a population register of some sort exists for the time period of case ascertainment. In a case-control study on brain cancers and exposure to cellular phones, exposure data could be based on secondary data, such as billing records. This data source may be preferable to collecting self-reported data on phone use, because recalled data are subject to differential recall. People with brain cancer will have searched their memories for potential causes of the disease. This search creates an asymmetry in exposure assessment that can be avoided if secondary data such as billing records are used.

In case-control studies the disease register (the secondary data source) may often be subject to closer scrutiny by adding primary data to the secondary data source. Assuming we want to estimate the association between use of cellular phones and brain cancer in a certain age stratum of the population, we may identify the cancer cases in an existing register. Once the cancer cases have been identified, we might ask an expert pathologist to review all clinical documents according to a set of commonly accepted diagnostic criteria. Usually these criteria are set at strict levels in order to exclude noncases from the case group. By restricting the study to definitive cases, some true cases may be missed, which may reduce the precision of the study but does not necessarily lead to biased relative effect estimates (see Chapter 8).

EPIDEMIOLOGIC STUDIES BASED FULLY ON EXISTING REGISTERS

Generating new data is often expensive and time-consuming, and furthermore may raise concerns about privacy and unwanted disclosure of data (any new data set carries a new risk of disclosure). Before starting new data collection, one should therefore assure that the required data do not already exist in a form that allows one to address the research question either fully or partly. At present, it may be difficult to determine whether this is the case in most countries, because research data or administrative data are not registered nearly as well as books or scientific papers. In addition, those who collect and maintain these data do not always comply with proper principles of data documentation or permit open access to data. Sometimes being in custody of data is taken to be ownership of data, which can then subsequently be sold for money or for co-authorships. Furthermore, because administrative registers may be used to examine how public laws influence health or how well health care systems perform, in some countries their identification may be considered by the government to be undesirable. That is one reason why many nondemocratic states have little epidemiologic research.

Access to public registers in order to do research has been—and still is—impossible in many countries. This lack of access may have severe consequences: If the registers cover long time periods, they may provide research options that can seldom be realized in ad hoc studies. This option is especially important for diseases that have an etiologic period that spans decades, such as when exposures early in life produce susceptibility that manifests itself in an increased disease risk much later.

EXAMPLES OF THE USE OF SECONDARY DATA

MULTIGENERATION REGISTERS

The mapping of the human genome brings new research opportunities, but it does not eliminate the need for empirical data related to family clustering of diseases. One often needs family data to show that a disease is inherited, occurrence data are needed to show the penetrance and mode of transmission, and family data are needed to evaluate whether the disease shows genetic anticipation. Using existing population registers—rather than patient records—to establish a family history of a disease will make it easier to ensure that the families are ascertained independently of their disease profile, that family size is taken into consideration, and with known follow-up periods for all the members of the families. The limitations lie in the fact that population registers may not have been in operation long enough to cover two or more generations. Longevity of family members will then determine whether, for example, grandparents were alive and registered at the time when a given register started. The probability of identifying a grandparent or great-grandparent generation will depend on their life expectancy, a fact that may have implications for the study designs. Furthermore, the family history is constructed backwards in time, whereas disease occurrence is studied forward in time. It is thus possible to use the disease experience to place cohorts in different risk strata according to the information already available when the study is planned. Such a strategy, however, violates the principle of not analyzing longitudinal data conditionally on what happens in the future, and could lead to biased results.

The twins study is a special case of the family study that rests on a set of simple assumptions that, if fulfilled, allow a disentangling of the effects of nature from those of nurture. Discordant occurrence of a disease in monozygotic twins argues against a strong genetic component in the etiology of the disease, although it will not refute such a mechanism because subtle genetic differences may exist between monozygotic twins.

Concordant disease occurrence in monozygotic twins but not in dizygotic twins supports a genetic cause of the disease, although it could also be explained by environmental intra- and extrauterine factors that may be more compatible for monozygotic twins than for dizygotic twins. If a specific antibody induced by a certain infection cross-reacts with fetal proteins and causes tissue damage, such an effect will depend on cross-placental transfer and the developmental stage of the fetal tissue, which may be more closely correlated in monozygotic than in dizygotic twins. Finally, even in national registers the number of exposure-discordant or disease-concordant monozygotic twins may be small, thus limiting statistical power and precision. Nonetheless, twins registers still represent important sources of secondary data for epidemiologists.

SIBS AND HALF-SIBS

Another variant of family studies makes use of half-siblings. In some countries, men and women often change partners during their reproductive years. Should records of such events be computerized, and they are in many countries, we may use this data source to study genetic and environmental determinants of diseases. In the model we used, the arguments go as follows:

> Suppose that we identify the set of couples who had a child with the disease we want to study, such as febrile seizures. The causes of this event could be not only fever (a necessary cause by definition), but also other environmental and genetic factors. Families who had a child with febrile seizures present themselves with a sufficient set of causes to produce the event. When the mothers have another child, they may have less of these component causes, which would then prevent the disease. The mother may, for example, have a child by a different father. If paternal genes played a role, we expect the disease risk to be less for these second children compared with the risk in the offspring by the same mother and father. We may also check the disease risk in the offspring of mothers who had a new father for the second child and whose first child did not experience febrile convulsions. We would expect that the risk in the second child of these mothers would be comparable or slightly higher than for stable couples whose first child had no febrile seizures. An increased risk is expected if paternal genes play a role, and the increased risk will be a function of the frequency of these genes in the population in general. By using the same strategy, we could check the effect of changes in the families' environment (job, place of living, etc.)

These examples illustrate that family studies usually have to rely on already-existing data and these data sources often have to be population-based, i.e., cover all in a given country or region.

STRESS AND PREGNANCY

It is a common belief that stress during pregnancy may harm the unborn child, hence most countries provide some support for pregnant women that allows them to stop working, change working conditions, or work reduced hours during at least part of the pregnancy. Stress is, however, a difficult exposure to measure. Events that stress some may not stress others, and if data on stress are collected retrospectively, it is difficult to avoid recall bias. Ask mothers who had a child with severe congenital malformation if they felt distressed during pregnancy, and the answer could easily be influenced by their current stress situation.

The alternative is to get prospective data on stress, which is possible at least for frequent types of stress. Feeling distressed, or being exposed to stressful events, is, however, only to some extent associated with being exposed to stress hormones, because the ability to cope with stress modifies the biologic and psychologic stress response. It would be advantageous to study extreme stressors to address questions such as "Can stress cause congenital malformations in humans?" These extreme stressors are rare, and it may be difficult to find a sufficient number of pregnant women exposed to them without access to a large population that experiences an earthquake, an act of war, or other serious stressors that stress nearly all who experience it.

Losing a child is an extreme stressor. Using existing registers, it may be possible to identify a large cohort of pregnant women who lost a child while being pregnant. It may even be possible to identify a sufficiently large group that lost a child unexpectedly (by SIDS, accident, etc.) when the woman was pregnant in the second or third month during the time of organogenesis. To do so, one needs a cause-of-death register, a register of pregnancies and births, a register of congenital malformations, and perhaps a register for social conditions. All of this information must be identifiable at the individual level, and it must be possible to link the data from these registers. Given these conditions, we could assess the extent to which severe life events (and thus severe stressors) can increase the prevalence of birth defects. Should such a study show little or no relation between stress and birth defects, it would tend to refute studies that report such a relation based on milder forms of stress. Nonetheless, the possibility of confounding by factors related to both perinatal and childhood mortality should be borne in mind when taking death of a child as the stressful exposure.

This example illustrates that using existing secondary data makes this study feasible. In contrast, a primary data source would need to be very large to be informative, regardless of whether the study was designed as a follow-up or a case-control study (both the exposure and the outcome are rare).

VACCINES AND AUTISM

Autism is a serious mental disorder with an increasing reported incidence during childhood in many countries. The reasons for this rise are unknown, but vaccination against measles has been suggested as a cause. The documentation for this concern is meager but nevertheless sufficient to cause public alarm that may jeopardize vaccination programs. Wakefield et al. (1998) reported a case series of 12 children from a clinic of gastroentorologic diseases who showed signs of both developmental regression and gastrointestinal symptoms. Eight of these children had experienced the onset of developmental symptoms following their measles vaccination. The authors came to the conclusion that a new variant of inflammatory bowel disease was present in children with developmental disorders. Although the nature of the interaction between the gut lesion and the cognitive impairment is unclear, autoimmunity and toxic brain encephalopathy have been suggested. Because vaccination is often recommended at the age at which signs of autism first surface, a temporal relation is expected and often seen. None of these observations provided any strong arguments for a causal link between vaccination and autism, but strong negative empirical evidence is nevertheless needed to diminish public concern.

In Denmark, it was possible to identify all who had received the measles vaccination in a given time period based on reports from the general practitioners who prescribe the vaccination. The register is based on forms that the general practitioners send to local health authorities, and because payment depends on these registrations, there are reasons to believe that data are accurate and complete.

Using this register, we can define a vaccinated cohort of children and a nonvaccinated cohort, and study the incidence of autism in these two cohorts. If autism is also recorded in a linkable registry, such a study can be based on register linkage and cover the entire nation in the right age group with no loss to follow-up. The actual study showed no excess risk among those vaccinated compared with those not vaccinated, which seems to support strongly the null hypothesis that MFR (measles, mumps, and rubella) vaccination is not a cause of autism, or at least not a very strong determinant of autism. The study does not preclude that some autism is related to vaccination, however, because data are subject to misclassification for both the exposure and for autism, this form of misclassification will most likely tend to attenuate a possible effect, and adjustment for confounding factors is limited. The main confounding of concern is of a genetic nature. It is known that children with autism have more psychiatric problems in their families, and if families with psychiatric problems do not get their children vaccinated, the unvaccinated group will have a higher genetic (or at least familial) risk of autism. Such negative confounding could mask a true association. Nevertheless, even that possibility could and should be explored further by means of secondary data, if mental disorders can be identified for family members.

This example illustrates how secondary data sources can be activated within a short time to address a research question that could have a long-term effect on disease prevention. Collecting primary data would take so long that the entire vaccination program may be jeopardized before results become available.

LINKAGE OF DATA

In most studies, data from different sources have to be linked. Linkage is best done by using an unambiguous identification system such as a unique personal number. Most research data are linked by means of such a number. If data are linked by means of other sources of information, such as date of birth, name, addresses, or genetic markers, there is usually a greater risk of error.

When data are linked according to a set of criteria that translate into a probability for a match that is <1, the researcher has to think about the problems that uncertain linkage may generate. One effect is that the study size shrinks, which will reduce precision, perhaps to a prohibitive level. Perhaps a greater concern is the possibility of bias being introduced. Finding an address back in time is often more difficult for people who move often than for those who stay in the same place. Social conditions and health may well be related to how much people move around. If school data are needed, then one must often need to have the name given at birth. Some people may change this name later in life because they marry or because they want or need another name. Changing names may well correlate with social conditions, including health.

If the probability of getting a perfect match depends on both exposures and outcomes under study (or confounders), bias may result from incomplete linkage alone. Simulation studies may be the only way of analyzing whether a study based on probabilistic matching is worthwhile.

VALIDATION OF DATA

Using secondary data in research raises the issue of data quality. Are data good enough, and good enough for what, and what does "good enough" actually mean? Often there is a sentence or two in a paper stating that the questionnaires or registers used in the study have been validated. Usually it is unclear what that means, or if it means anything at all of relevance for the study in question.

On the other hand, requests for validation have to be put into context. Why is it important in this particular study, and how valid should data be (all data have errors)?

Epidemiologists study the phenotypes that clinicians call patients, people who are labeled according to a set of diagnostic criteria. These criteria are usually based not on etiologic profiles but on other features, such as anatomic characteristics or what responds to available treatment. Many conditions, such as hypertension or ADHD, represent extreme values of a distribution, and we should perhaps take more interest in what shapes the distribution rather than what determines the outliers. Thus, it may be equally or even more informative to know the determinants of cognitive skills in addition to the determinants of mental retardation.

A disease classification based on etiologic consideration will in many situations deviate from a clinical definition. It may be more appropriate to classify congenital malformations according to the time of organogenesis rather than using the current standard classification. We use epistemiologic criteria when we write the protocol; are the diseases classified according to standardized guidelines or not? Often, the answer is not clear. Even when guidelines are well known, they are not always used. Using medical diagnoses even within highly specialized categories involves uncertainties and some misclassification. An advantage of using existing medical records is that prediagnostic exposure misclassification is usually nondifferential. In most situations, the clinician is unaware of the putative causes of the disease when making a diagnosis, and so the disease misclassification will also be nondifferential. That may be bad for the patients but good for epidemiologists.

DATA QUALITY

Good data quality in a disease registry may mean that the data in the registry on a given disease actually describe the disease according to an agreed set of diagnostic criteria, and that all in the population with this set of criteria have this label in the registry. These two conditions are often called validity and completeness.

The validity can be examined if the patients, or at least their relevant records, are available for further study. If the disease has a short duration and leaves no specific traits (such as a specific antibody response), then medical records for the time period of treatment will be the only source. If available, the records must contain useful information on the diagnostic criteria. Validity may then be expressed as the probability of having the diagnostic criteria (D), given the presence of the diagnostic label ($\overline{D}$): $P\ (D|\overline{D})$. Using screening terminology, this probability is similar to the predictive value of a positive test, the "test" in this case being the code for disease in the registry file: $P(\text{D}|\text{test positive})$. As in screening, this predictive value is closely associated with specificity, which is the proportion of those without the disease who did not have the diagnostic label. The problem of low specificity is usually larger in secondary data coming from population surveys than in secondary data coming from hospital patients who have passed through several referral systems.

A more difficult question to answer is "How complete is the register, or what proportion of diseased people in the population can be found in the register?" It may be possible to take a sample of those without the diagnostic label in the register and call them in for examination to see if in fact they qualify for the diagnosis, but usually this approach is not feasible. Furthermore, if the disease is rare, the sample needs to be very large to be informative.

Another option may be to use the capture-recapture method, which uses two-stage sampling to estimate an unknown size of a population. It has been widely used by biologists to estimate the size of wild animal populations. Assume that a biologist wants to know the number of salmon in a given lake. She cannot empty the lake and count all salmon. She may, however, get permission to catch some salmon in the lake. Suppose she catches n_1 salmon on the first round, marks these salmon, throws them back into the lake; and then makes a second catch of n_2 salmon and counts how many of the salmon had a mark and were recaptured. Using the number n_3 caught in both samples and the number caught in either sample provides the data needed to estimate the total number of salmon in the lake. Assuming that (a) all those caught are marked and returned to the lake, (b) the salmon do not differ in their probability of being caught (e.g., there are no "smart salmon" that consistently avoid capture, and the capture method applies equally well to all the salmon), (c) being caught once does not influence the probability of being caught again (i.e., the salmon caught do not learn to avoid being caught again), so that the samplings are independent, and (d) N does not change between samplings, the argument goes as follows: The probability of being in the first sample, P_1, is n_1/N, where N is the total number of salmon in the lake and n_1 is the number caught in the first round. The probability of being in the second sample, P_2, is n_2/N, where n_2 is the number of fish caught in the second round. The number of salmon expected to be caught both times is $N \times P_1 \times P_2 = N \times n_1/N \times n_2/N$; this number is estimated by the number n_3 actually caught both times. Setting $n_3 = N \times n_1/N \times n_2/N$ and solving for N provides an estimate for N of $(n_1 \times n_2)/n_3$.

In a register-based search, this method is often applied to situations in which the assumptions are questionable. Imagine two registers, a hospital discharge register and a pathology register, covering the same population. There may be 100 patients in the hospital register and 75 in the pathology register, and 50 of these overlap. The estimate of the total number of patients is then $(100 \times 75)/50 = 150$. Because 100 out of 150 were in the hospital discharge register, the investigator might conclude that the degree of completeness in the hospital register was $100/150 = 67\%$. It is, however, difficult to imagine that the two registers are independent. Most likely, there will be an oversampling of severe patients in the two samples, because patients are referred to pathologists from the clinical departments. The result will be to underestimate the total number with disease.

Given a registry of vaccinations in children based on clinical records from those who gave the vaccination, one may get additional information from an independent source. For example, it may be possible to interview the mothers in a region or look for vaccination scars on children (for smallpox or tuberculosis, for example) and then calculate the overlap in those vaccinated between the two data sources. Because these data sources are independent, the estimate of the coverage rate of vaccinations in the register may be valid, provided that the data on vaccine status are accurate in both systems.

The capture-recapture method may also be used with fewer restrictions with access to a population survey covering the same catchment area as the hospital register. With access to more than two sources, a dependency between registers can be taken into account in the analyses.

QUANTIFICATION OF BIAS RELATED TO MISCLASSIFICATION

Larger follow-up or case-control studies are designed to permit quality control of key elements of crucial importance for the validity of the findings. Extensive pilot testing is done to make sure that the study is feasible and worthwhile. Substudies are usually implemented to examine selection bias related to nonresponders and misclassification of key exposures, endpoints, or confounders. For studies based on secondary data, substudies may not be an option. The only alternative may be to present sensitivity analysis (see Chapter 19) to show the likely effects of anticipated sources of bias. Such analyses have traditionally been overlooked in favor of a preoccupation with random error, although this convention may change if standard packages for analyzing data begin to incorporate sensitivity analyses.

MONITORING

Routine data may be generated to monitor events over time, and studying disease frequencies over time or between populations has been extremely useful in many respects. There is a concern that the use of cellular phones may increase brain cancer risk by some yet-unknown mechanism. If so, the brain cancer incidence should increase in the entire population with a given latency time, because the exposure is widespread. Many of the ideas we have on environmental causes of cancer stem from comparing cancer incidence from such data. We know that the burden of diseases is extremely unevenly distributed across the world. The "big picture" shows clearly that poverty is the main determinant of poor health worldwide and within countries with large social inequalities. Monitoring of diseases also demonstrates the importance of lifestyle factors such as smoking and physical inactivity. Monitoring has demonstrated that even mortality rates may change

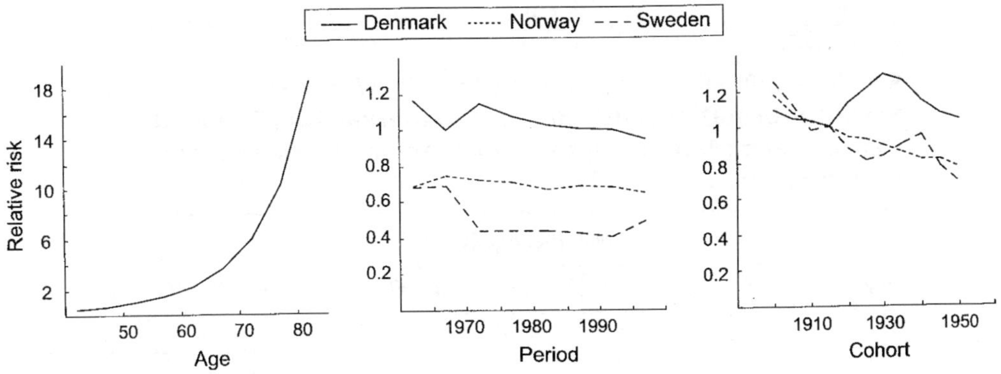

FIGURE 23–1 • Relative risk of death for women in each age, period, cohort, and country, when compared with Danish women born in 1915–1919 and aged 50 to 54 years in 1965–1969. (Reprinted with permission from Jacobsen R, Von Euler M, Osler M, et al. Women's death in Scandinavia—what makes Denmark different? *Eur J Epidemiol.* 2004;19:117–121.)

dramatically over short time periods, as seen in Russia after the fall of the communist regime. It also shows that emigrants often experience the disease patterns of their new homeland after one or two generations. Monitoring of occupational mortality in the United Kingdom has been a valuable source of information in understanding occupational diseases and social inequalities in mortality.

Longitudinal monitoring over time may also permit studies of changes in disease patterns that affect specific birth cohorts, which is what we would expect if we study exposures that operate only early in life and are restricted in calendar time. Age effects will be expected for most cancers, mortality, and many other diseases. Calendar effects are expected if exposures such as environmental pollution are localized in time and affect large segments in the population at once.

Given sufficient monitoring of a population over time, we may estimate these three effects, albeit with some limitations, because they are mathematically interdependent. If one knows the age of a person at a given point in calendar time, one can compute which birth cohort the person belongs to. And if one knows the time of birth, one can compute the age at given points in calendar time. Because of these linear dependencies, linear drifts can therefore not be attributed to a specific component of the age, time, birth-cohort model. Nevertheless, deviations from linearity can be identified. Figure 23–1 shows that mortality is, as expected, highly age-dependent among women in Denmark (and in most other countries). The figure also shows a higher mortality in Danish women compared with women in Norway and Sweden, attributable largely to a deviation from the linear decline in birth cohort mortality that started after 1910 and ended after 1930 in Denmark.

Fetal growth retardation may be key in understanding susceptibility to several diseases, and using secondary data may provide some indication if newborns who are small for their gestational age (SGA) come from certain birth cohorts, time periods, or maternal age groups. To overcome the linear dependency between age, period, and cohort effects, Ananth et al. (2004) constrained the effects of the last birth cohort (1981–1985) to zero. They analyzed SGA births in the United States by means of logistic regression of the form

$$\log\left[\frac{\Pr(Y_{ijk}=1)}{1-\Pr(Y_{ijk}=1)}\right] = \mu + \sum_{i=1}^{n}\alpha_i(age_i) + \sum_{j=1}^{m}\beta_j(period_j) + \sum_{k=j-1}^{m}\gamma_k(cohort_k)$$

Here Y denotes SGA status, μ is the baseline SGA rate, and the indices form age, period, and cohort groups in the analyses. Table 23–1 shows a U-shaped association between SGA and maternal age and a possible decline for younger birth cohorts.

In the field of asthma research, the ability to monitor diseases over time and between different populations led to the so-called hygiene hypothesis. This hypothesis posits that the asthma epidemic is partly a consequence of better hygienic standards—less crowding, better houses, more refrigerators for storing food, etc.

TABLE 23–1

Risk (per 100 births) of Singleton Term (≥ 37 weeks) Small-for-Gestational Age Births by Maternal Age, Period of Delivery, and Maternal Birth Cohorts among Black Women: United States, 1975—2000.

	Maternal Age (years)							
Period	15–19	20–24	25–29	30–34	35–39	40–44	45–49	Birth Cohort
							19.6	1926–30
						18.9	18.0	1931–35
					16.7	16.6	21.3	1936–40
				17.0	14.9	16.9	19.0	1941–45
			18.3	15.2	15.8	17.0	14.2	1946–50
		22.0	17.1	16.2	16.7	18.0	26.2	1951–55
	25.3	20.6	17.7	17.2	16.7	16.7		1956–60
1975 ↗	23.4	12.7	17.5	16.0	14.8			1961–65
1980 ↗	21.8	18.2	15.8	13.8				1966–70
1985 ↗	20.7	17.4	14.1					1971–75
1990 ↗	20.5	17.2						1976–80
1995 ↗	20.5							1981–85
2000 ↗								

From Ananth CV, Balasubramanian B, Demissie K, et al. Small-for-Gestational-Age Births in the United States. An Age-Period-Cohort Analysis. *Epidemiology*. 2004;15(1):28–35, Table 1.

These examples show the importance of basic descriptive morbidity and mortality. Although epidemiologists should provide new data on proximal determinants of disease, we should not forget to use and analyze data that illustrate the "big picture." Disease patterns change over time and vary greatly between different populations. To make substantial changes in health in the population it is often necessary to modify more distal social and environmental conditions.

ETHICS OF SECONDARY DATA ACCESS

The main concern in storing data with personal identifiers is the risk of political misuse. Although governments must collect data to govern effectively, political authorities have also used such data sources to identify subgroups of the population and violate their human rights, even in relatively recent times. Governments may be tempted to manipulate people or to limit their freedom to exercise democratic rights based on data collected and stored for seemingly legitimate government purposes. One solution is to place data sources that have this potential in the hands of independent research organizations rather than governmental institutions, although this solution has not been implemented in most countries with such data.

Research data should not be available for individual case administration. Thus, these data should not be accessible by insurance companies, employers, or public, social, or health administrative systems. People should be able to take part in research without running the risk of losing privileges, jobs, opportunities, or any other public benefits. It is even questionable whether the participants should have access to their own data, as suggested by some. First, a database that is constructed to facilitate personal access to data reduces data security as a result of the way the data file has to be organized. Second, open access makes it more difficult to deny access from other sources. Third, open access to data increases the risk of unwanted disclosure, because many research departments do not have the resources nor the training to make sure that people are who they claim to be.

Personal identifiers are needed only when data are to be linked, cleaned, and documented. Once that is done, analyses can be based on de-identified data. Ethical concerns are then limited to the problem of identifying risk groups that may be stigmatized by the reported findings. Reporting certain clustering of exposures or diseases in easily recognizable subgroups of this population should be avoided unless it has important public health implications. On the other hand, it is difficult to imagine how we can prevent the spread of HIV unless we deal with the characteristics of those who are infected, including their sexual orientation, use of drugs, and place of living.

It is usually in the best public interests that risk factors for disease and death are identified and that health care delivery systems are properly evaluated. For these reasons, one could argue for as much use as possible of secondary data. There are strong arguments for making not only secondary administrative data but also secondary research data freely available for all to use. Expensive new data collection may be avoided if existing data can address fully or partially the research questions posed. Primary data users rarely see all the potential for using their own data, and much of the public data is either neglected by researchers or inaccessible to them. Open access to data could not only generate more research but could also lead to more rapid corrections of mistakes. Open access to data requires not only procedures for data storage and data documentation but also the implementation of safeguards to avoid unacceptable risk of disclosure of personal data. Opponents of the open-access principle claim that data may be poorly analyzed by people who do not understand how the data were generated or even people who would not analyze data in good faith. These concerns are real but exist for all data analyses. These problems may in the long run best be addressed by openness and discussions based on data.

Research data collected with public resources should be made freely available for research once the primary aim of the study has been fulfilled for those who took the initiative to collect the data. Participants in research donate data for the public good, not for promoting researchers' career opportunities. For public registers the situation should be even more straightforward, because the data are in the public domain. This is not to say that all should have access to the data, but data must be made available on fair and equal terms. Given that researchers can meet the conditions necessary to secure unwanted disclosure of data and have worthwhile research ideas, they should have access. It is understandable that mediocre epidemiologists might want to protect the principle of ownership of data. It is more surprising, however, that similar attitudes are evinced by some first-rank epidemiologists. One hopes that open access to data would lead not only to more exhaustive use of the data sources but also better quality of reporting. Large data sources provide ample opportunities for making not only multiple comparisons but also multiple ways of classifying exposures, endpoints, and confounders. The proper way of analyzing data sources should be to explore how robust findings are in the light of these different classification options—to see if you can make the findings go away by using alternative analytical strategies. It is possible that the pressure to publish, the editorial desire for simple take-home messages, etc., lead to unjustified oversimplified presentations and underreporting of results that did not support the key message. This problem is a serious threat to the credibility of our discipline. Although time and expense may make it impossible or impractical to replicate findings from large epidemiologic studies, Peng et al. (2006) have argued for an "attainable minimum standard [of] 'reproducibility,' which calls for data sets and software to be made available for verifying published findings and conducting alternative analyses."

Open access to data sources would lead to a more cautious presentation of results, which is badly needed. From a practical and scientific point of view, open access to data cannot always be based on informed consent from the individuals. Withdrawal from the data source must therefore be an option. Should such a withdrawal reach high numbers, then the people themselves will cut off the option to conduct meaningful research. Though that would be regrettable, it would be a much more democratic procedure than the present political barriers to using data.

CONCLUSION

Secondary data may provide research resources that can be used in meta-analyses, new studies, or to reanalyze existing published reports. Not all secondary data have this potential, and the economic costs in preparing, storing, and maintaining data should of course be weighed against the potentials for use. Still, much has to be done before we have eliminated the obstacles of the use of valuable secondary data to expand knowledge and improve human health.

CHAPTER 24

Field Methods in Epidemiology

Patricia Hartge and Jack Cahill

Subject Identification and Recruitment 493
Variations among Study Populations 493
Recruitment to Intervention Studies 494
Subject Identification for Community Trials 494
Assembly of Cohorts 495
Identification of Subjects in Case-Control Studies 496
Cross-Sectional and Other Designs 497
Obtaining High Response Rates 497
Data Collection and Data Capture 499
Abstracting Records 499
Questionnaire Administration Method 500
Content and Wording of Questions 501
Questionnaires and Respondent Burden 503
Interviewing Techniques and Training 504
Physical Examinations 504
Biospecimen Collection 505
Environmental Samples and Global Positioning Systems 505
Tracing 507
Follow-up Techniques 507
Data Capture 508
Emerging Issues 509

To succeed in its goals, every epidemiologic study requires sound design, execution, and analysis. Field work encompasses all phases of study execution, from the selection and recruitment of subjects to the completion of the database for analysis. It is the bridge between the design and the analysis, and on it depend the validity and the precision of the effect measures to be estimated.

The underlying study population constrains or influences nearly every feature of the field methods. For example, field methods in studies in resource-poor nations will likely differ markedly from the methods in populations with complete population registries. Studies of multiple populations (multicenter studies) impose additional requirements. Language, culture, health status, and social class all may influence field design choices.

Once the study population is chosen, alternative methods for selecting and recruiting subjects can be considered. These will depend on whether the study is experimental or nonexperimental and on the need for either future contact or retrospective exposure assessment. Ethical requirements, privacy protections, and logistical considerations will constrain the choices. Incentives or other methods to increase motivation may be needed to achieve adequate response rates.

In many epidemiologic studies, data collection includes questioning the subject on the telephone, via the Internet, in writing, or in person. This questioning may be an inherent aspect of the study, or it may rely on records for which subjects were questioned for another purpose, such as birth certificates. Most studies also include some form of search and abstraction of data recorded in an external source, such as death certificates or banks of records from which eligible subjects are selected. A large and growing proportion of epidemiologic studies include the measurement of biomarkers, and a small but growing proportion includes measures of the environment.

Field work demands so much time in all but the smallest studies that the epidemiologist responsible for the study seldom does all of it, relying instead on study staff. In medium-sized studies, the daily operations of the study staff are directed by a field supervisor who is familiar with field methods but not necessarily trained in epidemiology. In large multicenter studies with a field staff of dozens, each center may have its own study manager as well. An experienced and capable study manager provides enormous benefit to the study but does not relieve the epidemiologist of responsibility for field work. The epidemiologist's job is also facilitated by the availability of management systems; these have improved dramatically over time, with more powerful and user-friendly software and smaller, lighter, varied hardware.

Epidemiologists can ensure the quality of the field work in many ways. For example, the investigators can often anticipate the potential weaknesses of the study, based on previous work, pretests, and other sources. They can use previous methodologic investigations, or conduct new ones, to compare alternative field methods to each other or, rarely, to a "gold standard." The findings of these methodologic investigations can help, first, in selecting the field methods and, later, in interpreting the likely direction and magnitude of potential study biases. In addition, the investigators ought to participate actively in testing the study instruments and procedures.

Finally, the investigators are responsible for documenting study operations and procedures and for incorporating quality control methods into each phase of the study. A documented quality control plan is ideal, addressing such issues as standardization and monitoring, protocol adherence, staff qualifications, training, data collection, procedures for ensuring the quality of biologic or environmental samples, coding, data editing, data entry, and data analysis. The study's level of complexity will dictate what quality assurance issues will apply, with a focus on enhancing the reliability and validity of the collected data.

SUBJECT IDENTIFICATION AND RECRUITMENT

VARIATIONS AMONG STUDY POPULATIONS

In typical studies conducted in industrialized countries, investigators rely on nearly universal telephone service, widespread access to the Internet, and high rates of literacy. Nevertheless, in most parts of the United States, no overall listing of the population within a defined geographic area is available for simple survey sampling, so approximations are attempted with samples drawn from motor vehicle registries (Titus-Ernstoff et al., 2002; Church et al., 2004), telephone directories or random-digit dialing (Casady and Leplowski, 1993; Brick et al., 2002), or census tracts (Montaquila et al., 1998). In contrast, in some developed countries (e.g., the Scandinavian countries), complete population rosters and various population registries have been used extensively for medical research purposes (Melbye et al., 1997; Laursen et al., 2004; Hall et al., 2004; Bergfeldt et al., 2002). Similar types of studies can sometimes be accomplished within closed populations that are completely covered by rosters, for example, within health maintenance organizations (Corley et al., 2002; Izurieta et al., 2000; Selby et al., 2004). Access to such databases is usually tightly restricted to prevent violation of privacy or other harm from the linkage of personal information across databases.

In limited-resource settings, study methods are adapted to the technologies that are locally accessible. Other factors to be addressed include cultural differences (language, traditions, beliefs) and global logistics (protocol approval, specimen shipment, specimen storage, training, local laws, communication). For example, if women give birth at home, study staff can measure birth outcomes by keeping close track of due dates and visiting the home on the birth date with a scale and measure (Christian et al., 2003). It may be necessary to adapt the study explanation and the process of obtaining consent to local levels of literacy and to cultural norms. A village elder may decide whether the entire community will participate in a study (Macintyre et al., 2003). Some devices that are not common in the community may be feasible to use for the study if they are portable and easily maintained. For example, laptop computers can reduce data recording errors and are feasible in limited-resource settings. In a study examining the validity of a telephone-administered 24-hour dietary recall interview in the rural Mississippi Delta region, households without telephones were randomized to receive either an in-person interview or a telephone interview. In the latter case, the subject used a cellular telephone, provided by the interviewer, to call a telephone research center interviewer. Thus, the dietary interviews were conducted in a standardized manner by a centralized facility (Bogle et al., 2001).

General principles govern the protection of human research subjects. Historical events that prompted concern about freedom of consent, disclosure of risks, and adequacy of treatment have spurred the evolution of principled statements such as the Nuremburg Code, the Declaration of Helsinki, the Belmont Report, and the Common Rule, which then yielded special regulations and guidelines for researchers to follow in the protection of human subjects. Although the adaptation of these principles and customs will vary among study populations, it is important that researchers be aware of them when designing and conducting studies involving human subjects.

RECRUITMENT TO INTERVENTION STUDIES

In intervention studies, subjects are ideally selected from existing lists of names, with current contact information, so that potential subjects can be approached individually. For example, in a trial to investigate the role of diet in the recurrence of adenomatous colon polyps, the investigators identified potential subjects by obtaining referrals from participating gastroenterologists and by reviewing the medical records of participating endoscopy services (Schatzkin et al., 1996). A trial of the preventive value of α-tocopherol and β-carotene against lung cancer targeted male smokers because of their high risk of disease (Virtamo et al., 2003). Physicians were targeted for a trial of the effect of low-dose aspirin and β-carotene on multiple health outcomes, not because of their risk of disease but because of their interest and likely compliance with the experimental regimen (Physicians' Health Study, 2004). In a trial of replacement hormones and diet in relation to breast cancer and other outcomes, investigators targeted women at elevated risk of developing breast cancer (Writing Group for the Women's Health Initiative Investigators, 2002; Women's Health Initiative, 2004).

When there is no list from which to recruit subjects for intervention studies, investigators use public notices, including the Internet, television, radio, newspapers, and posted advertising. Epidemiologists often solicit sponsorship or endorsement by prominent people and community or medical organizations to increase interest. Many trials offer reimbursement for parking or other minor costs of participating in the trial. If the time commitment or physical demands of the study are great (e.g., if the study involves multiple blood collections), financial compensation may be necessary. Ultimately, recruitment succeeds by persuading the subjects of the value of the trial to themselves (e.g., they may receive a free medical examination) and to society.

Randomization typically follows recruitment. After satisfying all of the eligibility criteria and consenting to participate, subjects are randomly assigned to one of the arms of the trial using a random-number simulator. Because randomization cannot guarantee a balance of risk factors across the experimental groups, the investigator typically uses a baseline questionnaire to measure the predictors of the main outcomes. The investigator also collects information for locating the subjects until the end of the follow-up period (e.g., names and location information for friends or relatives), because many intervention trials require annual or other regular follow-up by mailed questionnaire, with telephone calls to nonrespondents.

SUBJECT IDENTIFICATION FOR COMMUNITY TRIALS

With the community trial design, the investigator assigns exposure status to an entire community rather than to individuals. The outcome may be the risk of disease or the frequency of a health behavior. The field work for such community trials generally includes efforts to measure the potential confounders. Because the unit of observation is the community, the assessment of potential confounders can also occur at the community level. If the exposure is an education campaign aimed at changing knowledge, attitudes, and behaviors, the investigation may encompass more than the primary health outcome. Survey components might add measures of the effect of a smoking-cessation or weight-reduction campaign as well as measures of medical visits or hospitalizations. In general, community trials include public health education and other types of field work not typically involved in studies of individuals, even though the epidemiologic principles are the same (Glanz et al., 2002).

ASSEMBLY OF COHORTS

If a cohort study requires collecting the details of an exposure (timing, intensity, other exposures), the data sources used to characterize the exposure may be the same as those needed to assemble the cohort. Studies of occupational and medical cohorts typify the field methods used in cohort studies in general. Large cohort studies based in general populations have become increasingly common, and consortia that combine cohorts to produce very large study sizes have recently been formed (National Cancer Institute, 2004).

In an occupational cohort study, the investigator assembles the cohort from the records of a company, a union, or a professional or trade association. Many preliminary studies use union or association records alone. In retrospective studies, these records often permit assembly of a complete cohort but lack the detail on tasks and work locations essential to defining each individual's jobs and exposures. When both union and company records are available, both sources may be used to increase completeness. The investigator might also choose to form an inception cohort to follow prospectively. In such studies, the study staff first recruits employers, then recruits workers within defined job categories, interviews them to collect baseline information, and conducts follow-up over time to identify risk and disease incidence.

At the outset, the study team (typically an epidemiologist, an industrial hygienist, a study manager, and one or more abstractors) visits some of the plants and the headquarters or offices in which worker records are kept. The investigators inquire about every possible source of records, including occupation records, payroll ledgers, union rolls, medical records, and life and health insurance systems, both computerized and paper. Although the separate record systems will be incomplete, together they may provide a nearly complete enumeration of the cohort. Investigators can scan the records, creating an electronic file containing images of the documents. Files can then be compressed and downloaded to CDs for storage, saving time, space, and money.

To uncover as many record sources as possible, the investigator interviews many potential informants at different levels of authority, from clerical to managerial. It is necessary to ask about record systems no longer maintained and about groups of records stored separately, such as those from pensioners, workers terminated before pension eligibility, workers involved in litigation, or workers under medical care. It is also critical to determine whether lists or records were modified once created, for example, to remove decedents. Failure to recognize modifications to records that are related to the outcome can yield immortal person-time (see Chapter 6). Once the records are found, research staff abstract, photocopy, or scan them. Photocopying or scanning adds to the costs of data collection but allows the investigators to review the records at the study office, check on the quality of abstracting, and glean additional data. A modest cohort of 5,000 workers can yield 50,000 job lines (the combination of job title and department). Although straightforward in principle, the assembly of a complete occupational cohort requires considerable effort.

The research staff first captures the work history (progression through job titles and departments) and then classifies all job title/department combinations into jobs with common tasks and locations. The abstractors, supervised by the study manager, typically review the individual work histories from records and conversations with company personnel to resolve discrepancies. The industrial hygienist collapses the job lines into jobs, based on familiarity with the work environment (Stewart et al., 1992). In some studies, the third task is to impute exposure levels for jobs, based on current and historical environmental samples and details of job activities provided by workers and supervisors.

Medical cohorts are groups of people whose exposure of interest is a disease, medical condition, or medical treatment. The study staff selects cohort members from surveillance databases, hospital discharge diagnosis files, pharmacy records, medical insurance data, birth certificates, or routine activity logs kept by medical practices, clinics, and hospital departments such as pathology, surgery, or obstetrics. Cohort assembly may be complicated if some of the needed medical records have been destroyed, lost, or stored in inconvenient locations. Apart from logistical problems in obtaining the medical data, the classification of exposure often presents the greatest problem because medical records and medical exposures are complex and variable. Investigators generally make several preliminary visits to the hospital, clinic, or practice to investigate the sources and quality of data. Multiple record sources may be needed to determine whether a subject is eligible (e.g., surgical pathology logs to determine the diagnosis and hospital patient files to obtain demographic data).

Any procedures that will be used to confirm conditions or treatments should be specified in advance, for either the entire study group or a subset of the group.

IDENTIFICATION OF SUBJECTS IN CASE-CONTROL STUDIES

A case-control study derives from an underlying source population, with the protocol describing the population as explicitly as possible before field procedures are developed. This source population will be chosen in light of the frequency of the disease and exposures under study, the difficulties in diagnosing the disease, and the routine procedures for recording its occurrence. As both etiologic research and computerization of medical data have expanded, population-based disease registries have proliferated. Hospitals and clinics remain convenient and useful sources of cases, despite the challenge of understanding and sampling the underlying source population. Cohorts provide a source population for case-control studies when it would be expensive or unnecessary to acquire data from the entire cohort. The protocol for a case-control study might, for example, define the case group as encompassing all incident cases of ovarian cancer diagnosed in a specified period among residents of a specified region. The control group might be defined as a sample of women from the same population, stratified according to age and race.

Late changes in protocol occasionally occur in case-control studies (e.g., the addition of a specialty clinic as a source of controls in a hospital-based study), but investigators ought to avoid ad hoc changes in the composition of either the case or the control group. When logistical constraints force modifications to the study, such modification mandates consideration of whether the case and control group refer to the same source population. For instance, if the controls must be limited to people with little residential mobility because investigators must infer past residential exposures from current values, then cases must be so restricted.

Investigators can easily devise procedures for selecting cases in population-based studies if a disease registry has already collected much of the needed diagnosis data. On the other hand, such registries may not be suitable if the disease is rapidly fatal and collection of data from the subject is necessary. Sometimes registries that do not routinely collect data fast enough for the purposes of the study can accelerate ascertainment of cases.

Occasionally, a convenient population-based control group exists but there is no disease registry for case ascertainment. In this situation, the field work consists of locating all cases occurring in the base population. If the disease requires hospitalization or medical treatment, the study staff must create a disease registry by reviewing the records of hospitals, pathology laboratories, etc., while dealing with the problems of emigration, immigration, and medical care across boundaries. If the disease does not require hospitalization or medical treatment, the field work resembles the follow-up phase in a cohort study, with the use of questionnaires or interviews to determine who has had the disease of interest.

Sometimes a study can tap a fully enumerated source population from which the disease registry draws its cases, for instance, in several Scandinavian nations or in health maintenance organizations (see Chapter 24). More often, the source population is well defined but individual members are not readily identifiable by name and address (e.g., all residents of a geographic area in which cancers are reported to a central registry). In such circumstances, sampling frames are required to identify a sample of individuals from the source. Some frames work from lists of individuals, including listings of residents of municipalities, registered voters, licensed drivers, and persons eligible for Medicare in the United States (i.e., those aged 65 years or older). Municipal lists are accessible but not reliably current; licensed drivers provide an inexpensive and convenient, but incomplete, sample of the population.

Apart from list-based samples, two commonly employed frames use two-stage sampling schemes that begin by randomly sampling dwellings (area-based sampling) or telephone numbers (random-digit dialing, or RDD) (Waksberg, 1978; Hartge et al., 1984; DiGaetano and Waksberg, 2002; Brogan et al., 2001). RDD became a common technique in the 1980s, but response rates to RDD and all types of surveys have fallen substantially since the late 1990s. Furthermore, answering machines, mobile telephones, faxes, and data lines have added to the complexity of telephone sampling. For these reasons, the utility of RDD has diminished. Friend controls, an inexpensive and seemingly attractive alternative, can induce substantial bias (Flanders and Austin, 1986; Ma et al., 2004).

In studies based in hospitals, clinics, or medical practices, investigators gain access to a convenient list of potential cases (e.g., from hospital records) not linked to an enumerated underlying population. They must impute the source population and devise a control group to approximate it. Some studies compare hospital-based cases with controls selected from the neighborhoods of the cases' telephone exchanges, on the theory that such controls would be referred to the same hospitals if they developed the disease. Another common strategy is to select controls from among patients in other clinics within the same hospital. The protocol may specify which diagnoses are to be excluded from the control group because they are related to the exposures of interest. Additional exclusions often include psychiatric diagnoses or other conditions that compromise data collection. In one design variation, a few diagnostic categories are designated for inclusion rather than selecting from an unspecified mixture of diagnoses.

Procedures for case and control selection in hospital studies should be as precise as possible and should remain constant from day to day and from patient to patient. Study staff assigned to select a patient from a clinic on a certain day should, for example, be following an algorithm that dictates which particular patient ought to be picked. Such practices not only guard against deliberate or unconscious enrollment of particular patient types but also allow routine quality checks. Data on patients who are unavailable or unwilling to be studied ought to be recorded so that nonresponse can be characterized.

CROSS-SECTIONAL AND OTHER DESIGNS

Cross-sectional studies generally use a mixture of the selection and recruitment strategies needed for trials, cohort studies, and case-control studies. The sampling issues typify those of large population-based surveys. Smaller targeted cross-sectional studies of volunteers continue to play a key role in epidemiology. For example, a study of the relation between family cancer history and the presence of founder mutations in the *BRCA1* and *BRCA2* genes among Ashkenazi Jews began with a recruitment campaign typical of any study of volunteers (Struewing et al., 1997).

OBTAINING HIGH RESPONSE RATES

Many investigators believe that obtaining high response rates while maintaining high data quality has become the single largest obstacle to high-quality epidemiologic research. The specific threats depend on study design. For instance, loss of target population at recruitment into a cohort study does not threaten validity, but loss of follow-up of the recruited members can do so, because the rate of loss might differ by both disease and exposure. For every mode of interviewing, the barriers to contacting potential subjects are rising. In part, these barriers stem from changing societal perceptions of the value of participating in epidemiologic studies, and reluctant subjects who might have participated in the past may no longer choose to do so. The investigator needs multiple strategies for obtaining subject cooperation and maintaining a high response rate. Achievable interview response rates appear to be considerably higher in China (80% to 90%) than in Europe (70% to 80%) or in the United States (60% to 70%).

Generally, recruitment will succeed if the subjects are persuaded that the study has value to them or to society. At the outset, the investigators need a simple and clear statement of what participation entails and a persuasive argument for electing to participate. The reputation of the scientific institution sponsoring the study may be helpful in this endeavor but is seldom sufficient. Advance letters that come from subjects' physicians or include the names of key sponsors from community groups or government agencies are inexpensive aids; identifying readily available individuals who can speak for the study is critical. For example, case-control studies of a particular disease often include letters to the clinicians who are most likely to diagnose or treat cases.

At the beginning of the study, the investigator should consider whether an incentive will be used to gain cooperation and reduce nonresponse. As shown in the meta-analyses by Church (Church, 1993) and Singer (Singer, 2002), incentives do increase response rates on all kinds of surveys, although the percentage increase varies by questionnaire mode, the study population, and the difficulty of the study requirements. Increasingly, investigators conduct pretests to determine whether incentives offer promise. This pilot work can also help determine whether the incentive should be monetary or nonmonetary, what the value of the incentive should be, and whether the incentive is best paired

TABLE 24–1

Selected Studies Using Incentives

Name of Study (Reference)	Year	Type of Study	Value of Incentive	Comments
National Health and Nutrition Examination Survey[a]	1999	Cross-sectional, including a 3- to 4-h physical examination	Varied, $30–$100 depending on age and acceptance of appointment time	Effective in maintaining high response rates. In addition, expenses for transportation, interpreter, child care arrangements covered as necessary.
Observing Protein and Energy Nutrition (OPEN) Study (Subar et al., 2003)	1999	Methodologic dietary study requiring ingestion of doubly labeled water, 3 clinic visits, and a total commitment of 10 h	$200	Effective in maintaining high response rate after first visit. Remuneration reflected burden.
U.S. Radiologic Technologists Study (Doody et al., 2003)	1998	Cohort	$2/$5	$2 was most effective incentive.
Women's Health Questionnaire (Whiteman et al., 2003)	2000	Cross-sectional	$1/lottery ticket	Cash incentive worked best.
Park Nicollet Clinic Health Maintenance System Minnesota (Shaw et al., 2001)	2001	Community survey	$2/$5	$5 incentive resulted in higher response rate, but $2 incentive increased participation too.
Binational Cohort to Study *Helicobacter pylori* infection in children (Goodman et al., 2003)	2003	Cohort	Package of disposable diapers, baby books, educational toys	Study in U.S. and Mexico. Incentives represent effort to maximize compliance.

[a] Unpublished data, National Center for Health Statistics.

with an advance letter or a refusal-conversion letter. In some cultures, cash incentives work best and should be paid in advance. The value of the incentive should be determined by the level of respondent burden but should not be coercive. The literature shows enormous variation in the resulting response-rate increases. In all settings, participation is generally lower for blood collection than for interviewing. Studies in Europe and North America commonly use incentives of modest value to increase participation in the interview components (amounting to 1% or 2% of the overall cost of conducting an interview). These studies generally use either additional or slightly larger incentives for participation in blood collection. Ongoing studies in China, Ukraine, Japan, and Byelorussia offer small gifts, free physical examinations, and remuneration for transportation costs (Gail et al., 1998; Mobius Research, 2003). Table 24–1 presents examples of studies that have tested the effect of different types of monetary and nonmonetary incentives.

In addition to a clear and persuasive introduction of the study by a respected sponsor and the use of incentives, several other field procedures can help to minimize nonresponse. For example, initial response can be increased through callbacks, extended data collection periods, and face-to-face contacts. For subjects who refuse on the initial contact, the use of short questionnaires that capture the most critical data, the selection of proxy respondents, and changes in data collection mode or interviewer assignment can help salvage responses that would otherwise be lost. Of course, mail, telephone, Internet, and in-person surveys require different approaches. Similarly, cohort studies, case-control studies, clinical trials, and community-based studies demand different approaches to subject recruitment and nonresponse.

Pretesting is essential for gauging the likely level of nonresponse, but the pretest levels often overestimate the eventual response rate of the full-scale study. The effects of response-enhancement strategies vary greatly; in our experience in the United States, choice of primary data collection mode (e.g., telephone versus in-person interviewing) and length of instrument often change response rates by 10% to 30%. Incentives have enormously variable effects, from a trivial to a major increase in response. Callbacks and other field procedures designed to reduce first, or "soft," refusals can increase rates by 5% to 20%; effective refusal conversion, especially when initial refusals are high, can have the same large effect. Combining all of these changes raises response, but seldom by the sum of the maximum effect of each. In one common scenario, the early pretest shows a response rate of 40% to 60%, but the full-scale study response rates may be 10% lower, on average. Percentage-point gains may be achieved with a substantial change in data collection mode or instrument length (10 to 15 points), an added financial incentive (5 points or more), additional personnel and procedures to avoid initial refusal (5 points), and enhanced refusal conversion (5 points). Using the lower end of the percentage-point ranges in this hypothetical scenario, the eventual response rate would threaten the validity of the estimates. The potential selection biases are hard to overcome, because the many ways that respondents differ from nonrespondents cannot be known. In addition, effective study size declines with nonresponse (Groves et al., 2004; Dunn et al., 2004).

DATA COLLECTION AND DATA CAPTURE

ABSTRACTING RECORDS

Abstracts are used to distill information needed for the study from written records kept for other purposes, such as medical charts or employment records. The "abstract" itself may be a hardcopy form, a voice recording, an electronic Website entry using a laptop computer, or some other format. Personal digital assistants (PDAs) or notebook computers are increasingly used to simplify record abstraction, increase flexibility, and automate some quality control checks. The choice of such devices for a particular study depends on the budget and technology available, the complexity of the abstract instrument, and the skills and experience of the abstractors. Abstract design includes several key issues, regardless of the format of the abstract. To begin, all abstracts should provide spaces to record the subject's identification, the dates the abstract began and ended, and the abstractor's identification. When abstracts are collected on hardcopy, each page should record the subject's identification in case pages become separated.

The larger and more variable the original record, the harder the abstract is to design. The designer tries to make the layout clear, the wording consistent, and the path through the abstract evident. For hardcopy abstracts, the designer uses shading, indentation, arrows, and other formatting, especially for items that depend on an answer to another item. Typically, abstracts use closed-ended questions, which have a prerecorded set of responses from which to select (e.g., subject's sex). Open-ended questions may be used to capture uncommon or more detailed responses (e.g., subject's health insurance provider). The form may require the abstractor to distinguish between negative findings and absent findings for important items. For instance, some items can be grouped into one list, with an instruction to indicate all that apply; however, if it is important to know that the abstractor looked for and did not find mention of a particular clinical finding, the question ought to be formatted so that an answer must always be indicated (yes/no/not found).

Medical-record abstracts can be hard to design because medical charts are complex and idiosyncratic. Medical-record abstractors should receive training in the medical terminology pertinent to the study, but they cannot be expected to glean everything from the charts that a physician specialist would. The abstract form ought to be designed to reduce the need for interpretation, even at the expense of collecting items that may be redundant. Similarly, abstractors should be asked to complete items as similar as possible to the nature of the data found in the original record. For example, abstractors should record date of birth from medical records and should not be asked to calculate calendar age from the date of birth reported in the record.

Even if expert medical personnel will abstract the records, record-keeping practices vary among hospitals and clinics, so the investigator may need to review typical and atypical charts in the study sites before designing the abstract form. The designer may also need to interview some recording physicians or other health personnel to understand recording practices. When the analysis will exclude events before or after particular dates, the form may be designed to capture the relevant period only or the entire history, with exclusions made in the analysis.

Devising good abstract forms may be hard, but testing them is usually easy. The investigator abstracts several records, and then one or more of the abstractors independently abstracts the same records. This exercise can reveal gross errors or oversight in form design. A similar process can be used to measure interabstractor reproducibility during form development.

QUESTIONNAIRE ADMINISTRATION METHOD

Questionnaires remain the mainstay of epidemiologic investigations, but administration options have expanded greatly. As Groves et al. have noted, "with the proliferation of new data collection methods in recent years, largely associated with the introduction of computers to the survey process, survey mode now encompasses a much wider variety of methods and approaches, including combinations of different approaches or mix mode designs" (Groves et al., 2004). In addition to in-person, telephone, and self-administered surveys, modes of administration include computer-assisted personal interviewing (CAPI), computer-assisted telephone interviewing (CATI), audio computer-assisted self-interviewing (ACASI), interactive voice response (IVR), and Internet surveys.

The overarching consideration in deciding on the methods of questionnaire administration should be comparability between study groups, subject to the reservations regarding comparability of information quality raised in Chapter 7. Case-control studies comparing hospitalized cases and controls lend themselves to in-person interviews in the hospital. On the other hand, if cases are selected from hospitals and controls are selected from among neighbors or the general population (to approximate the referral network), interviews would be most comparable if they were conducted with all subjects at home. If biospecimens must be collected and an interview conducted, the protocol might specify one home visit to obtain both, home visits by two different field staff (e.g., an interviewer and a phlebotomist), a telephone interview and a home visit, and a home or telephone interview and the provision of respondent instructions and a mailer for collecting and shipping the specimen. If several modes of data collection are possible, the investigator may need to conduct a pilot study comparing them.

If a self-administered questionnaire is used, it may be mailed to the subject, sent by e-mail, provided at an Internet site, or delivered in person. Self-administered instruments generally cost less than interviewer-administered instruments, but they are also the least easily monitored and the most susceptible to misunderstood questions and skipped answers. One compromise is to rely on the self-administered forms for most respondents and, for the few cases that are incomplete, have study staff telephone the respondent for clarification. This approach keeps labor costs lower than they would have been with total interviewer administration.

Self-administered questionnaires offer advantages other than cost. They may yield more accurate data on sensitive or embarrassing topics because they are more anonymous. Because printed visual aids can be incorporated, some topics (e.g., self-perceived body morphology) are measured more easily in self-administered questionnaires than in telephone interviews. Self-administered questionnaires generally require a printed paper format. Optical scanning works with multiple-choice answers or free text. For smaller studies, however, the cost of developing the scanned forms may exceed the savings in coding and keying.

If the questions and answers are likely to need clarification, the questionnaire should be used as the basis for an interview, with a trained interviewer asking the questions and recording the responses. The choice between telephone and in-person surveys will be influenced by the subject's age, education, health, vision, and hearing; the budget; and the number and types of questions to be asked. Some epidemiology questionnaires are still printed as hardcopy booklets, but nowadays most are automated and administered using a computer-assisted interviewing program (CAPI,

CATI, ACASI, or IVR). Theoretically, computerization reduces the time between data collection and access to the data for analysis. For instruments with complex logical branching, computerization can reduce interviewer error (Fig. 24–1). The costs of developing and deploying such instruments continue to fall.

In-person interviews generally entail more labor costs than telephone interviews, because of the unavoidable need to schedule appointments and travel between one interview and the next. Nevertheless, the greater intimacy of in-person interviews may increase the subject's willingness to participate in the study. In-person interviewing typically increases the length of individual responses and of the total interview, but whether this increases accuracy is unknown (Groves et al., 1989).

In-person interviews can incorporate pictures, three-dimensional models, and other memory aids. If the questionnaire requires the respondent to recall distant events, such memory aids may be critical. For instance, photographs of medications help the respondent recognize individual formulations. Food models can be used to describe portion sizes in dietary interviews. Maps are used in questions pertaining to residence or travel. Diaries, timelines, or calendar grids can improve completeness and dating of lifetime residential, occupational, or reproductive histories. If there are no published evaluations of the contemplated memory aids in a similar setting, a small pilot test of such aids may help determine whether they are effective and feasible.

Telephone interviews typically elicit slightly shorter answers than in-person interviews (Groves et al., 1989). Also, respondents tend to favor the first answer when a list of possible answers is read to them on the telephone, but other differences between telephone and in-person interviews are modest (Groves et al., 2004). Supervisors can monitor interviewing more easily in telephone interviews than in-person interviews because they can listen to the conversation. Some sensitive topics can be difficult to query by telephone, because the respondent may become suspicious of the interviewer or the legitimacy of the study. On the other hand, once the respondent trusts the study and the interviewer, questions about socially undesirable behaviors may be answered more readily over the telephone than in person because of the greater social distance in a telephone call (Bradburn et al., 2004).

CONTENT AND WORDING OF QUESTIONS

Questionnaire designers grapple with the issues of cooperation, fatigue, meaning, memory, and honesty. Errors can be introduced by either the respondent or the interviewer, and the questionnaire should be designed to reduce both types of error. The design of epidemiologic questionnaires benefits from a vast body of survey research experience and literature (Groves et al., 2004; Bradburn et al., 2004; Biemer et al., 1991; Tanur, 1992). In addition, hundreds of questionnaires are available online or are easily obtained electronically. Parts of questionnaires, or modules, are readily available for topics that occur most frequently on epidemiologic questionnaires, including basic demographic data, common health problems, and major health-related behaviors, such as smoking, diet, and exercise (see, e.g., the Internet site of the National Cancer Institute's Division of Cancer Epidemiology at http://dceg2.cancer.gov/QMOD or the NHANES Internet site at www.cdc.gov/nchs/nhanes.htm).

After choosing the method of administration, the investigator focuses on framing the questions. This topic has appropriately received a large amount of attention in survey research literature (Bradburn et al., 2004; Clark and Schober, 1992). Wording matters in all surveys because people construe important and simple words such as *anyone, most, average, never,* or *fairly* in varied ways (Groves et al., 1989). Medical terms with precise meanings should be explained simply; therefore, "people related to you by blood" might be preferable to "family" and "Has a doctor ever told you that you had. . . ?" might be preferable to "Have you had. . . ?" On the other hand, vernacular expressions are not always preferred (e.g., "medications" ought to be used instead of "drugs" to avoid confusion with illicit drugs).

Question length also affects response. Short questions usually are clearer, but a longer question may improve respondent cognition. For instance, it is hard to absorb all the details of the question, "How many hours per week do you typically use this product in the summertime on weekdays?" The question may be more intelligible if it can be separated into specific questions to reduce the density of concepts (Tanur, 1992) or preceded with a description of some of the concepts (e.g., "I'd like you to think about the summertime. I will be asking you about weekdays separately from weekends.").

MCQ.160 Has a doctor or other health professional ever told {you/SP} that {you/s/he} . . . CAPI INSTRUCTION: TEXT OF QUESTION SHOULD BE OPTIONAL AFTER FIRST ITEM IS READ.	MCQ.170 {Do you/Does SP} still . . . ?	MCQ.180 How old {were you/was SP} when {you were/s/he was} first told {you/s/he} . . .	MCQ.190 Which type of arthritis was it?
a. **had arthritis?** YES .... 1 NO .... 2 (b) REFUSED ..... 7 (b) DON'T KNOW .. 9 (b)		had arthritis? |__|__|__| ENTER AGE IN YEARS REFUSED .... 777 DON'T KNOW 999	RHEUMATOID ARTHRITIS .... 1 OSTEOARTHRITIS .... 2 OTHER .... 3 REFUSED .... 7 DON'T KNOW 9
b. **had congestive heart failure?** YES .... 1 NO .... 2 (c) REFUSED ..... 7 (c) DON'T KNOW .. 9 (c)		had congestive heart failure? |__|__|__| ENTER AGE IN YEARS REFUSED .... 777 DON'T KNOW 999	
c. **had coronary heart disease?** YES .... 1 NO .... 2 (d) REFUSED ..... 7 (d) DON'T KNOW .. 9 (d)		had coronary heart disease? |__|__|__| ENTER AGE IN YEARS REFUSED .... 777 DON'T KNOW 999	
d. **had angina, also called angina pectoris?** YES .... 1 NO .... 2 (e) REFUSED ..... 7 (e) DON'T KNOW .. 9 (e)		had angina, also called agina pectoris? |__|__|__| ENTER AGE IN YEARS REFUSED .... 777 DON'T KNOW 999	
e. **had a heart attack (also called myocardial infarction)?** YES .... 1 NO .... 2 (f) REFUSED ..... 7 (f) DON'T KNOW .. 9 (f)		had a heart attack (also called myocardial infarction)? |__|__|__| ENTER AGE IN YEARS REFUSED .... 777 DON'T KNOW 999	

Available at { HYPERLINK "http://www.cdc.gov/nchs/data/nhanes/spq-mc1.pdf" }

FIGURE 24–1 ● Example of question branching in a computer-assisted interview. (From the National Health and Nutrition Examination Survey.)

How many questions does the investigator need to ask on a topic? One or two questions may not gather enough information for a thorough analysis, particularly if an unexpected association emerges. On the other hand, a long series of questions on a single topic bores the respondent and results in missing or inaccurate answers after the first few questions. Assessments of usual diet, lifetime occupational history, and lifetime residential history each take 10 to 20 minutes and are particularly prone to this problem.

The order of questions can also affect response. Many questionnaires begin with questions that are not threatening and not taxing to the memory and, if possible, are interesting to the respondent (Bradburn et al., 2004). Questions about sensitive topics usually follow questions about related but less sensitive topics. Some instruments precede such questions with a prologue that acknowledges the personal nature of the question, reiterates the subject's right not to answer, and states the importance of the question to the survey. The format of answers matters, too. For open-ended numerical responses (e.g., how many years), respondents often show digit preference (for 0 and 5). For closed-ended items with an ordered list (e.g., <5, 5 to 10, 11 to 19, ≥20), some respondents may favor a part of the range, often the central part.

Memory presents the most serious problem in epidemiologic questionnaires. First, many exposures under study did not seem interesting or important to the subject at the time they happened, let alone decades later Croyle and Loftus, 1992; Loftus et al., 1992. Second, many of the cognitive interviewing techniques (Fisher and Quigley, 1992) that can improve recollection dramatically (e.g., context reinstatement, focused retrieval, multiple representation) do not suit epidemiologic research. Standardization of instruments and techniques does not allow interviewers to pursue a topic as they would in an ordinary conversation or an investigative interview, but standardization does keep data collection comparable between cases and controls or exposed and unexposed subjects. Nonetheless, some recall-improving devices are applicable to epidemiology, such as using benchmarks in the subject's life to stimulate recall of a time period.

Standardization must be compromised at times to avoid losing data completely. For instance, a few telephone interviews may be conducted in an in-person interview study for subjects who would not participate otherwise. If a different data collection mode, source (e.g., a surrogate respondent), or setting is used, this fact must be recorded. Despite efforts to maintain comparability with standard instruments and training, differences in the quality of the data collection may arise. To detect such differences, the investigator may compare the rates and reasons for nonresponse, the length of the interview, the quality of understanding and response as assessed by the interviewer (poor, adequate, excellent), and the responses to questions that are expected not to differ between the groups (exposures or outcomes). For example, a substantially longer interview in one group raises the possibility of differential accuracy or completeness of information.

QUESTIONNAIRES AND RESPONDENT BURDEN

How much information can the questionnaire elicit? In-person interviews commonly last 50 to 90 minutes, telephone interviews typically last 30 to 60 minutes, and self-administered questionnaires typically take 10 to 20 minutes to complete. In our experience, interviewers and respondents report these times to be acceptable, and common sense suggests that much longer times are not feasible. The length of the interview does little to change the subject's willingness to agree to the interview. Usually, the subject continues with the interview to the end. On the other hand, longer interviews may increase the risk of breakoffs (Groves et al., 1989). Many epidemiologists find it hard to resist including as many questions as possible, even if the quality of the answers decreases as the interview lengthens. Some investigators place the least critical questions near the end in case of breakoff, but the effects of this practice are not known.

Some multipurpose studies (e.g., a complex case-control study with one control group and multiple case groups) use a modular questionnaire. A few core questions are asked of everyone, and many other questions are asked only of a subset of the subjects. This approach can keep the interview to a reasonable length but imposes logistical and training costs.

Special considerations arise with longitudinal studies that require repeated interviews. Timing questionnaire arrival on a strict annual schedule tied to the subject's birthday or the beginning of each calendar year may improve the likelihood that subjects report only events that occurred since the last contact. Otherwise, it is best to avoid questions that refer to "Since we asked you last. . ." because of the risk of events being forgotten or repeated.

INTERVIEWING TECHNIQUES AND TRAINING

Interviewers are trained to apply standard interviewing techniques to the particular questionnaire. In studies with components in addition to the interview, formal training sessions typically last 4 to 5 days and are followed by several weeks of practice. For a new interviewer, the interview supervisor checks many of the initial interviews, for instance, by attending the interview or reviewing an audio or video recording of it. After the interviewer has mastered the techniques, a fraction of his or her interviews may be audited at random throughout the study.

The interviewer's first job is to persuade the subject to participate. The introduction needs to convey the scientific importance of the study and of the subject's participation without making subjects with particular histories more or less likely to respond. If the subject refuses at first, the interviewer ought to make another effort to persuade the subject or learn the reason for the refusal. The interviewer may ask the subject to talk to the supervisor or someone else before the subject gives a firm refusal. Interviewers document nonresponses with notes that help the supervisor or another interviewer approach the subject.

After obtaining cooperation, the interviewer proceeds with the interview or arranges an appointment. Before an in-person interview, the interviewer arranges any equipment, memory aids, or materials. The interviewer tries to arrange the setting and timing to minimize interruptions and distractions to the respondent. Occasionally, interviews must be stopped and resumed later. The interviewer must note these and other deviations in the administration of the questionnaire, as well as an assessment of the quality of the responses.

Questions that the respondent does not understand are repeated slowly verbatim, not rephrased. If further clarification is needed, the interviewer follows the instructions given during training and in the study manuals. If the subject's answers are not clear or complete, the interviewer uses neutral probes, which are also covered in training and the manuals. Interviewers should be provided with scripted clarifications, such as definitions of medical terms. When respondents require clarifications that are not scripted, interviewers should offer to reread the question and ask participants to answer according to their best understanding. Nonscripted clarifications and interviewer prompts will almost certainly be directional and may therefore bias interview results. To conclude the interview, the interviewer quickly scans the questionnaire for omissions, thanks the respondent, and explains that the supervisor may call the respondent to review the interviewer's work. In some studies, the investigator offers the subjects the opportunity to be notified of the findings.

For paper-based studies, the study supervisor reviews completed questionnaires, querying the interviewer about any unclear entries. In many studies, the supervisor checks a small list of critical items to be sure they were not missed by the interviewer or the respondent. If any of these is missing, the supervisor or the interviewer attempts to retrieve the data by calling the respondent. In addition, many studies include a brief reinterview of a random subset of all respondents. The reinterview includes some of the questions in the questionnaire and elicits the respondent's impression of how long the interview took and his or her opinion of the interview.

PHYSICAL EXAMINATIONS

Epidemiologic studies can include physical examinations to measure blood pressure, count nevi, assess body fat distribution, and so on. The order and content of these examinations is much more explicitly prescribed than in a strictly clinical setting. Subjects with no abnormal findings whatsoever (including most controls in case-control studies) may be fully examined and described to ensure comparability in the epidemiologic study. If any of the findings is abnormal, the subject must be referred for clinical evaluation.

Examination forms often have complex logical branching, and the examiner has to be able to follow the flow and complete the form during the examination. Examination forms must usually be subjected to extensive pretesting to make sure they are easy to use during the examination. Variation among clinical observers remains a concern even with standardized instruments, so training and quality control are especially important. For example, training in blood-pressure measurement often uses a videotape test as an objective standard. Studies of interobserver variation may be necessary when the physical examinations are subtle or complex.

Physical examinations in epidemiologic studies may be conducted by medical or paramedical personnel, with oversight by a physician or other expert reviewer. If the expert reviewer does not see each subject, the examiner ought to record whether expert review occurred and distinguish the expert's evaluation from the original one.

BIOSPECIMEN COLLECTION

Epidemiologic studies increasingly involve laboratory components requiring collection of urine, blood, or tissue from subjects. A typical example of requirements for blood collection is shown in Figure 24–2. The biggest problems that arise often reflect unrecognized laboratory error. Indeed, epidemiologists usually need to investigate the reproducibility of the assay in a pilot study. Field problems may also arise in applying tests or assays to large-scale epidemiologic studies that previously have been conducted only on a small scale. For instance, laboratories that have developed an assay and can achieve high reproducibility with dozens of specimens may be unable to process the thousands of specimens required in a field study. Another typical problem arises when the investigator wishes to collect specimens for storage without a definite assay in mind, so the particular collection and storage requirements are not certain.

The protocol for collecting, processing, labeling, storing, and shipping the specimens ought to be documented in the manual of operations. The biospecimen collection forms record the subject, the specimen number, whether the specimen was collected at baseline or a subsequent encounter, results of the collection (e.g., number of tubes drawn, medical complications), and processing and storage details (e.g., in which freezer the specimen is stored). Bar-coded labels reduce handwriting or keying errors, and clear, detailed shipping and storage lists minimize losses in transit and aid in tracking those that occur.

ENVIRONMENTAL SAMPLES AND GLOBAL POSITIONING SYSTEMS

Epidemiologic studies sometimes include taking direct measurements of the subject's home or work environment, including chemicals in drinking water, air, soil, or carpet dust and levels of ionizing radiation, sunlight, or electromagnetic fields. These study components may dramatically improve the accuracy of exposure assessment, if the investigator can overcome the typical hurdles. Such issues include identifying a logistically feasible measurement technique, collecting and analyzing samples at an acceptable cost, obtaining the subject's permission and access to the environment for sampling, and (generally) limiting measurement to the current rather than a past environment.

Feasibility and cost are common challenges, even when toxicologists, industrial hygienists, radiation physicists, or other experts in the environmental exposure have developed reliable measurement techniques. Established exposure indicators are not necessarily suited to the size and settings of epidemiologic research. For example, a high-volume surface-sampler vacuum cleaner can extract carpet dust from which pesticide residues can be measured, but at a cost prohibitive to most studies. A convenient sample of the subject's own used vacuum cleaner bag provides an acceptable alternative (Colt et al., 1998). Finding feasible and inexpensive methods that produce valid and reliable environmental measures often requires pilot studies before the field protocol can be finalized. Because field conditions cannot always be tightly controlled in population studies, the sampling technician should record the conditions under which the monitoring occurred.

The timing of the relevant exposure often complicates the interpretation of environmental samples in epidemiologic studies, which typically measure current environments. The levels of exposure at a particular place may have changed over time. The subject may have moved or changed jobs. Occasionally, multiple old sites can be monitored. Sometimes, a cumulative environmental measure can be obtained, such as radiation decay products that leave behind traces on glass mirrors or picture frames. More commonly, the investigator has interview or other data on the lifetime or other long span of exposure and links those to the current environmental measures to form various measures of exposure status.

As awareness of environmental hazards has increased, investigators have encountered both a greater willingness to permit environmental sampling and heightened interest in the levels found

Venipuncture

Public Health Objectives:

Venipuncture is performed to obtain laboratory results that provide prevalence estimates of disease, risk factors for exam components, and baseline information on health and nutritional status of the population.

Staff:

Certified Phlebotomist

Protocol:

Methods:

Blood is drawn from the examinee's arm. In the laboratory the blood is processed, stored and shipped to various laboratories for analysis. The complete blood count (CBC) results are reported in the MEC and all other results are reported from NCHS to the participant. The volume of blood drawn by age follows.

- 1–2 years, 9 ml (0.3 ounces), 0.6 tablespoons
- 3–5 years, 22 ml (0.7 ounces), 1.5 tablespoons
- 6–11 years, 38 ml (1.2 ounces), 2.5 tablespoons
- 12 + 89–92 ml (3.0 ounces), 6.0 tablespoons

Time Allotment:

Depending on age of participant. Range 5–10 minutes

Health Measures:

Laboratory test results.

Eligibility:

Sample persons aged 1 year and older who do not meet any of the exclusion criteria

Exclusion Criteria:

- Hemophiliacs
- Participants who received chemotherapy within last 4 weeks
- The presence of the following on both arms: rashes, gauze dressings, casts, edema, paralysis, tubes, open sores or wounds, withered arms or limbs missing, damaged, sclerosed or occluded veins, allergies to cleansing reagents, burned or scarred tissue, shunt or IV.

Justification for using vulnerable populations:

- Minors are included in this component because they are an important target population group. Laboratory data are linked to other household interview and health component data and are used to track changes that occur in health over time.
- There is no reason to exclude mentally impaired or handicapped individuals because there is no contraindication.

Risks:

The following are known risks associated with venipuncture:

- Hematoma
- Swelling, tenderness and inflammation at the site
- Persistent bleeding
- Vasovagal response—dizziness, sweating, coldness of skin, numbness and tingling of hands and feet, nausea, vomiting, possible visual disturbance, syncope and injury fall from fainting.
- Rare adverse effects:
  Thrombosis of the vein due to trauma
  Infection which results in thrombophlebitis

Special precautions:

- Sterile equipment issued with all sample persons.
- Physician on call in case an adverse affect occurs.

Report of Findings:

Reported in the MEC:

Complete Blood Count (CBC)

Reported from NCHS:

Other laboratory results

Available at: www.cdc.gov/nchs/data/nhanes/blood.pdf

FIGURE 24–2 • Sample protocol for blood collection. (From the National Health and Nutrition Examination Survey.)

and their meaning. Epidemiologic investigations routinely notify subjects with levels above any existing standards. Most also report levels of any compound to a subject who requests the data, accompanied by a clear statement of any known risks and the level of uncertainty.

Increasingly, epidemiologic studies include the use of inexpensive global positioning systems (GPS) devices to record the latitude and longitude of the subject's home or workplace. The position can be linked to geographic information systems (GIS). Using GIS, the investigator can spatially display environmental and epidemiologic data. Applications for GIS in epidemiologic research include locating subjects' addresses through geocoding, mapping the source contaminants, and integrating environmental data with disease outcome. Sometimes it is possible to reconstruct historical exposures. With the availability of an increasing number of environmental databases, GIS and GPS technology allow the investigator to link environmental monitoring data with the study population, providing a better understanding of the environmental contaminants and disease outcomes (Nuckols et al., 2004).

TRACING

Some studies do not require contact with the subject but only a determination of vital status or date and cause of death. In the United States, relevant resources include the National Death Index (NDI), NDI Plus, Social Security Administration files, state mortality data tapes, Pension Benefit Information Services, driver's license and car registration records, and Internet mortality tracing. NDI provides the state where the death was recorded, the date of death, and the death certificate number. NDI Plus provides cause of death in addition to the other information. Cost, coverage, and quality vary among these sources (Doody et al., 2001).

In some Western countries, complete population, birth, and death registries greatly simplify tracing. In some resource-poor settings (e.g., rural China), local governments have established a vital registration system to track people for births, deaths, marriage, and migration. Specific study follow-up tracking systems have also been established to trace participants in the Nutrition Intervention Trial and the Shandong Intervention Trial. In these instances, the field station staff worked closely with the local governments to ensure that all endpoints were reported and documented in a timely manner (Li et al., 1986).

If subjects are to be questioned about outcomes or exposures (active follow-up), they must first be located. With recent, accurate, detailed information on the subject's name, address, telephone number, Social Security or other identification number, parents' names (for a child), and spouse's name and employer, the investigator may begin by mailing information to the last address or by telephoning the subject. Without such detailed information, the investigator uses methods described below to locate the subject. If many subjects have died, a vital-status search may be the first step.

The more out of date the last known address is, the more difficult the tracing will be. On the other hand, in many countries, tracing is easier if many cohort members have died. The algorithm for tracing depends on the composition of the cohort. In occupational cohort studies, the investigator often knows the subject's Social Security or other national identification number, which helps in matching to mortality registries and other files. With medical cohorts (Griem et al., 1994; Inskip et al., 1990, identifying data are often sparser and less accurate, so many sources may be needed to find a large proportion of the cohort. Additional problems arise in following cohorts of women (e.g., because of changes in surname) (Boice, 1978) or cohorts exposed before or at birth (Nash et al., 1983).

FOLLOW-UP TECHNIQUES

For studies requiring active follow-up, subject tracing and collection of outcome data are usually conducted in tandem. Procedures for mailing the questionnaires or interviewing by telephone or in person are similar to those in case-control studies. One typical procedure is to mail the follow-up questionnaire once, wait a few weeks for its return, mail a second questionnaire to nonrespondents, and then telephone the remaining nonrespondents. The second mailing and the telephone call both increase response markedly in most studies.

Longitudinal studies require repeated follow-ups and present special problems. In some circumstances, nonrespondents in one wave can be approached in subsequent waves. These subsequent waves are likely to achieve a greater response than the initial contact, because subjects who are not inclined to participate usually refuse the first time. On the other hand, if the cohort has been followed several times, motivation to answer more questions may flag. Subjects' willingness to participate can be enhanced with study newsletters sent before, and after, each round of follow-up, describing findings and progress of the study. Increasingly, investigators develop Internet sites to disseminate study findings, in the hope of encouraging subject participation in the next wave of follow-up. In some studies, subjects who refuse are not contacted in subsequent waves. Even with excellent response rates in each wave, the multiple opportunities for nonresponse lower the cumulative response rate.

Often, investigators design a study that requires using data from other sources to confirm outcomes reported by subjects or their next of kin on follow-up questionnaires. For instance, once the fact of death is known, the cause of death can be collected from the death certificate. Serious illnesses can also be confirmed and detailed by obtaining additional records. For cancers among residents of an area covered by a tumor registry, the registry can often confirm a cancer reported by the subject or next of kin (Wasserman et al., 1992). For other conditions requiring hospitalization, records can be requested from the hospital with permission from the patient. Timing is critical because some hospitals do not honor permission forms that were signed beyond a certain period of time.

DATA CAPTURE

Data capture means transforming the research data collected in the field into clean tables for data analysis. In outline, the steps are receipt of data by the study center (hardcopy forms or electronic files), followed by coding (if applicable), data entry (if applicable), and computer editing. Whether coding, data entry, and computer editing occur during the post–data collection phase depends on the type of data collection and whether these functions have occurred within the data collection phase itself. With the evolution of survey technology such as CATI, CAPI, IVR, ACASI, Internet-based, and scanning techniques, the degree of data capture or data preparation required for studies is changing. New technology has affected the operation and data collection activities of both the household in-person interview and the physical-examination phase of the survey. Data collection, data editing, data cleaning, and data release can now occur nearly simultaneously (Berman et al., 2002). With the decreasing expense of development, similar approaches are expected to be used in the smaller epidemiologic studies of the future.

Coding, or data reduction, occurs in virtually all studies. Regardless of whether the questionnaires, abstracts, and other data collection instruments are hardcopy or computer-assisted applications, they will include items that require the assignment of codes either during or after data collection. Whenever possible, coding should be restricted to judgmental tasks. For example, age at interview can be coded, but can also be calculated analytically from the recorded date of birth and recorded date of interview. Allowing age to be calculated analytically, rather than by coding, will reduce errors in the data set. When coding is necessary, the codes may be based on coding schemes in general use (e.g., International Classification of Diseases, Standard Industrial Classification codes) or schemes devised for the study. Standard practices for coding data are described in detail in other texts (Groves et al., 2004). Selection of coding schemes depends on the utility of the scheme in analysis and the ease of use in coding. The coding manual documents the schemes used to encode the data. If the data were collected using computer-assisted instruments, a mixed-mode approach for data capture may be warranted during the post–data collection phase, with "other specify" responses coded and the comments reviewed and coded as appropriate. A coding decision log documents decisions not covered by the general rules. For many types of information, computer-assisted coding systems are available (Speizer and Buckley, 1998). Available occupational, medical, and dietary coding systems provide the investigator with different coding options. It is up to the investigator to decide if these automated systems are a cost-effective approach to this data preparation activity. The literature details some decision criteria that may help the investigator decide whether to use automated coding in particular situations (Gillman, 2002). Nonautomated coding should be performed by a person blinded to the exposure (if coding disease) or disease (if coding exposure) status of subjects.

After the survey instruments have been coded, coded hardcopy forms are keyed. In some studies, all forms are keyed twice, with the second data entry clerk blind to the already-keyed data. This practice ensures against data-entry errors but costs more than single data entry. For identifiers and other critical items, double entry usually warrants the extra expense. Computer-assisted and optically scanned forms do not need coding but require care in handling. Keyed, computer-assisted, and scanned data are "cleaned" by checking the answers to be sure they fall within a range of plausible answers (which are overridden after an out-of-range answer has been verified) and that they are mutually consistent ("logic checks"). Inconsistent answers given by the respondent may be flagged but not changed. Errors in recording, coding, and keying are corrected.

Finally, the numbers of respondents and nonrespondents (overall and within specific groups) tracked by the management system during the field phase are compared and reconciled to the numbers in the data file to be used for analysis. The response counts and rates, manuals used during the field phase, study logs, and data collection instruments serve as essential reference documents throughout analysis and presentation of findings.

EMERGING ISSUES

Epidemiologists will encounter three challenges in the near term: pooling and comparison of data across sources, the growing concern for privacy and great uncertainty about how to protect it, and the need to work in an environment that is increasingly characterized by multidisciplinary teams. Other challenges doubtless will arise, but these three seem likely to affect the field methods applied in modern epidemiologic research.

Data pooling, meta-analysis, multicenter studies, and research consortia all require common data elements, and epidemiologists have typically championed efforts to standardize data collection. In recent years, government agencies and private organizations have pushed for greater standardization of data collection and storage, prompted by the increasing volume of health data captured in a variety of surveys or as part of routine health care or health insurance and by advances in computing and informatics. Epidemiologists already routinely use standard schemes for representing variables such as sex, race, dates, residence, occupation, disease, and cause of death. Further standardization of these variables and development of standards for many others can be expected.

When data standards can be used in specific epidemiologic studies, they offer advantages of efficiency, for instance, in software for variable manipulation. They also allow for instructive comparison to other data sets. How does the distribution of disease, or social class, or ethnicity within a study compare to the regional patterns? How do two study populations compare with each other? On the other hand, data standards can impede research progress if the investigator uses categories that may be appropriate for many uses but not for the hypothesis at hand.

For many studies based on interviews, recruitment has become so difficult that response rates seriously threaten the interpretation of results. Although privacy and confidentiality concerns seem certain to grow, it is hard to predict how legal developments and cultural shifts will influence the epidemiologic research climate. The problems will grow if access to records becomes further encumbered, or if public inclination to participate in research declines further. At the same time, unprecedented research opportunities may arise from the possible linking of health and other databases, provided that the governing agents can be assured that privacy and confidentially will be protected.

Research into genetic susceptibility poses some novel privacy and confidentiality challenges, inasmuch as the combination of data from a handful of genes can, in principle, identify a subject. Epidemiologists have typically shown appropriate restraint, but new public concerns in this area may emerge. Standards for protecting genetic data are being developed in many countries and ought to help assure both personal protection and population research.

Compared with their peers who used the first and second editions of this text, epidemiologic investigators are now more likely to work on teams that encompass other disciplines. The team approach often accompanies an expanded study scope or size. In addition, there may be more than one epidemiologist responsible for overall study design, conduct, and analysis. Indeed, many immensely informative epidemiologic studies, especially cohort studies, have passed to their second generation of investigators, with key design decisions having been made decades ago.

If the epidemiologists are pulled in many directions, the field effort may be the phase most likely to be given short shrift. Fortunately, more survey researchers, clinical collaborators, and laboratory scientists have some specialized training and experience in health studies in general and in epidemiology in particular. Researchers in these disciplines typically have a strong interest in some or all of the field methods of a study. The epidemiologists need to work closely with the rest of the team, and they need to maintain responsibility for the conduct of the study. The "field methods"—as outlined in the study protocol, detailed in the manuals of operations and procedures, and buttressed by quality control activities—still form the central bridge between sound design and credible analysis.

CHAPTER 25

Ecologic Studies

Hal Morgenstern

Concepts and Rationale 511
Levels of Measurement 512
Levels of Analysis 512
Levels of Inference 513
Rationale for Ecologic Studies 513
Study Designs 514
Multiple-Group Designs 514
Time-Trend Designs 515
Mixed Designs 517
Effect Estimation 517
Confounders and Effect Modifiers 518
Methodologic Problems 519
Ecologic Bias 519
Problems of Confounder Control 522
Within-Group Misclassification 526
Other Problems 527
Interpreting Ecologic Associations 528
Multilevel Analyses and Designs 528
Conclusion 530

An ecologic or aggregate study focuses on the comparison of groups rather than individuals. The underlying reason for this focus is that individual-level data are missing on the joint distribution of at least two and perhaps all variables within each group; in this sense, an ecologic study is an "incomplete" design (Kleinbaum et al., 1982). Ecologic studies have been conducted by social scientists for more than a century (Dogan and Rokkan, 1969) and have been used extensively by epidemiologists in many research areas. Nevertheless, the distinction between individual-level and group-level (ecologic) studies and the inferential implications are far more complicated and subtle than they first appear. Before 1980, ecologic studies were usually presented in the first part of epidemiology textbooks as simple "descriptive" analyses in which disease rates are stratified by place or time to preliminarily test hypotheses; little attention was given to statistical methods or inference—for example, see MacMahon and Pugh (1970). In the past two decades, the methods and conduct of ecologic studies have expanded considerably, and a dominant part of this field is now often labeled "spatial epidemiology" (Elliott et al., 2000; Lawson, 2001). The purpose of this chapter is to provide a methodologic overview of ecologic studies that emphasizes study design and causal inference. Although ecologic studies are easily and inexpensively conducted, the results are often difficult to interpret.

CONCEPTS AND RATIONALE

Before discussing the design and interpretation of ecologic studies, we must first define the concepts of ecologic measurement, analysis, and inference.

LEVELS OF MEASUREMENT

The sources of data used in epidemiologic studies typically involve direct observations of individuals (e.g., age and blood pressure); they may also involve observations of groups, organizations, or places (e.g., social disorganization and air pollution). These observations are then organized to measure specific variables in the study population: Individual-level variables are properties of individuals; and ecologic variables are properties of groups, organizations, or places. To be more specific, ecologic measures may be classified into three types:

1. *Aggregate measures* are summaries (e.g., means or proportions) of observations derived from individuals in each group (e.g., the proportion of smokers and median family income).
2. *Environmental measures* are physical characteristics of the place in which members of each group live or work (e.g., air-pollution level and hours of sunlight). Note that each environmental measure has an analog at the individual level, and these individual exposures (or doses) usually vary among members of each group (though they may remain unmeasured).
3. *Global measures* are attributes of groups, organizations, or places for which there is no distinct analog at the individual level, unlike aggregate and environmental measures (e.g., population density, level of social disorganization, the existence of a specific law, or type of health care system).

LEVELS OF ANALYSIS

The unit of analysis is the common level for which the data on all variables are reduced and analyzed. In an *individual-level analysis,* a value for each variable is assigned to every subject in the study. It is possible, even common in environmental epidemiology, for one or more predictor variables to be ecologic measures. For example, the average pollution level of each county might be assigned to every subject who is a resident of that county.

In a *completely ecologic analysis,* all variables (exposure, disease, and covariates) are ecologic measures, so the unit of analysis is the group (e.g., region, worksite, school, health care facility, demographic stratum, or time interval). Thus, within each group, we do not know the joint distribution of any combination of variables at the individual level (e.g., the frequencies of exposed cases, unexposed cases, exposed noncases, and unexposed noncases); all we know is the marginal distribution of each variable (e.g., the proportion exposed and the disease rate), i.e., the T frequencies in Figure 25–1.

In a *partially ecologic analysis* of three or more variables, we have additional information on certain joint distributions (the M, N, or A/B frequencies in Fig. 25–1); but we still do not know the full joint distribution of all variables within each group (i.e., the ? cells in Fig. 25–1 are missing). For example, in an ecologic study of cancer incidence by county, the joint distribution of age (a covariate) and disease status within each county (the M frequencies in Fig. 25–1) might be obtained from the census and a population tumor registry. From these sources, the investigator would be able to estimate age-specific cancer rates for each county.

	z = 1			z = 0			Total		
	x=1	x=0		x=1	x=0		x=1	x=0	
y=1	?	?	M_{11}	?	?	M_{10}	A_{1+}	A_{0+}	T_{+1}
y=0	?	?	M_{01}	?	?	M_{00}	B_{1+}	B_{0+}	T_{+0}
	N_{11}	N_{01}	T_1	N_{10}	N_{00}	T_0	T_{1+}	T_{0+}	T_{++}

FIGURE 25–1 • Joint distribution of exposure status ($x = 1$ vs. 0), disease status ($y = 1$ vs. 0), and covariate status ($z = 1$ vs. 0) in each group of a simple ecologic analysis: T frequencies are the only data available in a completely ecologic analysis of all three variables; M frequencies require additional data on the joint distribution of z and y within each group; N frequencies require additional data on the joint distribution of x and z within each group; A and B frequencies require additional data on the joint distribution of x and y within each group; and ? cells are always missing in an ecologic analysis.

Multilevel analysis is a special type of modeling technique that combines data collected at two or more levels (Wong and Mason, 1985, 1991; Bryk and Raudenbush, 1992; Goldstein, 2003; Kreft and de Leeuw, 1998). For example, an individual-level analysis might be conducted in each group, followed by an ecologic analysis of all groups using the results from the individual-level analyses. This approach is described in a later section.

LEVELS OF INFERENCE

The underlying goal of a given epidemiologic study or analysis may be to make *biologic* (or biobehavioral) *inferences* about effects on individual *risks* or to make *ecologic inferences* about effects on group *rates* (Morgenstern, 1982). The target level of causal inference, however, does not always match the level of analysis. For example, the explicit or implicit objective of an ecologic analysis may be to make a biologic inference about the effect of a specific exposure on individual disease risk. As discussed later in this chapter, such *cross-level inferences* are particularly vulnerable to bias.

If the objective of a study is to estimate the *biologic (individual) effect* of wearing a motorcycle helmet on the risk of motorcycle-related mortality among motorcycle riders, the target level of causal inference is biologic. On the other hand, if the objective is to estimate the *ecologic effect* of helmet-use laws on the motorcycle-related mortality rate of riders in different states, the target level of causal inference is ecologic. Note that the magnitude of this ecologic effect depends not only on the biologic effect of helmet use, but also on the degree and pattern of compliance with the law in each state. Furthermore, the validity of the ecologic-effect estimate depends on our ability to control for differences among states in the joint distribution of confounders, including individual-level variables such as age and amount of motorcycle riding.

We might also be interested in estimating the *contextual effect* of an ecologic exposure on individual risk, which is also a form of biologic inference (Valkonen, 1969; Boyd and Iversen, 1979). If the ecologic exposure is an aggregate measure, we would generally want to separate its effect from the effect of its individual-level analog. For example, we might estimate the contextual effect of living in a poor area on the risk of disease, controlling for individual poverty level (Humphreys and Carr-Hill, 1991). Contextual effects can be profound in infectious disease epidemiology, where the risk of disease depends on the prevalence of the disease in others with whom the individual has contact (Von Korff et al., 1992; Koopman and Longini, 1994).

In evaluating motorcycle helmet laws in the United States, we would probably not expect a contextual *effect* of living in a state that mandates helmet use on the risk of motorcycle-related mortality in riders, controlling for individual helmet use. If a rider's helmet use does not change after the helmet law takes effect, we would not expect his risk of motorcycle-related mortality to change. Nevertheless, we might expect to observe a contextual *association* between the same variables after the law because of differential compliance with the law within states. That is, those riders who comply with the law, but who would not have worn helmets without the law, may be at lower risk than are riders who do not comply with the law. Consequently, the risk of motorcycle-related mortality among riders who do not wear helmets will be higher in states with a helmet law than in states without such a law.

RATIONALE FOR ECOLOGIC STUDIES

There are several reasons for the widespread use of ecologic studies in epidemiology, despite frequent cautions about their methodologic limitations:

1. *Low cost and convenience.* Ecologic studies are inexpensive and take little time because various secondary data sources, each involving different information needed for the analysis, can easily be linked at the aggregate level. For example, data obtained from population registries, vital records, large surveys, and the census are often linked at the state, county, or census-tract level.
2. *Measurement limitations of individual-level studies.* In environmental epidemiology and other research areas, we often cannot accurately measure relevant exposures or doses at the individual level for large numbers of subjects—at least not with available time and resources. Thus, the only practical way to measure the exposure may be ecologically (Morgenstern, 1982; Morgenstern and

Thomas, 1993). This advantage is especially true when investigating apparent clusters of disease in small areas (Walter, 1991a). Sometimes individual-level exposures, such as dietary factors, cannot be measured accurately because of substantial within-person variability; yet ecologic measures might accurately reflect group averages (Hiller and McMichael, 1991; Prentice and Sheppard, 1995).

3. *Design limitations of individual-level studies.* Individual-level studies may not be practical for estimating exposure effects if the exposure varies little within the study area. Ecologic studies covering a much wider area, however, might be able to achieve substantial variation in mean exposure across groups—for example, see Rose (1985), Prentice et al. (1988), and Plummer and Clayton (1996).
4. *Interest in ecologic effects.* As noted earlier, the stated purpose of a study may be to assess an ecologic effect; i.e., the target level of inference may be ecologic rather than biologic—to understand differences in disease rates among populations (Rose, 1985; McMichael, 1995). Ecologic effects are particularly relevant when evaluating the effects of social processes or population interventions such as new programs, policies, or legislation. As discussed later in this chapter, however, an interest in ecologic effects does not necessarily obviate the need for individual-level data.
5. *Simplicity of analysis and presentation.* In large, complex studies conducted at the individual level, it may be conceptually and statistically simpler to perform ecologic analyses and to present ecologic results than to do individual-level analyses. For example, data from large periodic surveys, such as the National Health Interview Survey, are often analyzed ecologically by treating some combination of year, region, and demographic group as the unit of analysis. As discussed later in this chapter, however, such simplicity of analysis and presentation often conceals methodologic problems.

STUDY DESIGNS

In an ecologic study design, the planned unit of analysis is the group. Ecologic designs may be classified on two dimensions: the method of exposure measurement and the method of grouping (Kleinbaum et al., 1982; Morgenstern, 1982). Regarding the first dimension, an ecologic design is called *exploratory* if there is no specific exposure of interest or the exposure of potential interest is not measured, and it is called *etiologic* if the primary exposure variable is measured and included in the analysis. In practice, this dimension is a continuum, because most ecologic studies are not conducted to test a single hypothesis. Regarding the second dimension, the groups of an ecologic study may be identified by place (multiple-group design), by time (time-trend design), or by a combination of place and time (mixed design).

MULTIPLE-GROUP DESIGNS

Exploratory Study

In an exploratory multiple-group study, we compare the rate of disease among many regions during the same period. The purpose is to search for spatial patterns that might suggest an environmental etiology or more specific etiologic hypotheses. For example, the National Cancer Institute (NCI) mapped the age-adjusted cancer mortality rates in the United States by county for the period 1950–1969 (Mason et al., 1975). For oral cancers, they found a striking difference in geographic patterns by sex: Among men, the mortality rates were greatest in the urban Northeast; but among women, the rates were greatest in the Southeast. These findings led to the hypothesis that snuff dipping, which is common among rural Southern women, is a risk factor for oral cancers (Blot and Fraumeni, 1977). The results of a subsequent case-control study supported this hypothesis (Winn et al., 1981).

Exploratory ecologic studies may also involve the comparison of rates between migrants and their offspring and residents of their countries of emigration and immigration (MacMahon and Pugh, 1970; Hiller and McMichael, 1991). If the rates differ appreciably between the countries of emigration and immigration, migrant studies often yield results suggesting the influence of certain types of risk factors for the disease under study. For example, if U.S. immigrants from Japan have rates of a disease similar to U.S. whites but much lower than Japanese residents, the difference may be due to environmental or behavioral risk factors operating during adulthood. On the other hand, if U.S. immigrants from Japan and their offspring have rates much lower than U.S. whites but similar to Japanese residents, the difference may be due to genetic risk factors. Such interpretations, however, especially in the first instance, are often limited by differences between countries in the classification and detection of disease or cause of death.

In mapping studies, such as the NCI investigation, a simple comparison of rates across regions is often complicated by two statistical problems. First, regions with smaller numbers of observed cases show greater variability in the estimated rate; thus, the most extreme rates tend to be observed for those regions with the fewest cases. Second, nearby regions tend to have more similar rates than do distant regions (i.e., autocorrelation), because unmeasured risk factors tend to cluster in space. Statistical methods for dealing with both problems have been developed by fitting an autoregressive spatial model to the data and using empirical-Bayes techniques to estimate the smoothed rate for each region (Clayton and Kaldor, 1987; Mollie and Richardson, 1991; Devine et al., 1994; Moulton et al., 1994; Elliott et al., 2000; Banerjee et al., 2004). The degree of spatial autocorrelation or clustering can be measured to reflect environmental effects on the rate of disease (Walter, 1992a, 1992b). The empirical Bayes approach can also be applied to data from etiologic multiple-group studies (described next) by including covariates in the model—for example, see Clayton et al. (1993) and Cressie (1993).

Etiologic Study

In an etiologic multiple-group study, we assess the ecologic association between the average exposure level or prevalence and the rate of disease among many groups. This ecological design is the most common; typically, the unit of analysis is a geopolitical region. For example, Hatch and Susser (1990) examined the association between background gamma-radiation and the incidence of childhood cancers between 1975 and 1985 in the region surrounding a nuclear plant. Average radiation levels for each of 69 tracts in the region were estimated from a 1976 aerial survey. The authors found positive associations between radiation level and the incidence of leukemia (an expected finding) as well as solid tumors (an unexpected finding).

Data analysis in this type of multiple-group study usually involves fitting a mathematical model to the data. Ordinary least-squares procedures, however, may be inadequate because the groups typically vary in size and much of the unexplained variability in rates across groups cannot be attributed to sampling error alone. To address these concerns, Pocock et al. (1981) proposed a linear model in which the unexplained variation is treated as a random effect. Model parameters were estimated by an iteratively reweighted least-squares procedure. A similar procedure was used by Breslow (1984) to fit log-linear models. Prentice and Sheppard (1989) proposed a linear relative rate model, which leads readily to the estimation of rate ratios (assuming the model is properly specified). Prentice and Thomas (1993) considered an exponential relative rate model, which they argue may be more parsimonious than the linear-form model for specifying covariates. These methods can be applied to data aggregated by place and/or time (to be discussed later). Recent statistical developments in the analysis of multiple-group ecologic data emphasize the inclusion of supplementary data and/or prior information to improve effect estimation (Chambers and Steel, 2001; Wakefield, 2004). Use of ecologic modeling to estimate exposure effects (rate ratios and differences) is described in the next section.

TIME-TREND DESIGNS

Exploratory Study

An exploratory time-trend or time-series study involves a comparison of the disease rates over time in one geographically defined population. In addition to providing graphical displays of temporal trends, time-series data can also be used to forecast future rates and trends. This latter application, which is more common in the social sciences than in epidemiology, usually involves fitting autoregressive integrated moving-average (ARIMA) models to the outcome data (Box and Jenkins, 1976; Ostrom, 1990; Helfenstein, 1991; Chatfield, 2001; Zeger et al., 2006). The autoregressive component of this model accounts for the correlation among repeated outcome observations over time in the population by allowing the outcome observed at one time to depend on past outcome observations. The net result is that the correlation between observations decays with increasing lag between observations. The moving-average component allows for the outcome observed at one time to depend on random disturbances in the outcome at previous times. This process allows the correlation between observations to be large for a given lag and then drop to zero for larger lags. The integrated (nonstationary) component of the model allows for long-term trends in the outcome. ARIMA modeling can also be extended to evaluate the effect of a population intervention (McDowall et al., 1980; Helfenstein, 1991), to estimate associations between two or more time-series variables (Catalano and Serxner, 1987; Ostrom, 1990; Chatfield, 2001), and to estimate associations in a mixed ecologic design (Sayrs, 1989; Zeger et al., 2006; and see later).

A special type of exploratory time-trend analysis that is often used by epidemiologists is age–period–cohort analysis (or simply, cohort analysis). This approach typically involves the collection of retrospective data from a large population over a period of 20 or more years. Through graphical or tabular displays (e.g., Frost, 1939; Glenn, 1977) or formal modeling techniques (e.g., Mason et al., 1973; Holford, 1991), the objective is to estimate the separate effects of three time-related variables on the rate of disease: age, period (calendar time), and birth cohort (year of birth). By describing the occurrence of disease in this way, the investigator attempts to gain insight about temporal trends, which might lead to new hypotheses.

Lee et al. (1979) conducted an age–period–cohort analysis of melanoma mortality among white men in the United States between 1951 and 1975. They concluded that the apparent increase in the melanoma mortality rate was due primarily to a cohort effect. That is, persons born in more recent years experienced throughout their lives a higher rate than did persons born earlier. In a subsequent paper, Lee (1982) speculated that this cohort effect might reflect increases in sunlight exposure or sunburning during youth, which he hypothesized is a risk factor for melanoma.

From a purely statistical perspective, there is an inherent problem in making inferences from the results of age–period–cohort analyses because of the linear dependency among the three time-related variables (Glenn, 1977; Goldstein, 1979; Holford, 1991). Thus, we cannot allow the value of one variable to change when the values of the other two variables are held constant. As a result of this "identifiability" problem, each data set has alternative interpretations with respect to the combination of age, period, and cohort effects; there is no unique set of effect parameters when all three variables are considered simultaneously. The only way to decide which interpretation should be accepted is to consider the findings in light of prior knowledge and, possibly, to constrain the model by ignoring one effect.

Etiologic Study

In an etiologic time-trend study, we assess the ecologic association between change in average exposure level or prevalence and change in disease rate in one geographically defined population. As with exploratory designs, this type of assessment can be done by simple graphical displays or by time-series regression modeling—for example, see Ostrom (1990), Chatfield (2001), and Zeger et al. (2006).

In their etiologic time-trend study, Darby and Doll (1987) examined the associations between average annual absorbed dose of radiation fallout from weapons testing and the incidence rate of childhood leukemia in three European countries between 1945 and 1985. Although the leukemia rate varied over time in each country, they found no convincing evidence that these changes were attributable to changes in fallout radiation.

Causal inference from time-trend studies is often complicated by two problems. First, changes in disease classification and diagnostic criteria can produce distorted trends in the observed rate of disease, which can lead to substantial bias in estimating exposure effects. Second, there may be an appreciable induction/latent period between first exposure to a risk factor and disease detection. To deal with the latter issue in an ecologic time-trend study, the investigator can lag observations between average exposure and disease rate by a duration assumed to reflect the average induction/latent period of exposure-induced cases. There are two approaches for selecting the lag: (a) an *a priori* method based on knowledge of the disease; and (b) empirical methods that maximize the observed association of interest or optimize the fit of the model that includes a lag parameter. Unfortunately, the first method is often problematic because adequate prior knowledge is lacking, and the second method can produce results that are biologically meaningless and very misleading (Gruchow et al., 1983).

MIXED DESIGNS

Exploratory Study

The exploratory mixed design combines the basic features of the exploratory multiple-group study and the exploratory time-trend study. Time-series (ARIMA) modeling or age–period–cohort analysis can be used to describe or predict trends in the disease rate for multiple populations. For example, to test the hypothesis of Lee (1982) that changes in sunlight exposure during youth can explain the observed increase in melanoma mortality in the United States, we might conduct an age–period–cohort analysis, stratifying on region according to approximate sunlight exposure (without measuring the exposure). Assuming the amounts of sunlight in the regions have not changed differentially over the study period, we might expect the cohort effect described earlier to be stronger for sunnier regions.

Etiologic Study

In an etiologic mixed design, we assess the association between change in average exposure level or prevalence and change in disease rate among many groups. Thus, the interpretation of estimated effects is enhanced because two types of comparisons are made simultaneously: change over time within groups and differences among groups. For example, Crawford et al. (1971) evaluated the hypothesis that hard drinking water (i.e., water with a high concentration of calcium and magnesium) is a protective risk factor for cardiovascular disease (CVD). They compared the absolute change in CVD mortality rate between 1948 and 1964 in 83 British towns, by water-hardness change, age, and sex. In all sex–age groups, especially for men, the authors found an inverse association between trends in water hardness and CVD mortality. In middle-aged men, for example, the increase in CVD mortality was less in towns that made their water harder than in towns that made their water softer.

EFFECT ESTIMATION

A major quantitative objective of most epidemiologic studies is to estimate the effect of one or more exposures on disease occurrence in a well-defined population at risk. A measure of effect in this context is not just any measure of association such as a correlation coefficient; rather, it reflects a particular causal parameter, i.e., a counterfactual contrast in disease occurrence (Rubin, 1978, 1990a; Greenland et al., 1986, 1991; Greenland, 1987a, 2000a, 2005a; Morgenstern and Thomas, 1993; Maldonado and Greenland, 2002; see Chapter 4). In studies conducted at the individual level, effects are usually estimated by comparing the rate or risk of disease, in the form of a ratio or difference, for exposed and unexposed populations (see Chapter 4). In multiple-group ecologic studies, however, we cannot estimate effects directly in this way because of the missing information on the joint distribution within groups. Instead, we regress the group-specific disease rates (Y) on the group-specific exposure prevalences (X). (Note that, throughout this chapter, uppercase letters are used to represent ecologic variables and their estimated regression coefficients; lowercase letters are used to represent individual-level variables and their estimated regression coefficients.)

The most common model form for analyzing ecologic data is the linear model. Ordinary least-squares methods can be used to produce the following prediction equation: $\hat{Y} = B_0 + B_1X$, where B_0 and B_1 are the estimated intercept and slope. An estimate of the biologic effect of the exposure (at the individual level) can be derived from the regression results (Goodman, 1959; Beral et al., 1979). The predicted disease rate ($\hat{Y}_{x=1}$) in a group that is entirely exposed is $B_0 + B_1(1) = B_0 + B_1$, and the predicted rate ($\hat{Y}_{x=0}$) in a group that is entirely unexposed is $B_0 + B_1(0) = B_0$. Therefore, the estimated rate difference is $B_0 + B_1 - B_0 = B_1$, and the estimated rate ratio is $(B_0 + B_1)/B_0 = 1 + B_1/B_0$.

Alternatively, fitting a log-linear (exponential) model to the data yields the following prediction equation: $\ln(\hat{Y}) = B_0 + B_1X$ or $\hat{Y} = \exp(B_0 + B_1X)$. Applying the same method as used for linear models, the estimated rate ratio is $\hat{Y}_{x=1}/\hat{Y}_{x=0} = \exp(B_1)$.

As an illustration of rate-ratio estimation in an ecologic study, consider Durkheim's (1951) examination of religion and suicide in four groups of Prussian provinces between 1883 and 1890 (Fig. 25–2). The groups were formed by ranking 13 provinces according to the proportion (X) of the population that was Protestant. Using ordinary least-squares linear regression, we estimate the suicide rate ($\hat{Y}$, events per 10^5 person-years) in each group to be $3.66 + 24.0(X)$. Therefore, the estimated

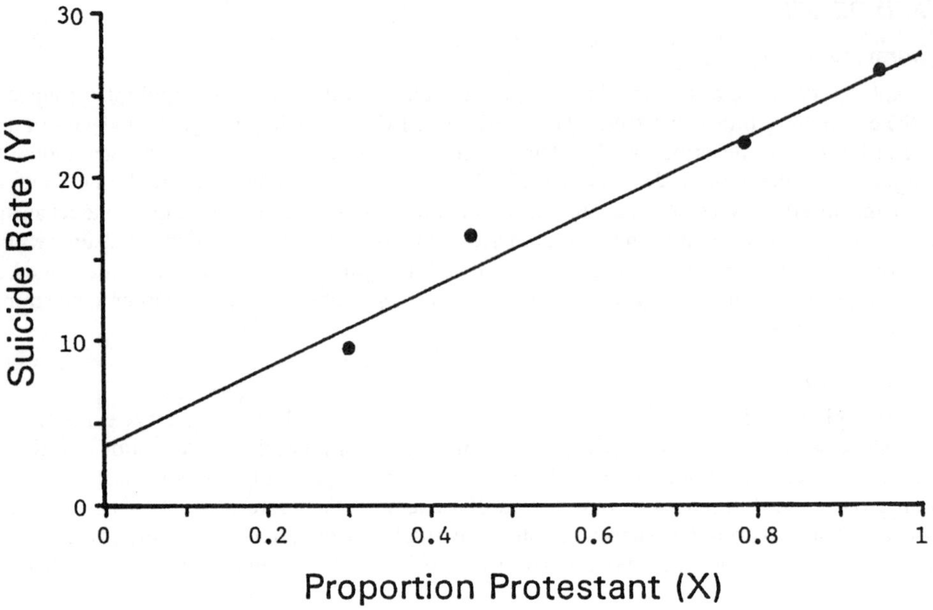

FIGURE 25–2 • Suicide rate (Y, events per 10^5 person-years) by proportion Protestant (X) for four groups of Prussian provinces, 1883–1890. The four observed points (X, Y) are (0.30, 9.56), (0.45, 16.36), (0.785, 22.00), and (0.95, 26.46); the fitted line is based on unweighted least-squares regression. (Adapted from Durkheim E. *Suicide: A Study in Sociology.* New York: Free Press; 1951.)

rate ratio, comparing Protestants with other religions, is $1 + (24.0/3.66) = 7.6$. Note in Figure 25–2 that the fit of the linear model appears to be excellent ($R^2 = 0.97$). In general, however, ecologic tests of fit can be misleading about the underlying model at the individual level that generated the ecologic data (Greenland and Robins, 1994).

The ecologic method of effect estimation requires that rate predictions be extrapolated to both extreme values of the exposure variable (i.e., $X = 0$ and 1), which are likely to lie well beyond the observed range of the data. It is not surprising, therefore, that different model forms (e.g., log-linear vs. linear) can lead to very different estimates of effect (Greenland, 1992b). Fitting a linear model, in fact, may lead to negative, and thus meaningless, estimates of the rate ratio. Other statistical methods for estimating exposure effects in ecologic studies are discussed by Chambers and Steel (2001), Gelman et al. (2001), and Wakefield (2004).

CONFOUNDERS AND EFFECT MODIFIERS

Two methods are used to control for confounders in multiple-group ecologic analyses. The first is to treat ecologic measures of the confounders as covariates (Z) in the model, e.g., percentage of men and percentage of whites in each group. If the individual-level effects of the exposure and covariates are additive (i.e., if the disease rates follow a linear model), then the ecologic regression of Y on X and Z will also be linear with the same coefficients (Langbein and Lichtman, 1978; Greenland, 1992b, 2002b). That is, the estimated coefficient for the exposure variable in a linear model can be interpreted as the rate difference adjusted for the covariates, provided the effects are truly additive and there are no other sources of bias. To estimate the adjusted rate ratio for the exposure effect, we must first specify values for all covariates (Z) in the model, because the effects of X and Z are assumed to be additive—not multiplicative. Thus, the estimated rate ratio, conditional on covariate levels (Z), is the predicted rate in a group that is entirely exposed ($\hat{Y}_{x=1|z}$) divided by the predicted rate in a group that is entirely unexposed ($\hat{Y}_{x=0|z}$).

Fitting a log-linear model to the ecologic data yields an estimate of the adjusted rate ratio that is independent of covariates—i.e., $\hat{Y}_{x=1|z}/\hat{Y}_{x=0|z} = \exp(B_1)$, where B_1 is the estimated coefficient for the exposure. Thus, the effects of X and Z are assumed to be multiplicative. Unfortunately, this ecologic estimate is a biased estimate of the individual-level rate ratio, even if the effects are multiplicative at the individual level and no other source of bias is present (Richardson et al., 1987; Greenland, 1992b).

The second method used to control for confounders in ecologic analyses is rate standardization for these confounders (see Chapters 3 and 4), followed by regression of the standardized rates as the outcome variable. Note that this method requires additional data on the joint distribution of the covariate and disease within each group (i.e., the M frequencies in Fig. 25–1). Nevertheless, it cannot be expected to reduce bias unless all predictors in the model (X and Z) are also mutually standardized for the same confounders (Rosenbaum and Rubin, 1984; Greenland and Morgenstern, 1989; Greenland, 1992b). Standardization of the exposure prevalences, for example, requires data on the joint distribution of the covariate and exposure within groups (i.e., the N frequencies in Fig. 25–1); unfortunately, this information is not usually available in ecologic studies.

As in individual-level analyses, product terms (e.g., XZ) are often used in ecologic analyses to model interaction effects, i.e., to assess effect modification. In ecologic analyses, however, the product of X and Z (both group averages) is not, in general, equal to the average product of the exposure (x) and covariate (z) at the individual level within groups. Assuming a linear model, XZ will be equal to the mean xz in each group only if x and z are uncorrelated within groups (Greenland, 1992b). Thus, as pointed out in the next section, interaction (nonadditive) effects at the individual level complicate the interpretation of ecologic results.

METHODOLOGIC PROBLEMS

Despite the many practical advantages of ecologic studies mentioned previously, there are several methodologic problems that may severely limit causal inference, especially biologic inference.

ECOLOGIC BIAS

The major limitation of ecologic analysis for making causal inferences is ecologic bias, which is usually interpreted as the failure of ecologic associations to reflect the biologic effect at the individual level (Goodman, 1959; Firebaugh, 1978; Morgenstern, 1982; Richardson et al., 1987; Greenland and Morgenstern, 1989; Greenland and Robins, 1994). More generally, ecologic bias can be interpreted as the failure of associations seen at one level of grouping to correspond to effect measures at the grouping level of interest. For example, relations seen in county-level data may poorly track relations that exist at the individual level (no grouping) or at the neighborhood level (neighborhood grouping), and so would be biased if individual-level or neighborhood-level relations were of interest (Openshaw and Taylor, 1981; Greenland, 2001a). This failure to capture desired effects applies also to estimating confounder effects at the level of interest, and hence threatens validity both directly and by undermining control of confounding (Greenland, 2001a, 2004b).

In addition to the usual sources of bias that threaten individual-level analyses (see Chapter 8), the underlying problem of ecologic analyses for estimating biologic effects is heterogeneity of exposure level and covariate levels within groups. As noted earlier, this heterogeneity is not fully captured with ecologic data because of missing information on joint distributions (Fig. 25–1). Robinson (1950) was the first to describe mathematically how ecologic associations may differ from the corresponding associations at the individual level within groups of the same population. He expressed this relation in terms of correlation coefficients, which was later extended by Duncan et al. (1961) to regression coefficients in a linear model. The phenomenon became widely known as the *ecologic* (or ecological) *fallacy* (Selvin, 1958), and researchers came to recognize that the magnitude of the ecologic bias may be severe in practice (Stavraky, 1976; Connor and Gillings, 1984; Feinleib and Leaverton, 1984; Richardson et al., 1987; Stidley and Samet, 1994).

As an illustration of ecologic bias, consider again Durkheim's (1951) data on religion and suicide (Fig. 25–2). The estimated rate ratio of 7.6 in the ecologic analysis may not mean that the suicide rate was nearly eight times greater in Protestants than in non-Protestants. Rather, because none of the regions was entirely Protestant or non-Protestant, it may have been non-Protestants (primarily Catholics) who were committing suicide in predominantly Protestant provinces. It is certainly plausible that members of a religious minority might have been more likely to take their own lives than were members of the majority. The implication of this alternative explanation is that living in a predominantly Protestant area has a contextual effect on suicide risk among non-Protestants; i.e., there is an interaction effect at the individual level between religion and religious composition of one's area of residence.

Interestingly, Durkheim (1951) compared the suicide rates (at the individual level) for Protestants, Catholics, and Jews living in Prussia, and from his data, we find that the rate was about twice as great in Protestants as in other religious groups. Thus, there appears to be substantial ecologic bias (i.e., comparing rate-ratio estimates of about 2 vs. 8). Durkheim (1951), however, failed to notice this quantitative difference because he did not actually estimate the magnitude of the effect in either analysis.

Greenland and Morgenstern (1989) showed that ecologic bias can arise from three sources when using simple linear regression to estimate the crude exposure effect; the first may operate in any type of study, the latter two are unique to ecologic studies (i.e., *cross-level bias*) but are defined in terms of individual-level parameters.

1. *Within-group bias*. Ecologic bias may result from bias within groups due to confounding, selection methods, or misclassification, even though within-group effects are not estimated. Thus, for example, if there is positive confounding of the crude effect parameter in every group, we can expect the crude ecologic estimate to be biased as well.
2. *Confounding by group*. Ecologic bias may result if the background rate of disease in the unexposed population varies across groups. More specifically, bias results if there is a nonzero ecologic correlation between mean exposure level and the background rate.
3. *Effect modification by group (on an additive scale)*. Ecologic bias may also result if the rate difference for the exposure effect at the individual level varies across groups.

Confounding and effect modification by group (the sources of cross-level bias) can arise in three ways: (a) extraneous risk factors (confounders or modifiers) are differentially distributed across groups; (b) the ecologic exposure variable has a contextual effect on risk separate from the biologic effect of its individual-level analogue, e.g., living in a predominantly Protestant area versus being Protestant (in the suicide example); or (c) disease risk depends on the prevalence of that disease in other members of the group, which is true of many infectious diseases (Koopman and Longini, 1994).

To appreciate the sources of cross-level bias, it is helpful to consider simple numerical illustrations involving both individual-level and ecologic analyses with the same population. The hypothetical example in Table 25–1 involves a dichotomous exposure (x) and three groups. At the individual level, both the rate difference and rate ratio vary somewhat across the groups, but the effect is positive in all groups; the crude and group-standardized rate ratio is 2.0. Fitting a linear model to the ecologic data, however, we find that the slope for the exposure variable (X) is negative and the rate ratio is 0.50, suggesting a protective effect. The reason for such large ecologic bias is heterogeneity of the rate difference across groups (effect modification by group). In this example, there is no confounding by group because the unexposed rate is the same (100 events per 10^5 person-years) in all three groups.

The example in Table 25–2 illustrates the conditions for no cross-level bias. First, group is not a modifier of the exposure effect at the individual level because the rate difference (100 events per 10^5 person-years) is uniform across groups (even though the rate ratio varies). Second, group is not a confounder of the exposure effect because there is no ecologic correlation between the percentage of exposed ($100X$) and the unexposed rate. Thus, the individual-level and ecologic estimates of the rate ratio are the same (1.8) and unbiased, even though the R^2 for the fitted model is very low (0.029).

Unfortunately, the two conditions that produce cross-level bias cannot be checked with ecologic data because those conditions are defined in terms of individual-level associations. This inability to check the validity of ecologic results seriously limits biologic inference. Furthermore, the fit of the ecologic regression model, in general, gives no indication of the presence, direction, or magnitude of ecologic bias. Thus, a model with excellent fit may yield substantial bias, and one model with a better fit than another model may yield more bias. For example, there was substantial bias when fitting a linear model to Durkheim's (1951) suicide data in Figure 25–2, despite an excellent-fitting model ($R^2 = 0.97$). Recall that the estimated rate ratio was 7.6, compared with a "true" rate ratio of approximately 2. If we fit a log-linear model to the same data, we get $\hat{Y} = \exp(1.974 + 1.418X)$

TABLE 25–1

Number of New Cases, Person-Years (P-Y) of Follow-up, and Disease Rate (*Y*, per 100,000y), by Group and Exposure Status (*x*) (top); Summary Parameters for Each Group (middle); and Results of Individual-Level and Ecologic Analyses (bottom): Hypothetical Example of Ecologic Bias due to Effect Modification by Group

Exposure Status (*x*)	Group 1			Group 2			Group 3		
	Cases	P-Y	Rate	Cases	P-Y	Rate	Cases	P-Y	Rate
Exposed ($x = 1$)	20	7,000	286	20	10,000	200	20	13,000	154
Unexposed ($x = 0$)	13	13,000	100	10	10,000	100	7	7,000	100
Total	33	20,000	165	30	20,000	150	27	20,000	135
Percentage of exposed (100*X*)			35			50			65
Rate difference (per 10^5y)			186			100			54
Rate ratio			2.9			2.0			1.5

Individual-level analysis	Ecologic analysis: linear model
Crude rate ratio[a] = 2.0	$\hat{Y} = 200 - 100X$ ($R^2 = 1$)
Adjusted rate ratio (SMR)[b] = 2.0	Rate ratio = 0.50

[a] Rate ratio for the total population, unadjusted for group.
[b] Rate ratio standardized for group, using the exposed population as the standard.

TABLE 25–2

Number of New Cases, Person-Years (P-Y) of Follow-up, and Disease Rate (*Y*, per 100,000y), by Group and Exposure Status (*x*) (top); Summary Parameters for Each Group (middle); and Results of Individual-Level and Ecologic Analyses (bottom): Hypothetical Example of No Ecologic Bias

Exposure Status (*x*)	Group 1			Group 2			Group 3		
	Cases	P-Y	Rate	Cases	P-Y	Rate	Cases	P-Y	Rate
Exposed ($x = 1$)	16	8,000	200	20	10,000	300	24	12,000	200
Unexposed ($x = 0$)	12	12,000	100	10	10,000	200	8	8,000	100
Total	28	20,000	140	50	20,000	250	32	20,000	160
Percentage of exposed (100*X*)			40			50			60
Rate difference (per 10^5y)			100			100			100
Rate ratio			2.0			1.5			2.0

Individual-level analysis	Ecologic analysis: linear model
Crude rate ratio[a] = 1.8	$\hat{Y} = 133 + 100X$ ($R^2 = 0.029$)
Adjusted rate ratio (SMR)[b] = 1.8	Rate ratio = 1.8

[a] Rate ratio for the total population, unadjusted for group.
[b] Rate ratio standardized for group, using the exposed population as the standard.

and $R^2 = 0.91$; therefore, the estimated rate ratio is $\exp(1.418) = 4.1$. Thus, the log-linear model produces less bias even though it has a smaller R^2 than the linear model. In general, we cannot expect to reduce bias by using better fitting models in ecologic analysis.

A potential strategy for reducing ecologic bias is to use smaller units in an ecologic study (e.g., counties instead of states) to make the groups more homogeneous with respect to the exposure. On the other hand, this strategy might not be feasible because of the lack of available data aggregated at the same level, and it can lead to another problem: greater migration between groups (see later) (Morgenstern, 1982; Walter, 1991b).

Other methods for reducing ecologic bias rely on statistical modeling techniques that incorporate external information, i.e., supplementary data or prior information (Elliott et al., 2000; Gelman et al., 2001; Guthrie and Sheppard, 2001; Wakefield and Salway, 2001; Banerjee et al., 2004; Wakefield, 2004). For example, Best et al. (2001) used a Bayesian hierarchical modeling approach to estimate the effect of environmental exposure to benzene on the incidence of childhood leukemia in Greater London. These investigators employed three units of analysis: local authority districts, census wards, and 1-km^2 grid squares. Although Best et al. found consistent positive associations between benzene exposure and childhood leukemia, the authors acknowledged several methodologic problems that limited their ability to make causal inferences.

A widely cited method for eliminating ecologic bias without the use of external information was proposed by King (1997). His approach combined the linear-regression method described previously (Goodman, 1959) and the method of "bounds" proposed by Duncan and Davis (1953). Early critics of King's method maintained that it does not provide accurate estimates of individual effects in certain datasets and that the diagnostics provided by King are not sensitive to the errors (Freedman et al., 1998). One key problem of King's model, in its original form, is that it assumes no contextual effects (Wakefield, 2004). These claims have been debated in the literature (King, 1999; Freedman et al., 1999), and the method remains controversial (Cho, 1998; McCue, 2001; Wakefield, 2004). One critic, for example, has concluded that King's method is unlikely to reduce ecologic bias relative to simpler models (McCue, 2001).

PROBLEMS OF CONFOUNDER CONTROL

As indicated in a previous section, covariates are included in ecologic analyses to control for confounding, but the conditions for a covariate being a confounder are different at the ecologic and individual levels (Greenland and Morgenstern, 1989; Greenland and Robins, 1994; Greenland, 2001a; Darby et al., 2001). At the individual level, a risk factor must be associated with the exposure to be a confounder. In a multiple-group ecologic study, in contrast, a risk factor may produce ecologic bias (e.g., it may be an ecologic confounder), even if it is unassociated with the exposure in every group, if the risk factor is ecologically associated with the exposure across groups (Greenland and Morgenstern, 1989; Greenland, 1992b). Conversely, a risk factor that is a confounder within groups may not produce ecologic bias if it is ecologically unassociated with the exposure across groups. For example, there is some evidence that confounding by indication in the estimation of intended treatment effects is less severe in ecologic studies than in observational studies conducted at the individual level (Wen and Kramer, 1999; Johnston, 2000).

In general, however, control for confounders is more problematic in ecologic analyses than in individual-level analyses (Greenland and Morgenstern, 1989; Greenland, 1992b, 2001a, 2002b; Greenland and Robins, 1994). Even when all variables are accurately measured for all groups, adjustment for extraneous risk factors may not reduce the ecologic bias produced by these risk factors. In fact, it is possible for such ecologic adjustment to increase bias (Greenland and Morgenstern, 1989; Greenland and Robins, 1994).

It follows from the principles presented in the previous section that there will be no ecologic bias in a multiple-linear-regression analysis if all the following conditions are met:

1. There is no residual within-group bias in exposure effect in any group because of confounding by unmeasured risk factors, selection methods, or misclassification.
2. There is no ecologic correlation between the mean value of each predictor (exposure and covariate) and the background rate of disease in the joint reference (unexposed) level of all predictors (so that group does not confound the predictor effects).

3. The rate difference for each predictor is uniform across levels of the other predictors within groups (i.e., the effects are additive).
4. The rate difference for each predictor, conditional on other predictors in the model, is uniform across groups (i.e., group does not modify the effect of each predictor on the additive scale at the individual level).

These conditions are sufficient, but not necessary, for the ecologic estimate to be unbiased; i.e., there might be little or no bias even if none of these conditions is met. On the other hand, minor deviations from the latter three conditions can produce substantial cross-level bias (Greenland, 1992b). Because the sufficient conditions for no cross-level bias cannot be checked with ecologic data alone, the unpredictable and potentially severe nature of such bias makes biologic inference from ecologic analyses particularly problematic.

The conditions for no cross-level bias with covariate adjustment are illustrated in the hypothetical example in Table 25–3. Both the exposure (x) and covariate (z) are dichotomous variables, and there are three groups. At the individual level, the covariate is not a confounder of the exposure effect because there is no exposure–covariate association within any of the groups. Thus, the crude and adjusted estimates of the rate ratio are nearly the same (1.3). In the ecologic analysis, however, the covariate is a confounder because there is an inverse association between the exposure (X) and the covariate (Z) across groups. Thus, although the crude ecologic estimate of the rate ratio (0.32) is severely biased, the adjusted estimate (1.3) is unbiased. The reasons for no cross-level bias with covariate adjustment are: (a) the rate (100 events per 10^5 person-years) in the joint reference group ($x = z = 0$) does not vary across groups, i.e., the second condition is met; and (b) the rate difference (100 events per 10^5 person-years) is uniform within groups and across groups—i.e., the third and fourth conditions are met.

The example in Table 25–4 illustrates cross-level bias when the null hypothesis is true. At the individual level, the covariate (z) is a strong confounder because it is a predictor of the disease in the unexposed population and it is associated with exposure status (x) within groups. Thus, the crude rate ratio (2.1) is biased. At the ecologic level, however, there is no association between the exposure (X) and the covariate (Z), so the covariate is not an ecologic confounder. Nevertheless, both the crude and adjusted rate ratios (8.6) are strongly biased because the rate in the joint reference category ($x = z = 0$) is ecologically associated with both the exposure (X) and the covariate (Z)—i.e., the second condition is not met.

Lack of additivity at the individual level (refer to the third condition) is common in epidemiology, but unmeasured modifiers do not bias results at the individual level if they are unrelated to the exposure (Greenland, 1987a). Furthermore, statistical interactions may be readily assessed at the individual level by including product terms as predictors in the model (e.g., xz). In ecologic analyses, however, lack of additivity within groups is a source of ecologic bias, and this bias cannot be eliminated by the inclusion of product terms (e.g., XZ) unless the effects are exactly multiplicative and the two variables are uncorrelated within groups (Richardson and Hémon, 1990). If x and z are correlated within groups, additional data on the x–z associations (the N frequencies in Fig. 25–1) can be used to improve the ecologic estimate of each predictor effect controlling for the other (Prentice and Sheppard, 1995; Plummer and Clayton, 1996; Guthrie and Sheppard, 2001; Wakefield and Salway, 2001; Wakefield, 2004).

Another source of ecologic bias is misspecification of confounders (Greenland and Robins, 1994). Although this problem can also arise in individual-level analyses, it is more difficult to avoid in ecologic analyses because the relevant confounder may be the distribution of covariate histories for all individuals within each group. In ecologic studies, therefore, adjustment for covariates derived from available data (e.g., proportion of current smokers) may be inadequate to control confounding. It is preferable, whenever possible, to control for more than a single summary measure of the covariate distribution (e.g., the proportions of the group in each of several smoking categories). In addition, because it is usually necessary to control for several confounders (among which the effects may not be linear and additive), the best approach for reducing ecologic bias is to include covariates for categories of their joint distribution within groups. For example, to control ecologically for race and sex, the investigator might adjust for the proportions of white women, nonwhite men, and nonwhite women (treating white men as the referent), rather than the conventional approach of adjusting for the proportions of men (or women) and whites (or nonwhites).

(text continues on page 526)

TABLE 25–3

Number of New Cases, Person-Years (P-Y) of Follow-up, and Disease Rate (*Y*, per 100,000y), By group, Covariate Status (*z*), and Exposure Status (*x*) (top); Summary Parameters for Each Group (middle); and Results of Individual-Level and Ecologic Analyses (bottom): Hypothetical Example of No Ecologic Bias; Covariate Is an Ecologic Confounder but Not a Within-Group Confounder

Covariate Status (*z*)	Exposure Status (*x*)	Group 1			Group 2			Group 3		
		Cases	P-Y	Rate	Cases	P-Y	Rate	Cases	P-Y	Rate
1	Exposed	18	3,000	600	24	4,000	600	24	4,000	600
	Unexposed	60	12,000	500	40	8,000	500	30	6,000	500
	Total	78	15,000	520	64	12,000	533	54	10,000	540
0	Exposed	4	2,000	200	8	4,000	200	12	6,000	200
	Unexposed	8	8,000	100	8	8,000	100	9	9,000	100
	Total	12	10,000	120	16	12,000	133	21	15,000	140
Total	Exposed	22	5,000	440	32	8,000	400	36	10,000	360
	Unexposed	68	20,000	340	48	16,000	300	39	15,000	260
	Total	90	25,000	360	80	24,000	333	75	25,000	300
Percentage exposed ($100X$)				20			33			40
Percentage with $z = 1$ ($100Z$)				60			50			40

Individual-level analysis	Ecologic analysis: linear models
Crude rate ratio[a] = 1.3	Crude: $\hat{Y} = 420 - 286X$ ($R^2 = 0.94$); rate ratio = 0.32
Adjusted rate ratio (SMR)[b] = 1.3	Adjusted: $\hat{Y} = 100 + 100X + 400Z$ ($R^2 = 1$); rate ratio[c] = 1.3

[a] Rate ratio for the total population, unadjusted for group or the covariate.
[b] Rate ratio standardized for group and the covariate, using the exposed population as the standard.
[c] Setting $Z = 0.50$ (the mean for all three groups).

TABLE 25–4

Number of New Cases, Person-Years (P-Y) of Follow-up, and Disease Rate (*Y*, per 100,000y), by Group, Covariate Status (*z*), and Exposure Status (*x*) (top); Summary Parameters for Each Group (middle); and Results of Individual-Level and Ecologic Analyses (bottom): Hypothetical Example of Ecologic Bias due to Confounding by Group; Covariate Is a Within-Group Confounder but Not an Ecologic Confounder

Covariate Status (z)	Exposure Status (x)	Group 1			Group 2			Group 3		
		Cases	P-Y	Rate	Cases	P-Y	Rate	Cases	P-Y	Rate
1	Exposed	40	8,000	500	195	13,000	1,500	140	14,000	1,000
	Unexposed	60	12,000	500	180	12,000	1,500	60	6,000	1,000
	Total	100	20,000	500	375	25,000	1,500	200	20,000	1,000
0	Exposed	2	2,000	100	6	2,000	300	12	6,000	200
	Unexposed	28	28,000	100	69	23,000	300	48	24,000	200
	Total	30	30,000	100	75	25,000	300	60	30,000	200
Total	Exposed	42	10,000	420	201	15,000	1,340	152	20,000	760
	Unexposed	88	40,000	249	249	35,000	711	108	30,000	360
	Total	130	50,000	450	450	50,000	900	260	50,000	520
Percentage exposed ($100X$)				20			30			40
Percentage with $z = 1$ ($100Z$)				40			50			40

Individual-level analysis	Ecologic analysis: linear models
Crude rate ratio[a] = 2.1	Crude: $\hat{Y} = 170 - 1,300X$ ($R^2 = 0.16$); rate ratio = 8.6
Adjusted rate ratio (SMR)[b] = 1.0	Adjusted: $\hat{Y} = 2,040 + 1,300X + 5,100Z$ ($R^2 = 1$); rate ratio[c] = 8.6

[a] Rate ratio for the total population, unadjusted for group or the covariate.
[b] Rate ratio standardized for group and the covariate, using the exposed population as the standard; also the common rate ratio within each group.
[c] Setting $Z = 0.433$ (the mean for all three groups).

WITHIN-GROUP MISCLASSIFICATION

The principles of misclassification bias with which epidemiologists are familiar when interpreting the results of analyses conducted at the individual level do not apply to ecologic analyses. At the individual level, for example, nondifferential independent misclassification of a dichotomous exposure biases the effect estimate toward the null (see Chapter 8). In multiple-group ecologic studies, however, this principle does not hold when the exposure variable is an aggregate measure. Brenner et al. (1992b) have shown that nondifferential misclassification of a dichotomous exposure within groups usually leads to bias away from the null and that the bias may be severe.

As an illustration of this distinct feature of ecologic analysis, consider the two-group example in Table 25–5, which contrasts analyses with correctly classified and misclassified exposure data at both the individual and ecologic levels. The sensitivity and specificity of exposure classification are assumed to be 0.9 for both cases and noncases in the population. The correct rate ratio at the individual level is 5.0. With nondifferential exposure misclassification, the observed rate ratio would be 3.4, which is biased toward the null. Although an ecologic analysis of the correctly classified data yields an unbiased estimate of the rate ratio (5.0), an analysis with misclassified data would yield an observed rate ratio of 11.0, which is strongly biased away from the null. To appreciate the direction of the misclassification bias in this ecologic analysis, notice that the difference in the percentage exposed ($100X$) between the two groups decreases from 40 – 20 = 20% to 42 – 26 = 16% when the exposure is misclassified (Table 25–5). Thus, the slope in the misclassified analysis increases from 200 to 250 events per 10^5 person-years. In addition, the intercept decreases from 50 to 25 events per 10^5 person-years. Each of these changes causes the observed rate ratio with the misclassified data to increase (away from the null).

TABLE 25–5

Number of New Cases, Person-Years (P-Y) of Follow-up, and Disease Rate (Y, per 100,000y), by Group, Type of Exposure Classification (correct vs. misclassified[a]), and Exposure Status (top); Percentage of Exposed by Group (middle); and Results of Individual-Level and Ecologic Analyses (bottom): Hypothetical Example of Ecologic Bias away from the Null due to Nondifferential Exposure Misclassification within Groups

Exposure Classification	Exposure Status	Group 1			Group 2		
		Cases	P-Y	Rate	Cases	P-Y	Rate
Correctly classified	Exposed ($x = 1$)	50	20,000	250	100	40,000	250
	Unexposed ($x = 0$)	40	80,000	50	30	60,000	50
	Total	90	100,000	90	130	100,00	130
Misclassified[a]	Exposed ($x' = 1$)	49	26,000	188	93	42,000	221
	Unexposed ($x' = 0$)	41	74,000	55	37	58,000	64
	Total	90	100,000	90	130	100,000	130
Percentage exposed, correctly classified ($100X$)				20			40
Percentage exposed, misclassified ($100X'$)				26			42

Individual-level analysis	Ecologic analysis: linear models
Correct: rate *ratio*[b] = 5.0	Correct: $\hat{Y} = 50 + 200X$; rate ratio = 5.0
Misclassified: rate *ratio*[c] = 3.4	Misclassified: $\hat{Y} = 25 + 250X'$; rate ratio = 11.0

[a] Sensitivity = specificity = 0.9 for both cases and noncases (nondifferential misclassification).
[b] Common rate ratio within each group.
[c] Common rate ratio, using the Mantel-Haenszel method

It is possible to correct for nondifferential misclassification of a dichotomous exposure or disease in ecologic analyses, based on prior specifications of sensitivity and specificity (Brenner et al., 1992a, app. 1; Greenland and Brenner, 1993). Suppose, for example, that we wish to correct for nondifferential exposure misclassification when using simple linear regression (no covariates) to estimate the exposure effect. The corrected estimator of the rate ratio derived from the model results is $(B_0 + B_1\text{Se})/[B_0 + B_1(1 - \text{Sp})]$, where B_0 and B_1 are the estimated intercept and slope from the misclassified data, Se is the sensitivity of exposure classification, and Sp is the specificity. Greenland and Brenner (1993) also derived a corrected estimator for the variance of the estimated rate ratio.

In studies conducted at the individual level, misclassification of a covariate, if nondifferential with respect to both exposure and disease, will usually reduce our ability to control for that confounder (Greenland, 1980; Savitz and Baron, 1989). That is, adjustment will not completely eliminate the bias due to the confounder. In ecologic studies, however, nondifferential misclassification of a dichotomous confounder within groups does not affect our ability to control for that confounder, provided there is no cross-level bias (Brenner et al., 1992a). More generally, however, misclassification of confounders will reduce control of confounding at the ecologic as well as the individual level.

If the outcome and all but one predictor (i.e., the exposure or a covariate) in a given analysis are measured at the individual level, this partially ecologic analysis may also be regarded as nonecologic with the ecologic variable misclassified. Thus, the resulting bias may be understood in terms of misclassification bias operating at the individual level. Künzli and Tager (1997) have labeled this type of design a "semi-individual study," which they have shown to yield more valid estimates of air-pollution effects than do pure ecologic studies (where no joint distributions are known).

OTHER PROBLEMS

Lack of Adequate Data

Certain types of data, such as medical histories, may not be available in aggregate form; or available data may be too crude, incomplete, or unreliable, such as sales data for measuring behaviors (Morgenstern, 1982; Walter, 1991b). In addition, secondary sources of data from different administrative areas or from different periods may not be comparable. For example, disease rates may vary across countries because of differences in disease classification or case detection. Furthermore, because many ecologic analyses are based on mortality rather than incidence data, causal inference is further limited because mortality reflects the course of disease as well as its occurrence (Kleinbaum et al., 1982).

Temporal Ambiguity

In a well-designed cohort study of disease incidence, we can usually be confident that disease occurrence did not precede the exposure. In ecologic studies, however, use of incidence data provides no such assurance against this temporal ambiguity (Morgenstern, 1982). The problem is most troublesome when the disease can influence exposure status in individuals (reverse causation) or when the disease rate can influence the mean exposure in groups (through the effect of population interventions designed to change exposure levels in areas with high disease rates).

The problem of temporal ambiguity in ecologic studies (especially time-trend studies) is further complicated by an unknown or variable induction and latent periods between exposure and disease detection (Gruchow et al., 1983; Walter, 1991b). The investigator can only attempt to deal with this problem in the analysis by examining associations for which there is a specified lag between observations of average exposure and disease rate. Unfortunately, there may be little prior information about induction and latency on which to base the lag, or appropriate data may not be available to accommodate the desired lag.

Collinearity

Another problem with ecologic analyses is that certain predictors, such as sociodemographic and environmental factors, tend to be more highly correlated with each other than they are at the individual level (Stavraky, 1976; Connor and Gillings, 1984). The implication of such collinearities is that it is very difficult to separate the effects of these variables statistically; analyses yield model coefficients with very large variances so effect estimates may be highly unstable. In general, collinearity is most problematic in multiple-group ecologic analyses involving a small number of large, heterogeneous regions (Duncan et al., 1961; Valkonen, 1969).

Migration across Groups

Migration of individuals into or out of the source population can produce selection bias in a study conducted at the individual level because migrants and nonmigrants may differ on both exposure prevalence and disease risk. Although it is clear that migration can also cause ecologic bias (Polissar, 1980; Kliewer, 1992), little is known about the magnitude of this bias or how it can be reduced in ecologic studies (Morgenstern and Thomas, 1993).

INTERPRETING ECOLOGIC ASSOCIATIONS

Knowing the severe methodologic limitations of ecologic analysis for making biologic inferences, many epidemiologists who report ecologic results argue that there can be no cross-level bias when their primary objective is to estimate an ecologic effect (e.g., Centerwall, 1989; Casper et al., 1992; Stewart et al., 1994). For example, we might want to estimate the ecologic effect (effectiveness) of state laws requiring smoke detectors by comparing the fire-related mortality rate in those states with the law versus other states without the law (Morgenstern, 1982). Although this is a reasonable objective, the interpretation of observed ecologic effects is complicated by several issues.

First, outcome events (disease or death) occur in individuals; thus, the disease or mortality rate in a population is an aggregate, not a global, measure. Consequently, biologic inference may be implicit to the objectives of an ecologic study unless the underlying biologic and contextual effects are already known from previous research. Can smoke detectors placed appropriately in homes reduce the risk of fire-related mortality in those homes by providing an early warning of smoke? Does living in an area where most homes are properly equipped with smoke detectors reduce the risk of fire-related mortality in homes with and without smoke detectors? The first question refers to a possible biologic (individual) effect; the second question refers to a possible contextual effect. The ecologic effect of smoke-detector laws depends on these biologic and contextual effects as well as other factors, e.g., the level of enforcement, the quality of smoke-detector design and construction, the cost and availability of smoke detectors, and their proper placement, installation, operation, and maintenance. In an ecologic study without additional information, the ecologic effect completely confounds biologic and contextual effects (Firebaugh, 1978; Greenland, 2002b).

Another complicating issue in interpreting observed ecologic effects as contextual effects is that there may be a need to control for confounders measured at the individual level (Greenland, 2001a, 2004b). Even if the exposure is a global measure, such as a law, groups are seldom completely homogeneous or comparable with respect to confounders. To make a valid comparison between states with and without smoke-detector laws, for example, we would need to control for differences among states in the joint distribution of extraneous risk factors, such as socioeconomic status of residents, firefighter availability and access, building design and construction.

When contextual effects are of interest, rarely are the available ecologic data grouped in a way that is closely relevant to the effect of interest. Typical vital statistics data on disease occurrence are aggregated by county or another convenient geopolitical unit, which may be far too coarse to allow valid estimation of small-area effects, e.g., at the neighborhood level. Unfortunately, ecologic associations can be extremely sensitive to the grouping level, making claims about relations seen at one level dubious when applied to another level of interest (Openshaw and Taylor, 1981; Greenland, 2001a, 2002b, 2004b).

MULTILEVEL ANALYSES AND DESIGNS

One solution to the problem of separating individual and contextual effects is to incorporate both individual-level and ecologic measures in the same analysis. This approach might include different measures of the same factor; e.g., each subject would be characterized by his or her own exposure level as well as the average exposure level for all members of the group to which he or she belongs (aggregate measure). Not only would this approach help to clarify the sources and magnitude of ecologic and cross-level bias, it would also allow us to separate biologic, contextual, and ecologic effects. It is especially appropriate in social epidemiology, infectious-disease epidemiology, and the evaluation of population interventions.

There are various statistical methods for including both individual-level and ecologic measures in the same analysis; two related methods are discussed here. The first method, often called *contextual analysis* in the social sciences, is a simple extension of conventional (generalized linear) modeling such as multiple linear regression and logistic regression (Boyd and Iversen, 1979; Iversen, 1991). The model, which is fitted to the data at the individual level, includes both individual-level and ecologic predictors. For example, suppose we want to estimate the effect of "herd immunity" on the risk of an infectious disease. The risk (y) of disease might be modeled as a function of the following linear component: $b_0 + b_1x + b_2X + b_3xX$, where x is the individual's immunity status and X is the prevalence of immunity in the group to which that individual belongs (Von Korff et al., 1992). Therefore, b_2 represents the contextual effect of herd immunity, and b_3 represents the interaction effect, which allows the herd-immunity effect to depend on the individual's immune status. The interaction term is needed in this application because we expect no herd-immunity effect among immune individuals. Note, however, that the interpretation of the interaction effect depends on the form of the model (see Chapter 20).

An important limitation of contextual analysis is that outcomes of individuals within groups are treated as independent. In practice, however, the outcomes of two individuals are more likely to be similar if they come from the same group (region) than if they come from different groups, because individuals in the same group tend to share risk factors for the outcome. Ignoring such within-group dependence ("clustering") generally results in estimated variances of contextual effects that are biased downward, making confidence intervals too narrow. To handle this problem of within-group dependence, we can add random effects to the conventional (contextual) model described earlier; this approach is called *mixed-effects modeling, multilevel modeling,* or *hierarchical regression* (Wong and Mason, 1985, 1991; Bryk and Raudenbush, 1992; Goldstein, 2003; Kreft and de Leeuw, 1998; Banerjee et al., 2004; Wakefield, 2004; and see Chapter 21).

Multilevel modeling is a powerful technique with many potential applications and statistical benefits (Greenland, 2000c, 2000d; Witte et al., 2000). It can be used to estimate contextual and ecologic effects and to derive improved (empirical-Bayes) estimates of individual-level effects. It can also be used to determine how much of the difference in outcome rates across groups (ecologic effect) can be explained by differences in the distribution of individual-level risk factors (biologic effects). For example, a two-level analysis is often used to examine individual-level and ecologic predictors. At the first level of analysis, we might predict individual risk or health status within each group as a function of several individual-level variables. At the second (ecologic) level, we predict the estimated regression parameters (e.g., the intercept and slopes) from the first level as a function of several ecologic variables. The underlying assumption is that the group-specific regression parameters are random samples from a population of such parameters. By combining results from both levels, we can predict individual-level outcome as a function of individual-level predictors, ecologic predictors, and their interaction terms.

For example, Humphreys and Carr-Hill (1991) used multilevel modeling to estimate the contextual effect of living in a poor area (electoral ward) on several health outcomes, controlling for the individual's income and other covariates. In a conventional ecologic analysis, the effects of living in a poor area and personal income would be confounded, and ecologic estimates of effect would be susceptible to cross-level bias. Similar findings for the effects of "neighborhood" socioeconomic status have been reported recently by several other investigators (Pickett and Pearl, 2001).

Despite many new insights generated by multilevel analysis about the social determinants of disease and health, this approach for analyzing observational data also poses new challenges. First, because there are many selection factors influencing the distribution of people among neighborhoods, it is difficult to control for these factors by covariate adjustment at the individual level. Thus, estimated effects of neighborhood (ecologic) factors, especially aggregate measures, may be confounded by unmeasured risk factors (Oakes, 2004). Second, it is often difficult to distinguish *a priori* whether a given individual-level risk factor affects the ecologic exposure of interest and is therefore a confounder that should be controlled, or whether the risk factor is an intermediate variable in the hypothesized causal pathway between the ecologic exposure and disease occurrence and therefore should not be controlled (Diez Roux, 1998, 2004). Third, estimated ecologic and contextual effects may be severely distorted when population interventions (related to the ecologic factor) are implemented in those groups with high outcome rates (reverse causation). Fourth, the ecologic units used in most multilevel analysis are administrative areas (e.g., census tracks), which may not correspond to relevant social contexts for estimating neighborhood effects (Diez Roux, 1998; Greenland, 2001a). Fifth, an assumption of most multilevel analyses, based on individual surveys, is that exposure and covariate distributions are stable over time, and this assumption will be suspect when important trends are known to exist (Greenland, 2001a). Sixth, to the extent that neighborhood characteristics (context) are determined (endogenously) by aggregating characteristics of individuals within neighborhoods, and not by global (exogenous) interventions, causal (counterfactual) interpretations of contextual and individual effects are problematic (especially when the neighborhoods are small), because we cannot change an individual's exposure status, holding constant the mean exposure status (context) of the neighborhood in which that individual resides—i.e., individual and contextual effects are not identifiable (Greenland, 2002b; Oakes, 2004).

Multilevel analysis can be extended to more than two levels. For example, we might want to predict certain health outcomes in nursing home residents as a function of characteristics of the residents (e.g., age and health status), their physicians (e.g., type of specialty and country of medical training), and the nursing homes (e.g., size and doctor-to-patient ratio). In this type of analysis, residents are grouped by their physician (who might provide care to many residents in one home) and by their nursing home affiliation.

The simplest design for generating multilevel analyses is a single survey of a population that is large and diverse enough so that multiple groups (e.g., counties or ethnic groups) can be defined for ecologic measurement and analysis. In addition to environmental and global variables for regions or organizations, ecologic measures are derived by aggregating all subjects in each group. An alternative, more efficient, approach is a *multilevel* or *hybrid design* in which a two-stage sampling scheme is used first to select groups (stage 1), followed by the selection of individuals within groups (stage 2) (Humphreys and Carr-Hill, 1991; Navidi et al., 1994; Wakefield, 2004). A hybrid design might involve conducting a conventional multiple-group ecologic study by linking different data sources, then obtaining supplemental data from individuals sampled randomly from each group. For example, by estimating the exposure–covariate association in each subsample, this approach can be used to improve the control of confounders in an ecologic analysis (Prentice and Sheppard, 1989, 1995; Navidi et al., 1994; Plummer and Clayton, 1996; Guthrie and Sheppard, 2001; Wakefield and Salway, 2001; Wakefield, 2004). A variation of this hybrid design might involve a case-control study as the second stage. Cases would be identified in the first (ecologic) stage, and controls would be matched to cases on group affiliation and possibly other factors.

CONCLUSION

There are several practical advantages of ecologic studies that make them especially appealing for doing various types of epidemiologic research. Despite these advantages, however, ecologic analysis poses major problems of interpretation when making ecologic inferences and especially when making biologic inferences (because of ecologic bias, etc.). From a methodologic perspective, it is best to have individual-level data on as many relevant nonglobal measures as possible. Just because the exposure variable is measured ecologically, for example, does not mean that other variables should be as well. The accuracy of effect estimates from ecologic studies can often be improved by obtaining additional data on the within-group associations between covariates, between the exposure and covariates, or between the disease and covariates, and by incorporating prior information.

Several epidemiologists have recently called for greater emphasis on understanding differences in health status between populations—a return to a public-health orientation, in contrast to the individual (reductionist) orientation of modern epidemiology (Rose, 1985; Krieger, 1994; Link and Phelan, 1995; McMichael, 1995; Pearce, 1996; Susser and Susser, 1996; Schwartz and Carpenter, 1999). This recommendation represents an important challenge for the future of epidemiology, but it cannot be met simply by conducting ecologic studies. Multiple levels of measurement and analysis are needed, and additional methodologic and conceptual issues must be addressed

(Greenland, 2001a). Even when the purpose of the study is to estimate ecologic effects, individual-level information is often essential for drawing valid inferences about these effects. Thus, to address the underlying research questions, we typically want to estimate and control for biologic and contextual effects, preferably using multilevel analysis. In contemporary epidemiology, the "ecologic fallacy" reflects the failure of the investigator to recognize the need for biologic inference and thus for individual-level data. This need arises even when the primary exposure of interest is an ecologic measure and the outcome of interest is the health status of entire populations.

CHAPTER 26

Social Epidemiology

Jay S. Kaufman

Causation and Confounding in Social Epidemiology 533
Exposure and Covariate Assessment in Social Epidemiology 534
Social Factors Defined and Measured at the Individual Level 534
Social Factors Defined and Measured at the Aggregate Level 538
Analytic Approaches 542
Multilevel Modeling 542
Marginal Models 544
Effect Decomposition 545
Life-Course SES Concepts 546
Experiments and Quasi-Experiments 547
Narrative Historical Approach 548

Social epidemiology is the study of relations between social factors and disease in populations. It may be broadly interpreted to subsume differential occurrence of any risk factor or health outcome across groups categorized according to any of a number of socially defined dimensions. Primary among the axes of social distinction in contemporary Western societies are race/ethnicity, gender, and socioeconomic class/position (Krieger et al., 1993; Lynch and Kaplan, 2000). Social epidemiology therefore embraces a large number of questions about exposures and outcomes, and indeed one might question whether there is any epidemiology that is *not* social epidemiology. The practical distinction appears to be that social epidemiology is characterized by explicit inclusion of social, economic, or cultural quantities in the exposure definition or the analytic model, or by explicit reference to social science theory in the interpretation. Therefore, any exposure–disease relation can be studied from the point of view of social epidemiology to the extent that the relation is modeled in light of social variation in the quantities under study, or interpreted in the context of a social theory or sociohistorical paradigm such as "social stratification," "urbanization," or "colonialism."

There are two distinct types of general epidemiologic activity, both well represented in the social epidemiologic literature: surveillance and etiologic inference. In surveillance, we merely seek to describe accurately what the world looks like (see Chapter 22). A typical social epidemiologic example describes the racial and social class distribution of coronary disease (Barnett et al., 1999). Although we often seek to generalize beyond our observed sample, the purpose is entirely descriptive. The focus is on occurrence of an outcome, perhaps in relation to a scaled axis—such as time, age, or social class—but without regard to a specific exposure. The epidemiologic quantity of interest is generally an occurrence measure itself, such as prevalence or incidence, rather than a causal effect.

The second class of epidemiologic activity is etiologic inference, in which we seek to understand the *causal* relation between a defined exposure and outcome. This activity is designed not to describe the world as it exists, but rather how it would change under some defined, generally hypothetical, intervention (Greenland, 2002a, 2005a; see Chapter 4). A typical social epidemiologic example estimates the causal effect of changes in wealth on risk of mortality in the elderly (Kington and Smith,

1997; Adams et al., 2003). Despite the many philosophic and methodologic dilemmas associated with causal inference, etiologic investigations constitute the bulk of published epidemiologic work. This result follows naturally from the fact that epidemiology is situated within the larger domain of public health, a disciplinary identity that fixes intervention as the primary focus of epidemiologic research (Breslow, 1998).

CAUSATION AND CONFOUNDING IN SOCIAL EPIDEMIOLOGY

Because a causal effect is defined on the basis of contrasts between potential outcomes under different intervention regimens, many authors argue that we must immediately exclude nonmanipulable factors, such as individual race/ethnicity and gender, from consideration as causes in this sense (Holland, 1986; Kaufman and Cooper, 1999). This conclusion does not imply that a construct such as race/ethnicity is not a valid focus of social epidemiologic research, only that the study design and analytic approach must correspond to a substantively meaningful conceptualization of the exposure and of the hypothesized intervention. For example, the effect of a patient's racial/ethnic classification on a clinician's diagnostic judgment is a well-defined causal quantity because the exposure can be physically manipulated in a real or imagined experiment (e.g., Loring and Powell, 1988; Schulman et al., 1999). In contrast, the effect of a patient's racial/ethnic classification on that same patient's risk of incident coronary disease is not a well-defined causal quantity in this sense and therefore has no obvious implications for intervention. Nonetheless, nonmanipulable quantities such as individual race/ethnicity and gender can be employed sensibly as stratification variables or effect-measure modifiers (Holland, 2001) or may be adjusted for as confounders in order to reduce error in the estimated exposure effects of interest (Kaufman and Cooper, 2001).

Common modifiable exposures of interest in social epidemiology include factors such as income, education, and housing quality. Although these exposures usually result from complex interactions of social stratification and individual volition, they are potentially modified through public policy via governmental programs of income supplementation, educational loans, and housing assistance. Etiologic interest then lies in the contrast between outcome distributions under various intervention regimens that fix the level (or distribution) of the exposure in the target population (Maldonado and Greenland, 2002). For example, consider binary outcome $Y = 1$, defined as an incident asthma attack within the period of observation, and the social exposure of interest, defined as residence in privately owned housing ($X = 1$) versus residence in a public housing project ($X = 0$) during a defined exposure period (a simple generalization would allow X to represent the proportion of the population assigned to privately owned housing, rather than just the extremes of 1 and 0). One causal effect of housing type on asthma would be the contrast (e.g., difference, ratio) between the average risks of an asthma attack in the target population during the specified time period if all households were assigned to public housing versus if all were assigned to private housing. In the notation of Chapter 21, the first risk would be $\Pr[Y = 1|\text{Set}(X = 1))$ and the second would be $\Pr(Y = 1|\text{Set}(X = 0)]$.

As discussed in Chapter 4, confounding arises when the association measure in the source population, $\Pr(Y = 1|X = 1)$ versus $\Pr(Y = 1|X = 0)$, does not correspond to the effect measure that would be observed under hypothetical manipulations of the social exposure in that population, $\Pr[Y = 1|\text{Set}(X = 1)]$ versus $\Pr[Y = 1|\text{Set}(X = 0)]$. For example, the hypothesis of a causal relation between housing type and asthma attacks is plausible, but subject-matter knowledge suggests other influences on this health outcome from quantities—such as poverty—that also potentially influence residential housing type. This prior knowledge implies that some part of the empirical association observed between housing type and incident asthma attack may arise not from the causal link between them, but rather from their mutual response to other material or psychosocial manifestations of poverty. The crux of the problem in observational data is that we do not have the opportunity to carry out any "settings" of the population, and so we must employ the observed quantities in some way to estimate more validly the causal effect of interest.

One solution is to condition on measured aspects of poverty status. The logic behind this strategy is that within the categorizations of poverty (e.g., poor and nonpoor if poverty is dichotomous and homogeneous within categories), there can be no confounding by this quantity (Greenland and Morgenstern, 2001; see Chapter 15). To the extent that we have enumerated and accurately measured a sufficient set of common causes of exposure and outcome, this conventional epidemiologic solution is adequate for the specification of the desired causal effect from observational data in point-exposure studies. Indeed, this strategy for the estimation of causal effects dominates epidemiologic analysis of observational data, and has enjoyed some success. For social exposures, however, the prospects are not always as hopeful, because the enumeration and accurate measurement of common causes for multifactorial disease outcomes and complex behaviors such as residential housing choices is a daunting task. Behaviors with dominating economic and social inputs have often proven quite difficult to model in the social sciences (McKim and Turner, 1997). Even if we know all the factors that determine where a person would choose to live, the task of obtaining accurate measures of these many variables in a real dataset is formidable. For example, one must decide on some measurable characterization of "poverty" in the preceding example, by obtaining reported information on a limited number of material factors considered likely to influence both housing type and exposure to other causes of an asthma attack.

EXPOSURE AND COVARIATE ASSESSMENT IN SOCIAL EPIDEMIOLOGY

Social epidemiology is characterized primarily by the nature of the exposures that are investigated, and techniques for defining and measuring exposures and covariates are therefore a major component of social epidemiologic methodology. Throughout the history of the subfield, measurement has involved a wide array of constructs. The majority of studies have considered exposures related in some way to the primary axes of social discrimination cited previously (race/ethnicity, gender, and social class/position), but many other studies have explored alternative quantities at the individual level, such as marital status, material deprivation, social support, or status incongruity. Additionally, many social epidemiologic exposures have also been defined at the aggregate level, including constructs such as social networks, economic inequality, social capital, and neighborhood deprivation. Not only have a staggering number of exposures been considered, many of these have in turn been defined and assessed in myriad different ways in different studies. Some representative and popular methodologic approaches are described in the following.

SOCIAL FACTORS DEFINED AND MEASURED AT THE INDIVIDUAL LEVEL

Race/Ethnicity

Racial/ethnic status is central to personal and social identity in many societies and serves as an important determinant of material and social status as well as influencing social networks, residential patterns, and behaviors. Although race and ethnicity are ostensibly designated in terms of ancestry and physical characteristics, the nature of these quantities as aspects of personal identity means that ultimately the "gold-standard" assessment is based on self-report (Kaufman, 1999). Although analysis of highly variable regions of DNA can apportion continental ancestry with considerable accuracy (Shriver et al, 1997), this quantity is not of social epidemiologic interest. The dominating influences on life chances and social status arise not from biologic ancestry, but rather from the racial/ethnic categorization recognized by others, and as a consequence, adopted by the individual as a foundation for social affiliation and self-definition.

The continual evolution of these categorizations and their administrative management is itself a methodologic morass (Williams, 1997). Epidemiologic studies in the United States have traditionally accepted the binary classification system of "white" and "black" that reflects the history of slavery and *de jure* segregation in these terms. More recently, categorization has generally followed definitions established for administrative purposes by the U.S. government for census data and other demographic monitoring (Office of Management and Budget, 1977, 1997). For the year 2000 U.S. census, respondents were for the first time permitted to report two or more racial identities, leading to 63 possible combinations of six basic racial categories: American Indian and Alaska Native, Asian, Black or African American, Native Hawaiian and Other Pacific Islander, White and "Some Other Race." In addition, individuals could define their ethnicity as Hispanic or Non-Hispanic (Mays and Ponce, 2003).

Sex/Gender

As in the case of race/ethnicity, gender serves as an important determinant of social, environmental, and material circumstances in all human societies and is therefore a key quantity in any social epidemiologic analysis as a covariate, effect-measure modifier, or stratification variable. Although gender is the social realization of biologic sex, which is ostensibly designated in terms of genotypic and phenotypic traits, its social implications are highly dependent on culture and therefore vary substantially with time and place (Krieger, 2003). Nonetheless, common practice for assessment of gender is self-report into a binary categorization, although recent decades have witnessed the increasing tendency to refer to this quantity more accurately as "gender" as opposed to "sex." Both theoretical work and increased awareness of substantial natural variability in physiology and behavior have also led to growing recognition that this strict dichotomy is a convenient fiction originating in historical convention (Dreger, 1998).

Educational Attainment

Level of achieved education is one of the oldest and most commonly used social epidemiologic quantities and has the practical advantages of having a naturally ordered scaling and a value that is often fixed early in adult life and reported consistently. The widespread use of this quantity also derives from its presence in a great variety of administrative databases and other common data sources. Educational attainment also has substantive relevance as a mechanism for achievement of social position, as it facilitates advantageous behaviors and occupational advancement and is therefore highly predictive of income and wealth (Miech and Hauser, 2001).

Nonetheless, the variable also has several disadvantages, both practical and theoretical. Typical educational attainment and the economic and social benefits that accrue as a result have changed over time, so comparison between age cohorts or across geographic regions is difficult (Liberatos et al., 1988). Similar incommensurabilities also complicate comparisons across gender and racial/ethnic groups (Kaufman et al., 1997). There are also inherent discontinuities in the education scale corresponding to completion of degrees and certifications (Oakes and Kaufman, 2006, pp. 56–58). For example, completion of an additional year of high school beyond tenth grade may confer little social advantage, whereas completion of an additional year beyond eleventh grade may confer substantial advantage. This distinction leads some analysts to categorize education according to these milestones—for example, into three categories corresponding to less than, equal to, or greater than 12 years of education (i.e., the U.S. standard for a high school diploma). Given the uncertain connection between educational content and years of schooling, as well as the overriding socioeconomic significance of degree completion, the graded relationship that can be observed for many health outcomes with years of completed education may be interpreted as evidence of the endogenous assignment of years of schooling as a function of family resources and other personality and environmental factors (Bowles et al., 2004).

Annual Individual or Family Income

Annual individual income is a key variable in social epidemiologic analyses for the obvious reason that health is a commodity in market economies, and therefore financial resources are logically expected to have a causal effect on health outcomes. Income also functions, like education, as a sensitive marker of social position and therefore as an indicator not only of financial resources but also of status and its social and material consequences, such as access to institutions and connections to individuals with power and influence (Oakes and Rossi, 2003). Unlike education, income is also fluid over time, and is therefore more responsive to changes in status over the life course. The fluid nature of annual income also presents an analytic challenge, however, especially for measuring the status and resources of the retired (Robert and House, 1996). It also makes income sensitive to "reverse causality"; whereas low income facilitates negative health transitions, it is also true that failing health lowers earnings (Smith, 1999). Indeed, the volatility of annual income itself has been an exposure of interest, under the hypothesis that drastic changes in financial resources, such as those associated with job loss or divorce, may be more salient for health outcomes (McDonough et al., 1997).

Measurement of income is often by self-report in surveys, although the data may also be drawn secondarily from administrative records (Rogot et al., 1992). For self-reported data, the data are often queried in broad categories in order to minimize respondent discomfort. Even so, item non-response for income is considerably higher than for education or occupation, with roughly 10% typically declining to answer (Liberatos et al., 1988). Use of empirical categories may limit the ability to compare studies if these categorization boundaries differ, but the implications of absolute income values are contextually dependent in any case, so comparison across populations may often be tenuous, even for studies with common categorizations. For statistical analysis, natural-log transformation of income is often warranted because of the rightward skew of the distribution, and the observation that effects on health outcomes appear more log-linear than linear (Backlund et al., 1996). Nonlinearity in this relation is intuitively reasonable, because income changes are inherently relative: A change of $1,000 has a much bigger effect on someone who is destitute than it does on a millionaire.

Because families tend to share both material resources and social prestige, it is common practice to assess not individual income, but rather household income (Oakes and Kaufman, 2006, pp. 58–60). This quantity could be construed to subsume all financial compensation received during the relevant period, including paid employment and value of employee benefits. Survey respondents may need to be specifically directed to consider less obvious sources of income, including Social Security payments, capital gains from sales of assets, interest and dividends received, receipt of rent payments, child support and alimony payments, and receipts from government aid programs. Measurement error can be substantial, and the error cannot be assumed to be uncorrelated with the true value (Pedace and Bates, 2001). The ascertained value may often be scaled to the number of people relying on the specified income, although "economies of scale" exist such that the accounting for family size might not involve a simple division (Buhmann et al., 1988).

A related concept is "poverty," a state of insufficient income to meet basic material needs. This designation is a dichotomization of household income on the basis of some assessment of what is a minimally sufficient quantity for sustaining the dependent individuals. The determination of this value has been controversial. In the United States it has relied heavily on a method devised in 1963 by an economist at the Social Security Administration (Fisher, 1992). This definition was revised in 1969 to allow the threshold to be linked to the Consumer Price Index, and has been subject to further incremental modifications in subsequent years. The definition accounts for household income, household size, and ages of individuals in the household, creating 48 distinct threshold values. Although many critics maintain that the definition remains inadequate, it has remained a fixture of government and public health statistics for four decades (Citro and Michael, 1995). In addition to modeling income as a continuous quantity or as a dichotomy at the poverty line, this definition also allows each income to be modeled in proportion to the poverty line with respect to the specific household size and composition, solving the problem of having to scale the income to the number of people supported. On the other hand, poverty thresholds remain undefined for many individuals outside of households, including those in prisons, nursing homes, college dormitories, and military barracks.

Household Wealth

Whereas income represents a flow of material resources to an individual or family, wealth represents the accumulated stock of these resources and therefore has relevance to health outcomes as both an indicator of achieved social position as well as a measure of the total resources that can be mobilized in the service of health and well-being. Lower levels of assets also make individuals and families vulnerable to income fluctuations, periods of unemployment that disrupt insurance coverage, and so forth. Incommensurabilities between income and wealth are particularly striking when comparing men and women, or when comparing racial/ethnic groups (Oliver and Shapiro, 1995). For example, models that contrast outcome risks between racial/ethnic groups while adjusting for income and education in order to control for social position leave the racial/ethnic contrast heavily confounded by wealth (Lynch and Kaplan, 2000; Kaufman et al., 1997).

Though traditionally absent from many health surveys, wealth data are now increasingly available, albeit often in the form of a few crude indicators. Whereas assets may exist in a variety of financial instruments (e.g., stocks, bonds, retirement accounts) and material repositories (e.g., home, vehicles, jewelry), the largest amount of wealth in the United States is held in the value of real estate and vehicles, comprising >50% of privately held assets in 2000 (Orzechowski and Sepielli, 2003). Therefore, questions as simple as "Do you own your home?" can be quite informative for distinguishing low from high asset levels. Surveys that query the home value are even more useful in this regard, although respondents are unlikely to distinguish between home value and equity actually held. An increasing proportion of personal wealth is held in individual retirement accounts, stocks, and mutual fund shares, but survey protocols for the accurate collection of these data are laborious and exist in only a few large health surveys. Where these have been analyzed with respect to health outcomes, however, they have been shown to be highly predictive of endpoints, even after conditioning on education and income and other socioeconomic covariates (e.g., Kington and Smith, 1997). Methodologic obstacles include the potential for substantial measurement error and item nonresponse, as well as the challenges posed by the large proportion of households with no assets, and the very extended right tail of the distributions. For example, median household assets for blacks and non-Hispanic whites in 2000 were $6,200 and $67,000, respectively, whereas mean household assets for the same two groups were $35,000 and $198,000 (Orzechowski and Sepielli, 2003).

Occupation/Unemployment

Another historically important indicator of social class or social position has been an individual's current employment status, occupation, or occupational class. These measures provide not only an indication of social prestige and the functional consequences of education and social connections, but also a direct reflection of the circumstances relevant to health through the physical and psychologic environment of the workplace itself (Oakes and Kaufman, 2006, pp. 49–56). Many countries, such as the United Kingdom, continue to base their standard socioeconomic position measure on occupational class, as opposed to the education and income measures that dominate in the United States. The British Registrar General's Scale, used for almost 100 years, was a hierarchy of six categories: Social Class I (professional), Social Class II (intermediate), Social Class III-NM (skilled nonmanual), Social Class III-M (skilled manual), Social Class IV (partly skilled), and Social Class V (unskilled) (Marmot et al., 1991). As of 2001, this schema has been revised to include eight categories, including a new category for the long-term unemployed, a subdivision of professionals into higher and lower managerial positions, and a change in terminology from "unskilled" to "routine" occupations (Elias et al., 2000).

Previously in the United States, occupational categories were commonly combined with achieved educational level or other socioeconomic quantities to generate a summary socioeconomic index. Various of these indices, such as the one developed by Hollingshead, experienced periods of popularity in sociology and epidemiology (Liberatos et al., 1988), although they are used to a much lesser extent in the contemporary epidemiologic literature. Among the most influential of these combined measures was the Duncan Socioeconomic Index (SEI), which required analysts to map all reported occupations onto U.S. census occupation score codes, a laborious and often frustrating task because of the ambiguity of many self-reported job descriptions (Hauser and Warren, 1997).

Like income, occupation and employment status can by dynamic throughout the life course, and therefore these measures share the advantages and disadvantages of this potential volatility, including the "reverse causality" of declining health leading to a diminution in occupational prestige. Occupation also shares the problem of incommensurability of prestige and remuneration across gender or racial/ethnic groups or across geographically distinct populations, as well as changes over time in the social and material significance of various occupations. Furthermore, occupational category is difficult to assign for individuals functioning outside of the wage economy, including unpaid domestic labor and those performing informal or illegal activities (Krieger et al., 1997).

One distinct conceptualization of occupation is as an indicator of economic relations between groups of people rather than as a measure of the characteristics of individuals considered in terms of a continuous social hierarchy. A contemporary operationalization of this approach is to categorize occupations in relation to the economic classes that define capitalist production (Wright, 1996). This entails collection of information about power relations in the workplace, as well as the assets that allow individuals to control their own production (e.g., in the case of craftspersons and artisans) or to control the process of production involving larger groups of workers in factories or office blocks.

Discrimination and Racism

Whereas dimensions of individual identity such as race/ethnicity, gender, and sexual orientation are not manipulable through public health interventions, the consequences of these categories as social labels are entirely malleable and therefore have causal meaning as exposures in the sense described previously (Kaufman and Cooper, 2001). The key distinction is that the causal quantity is not the identity of the individual per se, but rather the perception of this identity by others, and the role this perception plays in influencing the behavior of individuals and institutions that the person encounters. Differential behavior of individuals and the institutions on the basis of perceived social categorization is broadly described as "discrimination," including the forms of discrimination corresponding to specific dimensions of identity, such as "racism," "sexism," and so forth (Krieger, 1999).

Methodology for assessment of discrimination in surveys has most often focused on self-report of interpersonal affronts and experiences of perceived injustice (e.g., McNeilly et al., 1996). An obvious limitation of this approach is that discrimination need not be perceived by the respondent in order to be consequential, and indeed, structural and institutional discrimination may often be invisible to the individual. One innovation to achieve greater sensitivity in this regard is to query individuals not about their own experiences, but rather about the experiences faced by others who share their identity (Taylor et al., 1990).

Another approach is to use experimental or quasi-experimental designs to isolate the effect of perceived identity on the decision making of an individual or institutional process. For example, "audit studies" of medical or economic encounters, such as referral for surgical procedures or application for employment, involve comparison of cases matched (observationally or experimentally) on individual characteristics with the exception of social category of interest (usually race and/or gender) in order to isolate the causal effect of perceived group membership on the decision process (Yinger, 1986; Darity, 2003). When real subjects are matched on observed covariates, the possibility exists that imbalance persists in unmeasured attributes (Heckman, 1998). When actors are used in place of real subjects, or when case vignettes or medical charts or job applications are artificially created to be completely identical except for the group identifier, then the causal discrimination effect is directly identifiable (Blank et al., 2003).

SOCIAL FACTORS DEFINED AND MEASURED AT THE AGGREGATE LEVEL

A number of important quantities in social epidemiology are defined not at the individual or household level, but at the level of some larger aggregation, often neighborhoods, counties, states, or nations. Neighborhoods, in particular, have been of long-standing interest in social epidemiology (Kawachi and Berkman, 2003), despite the fact that no consensus on an operational definition for what constitutes a neighborhood has been achieved (O'Campo, 2003). Because of the frequent dependence on routine census data for characterizing aggregations of individuals, administrative boundaries such as census block groups and tracts in the United States (and census enumeration districts in the United Kingdom) are the most widely used proxies for neighborhood boundaries, even though the locations of these boundaries are generally unknown to the inhabitants.

Deprivation

Just as the material resources of individuals and households characterize their socioeconomic position, a neighborhood's material resources may be used to characterize the community's degree of deprivation. These material resources may be aggregates of individual-level data, such as the average income or average educational level, or they may be resources that are defined only at the neighborhood level, such as population density, the presence of health clinics or sidewalks, the prevalence of broken windows or graffiti, or the magnitude of some summary quantity such as "social disorganization" or "neighborhood efficacy" (Haan et al., 1987). When summary scores are created from a number of social variables, factor-analytic or latent-variable methods are often employed in order to find weights for the component quantities (Raudenbush and Sampson, 1999; Oakes and Kaufman, 2006, pp. 216–226). Several scales have been defined in the literature and have gained widespread use, such as the Townsend and Carstairs deprivation indices that were developed in the United Kingdom. The variables employed to characterize neighborhoods are most often those available from census and other administrative data, but direct observation of neighborhoods has also been employed in various studies in order to provide a richer assessment of the social and material environment (Caughy et al., 2001; Oakes and Kaufman, 2006, pp. 193–202).

Segregation

Residential segregation is a measure of the systematic physical arrangement of individuals with respect to some dimension of social identity, most often race/ethnicity, within communities or larger spatial units such as cities or counties (Oakes and Kaufman, 2006, pp. 169–192). Segregation emerges from a complex mix of factors, including voluntary choices and involuntary constraints such as discrimination in the housing market and economic barriers to mobility. Massey and Denton (1988) identified 20 statistical indices of residential segregation and grouped these into five distinct dimensions: evenness, exposure, concentration, centralization, and clustering.

Evenness is simply the degree to which a minority group is distributed uniformly over space and can be assessed statistically by the *dissimilarity index*:

$$\frac{\sum_{i=1}^{n}(t_i|p_i - P|)}{2TP(1-P)}$$

where n is the number of spatial units, t_i is the population of unit i, T is the total population of all spatial units combined, p_i is the proportion of unit i's population that is minority, and P is the proportion of the total population that is minority. The dissimilarity index therefore measures the percentage of the minority group's population that would have to change residence for each spatial unit to have the same percentage of that group as the population has overall, with the index ranging from 0 (no segregation) to 1 (complete segregation).

An alternative index of evenness is the Gini coefficient, which is the average absolute difference between minority-group proportions weighted across all pairs of spatial units, expressed as a proportion of the maximum weighted average difference:

$$\frac{\sum_{i=1}^{n}\sum_{j=1}^{n}\left(t_i t_j\left|p_i - p_j\right|\right)}{2T^2P(1-P)}$$

where i and j are indices for spatial units, and therefore the Gini coefficient also varies from 0 to 1. There are additional evenness measures, including Theil's entropy (or information index), and the Atkinson index (Iceland et al., 2002).

Exposure is the dimension of segregation that pertains to the extent of potential contact or interaction between members of diverse social groups. Evenness and exposure are correlated but distinct, because unlike evenness measures, exposure measures take into account the relative sizes of the groups being compared. The two measures of exposure that were identified by Massey and Denton (1988) represent the probability that a minority chosen at random will share a spatial unit with a majority person (interaction index) or another minority person (isolation index). When only two groups are considered, these two measures sum to unity.

Concentration describes the relative amount of physical space occupied by each social group. In considering two minority groups that have equal representation in the total population, the group that occupies the smaller physical space may be considered more highly segregated. Of the three concentration measures identified by Massey and Denton (1988), the oldest is Hoover's "delta," which represents the proportion of minorities in spatial units that have above-average density of minorities:

$$\frac{\sum_{i=1}^{n}|(x_i/X) - (a_i/A)|}{2}$$

where x_i is the minority group population and a_i is the land area in spatial unit i, and X is the total minority population and A is the total land area of all spatial units combined.

The fourth dimension of segregation is centralization, which refers to the location of the minority population with respect to the geographic center of the larger area under consideration. A relative measure of centralization represents the proportion of the minority population that would have to change spatial units in order to be distributed like the majority population, whereas an absolute measure of centralization considers the spatial distribution of the minority group alone, without reference to the distribution of the majority group. Both relative and absolute measures range from -1 to 1, with negative numbers indicating residence distant from the geographic center of the larger area and positive numbers indicating residence near the center. Some authors consider the centralization dimension to be increasingly irrelevant, as U.S. cities continue the trend of suburban growth and economic development, making a residential location that is close to or distant from the geographic center of the metropolitan area less significant.

Finally, clustering is the dimension of segregation that represents whether or not minorities live in contiguous spatial units. An absolute index of clustering measures the average number of minorities in adjacent spatial units as a proportion of the total denominator population of these units. Alternatively, a relative clustering measure compares the expected distance between any two minority individuals chosen at random with the expected distance between any two majority members chosen at random. Massey and Denton (1988) also propose "distance-decay interaction" and "distance-decay isolation" measures, which represent the probabilities that the person a minority next encounters is also member of the majority or minority group, respectively.

Inequality

Residential segregation is merely one dimension of inequality, but the differential distribution of social and material resources in the society may be considered along any of a number of other dimensions as well. Greatest interest has centered on economic inequality—for example, the unequal distribution in a population of income or wealth. A research agenda relating economic inequality to population health has been a primary focus of social epidemiologic activity for the last two decades (Lynch et al., 2004; Oakes and Kaufman, 2006, pp. 134–168), spurred in part by increasing levels of income and wealth inequality in industrialized societies since the 1970s. Whereas earlier papers focused on variation in income distribution between wealthy nations, the literature quickly expanded to include comparisons of smaller political entities such as states and provinces, as well as counties and metropolitan areas. These studies pursued a wide variety of health outcomes, with an emphasis on various measures of all-cause or cause-specific mortality risk. Most studies also adjusted for some measure of absolute wealth or poverty, such as per-capita income. This adjustment was motivated by the concern that if individuals with low incomes have higher risk of adverse outcomes and live disproportionately in areas with greater income inequality, then the causal effect of inequality may be confounded. This potential confounding has been described as a problem of disentangling the "compositional" from the "contextual" effects of income inequality, and has led in the last decade to widespread use of multilevel regression modeling in order to address this concern (Greenland, 2001a; Subramanian and Kawachi, 2004). Nonetheless, misspecification of the model (e.g., using linear regression though the true relationship is nonlinear) will still leave inequality and health outcomes associated, even if there is no true causal effect of inequality (Gravelle, 1998)

Several popular measures of income or wealth inequality are derived from the well-known curve introduced by Lorenz in 1905 (Cowell, 1995). To construct the Lorenz curve, rank-order the n individuals in the population according to the quantity of interest y—say, income—such that $y_1 \leq y_2 \leq y_3 \leq \ldots \leq y_n$, and pass through the population from smallest income value to largest value. The horizontal axis of the Lorenz curve measures the cumulative proportion of individuals passed at any point, $F(y)$, so it runs from 0 at the left to 1 at the right. The cumulative share of income accounted for by the ranked individuals, $\Phi(y)$, is similarly recorded on the vertical axis: as one reaches an income y_i while passing from left to right across the income values, the corresponding cumulative income proportion, p, held by the individuals to the left of y_i is plotted. The resulting graph of $F(y)$ versus $\Phi(y)$ is the Lorenz curve (Fig. 26–1). Because the individuals are rank-ordered, the curve must always lie along the 45° diagonal (in the case of perfect equality) or be strictly convex under the diagonal (if there is any inequality).

The Gini coefficient defined in the previous section is the most common inequality measure, and it has the attractive property of being the proportion of the area under the diagonal that is above the Lorenz curve. Therefore, when there is perfect equality, this area disappears, and the Gini coefficient is 0. When there is complete inequality (the richest unit y_n holds 100% of the income in the population), then 100% of the area under the diagonal is above the Lorenz curve, and the Gini coefficient equals unity. Despite its widespread use, the Gini coefficient has the notable disadvantage that it entails differential weighting of transfers that occur at various locations in the distribution. For example, a transfer of a fixed amount of income that occurs between a richer and a poorer individual has a much larger effect on the Gini coefficient if the two individuals are near the center of the rankings than if they are at the extremes.

A few other inequality measures have been applied in the social epidemiologic literature, including the Robin Hood index, Atkinson's index, and Thiel's entropy (Cowell, 1995). The Robin Hood

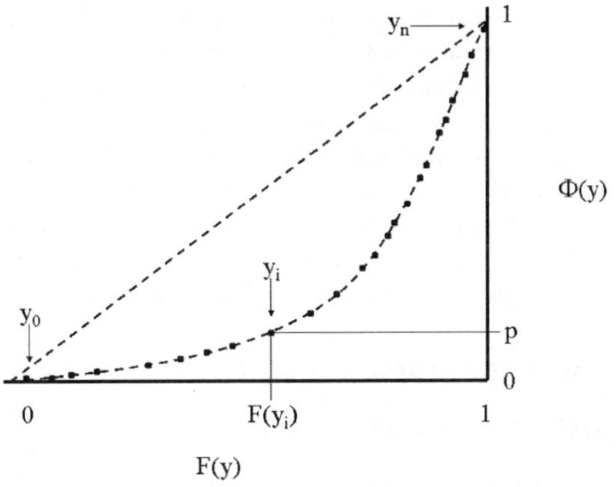

FIGURE 26–1 • The Lorenz Curve showing the cumulative share of income accounted for by ranked individuals.

index is the maximum vertical distance between the 45° diagonal representing perfect equality and the Lorenz curve. This can be interpreted as the proportion of the total income in the population that would have to be transferred from individuals above the mean to individuals below the mean in order to achieve equality in the distribution of incomes. Computation of Atkinson's index requires specification of a social-welfare constant representing the society's aversion to inequality, and therefore is perhaps less widely applied because of the difficulty in ascertaining this value. Theil's entropy index was introduced in the late 1960s and is based on information theory. Consider an individual's share of the total income $= s_i = y_i/n\overline{y}$. So, for example, if $s_i = 1/n$, everyone gets an equal share. Then Theil's inequality measure is

$$\sum\nolimits_{i=1}^{n} s_i \left[\ln(s_i) - \ln\left(\frac{1}{n}\right) \right] = \frac{1}{n} \sum\nolimits_{i=1}^{n} \frac{y_i}{\overline{y}} \ln\left(\frac{y_i}{\overline{y}}\right)$$

This index therefore has a range from 0 to ∞, with higher values representing greater entropy and thus a more equal distribution of income.

Social Capital

Another characteristic of a community, neighborhood, or other natural aggregation of individuals is the level of "social capital": the totality of social organization, including networks and relationships of trust and obligation that function to the mutual benefit or detriment of the inhabitants. This communitarian conceptualization, which dominates contemporary epidemiologic applications, is often attributed to work by Putnam, and contrasts with an alternate conceptualization attributed to Bourdieu that sees social capital primarily as an attribute of individuals (Portes, 2000). According to the dominant interpretation of social capital in public health research, bonding between individuals, and the bridging and linking of subgroups within the larger community, act to produce society-wide attributes of collective trust and result in an elevated level of functionality and cohesion. Commensurate with this viewpoint, the common measures of social capital in health research have involved measures of civic participation such as voting, or survey responses concerning the levels of membership in voluntary organizations and levels of reported "interpersonal trust" (Baum and Ziersch, 2003).

Closely linked to the concept of social capital is the study of social networks, which has established methodology within sociology and yet has been applied less consistently in public health research (Wasserman and Faust, 1994). This analytic approach adopts a view of social capital more heavily influenced by Coleman, focusing on social structure and exchange of material and information. Related concepts can be found in earlier work in psychosocial epidemiology around constructs such as "social support" and "instrumental support," based on scales summed from Likert-scale survey questions (Berkman, 1984). But in contrast to these earlier methods, analysis of social networks is at the aggregate level, considering the structure of the links between individuals in the population and how they function to transmit information, material assistance, or even infectious agents (Oakes and Kaufman, 2006, pp. 267–286). Networks are represented as directed arcs between nodes, which give rise to parameters such as density, centralization, and clustering (or segmentation), and facilitate statistical modeling for static or dynamic networks, such as decision-making structures, patterns of mutual assistance, or sexual relationship structures (Morris, 2004). Notably, social network analysis explicitly permits the potential responses of a unit to an exposure to depend on the treatments assigned to other units, thus allowing violations of the "stable-unit-treatment-value assumption" (Rubin, 1978, 1990a, 1991) used in most applications of potential-outcome models. Such analyses require significantly greater investment in data collection, but they are obviously much better suited to the task of providing realistic models of social phenomena than are the static, individually focused survey questions of past eras (Koopman and Lynch, 1999)

ANALYTIC APPROACHES

MULTILEVEL MODELING

Of the statistical innovations of the past decades, none has been more intimately tied to social epidemiology than multilevel regression modeling, also known as hierarchical regression (Chapter 21). This marriage of method and application arose in the early 1990s with roughly coincident revolutions in theory and technology. The theoretical revelation was that social epidemiology could not move forward without explicit accounting for hierarchical structures, a need articulated forcefully by Susser's metaphor of "Chinese boxes" (Susser and Susser, 1996). The "Chinese boxes" paradigm was intended to extend the traditional epidemiologic "black box" to encompass multiple and nested levels of organization, from the molecular to the individual to the societal. On the technology side, the innovation was the advent of regression methods for clustered data in popular statistical software, with rapid progress in the 1980s in the development and implementation of both random-coefficient and population-average models. Early work by Mason et al. (1983) introduced these methods to sociology, although it was another decade or more before they became common in social epidemiologic applications (O'Campo et al., 1997).

The term *multilevel model* is now used so broadly as to include any statistical technique that accommodates clustered data, but the random-coefficient model has become a common form in social epidemiologic applications (Subramanian and Kawachi, 2004; Oakes and Kaufman, 2006, pp. 316–340). The fundamental statistical dilemma is that epidemiologic analysts have come to rely heavily on regression methods to condition on multiple covariates without creating sparse cells. But standard model-fitting methods assume independent observations, an assumption that will be false under study designs such as cluster randomized trials or cohort studies with repeated measures, or when data are collected at several levels of a natural hierarchy, such as individuals within neighborhoods. If, after control of covariates, the cluster variable (such as neighborhood) still predicts the outcome, then an analysis that ignores this variable will produce biased variance estimates for estimated coefficients of neighborhood-level predictors, and therefore lead to invalid tests and intervals.

To illustrate the multilevel concept, consider continuous outcomes Y_{ij} for $i = 1, \ldots, n$ individuals living in $j = 1, \ldots, m$ neighborhoods, where Y is normally distributed within each neighborhood with mean β_{0j} and variance σ^2. The random-coefficient concept applied to the intercept (i.e., a random-intercept model) is to assume that the neighborhood-specific means β_{0j} can also be described by a random distribution of known form—for example, that they are normally distributed with mean γ_{00} and variance τ_{00}. These assumptions give rise to a two-level model:

$$Y_{ij} = \beta_{0j} + \varepsilon_{ij} \quad \text{(Level 1)}$$

$$\beta_{0j} = \gamma_{00} + \mu_{0j} \quad \text{(Level 2)}$$

where $\varepsilon_{ij} \sim N(0, \sigma^2)$, $\mu_{0j} \sim N(0, {\tau_{00}}^2)$, and $\text{COV}(\varepsilon_{ij}, \mu_{0j}) = 0$.

The combined model, replacing β_{0j} in Level 1 with its components from Level 2, is

$$Y_{ij} = \gamma_{00} + \mu_{0j} + \varepsilon_{ij}$$

which expresses each outcome as the sum of an individual deviation (ε_{ij}) and a neighborhood-specific deviation (μ_{0j}) from a grand mean (γ_{00}). This model is also known as a one-way random-effects ANOVA because it partitions variability into a component due to individuals and a component due to neighborhoods. The relative contribution of the variance components to the total variance may be represented by the intraclass (or intracluster) correlation coefficient, the proportion of the variability in Y that occurs between neighborhoods, rather than between individuals within neighborhoods:

$$\text{ICC} = \rho = \frac{\tau_{00}^2}{\sigma^2 + \tau_{00}^2}$$

(Bingenheimer and Raudenbush, 2004).

Multilevel models can be expanded to include fixed-coefficient and random-coefficient terms at the individual level, at the neighborhood level, or both. A fixed coefficient takes the same value for all neighborhoods. For example, the model

$$Y_{ij} = \beta_{0j} + \beta_1 X_{ij} + \varepsilon_{ij} \quad \text{(Level 1)}$$

$$\beta_{0j} = \gamma_{00} + \mu_{0j} \quad \text{and} \quad \beta_1 = \gamma_{10} \quad \text{(Level 2)}$$

implies that the expected change in Y per unit increase in X is $\beta_1$for all neighborhoods. A random coefficient for an individual-level covariate X, which allows a distribution of X effects rather than a single effect, could be modeled as

$$Y_{ij} = \beta_{0j} + \beta_{1j} X_{ij} + \varepsilon_{ij} \quad \text{(Level 1)}$$

$$\beta_{0j} = \gamma_{00} + \mu_{0j} \quad \text{and} \quad \beta_{1j} = \gamma_{10} + \mu_{1j} \quad \text{(Level 2)}$$

where $\mu_{0j} \sim N(0, \tau_{00})$, $\mu_{1j} \sim N(0, \tau_{11})$, and $\text{COV}(\mu_{0j}, \mu_{1j}) = \tau_{01}$.
One can also add neighborhood-level covariates to the Level 2 equations:

$$\beta_{0j} = \gamma_{00} + \gamma_{01} Z_j + \mu_{0j} \quad \text{and} \quad \beta_{1j} = \gamma_{10} + \gamma_{11} Z_j + \mu_{1j} \quad \text{(Level 2)}$$

This model implies cross-level product (interaction) terms between covariates X and Z, as well as a product between X and random effect μ_{1j}, as can be seen by replacing the coefficients in the Level 1 model with their equations in the Level 2 models to form a single combined equation:

$$\begin{aligned} Y_{ij} &= \gamma_{00} + \gamma_{01} Z_j + \mu_{0j} + (\gamma_{10} + \gamma_{11} Z_j + \mu_{1j}) X_{ij} + \varepsilon_{ij} \\ &= \gamma_{00} + \gamma_{01} Z_j + \gamma_{10} X_{ij} + \gamma_{11} Z_j X_{ij} + \mu_{1j} X_{ij} + \mu_{0j} + \varepsilon_{ij} \end{aligned}$$

Therefore, according to this model, the effect of X on the outcome Y in a given neighborhood j will depend on the level of Z in that neighborhood and on the random effect (Level 2 error term) μ_{1j}. For units with $Z = 0$, this random effect μ_{1j} is the deviation of the X effect in neighborhood j from the average X effect in all neighborhoods, γ_{10}. If only β_{0j} is treated as random, then the cross-level product involves only Z and X:

$$\begin{aligned} Y_{ij} &= \gamma_{00} + \gamma_{01} Z_j + \mu_{0j} + (\gamma_{10} + \gamma_{11} Z_j) X_{ij} + \varepsilon_{ij} \\ &= \gamma_{00} + \gamma_{01} Z_j + \gamma_{10} X_{ij} + \gamma_{11} Z_j X_{ij} + \mu_{0j} + \varepsilon_{ij} \end{aligned}$$

For example, for binary X, the expected difference between exposed ($X = 1$) and unexposed ($X = 0$) groups is $(\gamma_{10} + \gamma_{11} Z_j)$, and so depends on the value of Z in neighborhood j.

This framework may be applied to generalized linear modeling. For example, for binary Y_{ij}, the Level 1 model could be logistic while the Level 2 models could remain linear (see Chapter 21 for examples). More than two levels can be used, although applications with three or more levels are uncommon (Goldstein et al., 2002). Regardless of the model form or number of levels, however, a key point is that the regression coefficients in random-effects models represent within-cluster (i.e., cluster-conditional) relations. In this respect, their interpretation parallels those in stratified analysis and ordinary regression . For example, in the ordinary linear model $Y = \beta_0 + \beta_1 X + \beta_2 Z + \varepsilon$, the coefficient β_1 in the fitted model is interpreted as the expected change in Y per unit change in X, *holding Z fixed*. Similarly, in a model with a random effect such as μ_{0j} in $Y_{ij} = \gamma_{00} + \beta_1 X_{ij} + \mu_{0j} + \varepsilon_{ij}$, the interpretation of β_1 is similarly conditional on all other variables in the model held constant including μ_{0j}, a neighborhood-specific quantity that is not directly observable. Rearranging the model as $Y_{ij} = (\gamma_{00} + \mu_{0j}) + \beta_1 X_{ij} + \varepsilon_{ij}$, it can be more readily seen that within neighborhood

j, the regression of Y on X is linear with intercept $(\gamma_{00} + \mu_{0j})$ and X coefficient β_1. Note that this model assumes that the X coefficient is constant across neighborhoods. Considering the clusters as analysis strata, this assumption is just a regression version of the homogeneity (uniformity) assumption made by Mantel-Haenszel and other summary estimators discussed in Chapter 15. If we can interpret β_1 causally (and this requires absence of bias as well as correct specification of the model), this corresponds to assuming a uniform effect of X across clusters when effects are measured by estimated coefficients.

When a coefficient is treated as random, the cluster-specific estimates of effect are "shrunk" toward the mean value that corresponds to what would have been estimated had the coefficient been treated as fixed (Greenland, 2000d). For example, consider again the simplest model with a random intercept, $Y_{ij} = \gamma_{00} + \mu_{0j} + \varepsilon_{ij}$. We observe neighborhood-specific sample means $\widehat{\beta_{0j}} = \overline{Y}_j$, as well as the observed marginal (total) sample mean $\widehat{\gamma_{00}} = \overline{Y}$. In a valid cohort study, the neighborhood-specific sample means are unbiased estimates of the population values of β_{0j}, but fitting the random-intercept model instead produces estimates that are biased by being "shrunk" toward the grand sample mean $\widehat{\gamma_{00}} = \overline{Y}$. The extent to which they are shrunk is a function of their precision: A neighborhood with many observations has a stable estimate of its mean and therefore takes a value close to $\widehat{\beta_{0j}} = \overline{Y}_j$, whereas a neighborhood with fewer observations has an unstable estimate of its population mean and therefore takes a value close to $\widehat{\gamma_{00}} = \overline{Y}$. The inverse-variance weighted average of these two values produces estimates that minimize mean-squared error (between the estimates and population means), and are also known as empirical-Bayes estimates.

Frequently, the application of multilevel models in social epidemiology is oriented around the random-effects ANOVA interpretation, partitioning the variance that is due to community-level factors (contextual effects) from that due to individual-level factors (compositional effects). For example, the test of the null hypothesis that $\tau_{00}^2 = 0$, and thus that ICC $= 0$, is generally taken as evidence that the differences in outcome means observed between communities are accounted for by the covariates included in the model. This focus creates technical difficulties because τ_{00}^2 cannot be negative (Self and Liang, 1987). There is also the more fundamental problem that omitted covariates can account for residual variability at either level. For example, there can be large effects of neighborhood characteristics even when ICC is small (Bingenheimer and Raudenbush, 2004). Furthermore, if ICC > 0 even after inclusion of individual-level characteristics, there is no logical way to assert that the residual between-neighborhood variability is therefore contextual in nature (i.e., due to omitted neighborhood-level factors). Assertions of contextual effects should therefore be based on the estimated coefficients of measured neighborhood-level variables, rather than on variability that remains after individual-level variables have been included in the model (Oakes, 2004).

An important assumption of the multilevel model that is necessary for causal interpretation of the estimated coefficients is that there is no residual correlation between individual-level predictors and neighborhood-level random effects (i.e., Level 2 error terms), essentially an assumption of no-residual confounding. Interestingly, while concern over the validity of this assumption has preoccupied economists for decades (e.g., Hausman and Taylor, 1981), it receives considerably less attention in biostatistics and epidemiology. Econometricians generally test for violations of this assumption with a specification test due to Hausmann (Greene, 2003, pp. 301–303), and revert to a fixed-effects analysis if there is evidence of such a violation. The null hypothesis of this test is that there is no residual correlation between exposures and random effects. Under the null, both random-effects and fixed-effects models will be unbiased, but random-effects estimates will be more efficient (i.e., have smaller standard errors). If the null is false, however, then only the fixed-effects estimates remain unbiased and may be preferred despite their greater cost in terms of degrees of freedom.

MARGINAL MODELS

The models described so far exhibit the relation of Y to covariates among subjects *within* clusters and hence are sometimes called "subject-specific" or "cluster-specific" models. A different class of models, marginal models, describes the change in the mean of Y *across* clusters, and hence they are often described as "population-average" models. Instead of entering cluster effects as random terms, these models account for cluster effects by introducing parameters for within-cluster correlations, and by using a fitting method (generalized estimating equations, or GEE) that allows for these correlations. This method is available in major software packages (Diggle et al., 2002, pp. 70–80). Marginal models can be viewed as multilevel insofar as they permit inclusion of predictors from both levels of aggregation. Unlike within-cluster models, however, they do not directly model distributions of effects across clusters.

Suppose there are neighborhood effects beyond those captured by the modeled covariates, and one fits a model for the outcome that is neither linear nor log-linear (e.g., a logistic regression model). In this case, the parameters and hence estimates from marginal models will tend to differ from the corresponding parameters and estimates from within-cluster models, especially if the outcome Y is binary with $Y = 1$ common (Diggle et al., 2002, p. 131–137). The difference between the within-cluster and population-average parameters is just a general case of the noncollapsibility phenomenon for odds ratios illustrated in Chapter 4, and like that phenomenon it can lead to great confusion of interpretation and usage. The choice of approach should follow from consideration of the causal question at hand, however. Within-cluster models are suitable for estimating the effect on Y of changes in X within clusters, albeit they may assume that those effects are homogeneous across clusters. In contrast, marginal models are suitable for estimating the effect on Y of a change in X in the total population (i.e., the effect on the mean of Y of a unit change in X over all clusters), conditional on other covariates in the model. In this respect, marginal models are just generalizations of standardization (Sato and Matsuyama, 2003; see Chapter 21).

EFFECT DECOMPOSITION

A common analytic strategy in social epidemiology is the decomposition of effects by contrasting two adjusted effect estimates for the social exposure of interest: an estimate adjusted for potential confounders; and an estimate adjusted for the same set of potential confounders plus one or more additional variables hypothesized to be causal intermediates (i.e., to lie on pathway(s) through which the exposure exerts its effect). This contrast is then typically used to distinguish the exposure's *indirect* effect, through the specified intermediate variables, from its *direct* effect, transmitted via pathways that do not involve the specified intermediate variables (Fig. 26–2). If control of hypothetical causal intermediates greatly attenuates an exposure's estimated effect, it is usually inferred that the exposure's effect is mediated primarily through pathways involving these quantities; a small degree of attenuation is interpreted as evidence that other pathways predominate (Szklo and Nieto, 2000, pp. 184–187).

Recent work on the formal definitions of direct and indirect effects in a potential response framework casts some considerable suspicion on this approach, however (Robins and Greenland, 1992). One problem (described in Chapter 12) is that adjustment for an intermediate may introduce confounding where none existed before. Another problem is that direct effects need not be smaller in magnitude than total effects. Consider the simple example of a binary outcome of homelessness ($Y = 1$) for a young man as a function of education (high school dropout = 1; high school diploma = 0) and employment status ($Z = 1$ if unemployed; $Z = 0$ otherwise). We wish to consider the proportion of the total effect of dropping out of high school on homelessness that is due to the effect of dropping out on unemployment (often expressed as the extent to which unemployment "mediates" the education effect on homelessness). This task involves the decomposition of the total effect of X into that portion that is direct and that portion that is indirect (i.e., relayed through Z) (Fig. 26–2).

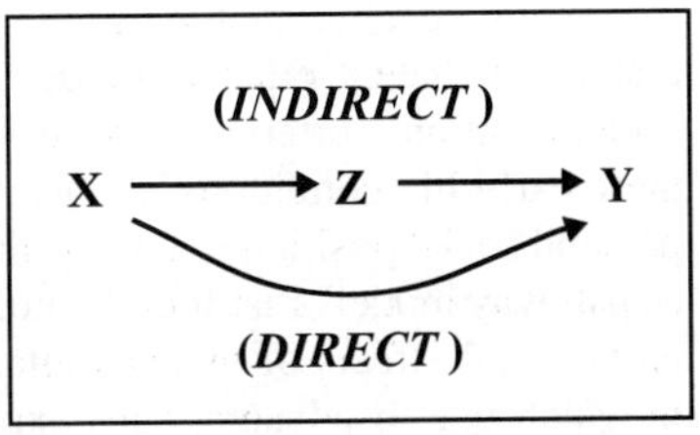

FIGURE 26–2 • A causal graph showing an indirect effect of X and Y, relayed through specified intermediate Z, and a direct effect of X and Y.

Now suppose that we have a population of young men who all have the same set of potential responses to interventions that encourage completion of high school education, or that facilitate employment through training or job placement: (a) whether induced to finish high school or not, they will become unemployed ($Z = 1$) if there is no intervention to provide training or job placement; (b) whether induced to finish high school or not, if denied employment ($Z = 1$) they will become homeless ($Y = 1$); and (c) if helped to become employed (by providing training and job placement) ($Z = 0$), then they will not become homeless ($Y = 0$) if they were induced to finish high school ($X = 1$), but they will become homeless ($Y = 1$) if they were not induced to finish high school ($X = 0$). In this population, therefore, the total effect of X is $\Pr[Y = 1|\text{ Set}(X = 1)] - \Pr[Y = 1|\text{Set}(X = 0)] = (1 - 1) = 0$. However, the direct effect in the employed stratum ($Z = 0$) is $\Pr[Y = 1|\text{Set}(X = 1, Z = 0)] - \Pr[Y = 1|\text{Set}(X = 0, Z = 0)] = (1 - 0) = 1$. The notion of partitioning the total effect into its constituent direct and indirect pathways is therefore deficient, because the null effect in this case must supposedly be partitioned into two parts, one of which is positive and the other null (Kaufman et al., 2004).

Effect decomposition is borrowed from the social sciences, where it has served as a foundation for path analysis and structural-equations modeling. The problem illustrated above arises when applying this method outside the models used by the original developers. Specifically, decomposition is interpretable when there is no additive-scale interaction between the exposure and the intermediate (i.e., when there is homogeneity of the risk difference in strata of Z), and when linear effect models are employed, such as linear structural equations models. The practice in social epidemiology of applying this approach to ratio measures of effect and over heterogeneous intermediate-stratum-specific effects, however, is not reliably valid.

Background knowledge is often available to investigators, and this should be used in order to specify structural models of socioeconomic exposures (Kaufman and Kaufman, 2001). When identifiable from the specified structure, both total and controlled direct effects of exposure on an additive scale may be estimated (Pearl, 2000, pp. 163–165). The preceding counterexample cautions against considering the ratio between the controlled direct and total effects as the "proportion explained" by the specified intermediate. Likewise, their difference is not generally the indirect effect, except in the narrowly defined conditions listed above. Rather, the controlled direct effect is the average causal effect obtained by setting the target population to different exposure states while at the same time holding the intermediate fixed at a specified value. Unless these stratum-specific direct effects are assumed to be homogeneous, the value at which the intermediate is to be fixed must also be specified, because there may be as many controlled direct effects as there are strata of the intermediate (Petersen et al., 2006).

LIFE-COURSE SES CONCEPTS

Another key social epidemiologic concept that has evolved rapidly over the last decade is the life-course model, which seeks to account for the dynamic trajectory of social exposures over the lifetime of the individual, rather than the simple cross-sectional association between adult social status and adult health that is so often modeled (Kuh et al., 2004). Interest in this model was spurred by accumulating evidence of social conditions in early life having an effect on adult risk for chronic disease, as posited, for example, by Barker's hypothesis, which suggests that deprivation during the fetal or infant periods of life "programs" the individual to a higher level of susceptibility to cardiovascular and metabolic diseases in adulthood (Barker, 1992). The life-course model soon expanded, however, to include not just a consideration of perinatal and adult conditions, but combinations, accumulation, and interactions of different conditions and experiences throughout all phases of life.

Several specific analytic models to address life-course effects have been described in the literature. A "latent effects" model focuses on early-life social exposures—for example, parental social position—often with control for adult social status, in order to estimate the direct effect of these early life conditions on later outcomes (i.e., ignoring the indirect effect that occurs because parental social position is a determinant of offspring's social position). Another conceptualization is a "pathway model" that focuses not merely on the direct effects of early-life deprivation, but rather on the total effects of this advantage by precipitating a "social chain of risk" or "life trajectory" in which one disadvantageous exposure predisposes to another through the life course (Marmot and Wilkinson, 1999). Sometimes this "life trajectory" total effect is modeled through a "social mobility model" in which the analysis considers contrasting patterns of upward or downward social movement, such as the contrast between those who are at a lower category of social position at each measured point in the life course contrasted with those who rose from a lower category to a higher category, or alternatively from a higher category to a lower category. This analytic design allows the consideration of health selection (i.e., sick individuals declining in their social position as a consequence of their illness) and of interaction between time points, such as in Forsdahl's hypothesis that the joint exposure to early-life deprivation and adult overnutrition is a particularly potent determinant of cardiovascular disease (Forsdahl, 1978). The "social mobility" model may be contrasted with a "cumulative model" that, like the "pathway model" described above, considers the total cumulative effect of deprivation throughout the life course, without regard to critical periods or specific patterns of mobility (Stansfeld and Marmot, 2002).

EXPERIMENTS AND QUASI-EXPERIMENTS

Given the potential for strong confounding in observational social epidemiology, it is natural to consider randomization study designs. A number of successful randomized social interventions have been conducted and reported, such as the Moving To Opportunity (MTO) study, in which residents in poverty housing were randomly assigned to receive vouchers for nonpoverty housing (Leventhal and Brooks-Gunn, 2003). Researchers may reap the benefits of randomization through a variety of designs other than traditional controlled experiments, however. For example, investigators may take advantage of a random assignment that is predictive of the exposure, even when the exposure of interest has not been randomly assigned. Hearst and colleagues used such an approach to estimate the effect of military service during the Vietnam War era on veterans' mortality in the postwar period, avoiding the selection bias associated with unmeasured determinants of service by capitalizing on the fact that birth dates were randomly selected in a lottery in order to determine draft eligibility (Hearst et al., 1986). This technique is referred to as "instrumental variable analysis" and has a long tradition in econometrics (Oakes and Kaufman, 2006, pp. 429–460; see Chapter 12). In other examples, investigators were able to find data in which nature had been so kind as to assign the exposure of interest in an essentially random fashion, as when Costello et al. tested competing theories of social causation versus social selection in the etiology of child psychopathology by making use of a fortuitous financial windfall that affected a portion of the children in a longitudinal study (Costello et al., 2003).

As discussed in Chapter 6, a primary weakness of randomized designs is one of generalizability, because participants in trials usually differ from nonparticipants. For example, studying lottery winners may be an ideal way to estimate the effects of income supplementation because the winners and losers will differ only randomly with respect to potential confounders. Nonetheless, individuals self-select to be in the experiment by purchasing a lottery ticket, and so any generalization to a population that includes nonparticipants may be faulty. Interpretation is further complicated if there is "noncompliance," meaning that some participants elect not to adhere to their assigned treatment regimen, or if the random assignment changes the behavior of the participants in other ways besides the receipt of treatment of interest (Kaufman et al., 2003). These problems can to some extent be addressed analytically if information on all those assigned is available, but often that is not the case. For example, if a substantial proportion of lottery winners fail to claim their prizes, this noncompliance is likely to introduce bias in the comparison of interest (because we expect behaviors such as losing a ticket or failing to be aware of having won to be associated with personality traits), and we will not likely have any idea who these noncompliers are.

In the case of randomized social interventions, changes in individual conditions may affect the entire social context, thus violating the assumption made by most statistical methods that one individual's treatment does not affect others. Such a violation would occur, for example, if an intervention such as randomly assigning individuals in poverty housing to receive vouchers for nonpoverty housing were to change the characteristics of the various neighborhoods involved in ways that would affect the outcomes (Sobel, 2006). There are numerous other limitations to the conduct and interpretation of randomized studies, especially for the complex interventions of interest to social epidemiology. Therefore, observational studies will undoubtedly remain a mainstay of social epidemiology (Kaufman et al., 2003).

NARRATIVE HISTORICAL APPROACH

The oldest and most widely used approach for examining the effect of social exposures on health is the one that is least often used by epidemiologists: the narrative historical approach. This method involves telling the story about exposures and outcomes in the specific sociohistorical context in which they actually occurred, rather than in the abstract and idealized context defined by statistical models. Narrative historical depictions can be quantitative, in that they may involve numerical summaries of what happened. They may involve causal assertions, in arguing that events are the results of specific conditions that, had these conditions not pertained, would have come out differently. What this method avoids, however, is the seductive generality of statistical models, the results of which are often described in universal terms, devoid of the specific context in which the data were realized. Narrative historical accounts also present causal assertions qualitatively as opposed to quantitatively, which avoids the illusion of numerical precision for observations that fall outside the realm of the observed data (King and Zeng, 2007).

For example, Randall Packard's *White Plague, Black Labor* (1989) describes how South African labor policies created epidemics of tuberculosis that differentially affected black and white communities. The arguments are quantitative, but no regression models are used and no statistical tests are conducted, and to the extent that causality is asserted, it is argued substantively rather than statistically. Many other deeply insightful and persuasive works of this nature have made great contributions to the social epidemiology of a variety of conditions, from the racial disparity in sexually transmitted diseases in the U.S. South (Thomas and Thomas, 1999) to the social class disparity in deaths during the 1995 Chicago heat wave (Klinenberg, 2002).

Regrettably, this approach appears to suffer a distinct lack of respect within epidemiology as a whole, as judged, for example, by the dearth of this sort of work in epidemiologic journals, which enforce formatting and length standards that are inconsistent with this methodology. Other social sciences recognize the narrative historical approach as an essential tool in understanding the complex relations between human social arrangements and their biologic consequences (King et al., 1994). If social epidemiology is to thrive in the 21st century, we must also accept that some scientific questions will not be answered best by treating observational data as though they arose from an experimental trial. The complexity of social arrangements may often surpass our ingenuity to model these arrangements with the quantitative precision demanded by statistical methodology, while at the same time validly reflecting the social system under study. Narrative methods provide a source of theories whose richness provides a valuable counterpoint to the Spartan oversimplifications that typify the parsimony-driven models of statistics.

CHAPTER 27

Infectious Disease Epidemiology

C. Robert Horsburgh, Jr., and Barbara E. Mahon

Epidemiologic Issues in Progression-Related Studies 553
Measures of Frequency of Infection and Disease 553
Assessing Risk of States of Infection 555
Epidemiologic Issues in Transmission-Related Studies 560
Measures of Frequency of Infectiousness and Transmission 560
Assessing Risk of States of Infectiousness 561
Conclusions 563

Infectious diseases are caused by transmissible agents that replicate in the affected host. Infection occurs when a susceptible host is exposed to and acquires the agent. Agents can be acquired from environmental sites or from other hosts that harbor the infectious agent. Many agents can be transmitted from one host to another, leading to chains of transmission through a population, the most distinctive feature of infectious disease epidemiology. As we shall see, the occurrence of chains of transmission through a population over time leads to dynamic changes in rates of, and risk factors for, transition through the states of the infectious process. These changes are known as "time-dependent happenings." Consequently, the outcomes of infection can be conceptualized as occurring on two separate axes. The first is the progression axis, the events leading from exposure to an infectious agent to clinical outcomes such as disease, cure, and death, with implications for the personal health of the infected person. Dealing with these issues is traditionally the realm of medicine. The second is the transmission axis, the events leading from exposure to transmission to others, with implications for others in the community whose health may be affected by transmission from the infected person. Dealing with transmission issues is traditionally the realm of public health.

On the progression axis, a series of events must take place for an infectious disease to occur. This series is shown schematically in Figure 27–1A. First, the human host must be exposed to the infectious agent. Next, exposure must lead to infection with the agent, defined as invasion into host tissues. Finally, infection must lead to the development of the clinical signs, symptoms, and laboratory findings that we recognize as the disease. In turn, disease is followed by cure, death, or persistent infection or disease. For some infectious diseases, some of these stages may be transient or may not occur; in such cases, the sequence is abbreviated. Also, in some situations, exposure may not lead to infection, but the agent may persist on the surface of the host without causing tissue invasion. This state is called colonization.

Similarly, on the transmission axis, a series of events must take place for an infected host to transmit the agent to others. This series is shown schematically in Figure 27–1B. First, exposure to the infectious agent must occur, and it must lead to colonization or infection. Next, colonization or infection must lead to the development of infectiousness. Infectiousness may or may not coincide with colonization, infection, or disease; the relationship of events on the transmission and progression axes varies for different infectious agents and hosts. Second, effective contact, meaning contact

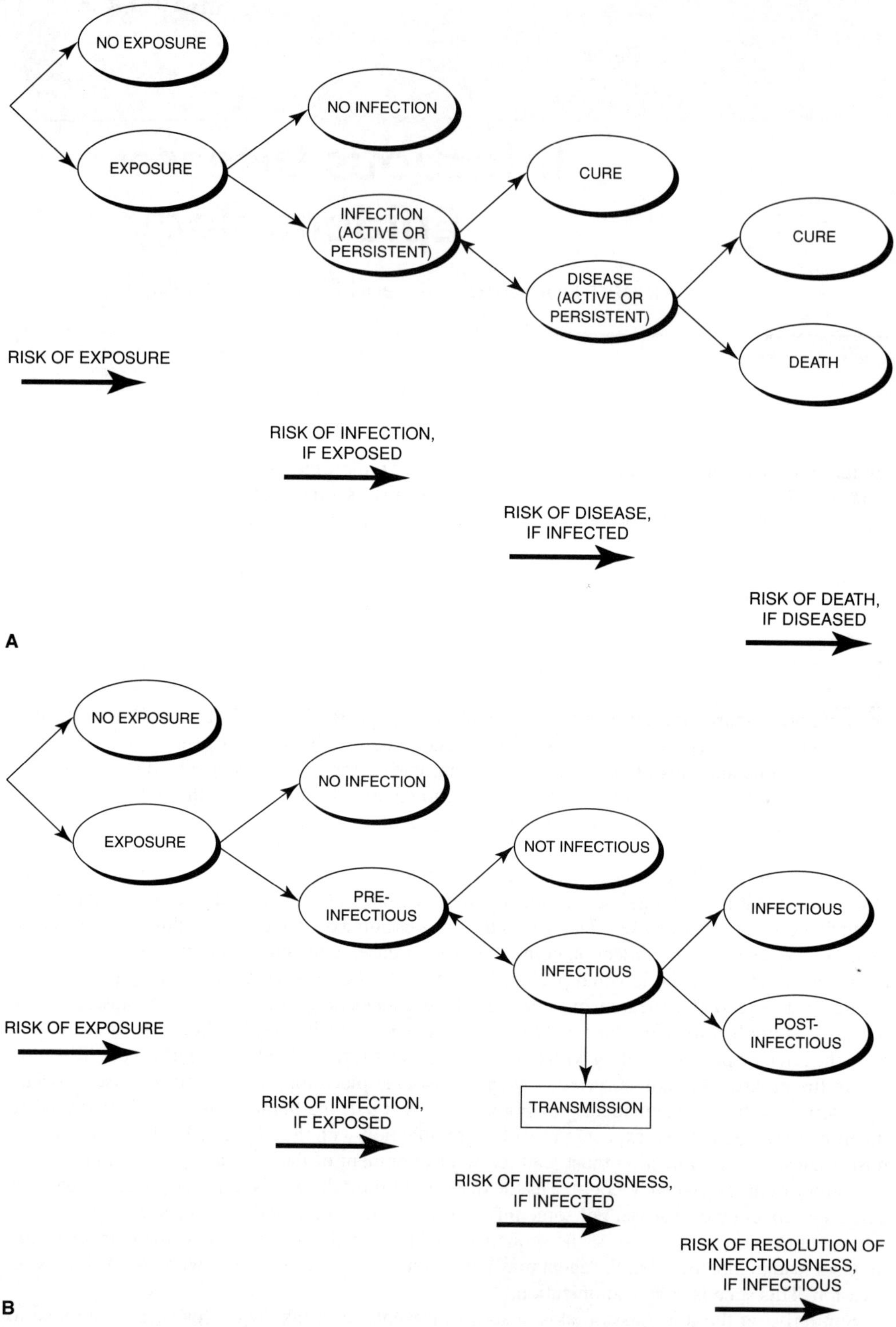

FIGURE 27–1 • **(A)** Schematic time course of stages of progression through the infectious process from exposure to death. **(B)** Schematic time course of states of transmission potential from exposure to postinfectiousness.

TABLE 27–1

Terminology for States of the Infectious Process

State of Infection	Definition	Alternative Terms
Progression-Related		
Colonization	Agent persists on host surface without tissue invasion	Transient colonization
Infection	Agent is present in host tissues without signs, symptoms, or laboratory evidence of tissue damage	Subclinical infection, asymptomatic infection
Persistent infection	A state of infection that does not lead promptly to disease or cure	Chronic infection, carrier state, chronic carrier state
Latency	A type of persistent infection in which the agent has invaded the host and is in a nonreplicating, noninfectious, but viable state	Latent infection, persistent infection, chronic infection
Disease	Agent is replicating in host tissues with signs, symptoms, or laboratory evidence of tissue damage	Clinical disease, symptomatic infection
Cure	Agent has been eliminated from host tissue (may persist on surface)	Resolution
Transmission-Related		
Preinfectious	Host is infected but has not become infectious	Latency, preinfective period
Infectious	Host is capable of transmitting agent to others	Contagiousness, infective period
Postinfectious	Host is no longer capable of transmission	Cure, postinfective period

that leads to transmission, must occur with a susceptible host. In turn, infectiousness may or may not resolve. For infections with agents that are not transmissible either directly or indirectly from person to person, there is no infectious state. Table 27–1 gives definitions of both the progression-related and transmission-related states of the infectious process.

Many terms have been used to describe the stages of progression of the infectious process. This inconsistent vocabulary can lead to considerable confusion. For many infectious agents, the terms *infection* and *disease* have been used interchangeably. This equivalence may be appropriate when all infected hosts progress to disease in a brief time, but for many agents this is not the case. For most epidemiologic studies it is important to distinguish invasion and replication of the infectious agent *without* signs, symptoms, or laboratory evidence of tissue damage from replication of the infectious agent *with* signs, symptoms, or laboratory evidence of tissue damage. We therefore use the term *infection* exclusively to refer to the state of tissue invasion without disease and use the term *disease* to refer to the state of clinical signs, symptoms, and abnormal laboratory findings, even though "infection" is usually also present in the disease state. The terms *subclinical infection* and *clinical disease* are sometimes used to describe what we call here *infection* and *disease,* but these cumbersome terms imply that there are two distinct additional states, "clinical infection" and "subclinical disease," which do not exist. The agent usually replicates in the host during both infection and disease, which are distinguished from each other by the absence or presence of signs, symptoms, or laboratory evidence of tissue damage. The term *latency* can also be confusing, as it has been used both for the progression-related state in which the agent is present in the host in a nonreplicating but viable state and also for the transmission-related state that precedes infectiousness; in this chapter we use *latency* for the progression-related state and *preinfectiousness* for the transmission-related state.

The terms *incubation period* and *persistent infection* are used to describe specific aspects of the basic progression-related states in Table 27–1. The *incubation period of a disease* is the time from an exposure resulting in infection until the onset of disease. Because infection usually occurs immediately after exposure, the incubation period is generally the duration of the period from the onset of infection to the onset of disease. If infection does not lead to disease, there is no incubation period of disease. If infection does not occur directly after exposure but rather at some later time, then the time from exposure to infection is the *incubation period of infection* and the incubation period of disease is the period from the time of exposure to the onset of disease. For example, meningococcal infection occurs after a variable period of meningococcal colonization of the nasopharynx; once infection has occurred, it can proceed rapidly to meningococcal disease. *Persistent infection* (also known as *chronic infection*) is a state of infection that does not lead promptly to disease or *cure*, whereas *persistent disease* (also known as *chronic disease*) occurs when signs, symptoms, and/or laboratory abnormalities continue without resolution. *Cure* is the state of elimination of the infectious agent from the host, either through a successful immune response or antimicrobial therapy. Cure usually implies elimination of both infection and disease, but in some situations a host can be cured of disease but have persistent infection. *Latency* is a unique type of persistent infection in which an organism is in a nonreplicating state but remains viable within host tissues. This state occurs when the host immune system forces the agent into the nonreplicating state, a state from which it may later reactivate. It is distinguished from *colonization*, in which the agent may replicate on the surface of the host without eliciting an immune response. There are also specific terms describing transmission-related states. The *preinfectious period,* the time from exposure to the agent until the onset of infectiousness, is the transmission-related analog of the incubation period, and the period from the onset of infectiousness until the person is no longer infectious is the *duration of infectiousness*.

Transitions between progression-related states and transmission-related states may or may not occur at the same time; persons with infection or disease may be infectious, noninfectious, or intermittently infectious. States of persistent infection can be distinguished based on their infectiousness. In latency, persistently infected persons are not infectious. When latent infection reactivates, infectiousness may return, leading to secondary periods of infectiousness. For example, persons with *Herpes simplex* infection are infectious during primary disease, noninfectious during latency, and again become infectious when disease recurs. By contrast, the *carrier state* occurs when a host is cured of disease but has persistent infection and the infectious agent continues to replicate, leading to continued infectiousness. The relative length of the incubation and preinfectious periods has important implications for the effectiveness of isolation of diseased persons in controlling transmission. When the incubation period is shorter than the preinfectious period, as for smallpox, isolation of diseased persons can prevent contact with susceptible persons during the infectious period. On the other hand, when the preinfectious period is shorter, as for varicella, the potential effectiveness of quarantine is limited because the infected host has already had a period of infectiousness by the time of disease onset.

The focus of epidemiologic studies of infectious diseases varies for different agents and changes over time as public health problems evolve and knowledge accrues. In the field of emerging infectious diseases, identifying the causative agent, the reservoir, and the factors that have led to introduction into the human population are paramount. For known agents, the most important epidemiologic questions concern identification of risk factors for exposure, for infection given exposure, for disease given infection, and for morbidity and mortality given disease. Intervention studies can be performed to identify ways to prevent exposure (behavior change, vector control, etc.), to prevent infection (prophylactic antimicrobial therapy, preventive vaccines, etc.), to prevent disease (therapeutic antimicrobial therapy, therapeutic vaccines, etc.), or to prevent death or chronic infection (therapeutic antimicrobial therapy). Some interventions may function at several points in this series. For example, antiretroviral human immunodeficiency virus (HIV) therapy has been studied as an intervention to prevent infection in exposed persons, to prevent disease in infected persons, and to prevent death in diseased persons. Integration of these parameters into models of disease transmission can then be used to predict the effect of preventative strategies on the dynamics of transmission of infectious agents and the burden of infectious diseases in a population.

The occurrence of outbreaks or epidemics is a distinctive feature of many infectious diseases. Outbreaks fueled by person-to-person transmission are called *propagated* outbreaks. Outbreaks can also occur as a result of mass exposure to a source of contamination, such as commonly occurs in food-borne outbreaks. These outbreaks can be *point-source* outbreaks if the exposure is limited to one place and time or *ongoing exposure* outbreaks if exposure is not limited. Outbreaks often require a rapid public health response with emergency control measures, but they can also present opportunities to expand knowledge regarding the infectious agent and its spread through a population.

Outbreak investigations can lead to the identification of infectious agents and diseases that were not previously recognized; these are known as *emerging infectious diseases*. Outbreak investigations have produced much information on risk factors for progression-related and transmission-related states for many infectious agents. During an infectious disease outbreak, the incidence of disease is by definition much greater than is normally expected. Thus, diseases that may be too rare to be studied feasibly at normal times can become accessible to epidemiologic investigation during an outbreak. However, outbreaks are also by definition unusual, so information on, for example, risk factors for infection, may not be applicable to nonoutbreak infections. For example, investigations of vaccine effectiveness conducted during outbreaks may be subject to *outbreak bias*. This bias occurs because vaccine failures may be clustered in space and time (either because of problems with vaccine storage or for other reasons) and because clusters of vaccine failure tend to lead to outbreaks. When these outbreaks are investigated, the vaccine effectiveness measures will tend to be biased toward the null (Fine and Zell, 1994).

EPIDEMIOLOGIC ISSUES IN PROGRESSION-RELATED STUDIES

MEASURES OF FREQUENCY OF INFECTION AND DISEASE

For several reasons, infection and disease caused by a given infectious agent may have characteristics that influence measurement of incidence and prevalence. First, the diagnosis of infection or disease may require tests that yield conclusive results only at some time after the onset of infection or disease; thus there may be a time lag in recognition of the state and some uncertainty about the true time of onset. Second, diagnosis of infection or disease may be uncertain. Accurate laboratory tests are available to establish the presence or absence of many infectious agents, but there are some notable exceptions. *Mycobacterium leprae*, the cause of leprosy, which has plagued humanity for millennia, is still not readily recovered by culture techniques. Diagnosis of early leprosy is therefore based on clinical criteria, and a firm diagnosis is often uncertain until the late stages of disease. Lyme disease has diverse and often nonspecific clinical manifestations, and serologic tests are also nonspecific. Therefore, the diagnosis of Lyme disease is often uncertain. Endocarditis, a disease in which heart valves are damaged by infectious agents, is difficult to identify directly, particularly in its early stages. Therefore, it is usually diagnosed by applying a clinical scoring system in which patients with higher scores are more likely to have the disease (Von Reyn et al., 1981; Durack et al., 1994). These scoring systems reflect the reality of imperfect diagnostic capability and thus represent a potential source of misclassification. Third, repeated episodes of an infectious disease can cause problems in estimating disease frequency, because reported incidence rates often do not distinguish between first episodes and repeat episodes. Some infectious diseases, such as measles, generate protective immunity such that they can only be acquired once in a lifetime, whereas others, such as rhinoviruses that cause the common cold, generate little immunity and can be acquired many times. Other agents, such as *Streptococcus pneumoniae,* the agent that causes pneumococcal pneumonia, have multiple serotypes; infection generates protective immunity that is serotype-specific. However, serotyping is not usually performed in the course of clinical care. As a result, recurrent episodes of pneumoccocal pneumonia may be categorized as recurrent disease when they are actually due to a different serotype against which the host does not have immune protection. In the extreme situation, a single person with multiple episodes of infection or disease could theoretically account for all the occurrences in a population.

The *attack rate* is defined as the risk of infection among exposed susceptible hosts. Like any risk measure, the attack rate always refers to a period of time, usually a year if not otherwise specified, but it does not have the dimension of inverse time, so it is not a true rate. In practice, it is often used for the risk of disease, thus combining the risk of infection among exposed hosts and the risk of disease among infected hosts. For situations in which nearly all infected persons develop disease, there is little distinction between the two risks, but when considering agents for which a high proportion of infections do not progress to disease, the alternative usage can be misleading. For example, Figure 27–2 shows the evolution of typhoid fever, the disease caused by *Salmonella* serotype Typhi infection, in experimental volunteers (Hornick et al., 1970). In this situation, all exposed hosts were known to be susceptible. The incubation period was measured from the time of exposure to the time of occurrence of fever, but some individuals became infected without progressing to disease. These

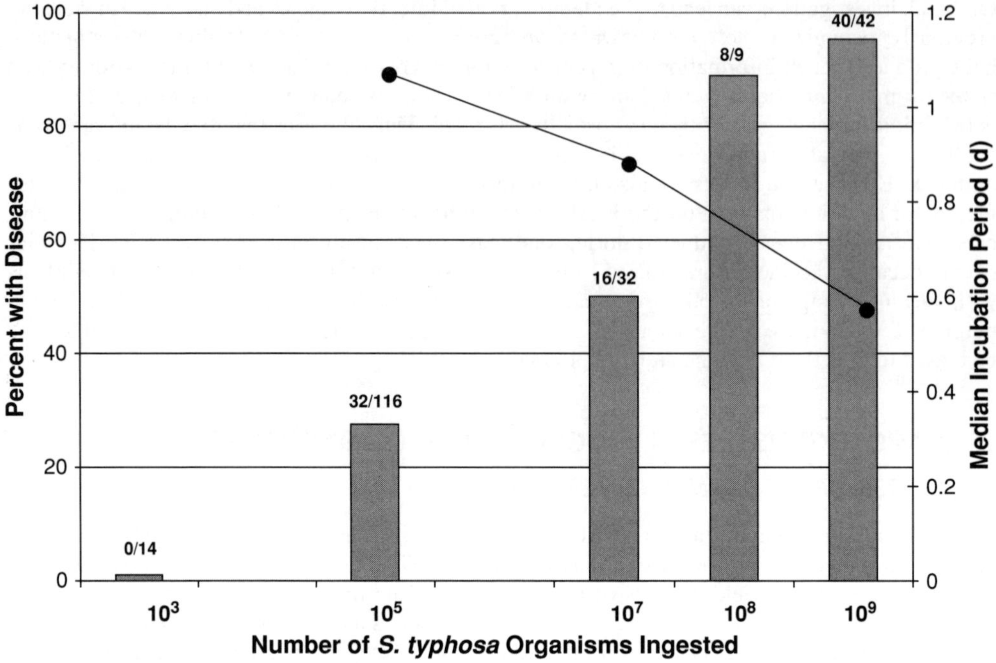

FIGURE 27–2 • Relationship among infectious dose, attack rate, and duration from infection to disease for *Salmonella typhosa*, Quailes strain, in volunteers (Data from Hornick et al., 1970). Percent of exposed persons developing disease is shown by bars; the line indicates mean incubation period of those in each category who develop disease.

subjects were not included in the numerator in calculating the attack rate. If, as is likely, different factors govern the risk of infection, given exposure, and the risk of disease, given infection, then conclusions about the effect of the ingested dose of *Salmonella* Typhi on occurrence of infection may have been flawed because of the exclusion of these asymptomatically infected subjects. A subsequent analysis suggested that this was the case (Blaser and Newman, 1982).

Excluding immune hosts from the denominator of the attack rate makes intuitive sense, as inclusion of persons who could not become infected if they were exposed would lead to an underestimate of the infectivity of the agent. However, susceptibility often has a continuous rather than a dichotomous distribution, so stratification of the population into susceptibles and nonsusceptibles can be a substantial oversimplification. The consequences of this oversimplification are particularly important among HIV-infected populations, in which immune competence of members of the population can vary over a wide spectrum.

Uncertainty about when an infectious disease is cured can complicate estimation of disease prevalence. For diseases of short duration this problem is minimal, but for chronic diseases it can be substantial. A person with hepatitis C infection, detectable hepatitis C virus DNA in serum, and persistent elevation of liver enzymes in serum for 6 months or more is considered to have chronic disease. Treatment for hepatitis C has recently become available (Kim and Saab, 2005). If treatment leads to elimination of the serum hepatitis C DNA and resolution of liver abnormalities, yet hepatitis C antibody persists, the patient may be presumed to be free of disease, but is the patient free of infection? Persistent antibody could indicate persistent infection or could merely be a marker of prior infection. Which it represents in this case is not currently known and likely will not be known until years of follow-up have accrued, allowing for observation of possible recrudescence of viral DNA in treated persons.

Barriers to case identification also complicate determination of the frequency of infection and disease. Such barriers include stigma, fear of economic loss, and limited access to diagnostic testing. For infections and diseases that have socially disadvantageous consequences, individuals may not present for clinical evaluation or may refuse diagnostic testing, and clinicians may be reluctant to report diagnosed patients to public health authorities even when reporting is legally mandated. Patients who are diagnosed with the condition may not participate in epidemiologic studies, either because they do not know they are eligible or because they fear discrimination as a result of participation. Such underascertainment because of stigma is an important potential source of bias in studies of leprosy, tuberculosis, and HIV/AIDS. Infections and diseases whose presence in a community could have negative economic consequences, such as reduced tourism or travel restrictions, may be downplayed or denied by government authorities. Underestimation of disease incidence also occurs if people with mild disease do not seek medical care. Lastly, many infections and diseases require diagnostic tools that are not generally available in much of the developing world; thus, even as common a condition as tuberculosis disease is underdiagnosed in the majority of the world's population.

ASSESSING RISK OF STATES OF INFECTION

This section addresses challenges in identifying and quantifying states of the progression-related infectious process shown in Figure 27–1A. The risk of infection is the product of the risk of exposure and the risk of infection if exposed. Similarly, the risk of disease is the product of the risk of exposure, the risk of infection if exposed, and the risk of disease if infected. Likewise, the risk of death if infected is the product of the risk of disease if infected and the risk of death if diseased. When a state, such as disease or cure, can be entered from more than one state of the infectious process, the overall risk is the sum of the risk from each state. Thus, the overall risk of cure is the risk of cure if infected among those who do not progress to disease plus the risk of cure if diseased times the risk of disease if infected.

Factors Influencing the Occurrence of Exposure to Infectious Agents

Infectious agents are present in specific locations, or reservoirs, and are acquired by human hosts through exposure to the reservoir in a manner that facilitates infection. The reservoir can be environmental sources, such as freshwater ponds (amebae), animals (Lyme disease in white-tailed deer, plague in prairie dogs) or humans (tuberculosis, sexually transmitted diseases). It is important to distinguish between exposure to a reservoir and exposure to the infectious agent. In the simplest situation, exposure to the reservoir is synonymous with exposure to the infectious agent, as in the case of swimming in a freshwater pond and being exposed to freshwater amebae, which are almost always present to some degree in freshwater ponds. In other situations, reservoir exposures may or may not pose risk for infection, depending on whether the reservoir exposure leads effectively to exposure to the infectious agent. Reservoirs may not harbor the agent at all times, or the intervention of a vector may be necessary. For example, eating undercooked chicken is an important source of exposure to *Campylobacter jejuni,* but not all poultry is contaminated with this organism, so some undercooked chicken does not provide exposure to *Campylobacter*. Exposure to prairie dogs carrying plague will not result in human exposure to plague unless the prairie dogs have fleas, the necessary vector, and a person is also exposed to those fleas. Exposure to mosquitoes can lead to exposure to malaria only if the mosquitoes have previously bitten a person with malaria. When humans are the reservoir, exposure to the agent occurs only when the infected person harbors viable organisms that can be presented to another person. For example, sexual contact does not lead *per se* to exposure to an agent of sexually transmitted infection; the sexual contact must be with a person harboring the infectious agent and in the infectious state.

Infectious agents can invade a human host following inhalation, ingestion, or direct penetration of skin or mucous membranes. Any activity that facilitates contact between a host and an environmental reservoir, vector, or infectious person can result in exposure. Exposure to sources of infectious agents is notoriously difficult to quantify, though, particularly because most infectious agents are too small to be visible. As a result, surrogates for exposure are commonly used—living in the same house as an infectious patient with tuberculosis instead of number of organisms inhaled, or time spent in a malarious area rather than number of bites by malaria-carrying mosquitoes. Individuals are unlikely to know the infectious status of the mosquitoes that bite them, or the sexually transmitted infection status of their sexual contacts, so misclassification of exposure to infectious disease agents is common.

The state of colonization is usually brief and can often be ignored in epidemiologic studies, but when it is prolonged, it may obscure the factors leading to infection, because the risk factors for colonization given exposure may be different for those for infection given colonization. Colonization with *Neisseria meningitidis* lasts for days to weeks and may or may not progress to infection and disease. Epidemiologic information about risk factors for colonization has been essential in developing control methods for *N. meningitidis*. In contrast, *Candida* species can have a colonization period that lasts months to years. *Candida* infection occurs when fungal organisms that are normally only asymptomatic colonizers of the host invade tissues, often leading to the diseases pharyngitis or vaginitis. In such cases, the exposure to an outside reservoir may have occurred well before infection is apparent, and epidemiologic studies are likely to focus on risk factors for progression from colonization to infection rather than from exposure to colonization.

Factors Influencing the Occurrence of Infection, Given Exposure

Once exposure has occurred, the next stage of the infectious process is infection. Factors that influence this transition can be categorized as dose-related, agent-related, and host-related.

Dose-related factors are usually strong predictors of the risk of infection, given exposure, because exposure to a larger number of organisms increases the likelihood of infection. The number of organisms to which the host is exposed is rarely measured, for the same reasons discussed in the section on risk factors for exposure. Therefore, surrogate markers of dose are commonly used, such as amount of time in the same room as an infectious person, amount of contaminated food consumed, or number of sexual contacts with an infected person. Behavioral characteristics of the exposure can alter the risk of infection by reducing the dose of infectious agent to which the host is exposed. Cooking eggs contaminated with *Salmonella* reduces the number of viable organisms to which the host is exposed, reducing the risk of infection that could lead to diarrheal disease. The use of insecticide-impregnated bed nets reduces the number of mosquito bites and thus the dose of malaria parasites, reducing the risk of malaria. Washing hands reduces the number of respiratory virus particles that are brought into contact with the nasopharynx, decreasing the risk of the common cold. There is also substantial variability in the number of organisms produced by individual infectious sources. So-called superspreaders of HIV infection, severe acute respiratory syndrome (SARS), and tuberculosis have been identified (Clumeck et al., 1989; Fennelly et al., 2004). In such cases, the infectious source case excretes an unusually large number of organisms. The contacts of "superspreaders" are exposed to a higher dose of the infectious agent than the contacts of other source cases with equivalent duration of exposure. The dose of an infectious agent excreted by an individual may also vary substantially over time (Pilcher et al., 2004).

Agent-related factors influencing the occurrence of infection, or *infectivity factors,* are characteristics of the agent that promote its ability to invade and establish infection in the human host. Most infectivity factors, which are usually determined by the genetic composition of the agent, promote attachment of the pathogen to host cells and penetration into these cells. Production of adhesins, surface molecules that facilitate binding to host target cells, is the most common infectivity factor. Examples include the hemagglutinin protein of the influenza virus, the GP120 protein of HIV, and the galactose adhesin of the parasite *Entamoeba histolytica,* a parasite that causes diarrhea. Influenza viruses that do not have the requisite hemagglutinin, or *Entamoebae* that do not have the galactose adhesin, cannot infect humans.

Many *host-related factors,* also called *susceptibility factors,* influence the occurrence of infection. One of the most important host-related factors is immunity. Vaccination or previous infection with a pathogen may provide full or partial immune protection. Persons who have previously had measles, mumps, or hepatitis A infection have complete immune protection and will not become infected if they are re-exposed to those agents. Persons with previous tuberculosis infection are partially protected against reinfection with *Mycobacterium tuberculosis.* However, persons whose immune system deteriorates (as happens in AIDS or with administration of immunosuppressive medications) may lose immune protection. Malnutrition may also decrease immune defenses (Corman, 1985). Cross-protection by immunity to a similar organism can also occur; persons with previous infection with nontuberculous *Mycobacteria* have partial protection from tuberculosis infection even if they have not previously had tuberculosis (Fine, 1995).

Host-related factors other than specific immunity may also influence susceptibility. Hosts may have variants of receptors that pathogens use for invasion, such as the CCR5 receptor for HIV and the Duffy blood group antigen for *Plasmodium vivax* malaria. Persons who lack these receptors have markedly reduced susceptibility to HIV and malaria, respectively (Luzzi et al., 1991; Fauci, 1996). Physiologic conditions that impair host clearance of microorganisms may also increase risk of infection. For example, impaired gastric acid secretion decreases killing of *Salmonella* in the stomach, leading to increased risk of *Salmonella* infection, whereas impaired mucus clearance from the lungs decreases elimination of bacteria from the tracheobronchial tree, leading to increased risk of infection with respiratory bacterial pathogens.

With recent advances in human genetics and genomics, the role of the genetic constitution of the host in determining progress through the states of infection has received increased attention. We discuss host genetics here in the context of risk for infection given exposure, but host genetics can also influence all stages of progression and transmission. A number of inherited immune defects, such as those associated with hypogammaglobulinemia, chronic granulomatous disease, and Job syndrome, can predispose to infection (and disease) with many infectious agents. More recently, specific host genetic defects that predispose to infection with particular pathogens have been recognized, such as defects in the interferon-gamma gene and the interferon-gamma receptor gene that predispose to mycobacterial infection (Newport et al., 1996; Holland et al., 1998; Dorman and Holland, 1998). These inherited defects of host immunity are severe but also rare; more subtle host immune defects may also play a role in determining progression through both the states of the infectious process and the states of transmissibility. Susceptibility to some infections may also be modulated by nonimmune host genetic factors, such as the structure of receptors needed for replication by infectious agents. Examples include resistance of persons with thalassemia to *P. vivax* malaria and resistance to HIV infection among persons without the CCR5 receptor.

Factors Influencing the Occurrence of Disease, Given Infection

As mentioned earlier, the proportion of infected hosts who progress from infection to disease varies substantially for different infectious agents. After infection with poliovirus, as few as 1 in 1,000 infected people progress to poliomyelitis disease (Melnick and Ledinko, 1951; Nathanson and Martin, 1979). In contrast, without antiretroviral therapy, nearly all persons infected with HIV eventually progress to AIDS. Progression from infection to disease may occur over a few days or weeks, so that the proportion of persons progressing is readily apparent, but for infections with incubation periods of months to years, such as HIV and hepatitis C, this proportion is more difficult to measure. For agents with long incubation periods, a cohort study with extended follow-up, as shown in Figure 27–3, is often necessary to determine the risk and rate of progression from infection to disease (Hessol et al., 1994). On the other hand, for infectious agents for which most infections lead to disease after a short incubation period, such as *Salmonella* and *Campylobacter,* cross-sectional or case-control designs can be used with little risk of misclassification of infection or disease status. Age can be an important factor in the risk of progression from infection to disease. Children with hepatitis A virus infection rarely develop symptomatic disease, whereas adults frequently have prolonged illness including severe fatigue, jaundice, and occasionally death (Hadler et al., 1980).

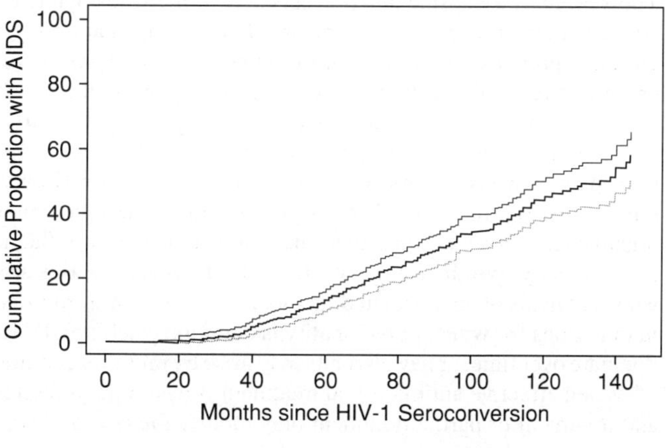

FIGURE 27–3 • Time from HIV infection to disease (AIDS) in a cohort of homosexual men. The dark line represents the cumulative proportion of men with AIDS, and the upper and lower lines represent the 95% confidence limits (Reproduced from Hessol et al., 1994).

For some infectious diseases, difficulty in establishing that disease has occurred can lead to failure to appreciate the true risk of progression from infection to disease. For example, *Chlamydia trachomatis* infection of the female genital tract can cause chronic inflammation and scarring that leads to infertility without causing symptoms. Although tissue damage is present, it can only be observed with invasive procedures that are not routinely performed. Thus, the risk of progression from *Chlamydia trachomatis* infection to disease has often been underestimated.

Accurate assessment of the effect of risk factors for disease, given infection, requires distinguishing the various components of the stages of the infectious process, as shown in Figure 27–1A. Failure to appreciate the inherent complexity of the infectious process can lead to confounding when intermediate transition risks are not measured. An example is the risk of tuberculosis disease attributed to diabetes mellitus. Studies performed in the 1950s showed that persons with uncontrolled diabetes had substantially greater risk of tuberculosis disease than the general population (Oscarsson and Silwer, 1958; Opsahl et al., 1961; Boucot et al., 1952). This increased risk was attributed to impaired immunity resulting from diabetes. Persons with uncontrolled diabetes, however, are frequently hospitalized, and being hospitalized in the 1950s meant increased risk of exposure to persons with active tuberculosis, who were also often hospitalized. Thus, because of their increased risk of hospitalization, the risk for exposure to *M. tuberculosis* was greater for diabetics than for the general population. Increased exposure resulting from hospitalization rather than diabetes itself could have accounted for the increased risk of tuberculosis in diabetics. Ideally, risk factors for each stage transition shown in Figure 27–1A should be studied independently.

Host immunity can influence the transition from infection to disease, because specific immunity is frequently the mechanism for controlling infection sufficiently to prevent the development of disease. Conversely, decreased immune system effectiveness usually increases the risk of disease, given infection. The clearest example of this phenomenon is AIDS. Because HIV infection progressively impairs the ability of the immune system to respond to infection, patients become more likely to progress from infection to disease with organisms such as *Mycobacterium avium,* which frequently causes infection but rarely causes disease in normal hosts. Although it at first seems counterintuitive, effective host immunity can also in some cases actually predispose to the occurrence of disease. For example, dengue hemorrhagic fever occurs when a host with immunity due to a previous dengue virus infection acquires a second infection with a different viral serotype. In immunocompetent hosts, the pre-existing immunity results in an antibody response that leads to hemorrhagic disease (Kliks et al., 1989; Halstead and O'Rourke, 1977).

Infectious agents can have endogenous properties influencing the occurrence of disease that are analogous to the infectivity factors that influence the risk of infection, given exposure. These properties are called *virulence factors,* a term that encompasses not only factors involved in pathogenesis—the development of disease—which is our focus here, but also factors that determine disease severity, which are discussed in the next section. Toxins, proteins secreted by an organism that lead directly to the manifestations of disease, are the most common virulence factors affecting the risk of disease given infection. For example, strains of *Corynebacterium diphtheriae* that do not secrete diphtheria toxin may cause infection but do not lead to diphtheria disease. Other virulence factors of microorganisms lead to disease by facilitating evasion of host immune defenses: Some organisms produce a polysaccharide capsule that prevents ingestion by host white blood cells (e.g., *Pneumococci*), others vary their surface antigen expression to avoid host antibody binding (*Borreliae,* trypanosomes), secrete a protease that cleaves host antibody (*Haemophilus influenzae*), or produce enzymes that prevent intracellular killing of the infectious agent by the host's immune system (*Legionella, Listeria*). Strains of these organisms that do not produce the virulence factor are less able or unable to cause disease even after establishing infection. Some organisms, such as *Staphlococcus aureus,* have pathogenesis factors with intermittent expression (Lowy, 1998); the factors that influence this expression must therefore also be considered in epidemiologic analysis. For some infectious organisms, more than one gene or gene product may influence infectivity, immunogenicity, or pathogenicity. Within a single host, most infectious diseases are caused by a single clone of organisms. Analysis of agent-related factors in progression from infection to disease can be complicated in infections for which polyclonality is common, such as HIV infection. The dominant variant may fluctuate over time, or new variants may arise by mutation, adding further complexity to the analysis.

When effective antimicrobial treatment is available, infection can be treated to prevent disease, and treatment or partial treatment may modify the risk of disease, given infection. Such treatment is effective for acute infections such as pertussis and hepatitis B virus infection, in which antibiotic treatment of recently infected persons can prevent progression to disease. Similarly, treatment can be effective in chronic infections such as HIV, for which antiretrovirals can prevent AIDS, and in hepatitis C, for which interferon and ribavirin treatment can prevent cirrhosis and liver cancer. Antimicrobial drug resistance is an important agent-related genetic characteristic of infectious agents that must be considered in epidemiologic studies of infectious diseases whenever effective antibiotic therapy exists. Drug resistance has a profound effect on the ability to treat infection and disease successfully and thus may alter the course of the infectious process by extending the duration and severity of states on both the progression-related and transmission-related axes. As a result, drug resistance is a major problem in controlling infectious diseases.

Most infectious agents do not have the potential for persistent infection. For those that do, clinical features of recurrent disease and its risk factors are often distinct from those for disease following initial infection. For infections that can establish latency, such as human herpesviruses and *M. tuberculosis,* disease occurring after latency is called *reactivation disease.* In some cases, reactivation disease is easily differentiated from primary disease occurring after an exposure that results in infection. For example, chicken pox is the primary disease that occurs directly after infection with *Varicella zoster* virus, and shingles is the reactivation disease that occurs after a period of latency. In contrast, tuberculosis disease that occurs soon after an exposure resulting in infection cannot be differentiated clinically from reactivation tuberculosis disease. Because risk factors for the two tuberculosis disease states are different, cohort studies that enroll persons with tuberculosis infection but no history of tuberculosis disease are essential to minimize misclassification of disease state. Most risk factors for reactivation disease are conditions that impair host immunity, because immunocompetence is the major determinant in keeping organisms from returning to the replicating state. HIV-mediated immune suppression is the strongest risk factor for progression from latent tuberculosis to tuberculosis disease; other major risk factors include immune impairment from chronic renal disease or exogenously administered immunosuppressive medications (Horsburgh, 2004). Treatment of latent tuberculosis infection can reduce the risk of subsequent reactivation disease by 60% to 90% (Cohn et al., 2000).

Factors Influencing the Occurrence of Cure, Death, or Persistent Infection, Given Disease

The host may progress from disease to cure or death from the disease or may develop persistent infection, thus returning to the state of infection (without disease). For diseases that have high mortality, death is the most important outcome, and studies to identify risk factors for this outcome predominate. When death is less common or occurs after a long period of disease and cure is not possible, such as currently is the case with HIV and hepatitis C, studies focus on identifying factors that prolong survival of the diseased person or factors that reduce morbidity (signs, symptoms, and laboratory evidence of ongoing tissue damage), resulting in a return to the state of infection. Surrogate markers are frequently used as endpoints in studies of such infectious processes. The use of such markers in epidemiologic studies has been controversial because, in addition to being outcomes, the markers are also the result of the underlying disease process and may be affected by other variables that affect the outcome of interest (Cole et al., 2003; Robins et al., 2000). Confounding can result. Thus, CD4 cell counts are not only a manifestation of the extent of immune destruction caused by HIV infection but also an indicator of the receipt of effective antiretroviral therapy and a predictor of future survival. Histologic grading of liver tissue in hepatitis C infection is both a manifestation of the extent of hepatic damage and a predictor of survival. Despite the theoretical disadvantage of such markers as outcome measures, surrogate markers have been widely used in epidemiologic and interventional studies.

A number of factors can influence the probability of cure, death, or persistent infection, with pathogen virulence and host immunity playing important roles. Prominent examples of virulence factors that affect the severity and outcome of disease are the Group A Streptococcal toxin associated with toxic-shock syndrome (Cone et al., 1987), the Shiga-like toxin of some *Escherichia coli* that leads to hemolytic uremic syndrome (Riley et al., 1983), and the Panton-Valentine leukocidin of *S. aureus*, which has been associated with a high mortality rate in patients with pneumonia caused by this organism (Gillet et al., 2002)

One of the most important factors influencing the probability of cure or death is antimicrobial therapy. Since the introduction of sulfonamides in the late 1930s, many antimicrobial agents have become available, and many infectious diseases are now treatable with therapeutic agents that can achieve cure or that have a substantial ameliorating effect on the outcome of the disease. In the case of tuberculosis, approximately 30% of patients with disease self-cured in the preantibiotic era, while 50% died and 20% developed chronic disease (Mitchell, 1955). Current antituberculosis antibiotic regimens can reduce deaths to less than 1%, with over 95% of subjects cured. Unfortunately, emergence of antibiotic resistance in *M. tuberculosis* is common, and it is frequently associated with decreased cure rates and shortened survival.

For infectious agents that can establish persistent infection, either with or without latency, it can sometimes be difficult to distinguish which state the subject is in. When latency is known to be common, such as for human herpesviruses and tuberculosis, distinguishing between cure and persistent infection with latency can be difficult. Latency may be firmly identified only after reactivation disease has occurred. For practical purposes, all untreated persons who have evidence of prior infection with agents known to have a latent state—whether laboratory evidence of infection or a clinically recognized episode of disease—but no evidence of ongoing replication are assumed to have persistent infection with latency. However, a substantial fraction of such persons will never have recurrent disease, suggesting that at least some of them may never have established latency, or may have progressed from latency to cure at some time after establishing latency. For agents that can establish persistent infection but do not have a latent state, such as hepatitis B and C, laboratory testing can often be used to distinguish between persistent infection and cure.

EPIDEMIOLOGIC ISSUES IN TRANSMISSION-RELATED STUDIES

MEASURES OF FREQUENCY OF INFECTIOUSNESS AND TRANSMISSION

The state of infectiousness, shown in Figure 27–1B, is neither constant nor synonymous with any of the states of the progression-related infectious process shown in Figure 27–1A. In fact, infectiousness is commonly greatest just before the onset of disease and frequently wanes well before disease resolution. For different infectious agents, however, infected hosts can be infectious at various progression-related stages of the infectious process. For example, the infected host may transmit infection when colonized (*Candida*), infected without disease (hepatitis B), or diseased (most infectious agents). By definition, transmission cannot occur during persistent infection with latency or in the "cured" state, because replicating organisms are not present in either state, but there are numerous examples of infections in which clinical cure is followed by a prolonged period of asymptomatic infection or colonization during which continued transmission is possible. The typhoid carrier state is the classic example. Defining the degree and duration of the infectious state is therefore an essential feature of describing an infectious process and is a critical parameter in explaining and predicting the spread of an infectious agent through a population. Studies of infectiousness are complicated by the inherent difficulty in discerning whether an infected person is, in fact, infectious. Infectiousness cannot be observed by direct observation of the infected person. It can only be inferred indirectly, when transmission to another susceptible host occurs. However, transmission depends on a number of factors in addition to infectiousness; infectiousness is a necessary but not sufficient condition. Surrogates for infectiousness, such as the recovery of the organism from the infected host, are often used in epidemiologic studies, even though they may not be completely accurate proxies for infectiousness.

Because infectiousness cannot be measured directly in the absence of exposure to susceptible hosts, the duration of the preinfectious and infectious periods can be difficult to define. However, when chains of transmission occur, the time between the onset of disease of successive generations of infected persons, termed the *serial interval,* can shed light on the onset of infectiousness. Assuming average incubation periods, the serial interval reflects the amount of time elapsed between exposure from one generation of spread to the next. Thus, the serial interval cannot be shorter than the preinfectious period; observation of the minimum serial interval gives information about when the preinfectious period ends.

In studies of infectiousness, a specific kind of attack rate known as the *secondary attack rate* is often calculated. The secondary attack rate is the risk of infection among susceptible contacts of an infectious host and thus encompasses factors that affect both infectiousness and transmission given infectiousness. It is often measured among susceptible household contacts but can be measured among contacts of any type—community, workplace, sexual, etc. The *basic reproductive number,* or R_0, is a related concept that is widely used in mathematical modeling of transmission within populations. R_0 is the average number of secondary cases of an infection that occur in a completely susceptible population following introduction of a single infectious case. Like the secondary attack rate, R_0 reflects both the inherent infectiousness of a case of infection and the factors that lead to transmission given infectiousness.

ASSESSING RISK OF STATES OF INFECTIOUSNESS

Factors Influencing the Occurrence of Infectiousness

The occurrence and degree of infectiousness are influenced by biologic characteristics of the infectious agent and by both physical and behavioral characteristics of the infected person. For example, persons with pulmonary tuberculosis are minimally infectious unless they cough, whereas persons with extrapulmonary tuberculosis disease are essentially noninfectious, because other persons are very unlikely to come into contact with organisms that are sequestered in an internal tissue compartment. Persons with diarrhea due to Hepatitis A, which is spread primarily through fecal–oral contact, are much more likely to be infectious than persons without diarrhea, because diarrhea is both a marker for increased numbers of infectious organisms in the stool and a condition that increases the risk of exposing others to the virus. There is also substantial variability in the number of organisms produced by individual infectious sources. As noted earlier, "superspreaders" of some infectious agents have been identified who excrete an unusually large number of organisms, with the result that the superspreader's contacts are exposed to a higher dose of the infectious agent than the contacts of other source cases with equivalent duration of exposure. This can lead to a higher secondary attack rate among contacts of these cases.

Factors Influencing the Occurrence of Transmission, Given Infectiousness

Transmission, given infectiousness, depends on both the duration of infectiousness and the number of susceptible contacts exposed during the infectious period. Thus, for a given degree of infectiousness, transmission can vary widely depending primarily on behavioral host factors and on the immunity of the host's contacts. Factors that prolong the infectious period can increase transmission. For example, antibiotic treatment of salmonellosis is thought to prolong the shedding of *Salmonellae* in stool, increasing the risk of transmission. Host behaviors that increase the contact rate during the infectious period can also increase transmission; once they are infectious, commercial sex workers, who have sexual contact with multiple partners, are more likely to transmit sexually transmitted diseases (STDs) than equally infectious persons who have few sexual partners. Other host behaviors, such as using condoms in this example, may decrease STD transmission, given infectiousness. The susceptibility of the infectious host's contacts is also a critical factor in determining whether transmission occurs. When contacts are immune to the infectious agent, either through previous infection or because of vaccination, transmission will not occur.

The parameters that influence transmission may vary over time. Such factors are known as *dependent happenings*. Epidemiologic studies that treat these factors as static may fail to identify important risk factors for exposure, infection, or disease. An example of the importance of dependent happenings in transmission of infectious disease is the phenomenon known as *herd immunity*. As an infection that produces protective immunity moves through a population, the proportion of the population that is susceptible declines. Thus, the pool of susceptible persons dwindles. Eventually, if the contact rate remains constant, the risk of encounters between infectious hosts and susceptible persons drops to a point at which transmission ceases, even if there is no change in the transmission-related behavior of infectious persons. When a high proportion of the population is immune, remaining susceptibles are protected from infection to some degree, not by personal immunity but because the likelihood of exposure to the infectious agent decreases. An excellent example of herd immunity and cholera is shown in Table 27–2. In this analysis, the risk of cholera among unvaccinated, and presumably susceptible, people living in an area where cholera is endemic

TABLE 27–2

Risk of Cholera by Level of Cholera Vaccine Coverage in a Community, Showing Decreased Risk in Nonimmune (Unvaccinated) Persons, Associated with Increased Levels of Protective Immunity in the Population (Herd Immunity)

Level of Vaccine Coverage Achieved in Population from Which Placebo Vaccine Recipients Were Drawn	Number of Placebo Recipients (Nonimmune)	Number of Placebo Recipients Developing Cholera	Risk per 1,000 Placebo Recipients
<28%	2,852	20	7.01
28%–35%	4,429	26	5.87
36%–40%	5,503	26	4.72
41%–50%	5,801	27	4.65
>51%	6,082	9	1.47

was inversely related to the level of vaccine coverage in the household, with 7.01 cases per 1,000 in the lowest quintile of coverage and 1.47 cases per 1,000 in the highest quintile (Ali et al., 2005).

Factors Influencing the Resolution of Infectiousness

Because the infectious period is not synonymous with the progression-related stages of colonization, infection, or disease, specific assessment of factors that lead to cessation of infectiousness is also important. However, factors that lead to resolution of colonization, infection, and disease on the progression axis often also influence resolution of infectiousness. Such factors include pathogenicity of the organism, host immunity, and antimicrobial therapy. Somewhat paradoxically, virulence factors that increase acute mortality may decrease transmission by shortening the duration of the infectious period. For other infections, such as hepatitis B virus, the infectious period is bimodal; the majority of cases have a brief infectious period, whereas a prolonged infectious carrier state can occur in as many as 10% of infected individuals.

For some infectious agents, it is also possible for a single individual to have multiple periods of infectiousness. This situation can occur when disease that is infectious resolves and then relapses, as can happen in tuberculosis. Often, but not always, this return to infectiousness is the result of failure of antibiotic therapy; retreatment can then lead to resolution of the second period of infectiousness. For infectious agents that have a latent state, periods of activity of the infection between latent periods can produce recurrent periods of infectiousness, as in the case of herpesvirus reactivations.

Infectious Disease Transmission Models

Infectious disease transmission models are dynamic analytic systems that incorporate dependent happenings to explain and predict the movement of infection through populations over time (Halloran, 2003). The conceptual basis of such models was developed by Sir Ronald Ross to explore the transmission dynamics of malaria. Early mathematical formulations of transmission models were developed by Kermack and Reed and Frost in the 1920s (Abbey, 1952; Fine, 1977). These models consider the members of the population to fall into "compartments," or transmission-related states, such as "susceptible," "infectious," and "recovered and immune." The simplest models use only two or three compartments, but many compartments can be used in models of complex situations. Parameters describing the movement between compartments are used to produce a model of transmission over time. Thus, in a simple model, the number of persons becoming infectious at time $t + 1$ is calculated as a function of the number of infectious persons at time t, the contact rate between infectious persons and others in the population, the probability that contact at time t is with a susceptible person, and the probability of transmission per contact with a susceptible. Similarly, the number of people who have recovered and are immune and noninfectious at time $t + 1$ is calculated from the number of infectious people at time t and the duration of infectiousness. The number of people in the population who are susceptible, infected, and recovered are then calculated over time to depict the dynamics of transmission at the population level. This simple model assumes a number of conditions that are not usually realistic, such as that the contact rate is constant for all people and that no one enters or leaves the population. More sophisticated transmission models have been developed to include the possibilities of unequal mixing, varying infectiousness, varying susceptibility over time, and migration into and out of the cohort (Longini et al., 1988). Because of dependent happenings, it is important to avoid assumptions that transmission parameters are either static or independent of each other.

Infectious disease transmission models are often used to predict the course of epidemics, and they also allow investigation of the effects of changes over time in the parameters that determine the transition from one state to another. For example, to aid in preparation for future influenza pandemics, detailed models have been developed to predict the anticipated effects of various public health responses, including treatment of influenza disease, distribution of prophylactic antiviral medications, mass immunization with vaccines of varying effectiveness, school closures, travel restrictions, and social distancing measures on transmission of influenza strains with varying R_0 (Germann et al, 2006). In order to construct such models, precise measurement of the factors that influence the transition from one stage to another is needed. The resulting transition probabilities are then incorporated into the dynamic system and varied to identify which ones have the greatest influence on infection and disease incidence and prevalence. Thus, construction of useful dynamic transmission models requires a substantial amount of information about specific factors that influence the progression from one stage of infection to the next. A common goal of such a model is estimation of the *effective reproductive number* of an infection. The effective reproductive number, R, is the average number of transmissions of infection that occur from each infectious case. In contrast to R_0, which refers to a completely susceptible population, R reflects the actual level of immunity in the population. Thus, R can vary over time as immunity changes in the population. If susceptibles are introduced into the population, R will increase, and if the proportion of susceptibles decreases, through vaccination or the spread of infection with subsequent immunity, R will decrease. If $R < 1$, then transmission will not be sustained, and infection will die out over time as each infected person transmits the infection, on average, to fewer than one person who can subsequently transmit. If $R > 1$, then transmission increases and the epidemic spreads until the proportion of immune persons increases to the point at which R falls below 1. A major difficulty with modeling the course of epidemics is the variability in infectiousness among transmitters; rare events, such as the occurrence of a highly efficient transmitter or migration of an infectious host into a nonimmune population, as can easily occur with international air travel, can cause an epidemic to blossom.

CONCLUSIONS

Infectious diseases result from human encounters with a wide variety of organisms that cause both acute and chronic infection and disease. This diversity leads to a wide variety of approaches to the study of infectious disease epidemiology. Identification of the causal agent of a given disease is usually straightforward, although when previously unrecognized agents present as emerging infectious diseases, identification can be challenging. *Legionella* pneumonia ("Pontiac fever," "legionnaire's disease"), HIV infection ("GRID," "AIDS"), and coronavirus pneumonia ("SARS") all remained elusive for long enough that the diseases they cause acquired one or, in some cases, multiple eponyms.

Once the causal agent is identified, epidemiologic attention turns to defining risk factors for acquisition, progression or recovery, and transmission. Interventions to modify acquisition and clinical course and decrease transmission are also explored through interventional studies, both controlled and uncontrolled. Once these factors are reasonably well understood, models can be constructed that allow exploration of the dynamic epidemiology of infectious agents in both human and nonhuman populations. These analyses constitute the tools for arriving at a full understanding of the interplay between exposures and outcomes in the study of infectious diseases.

CHAPTER 28

Genetic and Molecular Epidemiology

Muin J. Khoury, Robert Millikan, and Marta Gwinn

Multidisciplinary Approaches to the Evaluation of Biomarkers 566
Analytic Validity 566
Clinical Validity 566
Clinical Utility 567
Ethical, Legal, and Social Issues 567
Conventional Epidemiologic Studies 568
Case-Control Studies 568
Cohort Studies 568
Cross-Sectional Studies 569
Methodologic Issues 570
Confounding 570
Genotype and Exposure Misclassification 570
Gene–Environment Interaction 570
Emerging Analytic Complexity 571
Nonconventional Epidemiologic Studies 573
Case-Only Studies 573
Case-Parent Studies 575
Example 1: Colorectal Cancer 575
Exposure Assessment 576
Genetic Susceptibility 576
Cancer Screening 577
Tumor Heterogeneity 577
Example 2: Inflammatory Bowel Disease 577
Genetic Susceptibility and Gene Discovery 577
Generating New Hypotheses 578
Epidemiology and Complexity 579

Since the chapter on "genetic epidemiology" was published in the second edition of *Modern Epidemiology* (Khoury, 1998), rapid developments in genetic and molecular technologies have occurred, including the completion of the human genome project (Collins et al., 2003; Collins and Guttmacher, 2003). The term *genomics* is now used regularly with reference to "the study of the functions and interactions of all the genes in the genome" (Guttmacher and Collins, 2002). Moreover, new "omic" disciplines have emerged to study gene expressions, products, and interactions (e.g., proteomics [Sellers and Yates, 2003], transcriptomics [Kiechle and Holland-Stanley, 2003], metabonomics [Nicholson et al., 2002], nutrigenomics [van Ommen and Stierum, 2002], pharmacogenomics [Sweeney, 2004], and toxicogenomics [Tugwood et al., 2003]). The pace of gene discovery has accelerated markedly in 2006 and 2007 with a number of large scale case-control studies of several common chronic diseases that used genome-wide association (GWA) analyses that provide impressive results in finding new genetic variations related to these diseases.

Before the "omic" era, epidemiology had a long history of using biologic markers (Schulte, 1993), such as antibody titers in infectious disease epidemiology, blood lipids in cardiovascular disease epidemiology (Truett et al., 1967), and blood levels of potential toxins in environmental epidemiology. The integration of biologic markers of exposures, susceptibility, and outcomes into epidemiologic research has been referred to as "molecular epidemiology" (Schulte and Perera, 2003). The term *genetic epidemiology* has been often used to denote the study of the role of genetic factors in the occurrence of disease in populations (Khoury, 1993), focused largely

TABLE 28–1

Fields of Biomarker Epidemiology: The Continuum of Epidemiologic Approaches to the Genome, Its Products, and Interactions with the Environment[a]

Field	Application	Types of Studies
Genetic epidemiology	Gene discovery	Linkage analysis, family-based association studies
Molecular epidemiology	Gene characterization Use of other biomarkers of exposures, susceptibility, and outcomes	Research to characterize gene–disease associations and gene–environment interactions using biomarkers
Applied epidemiology/ health services research	Evaluating health effects	Studies to evaluate clinical validity and utility of genetic information in practice

[a] We have used the term *human genome epidemiology* to refer to the continuum of epidemiologic approaches to the human genome (2004).

on statistical methods for gene discovery in family studies. We are now using the term *human genome epidemiology* to refer to the continuum of epidemiologic approaches to the human genome from gene discovery to applications in medicine and public health (Khoury, 2004a) (see Table 28–1 for definitions and scope). In the next decade, the use of biomarkers in epidemiology will reach a new level of complexity (Table 28–2), with the simultaneous study of hundreds and even thousands of data points (e.g., DNA variants, mRNA expressions, protein patterns) for each person. Increasing complexity will require rigorous approaches to study design, analysis, and interpretation.

Thus, it seems natural to combine the topics of genetic and molecular epidemiology. We start with a general section about the validation of biomarkers, followed by epidemiologic approaches to the study of gene–disease associations and gene–gene and gene–environment interactions using conventional epidemiologic study designs. We discuss analytic and methodologic issues applicable to these studies, as well as emerging nonconventional epidemiologic methods that can be used as adjuncts to traditional approaches. We present two current examples on the use of biomarkers, in colorectal cancer and inflammatory bowel disease. We do not cover traditional genetic analyses of human pedigrees to assess Mendelian transmission (segregation analysis) or to locate human genes (linkage analysis/gene mapping) but rather cover emerging key areas central to the practice of epidemiology in the 21st century. For additional information, readers are referred to the recent book by Thomas (2004a).

TABLE 28–2

Examples of Conventional Markers and New "Omic" Markers Used in Epidemiologic Research, by Type of Biomarker

Type of Biomarker	Conventional Biomarkers	"Omic" Biomarkers
Exposure	Blood levels of chemical agents	Changes in gene expression in tissues as signatures of exposure
Susceptibility	DNA variant at one or more loci	Genomic profile of variation in numerous genes
Outcomes	Estrogen receptor status in breast cancer	Gene expression profiles for breast cancer prognosis

MULTIDISCIPLINARY APPROACHES TO THE EVALUATION OF BIOMARKERS

Whether we are dealing with traditional biomarkers such as biochemical indices of exposure, early biologic effects (such as DNA adducts), or new "omic" approaches to genetic variants or their products, biomarkers need validation using laboratory, epidemiology, and clinical studies. As shown in Table 28–3, we use general terminology developed by two national genetic testing committees (Task Force on Genetic Testing, 1997; Secretary's Advisory Committee on Genetic Testing, 2000; Haddow and Palomaki, 2003). Although these parameters were developed for tests in clinical practice, they also apply to epidemiologic research.

ANALYTIC VALIDITY

The analytic validity of a biomarker refers to its accuracy in measuring what it is supposed to measure. As in other areas of epidemiology, this includes its sensitivity and specificity, illustrated in Table 28–4 for binary biomarkers; for continuously measured biomarkers, additional work is needed to establish cutoffs to maximize predictive value. Genetic markers encompass a range that includes a single nucleotide polymorphism (SNP) in one gene, a collection of SNPs on a chromosome (haplotype), a whole collection of SNPs on a gene chip, or mRNA expression profiles or proteomic patterns. The overall analytic validity of biomarkers depends on sample type, processing, storage, and assay variability. Biomarkers themselves may have inherent variability (e.g., by time of day). Initial efforts to characterize biomarkers for use have been called "transitional studies" (Hulka and Margolin, 1992; Schulte and Perera, 1997).

In the genomics age, bundling many variants together can complicate the analytic validation process. In addition, biomarker reliability, laboratory quality assurance, and proficiency testing are crucially important. All in all, we are still in the infancy of a rapidly changing field of new biomarkers.

CLINICAL VALIDITY

Once the analytic validity of a biomarker has been established, its clinical validity needs to be assessed in clinical and epidemiologic studies. Clinical validity of a biomarker includes its sensitivity and specificity for measuring a clinical (or subclinical) endpoint. If the biomarker is to be analyzed as a risk factor, its validity is first established using epidemiologic study designs (as explained later). For use as a clinical tool (e.g., for early diagnosis of a condition), its clinical sensitivity, specificity and predictive values must be documented (for illustrations with simple biomarkers, see Table 28–4; also see Manolio [2003] for further discussion).

TABLE 28–3

Multidisciplinary Approaches to the Evaluation of Biomarkers

Type of Evaluation[a]	Terms/Variables	Types of Studies
Analytic validity	Analytic sensitivity, specificity and predictive values	Laboratory studies "Transitional" studies
Clinical validity	Risk of current or future health outcomes for people with/without marker	Conventional and nonconventional study designs
Clinical utility		Risk of disease with and without using biomarker and accompanying interventions

[a] Adapted from the Task Force on Genetic Testing (1997) and the Secretary's Advisory Committee on Genetic Testing (2000).

TABLE 28–4

Multidisciplinary Evaluation of Biomarkers[a]

I. Analytic validity

	Biomarker	
Test	**Present**	**Absent**
+	A	B
–	C	D

Analytic sensitivity: A/A + C
Analytic specificity: D/B + D

II. Clinical validity of biomarkers as risk factors and as clinical tests

	Clinical Outcome	
Biomarker	**Present**	**Absent**
+	A	B
–	C	D

As risk factor: analysis to proceed as part of case-control analysis
Odds ratio = AD/BC
For cohort analysis: risk ratio = (A/A + B)/(C/C + D)
As a clinical tool: analysis assesses sensitivity, specificity, and predictive value.
Clinical sensitivity: A/A + C; clinical specificity: D/B + D
Positive predictive value (PPV) = A/A + B (assuming total population tested)
Negative predictive value (NPV = D/C + D) (assuming total population tested)

III. Clinical utility (an example) among persons with a + biomarker

	Outcome	
Intervention	**Sick**	**Not**
1	A	B
2	C	D

Analysis in the context of controlled clinical trial comparing different interventions among persons with the biomarker
Risk ratio = (A/A + B)/(C/C + D) (comparing two hypothetical interventions)

[a] These tables are for illustration purposes only and apply to dichotomous biomarkers (present/absent). Additional analyses involve stratification, person-time analysis in cohort studies (see text), adjustment for confounding, and assessment of effect-measure modification.

CLINICAL UTILITY

Biomarkers proposed for use in practice should first be evaluated for clinical utility, i.e., the complete set of positive and negative outcomes accruing from their use. For example, although tests for genetic variants of clotting factors *F5* (Factor V Leiden) and *F2* (prothrombin 20210G-A) are in widespread use, their clinical utility has yet to be established in most settings. Clinical utility is first assessed in the context of controlled clinical trials combining use of biomarker and various interventions (see Table 28–4 for simple illustration). For additional readings, consult Burke et al. (2002) and Pinsky et al. (2004).

ETHICAL, LEGAL, AND SOCIAL ISSUES

The use of biomarkers in epidemiologic research raises a number of ethical, legal, and social (ELSI) issues (Schulte et al., 1999; Schulte, 2004). The acronym ELSI has been used extensively in the context of genetics research and genomic medicine (Meslin et al., 1997). Ethical, legal, and social issues around genetic information have been raised in a number of areas, including informed consent, recruitment of subjects, returning information about study results, and the potential for discrimination against or stigmatization of individuals and groups. Issues related to proper informed consent in the study of genetic variants with low disease risks in population-based epidemiologic settings have been described (Beskow et al., 2001). In consultation with a multidisciplinary group, the Centers for Disease Control and Prevention (CDC) has published an online consent form template and supplemental information that can be adapted by researchers for genetic epidemiologic studies (Beskow et al., 2001; Centers for Disease Control and Prevention, 2001a, 2001b).

CONVENTIONAL EPIDEMIOLOGIC STUDIES

Biomarkers of genetic and environmental factors involved in human disease have been used in case-control, cohort, and cross-sectional studies.

CASE-CONTROL STUDIES

The case-control approach is particularly well suited for studies of genetic variants because (a) unlike other biologic markers of exposures (e.g., hormonal levels, DNA adducts), genetic markers are stable indicators of host susceptibility; (b) case-control studies can provide an opportunity to do a comprehensive search for the effects of several genes, along with other risk factors, and to look for gene–environment interaction; and (c) case-control studies are suitable for many uncommon disease endpoints such as birth defects and specific cancers. On the other hand, because of changes in environmental exposures over time, cohort studies with repeated biomarkers of exposures and intermediate outcomes may be preferable to case-control studies, unless case-control studies are nested in an underlying cohort of a well-defined population for which biologic samples stored at the beginning of the study are later analyzed for exposures.

Case-control studies can simultaneously support gene discovery and population-based risk characterization. For example, registries of population-based incident disease cases and their families provide a platform for conducting family-based linkage and association studies (Thomas, 2004b). The National Cancer Institute (NCI) sponsors Cooperative Family Registries for Breast and Colorectal Cancer Research that reflect this philosophy (Daly et al., 2000; Hopper, 2003). Population-based case registries can support a number of study designs, including extended family studies, case-parent trios (Thomas, 2004b), and case-control-family designs (Peel et al., 2000). One type of family-based association study is the kin-cohort design in which researchers estimate the genotype-specific risk of disease occurrence in first-degree relatives of study participants (probands), inferring genotypes of relatives from genotypes measured in probands (Wacholder et al., 1998).

COHORT STUDIES

Efforts are now being made to integrate genomics into population-based epidemiologic cohort studies initiated in the pregenomic era to study disease incidence and prevalence, natural history, and risk factors. Well-known cohort studies include the Framingham study (National Heart, Lung, and Blood Institute, 2004), the Atherosclerosis Research in Communities study (ARIC Investigators, 1989), the European Prospective Investigation on Cancer (Riboli et al., 2002), and the newly designed National Children Study (National Institutes of Health, 2004), a planned U.S. cohort study of 100,000 pregnant women and their offspring to be followed from before birth to age 21 years. In addition, the genomics era is inspiring the development of very large longitudinal cohort studies and even studies of entire populations to establish repositories of biologic materials ("biobanks") for discovery and characterization of genes associated with common diseases. Table 28–5 shows a partial listing of such studies, which range from large random samples of adult populations such as the UK Biobank ($N = 500{,}000$; Wright et al., 2002) and the CartaGene (2004) project in Quebec ($N = 60{,}000$) to populations of entire countries such as Iceland ($N = 100{,}000$; Hakonarson et al., 2003) and Estonia ($N = 1{,}000{,}000$; Estonian Genome Project, 2004), to a cohort of twins in multiple countries (GenomeEUtwin, 2004). These biobanks may also help epidemiologists to quantify the

TABLE 28–5

Examples of Ongoing Large-Scale Population-Based Genomics Studies[a]

Study	Sample Size	Population	Study Objectives
Decode Genetics	>100,000	Iceland	"To identify genetic causes of common diseases and develop new drugs and diagnostic tools." Measures genes, health outcomes, and links with genealogy database.
UK Biobank	500,000	Population sample of persons aged 45–69 y	"To study the role of genes, environment and lifestyle." Link with medical records
CartaGene (Quebec)	>60,000	Population sample of persons aged 25–74 y	"To study genetic variation in a modern population." Link with health care records, and environmental and genealogy databases.
Estonia Genome Project	>1,000,000	Estonian population	"To find genes that cause and influence common diseases." Link with medical records.
GenomeEUtwin	~800,000 twin pairs	Twin cohorts from 7 European countries + Australia	"To characterize genetic, environmental and lifestyle components in the background of health problems"

[a] The last three projects are part of the global P3G collaboration (Public Population Project in Genomics).

occurrence of diseases in various populations and to understand their natural histories and risk factors, including gene–environment interactions.

Longitudinal cohort studies permit repeated phenotypic and outcome measures on individuals over time, including intermediate biochemical, physiologic, and other precursors and sequels of disease. Cohort studies can also be used for nested case-control studies or even as an initial screening method for case-only studies (as explained later). Such studies will produce a large amount of data on disease risk factors, lifestyles, and environmental exposures, and provide opportunities for data standardization, sharing, and joint analyses. An example of data standardization across international boundaries is the global P3G (Public Population Project in Genomics, 2004), which to date includes three international studies from Europe and North America (see Table 28–5). "Harmonization" is crucial to create comparability across sites on measures of genetic variation, environmental exposures, personal characteristics and behaviors, and long-term health outcomes.

CROSS-SECTIONAL STUDIES

Cross-sectional epidemiologic studies can be used to estimate allele and genotype frequencies, exposure levels in the population, and the relationships among genotypes, exposures, and phenotypes. Although cross-sectional studies cannot distinguish between incidence and natural history for the purpose of causal inference, they can provide population-level data on genetic variants and environmental exposures that may be useful for guiding research and health policy. An example of a population-based prevalence study is the analysis of two common mutations in the hemochromatosis gene (*C282Y* and *H63D* variants of *HFE)* in the U.S. population. Steinberg et al. genotyped 5,171 samples from the CDC's Third National Health and Nutrition Examination Survey (NHANES III), a nationally representative survey conducted in the United States from 1992 to 1994. Genotype and allele frequency data were cross-classified by sex, age, and race/ethnicity (Steinberg et al., 2001). The NHANES surveys have also been analyzed by the CDC to provide an ongoing assessment of the U.S. population's exposure to environmental chemicals. The first National Report on Human Exposure to Environmental Chemicals was issued in 2001 and presented exposure data for 27 chemicals from NHANES 1999–2001. The second report, released in 2003, presented exposure data for 116 environmental chemicals stratified by age, gender, and race/ethnicity (Centers for Disease

Control and Prevention, 2003). Currently, in collaboration with the National Cancer Institute, the CDC is using the NHANES III survey to measure prevalence of variants in 57 genes and correlate the resulting genotypes with medical history, clinical, and laboratory data (Lindegren and the CDC NHANES Working Group, 2003). When completed, such studies will provide valuable information on the association between genetic variation and numerous health endpoints.

METHODOLOGIC ISSUES

CONFOUNDING

A crucial consideration in studies of genetic susceptibility is the choice of an appropriate comparison group. The use of convenient comparison groups may lead to spurious findings as a result of confounding caused by unmeasured genetic and environmental factors. Race/ethnicity can be an important confounding variable in such studies (often referred to as population stratification) (Thomas and Witte, 2002). One example is the reported association between the genetic marker Gm3;5;13;14 and non–insulin-dependent diabetes mellitus (NIDDM) among Pima Indians (Knowler et al., 1988). In this cross-sectional study, individuals with the genetic marker had a higher prevalence of diabetes than those without the marker (29% vs. 8%). This marker, however, is an index of white admixture. When the analysis was stratified by degree of admixture, the association all but disappeared. Failure to account adequately for ethnicity in the study design or analysis can bias estimates of genetic effects on disease risk when both the occurrence of disease and the genotype distribution vary across groups and correlate with each other. Another way to adjust for hidden population stratification is to use several genetic markers to index population groups (such as the genomic control approach; Lee, 2004). Generally, in well-conducted epidemiologic studies that control for self-reported ethnicity, the bias from population stratification in estimating genetic effects is likely to be small, especially when there are many subgroups of the population (Wacholder et al., 2002).

GENOTYPE AND EXPOSURE MISCLASSIFICATION

As discussed earlier, the analytic validity of a biomarker must be established before it can be used in epidemiologic research. Unless errors are systematic (e.g., because the biomarker is related to the outcome as well as the exposure), misclassification is likely to dilute the association between a dichotomous biomarker and outcomes. Indirect methods have sometimes been used to classify individual genotypes. For example, Cartwright et al. (1982) used dapsone loading followed by urinary measurements of various metabolites in a case-control study of bladder cancer, a method for classifying subjects as slow or fast acetylators. Nondifferential, independent misclassification by indirect measures can bias the relative risk toward unity.

When a genotype is measured at the DNA level, misclassification can also be caused by linkage disequilibrium. Ideally, if the gene of interest has been sequenced, the presence of one or more mutations within the gene can be correlated with an altered gene product/function and case-control status. Many markers, however, are linked with other markers in the same chromosomal region (haplotypes). Investigators thus measure these markers instead of the disease susceptibility mutation itself. Marker alleles may be in linkage disequilibrium with disease alleles if the mutation has arisen relatively recently or if there are selective advantages of specific haplotypes. After several generations, genetic recombination generally leads to complete independence between a marker allele and a disease allele in the same region. In the meantime, under linkage disequilibrium, a marker allele and disease allele occur more often together. Thus, the use of a marker allele as a proxy for the disease allele in a case-control study presumably leads to nondifferential misclassification and a dilution of the odds ratio. Thus, a weak association of a marker with disease may obscure a potentially important association with the gene locus of interest.

GENE–ENVIRONMENT INTERACTION

Essentially, all human disease is caused by the interaction between genetic and environmental factors (see Chapter 2). Thus, in the design and analysis of epidemiologic studies, gene–environment and

TABLE 28–6

Gene–Environment Interaction Analysis in a Case-Control Study

Exposure	Genotype	Cases	Controls	Odds Ratio (OR)[a]
−	−	A_{00}	B_{00}	$OR_{00} = 1.0$
−	+	A_{01}	B_{01}	$OR_{01} = A_{01}B_{00}/(A_{00}B_{01})$
+	−	A_{10}	B_{10}	$OR_{10} = A_{10}B_{00}/(A_{00}B_{10})$
+	+	A_{11}	B_{11}	$OR_{11} = A_{11}B_{00}/(A_{00}B_{11})$

+, present; −, absent.
Interaction contrast (IC): $OR_{11} - OR_{10} - OR_{01} + 1$
Departure from odds ratio homogeneity: $OR_{11}/(OR_{10} \times OR_{01})$
[a] Case-only odds ratio OR: $(A_{11}A_{00})/(A_{10}A_{01}) = OR_{11}/(OR_{10} \times OR_{01}) \times OR_{co}$, where $OR_{co} = (B_{11}B_{00})/(B_{10}B_{01})$ (control-only odds ratio).

gene–gene interaction need to be considered explicitly. Examining the marginal association between a genotype and disease (or between exposure and disease) may mask the effect of biologic interaction between the genotypes and exposures (Khoury et al., 1993).

To assess gene–environment interaction at the simplest level, researchers can display data in a 2 × 4 table (Table 28–6). Here, we assume that an exposure is classified as being either present or absent and that the underlying susceptibility genotype is also classified as being present or absent. This genotype may reflect the presence of one or two alleles at one locus or a combination of alleles at multiple loci. Using unexposed subjects with no susceptibility genotype as the reference group, one can compute odds ratios for all other groups. As discussed by Botto and Khoury (2001), such presentation has several advantages. The role of each factor is independently assessed in terms of both association and potential attributable fraction. In addition, the odds ratios can be examined in terms of departure from specified models of independence (based ideally on additivity of excess relative risk—see Chapter 5). The table also provides the distribution of the exposures among controls, and helps evaluate the dependence of factors in the underlying population (provided the controls are representative). Finally, a case-only odds ratio can be derived (as explained later). The 2 × 4 table approach to presenting gene–environment interactions essentially summarizes seven 2 × 2 tables (Botto and Khoury, 2001). It underscores study-size issues because cell sizes are presented. It also favors effect estimation over statistical significance testing (see Chapter 10). To illustrate, we use data from a case-control study of venous thromboembolism in relation to Factor V Leiden and oral contraceptive use to show key aspects of gene–environment interaction (See Table 28–7), including marginal and joint effects and potential population-attributable fractions and calculation of case-only and control-only odds ratios.

From an efficiency perspective, case-control studies could be used to evaluate gene–environment and gene–gene interactions, particularly for common exposures and genotypes. Desirable study sizes depend on the underlying model of interaction between the genotype and the exposure. In specific types of biologic interactions—such as when the exposure and the genotype alone do not increase disease risks per se—the study sizes needed to assess the marginal effects of the exposure (in a 2 × 2 table) will be more than adequate to estimate interaction between the exposure and the interacting genotype.

EMERGING ANALYTIC COMPLEXITY

The potential use of thousands of genetic variants in epidemiologic studies creates increased potential for Type I and Type II errors, especially when significance testing is overemphasized. Large-scale data mining will unavoidably lead to numerous positive associations that are not replicated. One reason for Type I errors is simply reliance on statistical significance testing. Wacholder et al. (2004) has developed a Bayesian approach to assess the probability that—given a statistically significant finding—no true association exists between a genetic variant and disease. This approach incorporates not only the observed *P*-value but also the prior probability of the gene–disease association

TABLE 28–7

Analysis of Oral Contraceptive Use, Presence of Factor V Leiden Mutation, and Risk for Venous Thromboembolism[a]

Factor V Leiden	OC	Cases	Controls	Odds Ratio		95% CI	AF-Exp (%)
−	−	36	100	OR_{00}	1.0	reference	
−	+	10	4	OR_{01}	6.9	1.83, 31.80	85.6
+	−	84	63	OR_{10}	3.7	2.18, 6.32	73.0
+	+	25	2	OR_{11}	34.7	7.83, 310.0	97.1
Total		155	169				

OC, oral contraceptives; AF-Exp (%), attributable fraction (percent) among exposed.
Interaction contrast (IC): $OR_{11} - OR_{10} - OR_{01} + 1 = 34.7 - 3.7 - 6.9 + 1 = 25.1$
Departure from odds ratio homogeneity: $OR_{11}/(OR_{10} \times OR_{01}) = 34.7/(3.7 \times 6.9) = 1.4$
[a] Case-only odds ratio OR: $(A_{11}A_{00})/(A_{10}A_{01}) = OR_{11}/(OR_{10} \times OR_{01}) \times OR_{co}$, $(25 \times 36)/(63 \times 4) = 1.1 = 1.4 \times 0.8$
where $OR_{co} = (B_{11}B_{00})/(B_{10}B_{01})$ (control-only odds ratio) $(2 \times 100)/(63 \times 4) = 0.8$
From Botto and Khoury (2002); data from Vandenbroucke et al. (1994).

and the statistical power of the test. The problem of false positives is compounded by the obvious tendency of authors and journals to publish statistically significant "positive" or interesting findings (publication bias), and for all stakeholders to overemphasize results of an individual study, even when the prior probability of the hypothesis is very low.

On the other hand, let us consider for a moment the staggering implication for epidemiology of identifying numerous genetic risk factors. Imagine that, for a common disease, only 10 genes contribute a substantial population-attributable fraction. Even if variation at each locus can be classified in a dichotomous fashion (e.g., susceptible genotype vs. not), this classification will create 2 to the power 10, or over a thousand possible strata. Dichotomous classification based on just 20 genes will produce over a million strata. The analysis can get even more complicated when we consider the interactions of these genes with other genes and with environmental factors. Emerging technology will allow us to measure simultaneously hundreds and thousands of genome variations, gene expression profiles, and protein patterns. Our epidemiologic analysis of 2 × 4 tables, stratified analyses, and even logistic regression analysis will quickly face the limitations of small study size in an age when a large amount of data on each individual is the rule rather than the exception (Hoh and Ott, 2003).

As a result of increasing complexity, novel analytic strategies are emerging, including hierarchical regression and Bayesian methods (Dunson, 2001; Greenland, 2007a; see Chapter 21). These methods may be suited to address the problem of false-positive associations resulting from multiple comparisons. Another approach to joint analysis of multiple genes for quantitative traits is the combinatorial partitioning method (CPM; Nelson et al., 2001), which represents an extension of traditional analysis of variance between and within genotypes at one gene locus. An excess of variability between the genotypes, relative to within genotypes, represents an association between the gene and the trait. The CPM extends this concept to many genes by genotypic partitioning based on multiple loci. An extension of CPM is the multifactor dimensionality-reduction (MDR) method (Hahn et al., 2003). Using this approach, genotypes at multiple loci are grouped into a few categories to create high-risk and low-risk groups. This method reduces the number of genotypes from many dimensions to one (Ritchie, 2001; Zhang et al., 2001). For example, these methods may be able to classify persons into two or more distinct groups with respect to their propensity to "bleed' or "coagulate" based on the combination of genotypes at multiple loci involved in maintaining a delicate balance between bleeding and thrombosis (e.g., the cascade of Factors I through X). When based on understanding of underlying biology, it is possible that these composite complex genotypes may be useful for predicting disease outcomes or response to treatment. Although these methods continue to evolve, they are still vulnerable to the problems of nonreproducibility and false positive findings. Further research and application is needed for these methods to be useful to practicing epidemiologists.

NONCONVENTIONAL EPIDEMIOLOGIC STUDIES

Here, we highlight two nonconventional approaches that have recently emerged in epidemiologic studies of genetic factors and gene–environment interaction in disease: the case-only study and the case-parent study. These approaches involve the use of an internal control group rather than an external one.

CASE-ONLY STUDIES

As in other areas of epidemiology, a case-series design has been gradually recognized as an approach that can be used for multiple purposes: to evaluate gene–gene and gene–environment interaction in disease etiology, to scan for the contribution of complex genotypes, and to assess heterogeneity in outcomes (Botto and Khoury, 2004; Begg and Zhang, 1994; Piegorsch et al., 1994). Although the case-only method is best known for the analysis of interactions, it may have the most limitations in this area, and the other two applications may become more prominent, as will be discussed.

For estimating interaction effects, investigators use case subjects only to assess the magnitude of the association between a genotype and an exposure (or another genotype). The basic setup for analysis is a 2 × 2 table relating exposure to genotype in cases only (Table 28–6). If the genotype and the exposures are independent in the source population from which cases arose, the expected value of OR_{co} becomes unity; thus the odds ratio obtained from a case-only study measures the departure from multiplicative joint effect of the genotype and the exposure. Under the null hypothesis of multiplicative effects, the expected value of OR_{ca} is unity; if the joint effect is more than multiplicative, OR_{ca} is expected to be more than 1. This approach provides a simple tool with which to screen for gene–gene and gene–environment interaction in disease etiology. It can be used in the context of crude analysis of a 2 × 2 table or in the context of regression models adjusted for other covariates. Several methodologic issues should be considered when applying the case-only approach (Liu et al., 2004):

1. The choice of cases is still subject to the usual rules of valid case selection for any case-control study. Ideally, incident cases from a well-defined population will enhance etiologic inference of findings
2. Researchers must assume independence between exposure and genotype in the underlying source population to apply this method. This assumption may seem reasonable for a wide variety of genes and exposures. There are some genes, however, whose presence may lead to a higher or lower likelihood of the exposure on the basis of some biologic mechanism. For example, genetic variations in alcohol and aldehyde dehydrogenases, the main enzymes involved in alcohol metabolism, are suspected risk factors for alcoholism and alcohol-related liver damage. Individuals with delayed alcohol metabolism as a result of particular genetic variants may have an increased flushing response after alcohol ingestion and thus be less likely to use alcohol, which could lead to a negative correlation between alcohol exposure and alcohol dehydrogenase polymorphisms in some populations (Sherman et al., 1994).
3. The case-only approach does not allow investigators to evaluate the independent effects of the exposure alone or the genotype alone, merely departure from multiplicative effects.
4. The measure obtained from this analysis can only be interpreted as a departure from a multiplicative relation, whereas departure from additivity may be of greater interest (see Chapter 5).

In addition to the study of gene–gene and gene–environment interaction, the case-only approach has two other relevant applications (see Table 28–8) that are especially suited for population-based disease registries (e.g., cancer, birth defects) (Botto and Khoury, 2004):

1. One can scan for genotypes that potentially contribute most to disease occurrence in a population. By using the concept of population-attributable fraction, case-only studies can provide an upper estimate of the contribution of complex risk factors, including multiple genetic variants at different loci, for disease occurrence. Genotypes comprising combinations of multiple genetic variants have a low expected population frequency even when the variants are individually

TABLE 28–8

Illustration of the Contributions of the Case-Only Epidemiologic Study Design in the Genomics Era

I. Scan for complex genotypes that could have a significant attributable fraction

Gene variants at N loci			Cases (T)
1	2	3 . . . N	
−	−	− . . . −	A
+	−	− . . . −	B
.	.	. . .	. . .
+	+	+ . . . +	X

For complex genotypes at N loci, the expected proportion of the population with such a combination will decrease markedly with increasing number of loci, even if each variant is common in the population. For example, if we have genetic variants at 10 loci each with 50% prevalence in the population, about 1 in 1,000 or fewer people are expected to be positive for all 10. Therefore, we can use the ratio of X/T to derive an upper bound of population-attributable fraction for complex genotypes even in the absence of controls (for more details, consult Botto and Khoury, 2004).

II. Assess etiologic heterogeneity and genotype–phenotype correlation among cases

Risk factor	Cases	
(exposure/genotype)	Phenotype 1	Phenotype 2
Yes	A	B
No	C	D

Odds ratio = AD/BC = 1 if homogeneous subgroups

Phenotypes can be based on clinical classification, use of gene expression profiles, or protein expression markers (for examples, see text).

III. Screen for multiplicative gene–environment or gene–gene interaction

Risk factor	Cases	
(exposure/genotype)	Genotype 1	Genotype 2
Yes	A	B
No	C	D

Odds ratio = AD/BC = 1 if joint effects are multiplicative and >1 if supramultiplicative

common. Therefore, the case-only approach may be useful in identifying combinations of genes to evaluate further for potential etiologic importance (Botto and Khoury, 2004).

2. One can evaluate disease etiologic, diagnostic, and prognostic heterogeneity. Genotype–phenotype correlations can be examined among subsets of cases defined clinically, or by use of biologic markers based on genotype, gene expression, protein products, or other features. For

example, a recent study found that mutations of the *CARD15* gene known to be associated with Crohn disease were correlated with disease of the ileum but not the colon (Lesage et al., 2002). In another example, Le Marchand et al. conducted a population-based study to evaluate overall and stage-specific associations of the *870A* allele of the *Cyclin D1 (CCND1)* gene with colorectal cancer. They found that the allele was associated with colorectal cancer, and particularly with more severe forms of the disease that result in higher morbidity and mortality (LeMarchand et al., 2003). A third example is the analysis of genotype–phenotype correlation in cystic fibrosis, a common single-gene disorder in people of Northern European descent. More than 1,000 different mutations in the *CFTR* gene have been described (Mickle and Cutting, 2000), and genotypic heterogeneity explains in part the highly variable clinical expression of cystic fibrosis. Because lung function varies even among patients with similar *CFTR* genotype, other genetic and environmental determinants also have a role (Burke, 2003).

CASE-PARENT STUDIES

In the case-parent approach, persons with specific health outcomes and their parents are used as a triad to compare the genotypic distribution at one or more loci of the cases with the expected distribution of genotypes based on the parental genotypes. We considered this approach as equivalent to a matched case-control study (Khoury and Flanders, 1996), in which transmitted alleles among cases are compared with nontransmitted alleles from the parents. This approach can be appropriately described as equivelant to a case-cohort design (see Chapter 8). In either scenario, genetic markers associated with increased disease risk could reflect a causal role or could be in linkage disequilibrium with alleles at a neighboring locus (Schaid and Sommer, 1993; Spielman et al., 1993). The method requires the availability of genotypic information on the parents of case subjects. In its simplest form, the genotype of each case subject can be compared with the genotype of a fictitious control formed by the nontransmitted alleles from each parent. Because this is a matched analysis, one can construct a 2×2 table comparing case and control subjects with respect to the presence or absence of the allele (or genotype). Odds ratios can be simply obtained, with the analysis following that of a matched-pair design. This method can also be used to stratify case subjects according to the presence or absence of the pertinent interacting exposure, and odds ratios can be derived with or without the exposure.

Several methods of analysis have been have proposed for this type of study (Flanders and Khoury, 1996; Flanders et al., 2001; Sun et al, 1998). By and large, these methods are noniterative and lead to a closed estimate of the risk ratios, comparing risk among those with a specific genotype to the risk among those with a comparison genotype. Essentially, for each combination of parental genotypes, the observed distribution of the offspring (case) genotype is compared with the distribution expected on the basis of Mendelian transmission probabilities. Another analytic approach, suggested by Weinberg et al. (1998), is log-linear Poisson regression that is fitted using a standard software package, and that has the distinct advantage over matched analysis of using all information efficiently, including heterozygote parents and those with missing genotypic data.

As with the case-only design, the case-parent approach does not allow assessment of the independent effect of the environmental exposures, merely whether the effect of the genotype is different for persons with the exposure than for persons without the exposure. As in the case-only design, this effect-measure modification is also measured on a multiplicative scale. Nevertheless, the case-parent design permits assessment of the effect of the genotype (with and without the exposure), whereas the case-only approach does not. Case-parent studies have also been suggested to look for gene–environment interactions (Lake and Laird, 2004), imprinting effects (Weinberg et al., 1998), and parent-of-origin effects (Weinberg et al., 1998; Weinberg, 1999).

EXAMPLE 1: COLORECTAL CANCER

Colorectal cancer provides a useful illustration of new "omic" tools in epidemiology. These illustrations include the use of biomarkers for improved exposure assessment, markers of genetic susceptibility appropriate for large populations, new methods for cancer screening, and molecular profiles of tumors that can predict response to therapy. The following examples illustrate how "omic" tools can strengthen and enhance (rather than detract from or replace) conventional epidemiologic studies.

EXPOSURE ASSESSMENT

For decades, epidemiologic studies implicated high levels of meat consumption as a risk factor for colorectal cancer (Potter et al., 1993). Improved exposure assessment using biomarkers has revealed many of the relevant causal pathways. Specific methods of cooking, including grilling or frying meat to high internal temperatures, produce heterocylic amines (HCAs). HCAs are identified using a combination of liquid chromatography and mass spectrometry (Felton et al., 2004), and can be detected in food as well as human blood and urine. HCAs cause tumors in laboratory animals and are classified as suspected human carcinogens (Dashwood, 2003). Toxicologists and epidemiologists collaborated to develop an index to correlate HCA levels in food with types and cuts of meat, method of cooking, and degree of doneness (Sinha et al., 1998). Exposure to dietary HCAs can now be estimated in epidemiologic studies using standardized photographs of cooked meat and food-frequency questionnaires. Using these methods, increased HCA exposure was associated with increased risk of colorectal polyps (Sinha et al., 1999) and colon cancer (Butler et al., 2003).

HCAs as biomarkers of exposure help to address diet as a complex mixture. In human volunteers, intake of broccoli increased urinary excretion of one particular HCA, 2-amino-1-methyl-6-phenylimidazo[4,5-*b*]pyridine or PhIP, and certain types of tea inhibit the mutagenicity of PhIP in bacterial assays (Felton et al., 2004; Dashwood, 2003). Unraveling the complexity of dietary exposures at the molecular level has provided important insights into the etiology of colon and other cancers (Ketterer, 1998). Because HCA content can be lowered by changing methods of cooking and preparing meat, HCAs as biomarkers have helped to design interventions to reduce risk of colon and other cancers.

Previously, biomarkers such as HCAs were the province of molecular epidemiology and toxicologists. But these markers have entered mainstream epidemiology through their incorporation into conventional epidemiologic studies (Felton et al., 2004, p. 142). In addition, because metabolism of HCAs, isothiocyanates in broccoli, and other dietary constituents is under genetic regulation, polymorphisms in genes involved in metabolism of HCAs and compounds (Houlston and Tomlinson, 2001) may help to uncover additional information about the role of diet in colon cancer risk.

GENETIC SUSCEPTIBILITY

Approximately 10% of colorectal cancer patients report a history of the disease among first-degree relatives (Lynch and de la Chapelle, 2003), and family history is associated with a two- to threefold increase in risk of colorectal cancer (Potter et al., 1993). A portion of colorectal cancer patients with multiple affected relatives carry rare, inherited mutations in genes that confer high lifetime risk of colorectal cancer and are called high-penetrance mutations (Lynch and de la Chapelle, 2003). Genetic testing followed by specific clinical interventions (including increased screening and prophylactic surgery) can lower risk of colorectal cancer in mutation carriers. These interventions, however, apply to only a small percentage of persons in the general population. With the sequencing of the human genome, more common sources of genetic variation (polymorphisms) have been discovered. These inherited genetic variants have a much weaker effect, often acting in combination with other genes and environmental factors (Vineis et al., 1999).

Colorectal cancer illustrates how molecular and genetic tools can uncover new clues about the biologic basis of cancer, and provide insight into the multicausal nature of disease. Epidemiologic studies incorporating genetic polymorphisms have helped to clarify the role of dietary supplements and medication use in the etiology of colorectal cancer. Conventional epidemiologic studies of the risk of colon cancer associated with calcium and vitamin D supplementation, and aspirin and other nonsteroidal anti-inflammatory drugs (NSAIDs) such as ibuprofen and acetaminophen, have yielded inconsistent results (Potter et al., 1993). A major limitation has been the potential for confounding by lifestyle, including diet and physical activity. By genotyping participants from epidemiologic studies, researchers showed that polymorphisms in prostaglandin synthase 2 (*PTGS2*) (Lin et al., 2002), ornithine decarboxylase (*ODC*) (Martinez et al., 2003), cytochrome P450 2C9 (*CYP2C9*) and uridine diphospho-glucuronosyltransferase IA6 (*UGTIA6*) (Bigler et al., 2001) modified the protective effect of NSAIDS and aspirin on risk of colon polyps. Genotypes for the methylenetetrahydrofolate reductase (*MTHFR*) gene modified the effects of folic acid intake on colorectal cancer (Chen et al., 1996; Keku et al., 2002), and the protective effects of calcium supplements and vitamin D intake were modified by genotypes at the vitamin D receptor (*VDR*) locus (Kim et al., 2001). The protein products of these genes are known to play key roles in metabolism of dietary supplements or medications. Therefore, the presence of effect-measure modification provides evidence that the observed protective effects of these compounds may have a biologic foundation.

CANCER SCREENING

To improve the sensitivity and specificity of colorectal cancer screening and to increase acceptability and affordability for patients, researchers are seeking to identify stool-based genetic screening tests for colorectal cancer. The procedures use molecular biology techniques to isolate, amplify, and characterize specific genetic alterations in epithelial cells in stool. The genetic alterations are acquired somatic changes that are present in tissues undergoing malignant transformation and are not present elsewhere in the body (Hanahan and Weinberg, 2000). By developing tests for key mutations in these genes, researchers hope to be able to detect colon cancer at an earlier stage, when it can be more effectively treated. Stool-based genetic tests are noninvasive (do not require endoscopy, biopsy, or sedation/anesthesia) and thus do not require specialized health care personnel. The tests also do not require patients to maintain a controlled diet before the test. Stool samples can be collected in a patient's home, using procedures similar to fecal occult blood testing.

Examples of stool-based genetic tests under development for colorectal cancer screening include somatic mutations in the *APC* gene (Traverso et al., 2002), *K-ras* (Tobi et al., 1994), P53, and BAT26 (Dong et al., 2001). Stool-based genetic tests that use multiple genetic targets may be more effective than those based on single alterations. Comparisons need to be made of the sensitivity, specificity, and predictive value of stool-based genetic screening tests for colorectal cancer versus fecal occult blood testing and endoscopy. These comparisons need to be made in population-based settings, using realistic estimates of the prevalence of disease. Estimates of predictive value derived from matched sets of cases and controls are invalid, because the prevalence is preset ahead of time by the investigator and cases are often detected on the basis of symptoms. As an example for another cancer, Petricoin et al. (2003) developed a potential proteomic test for early detection of ovarian cancer. Proteomics uses a variation of mass spectroscopy to detect and differentiate small-molecular-weight proteins in serum. The authors found a protein fragment at higher concentration in 50 ovarian cases compared to 66 hospital controls, and claimed a predictive value of 94%. As shown by Rockhill (2002), a test with identical sensitivity and specificity would yield a predictive value of only 1% when used as a screening tool in populations in which the prevalence of ovarian cancer is only 50 per 100,000. Ultimately, randomized trials using mortality as the endpoint will be needed to determine whether stool-based genetics tests offer any advantages over conventional screening methods.

TUMOR HETEROGENEITY

Gene expression can be monitored using nucleotide arrays or gene chips (King and Sinha, 2001). Tumors show increases and decreases in levels of gene expression compared with normal tissue, and expression profiles can be used to categorize tumors into subtypes with clinical relevance. For examples, gene expression profiling can be used to identify subtypes of colon cancer that respond to specific forms of chemotherapy (Mariadason et al., 2003). In the future, it may be possible to choose therapeutic regimens based on tumor expression profiles and design new treatments based on the types of biologic changes that occur in cancer, but randomized trials will be needed. In the meantime, epidemiologists can use these new tools to determine whether subtypes of cancer based on expression profiles have different underlying etiologies.

EXAMPLE 2: INFLAMMATORY BOWEL DISEASE

GENETIC SUSCEPTIBILITY AND GENE DISCOVERY

Inflammatory bowel disease (IBD) encompasses a spectrum of chronic, relapsing intestinal diseases that require lifelong medical and surgical management. The two major forms of IBD—ulcerative colitis and Crohn disease—are distinguished on clinical grounds, although considerable overlap exists and no system of diagnostic criteria has been universally adopted. Both conditions cluster in families without a clear pattern of inheritance, suggesting that multiple familial factors—genetic and environmental—may influence susceptibility (Podolsky, 2002). Because relatives of people with either Crohn disease or ulcerative colitis are at increased risk for both conditions, it appears likely that some risk factors are shared while others are distinct (Bonen and Cho, 2003).

The inflammatory response to infection is a paradigm for gene–environment interaction, and intestinal bacteria have long been suspected as environmental triggers for IBD. For many years, etiologic studies focused on specific pathogens and on the immune system—especially the major histocompatibility complex—without identifying specific causes. More recently, advances in molecular biology have intensified the search for underlying mechanisms by investigating genetic determinants of the immune response (Podolsky, 2002; Hugot, 2004).

In 1996, Hugot et al. reported that a genome-wide linkage study had found a susceptibility region for Crohn disease on chromosome 16, which they termed *IBD1* (Hugot et al., 1996). In 2001, Ogura et al. identified the *NOD2* gene (subsequently renamed *CARD15*), mapped it to chromosome 16, and demonstrated that the corresponding protein has a role in innate immunity (Ogura et al., 2001a). Later that year, both groups of investigators reported that *CARD15/NOD2* variants were implicated in Crohn disease (Hugot et al., 2001; Ogura et al., 2001b).

Ogura et al. selected *CARD15/NOD2* as a candidate gene for Crohn disease because it mapped to the *IBD1* region and its function was consistent with etiologic hypotheses (Ogura et al., 2001b). After identifying a single-base insertion mutation (*3020insC*) in three cases, they demonstrated its association with inherited susceptibility to Crohn disease in a study of multiply affected families using the transmission disequilibrium test. An association study found the *CARD15/NOD2* (*3020insC*) variant in 14% (57/416) of unrelated cases and 8% (23/287) of samples obtained previously from people without Crohn disease; 3% (11/416) of cases—but no controls—were homozygous. The authors reported "genotype-relative risks" (estimated by odds ratios) of 1.5 for heterozygotes and 17 for homozygotes (estimating the expected number among controls by assuming Hardy-Weinberg equilibrium). Functional studies of the *CARD15/NOD2 3020insC* variant found that the corresponding protein had reduced ability to react with bacterial components.

Hugot et al. had already examined and rejected two other candidate genes in the *IBD1* region; they turned instead to a positional cloning strategy, which ultimately yielded three SNPs associated with Crohn disease in 235 families (Hugot et al., 2001) All three SNPs proved to be variants of the *CARD15/NOD2* gene, and the SNP with the strongest association was identical to the single-base-pair insertion found by Ogura et al. The genotypes of 468 people with Crohn disease were compared with those of 159 people with ulcerative colitis; 103 unaffected people were recruited among spouses and other nonblood relatives of patients. Overall, 43% of people with Crohn disease had at least one of the three SNPs, compared with 9% of those with ulcerative colitis and 15% of controls; homozygous and compound heterozygous genotypes were found only in people with Crohn disease (68/468, 15%), except for one person with ulcerative colitis. The authors reported relative risks of 3 for simple heterozygotes and approximately 40 for compound heterozygotes and homozygotes (estimating the expected numbers among controls by assuming Hardy-Weinberg equilibrium).

GENERATING NEW HYPOTHESES

Within 3 years, more than 150 scientific articles had elaborated on this discovery (National Library of Medicine, 2004), offering insights into the pathobiology of Crohn disease and suggesting potential new approaches to therapy (Elson, 2002). Published studies examined the association of *CARD15/NOD2* variants with Crohn disease in other countries and ethnic groups; documented genotype–phenotype correlations; reported genotype-specific results of therapeutic trials; and analyzed gene–gene and gene–environment interactions.

For example, several studies quickly documented that *CARD15/NOD2* variants were virtually absent in Asian patients with Crohn disease, but were common among those of European descent (Yamazaki et al., 2002; Croucher et al., 2003). Genotype–phenotype studies established that *CARD15/NOD2* variants were associated with Crohn disease of the ileum in both sporadic and familial cases (Hampe et al., 2002; Lesage et al., 2002). Clinical trials swiftly dismissed the hypothesis that *CARD15/NOD2* variants would predict response to therapy with infliximab (monoclonal antibody directed against tumor necrosis factor [TNF]) (Vermeire, 2002; Mascheretti et al., 2002).

Investigators searched for additional clues to the pathogenesis of Crohn disease by examining potential interactions between *CARD15/NOD2* genotype and environmental exposures (e.g., tobacco use; Brant et al., 2003) or biomarkers (e.g., anti-*Saccharomyces cerevisiae* antibodies [ASCA]; Walker et al., 2004). Others explored potential interactions between *CARD15/NOD2* variants and additional susceptibility loci for Crohn disease (Newman et al., 2004; Negoro et al., 2003; Mirza et al., 2003). Still others examined associations of *CARD15/NOD2* variants with other forms of bowel disease (e.g., colorectal cancer; Kurzowski et al., 2004) and other disorders related to immune dysregulation (e.g., psoriatic arthritis; Rahman et al., 2003).

EPIDEMIOLOGY AND COMPLEXITY

The association of *CARD15/NOD2* with Crohn disease in European populations provides an unusually striking example of genetic susceptibility to complex disease. Not only are implicated variants common among cases, the association is strong and consistent among studies. Nonetheless, the implications of this discovery cannot be fully assessed without additional population-based information. Perhaps most important, the population-attributable fraction cannot be estimated with confidence because population-level genotype prevalence data are not available. Most association studies have employed convenience samples of cases and controls, and although several have addressed potential gene–gene interactions, very few have examined interactions with potential environmental factors. Thus, the epidemiology of *CARD15/NOD2* variants remains an important area for additional research.

New insights into the pathobiology of Crohn disease have also revealed further complexity. Associations were found with genetic variants at the 5q31 locus known as *IBD5*, which contains the cytokine gene cluster (Rioux et al., 2001). Subsequent analysis identified these with a susceptibility haplotype containing variants of the *OCTN1* and*OCTN2* genes (also known as *SLC22A4* and*SLC22A5*), which code for organic cation transporters, not cytokines. It has been suggested that *SLC22A4*, *SLC22A5*, and *CARD15* act in a common pathogenic pathway to cause Crohn disease (Peltekova et al., 2004).

Molecular methods have advanced understanding of the genetics of IBD, but environmental influences remain poorly understood. Since the 1930s, incidence of both ulcerative colitis and Crohn disease has increased steadily in Europe and North America, with evidence for recent leveling in high-incidence areas (Loftus, 2004; Timmer, 2003). Environmental factors are clearly responsible, yet decades of active investigation have identified only a single definitive association: smoking, which paradoxically increases the risk and severity of Crohn disease but appears to reduce the risk of ulcerative colitis. Many epidemiologic studies have found associations with factors such as diet, stress, and socioeconomic status that are difficult to measure but are often shared within families and are more generally associated with the modern Western lifestyle (Timmer, 2003). Thus, epidemiologic evidence suggests that the current causal model for IBD—immune dysregulation producing a hyperactive inflammatory response to intestinal bacteria—is necessarily incomplete (Timmer, 2003). Advances in molecular biology may yet uncover additional clues in studies of bacteria, whose genomes are under selection pressures that change with manipulation of the environment that humans and microbes share (Hugot et al., 2003).

A comprehensive explanation of the etiology of IBD is likely to emerge only from a wide-ranging research agenda coupled with an inclusive approach to synthesis of knowledge from diverse fields. This challenge requires extending the scientific horizon beyond systems biology to an ecology of interactions among humans, microbes, and their environments (Hugot et al., 2003), occurring not only as "gene–environment interactions" at the molecular level but within families and populations. Epidemiologists have much to contribute and to learn from this endeavor.

CHAPTER 29

Nutritional Epidemiology

Walter C. Willett

Epidemiologic Studies of Nutritional Exposures 581
Ecologic Studies 581
Special Exposure Groups 582
Migrant Studies and Secular Trends 582
Case-Control and Cohort Studies 582
Experimental Studies 585
Measurement of Diet in Epidemiologic Studies 586
Nutrients, Foods, and Dietary Patterns 586
Dimension of Time 588
General Methods of Dietary Assessment 588
Methods Based on Food Intake 589
Validity of Dietary Assessment Methods 591
Biochemical Indicators of Diet 592
Choice of Tissues for Analysis 594
Limitations of Biochemical Indicators 594
Anthropometry and Measures of Body Composition 594
Methodologic Issues in Nutritional Epidemiology 595
Between-Person Variation in Dietary Intake 595
Implications of Total Energy Intake 596
Conclusion 597

The discipline of nutritional epidemiology uses epidemiologic approaches to determine relations between dietary factors and the occurrence of specific diseases. For many years, many nutritionists and epidemiologists thought that the difficulties of assessing the diets of free-living human beings over extended periods of time made large-scale studies impossible. Recently, however, methods for assessing dietary intake have been developed and validated, thus providing the underpinning for this rapidly expanding field. Largely as a result of this effort, the potential importance of diet in the cause and prevention of nearly all major diseases has come to be appreciated. For example, diseases as diverse as birth defects, most forms of cancer, cardiovascular diseases, infertility, and cataracts have important dietary determinants. Moreover, the definition of *nutrient* has become increasingly unclear as the role of food constituents not normally considered to be nutrients for maintaining long-term health has become evident. In general, nutritional epidemiologists have not felt constrained by any formal definition of nutrition and are broadly concerned about health as it is related to food and its components, whether they be essential nutrients, other natural constituents of food, chemicals created in the cooking and preservation of food, or noninfectious food contaminants. Because the major distinction between nutritional epidemiology and other areas of epidemiology is that the exposures are aspects of diet—an extremely complex set of variables—much of this chapter is devoted to the measurement of dietary intake. Before doing so, however, the classic epidemiologic approaches—ecologic, case-control, and cohort studies—are discussed in the context of issues that are particularly germane to the study of nutritional exposures.

As many of the topics considered in this chapter can be discussed only briefly, readers are referred to a full text on the topic of nutritional epidemiology (Willett, 1998) and to cited references for more detailed treatment.

EPIDEMIOLOGIC STUDIES OF NUTRITIONAL EXPOSURES

ECOLOGIC STUDIES

With few exceptions (Dawber et al., 1961), epidemiologic investigations of diet and disease before 1980 consisted largely of *ecologic* or *correlational* studies; that is, comparisons of disease rates in populations with the population per-capita consumption of specific dietary factors. Usually, the dietary information in such studies is based on "disappearance" data, meaning the national figures for food produced and imported minus the food that is exported, fed to animals, or otherwise not available for humans. Many of the correlations based on such information are remarkably strong; for example, the correlation between meat intake and incidence of colon cancer is 0.85 for men and 0.89 for women (Armstrong and Doll, 1975).

The use of international ecologic studies to evaluate the relation between diet and disease has several strengths. Most important, the contrasts in dietary intake are typically very large. For example, in the United States, most individuals consume between 30% and 45% of their calories from fat (Willett, 1987), whereas the *mean* fat intake for populations in various other countries has varied from approximately 15% to 42% of calories (Goodwin and Boyd, 1987). Also, the average of diets for persons residing in a country are likely to be more stable over time than are the diets of individual persons within the country; for most countries, the changes in per-capita dietary intakes over a decade or two are relatively small. Finally, the disease rates on which international studies are based are usually derived from relatively large populations and are therefore subject to only small random errors.

A major limitation of such ecologic studies is that many potential determinants of disease other than the dietary factor under consideration may vary between areas with a high and low incidence of disease (see Chapter 23). Such confounding factors can include genetic predisposition, other dietary factors, including the availability of total food energy, and other environmental or lifestyle practices. For example, with few exceptions, such as Japan, countries with a low incidence of colon cancer tended to be economically undeveloped. Therefore, any variable related to industrialization will be similarly correlated with incidence of colon cancer. Indeed, the correlation between gross national product and colon cancer mortality rate is 0.77 for men and 0.69 for women (Armstrong and Doll, 1975). More complex analyses of such ecologic data can be conducted that control for some of the potentially confounding factors. For example, McKeown-Eyssen and Bright-See (1985) found that an inverse association of per-capita dietary fiber intake and national colon cancer mortality rates decreased substantially after adjustment for fat intake.

Another major limitation of ecologic studies is their reliance on population rather than individual characteristics (see Chapter 23). Aggregate data for a geographic unit as a whole may be only weakly related to the diets of those individuals at risk of disease. As an extreme example, the interpretation of ecologic data regarding alcohol intake and breast cancer is complicated because, in some cultures, most of the alcohol is consumed by men, but it is the women who develop breast cancer. In addition, ecologic studies of diet are often limited by the use of disappearance data that are only indirectly related to intake and are likely to be of variable quality. For example, the higher "disappearance" of calories per capita for the United States compared with most countries is probably related largely to wasted food. These problems of ecologic associations and issues of data quality can potentially be addressed by collecting information on actual dietary intake in a uniform manner from the population subgroups of interest (Navidi et al., 1994; Sheppard and Prentice, 1995). This strategy separates groups at a level sufficiently fine for the study objectives, and has been applied in a study conducted in 65 geographic areas in China (Chen et al., 1990).

Another serious limitation of the international ecologic studies is that they cannot be reproduced independently, which is an important part of the scientific process. Although the dietary information can be improved and the analyses can be refined, the data will not really be independent even as more information becomes available over time; the populations, their diets, and the confounding variables will be similar. Thus, it is not likely that many new insights will be obtained from further ecologic studies among countries.

The role of ecologic studies in nutritional epidemiology is controversial. Clearly, these analyses have stimulated much of the current research on diet in relation to cancer and cardiovascular disease, and in particular they have emphasized the major differences in rates of these diseases among countries. Traditionally, such studies have been considered the weakest form of evidence, primarily owing to the potential for confounding by factors that are difficult to measure and control (Kinlen, 1983). Others have felt that such studies provide the strongest form of evidence for evaluating hypotheses relating diet to cancer (Hebert and Miller, 1988; Prentice et al., 1988). On balance, ecologic studies have clearly been useful, but they are far from conclusive regarding the relations between dietary factors and disease and may sometimes be totally misleading (Greenland and Robins, 1994; see Chapter 25).

SPECIAL EXPOSURE GROUPS

Subgroups within a population that consume unusual diets provide an additional opportunity to learn about the relation of dietary factors and disease. These groups are often defined by religious or ethnic characteristics and provide many of the same strengths as ecologic studies. In addition, the special populations often live in the same general environment as the comparison group, which may somewhat reduce the number of alternative explanations for any differences that might be observed. For example, the observation that colon cancer mortality in the largely vegetarian Seventh-Day Adventists is only about half that expected (Phillips et al., 1980) has been used to support the hypothesis that meat consumption is a cause of colon cancer.

Findings based on special exposure groups are subject to many of the same confounding issues as ecologic studies. Many factors, both dietary and nondietary, are likely to distinguish these special groups from the comparison population. Thus, another possible explanation for the lower colon cancer incidence and mortality among the Seventh-Day Adventist population is that differences in rates are attributable to a lower intake of alcohol and rates of smoking or higher intake of vegetables. Given the many possible alternative explanations, such studies may be particularly useful when a hypothesized association is *not* observed. For example, the finding that the breast cancer mortality rate among the Seventh-Day Adventists is not appreciably different from the rate among the general U.S. population provides fairly strong evidence that eating meat is not a major cause of breast cancer.

MIGRANT STUDIES AND SECULAR TRENDS

Migrant studies have been particularly useful in addressing the possibility that the correlations observed in the ecologic studies are due to genetic factors. For most cancers, populations migrating from an area with its own pattern of cancer incidence rates acquire rates characteristic of their new location (Staszewski and Haenszel, 1965; Adelstein et al., 1979; McMichael and Giles, 1988; Shimizu et al., 1991), although for a few tumor sites this change occurs only after several generations (Haenszel et al., 1972; Buell, 1973). Therefore, genetic factors cannot be primarily responsible for the large differences in cancer rates among these countries. Migrant studies may also be useful for examining the latency or relevant time of exposure.

Major changes in the rates of a disease within a population over time provide evidence that nongenetic factors play an important role in the etiology of that disease. In Japan, for example, rates of colon cancer have risen dramatically since 1950 (Ferlay et al., 2001). These secular changes clearly demonstrate the role of environmental factors, possibly including diet, even though genetic factors may influence who becomes affected within a population.

CASE-CONTROL AND COHORT STUDIES

Many weaknesses of ecologic studies are potentially avoidable in case-control studies or cohort investigations. In such studies, the confounding effects of other factors can be controlled either in the design or in the analysis if good information has been collected on these variables. Furthermore, dietary information can be obtained for the individuals actually affected by disease, rather than using the average intake of the population as a whole.

Unfortunately, consistently valid results are difficult to obtain from case-control studies of dietary factors and disease because of the inherent potential for methodologic bias in those of retrospective design. This potential for bias is not unique for diet, but is likely to be unusually serious for several reasons. Owing to the limited range of variation in diet within most populations and some inevitable error in measuring intake, realistic relative risks in most studies of diet and disease are likely to be modest, within the range of 0.5 to 2.0, even for extreme categories of intake. These relative risks may seem small but would be quite important because the prevalence of exposure is high. Given typical distributions of dietary intake, these relative risks are usually based on differences in means for cases and controls of only about 5% (Willett, 1998). Thus, a systematic error of even 2% or 3% can seriously distort such a relation. In retrospective case-control studies, biases (due to selection or recall) of this magnitude could easily occur, and it is extremely difficult to exclude the possibility that this degree of bias has occurred in any specific study. Hence, it would not be surprising if retrospective case-control studies of dietary factors provide inconsistent findings.

The selection of an appropriate control group for a study of diet and disease is also usually problematic. One common practice in hospital-based studies is to use patients with another disease to provide the controls, with the assumption that the exposure under study is unrelated to the condition of this control group. Because diet may influence the incidence of many diseases, however, it is often difficult to identify, with confidence, disease groups that are unrelated to the aspect of diet under investigation. A common alternative is to use a sample of persons from the general population as the control group. In many areas, particularly large cities, participation rates are low; it is common for only 60% or 70% of eligible population controls to complete an interview (Hartge et al., 1984). Since diet is particularly associated with the level of general health consciousness, the diets of those who participate are likely to differ substantially from those who do not.

The potential opportunities for bias in case-control studies of diet raise a concern that incorrect associations may frequently occur. So far, direct empiric evidence regarding the magnitude of these biases is limited. In two large prospective cohort studies of diet and cancer, the diets of breast cancer cases and a sample of controls were also assessed retrospectively. In one study, no evidence of recall bias was observed (Friedenreich et al., 1991), but in the other the combination of recall and selection bias seriously distorted associations with fat intake (Giovannucci et al., 1993). Even if many studies arrive at correct conclusions, distortion of true associations in a substantial percentage would produce an inconsistent body of published data, making a coherent synthesis difficult or impossible for a specific diet-and-cancer relation. Additional sources of inconsistency may also be particularly troublesome in nutritional epidemiology owing to the inherent biologic complexity resulting from nutrient–nutrient interactions. Because the effect of one nutrient may depend on the level of another (which can differ between studies and may not have been measured), interactions may result in apparently inconsistent findings in epidemiologic studies. Thus, compounding biologic complexity with methodologic inconsistency may result in a literature that is a challenge to interpret.

Prospective cohort studies reduce most of the potential sources of methodologic bias associated with retrospective case-control investigations. Because the dietary information is collected before the diagnosis of disease, illness cannot affect the recall of diet. Although losses to follow-up that vary by level of dietary factors can result in distorted associations in a cohort study, follow-up rates tend to be high because participants have already provided evidence of willingness to participate. Also, in prospective studies participants may be followed passively by means of disease registries and vital statistics listings (Stampfer et al., 1984), although information on time-dependent variables (which might include diet) would be lost even with registry-based follow-up. In the last several years a sufficient number of prospective cohort studies have been published to compare their results with those of retrospective case-control investigations of the same relations. For total dietary fat and breast cancer, the associations in retrospective case-control studies have been heterogeneous, but in a meta-analysis (Howe et al., 1990), a small but precisely estimated positive association was seen (see Fig. 29–1a). In contrast, prospective cohort studies on the same topic have consistently found little relation between total fat intake and breast cancer risk, and a meta-analysis showed no association (Hunter et al., 1996). Even more strikingly, total fat intake had been positively associated with risk of lung cancer in several retrospective case-control studies, but the findings were highly inconsistent (see Fig. 29–1b). In contrast, findings from prospective cohort studies have been consistently null (Smith-Warner et al., 2002). As another example, an apparent protective effect of fruits and vegetables had been seen so frequently in retrospective case-control studies and lung cancer that this relation was thought to be established (World Cancer Research Fund, 1997). In prospective cohort studies, however, the findings have been far weaker, and in a pooled analysis there was little overall association (Smith-Warner et al., 2003). The available evidence now strongly suggests that retrospective case-control studies of the effects of dietary factors on the risks of disease are often misleading.

In addition to being less susceptible to bias, prospective studies provide the opportunity to obtain repeated assessments of diet over time and to examine the effects of diet on a wide variety of diseases,

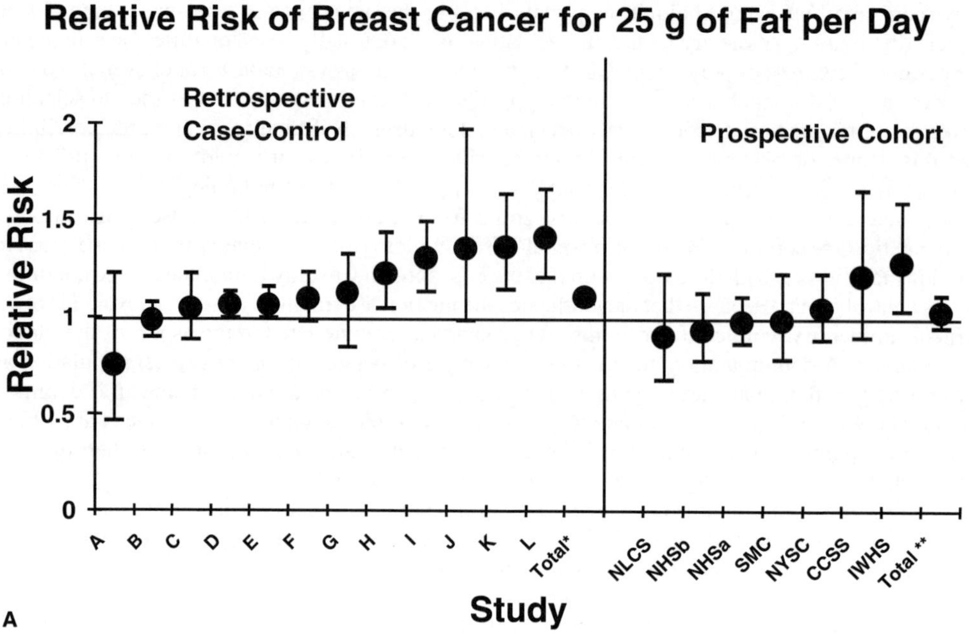

A

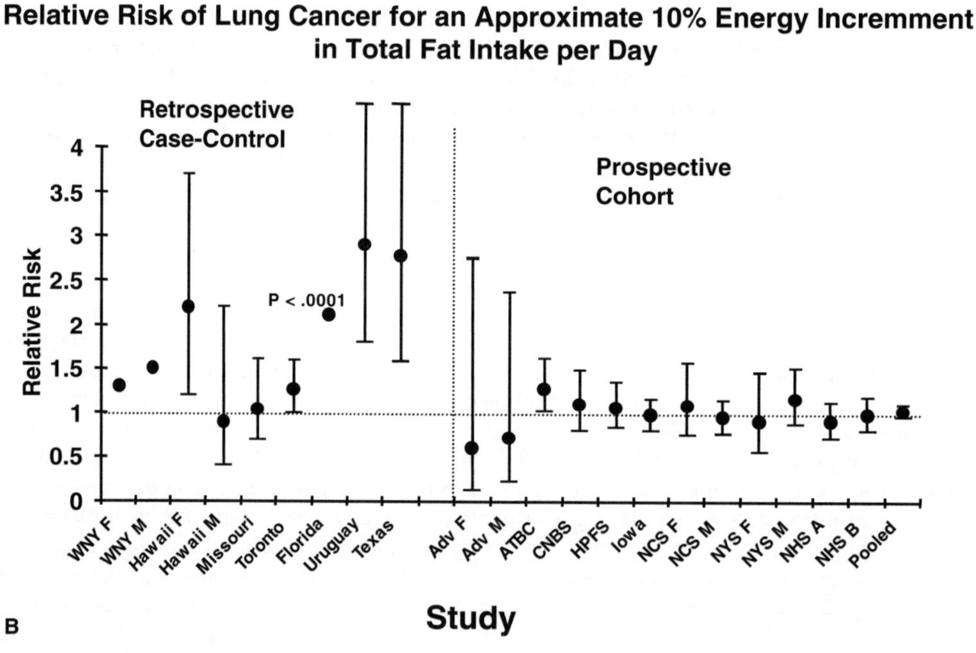

B

FIGURE 29–1 • Comparison of results for retrospective case-control studies of total dietary fat and breast cancer **(A)** and of dietary fat and lung cancer **(B)**. Retrospective case-control studies of breast cancer were summarized by Howe et al. (1990), and prospective cohort studies were summarized by Hunter et al. (1996). Retrospective case-control studies of lung cancer included those by Byers et al. (1987), Goodman et al. (1988), Mohr et al. (1999), De Stefani et al. (1997), and Alavanja et al. (1993). Prospective cohort studies of lung cancer were summarized by Smith-Warner et al. (2002).

including total mortality, simultaneously. The primary constraints on prospective cohort studies of diet are practical. Even for common diseases such as coronary heart disease or breast cancer, it is necessary to enroll tens of thousands of subjects to have reasonable precision to measure effects. The use of structured, self-administered questionnaires has made studies of this size possible, although still expensive. For diseases of somewhat lower frequency, however, even very large cohorts will not accumulate a sufficient number of cases within a reasonable amount of time. Therefore, case-control studies will continue to play some role in nutritional epidemiology, but should be designed and interpreted with the preceding limitations in mind.

EXPERIMENTAL STUDIES

The most rigorous evaluation of a dietary hypothesis is the randomized trial, optimally conducted as a double-blind experiment. The principal strength of a randomized trial is that potentially distorting variables should be distributed at random between the treatment and control groups, thus permitting reliable calculation of the probability that a test statistic as large as observed or larger could have been produced by random error alone (see Chapter 10). The investigator can reduce this probability below any threshold he or she desires by increasing the size of the trial. In addition, it is sometimes possible to create a larger dietary contrast between the groups being compared by use of an active intervention. Such experiments among humans, however, are best justified after considerable nonexperimental data have been collected to ensure that benefit is reasonably probable and that an adverse outcome is unlikely. Experimental studies are particularly practical for evaluating hypotheses that minor components of the diet, such as trace elements or vitamins, can prevent cancer, because these nutrients can be formulated into pills or capsules.

Even if feasible, randomized trials of dietary factors and disease are likely to encounter several limitations. The time between change in the level of a dietary factor and any expected change in the incidence of disease is typically uncertain. Therefore, trials must be of long duration, and if an effect is not found, it will usually be difficult to eliminate the possibility that the follow-up was of insufficient duration. Compliance with the treatment diet is likely to decrease during an extended trial, particularly if treatment involves a real change in food intake, and the comparison group may well adopt the dietary behavior of the treatment group if the treatment diet is thought to be beneficial. Such trends, which were found in the Multiple Risk Factor Intervention Trial of coronary disease prevention (Multiple Risk Factor Intervention Trial Research Group, 1982), may obscure a real benefit of the treatment.

The more recent case of the Women's Health Initiative low-fat dietary trial provides an additional example of the difficulty of maintaining a substantial contrast in diet between groups (Prentice et al., 2006). The investigators expected a 14% of energy difference in fat intake between groups, but the difference based on self-reported intake was only 9% of energy. Further, this difference is almost certainly greater than the reality because of the general tendency of humans to overreport compliance with interventions (Willett, 1998). Notably, two biomarkers that would be expected to change with reductions in dietary fat, plasma levels of triglycerides and high-density lipoprotein (HDL) cholesterol, differed little between the dietary groups during follow-up, which raises even more serious concerns about compliance.

A related potential limitation of trials is that participants who enroll in such studies tend to be highly selected on the basis of health consciousness and motivation. Therefore, it is likely that the subjects at highest potential risk on the basis of their dietary intake, and who are thus susceptible to intervention, are seriously underrepresented. For example, if low β-carotene intake is thought to be a risk factor for lung cancer and a trial of β-carotene supplementation is conducted among a health-conscious population that includes few individuals with low β-carotene intake, one might see no effect simply because the study population was already receiving the maximal benefit of this nutrient through its usual diet. In such an instance, it would be useful to measure dietary intake of β-carotene before starting the trial. Because the effect of supplementation is likely to be greatest among those with low dietary intakes, it would be possible either to exclude those with high intakes (for whom supplementation would likely have little effect) either before randomization or in subanalyses at the conclusion of the study. This approach requires a reasonable measurement of dietary intake at the study's outset.

It is sometimes said that trials provide a better quantitative measurement of the effect of an exposure or treatment because the difference in exposure between groups is better measured than in a nonexperimental study. Although this contrast may at times be better defined in a trial (it is usually clouded by some degree of noncompliance), trials still usually produce an imprecise measure of the effect of exposure owing to marginally adequate study sizes and ethical considerations that require stopping a trial after interim analyses (see Chapter 5). For example, were a trial stopped with a P-value close to 0.05, the corresponding 95% confidence interval would likely extend from a lower bound of a near zero effect to an upper bound indicating an implausibly strong effect. In a nonexperimental study, interim analyses do not yield an ethical imperative to stop the study early so long as the interim results are published. Continued accumulation of data can therefore improve the precision of the estimated relation between exposure and disease. On the other hand, a trial can provide information on the induction period between change in an exposure and change in diet, whereas estimation of induction periods for dietary effects will usually be difficult in nonexperimental studies because spontaneous changes in diet are typically not clearly demarcated in time.

Practical or ethical reasons often preclude randomized trials in humans. For example, our knowledge of the effects of cigarette smoking on risk of lung cancer is based entirely on observational studies, and it is similarly unlikely that randomized trials could be conducted to examine the effect of alcohol use on human breast cancer risk. It is unlikely that cancer-prevention trials of sufficient size, duration, and degree of compliance can be conducted to evaluate many hypotheses that involve major behavioral changes in eating patterns. For these hypotheses, nonexperimental studies will continue to provide the best available data to understand the relation between diet and disease.

MEASUREMENT OF DIET IN EPIDEMIOLOGIC STUDIES

The complexity of the human diet represents a daunting challenge to anyone contemplating a study of its relation to chronic diseases such as cancer. The foods we consume each day contain literally thousands of specific chemicals, some known and well quantified, some characterized only poorly, and others completely undescribed and presently unmeasurable. In human diets, intakes of various components tend to be correlated. With few exceptions, all individuals are exposed; for example, everyone eats fat, fiber, and vitamin A. Thus, dietary exposures can rarely be characterized as present or absent; rather, they are continuous variables, often with rather limited range of variation between persons with a common culture or geographic location. Furthermore, individuals are generally not aware of the composition of the foods that they eat; hence, the consumption of nutrients is usually determined indirectly.

NUTRIENTS, FOODS, AND DIETARY PATTERNS

Throughout nutrition in general and in much of the existing nutritional epidemiology literature, diet has usually been described in terms of its nutrient content. Alternatively, diet can be described in terms of foods, food groups, or overall dietary patterns. The primary advantage of representing diets as specific compounds, such as nutrients, is that such information can be related directly to our fundamental knowledge of biology. From a practical perspective, the exact structure of a compound must usually be known if it is to be synthesized and used for supplementation. In epidemiologic studies, measurement of total intake of a nutrient (as opposed to using the contribution of only one food at a time) provides the most powerful test of a hypothesis, particularly if many foods each contribute only modestly to intake of that nutrient. For example, in a particular study, it is quite possible that total fat intake could be clearly associated with risk of disease, whereas none of the contributions to fat intake by individual foods would be strongly related to disease on their own.

The use of foods to represent diet also has several practical advantages when examining relations with disease. Particularly when suspicion exists that some aspect of diet is associated with risk but a specific hypothesis has not been formulated, an examination of the relations of foods and food groups with risk of disease will provide a means to explore the data. Associations observed with specific foods may lead to a hypothesis relating to a defined chemical substance. For example, observations that higher intakes of green and yellow vegetables were associated with reduced rates of lung cancer led to the hypothesis that β-carotene might protect DNA from damage due to free radicals and singlet oxygen (Peto et al., 1981). The finding by Graham et al. (1978) that intake of cruciferous vegetables was inversely related to risk of colon cancer suggested that indole compounds contained in these vegetables may be protective (Wattenberg and Loub, 1978).

A problem even more serious than the lack of a well-formulated hypothesis, the premature focus on a specific nutrient that turns out to have no relation with disease, may lead to the erroneous conclusion that diet has no effect. Mertz (1984) pointed out that foods are not fully represented by their nutrient composition, noting as an example that milk and yogurt produce different physiologic effects despite a similar nutrient content. Furthermore, the valid calculation of a nutrient intake from data on food consumption requires reasonably accurate food composition information, which markedly constrains the scope of dietary chemicals that may be investigated, because such information exists for only several dozen commonly studied nutrients. Even then, there can be considerable variation in nutrient composition that is not captured in standard food tables. If extreme, as in the case of selenium, which can vary in concentration several hundred-fold in different samples of the same food, calculated intake may be of no value (Willett, 1998).

Epidemiologic analyses based on foods, as opposed to nutrients, are generally most directly related to dietary recommendations because individuals and institutions ultimately determine nutrient intake largely by their choice of foods. Even if the intake of a specific nutrient is convincingly shown to be related to risk of disease, this relation is not sufficient information on which to make dietary recommendations. Because foods are an extremely complex mixture of different chemicals that may compete with, antagonize, or alter the bioavailability of any single nutrient contained in that food, it is not possible to predict with certainty the health effects of any food solely on the basis of its content of one specific factor. For example, there is concern that high intake of nitrates may be deleterious, particularly with respect to gastrointestinal cancer. The primary sources of nitrates in our diets are green, leafy vegetables, however, which, if anything, appear to be associated with reduced risk of cancer at several sites. Similarly, because of the high cholesterol content of eggs, their avoidance has received particular attention in diets aimed at reducing the risk of coronary heart disease; per-capita consumption of eggs declined by 25% in the United States between 1948 and 1980 (Welsh and Marston, 1982). But eggs are more than cholesterol capsules; they provide a rich source of essential amino acids and micronutrients and are relatively low in saturated fat. It is thus difficult to predict the net effect of egg consumption on risk of coronary heart disease, much less the effect on overall health, without empiric evidence.

Given the strengths and weaknesses of using nutrients or foods to represent diet, an optimal approach to epidemiologic analyses will employ both. In this way, a potentially important finding is less likely to be missed. Moreover, the case for causality is strengthened when an association is observed with overall intake of a nutrient and also with more than one food source of that nutrient, particularly when the food sources are otherwise different. This situation provides, in some sense, multiple assessments of the potential for confounding by other nutrients; if an association was observed for only one food source of the nutrient, other factors contained in that food would tend to be similarly associated with disease. As an example, the hypothesis that alcohol intake causes breast cancer was strengthened not only by observing an overall association between alcohol intake and breast cancer risk but also by independent associations with both beer and liquor intake, thus making it less likely that some factor other than alcohol in these beverages was responsible for the increased risk.

One practical drawback of using foods to represent diet is their large number and complex, often reciprocal, interrelations that are due largely to individual behavioral patterns. Many reciprocal relations emerge upon perusal of typical datasets; for example, dark-bread eaters tend not to eat white bread, margarine users tend not to eat butter, and skim-milk users tend not to use whole milk. This complexity is one of the reasons to compute nutrient intakes that summarize the contributions of all foods.

An intermediate solution to the problem posed by the complex interrelations among foods is to use food groups or to compute the contribution of nutrient intake from various food groups. For example, Manousos et al. (1983) combined the intakes of foods from several predefined groups to study the relation of diet with risk of colon cancer. They observed increased risk among subjects with high meat intake and with low consumption of vegetables. The computation of nutrient intakes from different food groups is illustrated by a prospective study among British bank clerks conducted by Morris et al. (1977), who observed an inverse relation between overall fiber intake and risk of coronary heart disease. It is well recognized that fiber is an extremely heterogeneous collection of substances and that the available food composition data for specific types of fiber is incomplete. Therefore, these authors computed fiber intake separately from various food groups and found that the entire protective effect was attributable to fiber from grains; fiber from fruits or vegetables was not associated with risk of disease. This analysis circumvents the inadequacy of food composition databases and provides information in a form that is directly useful to individuals faced with decisions regarding choices of foods.

In general, maximal information will be obtained when analyses are conducted at the levels of nutrients, foods, food groups, and dietary patterns. Dietary patterns take into account the complex interrelations of food consumption and are usually derived by empirical methods such as factor analysis, or by creating *a priori* indices. The latter approach, for example, has been used to develop a Mediterranean diet index based on specific aspects of diet; this index was then found to predict lower mortality (Trichopoulou et al., 2003). Dietary patterns are potentially useful because they combine multiple aspects of diet into one or two variables, but they lack direct biologic interpretation. It is also possible to enter the distinct levels of nutrients, foods, food groups, and dietary patterns into the same analysis through the use of hierarchical (multilevel) analysis, which allows some degree of adjustment for effects at one level (e.g., the food level) when estimating effects at another level (e.g., the nutrient level) and which produces more stable effect estimates (Greenland, 2000c; see Chapter 21).

DIMENSION OF TIME

The assessment of diet in epidemiologic studies is further complicated by the dimension of time. Because our understanding of the pathogenesis of cancers and many other diseases is limited, considerable uncertainty exists about the period of time before diagnosis for which diet might be relevant. For some cancers and cardiovascular disease, diet may be important during childhood, even though the disease occurs decades later. For other diseases, diet may act as a late-stage promoting or inhibiting factor; thus, intake near the time before diagnosis may be important. Ideally, data on dietary intake at different periods before diagnosis could help to resolve these issues. Individuals rarely make clear changes in their diet at identifiable points in time; more typically, eating patterns evolve over periods of years. Thus, in case-control studies, epidemiologists often direct questions about diet to a period several years before diagnosis of disease with the hope that diet at this point in time will represent, or at least be correlated with, diet during the critical period in cancer development.

Fortunately, diets of individuals do tend to be correlated from year to year, so that some imprecision in identification of critical periods of exposure may not be serious. For most nutrients, correlations for repeated assessments of diet at intervals from 1 year to about 5 years tend to be of the order of 0.6 to 0.7 (Rohan and Potter, 1984; Willett et al.,1985; Byers et al., 1987), with decreasing correlations over longer intervals (Byers et al., 1983). For scientists accustomed to measurements made under highly controlled conditions in a laboratory, this correlation may seem like a low degree of reproducibility. Nevertheless, these correlations are similar to other biologic measurements made in free-living populations, such as serum cholesterol (Shekelle et al., 1983) and blood pressure (Rosner et al., 1977).

Even though diets of individuals have a strong element of consistency over intervals of several years, they are characterized by marked variation from day to day (Willett, 1998; Beaton et al., 1979). This variation differs from nutrient to nutrient, being moderate for total energy intake but extremely large for cholesterol and vitamin A. For this reason, even perfect information about diet on any single day or the average of a small number of days will poorly represent long-term average intake, which is likely to be more relevant to etiology of most diseases.

GENERAL METHODS OF DIETARY ASSESSMENT

Three general approaches have been used to assess dietary intake: information about intake of foods that can be used directly or to calculate intake of nutrients, biochemical measurements of blood or other body tissues that provide indicators of diet, and measures of body dimensions or composition that reflect the long-term effects of diet. Because the interpretation of data on diet and disease is heavily influenced by the methods used to assess diet, features of these methods and their limitations will be considered.

METHODS BASED ON FOOD INTAKE

Short-Term Recall and Diet Records

The 24-hour recall, in which subjects are asked to report their food intake during the previous day, has been the most widely used dietary assessment method. It has been the basis of most national nutrition surveys and numerous cohort studies of coronary heart disease. Interviews are conducted by nutritionists or trained interviewers, usually using visual aids such as food models or shapes to obtain data on quantities of foods, and are now often computer-assisted to standardize the technique and facilitate data entry. The 24-hour recall requires about 10 to 20 minutes for an experienced interviewer; although it is usually conducted in person, it has also been done by telephone using a two-dimensional chart that is mailed beforehand to assist in the estimation of portion sizes (Posner et al., 1982). This method has the advantages of requiring no training or literacy and minimal effort on the part of the participant.

Dietary records or food diaries are detailed meal-by-meal recordings of types and quantities of foods and beverages consumed during a specified period, typically 3 to 7 days. Ideally, subjects weigh each portion of food before eating, although doing so is frequently impossible for all meals, as many are eaten away from home. Alternatively, household measures can be used to estimate portion sizes. The method places a considerable burden on the subject, thus limiting its application to those who are literate and highly motivated. In addition, the effort involved in keeping diet records may increase awareness of food intake and induce an alteration in diet. Nevertheless, diet recording has the distinct advantages of not depending on memory and allowing direct measurements of portion sizes.

The validity of 24-hour recalls has been assessed by observing the actual intake of subjects in a controlled environment and interviewing them the next day. In such a study, Karvetti and Knuts (1985) observed that subjects both erroneously recalled foods that were not actually eaten and omitted foods that were eaten; correlations between nutrients calculated from observed intakes with calculations from the recalled information ranged from 0.58 to 0.74. In a similar study among elderly persons, Madden et al. (1976) found correlations ranging from 0.28 to 0.87. Relatively few validation studies have been conducted of diet recordings. In a comparison of nitrogen intake calculated by diet records kept by subjects consuming their usual diets while on a metabolic ward with analysis of replicate meals, Bingham and Cummings (1985) found a correlation of 0.97; however, the generalizability of this result to a free-living population is not clear.

The most serious limitation of the 24-hour-recall method is that dietary intake is highly variable from day to day. Diet records reduce the problem of day-to-day variation, because the average of a number of days is used. For nutrients that vary substantially, however, even a week of recording will still not provide an accurate estimate of an individual's intake (Beaton et al., 1979; Rimm et al., 1992a; Rimm, 1992b). The variability in intake of specific foods is even greater than for nutrients (Salvini et al., 1989; Geskanich et al., 1993), so that only very commonly eaten foods can be studied by this method. The problem of day-to-day variation is not an issue if the objective of a study is to estimate a mean intake for a population, as might be the goal in an ecologic study. In case-control or cohort investigations, however, accurate estimation of individual intakes is necessary.

Practical considerations and issues of study design further limit the application of short-term-recall and diet-record methods in epidemiologic studies. Because they provide information on current diet, their use will typically be inappropriate in case-control studies, because the relevant exposure will have occurred earlier and diet may have changed as a result of the disease or its treatment. A few exceptions may occur, as in the case of very early tumors or premalignant lesions. Although the average of multiple days of 24-hour recalls or diet recording could theoretically be used in prospective cohort studies of diet, the costs are usually prohibitive because of the large numbers of subjects required and the substantial expense involved in collecting this information and processing it. These methods, however, can play an important role in the validation or calibration of other methods of dietary assessment that are more practical for epidemiologic studies.

Food-Frequency Questionnaires

Because short-term-recall and diet-record methods are generally expensive, unrepresentative of usual intake, and inappropriate for assessment of past diet, investigators have sought alternative methods for measuring long-term dietary intake. Burke (1947) developed a detailed dietary history interview that attempted to assess an individual's usual diet; this assessment included a 24-hour recall, a menu recorded for 3 days, and a checklist of foods consumed over the preceding month. This method was time-consuming and expensive, because a highly skilled professional was needed for both the interview and processing of information. The checklist, however, was the forerunner of the more structured dietary questionnaires in use today. During the 1950s, Wiehl and Reed (1960), Heady (1961), Stephanik and Trulson (1962), and Marr (1971) developed food-frequency questionnaires and evaluated their role in dietary assessment. In diet records collected from British bank clerks, the *frequencies* with which foods were used correlated well with the total *weights* of the same foods consumed over a several-day period, thus providing the theoretical basis for the food-frequency method (Heady 1961). Similar findings were seen more recently in a U.S. population (Humble et al., 1987). Multiple investigators have converged toward the use of food-frequency questionnaires as the method of dietary assessment best suited for most epidemiologic studies. During recent years, substantial refinement, modification, and evaluation of food-frequency questionnaires have occurred, so that data derived from their use have become considerably more interpretable.

A food-frequency questionnaire consists of two main components: a food list and a frequency-response section for subjects to report how often each food was eaten (see Fig. 29–2). Questions related to further details of quantity and composition may be appended. A fundamental decision in designing a questionnaire is whether the objective is to measure intake of a few specific foods or nutrients or whether to obtain a comprehensive assessment of diet. A comprehensive assessment is generally desirable whenever possible. It is often impossible to anticipate at the beginning of a study all the questions regarding diet that will appear important at the end of data collection; a highly restricted food list may not have included an item that is, in retrospect, important. Furthermore, as described later in this chapter, total food intake, represented by total energy consumption, may confound the effects of specific nutrients or foods, or create extraneous variation in specific nutrients. Nevertheless, epidemiologic practice is usually a compromise between the ideal and reality, and it may simply be impossible to include a comprehensive diet assessment in a particular interview or questionnaire, especially if diet is not the primary focus of the study.

Because diets tend to be reasonably correlated from year to year, most investigators have asked subjects to describe the frequency of their using foods in reference to the preceding year. This

	Foods and amounts	Never or less than once per month	1–3 per mo	1 per wk	2–4 per wk	5–6 per wk	1 per day	2–3 per day	4–5 per day	6+ per day
A	Eggs (1)	O	O	(W)	O	O	●	O	O	O
B	Whole milk (8-oz glass)	O	O	(W)	O	O	(D)	●	O	O
C	Ice cream (½ cup)	O	O	(W)	O	●	(D)	O	O	O

FIGURE 29–2 • Section from a food-frequency questionnaire completed by several large cohorts of men and women. For each food listed, participants were asked to indicate how often, on average, they had used the amount specified during the past year. Example of calculation of daily cholesterol intake: From a food composition table, the cholesterol contents are: 1 egg = 274 mg; 1 glass of milk = 33 mg; 1/2 cup of ice cream = 29.5 mg. Thus, the average daily cholesterol intake for the person completing this abbreviated questionnaire would be: (274 mg × 1) + (33 mg × 2.5) + (29.5 mg × 0.8) = 380.1 mg/d. (Reproduced with permission from Sampson, 1985.)

interval provides a full cycle of seasons so that, in theory, the responses should be independent of the time of year. In retrospective case-control studies, the time frame could be in reference to a period of a specified number of preceding years.

Typically, investigators have provided a multiple-choice response format, with the number of options usually ranging from 5 to 10 (Fig. 29–2). Another approach is to use an open-ended format and provide subjects the option of answering in terms of frequency per day, week, or month (Block et al., 1986). In theory, an open-ended frequency-response format might provide for some enhanced precision in reporting, because the frequency of use is truly a continuous rather than a categorical variable. Nevertheless, it is unlikely that the overall increment in precision is large, because the estimation of the frequency of use of a food is inherently an approximation.

Several options exist for collecting additional data on serving sizes. The first is to collect no additional information on portion sizes at all—that is, to use a simple frequency questionnaire. A second possibility is to specify a portion size as part of the question on frequency—for example, to ask how often a glass of milk is consumed rather than only how often milk is consumed. This technique has been termed a *semiquantitative* food-frequency questionnaire. A third alternative is to include an additional question for each food to describe the usual portion size in words (Stephanick and Trulson, 1962), using food models (Morgan et al., 1978), or using pictures of different portion sizes (Hankin et al., 1983). Because most of the variation in intake of a food is explained by frequency of use rather than differences in serving sizes, several investigators have found that portion-size data are relatively unimportant (Samet et al., 1984; Pickle and Hartman, 1985; Block et al., 1990). Cummings et al. (1987) found that adding questions on portion sizes to a simple frequency questionnaire only slightly improved estimation of calcium intake, and others have found that the use of food models in an in-person interview did not increase the validity of a self-administered semiquantitative food-frequency questionnaire (Hernandez-Avila et al., 1988). These findings have practical implications, because the cost of data collection by mail or telephone is far less than the cost of personal interviews, which are necessary if food models are to be used for assessing portion sizes. Cohen et al. (1990) also found that the portion-size information included in the Block questionnaire added only slightly to agreement with diet records (average correlation of 0.41 without portion sizes and 0.43 with portion sizes).

Food-frequency questionnaires are extremely practical in epidemiologic applications because they are easy for subjects to complete, often as a self-administered form. Processing is readily computerized and inexpensive, so that their use in prospective studies involving repeated assessments of diet among many tens of thousands of subjects is feasible.

VALIDITY OF DIETARY ASSESSMENT METHODS

The interpretation of epidemiologic data on diet and disease depends directly on the validity of the methods used to measure dietary intake, particularly when no association is found, because one possible explanation could be that the method used to measure diet was not able to discriminate among persons. A substantial body of evidence has accumulated regarding the validity of food-frequency questionnaires.

In evaluating the validity of a dietary-assessment method, the choice of a standard for comparison is a critical issue, because no perfect standard exists. A desirable feature for the comparison method is that its errors be independent of the method being evaluated, so that an artificial correlation will not be observed. For this reason, biochemical indicators of diet are probably the optimal standard. Their greatest limitation is that specific markers of diet do not exist for most of the nutrients of current interest, such as total fat, fiber, and sucrose intake. Moreover, the available biochemical indicators of diet are likely to be imprecise measures of diet because they are influenced by many factors, such as differences in absorption and metabolism, short-term biologic variation, and laboratory measurement error. Nevertheless, for biochemical indicators that are sensitive to intake, a correlation between a questionnaire estimate of nutrient intake and the indicator can provide a useful measure of the validity of the questionnaire estimate. Such correlations have been reported for questionnaire estimates of a variety of nutrients (Willett et al., 1985; Willett et al., 1983; Russell-Briefel et al., 1985; Sacks et al., 1986; Stryker et al., 1988; Silverman et al., 1990; Coates et al., 1991; London et al., 1991; Ascherio et al., 1992; Hunter et al., 1992; Jacques et al., 1993; Selhub et al., 1993). For example, in controlled feeding studies, dietary fat reduces blood triglyceride levels;

thus, documentation that total fat intake assessed by a food-frequency questionnaire was inversely associated with blood triglycerides provides important support for the validity of the questionnaire assessment (Willett et al., 2001).

Relatively few validation studies of dietary questionnaires have been conducted by comparing computed intakes with biochemical indicators of diet because of the limitations of these indicators. Most validation studies have instead compared computed intakes with those based on other dietary assessment methods. Among the possible comparison methods, diet records are particularly attractive because they do not depend on memory and, when weighing scales are used to assess portion sizes, do not depend on perception of amounts of foods eaten. These characteristics tend to reduce correlated errors; because 24-hour recalls share many cognitive demands with food-frequency questionnaires, they are, in principle, less than ideal. Although the detail of questionnaires and the populations studied have varied substantially, the correlation between nutrients assessed by food-frequency questionnaires and the comparison methods, when adjusted for total energy intake, have consistently varied between 0.4 and 0.7 (Willett, 1998). Four comprehensive validation studies that compared questionnaires completed at about a 1-year interval, with multiple diet records collected during the intervening months, are summarized in Table 29–1 (Willett et al., 1985; Rimm et al., 1992a; Rimm, 1992b; Pietinen et al., 1988; Goldbohm et al., 1994). Roughly similar degrees of correlation were seen in these studies; for questionnaires completed at the end of the 1-year recording of diet (which corresponds to the time frame of the questionnaires), correlations adjusted for total energy intake tended to be mainly between 0.5 and 0.7.

Subar et al. (2003) used doubly labeled water and urinary nitrogen as biomarkers of energy and protein intake to assess the validity of a food-frequency questionnaire and 24-hour dietary recalls. The authors claimed that this study documented that errors in the 24-hour recalls and food-frequency questionnaires are correlated, and therefore that earlier studies using 24-hour recalls and food-frequency questionnaires as comparison methods have overstated validity. Subar et al. did not, however, obtain a realistic measure of the within-person variation in their biomarkers (e.g., at an interval of 6 to 12 months), and failure to account for this variation may have created the false impression of correlated error (Willett, 2003).

Although the degree of measurement error associated with nutrient estimates calculated from food-frequency questionnaires appears to be similar to that for many epidemiologic measures, errors in the nutrient of interest tend to lead to important underestimates of relative risks, and errors in other confounding nutrients tend to lead to loss of confounding control (see Chapter 9). Less commonly appreciated, the errors will also result in observed confidence intervals that are inappropriately narrow. To form inferences properly cautioned by data limitations, one should consider the entire range of possible relative risks that are reasonably compatible with the data, and overly narrow intervals tend to lead to overstated conclusions (see Chapters 11 and 19). In part, generated by the interest in diet and cancer and the recognized issue of measurement error in assessing dietary intake, considerable effort has been directed to the development of methods that provide corrected estimates of relative risks and confidence intervals based on quantitative assessments of measurement error (Spiegelman et al., 1997). Thus, validation studies of dietary questionnaires can provide important estimates of error that can be used to interpret quantitatively the influence of error on observed associations. Based on such analyses, it can be shown that important associations will generally not be missed by typical dietary questionnaires (Rosner et al., 1989; Rosner et al., 1990), although sample sizes for studies will need to be several times larger than those estimated assuming that measurement error did not exist (Walker and Blettner, 1985). One valuable way to improve measurement of diet in a longitudinal study is to repeat the dietary assessments over time. This will tend to dampen random (nonsystematic) error and will also account for true changes in intake (Hu et al., 1999).

BIOCHEMICAL INDICATORS OF DIET

The use of biochemical measurements made on blood or other tissues as indicators of nutrient intake is attractive because such measurements do not depend on the memory or knowledge of the subject. Furthermore, they can be made in retrospect, for example, using blood specimens that have been collected and stored for other purposes.

TABLE 29–1

Comparison of Food-Frequency Questionnaires with Other Dietary-Assessment Methods

Source	Population	Comparison Methods	Interval Between Methods	Reference Period	Range of Correlations	Comments
Willett et al. (1985)	Registered nurses ($n = 194$)	Diet record	1–12 mo	Previous year	0.36 vitamin A without supplements to 0.75 vitamin C	
Pietinen et al. (1988)	Finnish men ($n = 189$)	Twelve 2-day diet records (vs. 273-item questionnaire)	1–6 mo	1 yr	0.51 vitamin A to 0.73 polyunsaturated fat	Adjustment for energy had little effect on correlations
Block et al. (1990)	260	Three 4-day diet records	1–12 mo	6 mo	0.37 vitamin A to 0.74 vitamin C, with 5 supplements average = 0.55	Correlations were similar in low-fat and usual-diet groups. Variable portion sizes added little to correlation
Rimm et al. (1992a)	127 U.S. health professionals	Two 1-week diet records	1–12 mo	1 yr	0.28 for iron to 0.86 for vitamin C with supplements, average = 0.59	Mean correlation increased to 0.65 with adjustment for variation in diet records
Goldbohm et al. (1994)	59 men, 48 women	Three 3-day diet records	3–15 mo	1 yr	0.33 for vitamin B_1 to 0.75 for polyunsaturated fat; average = 0.64	Adjustment for sex and energy intake had little effect except for fat intake, changing from 0.72 to 0.52

CHOICE OF TISSUES FOR ANALYSIS

Most commonly, serum or plasma has been used in epidemiologic studies to measure biochemical indicators of diet. Consideration should also be given, however, to red blood cells, subcutaneous fat, hair, and nails. The choices should be governed by the ability of the tissue to reflect dietary intake of the factor of interest; the time-integrating characteristics of the tissue; practical considerations in collecting, transporting, and storing the specimen; and cost. These considerations are examined in detail elsewhere for a number of dietary factors (Hunter, 1998); some general comments are provided here.

Red Blood Cells

For some dietary factors, red cells are less sensitive to short-term fluctuations in diet than plasma or serum and may thus provide a better index of long-term exposure. Nutrients that can be usefully measured in red cells include fatty acids, folic acid, and selenium.

Subcutaneous Fat

Composed primarily of fatty acids, the adipose tissue turns over slowly among individuals with relatively stable weight. For at least some fatty acids, the half-life is of the order of 600 days, making this an ideal indicator of long-term diet in epidemiologic studies. Fat-soluble vitamins such as retinol, vitamin E, and carotenoids are also measurable in subcutaneous fat, but these measurements are generally not superior to food-frequency questionnaires as a measure of intake (Kabagambe et al., 2001).

Hair and Nails

Hair and nails incorporate many elements into their matrix during formation, and for many heavy metals these may be the tissues of choice because these elements tend to be cleared rapidly from the blood. Nails appear to be the optimal tissue for the assessment of long-term selenium intake owing to their capacity to integrate exposure over time (Longnecker et al., 1996). Because the hair and nails can be cut at various times after formation (a few weeks for hair close to the scalp and approximately 1 year for the great toe), an index of exposure can be obtained that may be little affected by recent experiences. This information can be a particular advantage in the context of a case-control study of diet and cancer. Contamination poses the greatest problem for measurements in hair owing to its intense exposure to the environment and very large surface area; these problems are generally much less for nails but still need to be considered.

LIMITATIONS OF BIOCHEMICAL INDICATORS

Although the use of biochemical indicators for assessing diet is attractive, no practical indicator exists for many dietary factors. Even when tissue levels of a nutrient can be measured, these levels are often highly regulated and thus poorly reflect dietary intake; blood retinol and cholesterol are good examples. Just as with dietary intake, the blood levels of some nutrients fluctuate substantially over time, so one measurement may not provide a good reflection of long-term intake. Furthermore, experience has provided sobering evidence that the tissue levels of many nutrients can be affected by the presence of cancer, even several years before diagnosis (Wald et al., 1986), rendering the use of many biochemical indicators treacherous in most retrospective case-control studies. Despite these limitations, careful application of biochemical indicators can provide unique information about dietary intake, particularly for nutrients or food contaminants that cannot be accurately calculated from data on food intake.

ANTHROPOMETRY AND MEASURES OF BODY COMPOSITION

Energy balance at various times in life has important effects on the incidence of many diseases. Energy balance is better reflected by measurements of body size and composition than by assessments based on the difference between energy intake and expenditure (largely physical activity), because both of these variables are measured with considerable error (Willett, 1998).

The most common use of anthropometric measurements is to calculate adiposity using either indices such as the Quetelet or body mass index (BMI) (weight in kilograms divided by the second power of height in meters) or relative weight (weight standardized for height). Remarkably valid estimates of weight and height can be obtained even by questioning (Stunkard and Albaum, 1981), including their recall several decades earlier (Rhoads and Kagan, 1983; Must et al., 1993). Thus, good estimates of adiposity can be obtained easily for large prospective investigations or retrospectively in the context of case-control studies. The major limitation of adiposity estimates based on height and weight is that they cannot differentiate between fat and lean body mass. Studies of the validity of the BMI as a measure of obesity have commonly used as a "gold standard" body fat expressed as a percentage of total weight, usually determined by underwater weighing, or more recently by dual x-ray absorptiometry (DEXA). BMI, however, is actually a measure of fat mass adjusted for height rather than a measure of percentage body fat. When fat mass determined from densitometry is adjusted for height and used as the standard, the correlation with BMI is approximately 0.90 among young and middle-aged adults, indicating a substantially higher degree of validity than has generally been appreciated (Spiegelman et al., 1992). Moreover, in the same study, fat mass adjusted for height correlated more strongly with biologically relevant variables such as blood pressure and fasting blood glucose than did percentage body fat. BMI may be less valid as an index of adiposity among the elderly, however, because variation in loss of lean body mass contributes more importantly to weight during this period of life.

The use of one or a small number of skin-fold thicknesses does not appear to be appreciably more accurate than weight and height in the estimation of overall adiposity among young and middle-aged adults, but it can provide additional information on the distribution of body fat. The ratio of waist-to-hip circumference, or waist circumference alone, provides information on adiposity that adds independently, beyond BMI alone, to predictions of obesity-related conditions (Snijder et al., 2004). This additional prediction may be, in part, because central fat functions metabolically differently from peripheral fat, and also because these circumference measurements help distinguish fat mass from muscle mass.

Height has often been ignored as a variable of potential interest in epidemiologic studies, perhaps because analysts fail to recognize that it is not addressed by control for BMI. Height can, however, provide unique information on energy balance during the years before adulthood, a time period that may be important in the development of some cancers that occur many years later. For example, in many studies height has been positively associated with risk of breast cancer (van den Brandt et al., 2000). Furthermore, this information can be valid even in the context of case-control studies, because height will usually be unaffected even if illness has caused recent weight loss. Therefore, one should not exclude height from consideration just because BMI or another weight-for-height-based index is included in the analysis (Michels et al., 1998).

METHODOLOGIC ISSUES IN NUTRITIONAL EPIDEMIOLOGY

BETWEEN-PERSON VARIATION IN DIETARY INTAKE

In addition to the availability of a sufficiently precise method for measuring dietary intake, an adequate degree of variation in diet is necessary to conduct observational studies within populations. If no variation in diet exists among persons, no association can be observed. Some have argued that the diets in populations such as the United States are too homogeneous to study relations with disease (Goodwin and Boyd, 1987; Hebert and Miller, 1988; Prentice et al., 1988). The true between-person variation in diet is difficult to measure directly, and generally cannot be measured by the questionnaires used by epidemiologists because the observed variation will combine true differences with those due to measurement error; more quantitative methods must be used for this purpose. The fat content of the diet varies less among persons compared with most other nutrients (Beaton et al., 1979); for women in one prospective study (Willett et al., 1987), the mean fat intake assessed by the mean of four 1-week diet records for those in the top quintile was 44% of calories, while for those in the bottom quintile it was 32% of calories. Although this range of fat intake is not large, and it is certainly smaller than the variation among countries, it is of considerable interest because this difference corresponds closely to the changes recommended by many organizations. Other nutrients vary much more among persons than total fat intake (Willett, 1998; Beaton et al., 1979).

Evidence that measurable and informative variation in diet exists within the U.S. population is provided by several sources. First, the correlations between food-frequency questionnaires and independent assessments of diet found in the validation studies noted previously would not have been observed if variation in diet did not exist. For the same reason, the correlations between questionnaire estimates of nutrient intakes and biochemical indicators of intake provide solid evidence of variation. In addition, the ability to find associations between dietary factors and incidence of disease (particularly when based on prospective data) indicates that measurable and biologically relevant variation exists. For example, reproducible relations have been observed between fiber intake and risks of coronary heart disease (Hu and Willett, 2002) and diabetes (Schulze and Hu, 2005).

Although accumulated evidence has indicated that informative variation in diets exists within the U.S. population and that these differences can be measured, it is important that findings be interpreted in the context of that variation. For example, a lack of association with fat intake within the range of 32% to 44% of energy should not be interpreted to mean that fat intake has no relation to risk of disease under any circumstance. It is possible that the relation is nonlinear and that risk changes at lower levels of fat intake (e.g., <20% of total energy) or that diet has an influence much earlier in life.

IMPLICATIONS OF TOTAL ENERGY INTAKE

Energy balance is likely to have important associations with some cancers; however, this relation cannot be studied directly because energy intake largely reflects factors other than over- or undereating in relation to requirements (Willett, 1998; Willett and Stampfer, 1986). The implications of total energy intake can be appreciated by realizing that variation among persons is to a large degree secondary to differences in body size and physical activity. Persons also appear to differ in metabolic efficiency (inefficient persons requiring higher energy intake for the same level of function); however, these differences in metabolic efficiency are not practically measurable in epidemiologic studies. Because virtually all nutrient intakes tend to be correlated with total energy intake, much of the variation in intake of specific nutrients is secondary to factors that may be unrelated to risk of disease. Nutrient intakes adjusted for total energy can be viewed conceptually as measures of nutrient composition rather than as measures of absolute intake. Measures of nutrient composition are more relevant to personal decisions and public health policy than are absolute intakes because individuals must alter nutrient intakes primarily by manipulating the composition of their diets rather than their total energy intake. Thus, for most purposes, measures of dietary composition are the appropriate focus of epidemiologic studies.

When total energy intake is related to risk of disease, failure to consider total energy intake in the analysis can be particularly serious because it can confound associations with specific nutrients. For example, total energy intake increases with physical activity, so when physical activity is protective, total energy intake will also be protective. The example of coronary heart disease is instructive. Risk of coronary heart disease is inversely related to physical activity and so also to total energy intake. Specific nutrients such as saturated fat also tend to be inversely related to risk of coronary heart disease. Several statistical methods can be used to adjust for total energy intake, which is necessary to avoid the misleading conclusion that saturated fat intake protects against coronary heart disease. The most common method, division of saturated fat intake by total energy intake, which is also called nutrient density, is not an adequate solution because the division can introduce confounding by the inverse of energy intake. Instead, total energy intake must be included in a multiple-regression model together with the nutrient density, Alternatively, nutrient intake residuals standardized for total energy intake will not be confounded by total energy intake. Appropriate adjustment for energy intake can be a nontrivial issue in some studies. Without such an adjustment, the direction of association with a specific nutrient can be reversed, such as with the relation between saturated fat intake and myocardial infarction (Gordon et al., 1981) and with the relation between fiber intake and risk of colon cancer (Lyon et al., 1987). If total energy intake has not been measured or adjusted appropriately, a useful interpretation of a finding may not be possible.

Although it is not the primary rationale for energy adjustment, this adjustment will often reduce measurement error, which can be seen as higher correlation in validation studies or stronger associations with biomarkers (Willett, 2002). The reason for the reduction in error can be appreciated by considering that the observed nutrient density is $(N + e_N)/(E + e_E)$. e_N and e_E will tend to be highly correlated because they are calculated from many of the same foods; for example, if meat is overreported, both fat and total energy will be overreported. Thus, these errors will largely cancel out, leaving an improved estimate of N/E. Jakes et al. (2004) have suggested that adjusting for physical activity and body size provides a better adjustment for total energy intake itself than measured energy intake. This approach will not, however, necessarily result in better control for confounding, and it will fail to reduce measurement errors that are correlated with those in total energy intake (Spiegelman, 2004).

CONCLUSION

The last two decades have seen enormous progress in the development of nutritional epidemiology methods. Work by many investigators has provided clear support for the essential underpinnings of this field. Substantial between-person variation in consumption of most dietary factors in populations has been demonstrated, methods to measure diet applicable to epidemiologic studies have been developed, and their validity has been documented. Based on this evidence, many large prospective cohort studies have been established that are providing a wealth of data on many outcomes that will be reported during the next decade. In addition, methods to account for errors in measurement of dietary intake have been developed and are beginning to be applied in reporting findings from studies of diet and disease.

Nutritional epidemiology has contributed importantly to understanding the etiology of many diseases. Low intake of fruits and vegetables has been shown to be related to increased risk of cardiovascular disease. Also, a substantial amount of epidemiologic evidence has accumulated indicating that replacing saturated and trans fats with unsaturated fats can play an important role in the prevention of coronary heart disease and type 2 diabetes. Many diseases—as diverse as cataracts, neural-tube defects, and macular degeneration—that were not thought to be nutritionally related have been found to have important dietary determinants. Nonetheless, much more needs to be learned regarding other diet and disease relations, and the dimensions of time and ranges of dietary intakes need to be expanded further. Furthermore, new products are constantly being introduced into the food supply, which will require continued epidemiologic vigilance.

The development and evaluation of additional methods to measure dietary factors, particularly those using biochemical methods to assess long-term intake, can contribute substantially to improvements in the capacity to assess diet and disease relations. Also, the capacity to identify those persons at genetically increased risk of disease will allow the study of gene–nutrient interactions that are almost sure to exist. The challenges posed by the complexities of nutritional exposures are likely to spur methodologic developments. Such developments have already occurred with respect to measurement error. The insights gained will have benefits throughout the field of epidemiology.

CHAPTER 30

Environmental Epidemiology

Irva Hertz-Picciotto

The Domain of Environmental Epidemiology 598
Exposure Assessment 600
Types of Exposure Data 600
Issues in Exposure Assessment 602
Study Designs for Environmental Epidemiology 604
Randomized Recruitment 604
Case-Crossover Design 605
Ecologic Studies 606
Time Patterns 606
Mapping 608
Comparison of Time-Trend and Spatial-Data Analysis 609
Analysis and Methodologic Challenges in Environmental Epidemiology 610
Time-Series Analyses: Confounding and Auto-Regression 610
Social Class as a Confounder in Intercommunity Comparisons 611
Analysis of Clusters 612
Analysis of Clustering around Point Sources 613
General Considerations in the Investigation of Clusters 613
Surveillance and Risk Assessment of Environmental Hazards 613
Environmental Health Surveillance 613
Risk Assessment 614
Historical Lessons in Environmental Epidemiology 615
Water Contamination 615
Air Pollution 615
Persistent Organic Pollutants 616
New Environmental Health Challenges 617
Future Needs 619

THE DOMAIN OF ENVIRONMENTAL EPIDEMIOLOGY

One of the earliest published environmental epidemiology studies was Baker's report on the "endemial colic of Devonshire" (1767). Physicians had puzzled for 50 years about why those who drank cider in Devonshire became seriously ill, experienced seizures, and sometimes died, whereas cider drinkers elsewhere drank with impunity. Baker concluded that "the cause of this Colic is not. . . in the pure Cyder; but in some, either fraudulent, or accidental adulteration." Inspections of the presses revealed abundant use of lead in Devonshire, but not elsewhere. Baker then chemically tested the cider and found lead precipitated only in Devonshire samples. Like many environmental epidemiology studies, the investigation began with observations of regional differences in disease rates, proceeded to a more careful examination of symptoms and circumstances and discovery of a suspect cause, and finally confirmed the cause acting in the high-incidence county but not the low-incidence counties.

For our purposes, the *environment* will be defined as factors that are exogenous to and nonessential for the normal functioning of human beings and that alter patterns of disease and health. It therefore includes physical, chemical, and biologic agents, as well as social, political, cultural, and engineering or architectural factors affecting human contact with such agents. Previously, environmental epidemiology focused on biologic agents and factors such as water distribution systems, sewage collection, and food handling. The delivery of sanitary water, construction of comprehensive sewage systems, and passage of laws governing the handling of food were environmental measures that substantially reduced morbidity and mortality from infectious agents. In many developing countries, these basic issues are still the primary environmental health concern.

Beginning around the 1960s and 1970s, the focus of environmental epidemiology shifted largely to chemical and physical agents such as volatile organic compounds, metals, particulate matter, pesticides, and radiation. Sources can be industrial and motor-vehicle emissions; hormones added to animal feed; pesticide residues in food and in runoff reaching drinking-water reservoirs; chemical spills during production or transportation; hazardous waste sites; radon from naturally occurring geologic sources; minerals in groundwater—both naturally occurring (e.g., arsenic) and added through human activity (e.g., lead, fluoride)—and household products contacting the skin, such as cleaning agents, cosmetics, and hair dyes. Environmental epidemiology also examines patterns of disease in populations struck by disasters, including war, floods, tsunamis, and earthquakes, and most recently has begun tackling the "built" environment and global climate change.

This chapter does not seek to cover a litany of exposures and what has been learned through epidemiology. Instead, it focuses on key methodologic issues currently facing the field, problems that feature more prominently in environmental epidemiology than in other substantive areas. In addition, it provides a flavor of how the field has made progress over time.

The focus on chemical and physical agents links environmental with occupational epidemiology. Adverse effects observed at high exposure levels in work settings (e.g., dust in mines) raise the possibility of analogous effects at community-level exposures. The continual introduction of new chemicals fuels concern by the lay and scientific communities.

Toxicology also interfaces with environmental epidemiology: Hypotheses are generated by animal experiments, but only an epidemiologic study can establish relevance to humans and determine the harmful doses. Alternatively, an epidemiologic association is reported, but plausibility is questioned until a controlled animal experiment demonstrates similar outcomes or an in vitro study uncovers a pathogenic mechanism. Limited human data may trigger molecular biologists to develop a knock-out strain using genetic engineering technology and to describe the full range of effects or pathways, opening new avenues for epidemiologic research.

Environmental epidemiology studies may seek to characterize the health effects of a known exposure. Conversely, a disease pattern is observed and the epidemiologist sets out to determine the causes. In either case, definitiveness of the findings will depend on the quality of the exposure assessment. Evidence can be strengthened by distinguishing persons receiving large versus small exposures or by identifying a susceptible time period when exposure can affect the relevant tissue.

Although *environment* can refer to all nongenetic factors, this chapter presumes the more commonly used, restricted definition given earlier. Dietary habits are excluded, even though they are often geographically circumscribed, some deficiency diseases are environmentally determined (cretinism caused by lack of dietary iodine; DeLong, 1993), and nutritional epidemiology (Chapter 29) may suggest effect modifiers of the environment/disease association (e.g., calcium deficiency increases lead absorption from the gastrointestinal tract; Goyer, 1995).

Exposure to environmental agents is frequently determined by where one lives, works, socializes, or obtains food. The social, political, and economic contexts are integral to most environmental epidemiology problems, aspects that have often been underappreciated. For purposes of this chapter, social class will be treated as a potential confounder, effect modifier, or antecedent and determinant of exposure.

Environmental exposures are often largely involuntary, e.g., noise pollution from a local airport or perchloroethylene in groundwater from a nearby dry-cleaning establishment. The presence or magnitude of such exposures may be subject to legal restrictions or influenced by political or economic pressures. Because an industrial or commercial party may be responsible for the pollution, policy implications of many environmental epidemiology studies are often immediate. Results may be used as evidence in litigation or as the basis for risk assessment and regulatory policy decisions. Epidemiologists may conduct quantitative risk assessments to assist policy makers (Hertz-Picciotto, 1995; Kunzli et al., 2000; Cifuentes et al., 2001). The need for the work to withstand intense scientific and public scrutiny thus underscores the importance of rigorous methodology.

The remainder of this chapter is organized as follows. The presentation begins with exposure assessment because of the critical role it plays in this field. Next, study designs and issues related specifically to investigations of environmental factors are discussed. Analytic methods for such investigations are addressed, including Poisson regression, time-space analyses, and clustering. The chapter continues with discussions of environmental health surveillance, some historical examples, and an exposition of new global environmental challenges, and concludes with brief remarks about future needs, both practical and conceptual.

EXPOSURE ASSESSMENT

The quality of exposure measurement is often the most critical determinant of the validity of an environmental epidemiology study. Moreover, the existing exposure data or the available and feasible methods for its collection are often the determinant of the design to be used. For this reason, exposure assessment is placed at the start of this exposition.

Exposure may be measured using sophisticated instruments, or it may be inferred from databases or questionnaires about the presence or use of the agents of concern. Crude categorization (yes/no or high/low) is often not adequate because of uncertainty in the assignment and the wide variability within groups. Ordinal categories provide the opportunity to assess dose–response relations. Optimally, the quantification on a continuous scale of exposure from the relevant time period will endow a study with the greatest sensitivity. Quantified measures also allow researchers to assess comparability across studies and can provide the basis for regulatory decision making.

It is useful to distinguish among an exposure setting, a complex mixture, and a single agent. An exposure setting involves a specific situation and a mix of exposures that may change over time or from place to place. Coal burning produces a different mix of air pollutants than combustion of automotive fuel. Pollutants from automotive exhaust vary by type of fuel, air temperature, and sunshine; the fuel composition has itself changed over time. Sidestream and mainstream smoke differ in composition, and both vary by source of tobacco and additives. The investigator should be clear on whether the hypothesis concerns a setting, a mix, or a single exposure, and needs to select the appropriate study design and exposure assessment strategy. Inferences about a mix of exposures or a specific setting can be equally valid as those pertaining to individual agents. They may also have more predictive and public health value, because interventions frequently affect an overall exposure scenario rather than a single agent. The potency of a mix may be greater or less than the sum of the potencies of the component parts owing to synergistic or antagonistic relations between the factors (Germolec et al., 1989; Hertz-Picciotto et al., 1992).

The relevant timing for an exposure assessment is specific to the etiologic hypothesis and disease outcome. Timing can be measured in relation to when a health effect should be observed or to when the organism is likely to be susceptible. The former is related to the induction period, the time between exposure and disease occurrence. This interval may be minutes or hours for acute poisonings, hours or days for respiratory conditions, months or years for developmental disorders, or decades for carcinogenic or cardiovascular effects. Susceptibility, on the other hand, is frequently related to a period in development, such as the time when neural networks are forming in the cerebral cortex, when infant production of IgG begins, or when an adolescent growth spurt is occurring. Timing may also be defined by presence of a cofactor that magnifies or reduces the effect of the exposure: physical activity (e.g., during exercise) or a health condition (viral infection).

TYPES OF EXPOSURE DATA

Instruments for exposure assessment include (a) databases on sales or use of products; (b) interviews, questionnaires, and structured diaries; (c) measurements in external media (macroenvironment) either from existing records or conducted expressly for the epidemiologic investigation (e.g., levels of chlorination by-products measured at the water company's reservoir); (d) concentrations in the personal or microenvironment (e.g., carbon monoxide in indoor air or trihalomethanes in tap water); (e) individual doses (e.g., using personal air monitors, or combining measurements at the tap with self-reported water consumption and hot shower use); (f) measurements of concentrations in human tissues (blood lead or polychlorinated biphenyls [PCBs] in breast milk) or metabolic products (dimethylarsinic acid in urine after arsenic exposure); and (g) markers of physiologic effects (e.g., protein adducts induced by β-naphthylamine in cigarette smoke).

All questionnaires and interviews rely on human knowledge and memory, and hence are subject to error. Personal or telephone interviews may also elicit underreporting of many phenomena and are susceptible to "desirability" of the activity being reported. Self-administered questionnaires avoid interviewer influences, but they typically have lower response rates and may not be suitable for obtaining complex information, whereas an interviewer can check that the respondent understands the questions and follows skip patterns (Armstrong et al., 1992). Use of proxy respondents results in greater errors.

A distinction is made between an *exposure* measured in the external environment and a *dose* measured either in human tissue or at the point of contact between the subject and the environment (e.g., using a personal monitor or breath sampler). The difference between the two depends on human activity patterns, physiologic characteristics, and variation in the external exposures themselves over time and space. Measurements in external media yield an ecologic measure and are useful when the exposures are widespread in some but not all geographic areas or time periods under study or, more specifically, when group differences outweigh interindividual differences. If trihalomethanes or arsenic in the drinking water are 10 times higher in one community than in other areas, interindividual variation in doses based on water consumption might be far outweighed by the between-community differences, and the benefit of collecting extensive water-consumption data would then be small. Macroenvironment measures are also useful when the overall exposure setting rather than individual pollutants are of concern, for instance, if regulatory action levels are to be determined. Direct methods of external exposure measurement must be validated through both a quality control or quality assurance program and a logical relation between the sampling strategy and the biodynamics of the pollutant in the environment (Seifert, 1995).

Duration of contact (or potential contact) may be employed as a surrogate quantitative exposure measure. This measure, however, can be problematic if intensity of exposure varies across individuals and across time, and is a strong determinant of the effect. In this case, real associations could be obscured (see "Issues in Exposure Assessment"). A lack of data on exposure changes over time is difficult to overcome. When external measurements are available, they can be combined with duration and timing of residence and activity-pattern information (time spent indoors and outdoors, quantity of water ingested, etc.) to assign quantitative or semiquantitative exposure estimates for individuals.

When measurements on each individual are infeasible, a surrogate can be constructed using dosimetric modeling (Lebret, 1995). Measurements at the source of exposure are combined with information about physicochemical properties and often also with field measurements in multiple locations. Examples include dispersion models for air pollutants, hydrogeologic modeling of waterborne exposures, and isopleth modeling of soil contaminants. Because a model is simply a set of structured assumptions, dosimetric models should be validated in the relevant locations before being introduced into epidemiologic studies (Seifert, 1995).

Estimated individual measures could be a poor surrogate for individual absorbed doses because of variability by breathing rate, age, sex, medical conditions, and so on. The pertinent dose at the target tissue further depends on pharmacokinetics, that is, distribution to various body compartments (bloodstream, kidney, brain, etc.), metabolic rates and pathways that could either produce the active compound or detoxify it, storage or retention times, and elimination rates. Individual differences in pharmacokinetics influence the dose at the target site and its time course. Tissue concentrations may be better than external measures and activity data, but in some situations could be a poor indication of long-term exposure. For advantages and disadvantages of various exposure measurement methods, see Armstrong et al. (1992) and Nieuwenhuijsen (2003).

Biologic markers, which are alterations at the cellular, biochemical, or molecular level, may provide clues about past exposure. These can indicate absorbed dose or be used to estimate target-tissue doses, hence supplementing personal recall data. Biologic markers are usually divided into markers of exposure, markers of susceptibility and markers of early disease, but the dividing lines are often blurry, as those with greater susceptibility may absorb or retain the compounds for longer, or may already be exhibiting early stages of disease. The investigation of biomarkers is focused largely on illuminating mechanisms of disease, beginning with exposure, through internal dose, bioactive dose (e.g., at the target tissue, or the metabolite believed to cause damage), evidence of altered physiology, and early signs of disease. To be useful for this purpose, links must be made both with exposure and with the disease outcome. For instance, C-reactive protein, produced in response to infection or local injury, has been hypothesized to be a causal risk factor for coronary heart disease (Pai et al., 2004). This result opens the door to determining environmental, genetic or nutritional factors that influence C-reactive protein levels.

Biomarkers are sometimes measured in tissue that is not involved in the causal pathway because organs of interest are inaccessible (brain, lung, liver, etc.): DNA adducts measured in white blood cells are surrogates for DNA damage in relevant tissue. Biomarkers are also useful for exploring gene–environment interactions. For instance, *GSTM1* genotype among breast cancer cases was associated with PAH adducts in those who drank alcohol but not in those who abstained (Rundle et al., 2003). Life stage appears to influence adduct frequency, as newborns have been reported to have higher adduct frequencies compared with their mothers, even though gene mutations at the *HPRT* locus were lower (Perera et al., 2002). This apparent paradox is explained by a longer lifetime of the adducts in the neonates, underscoring that the time frame of exposure reflected by any biomarker must be understood in order to avoid flawed conclusions.

ISSUES IN EXPOSURE ASSESSMENT

Whether planning a study or evaluating a body of literature, epidemiologists must grapple with uncertainty regarding the best exposure metric for the outcome under study. Cumulative exposures are often assumed to be the biologically relevant quantity, but this assumption is usually not verifiable. Cumulative exposure in case-control and some cohort studies requires reconstruction of past exposures, a process fraught with problems of recall, incomplete measurements in external media, or inaccurate records that can no longer be validated. Reproductive and developmental outcomes are frequently related to relatively short critical time windows. If the representation chosen is not the biologically relevant one, the resulting misclassification could cause biased estimates of association.

A measure of the misclassification that results from using too broad a time window is the ratio of overall exposure prevalence to prevalence within a specific time window, abbreviated as the overall:time-window (OTW) ratio (Hertz-Picciotto et al., 1996). This measure ranges, in the limit, from 1 to ∞. High values indicate variability in exposures over time; a value of 1 implies no such variability, i.e., those exposed at one point in time, or during a specific, possibly critical, window are exposed throughout the period in which exposure is assessed. In a study of fetal deaths, the low OTW for cigarette smoking (1.1 or 1.2) indicated that those who smoked tended to do so throughout the pregnancy, whereas the OTW for pesticide exposures at work ranged from 2.1 to 3.2, indicating that those exposed in one trimester tended not to be exposed in other trimesters, and that considerable misclassification would occur by assuming homogeneous exposures throughout pregnancy.

Exposures or residences at times in the past are more appropriate for studying diseases that have long induction periods or are caused by long-term chronic insults. Extensive investigations of leukemia clustering around the Sellafield nuclear facility in West Cumbria, England, found an excess among children born in the village but not among those who moved into the area, suggesting that if an exposure was responsible, it operated before the birth (Gardner et al., 1987). Cognitive function in the elderly might be related to lifetime lead exposure, which is better assessed by measurements of bone lead (with a half-life of 10 to 15 years) than blood lead (half-life of 45 days). In contrast, for a study of the effect of *in utero* lead exposure on the fetus, the mother's cumulative exposure is less relevant than the amount reaching fetal circulation; hence, maternal blood lead during pregnancy (which readily crosses the placenta) might be superior to a single measurement of bone lead.

For acute or moderately short-term effects (e.g., air pollution–induced asthma episodes, certain adverse reproductive outcomes), the critical period may be easier to identify, and the payoff from collection of detailed timing information may be great. Bell et al. (2001a, 2001b) found that the strength of association between pesticides and late fetal deaths from congenital anomalies was greatest for weeks 3 through 8, the period of organogenesis. This study took advantage of the known critical window for that outcome. When information on timing of exposure is collected but the critical time window is not known, analyses with several different choices may be instructive (see Chapter 16), as long as there is variability in exposure between time periods and across persons (Bell et al., 2001c).

A related issue is that of retention time. Even though external exposures may have ended years earlier, a compound with a long half-life will be present in certain organs. The tragic incidents known as Yusho ("oil disease") in Japan and Yu-Cheng in Taiwan involved consumption of cooking oil contaminated with PCB compounds (Kuratsune et al., 1972; Chen et al., 1994). Children born years later to women who had been poisoned suffered severe developmental deficits as a result of their prenatal exposures to the mother's body burden (Chen et al., 1994). The persistence of organochlorine pesticides in fat tissue enables inferences about exposures in earlier periods, an advantage for case-control studies.

More broadly, in developing a plan for exposure assessment, epidemiologists will need to consider the lengths of the induction and latency periods. Although there are different traditions in different specialty areas, for our purposes here, we consider that, when exposure occurs at only one point in time, the induction period represents the time between exposure and the initiation of disease. The latency period then represents the time from initiation to clinical detection of disease. For protracted exposures, the combined induction and latency periods span from the time when exposure reaches a critical threshold until the time when disease is clinically manifested. The point when exposure reaches a critical threshold will not usually be known: It occurs at some point when the cumulative exposure or exposure intensity surpasses the threshold that the organism can tolerate. It could even occur beyond the period of external exposure, if internal stores continue to "expose" the target tissues as a result of long retention times (Hertz-Picciotto et al., 2004). For protracted exposures, epidemiologists have often used the time between initiation of exposure and detection of disease, but this interval is only a proxy for the true combined induction and latency periods and may lead to misclassification bias.

For a substantial proportion of diseases, environment interacts with genetics (see Chapter 2). At the individual level, exposures affect those who are genetically susceptible, such that the sufficient set of causes includes both the exposure and genes. Thus, disease is caused jointly by both the genetic inheritance and the exogenous exposures the individuals encountered, and would not develop without both. For certain diseases, this will be true of all, or nearly all, cases, implying a (nearly) 100% attributable fraction for genetic causes and the same for environmental causes. Nevertheless, when epidemiologists attempt to measure the contribution of widespread environmental factors, the estimates can be very wrong. If exposures tend to be homogeneous (low variability), their effects will be underestimated or even completely obscured. All study designs may fail to detect an association with the environmental exposure and will primarily identify markers of susceptibility (Rose, 1985). Other scenarios could also produce this problem. For example, even if exposures are widespread and vary, exposure-induced disease may occur below the level at which most people are exposed (i.e., exposures exceed the threshold that influences disease risk). Here, studies will not be able to observe an association with exposure, even though it is omnipresent and universally causal, and even though the study was designed to assess gene–environment interactions.

The importance of exposure assessment in environmental epidemiology cannot be overstated. Not only are errors often substantial, additionally the researchers sometimes do not know what the toxic exposures are or what the route of exposure is (inhalation, ingestion, dermal absorption). Even when the exposure and route are known, personal exposure levels are often not assessed in spite of potentially high variability. Of course, expense is often a barrier.

Errors in measurement of exposure introduce both bias and imprecision into the estimates of their health effects (Brunekreef et al., 1987). Repetition of measurements can improve precision in exposure estimates, thereby reducing bias in effect measures (Brunekreef et al., 1987; Liu et al., 1978). Note also that when intraindividual variability is great, macro-level exposure measures may be preferred over personal or biologic measures, because the former will tend to give better estimates of average exposures (Rappaport et al., 1995). Sheppard and colleagues point out that in time-series studies of air pollution, when nonambient sources of pollution are ignored, if they are independent of the ambient sources, the resulting error in exposure assessment will not introduce bias in the estimation of effect (Sheppard et al., 2004). The literature on measurement error is abundant (Thurigen et al., 2000; Sturmer et al., 2002; Spiegelman et al., 2005), with entire textbooks devoted to this topic, ranging to levels that are highly technical (e.g., Carroll et al., 2006). Chapter 9 discusses basic concepts and consequences of such error.

Other perspectives on improving exposure assessment focus on integration of a wide range of variables through geographic information systems (GIS), software that provides data management, mapping, and statistical analysis capabilities for incorporating spatial attributes of data (Cromley and McLafferty, 2002). These systems can superimpose maps of topographic (e.g., land cover, soil type, watershed), meteorologic, sociodemographic, health services infrastructure, and other data. Applications have included determination of landscape elements that explain vector abundance of *Anopheles albimanus* in Chiapas, Mexico (Beck et al., 1994); analysis of childhood cancer incidence at the level of census tracts in relation to hazardous air-pollutant exposures from various sources (Reynolds et al., 2003); and identification of the areas within a county where children with high lead levels were concentrated, in order to plan targeted screening (Reissman et al., 2001).

In study planning, the utility of existing measurements from administrative or surveillance databases and the decisions of how many and what kind of measurements to make are critical. Both require a close examination of variability within and across individuals over time, as well as sources of error and uncertainty.

STUDY DESIGNS FOR ENVIRONMENTAL EPIDEMIOLOGY

Environmental epidemiology uses all of the standard study designs: cohort, cross-sectional, case-control, ecologic, community intervention, and occasionally, randomized trials. For example, early studies of chronic low-level lead exposure and mental development in children included cohort (de la Burde and Choate, 1975) and case-control (Youroukos et al., 1978) designs, and in a classic cross-sectional study, Needleman et al. (1979) estimated cumulative childhood exposure by measuring the dentin lead content of their deciduous teeth, establishing that, after adjustment for many confounders, higher lifetime lead exposure was associated with lower IQ and more behavior problems. Longitudinal follow-up showed further that early lead exposure predicted failure to complete high school, and poorer scores on reading, vocabulary, hand–eye coordination, and reaction-time tests (Needleman et al., 1990). Bellinger et al. (1994a) similarly found that dentin lead in deciduous teeth was associated with problem behaviors in 8-year-old children, whereas prenatal exposure, measured by cord blood lead, was not. In adolescents, executive function and self-regulation were found to be adversely affected by lead exposure (Bellinger et al., 1994b). Thus, a series of studies of different designs builds a compelling body of evidence.

Community intervention studies are exemplified by trials of fluoridation of public water supply systems. These trials demonstrated that addition of fluoride had the same effect as naturally occurring fluoride in the prevention of dental caries, reducing the number of decayed, missing, or filled teeth per child by 48% to 70% (Ast 1962).

Environmental epidemiology has provided impetus for methodologic development of two relatively new designs: two-stage, randomized recruitment in case-control studies (Weinberg and Sandler, 1991) and case-crossover studies (MacClure, 1991; Levy et al., 2001; Janes et al., 2005).

RANDOMIZED RECRUITMENT

Two-stage case-control designs (Walker, 1982a; White, 1982b; see Chapters 8 and 15) are useful (a) for studying rare exposures in relation to rare diseases (e.g., late fetal deaths and occupational exposures in a population-based cohort), or (b) whenever some cases are much more informative than others, as occurs when the majority of cases are attributable to a known risk factor that is not of interest to the investigators. An example of the latter is a case-control study of nonsmoking causes of lung cancer. In a two-stage design, some readily available variables are obtained on all potential subjects, while the costly collection of other data is limited to the second-stage subjects who are chosen on the basis of both disease status and other first-stage variables. The major advantage of the two-stage design is substantial reduction of data-collection costs.

In randomized recruitment, the desired second-stage probabilities for selection are applied to strata based on first-stage variables to determine if recruitment is attempted on the potential subject. These probabilities are precalculated to maximize efficiency (similar to a more standard matched design), for instance, by assigning a high probability to a nonsmoking case and a low probability to a smoking case or nonsmoking control. This design does not require that an enumeration of potential controls be available in advance, and thus controls can be recruited simultaneously as cases accrue. Further advantages are that the distribution of the matching factor in the general population need not be known in advance, and the effect of the "matching" or first-stage screening factors can be assessed.

CASE-CROSSOVER DESIGN

Case-crossover designs were introduced in the early 1990s (Maclure, 1991) for estimating a short-term, transient effect of intermittent exposures on acute-onset diseases. For each event occurrence, the exposure status in the period just preceding it (case period) is compared with exposures of the same person in one or more control or referent periods. Confounding from individual time-invariant characteristics is completely controlled, as the individual supplies his or her own referent periods. This design can be used for both one-time events (death) and recurrent events (asthma episodes, respiratory illnesses). The analysis may be done using person-time methods if exposure is recorded continuously, or by conditional logistic regression if exposure is known only at sampled times, given the matching of cases to their own "controls" (that is, self-matched control time periods); see Chapters 8 and 16 for further discussion of the design and its analysis. In the last decade, this design has been commonly applied to air-pollution health-effect studies.

Several sampling strategies for referent periods have been proposed and evaluated. Some of these are shown in Figure 30–1. The choice of an appropriate "referent" period will depend on the major sources of bias in a particular study. Challenges include time trends in exposure, seasonal variation, day-of-the-week effects, auto-correlation with nearby referent periods, and bias due to (incorrect) use of conditional maximum likelihood when symmetric bidirectional sampling is used. Levy et al. (2001) demonstrated that unidirectional sampling, i.e., selecting only referent periods before the event, produced biased estimates of exposure effects, primarily owing to the long-term trend of declining exposures. They also showed that the selection of a symmetric set of referent periods, for instance, 2 days, one occurring 7 days before and the other 7 days after the case event-day, rendered the conditional-likelihood function used for estimation of coefficients in a logistic regression incorrect (as the true likelihood function is constant and equal to 1). This design therefore yields biased results. A couple of solutions have been proposed. Navidi and Weinhandl (2002) proposed a "semisymmetric bidirectional design," using days both before and after, then randomly selecting only one of them, basing their derivation on the theory of risk-set sampling. Janes et al. (2005) refer to "overlap bias," when referent periods are not chosen *a priori* and are functions of the observed event times, and demonstrate for which referent-selection strategies conditional logistic regression will produce unbiased results. They recommend "time-stratified" referent periods, the solution proposed by Levy et al. (2001), in which the time period is divided into fixed strata (e.g., calendar months) and referent days are selected within each stratum. With this design, cases occurring early in the month will have most referent days later and cases near the end of the month will have most referent days earlier (Fig. 30–1C). Case-crossover designs can be very useful in environmental epidemiology of transient exposures, but they must be applied cautiously.

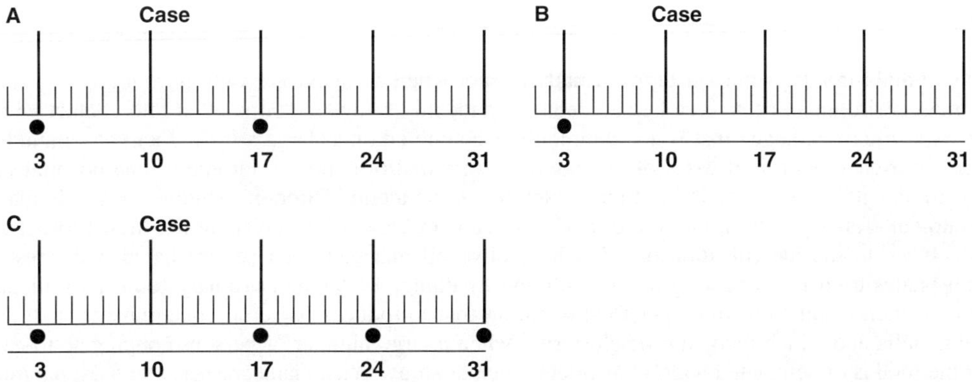

FIGURE 30–1 • Sampling strategies for referent times in case-crossover designs. **A:** Two referent days are selected for comparison with case-day exposures, one before and one after the case date, using the same day of the week (symmetric bidirectional). **B:** Referent day for exposure is 1 week preceding case date (restricted unidirectional). **C:** Referent days are all days in the calendar month that fall on the same day of the week (time-stratified). This design is recommended by Janes et al. (2005).

ECOLOGIC STUDIES

Ecologic studies have featured prominently in environmental epidemiology, because exposures are often already measured at the group level or because limited resources for conducting the study prohibit collection of individual-level data. Ecologic studies may be the best or only way to address many policy questions, which are sometimes at the heart of environmental epidemiologic investigations. That is, a policy affects the group as a whole: If technology reduces the emissions from tailpipes of motor vehicles, air mixing leads to changes in pollutant levels breathed throughout the state or country, and any health effects will be observed population-wide. If the policy is implemented at different time points in different locations, the effect of confounding from other changes will be reduced, so long as confounding variables do not change in parallel (e.g., because of similar staggering of policy or other changes).

Note that if only one variable is being measured at the group level, typically the exposure, the analysis can be considered an individual-level analysis with measurement error in the one variable. A detailed discussion of ecologic studies and associated biases is given in Chapter 25.

Susser (1994) presents a four-level hierarchy for ecologic studies and illustrates circumstances in which this design is (a) "obligate and apt," (b) "optional and apt," (c) "optional, not apt, but convenient," and (d) maladroit. At the top of this hierarchy are studies for which the goal is to determine the effectiveness of programs, policies, or regulations that are implemented at the ecologic level, such that the exposure is homogeneous across individuals and the outcomes are meaningful primarily for the group. In the second category, one might place studies in which exposure itself is defined at the group level and cannot be measured at the individual level, such as neighborhood density of liquor stores, or median income or percent employment in the census block, or type of hospital (teaching, referral, etc.). Ecologic studies can also be useful when a field is new and the goal is to screen hypotheses inexpensively (time trend, birth cohort, and mapping studies might apply) or when interindividual variation is outweighed by between-group differences (see, for example, the preceding discussion of trihalomethanes in drinking water). These examples might fall in Susser's third group, as it would be convenient to do such studies at the ecologic level, even though an individual level study would be more convincing.

Common ecologic approaches include exploration of regional variations through mapping, changes through time-trend or time-series analyses, and either differences in time trends across regions or changes in spatial patterns over time. In each of these, descriptive analyses can then proceed to the fitting of models that use regional or time-period attributes to predict disease rates. Tools that link space and time variation in exposure with space and time variation in health outcomes have undergone tremendous development; sophisticated geographic information systems (GIS) permit overlay of numerous, diverse databases with spatially linked variables.

TIME PATTERNS

There are three main types of time-related disease patterns: time clustering, cyclic patterns, and longitudinal trends. Time clustering usually occurs when an agent is newly introduced into the human environment or when a human behavior suddenly brings the population into contact with an exposure or pathogen that is not commonly encountered on as large a scale. Examples include the occurrence of several cases of an extremely rare malformation syndrome in one hospital in Australia within a short period of time, which led to the identification of thalidomide as a human teratogen (Taussig, 1962); an outbreak of thousands of cases of paralysis in Meknes, Morocco, which led to the identification of a batch of olive oil that had been contaminated with cresyl phosphates used in lubricating oils (Smith and Spalding, 1959); and ordinary food poisonings, which often result from improper food handling that introduces bacterial contaminants such as salmonella and which involve time clustering when a large number of persons congregate to eat or the food is disseminated widely. Accidents such as shipwrecks, plane crashes, and fires; natural disasters such as earthquakes, heat waves, floods, or tsunamis; and political and social upheavals such as wars and forced migration may also produce time (and space) clusters of injury and death. When the cause is known, the focus of epidemiologic studies may be on documenting the attributable fraction, or identifying cofactors associated with higher or lower than typical risk. An analysis of deaths from the 1999 earthquake in Taiwan demonstrated, for instance, that those with

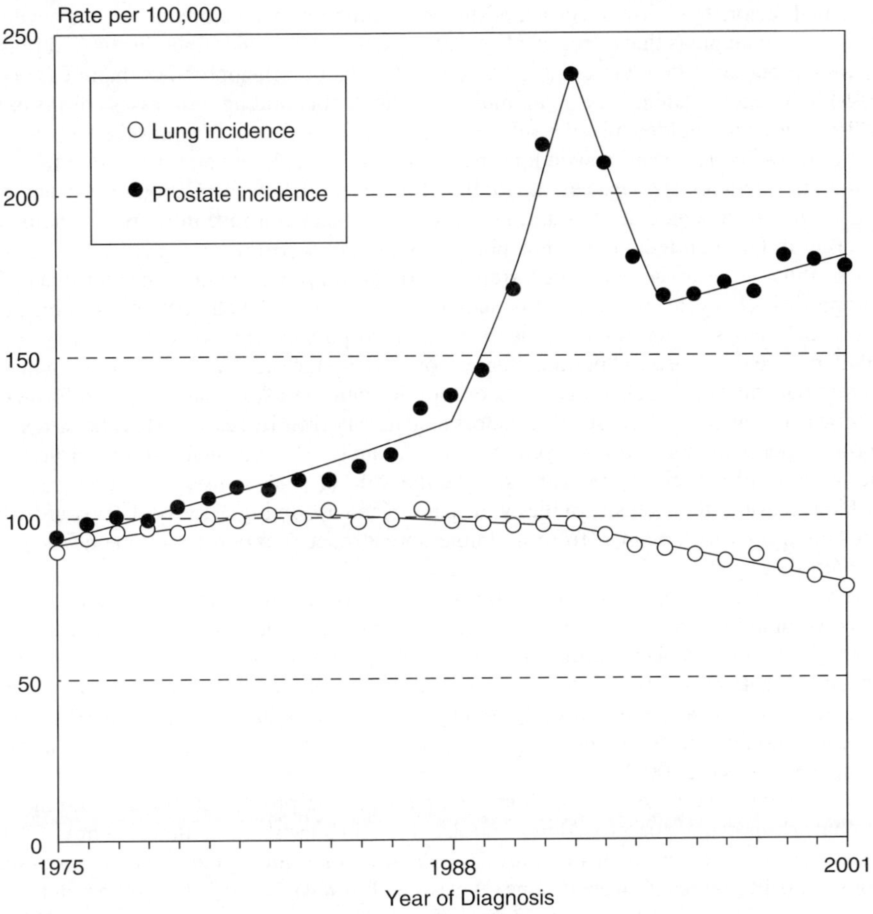

FIGURE 30–2 • Prostate versus lung cancer incidence, all races, males, 1975–2001. *Source:* SEER 9 areas. Rates are age-adjusted to the 2000 U.S. standard million population by 5-year age groups. Regression lines are calculated using the Joinpoint Regression Program Version 2.7, September 2003, National Cancer Institute.

mental illness, physical disability, or low socioeconomic status were at highest risk (Chou et al., 2004).

Clustering can also occur when a new diagnostic tool comes into medical practice, resulting in a surge in diagnoses, often at an earlier stage than was previously possible. After the introduction of a diagnostic test, the PSA (prostate-specific antigen), prostate cancer incidence showed a clear clustering (Fig. 30–2): a sharp rise and fall between 1989 and 1995 with a peak at 1992, overlaid above a steady increase (SEER Cancer Statistics Review, 1975–2001). The peak can be understood as the "iceberg" of undiagnosed preclinical cases detected by PSA; the linear slope before 1988 is similar to that after 1995, but the later one is higher (it has a larger intercept). This difference (the vertical distance between those two lines) represents the incidence of cases that went undiagnosed in the earlier period.

Cyclic patterns characterize a number of diseases. These patterns are not surprising, given well-known cycles in the size and activities of vector populations, in changes in the physical environment that influence exposure, and in many human physiologic functions and behaviors. Cardiovascular, cerebrovascular, and respiratory disease deaths rise in winter and decline in summer (Anderson and Le Riche, 1970; Bull and Morton, 1975), but extreme heat waves also cause increases in these deaths, usually peaking over only a few days (Gover, 1938; Poumadere et al., 2005). Finding a cycle in incidence implies a cyclic cause and is often viewed as evidence for a possible infectious etiology, although many potential causes, such as temperature, sunlight, behaviors, fertility, seasonal environmental factors (e.g., use of certain pesticides), and even magnetic fields are also cyclic. An interesting case example is that of seasonality and schizophrenia. Late-winter births (February and March) were reported to be more common among over 16,000 schizophrenics than in the general population in Sweden (Dalen, 1968). Attempts to replicate this finding or to assess births exposed to influenza epidemics yielded mixed results (e.g., Hare et al., 1974, vs. Krupinski et al., 1976), and by the 1980s, researchers were concluding that seasonality was likely an artifact due to errors in design and interpretation (Fananas et al., 1989). Most recently, however, serologic evidence from maternal serum specimens collected during pregnancy indicated a sevenfold higher incidence of first-trimester influenza infection in schizophrenics than others (Brown et al., 2004).

Most methods to evaluate cyclic occurrence involve fitting a sine curve to the frequencies or rates during a single cycle. If the cycle is annual, analysis of the cyclic pattern is often referred to as "seasonal analysis." Regression modeling that incorporates trigonometric terms to describe cyclic patterns are described as "periodic regression." Many factors that can confound other types of epidemiologic analysis, such as age, socioeconomic status, smoking habits, and so forth, do not confound seasonal analysis because these factors tend to vary little by season. This phenomenon and the stability of denominators during a cycle simplify the analysis of seasonal patterns. From monthly (or other periodic) frequencies, one can estimate the ratio of peak-to-trough occurrence during a cycle, which measures the intensity of the cyclic pattern and the timing of the peak (Edwards, 1961). These results are easily obtained from a simple spreadsheet program (http://members.aol.com/krothman/episheet.xls).

The examination of morbidity and mortality patterns over longer time periods (i.e., years or decades) is commonly used to generate hypotheses about nongenetic causal factors: in heart disease (Marmot, 1992), breast cancer (Tarone and Chu, 1992), and asthma (Arrighi, 1995). The increase in incidence of autism has been cited as evidence for an environmental contribution, although improved diagnosis and a changed attitude among parents in bringing their children to the attention of the medical community undoubtedly play a part in these statistics (California Department of Developmental Services, 2003).

Inferences about the causes of longitudinal trends can be problematic. Confounding factors include changes in diagnostic procedures and accuracy, in survival time due to more efficacious treatments (hence affecting studies of prevalence and of mortality), and in health care–seeking behavior for less life-threatening conditions (Devesa et al., 1984). Nevertheless, time trends provide a source of etiologic clues. When gender differences in time trends are seen, factors on which men and women tend to differ (e.g., occupations, smoking, alcohol, etc.) are more suspect. Conversely, when no gender difference is observed, exposures in common are more plausible.

Behavioral or other exposure changes that occur population-wide over calendar time give rise to a period effect; changes occurring across generations (persons born later behaving differently or being exposed to new environmental factors) result in a birth-cohort effect. Because age, period, and cohort are linearly dependent, a full model incorporating all three factors is nonidentifiable, meaning that there is no way to estimate uniquely all three effects at once without making further assumptions. Birth-cohort analysis is particularly useful when the exposures are short-lived or change nonmonotonically over time (e.g., Frost, 1939).

MAPPING

Mapping of disease rates serves a similar function as time-trend or birth-cohort analysis. As early as the 1790s, spot maps of yellow-fever cases along the eastern seaboard of the United States played a role in the debate between contagionists and anticontagionists (Howe, 1989). Snow's map of cholera cases surrounding the Broad Street pump illuminated the proximate cause (1855). Mapping of endemic disease came later. For a history of disease mapping and its use in the study of 19th- and 20-century epidemics, see Howe (1989).

Three important characteristics of a map are (a) whether the locations are points or regions, (b) if regions, whether they are regular or irregular, and (c) whether the variable being mapped is continuous or discrete. Constructing maps for continuous data, such as disease rates or mean life expectancies in states or counties, typically involves (a) dividing the geographic region of concern into discrete areas (often predefined by the administrative units that collect the data), (b) calculating standardized rates or means in each area, (c) categorizing these rates or means, and (d) associating a color or shading scheme to represent the ordered categories. The result is a chloropleth map of the rates or means.

Decisions must be made regarding the choices of boundaries, method of standardization, number of categories of rates, where to make the cutpoints, and whether cutpoints should vary among maps within a set (Smans and Esteve, 1992). See Chapters 3, 4, and 15 for methods of standardization. The number of categories should be chosen to maximize the information to be conveyed to the reader. See Chapters 13, 15, and 17 for discussions of choice of categories. Cromley and McLafferty (2002) discuss these and numerous other decisions that can either obscure or highlight information in environmental health maps.

A far more difficult problem is that of rare diseases. Because the size of the underlying population will almost always differ among the areas, many of the high-rate areas will have very few cases. The greater the instability of rates, the stronger is the likelihood of an extremely high rate. Maps of either crude or standardized disease rates will therefore predominantly draw attention to elevated but unstable risks in sparsely populated areas. An alternative is to map the P-values, but because P-values reflect both strength of association and precision, this approach tends to highlight large regions that have relatively small elevations in risk, focusing attention on population size rather than magnitude of risk.

The most viable solutions to this problem fall under the rubric of "shrinkage" or Bayes methods, which combine "prior" information with the empirical data to derive an improved posterior estimate. In the mapping application, the underlying rate in the total map serves as the prior information. Because this underlying rate is also unknown and it is replaced with an estimate from the data, the method is referred to as "empirical Bayes." The term "shrinkage" refers to replacing each rate with an adjusted rate that is closer to the mean rate for all locations—a shrinkage (or increase) toward the overall mean. For disease mapping, variation in population sizes is a nuisance source of heterogeneity, and empirical Bayes methods are smoothing techniques based on three assumptions: (a) the overall rate is unbiased and should not be altered; (b) shrinkage of an individual rate should increase as the variance increases; and (c) the distribution of incidence rates follows a probability distribution (Cromley and McLafferty, 2002). Elliott et al. (1992, see color plate 4) shows how mapping rates that have been stabilized via empirical Bayes techniques can filter out noise and highlight noteworthy geographic patterns of disease. Although not all artifacts of mapping can be removed (Gelman and Price, 1999), these methods offer major advantages over maps of crude rates (Moulton et al., 1994).

Maps can stimulate etiologic research, including focused case-control or cohort studies. The United States county-specific maps published by the National Cancer Institute (NCI) in the 1970s (Mason et al., 1976) were used for surveillance and led to targeted case-control studies that ultimately identified high mortality rates from nasal cancer in areas with furniture-manufacturing industries (Brinton et al., 1977), lung cancer in counties with petrochemical manufacturing (Blot and Fraumeni, 1976), bladder cancer where chemical industries were located (Hoover et al., 1975), and oral cancer in regions where snuff use was common (Blot and Fraumeni, 1977).

Even for studies of determinants of disease that are not obviously spatial in nature, geographic location may need to be controlled because important confounders that are hard or infeasible to measure may cluster spatially. Examples include physician diagnostic practices or local customs that propel persons to seek medical attention. Cressie (1991) demonstrated the use of techniques to remove spatial trends in data and thereby control spatially related confounders.

COMPARISON OF TIME-TREND AND SPATIAL-DATA ANALYSIS

Unlike spatial analyses, temporal comparisons may require only event data, if it is reasonable to assume no important temporal change in baseline risk factors or in the size of the population at risk. In contrast, spatial comparisons almost invariably require data on both the events and the population at risk—that is, its size, age, and sex distributions, etc.

Crucial to both temporal and spatial data is the scale of data. The time scale for tracking measles epidemics is days to weeks, whereas cardiovascular disease mortality shows trends covering decades (Uemura and Piša, 1988), as well as seasonal variation (Anderson and Le Riche, 1970). Obviously, both the exposure and the disease will dictate what time scale is important. Time-trend analyses, regardless of scale, are most useful when the exposures of concern are widespread, because one can aggregate over sizable regions to obtain time-specific rates. The stability of associations with disease will depend on the population size, the background disease rate, and the width of the time periods of interest. Studies of shorter time periods require larger population sizes or higher background rates.

For spatial data, however, the problem of scale frequently raises additional methodologic problems. When exposures are localized, the investigator will be interested in small areas where disease rates will tend to be unstable. Stability might be achieved if these localized exposures (e.g., chemicals migrating from a hazardous waste site) were present and documented for extended periods of time and appropriate outcome data could be obtained. Issues surrounding variable and small geographically defined populations are addressed by the literature on small-area analysis (Elliott et al., 1992; Richardson et al., 2004).

ANALYSIS AND METHODOLOGIC CHALLENGES IN ENVIRONMENTAL EPIDEMIOLOGY

When studying disease rates in relation to geography or time period, epidemiologists will want to adjust for multivariate confounding and may want to model exposure–response relations quantitatively. In longitudinal studies, repeated measures will require adjustment for auto-correlation, whereas geographic studies may require special methods such as empirical Bayes, or kriging, adjacency, and distance-based techniques. Generalized linear models provide an overall framework that can encompass both group-level and individual-level data, cross-sectionally, over time or across space. For group-level data, namely, disease rates, Poisson regression (see Chapter 21) is frequently the method of choice (Checkoway et al., 2004) and can be applied to data in which time and space are central factors defining the units of observation. When the disease is more common, binomial regression or survival analysis is more appropriate. The interrelationships among these three methods are discussed by Pearce et al. (1988). In Poisson regression, the counts or rates of events are described as a function of exposure, spatial, time-period, demographic, and other variables. The method is commonly used when the predictor variables (regressors) are categorical (nominal or ordinal) but need not be limited to such variables. Within cells constructed by cross-classification across predictor variables, events are enumerated, and in most cases it will also be necessary to obtain the person-time or expected count associated with each cell. The data collected from time series or geographic regions can be organized into cells such as days, weeks, years, etc., counties, states, regions of the world, etc., or space-time units such as county-years, etc.

In typical exponential (log-linear) Poisson regression models, assumptions include that (a) the logarithm of the disease rate changes linearly with equal-increment increases in the exposure variable; (b) changes in the rate from the combined effects of different exposures or risk factors are multiplicative; (c) at each level of the covariates, the number of cases has variance equal to its mean; and (d) observations are independent. Methods to detect and deal with violations of assumptions (a) and (b) are similar to those used for other exponential models (e.g., logistic, proportional hazards) (see Greenland, 1989b; McCullagh and Nelder, 1989; and Chapter 20). Methods to identify violations of assumption (c), that is, to determine whether there is overdispersion (variances are too large) or underdispersion (too small), include plots of residuals versus the mean at different levels of the predictor variable. Methods for dealing with violation of the Poisson assumptions are discussed by Breslow (1984) and by McCullagh and Nelder (1989).

In spatial or time-trend studies, the assumption of independence may be violated. In time series, the numbers of events (e.g., deaths, hospital admissions, etc.) occurring on a given day i may be correlated with the numbers of events on days $i - 1$, $i - 2$, etc., not because of the correlation in explanatory variables (cold weather, for instance) but for unknown or unmeasured reasons. Similar lack of independence can occur with spatial data. Similarity of disease rates in a given geographic region with rates in contiguous regions could be due to person-to-person transmission, the presence of the same vectors or sources of exposure, or the influence of physician diagnostic practices. Auto-correlation models can incorporate these nonindependent observations.

TIME-SERIES ANALYSES: CONFOUNDING AND AUTO-REGRESSION

Time series analyses follow a given community or region through time, usually without covariate data on individuals. Although outcomes can include means of continuous measures made on individuals, such as pulmonary function, they are often rates of binary events (death, hospital admission, symptom present, etc.) and are well suited for Poisson regression.

As stated earlier, within-community comparisons, in contrast to spatial comparisons, obviate the need for denominator data when the population composition and size do not change over the time period of interest. This approach is particularly advantageous where the catchment area is unclear, say, for hospital-based studies in densely populated areas where not all hospitals can be included, counts of admissions or outpatients might be comparable for high- versus low-pollution days. Thus, time-based comparisons within a population are convenient to assess acute effects from community-wide exposures and may provide more valid estimates than comparisons between communities.

Although individual-level confounders are not a problem in such studies, confounding can occur as a result of infectious agents, correlated pollutants, time trends in mortality, and meteorologic factors. Temperature, humidity, and seasonal fluctuations may correlate with both pollution and health outcomes. High correlations among individual pollutants (particulates, acid aerosols, ozone, etc.) are not a problem if the mixture is of interest but are a challenge if the goal is to identify the precise factor responsible for adverse health effects, or to distinguish the relative roles of different components of the mixture. In theory, these difficulties can be overcome by studying areas or time periods in which correlations are low or vary across regions. Borja-Aburto et al. (1997) focused on Mexico City, where ozone levels are not as highly correlated with sulfur dioxide, temperature, or total suspended particles as they are in most cities in the United States.

Long-term trends in mortality can also be a problem in a long time series. Adjustment for such trends, however, should be undertaken with caution. If there has been a long-term trend in the exposure (increases or declines in pollution levels), then adjustment could introduce bias toward the null in measures of pollution effects. On the other hand, time can be a true confounder. In particular, when longer time periods are being addressed, patterns of migration, shifting diagnostic practices, changes in behavior, and other important sources of drift or bias gain importance.

SOCIAL CLASS AS A CONFOUNDER IN INTERCOMMUNITY COMPARISONS

A common study design compares disease rates in communities that have high exposure with rates in low-exposure communities. This design is appropriate when exposures are spread throughout a community, but not where point sources pollute very small areas within a community. Although many intercommunity comparison studies are ecologic, a more valid design (not subject to ecologic biases) involves measuring covariates and outcome at the individual level, even if exposure can only be feasibly measured at the group level. Intercommunity comparisons are particularly useful for evaluating the effect of chronic ongoing exposures that vary primarily between rather than within communities. However, social, cultural, and economic factors may similarly vary across communities, introducing serious difficulty in achieving complete control for confounding.

Social class is strongly associated with a broad range of diseases (Krieger and Fee, 1994), and systematic inequities in environmental pollution with regard to poverty or race are well documented (United Church of Christ Commission on Racial Justice, 1987; United States Environmental Protection Agency, 1992; Evans and Kantrowitz, 2002). These disparities are not new, even if research has lagged behind. The concentrations of DDT, its metabolites, and PCBs in San Francisco Bay Area residents were substantially higher among African Americans than among whites during the 1960s (James et al., 2002). Similarly, data collected in 1976–1980 for the Second National Health and Nutrition Examination Survey (NHANES) demonstrated much higher levels of blood lead among African Americans and among those of low education, compared with whites and those of higher education (Mahaffey et al., 1982).

Given strong associations of socioeconomic status with both environmental exposures and health outcomes, the potential for confounding is great. Typically, because income is difficult to obtain, epidemiologists use education to capture social class, and occasionally, occupation. Adjustment for these factors may be inadequate owing to residual confounding arising in multiple ways, including the use of broad categories for education or socioeconomic status (Kaufman et al., 1997) and lack of data on resources or social capital, factors that operate at the individual, household/family, or neighborhood level and that influence host susceptibility and access to medical or preventive care;

see Chapter 26. Neighborhood characteristics appear to predict health even after controlling for individual-level factors. Potentially relevant census-derived neighborhood factors include percentage unemployed, percent owner-occupied housing, and median income; others are the availability of supermarkets with fresh produce (Fitzgibbon and Stolley, 2004), density of liquor stores (LaVeist and Wallace, 2000), and crime rates (Cinat et al., 2004).

Inadequately measured confounders can result in biased estimates of associations between the main exposure and outcome, even after adjustment for these confounders (see Chapter 9). Such errors can be substantial but would not be detectable in standard analysis that lacks data on the degree of measurement error of the confounder (social class). Moreover, even when the misclassification (of confounders) is nondifferential, the adjusted measure could be more biased than the crude one (Greenland, 1980; Brenner, 1993). Hence one may need to go beyond the usual surrogates for this important determinant of health status.

Although socioeconomic status is a profound predictor of health, treating it as a confounder could be incorrect if some of the disparities in health outcomes attributed to socioeconomics are actually a consequence of environmental exposures (Bellinger, 2004). Investigators need to address social class in the design, data-collection, and analysis phases of a study. Use of directed acyclic graphs (Hernan et al., 2002; Greenland et al., 1999a; Pearl, 2000) in conjunction with the existing literature can help clarify the factors involved and how they fit into a conceptual causal model; see Chapter 12 for further details.

ANALYSIS OF CLUSTERS

A disease cluster is defined as an unusual aggregation, in time or space or both, of occurrences of a disease. To understand what is *unusual,* one first needs to look outside the particular time, space, or time and space that is of interest to determine what is *usual*. These "usual" rates will come from the distribution of occurrences in the same location at other time periods, in one or more other similar locations at the same time periods, or in larger areas than the locale of interest. For spatial clustering, the distributions of noncases (or the population at risk) over the same time and space is needed. Deriving denominators may be a formidable task when the regions of homogeneous exposures may not correspond to the regions for which population or health data are available (Hertz-Picciotto, 1996).

Investigations of single clusters are usually not fruitful, whereas research on generalized clustering over large areas (Does this disease tend to occur in clusters? Where are the hotspots for this disease?) can serve as surveillance to provide information on what is "usual" and generate hypotheses when areas of high and/or low incidence are observed.

Some cluster investigation methods rely on case-only data. Others require either population denominators or a control group sampled randomly from the population. In general, the scale at which data are collected will often be a major determinant of what type of analysis can be used and of the ability to uncover meaningful patterns. Three classes of analytic approaches for studying geographic variation are cell count, adjacency, and distance or nearest-neighbor methods.

Cell-count methods compare observed counts of events in cells, usually defined by geographic areas, with expected counts of events, usually under the assumption of a Poisson distribution. Methods have recently been developed that do not suffer from the problems of arbitrary but fixed boundaries and regions or time intervals that are either too small or too large relative to the scale at which events cluster. One class of such methods is the "scan" statistics. Zones of cells for which the centroids fall within prespecified regions are examined, and likelihood-ratio statistics are calculated to identify the most likely clusters (Kulldorff, 1997).

An extension of cell-count approaches is adjacency methods, which examine whether areas of high rates of disease are likely to be adjacent to other high-rate areas. If exact locations of cases are not known and/or the scale of clustering is unknown or spans multiple cells, adjacency methods are appropriate. These techniques examine the degree to which areas with higher-than-expected counts tend to cluster, using tools from geography known as spatial auto-correlation statistics, which measure the extent to which the value of a variable at one location depends on values of this variable at nearby locations. "Nearby" can be defined in various ways, e.g., the number of residents in one region who work in the neighboring one, etc.

Distance or nearest-neighbor methods compare physical distances between cases to expected distances. These analyses intrinsically avoid imposing arbitrary regional boundaries, require no prespecification of how close cases need to be to constitute a cluster, and usually do not require denominator data. Distances between cases and nearest other cases can be used in a number of types of analyses (Besag, 1989; Besag and Newell, 1991). Nearest-neighbor analyses are useful for case-control studies; relative clustering can be defined using distances between cases versus distances between controls, with numerous elaborations (Rogerson, 2006).

ANALYSIS OF CLUSTERING AROUND POINT SOURCES

A conventional approach to address clustering around known pollutant sources is a variant of the cell-count method that involves drawing boundaries around the site to include a nearby exposed population, calculation of the disease rate, and comparison with state or national rates. Problems with this approach include (a) indeterminate population sizes, (b) arbitrariness of the boundaries, and (c) difficulties if the area chosen is too large (effect is swamped) or too small (low power) (Bithell and Stone, 1989). Another problem is the lack of sociodemographic comparability between the exposed and referent populations.

Some of these problems are overcome by distance-measure methods that avoid arbitrary definitions of the affected area and do not require equal population sizes. The method of Besag and Newell (1991) involves creation of zones ordered by distance from an exposure source. The source need not be a point; it could be a river or a coastline, with distance defined appropriately.

GENERAL CONSIDERATIONS IN THE INVESTIGATION OF CLUSTERS

Reports of perceived clusters are frequently made to local, state, and federal agencies by concerned citizens, physicians, or other health practitioners, sometimes overwhelming local, state, or federal agencies. The Centers for Disease Control (1990b) guidelines for investigation of clusters calls for an integrated approach that seeks to be responsive to community concerns, and at the same time recognizes that most such reports do not lead to identification of a common causal exposure for the events of interest. Frequently, there simply is no excess of cases. Second, the reported cases may be too diverse to be reasonably suspected of arising from the same cause. Third, even if there is an excess, the number of cases may be too small for meaningful statistical analysis. Fourth, there may be no identified suspect exposure, or the exposure(s) suggested by the community may not be a plausible cause or set of causes for the outcome reported.

In general, it is difficult to draw a conclusion regarding clustering from a single cluster, no matter how unusual. Cluster investigations are most fruitful when (a) the outcome is rare and occurs primarily by a single mechanism or (b) the rate of disease increases rapidly (Rothman, 1990b). Health professionals who communicate with the lay public need to recognize the culture gap between scientists and nonscientists regarding how evidence is evaluated. This gap can only be bridged through two-way communication: listening to the concerns and ideas of those outside the profession and respectfully explaining the rationale for choices made. Bringing the community into the process of evaluating health and exposure information will go a long way toward overcoming the differences in perspectives.

SURVEILLANCE AND RISK ASSESSMENT OF ENVIRONMENTAL HAZARDS

ENVIRONMENTAL HEALTH SURVEILLANCE

Environmental health surveillance involves the systematic collection, linkage, and analysis of both environmental and health data, in order to identify those exposures that are adversely affecting the well-being of the population so that rational public policy can be developed. Despite regulations governing chemicals introduced into the environment, not all functions or systems are studied for long-term chronic effects. Neurodevelopmental toxicity testing, for instance, is not required, even though it may occur at lower exposures than other toxicities. In the absence of adequate prerelease testing, systematic monitoring for adverse health effects is rational and appropriate. Disease surveillance is discussed extensively in Chapter 22, but surveillance for environmental hazards requires additional elements (Hertz-Picciotto, 1996).

An ideal surveillance system for environmentally induced disease would have the following elements: (a) high-quality mortality and morbidity data with residence information; (b) timely population data for denominators to calculate rates with adjustment for migration between censuses; (c) timely, high-quality emissions and environmental monitoring data for air, water, soil, food, and other exposure media, characterized geographically and temporally; (d) personal monitoring, biomonitoring, and exposure modeling data to capture transport and transmission; (e) tools to link these various types of data; (f) compatible standards across data sources and standardized vocabularies; (g) fine enough resolution to be useful for observing effects of localized exposures on small communities; and (h) systems for dissemination of such data (Hertz-Picciotto, 1996; McGeehin et al., 2004). Although costly, the benefits of such a surveillance system would include information on long-term trends; an early-warning capability, that is, the ability to detect unusually high incidence of diseases covered by the system; avoidance of public anxiety and costly investigations of situations in which no excess risk is ascertained; and the potential for increased public confidence in the commitment of government and health scientists to protect the population's health.

Recently, initiatives in the United States and other countries have begun to address the need for integrated surveillance systems. In the United States, the Pew Environmental Health Commission (2000) called for establishment of a Nationwide Health Tracking Network that would monitor and establish relations between environmental hazards and disease. The report cited the absence of information on auto-immune diseases, developmental disabilities, diabetes and other endocrinologic disorders, asthma, and birth defects. Initial steps appear to be underway, involving several health and environmental agencies (McGeehin et al., 2004). Given newer environmental health challenges described later, these systems will also need to integrate large-scale global changes, such as stratospheric ozone and climatic factors.

RISK ASSESSMENT

Risk assessment, an interface between environmental epidemiology and environmental health policy, involves estimation of risks for situations in which they cannot be measured or observed directly, either because the risks are too low, the population is too small, the exposures do not occur in isolation from other hazardous exposures, the exposure scenario is projected but has not yet occurred, or a sufficient induction period since exposure has not yet passed. The U.S. National Academy of Sciences (1983) defined risk assessment as "the use of the factual base to define the health effects of exposure of individuals or populations to hazardous materials and situations." This definition, however, falls short of depicting the true state of the art: The factual base is usually not fully adequate, and hence, some assumptions are made that are not directly testable. Because decisions may need to be made before the evidence is complete, policymakers and the public seek estimates of what the health costs are from certain societal actions or inactions. Without input from epidemiology (and toxicology), the regulatory approaches may be influenced by economic pressures alone.

The four steps in risk assessment are (National Research Council, 1983; U.S. Environmental Protection Agency, 1986)

1. *Hazard identification:* Is there evidence that the agent is capable of harming the health of the exposed population?
2. *Exposure assessment:* Who is exposed; through what medium, such as air, water, food, etc.; at what dose; and for how long?
3. *Dose–response:* What is the response rate for doses in the observable range, and what is the predicted response at the lower levels?
4. *Risk characterization:* Given the exposed population and their estimated or actual exposure and given the extrapolated dose–response relation, what is the predicted population health impact? Risk assessment has a long history of being used informally as a natural part of preventive health practice.

Epidemiologic data have been used to quantify risks for environmentally induced cancer and cardiorespiratory mortality (Hertz-Picciotto and Hu, 1994; Hertz-Picciotto, 1995; Kunzli et al., 2000, 2001) and for checking plausibility of animal-based risk extrapolations (Hertz-Picciotto and Hu, 1994; Hertz-Picciotto, 1995).

Faced with new challenges such as global transport of air pollutants, climate change, depletion of the ozone layer, and so forth, there may be much from "traditional" risk assessment that can be useful as we face unknown risks and scenarios that can be only partially predicted.

HISTORICAL LESSONS IN ENVIRONMENTAL EPIDEMIOLOGY

In its early period, environmental epidemiology was concerned largely with biologic agents and environmental factors that altered human contact with such agents. This section provides a few historical examples, beginning with lessons from Snow (1855) on water contamination, then turning to ambient air pollution and concluding with persistent organic pollutants.

WATER CONTAMINATION

The classic work of John Snow (1855), *On the Mode of Communication of Cholera,* presented an array of evidence that fecal matter from infected patients carried the "morbid poison," that ingestion of very small quantities was the mode of transmission, and that mixing of sewage and drinking-water sources enabled such transmission on a wide scale. The method proceeded from a case series tracing the introduction of the epidemic into a municipality to mapping of cases and ecologic comparisons among districts of London for the 1832, 1849, and 1853 outbreaks, to a natural experiment (a cohort design in which exposure is assigned as if at random, see Chapter 6). The ecologic intercommunity comparisons of districts in London were accompanied by property-value data to show the lack of correspondence between water source and wealth, thereby providing evidence that the association was not due to this potential confounder. The natural experiment was a serendipitous occurrence, but Snow strengthened the findings by incorporating individual confirmation of exposure. In fact, Snow himself (and one assistant) visited the homes of all cholera victims and asked the survivors for the name of their water company. If written documentation of the water supplier could not be found, Snow collected a vial of tap water. Although he could not test for the microorganism itself (because it had yet to be identified), the contaminated water from downstream, which contained London's sewage, had 40 times the quantity of sodium chloride. Addition of silver nitrate could distinguish the two sources of water, by precipitating a far greater amount of silver chloride in the contaminated water than in the cleaner water that was drawn farther upstream, beyond the reach of the sewage of London (Snow, 1855, p.78). Exposure of each case's household was thereby determined with high accuracy.

Snow's accounts examined in detail the consistency of a wide range of information with the hypothesized mode of transmission. He noted that wherever the general water supply was not contaminated, cholera was seen primarily in crowded areas where the poor and laboring classes lived, but that in districts near the Broad Street pump, the disease had struck the wealthier and poorer houses equally. Although it may be difficult for today's epidemiologists to appreciate the skepticism with which Snow's theory of epidemic transmission was received, Snow's clarity and unrelenting thoroughness as he sought to reconcile every detail of the cholera epidemics with an unpopular theory serve as a model for present-day environmental epidemiology.

AIR POLLUTION

Research on health effects of air pollution has progressed through several stages, each addressing the problem using distinct designs. Episodes with extremely high levels of air pollution produced by meteorologic inversions in the Meuse Valley of Belgium in 1930 (Firket, 1931), in Donora, Pennsylvania, in 1948 (Schrenk et al., 1949), and in London in the winter of 1952 focused attention on the dramatic effect on deaths from respiratory- and cardiovascular-related causes (Logan, 1953). These studies resembled the reports of infectious disease epidemics that filled the epidemiology and public health journals of the time: within-community comparisons using a before-and-after design. This within-community comparison is ideal for effects of short induction time, that is, as little as a few hours to a few weeks or months, where migration is not extensive, and when a clear line demarcates unexposed from exposed time periods.

Subsequent research in the 1950s and 1960s was concerned with less extreme levels of pollution and typically compared communities with higher versus lower pollutant levels (Lave and Seskin,

1970). The greatest problem in these between-community studies was the strong correlation between socioeconomic level and air pollution level. However, despite weaknesses, these air pollution studies contributed to the establishment of air standards, including the passage of the Clean Air Act of 1970 in the United States, which attempted to provide comprehensive protection to the general population from air pollution. (See Luneberg, 1995, for a historical account of the legal framework of environmental protection in the United States.)

The third set of air pollution studies used within-community time-series analyses to examine how fluctuations in pollutant levels over time in a single region influence mortality or morbidity. This design avoided problems from confounders that differ across individuals yet tend to remain constant over the time periods of interest. For instance, smoking prevalence or distributions of social class and age tend not to change markedly within a community over short time periods, and even if they do (e.g., for a 3-year study), the changes are unlikely to mirror short-term contrasts in air pollution that occur in a period of a few weeks. Similarity of findings across health outcomes (cardiopulmonary deaths, hospital admissions, self-reported symptoms, and exacerbations of asthma) in both intra- and intercommunity study designs strengthens the evidence for causality. The fourth generation of studies, largely cohorts in which individual-level data are integrated with community-based exposure data or in which more refined measures of exposure are made, will likely provide further understanding regarding mechanisms of susceptibility, effects related to developmental stages, and more specific indications of the pollutants that are most harmful.

PERSISTENT ORGANIC POLLUTANTS

In the 1990s, Theo Colborn published *Our Stolen Future* (Colborn, 1996) which eloquently made the case that certain classes of industrially produced chemicals are highly persistent, disrupt hormone regulation, and have permeated the environment, harming wildlife populations throughout the world. The possibility that human populations may also have been affected generated concern among the public and the media, and over the next few years, health and environmental agencies in the United States and Europe began funding expanded research into the effects of "endocrine-disrupting chemicals." Some of these studies focused on chemicals with estrogenic, antiestrogenic, androgenic, or antiandrogenic activity, and health outcomes such as breast and testicular cancer, cryptorchidism, sperm counts, and sex ratio of births. Standard designs, e.g., case-control studies of rare diseases or conditions, have sometimes used serum measures of body burdens that represent cumulative exposures over long time periods, in some cases, decades. For example, dozens of studies searched for differences in serum PCB concentrations between breast cancer patients and unaffected controls, but the findings have been largely null. A few meta-analyses reporting a decline in sperm counts over the period when endocrine-disrupting chemicals were increasing have been considerably debated. Causal inference is hampered by the inherent problems with documenting comparability of historical measurements when laboratory variability and interindividual variability are substantial.

Others have examined metabolic disorders such as diabetes (Longnecker and Daniels, 2001) or developmental deficits possibly mediated through thyroid hormone disruption (Winneke et al., 2002). The literature on these outcomes is growing but still inconclusive. In contrast, research in wildlife populations has uncovered striking associations. In Florida, alligators exposed to organochlorine pesticides from a chemical waste site showed developmental abnormalities of the reproductive tract, including reduced penis size in males (Guillette et al., 1999; Semenza et al., 1997). Snapping turtles in Ontario, Canada, displayed changes in sexually dimorphic characteristics such that males resembled females (de Solla et al., 1998). Intersex gonads and sex-ratio reversal were seen in PCB- and polychlorodibenzofuran PCDF)-exposed cricket frogs (Reeder et al., 1998). Laboratory studies in numerous species demonstrate that PCBs, dioxins, and other endocrine disruptors cause altered behavior, as well as structure and function changes, in several organ systems (Birnbaum and Tuomisto, 2000; Birnbaum and Fenton, 2003). Evidence from human studies is less conclusive, but again, the literature suggests involvement of multiple pathologic processes and organ systems (Longnecker et al., 1997; Hertz-Picciotto et al., 2003). Phthalates, which are present in a wide range of consumer products, may alter male reproductive-tract development, and several epidemiologic investigations suggest adverse effects on respiratory health (Hauser and Calafat, 2005).

Colborn (2004) outlines a number of reasons for the much stronger associations in wildlife than are observed in epidemiologic studies. Because the major effects from these chemicals arise in association with prenatal exposures, the much lower reproductive rate in human populations and much longer interval to sexual maturity render epidemiologic studies much less statistically powerful than wildlife investigations. Many wildlife species, for instance, reproduce annually, such that most or all females (as compared with ~1% in humans) produce offspring during a short period of time each year. Colborn hypothesizes that even with a high reproductive rate, if birds were continuous breeders such that the births were spread out over the year, many of the reproductive problems might never have been noticed.

The field of research on endocrine disruption is relatively young, and outcomes such as developmental deficits can be subtle. The parallels and differences between wildlife biology and epidemiology are instructive. Both involve nonexperimental research and hence must confront problems of confounding and mixtures of chemicals. Fortunately, experimental studies also supplement the work on wildlife, and studies can be designed to replicate the findings and identify the causal exposures as well as mechanisms of action. The field will also benefit from further work to identify tests for human behavioral and developmental effects that are sensitive to environmental toxins (Bellinger, 2003, 2004b).

NEW ENVIRONMENTAL HEALTH CHALLENGES

In recent years, "globalization" has become a buzzword throughout society; its ramifications for environmental epidemiology are not difficult to see. First, issues that were of high priority only in Western countries are now on the agendas of less industrialized nations (e.g., motor-vehicle exhaust). Second, pollution does not respect national borders, as the industrial waste poured into the rivers, lakes, and oceans of one country washes up on the shores of many others, and toxins released into the air (e.g., chlorinated hydrocarbons) are deposited thousands of miles away. Third, localized problems, such as overuse of fertilizers, are frequently repeated in one region after another. As for future directions, several themes are emerging for the 21st century.

Infectious diseases are re-emerging as major threats to public health, sometimes linked in com plex ways to problematic chemical toxins and physical hazards. For instance, hundreds of thousands of tube wells dug during the 1970s in India, Bangladesh, and elsewhere to combat water-borne diseases have resulted in high arsenic exposure for millions of people, at levels that increase risks for cancer, and possibly also respiratory and other adverse effects (Smith et al., 2000; Mazumder et al., 1998; Chowdhury, 2004; Wasserman et al., 2004; von Ehrenstein et al., 2005).

Major planetary changes with a potential for large-scale health effects are underway. The depletion of stratospheric ozone resulting from the dissemination of chlorofluorocarbons is expected to increase exposure to UV-B radiation, which in turn may bring about increased rates of skin cancer and cataracts, and changes in immune function over the next century (Armstrong, 1994; Lloyd, 1993). Already, short episodes of high radiation in areas of southern Chile have produced increased incidences of sunburn (Abarca et al., 2002), and scientists are predicting a combined effect of ozone depletion with climate change (van der Leun, 2002; Diffey, 2004).

Predictions of climatologists regarding global climate change may already have begun to surface (Fig. 30–3). A rise in global mean temperature of between 1 and 3.5°C by the year 2100, along with more frequent extreme events (heavy rains and storms, drought, and heat waves) in some latitudes are expected scenarios (Martens, 1998; Haines et al., 2000; Patz, 2000). Although current models cannot predict the precise geographic and temporal pattern of these changes, a 0.4°C increase has already occurred over the last 25 years. Was the summer 2003 heat wave in Europe that killed nearly 15,000 in France alone (Vandentorren et al., 2004; Ledrans et al., 2003) an episode in this trajectory or a random event? What about the 2002 flooding of the Danube and Vltava rivers, the latter being the worst in over 100 years for the city of Prague? Or the heavy storms that flooded Los Angeles in December 2003–January 2004, with more rain in 2 weeks than occurs on average in a year, based on data since the late 1800s? Was the intensity of Hurricane Katrina influenced by rising sea temperatures (Webster et al., 2005)?

Global warming is also predicted to cause changes in the distribution of vector-borne diseases such as malaria and tick-borne encephalitis (Lindsay and Martens, 1998; Kovats et al., 1999; Patz, 2000), alterations in food productivity, a possible rise in the oceans and a consequent flooding of

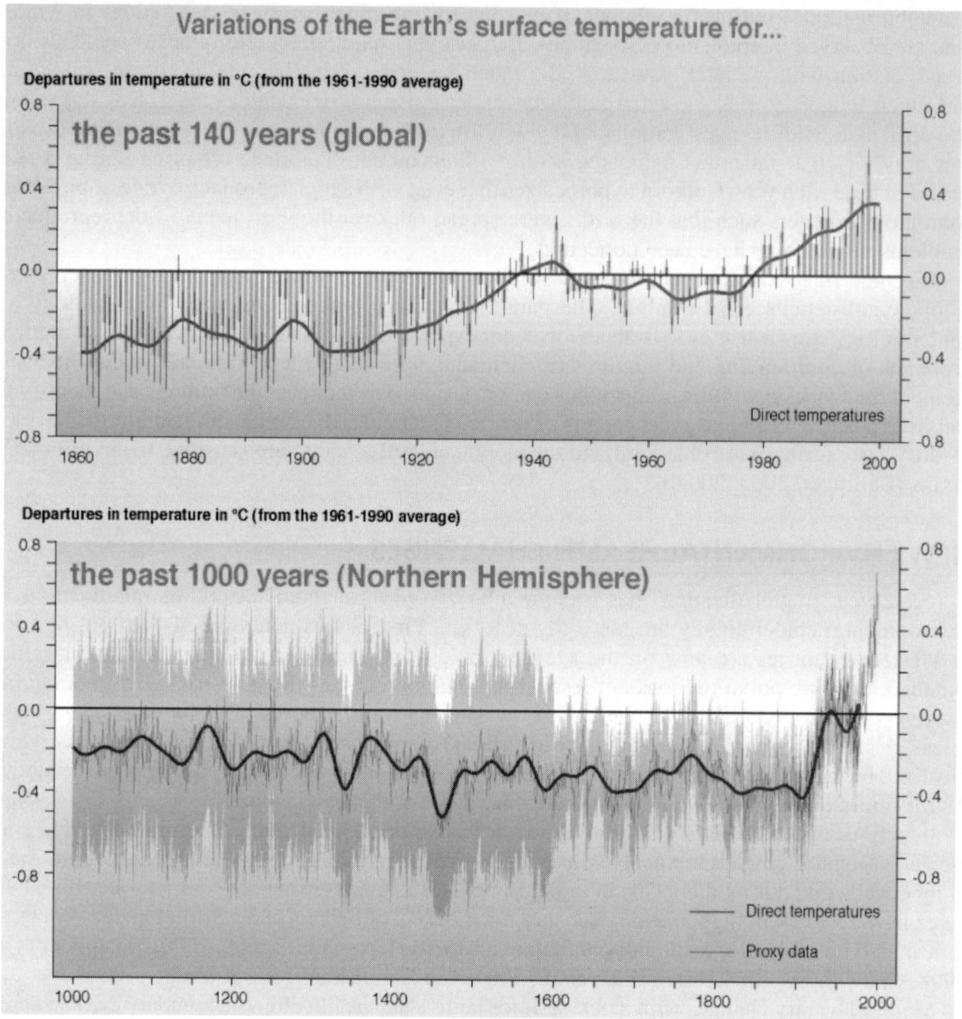

FIGURE 30–3 • Departures of the earth's surface temperature from average. (Copyright 2001, Intergovernmental Panel on Climate Change.)

coastal areas, where a substantial portion of the world's population resides, and numerous other indirect consequences of increased climatic variability (McMichael, 2001; Patz et al., 2000). Complex ecosystem relationships may compound the health consequences: A majority of water-borne disease outbreaks occurring between 1948 and 1994 in the United States were temporally related to heavy rains (Curriero et al., 2001). Similarly, population displacement may alter land-use patterns, which may bring about further changes in temperature and rainfall, and hence, distribution of disease vectors.

Deforestation of a large proportion of the earth's land mass is predicted to change weather patterns. Overuse of fresh water is lowering water tables in many areas of the world, potentially threatening sustainable food production. These environmental alterations are co-occurring with major demographic migrational shifts, in which the populations of cities in less developed regions of the world are swelling far beyond the capacity of the infrastructure to provide clean water, adequate housing, and sanitation (McMichael, 2000). Massive changes in both the physical and social environments may significantly alter patterns of health and disease (McMichael et al., 1998).

The appropriate epidemiologic and public health responses to these changes have yet to be delineated. One thing is clear, however: New scientific data are needed. Surveillance systems need to be created to document changes in time and space of both health outcomes and exposure, broadly defined to include not only the standard suspects of chemicals and radiation, but also climate and ecosystems (Intergovernmental Panel on Climate Change, 2001). In tandem with the development of extensive databases will be a second need: for creative epidemiologic methods that will enable us to both understand these phenomena and to devise policies that can prevent potentially catastrophic effects on human health and well-being. As some potential adverse health effects of "global change" cannot yet be observed, forward-looking strategies may include "scenario epidemiology" that will allow us to make reliable, quantitative estimates of the effects on population health from future global changes in climate, land use, and social conditions (Sieswerda et al., 2001; Cifuentes et al., 2001). Although future-oriented models are more frequently used in infectious-disease epidemiology, where they play a role in policy and planning by state and federal agencies, the time may be ripe for their incorporation into environmental epidemiology.

FUTURE NEEDS

Although the 21st century will herald new challenges, traditional environmental epidemiology will probably remain a major part of our field. Themes likely to be of continued importance include advances in environmental-exposure assessment, integration of biologic markers, and understanding of time-related issues such as critical windows, induction, and latency. Combined effects from mixed, multiple exposures raise the possibility of unpredictable interactions. An obstacle to analysis of multiple exposures is the near-impossibility of separating induction periods, dose–response, and interactive effects from one another (Thomas, 1983; Greenland, 1993a). Moreover, these multiple exposures include not only the traditional chemical and physical agents, they extend to social and population-level factors as potential effect modifiers. More interaction between epidemiology and several other disciplines would benefit all concerned. These would include toxicologists, wildlife biologists, environmental scientists, sociologists, climatologists, oceanographers, molecular biologists, and geneticists, to name a few.

At the same time, good public policies require scientific input from epidemiologists to help those outside our field distinguish real from imagined hazards and important from negligible risks and can pave the way for a more rational allocation of intervention resources to reduce environmentally induced disease. This chapter began with a description of George Baker's investigation of lead in the cider of Devonshire. Baker (1767) went on to disseminate his report to the people of Devonshire in order to provide them "the earliest intimation of their danger; in order that they may take the proper steps to preserve their health."

CHAPTER 31

Methodologic Issues in Reproductive Epidemiology

Clarice R. Weinberg and Allen J. Wilcox

General Considerations 620
Puberty and Menopause 622
The Menstrual Cycle 623
Semen Quality 623
Fertility 624
Time-to-Pregnancy Studies 625
Pregnancy Loss 628
Recognized Loss 628
Early (Subclinical) Pregnancy Loss 630
Pregnancy Complications 632
Birth Weight 632
Dichotomized Birth Weight 633
Paradoxes 633
Weight-Specific Mortality 633
Relative Birth Weight 635
Birth-Weight Summary 635
Perinatal Mortality 635
Birth-Weight or Gestational-Age-Specific Mortality 636
Birth Defects 636
Genetic Factors in Reproductive Epidemiology 637
Appendix 640

GENERAL CONSIDERATIONS

Reproductive epidemiology encompasses a wide range of topics, from the development of reproductive systems to conception and pregnancy, to delivery and health of the offspring, to reproductive senescence. The epidemiologic study of reproduction is complicated by some important methodologic problems that are not often seen in other areas of epidemiology. We begin by introducing some of the major practical and conceptual issues.

1. Reproductive function can be abnormal with no overt signs of disease. For instance, infertile couples are usually not ill in any easily identifiable sense, and they may not even be aware that they are infertile. Their inherently private problem may never come to medical attention. Selection bias in ascertainment of infertile cases can arise from self-selection related to the highly personal decisions people make about birth control and about when (and whether) to seek medical help.
2. As is often the case in epidemiology, phenomena that clinicians may tend to dichotomize (as in the diagnosis of "habitual abortors," see Gladen (1986)) can be described more accurately as falling on a continuum, with heterogeneity across individuals. Heterogeneity in risk is a general phenomenon in epidemiology, but it is especially important in reproduction because individuals (and couples) can have repeated opportunities to experience reproductive outcomes.
3. Heterogeneity in risk among couples can lead to population sorting in ways that can lead the investigator badly astray. For example, couples with a long history of using an unreliable method of contraception (such as spermicide) who then attempt conception may have lower fecundability than couples who have previously relied on oral contraception. This difference occurs because oral contraception is more effective than spermicides. If one carries out a

prospective comparative fertility study based on sampling couples who are currently attempting pregnancy, one should recognize that the cohort of couples with a history of spermicide use has already been depleted of its most fertile couples; they reached their desired family size by unintended pregnancies. If one ignores this sorting, one can conclude that history of spermicide use has a deleterious effect on fertility. This attrition-related bias can plague both retrospective and prospective studies of fertility (Baird et al., 1994).

4. Many of the endpoints of interest to the reproductive epidemiologist are not independent and may compete directly with one another. For example, approximately 25% of pregnancies are lost before clinical recognition (Wilcox et al., 1988). Suppose that an exposure increases the risk of very early pregnancy loss by accelerating the death of conceptuses that would otherwise have failed later in pregnancy as clinically recognized spontaneous abortions. If we were to study only recognized spontaneous abortions, such an exposure would mask some recognized losses by converting them to occult losses and could even appear to be *protective* against spontaneous abortion, when it only "protects" against *detection* of spontaneous abortion. The dose–response relation for this exposure could consequently show a paradoxical downturn at the higher levels (Selevan and Lemasters, 1987). This artifact can distort inference if we fail to recognize that studies of just one endpoint examine only one piece of a larger picture. As another example, birth defects can compete with spontaneous abortion: The reported "incidence" of trisomy is nearly always its prevalence at birth (and not its incidence measured from the time of conception) (Warburton et al., 1983; Khoury et al., 1989b), and trisomy 21 is more common than other trisomies primarily because it is unusually compatible with survival to delivery.
5. Because reproductive outcomes (e.g., pregnancy complications or spontaneous abortion) are relatively common, are incompletely ascertained, and often have a short time between exposure and effect, the usual advantages of case-control studies are less applicable for reproductive epidemiology, and cohort studies play a relatively more important role.
6. For many reproductive endpoints, the proper unit of study is the couple and not an individual person. The woman carries the pregnancy, but the father provides half of the nuclear genetic material. The paternal genome is especially important to the development of the placenta (Marx, 1988). Thus exposures and characteristics of both parents are relevant to reproductive studies. In particular, because of shared parental factors, the father's exposures can be strong confounders in studies of the mother's exposures, and vice versa. The role of genetics in the family introduces further complexities. During gestation, the genomes of mother and fetus can respond synergistically to exposures, which can influence the pregnancy outcome. (The genetic structure of families also provides new opportunities for studies—see later.)
7. Reproductive events are (to varying degrees) under the control of the person studied. The resulting dependencies can sometimes produce highly nonstandard forms of confounding. For example, time can be a confounder. If one studies a group of women of reproductive age using a cross-sectional design, the apparent risk of spontaneous abortion in their most recent pregnancy will be highest for pregnancies that ended closest to the time of interview (Weinberg et al., 1994a). This pattern arises because a spontaneous abortion that occurred a year ago or more is more likely than a live birth to have been followed by another pregnancy (and thus no longer be "most recent"). If the investigator fails to recognize the resulting pseudo-time effect and to adjust for it in the analysis, spurious associations can arise between risk of spontaneous abortion and any exposure that has itself changed over recent time. Another example involves women who change partners between pregnancies, which can be taken as a surrogate for changes in her environment, her immune system's new exposure to antigenically different sperm, or a relatively long interpregnancy interval (Basso et al., 2001).
8. Denominators can easily be miscounted in reproductive studies. For example, a study of early pregnancy loss ideally requires that all conceptions be identified, because the set of all conceptions is the risk set. This goal is not achievable, however, because present techniques cannot identify conceptions that fail before implantation. A more feasible goal is to identify all conceptions that survive long enough to implant and produce measurable levels of the pregnancy hormone, human chorionic gonadotropin (hCG). Unfortunately, algorithms that use hormonal assays to identify short-lived conceptions can yield many false positives and false negatives (Weinberg et al., 1992; Cho et al., 2002). As another example, in studies of recognized spontaneous abortions, the woman herself needs to be aware of the pregnancy to be able to report

a spontaneous abortion, and a woman's attentiveness to the possibility of conception may be associated with variables under investigation. There is also the problem of how induced abortions should be counted (Hilden et al., 1991).

9. Reverse causality readily distorts reproductive studies. For example, women with pregnancy complications may schedule more prenatal obstetric visits because of heightened concern, producing bias in assessing the effect of prenatal care. (Econometricians call this phenomenon *endogeneity*. It can also be thought of as confounding by indication.) As another example, women who have not had a successful pregnancy are more likely to remain in the workforce and may consequently have more opportunity for occupational exposure than women with young children who stay at home. This phenomenon, termed the *infertile worker effect* (or the *reproductively unhealthy worker effect*), can lead to spurious associations between occupational exposures and adverse reproductive outcomes (Joffe, 1985).
10. The availability of repeated outcomes for a woman or couple (or a family over multiple generations) offers research opportunities that are not seen in many other areas of epidemiology. One of the strongest risk factors for adverse reproductive outcomes is the occurrence of the same outcome in a woman's earlier pregnancy. This pattern opens new possibilities for analytic studies. For example, it is possible to explore the relative contributions of environmental and genetic causes in a given setting by studying recurrence risk in women who do or do not change partners between pregnancies, or who keep the same partner but do or do not change some crucial environmental exposure (Lie et al., 1994). Another opportunity lies in the conduct of clinical trials among high-risk women. Clinical trials of women who had earlier delivered a baby with a neural-tube defect provided efficient proof of the benefit of folic acid in preventing this defect (Laurence et al., 1981), leading eventually to changes in prenatal recommendations for all women. The strong patterns of recurrence risk also present analytic traps. Some investigators have adjusted for these prior outcomes in assessing etiologic associations. This adjustment itself can produce bias if the exposures under study influenced both current and past risk (Weinberg, 1993).

With these general problems in mind, we turn to specific reproductive endpoints. In this chapter, we discuss puberty and menopause, the menstrual cycle, fertility, pregnancy loss, pregnancy complications, birth weight, and birth defects.

PUBERTY AND MENOPAUSE

The age at puberty or menopause may be related to diet, exercise, genetics, and environmental toxicants. For example, the onset of puberty can be accelerated (e.g., by hormonally active chemicals) or retarded (e.g., by inadequate nutrition). Menopause can be accelerated by exposures that are toxic to the ovary (Gold et al., 2001). We consider menopause in some detail, but most of the issues apply to the onset of puberty as well.

Both milestones present the investigator with definitional problems. Puberty for girls involves a series of hormonal and physical changes, but the onset of menarche provides a convenient, though crude, marker. The timing of puberty for boys is more difficult to pinpoint. Both transitions can be studied by categorizing children according to Tanner stages (Marshall and Tanner, 1969; Marshall and Tanner, 1970; Rockette et al., 2004) as they progress through the successive levels of sexual maturation.

Though medically well defined (for a woman who has not had her uterus removed) as the time when the woman stops menstruating, menopause and age at menopause can also be hard to define in an epidemiologic study. The usual definition of menopause is that it has occurred following at least 1 year without a menstrual period. Menstruation can sometimes resume after a year of amenorrhea, however. Also, women who experience natural menopause remain unclassifiable for a full year. A woman who has a hysterectomy 11 months after her natural menopause may falsely be considered to have had a surgical menopause. If a woman is in a case-control study for myocardial infarction because she died of a heart attack at that 11-month point, she may be falsely coded as premenopausal at the time of death.

If the age distribution of any life event is estimated only with data from those who have already experienced the event, the result is biased by differential inclusion of those for whom the event was early. For example, in a cross-sectional study of age at menopause, premenopausal women who are over the mean age at menopause will not be able to contribute to the estimate, biasing the average age at menopause downward. Age at menopause for premenopausal women has been "censored" at their observed age. Hysterectomy, which serves as a competing risk, can also be a censoring mechanism. A premenopausal woman who has a hysterectomy at age 50 years was nonetheless at risk of natural menopause at each age up to 50. Information for women who are premenopausal or who were premenopausal at the time of hysterectomy needs to be included through survival-analytic methods. One can estimate the age distribution for natural menopause based on cross-sectional (Krailo and Pike, 1983; Gold et al., 2001) or prospective (Brambilla and McKinlay 1989) data. Both approaches depend on a parametric model for the distribution of age at natural menopause, and both presume a linear relation between age and risk of surgical menopause.

THE MENSTRUAL CYCLE

In women of reproductive age, the reproductive system goes through cyclic changes under neuroendocrine control. About once each month, one (or sometimes more) mature egg (ovum) is released from the ovary and picked up by the oviduct for transport to the uterus, in a process called *ovulation*. If it is not rapidly fertilized by a sperm, the egg dies, and menstruation begins about 2 weeks later. The recruitment and maturation of the egg and the development of the uterine lining are stimulated by pituitary and ovarian hormones under the neural oversight of the hypothalamus. The usual length of the menstrual cycle, defined for convenience as the number of days from the first day of one menstrual bleed to the first day of the next, is about a month.

Although the menstrual cycle is described in medical textbooks as lasting 28 days, with ovulation on day 14, there is considerable variability in its length and in the timing of ovulation (Baird et al., 1994). The extent of the variability in cycle length, both within and among women, has been well demonstrated in the extraordinary longitudinal study launched by Alan Treloar, who maintained a cohort of women throughout their reproductive life span (Treloar et al., 1967).

Certain exposures and physiologic states (such as intense physical training or emaciation) can produce anovulation (failure to ovulate). Less extreme forms of the same conditions would also be expected to produce measurable changes in the menstrual cycle, perhaps by lengthening it or increasing its variability. The menstrual cycle is fairly easy to study noninvasively and prospectively, and menstrual-cycle characteristics can be informative as a marker for female reproductive function (Harlow and Zeger, 1991; Hornsby et al., 1994). Characteristics of interest include the mean length of the menstrual cycle, the variability in the cycle lengths, the mean duration of menses, and the mean amount of blood lost (Harlow and Ephross, 1995).

The modeling of data based on "diary" menstrual-cycle data presents special statistical problems. One can apply longitudinal methods for studying cycle length, based on the occurrence or nonoccurrence of abnormally long cycles (Harlow and Zeger, 1991). Differences among women in their menstrual-cycle patterns create complex dependencies in the data. More methodologic work is needed to make full use of the cycle-length data for comparing exposed with unexposed women (Murphy et al., 1995; Lisabeth et al., 2004).

If diary data show that an exposure lengthens or increases the variability of the menstrual cycle, a study based on daily biologic samples may be warranted. Metabolites of luteinizing hormone, a pituitary hormone, and the ovarian hormones estrogen and progesterone can easily be assayed in daily urine specimens to study reproductive hormonal patterns (Baird et al., 1991, 1994). Saliva carries transudates of serum hormones (Lu et al., 1999), and current techniques also allow one to use saliva or urine to collect DNA for genetic assays (Taylor and Ilyia, 2002; vanNoord, 2003; Ng et al., 2004).

SEMEN QUALITY

While characteristics of the menstrual cycle and the onset of menarche and menopause can serve as convenient markers of female reproductive function, women provide no ready access to their gametes, except in unusual clinical settings such as in vitro fertilization. Male reproductive function, in contrast, can be assessed through studies of semen quality, men having a bountiful excess of gamete production, and automated methods are available to quantify semen quality. Semen characteristics are in turn related to a man's fertility (Larsen, Scheike et al. 2000). Care must be taken, however, to require that a few days have transpired since the man's previous ejaculation, because abstinence time can have a strong influence on the results. Additional sources of variability from specimen to specimen can be reduced by repeated sampling.

Because data on semen quality have been recorded for some time, e.g., at sperm banks, analyses have been carried out to look for trends over time, and these suggest a decline over recent decades (Carlsen et al., 1992; Swan et al., 2000). Although these trends can be questioned on the basis of changes in methods of analysis and sample selection over time, some investigators have related them to apparently parallel increases in cryptorchidism, hypospadias, and testis cancer in the developed world and have speculated that there may be environmental causes (Sharpe and Skakkebaek, 2003). The possible influence of environmental factors is supported by studies showing regional variation in measures of semen quality (Jorgensen et al., 2001), and recent evidence suggests a prenatal effect of maternal smoking on the male fetus (Storgaard et al., 2003; Jensen et al., 2004). Some have suggested that, in response to concern about evidence of deterioration in male reproductive health, we should systematically monitor semen quality as a method of population surveillance; concern in Denmark has risen to a level at which such a program has now been instituted (Jensen et al., 2002). For use in assessing possible reproductive effects of specific exposures encountered, for example, in an occupational setting, we caution that there are difficulties in persuading men to participate in the process of producing a specimen for research, and one can expect to encounter low recruitment rates (Selevan et al., 2000).

FERTILITY

The most direct indicator of reproductive health is the capacity of a couple to produce a healthy baby. The word *fertility* is used in different ways by clinicians, demographers, and the general public. Clinicians who refer to "involuntary infertility" as a syndrome imply the existence of voluntary infertility, that is, couples who have no children by choice. In a similar usage, demographers and health statisticians refer to "fertility" in a population, e.g., as the number of offspring per year per 1,000 women of child-bearing age. By contrast, "fertility" for the general public (and for most clinicians) means the biologic capacity to reproduce, with "infertility" and "subfertility" referring to the involuntary impairment of that capacity. We will use the terms in this way.

Reduced fertility as an endpoint integrates many possible reproductive impairments. Problems in gametogenesis, sperm transport, tubal patency, hormonal preparation of the uterine lining, implantation, and viability of the conceptus will all make it hard to achieve a recognized pregnancy. A couple in the United States is considered to be clinically infertile after at least 1 year without contraception and without pregnancy.

Traditional case-control methods can be used to study clinical infertility. One advantage of studying clinic-identified cases is that one can differentiate them by their proximal medical cause, such as ovulatory dysfunction, occlusion of the oviducts, or antisperm antibodies. Clinically distinct categories may be etiologically distinct, and aggregating them into a single "infertile" category may obscure disparate etiologies. In practice, however, the diagnoses are often derived from an incomplete medical evaluation and must be regarded as provisional, overlapping, and uncertain. The diagnostic process is often itself cut short by the occurrence of pregnancy.

While the case-control design can offer important practical advantages over other approaches, the method is not as useful here as in studies of rare and well-defined outcomes such as cancer (Weinberg, 1990). One problem involves defining clinically infertile "cases." This clinical categorization is based primarily on waiting time, with no requirement of any documented physiologic dysfunction. Thus, some couples may be diagnosed as infertile who are normal but unlucky, and others with low fertility but better luck might be miscategorized as normal. Spontaneous "cures" are common: Most couples who go for a year without conception do eventually achieve pregnancy, even without medical intervention. Thus case status in this context is an elusive concept.

The most serious issues with case-control studies of infertility involve validity. Such studies often rely on infertility clinics for case identification, and there is no convenient source of appropriate controls. Although almost all babies in the United States are delivered in hospitals, providing a ready population of normal couples to sample, only about half of infertile couples seek medical help (US Congress, 1988). Thus there is a strong potential for ascertainment bias in identifying "cases" through the medical system, particularly when studying lifestyle factors. For example, couples with a history of sexually transmitted disease may have become inured to medical interventions and consequently may be more willing to seek medical help when confronted with infertility.

To understand approaches other than the case-control design, one must first recognize that the clinical dichotomy of fertile and infertile is an oversimplification. Biologically, there is a wide range of reproductive capacity, even among couples who achieve pregnancy. The proportion of couples conceiving in a given cycle will be referred to as the conception *rate*. When couples who discontinue contraception in order to begin a pregnancy are followed prospectively, around one third conceive in the first menstrual cycle at risk. Among those remaining at risk in the second menstrual cycle, the proportion conceiving is lower, perhaps one fourth. As time goes on, the conception rate continues to decline (Tietze, 1968). This declining pattern is seen (albeit with higher conception rates) even if the couples who do not eventually conceive (including those who are simply sterile) are subtracted from all the denominators (Baird and Wilcox, 1985; Weinberg and Gladen, 1986). The declining conception rate is not a true time effect, but rather evidence of sorting among a population who are heterogeneous in their capacity to conceive: The most highly fertile couples conceive early and are therefore absent from subsequent risk sets. In this way, the successive cohorts remaining at risk are more and more dominated by relatively subfertile couples, and the conception rate inexorably declines.

Heterogeneity among couples raises the possibility that some of this variation may be explained by identifiable factors. If so, preventable causes of subfertility might be discovered by comparative studies of exposed and unexposed couples.

TIME-TO-PREGNANCY STUDIES

Studies of time to pregnancy, or waiting time to conception (Baird, Wilcox et al. 1986), have proved fruitful in identifying male and female exposures with adverse effects on fertility. Such studies make use of more detailed time information beyond the usual clinical dichotomy. Survival-analytic methods allow dropouts (e.g., those who change their mind about wanting a pregnancy) to contribute information appropriately.

Women who intend to become pregnant or who are currently attempting to become pregnant can be enrolled in a prospective cohort study, in which exposures are ascertained and then participants are followed until they become pregnant, change their mind and resume contraception, or reach a certain maximum follow-up time without pregnancy. Alternatively, women (or their partners) can be asked to reconstruct their time to pregnancy retrospectively for a particular pregnancy. In this retrospective approach, both the exposures and the time to an index (nonaccidental) pregnancy are based on recall. Certain biases, such as differential persistence in trying, can be a problem (Basso et al., 2000), but much has been learned from such studies. Women are evidently able to recall these durations many years later with surprising accuracy (Basso et al., 2000). Men are also able to provide usable data on time to most recent pregnancy (Nguyen and Baird, 2004). When the exposure of interest is rare, or the available population is fixed, as in an occupational study, the retrospective time-to-pregnancy study may be the only feasible way to study fertility, because it allows a much larger fraction of persons to contribute information than would a prospective cohort study.

Retrospective and prospective approaches do not, however, yield the same data for time to pregnancy. In a prospective cohort study, the sampling unit is the attempt at pregnancy; in the retrospective time-to-pregnancy study, the sampling unit is typically the pregnancy itself. If every attempt at pregnancy ended in pregnancy, the two designs would generate equivalent data. In fact, couples who are unknowingly sterile will be present in cohort studies but not in retrospective studies. Thus an exposure that caused complete sterility in a subpopulation and had no effect on the remainder would be missed by the retrospective time-to-pregnancy design. One way to allow sterile couples to contribute information is to base the sampling on couples rather than pregnancies, and to ascertain for each the length of the most recent waiting time (i.e., the interval during which the couple was having unprotected intercourse, whether or not the waiting time culminated in a pregnancy (Bolumar et al., 1996). If the couple had stopped trying or was still trying at the time of interview, the data would be considered right-censored at that point. Nonetheless, pregnancy-based retrospective time-to-pregnancy studies should be adequate for exploratory studies, because most reproductive toxicants can be expected to cause subfertility among the exposed who have not been rendered sterile.

Each menstrual cycle provides a single ovulatory opportunity for conception. Thus, time to pregnancy is inherently discrete (taking only integer values), with the menstrual cycle serving as the natural counting unit of time. In a prospective study, menstrual cycles are enumerated directly through diary records. Ideally, the method for diagnosing pregnancy would be objective and standardized (e.g., a commercially available home test kit, with a well-defined protocol).

In a retrospective time-to-pregnancy study (e.g. one based on the most recent nonaccidental pregnancy), the wording of the question can strongly affect the data. It is ambiguous to ask women how many menstrual cycles it took them to conceive. Some women who conceived in their first cycle may answer that they took zero cycles, and others may respond one (Joffe et al., 1993). This reporting inconsistency can be avoided by asking women whether the pregnancy occurred in the very first menstrual cycle after discontinuing contraception, and if not, whether it occurred in the second or third. For times longer than three cycles, one can ascertain the calendar time between when contraception was discontinued up to the last menstrual period preceding conception. One then must divide this interval by the usual cycle length and add 1, to allow for the cycle when conception actually occurred. Women can give credible answers (Baird et al., 1991) to a short series of questions about their time to the most recent pregnancy, and retrospective data agree reasonably well with data on the same pregnancies that have been gathered prospectively in a cohort study many years before (Joffe et al., 1993).

What are the options for analyzing such data? Each couple has a certain average probability of conception in a menstrual cycle during which they use no contraception. This probability is called their *fecundability*. Couple-specific fecundability varies across couples, as discussed earlier, and one can model the distribution of fecundabilities parametrically (Sheps and Mencken, 1973; Weinberg and Gladen, 1986).

If we assume simple random sampling, the fraction of couples who conceive in the first cycle after discontinuing contraception provides an unbiased estimate of the mean fecundability without parametric model assumptions (assuming that the method of contraception has had no residual effect). The very simplest comparative fecundability study would estimate the fractions for exposed and unexposed couples and compute a *fecundability ratio* (dividing one fraction by the other). The fecundability ratio defined in this way is simply a risk ratio, although the word *risk* is misleading in this setting, in which conception is a desired outcome.

This approach does not, however, take full advantage of the data. A natural extension is to use all cycles by stratifying on each cycle number (not just cycle 1) and assuming a fixed ratio of fecundabilities across strata of cycle time (Weinberg et al., 1994c). This model can be seen as a discrete analog of the Cox proportional hazards model (Cox and Oakes, 1984), in which one models the probability of conception and assumes that an exposure imposes a fixed multiplier on that probability, the *fecundability ratio*. The fecundability ratio is the cycle-specific probability of conception among the exposed divided by that among the unexposed. For example, a fecundability ratio of 0.3 means that the exposed are only 30% as likely as the unexposed to conceive in each menstrual cycle at risk. It is easy to extend such a model to incorporate adjustments for potential confounders. (See the Appendix at the end of this chapter for technical details.)

Practical issues arise in fitting and interpreting these models for time-to-pregnancy data. First, if a prospective cohort study is undertaken, it is usually inconvenient and too restrictive to limit participation to couples who are just about to discontinue contraception. Thus, investigators usually choose to include couples who have already been trying for a while. It is important to ascertain the prior attempt time for such couples, so that they can be delay-entered into the appropriate risk set for their first observed menstrual cycle in the study. The situation is analogous to the usual survival analyses, where those who enter late contribute "left-censored" data to the analysis. The biologically relevant time scale is time from when contraception was discontinued, and not time in the study. A couple who has already been trying for three cycles before recruitment should contribute data beginning at cycle 4 (not cycle 1). If prior-attempt time is not taken into account, bias can result. This issue is particularly important if the timing of joining the study cohort is related to exposure. For example, exposed individuals who have already been trying for some time may be more likely to participate than unexposed individuals who have been trying for a similar length of time.

A second practical problem in time-to-pregnancy studies is accounting for possible effects of medical interventions. Such interventions could be differential by exposures under study. In a prospective cohort study, one can determine at what point a couple seeks medical help and simply censor their data as of that cycle. Lacking such detailed information, it is customary to truncate the analysis at about a year because medical interventions typically begin after a year. With this truncation, couples who begin in the study at cycle 1 and do not conceive until 2 years later contribute their first 12 months of failures to the analysis; their higher cycle numbers are not included in the analysis.

Third, a prospective study of couples attempting pregnancy potentially allows collection of exposure data specific to the month or day. Such time-varying exposures can be used directly in fecundability modeling. In a retrospective time-to-pregnancy study, such precision is usually not possible. Exposures can be ascertained with reference to a single point in time, but one must choose this reference date carefully. If one asks about exposures around the time of conception, there could be bias from behavioral changes caused by a fertility problem. Thus, for example, a woman who has been trying to conceive for a long time might be motivated to give up smoking, reduce her consumption of caffeine, etc., which could bias the results for any modifiable factor that women regard as unhealthy. This problem can be avoided by instead choosing a reference date for exposures around the time when contraception was first discontinued.

In retrospective studies of time to pregnancy, there is a potential for bias if one of the exposures or confounders has changed in prevalence over calendar time. This problem was noticed in the context of a study of female dental assistants, in which the wearing of latex gloves was found to enhance fertility (Weinberg et al., 1993). This puzzling finding was presumably an artifact: The exposure reference dates for pregnancies in the study spanned the first decade of the acquired immune deficiency syndrome (AIDS) epidemic, during which time dental assistants rapidly adopted the use of latex gloves in response to concerns about infection. Women with long times to pregnancy tended to have begun their attempt at a time when glove use was relatively uncommon in dental offices; those with short times to pregnancy tended to have begun their attempt more recently, when glove use was common. There is not a ready-made solution to this problem in a retrospective time-to-pregnancy design: Adjustment for calendar time when the attempt began does not solve the problem (Weinberg et al., 1993). Treating the exposure as time-dependent does not solve it either, because the opportunity for exposure is still correlated with the outcome. If external data are available on exposure prevalence over time, certain *ad hoc* remedies can be employed (Weinberg et al., 1993). Otherwise, one must rely on sensitivity analyses that estimate the extent of the bias under plausible assumptions regarding changes in the exposure over calendar time.

Other, more subtle sources of bias in fertility studies can be equally damaging (Weinberg et al., 1994c; Juul et al., 2000). For example, there is evidence that smokers as a group have more accidental pregnancies than nonsmokers (Schwingl, 1992). If one were to compare the fertility of smokers and nonsmokers, smokers might appear to be less fertile than nonsmokers because relatively more of the highly fertile smokers have had all the pregnancies they want as birth-control failures and are consequently absent from the cohort of couples having planned pregnancies. This bias afflicts both retrospective and prospective studies of time to pregnancy (Baird et al., 1994). There is no secure protection against it; however, some reassurance can be gained in a retrospective study by ascertaining exposure information from women whose most recent pregnancy was unintended. Similarly, in a prospective cohort study, one can ask about unintended pregnancies in the past (e.g., as indicated by history of induced abortions). If the exposed and unexposed women have similar histories of contraceptive use and induced abortions, we may be justified in assuming that this bias is not important.

Another source of bias involves the definition of a birth-control failure in a retrospective study. Analysis is necessarily restricted to nonaccidental pregnancies. There may be systematic differences in how couples interpret a birth-control failure after the fact. Consequently, conceptions that reportedly occurred during the first menstrual cycle at risk may include pregnancies that another couple would have characterized as accidental. If misclassification of accidents as intentional cycle 1 conceptions is differential by exposure status, there may be bias in either direction. One way to protect against this bias is to reanalyze the data with all cycle 1 outcomes omitted (i.e., beginning the analysis at cycle 2). If results are similar to those with the entire data set, this "definitional bias" probably does not account for the results (Weinberg et al., 1994c).

Another source of bias alluded to earlier arises because of the reproductively unhealthy worker effect. Women who are reproductively healthy tend to have children, and women with young children tend to leave the salaried workforce. Women with underlying reproductive problems are more likely to remain in the workforce. Thus, the comparison of reproductive endpoints for employed and unemployed cohorts of women needs to account for this phenomenon. Even within a working population, the same selective process could cause job seniority (hence cumulative exposure) to be associated with poor reproductive capacity. In this way, working status and job seniority can become confounders in such studies. Further difficulties may arise because work status and seniority may have been indirectly affected by the exposure, via effects on fertility, in the kind of complex causal pathway with feedback discussed by Robins (1986, 1987, 1997, 1998) and Robins et al. (1992).

In summary, time-to-pregnancy studies may reveal a great deal about factors that affect human fertility, but there are unique pitfalls and sources of bias that must be taken into account in the interpretation of such studies.

PREGNANCY LOSS

Like infertility, pregnancy loss is not a rare event. About 10% to 15% of recognized pregnancies end in spontaneous abortion. If very early occult loss is included, the total is one third or more of all conceptions (Wilcox et al., 1988). There are doubtless additional losses due to conceptuses that fail to implant, but these cannot be detected by currently available methods. Although some couples may have markedly elevated risk for pregnancy loss, there is likely a continuum of risk across couples and not a simple dichotomy between high-risk and low-risk couples.

RECOGNIZED LOSS

Clinically recognized pregnancy loss in the first 20 or 24 weeks of pregnancy is referred to variously as spontaneous abortion, miscarriage, or (less commonly) early fetal loss. The design of studies to identify risk factors for miscarriage continues to be challenging. If a woman contributes several pregnancies in a study, these events are not statistically independent; a woman with one miscarriage is at increased risk for another, presumably reflecting heterogeneity in exposures and in innate risk across members of the population. Thus, methods that assume independence of outcomes are not strictly valid. Some investigators have solved this problem by studying a random pregnancy for each woman. Such strategies, however, are not practical for self-administered questionnaires, waste valuable information, and may seem odd and frustrating to the women being interviewed.

Methods have been proposed for analyzing reproductive history data based on "random effects" logistic regression models. In this approach, which can be applied using commercially available software, the logit of the risk depends on a linear function of covariates plus a "random" intercept specific to the woman. Another approach available in commercial software is GEE logistic regression, which explicitly allows dependent outcomes within each woman's history. For mathematical reasons, the latter approach generally gives odds-ratio estimates closer to 1, but both methods tend to give similar P-values (Diggle et al., 2002). However, GEE becomes invalid if the cluster size is "informative" (Hoffman et al., 2001). This informativeness would hold, for example, if women with a higher risk of loss have more pregnancies in order to achieve their desired family size. Thus, despite its continuing use (Louis et al., 2006), GEE has limited application in this setting. Furthermore, random-effects and GEE methods can both be misleading if earlier pregnancy outcomes affect later outcomes, for example because earlier outcomes influenced later exposures (Robins et al., 1999b).

Case-control approaches to the study of miscarriage risk raise questions about case definition and sampling strategy. If one compares hospitalized cases of spontaneous abortion with hospitalized live births, one must recognize that many women with spontaneous abortion are not hospitalized, whereas most women delivering an infant are. Thus, there is potential for case self-selection, and study validity can be called into question. One innovative design in which chromosomally abnormal hospitalized miscarriages serve as "controls" for chromosomally normal hospitalized miscarriages avoids this problem (Kline et al., 1989).

The investigator designing a study of spontaneous abortion must have a particular biologic entity in mind. If the unit of study is the pregnancy (as in a hospital-based study), then usual methods can be applied to evaluate the influence of particular exposures experienced early in that pregnancy. Alternatively, if the unit of study is the woman (or the couple), then case definition could take the whole reproductive history into account, rather than the outcome of a single pregnancy. The couple having a spontaneous abortion whose previous two pregnancies ended in live birth has far less evidence for disability than the couple having their third spontaneous abortion, with no previous live births. As with infertility, case definition is unavoidably related to chance. A couple with two spontaneous abortions may have the same intrinsic risk as another couple with two live births. There may be no meaningful dichotomy between normal and abnormal (despite the clinical entity of "habitual aborters"), and epidemiologic methods premised on the existence of a definable dichotomous disease are unavoidably problematic.

A third issue with miscarriage studies involves possible bias related to the gestational age at which the woman would first consider herself to be pregnant. Some women, perhaps especially those who have a history of spontaneous abortion or have been trying to conceive for some time, tend to recognize their pregnancies early. Sensitive home diagnostic test kits are now widely available. Because most pregnancy loss occurs early in pregnancy, women who test themselves early will appear to have higher rates of loss than women who wait. Variations in self-testing behavior can be an important source of bias if time of recognition is not taken into account.

If time of recognition is ascertained in a prospective study, then survival-analytic methods (see Chapter 16) can be used to include only woman-weeks when the woman was at risk of a recognized loss during follow-up. In this way, a woman who did not realize she was pregnant until the eighth week will not inappropriately contribute earlier weeks to the analysis. The prospective cohort study also allows pregnancies that end in induced abortion to contribute information from the time of recognition to the time of censoring at abortion. Exposure information can also be collected repeatedly, allowing exposure effects to be targeted to the corresponding time in gestation. Finally, exposures can be ascertained before the outcomes, avoiding potential for differential recall.

Alternatively, if one can identify a cohort of pregnancies at the time of diagnosis (for example, through a health maintenance organization), then a case-cohort approach (Chapter 8) can be used, although this requires special analysis methods (see Chapters 14 and 21). Pregnancies that end in spontaneous abortion are identified as cases, and a random sample of the cohort as a whole serves as the "subcohort" pregnancies. Unless exposure information is available from prospectively recorded records (e.g., medical records), the information must be ascertained retrospectively (Hertz-Picciotto et al., 1989).

An alternative retrospective type of study ascertains the outcome of the most recent pregnancy and relates this outcome to exposures at that time. This outcome is a particularly convenient endpoint for studies of a rare exposure or a small fixed population, such as an occupational cohort, in which few women will be currently pregnant and available for a prospective cohort study. A problem with this design arises because a wanted pregnancy ending in loss is likely to be replaced by other pregnancies until a viable one is conceived (Weinberg et al., 1994a). This selective masking can produce the appearance of change of risk over time (see point 7 "General Considerations"). Thus, the interval of time between conception and interview can act as a confounder and must be taken into account when studying an exposure that may have changed in prevalence over time.

Pregnancy replacement can also produce biases when comparing groups of women. For example, couples who use contraception fastidiously and who carefully plan all their pregnancies will appear to have a lower risk of spontaneous abortion than couples with similar inherent risk who use contraception sporadically and have most of their pregnancies unintentionally. This difference arises because the planners very quickly replace a spontaneous abortion, and thus such outcomes retain their "most recent" status for only a relatively short time. If related to the exposure under study, the bias produced by this kind of differential history can be almost impossible to control in a study that collects information related only to the most recent pregnancy.

Finally, in deciding what to include as potential confounders in the analysis of spontaneous abortion data, it may seem natural to include gravidity, which is often associated with risk in the current pregnancy. Nonetheless, adjustment or stratification on gravidity can introduce serious distortions (Wilcox and Gladen, 1982; Gladen, 1986; Weinberg, 1993). Similarly, prior spontaneous abortion is also a "risk factor," in the sense that women who have a spontaneous abortion are at increased risk of a recurrence in subsequent pregnancies. If the earlier spontaneous abortion was caused in part by earlier exposure to the factor under study, adjusting for it can seriously distort the estimated risk ratio based on the current pregnancy (Weinberg 1993). Causal diagrams can be particularly useful in this context (Greenland et al., 1999a; Howards et al., 2007; see Chapter 12).

One feature to keep in mind when studying pregnancy loss is that not only the time of exposure but the time of loss in gestation may be closely related to the cause of loss. Thus the time of loss can help differentiate distinct mechanisms of loss. Chromosomal abnormalities may represent a much higher fraction of early losses than of later losses, for example (Kline, Stein et al. 1989). Exposures that are spindle poisons and cause aneuploidy may cause losses that occur right around the time of failed implantation and are accordingly impossible to detect without preconception enrollment.

Returning to the multiple-outcomes issue, suppose that one has access to reproductive and exposure history data that can be linked, and one wants to estimate odds ratios in a way that uses all the pregnancies but does not need to assume independence among pregnancies within the same woman. Hierarchical mixed-model methods can serve well to address dependencies among reproductive outcomes (Watier et al., 1997). This approach has been criticized, however, because reproductive decisions that couples (and their physicians) make are highly dependent on their experiences, implying that the within-couple dependency structure may not be adequately captured by a mixed model (Olsen and Andersen, 1998) and that it may be preferable to focus instead on a single pregnancy, e.g., the first.

Other methods for handling clustered binary outcomes have since been developed, which can handle complex dependency structures and *informative* cluster size. One approach is to sample one pregnancy from each woman, fit a risk model, e.g., using logistic regression, save the estimated coefficients and standard errors, and then repeat the same sampling and analysis many times. To estimate a coefficient, β, and its standard error SE, using all ($I = 1, \ldots, I$) of the I resample-specific estimates, $\hat{\beta}_i$ and SE_i, one takes the mean of the $\hat{\beta}_i$ and estimates the variance as follows (Hoffman et al., 2001):

$$\frac{\sum_i (SE_i)^2}{I} - \frac{(I-1)}{I} S^2$$

where S^2 is the estimated variance among the resample-based $\hat{\beta}_i$. The resampling approach is robust to informative cluster size (as may occur, for example, if a couple susceptible to miscarriage requires many pregnancies to achieve their desired family size) and complex dependencies among the outcomes. A weighted estimating equation approach (Williamson et al., 2003) is equivalent to the resampling approach asymptotically, but may work better when studies are small. As with random-effects models, however, effect estimation may be somewhat biased if earlier outcomes influence later exposures (Robins et al., 1999b).

EARLY (SUBCLINICAL) PREGNANCY LOSS

Pregnancy can be detected as early as 6 to 9 days following ovulation, using highly sensitive and specific urinary assays for the pregnancy hormone, human chorionic gonadotropin (hCG) (Wilcox et al., 1999). This period corresponds to the time when the developing conceptus is invading the uterine wall and first establishing its vascular interchange with the mother. In an idealized 28-day menstrual cycle, this time corresponds to day 21–24, several days before the next period is expected. For pregnancy to be detected at this stage, women who are trying to conceive must collect daily first-morning urine specimens, a demanding protocol that is feasible only in some populations. Such studies can provide a detailed record of the hormonal events corresponding to the initial establishment of pregnancy (Wilcox et al., 1988). Bleeding that accompanies very early losses begins around the time of the expected menstrual period, an experience seldom recognized by the woman as a lost pregnancy. Figure 31–1 shows an example of early loss.

Studies of spontaneous abortion (recognized pregnancy loss) necessarily overlook such short-lived pregnancies altogether, as do fertility studies based on time to recognized conception. Although each early loss will prolong the time to recognized conception, fertility studies may not be efficient for detecting group differences in risk of such events. For example, a doubling of the risk of unmeasured early loss (say, from 0.2 to 0.4) would cause a couple's apparent fecundability to be reduced by only 25% (relative fecundability $= (1 - 0.4)/(1 - 0.2) = (0.6)/(0.8) = 0.75$).

Direct studies of early pregnancy loss are difficult to carry out. For the sake of study efficiency (i.e., a high yield of pregnancies for a given number of couples), women should be recruited early in their attempt at conception, ideally at the time they first stop their use of birth control. Later enrollment produces a lower yield of pregnancies per observed cycle. Current methods require the daily collection of urine specimens, which must be refrigerated or frozen for later assay. This kind of study can be done only with a well-motivated group of participants.

Because the pattern of rise and fall of hCG levels with an early loss usually brackets the onset of the accompanying bleeding (as in Fig. 31–1), one can detect most early losses by analyzing

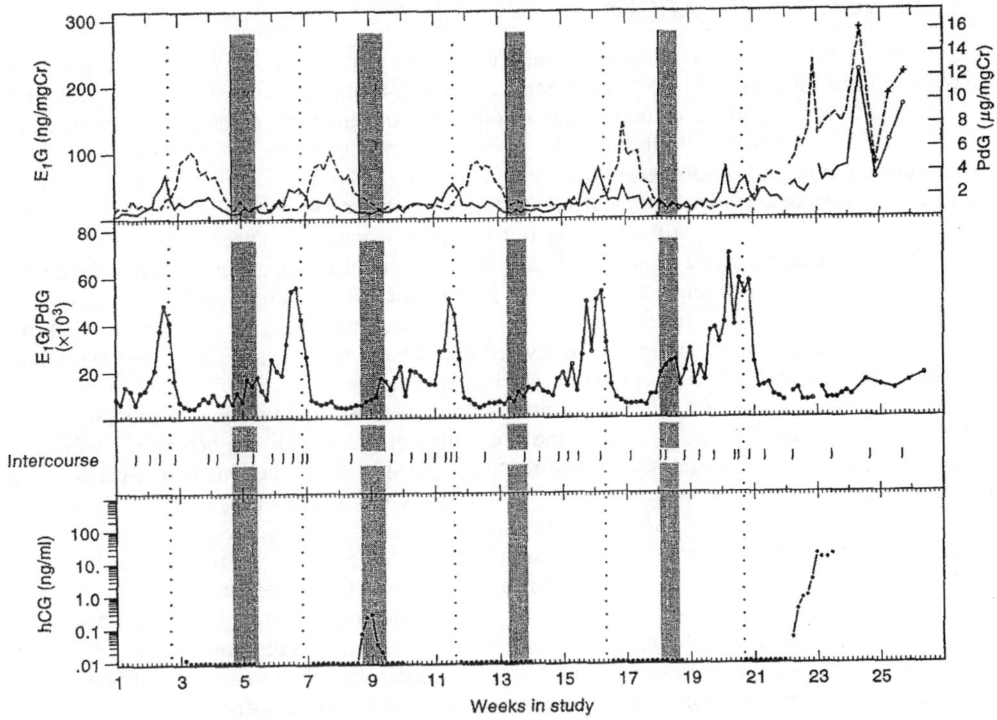

FIGURE 31–1 • Hormonal data for a woman who participated in the Early Pregnancy Study (Wilcox et al., 1988) for 25 weeks. The vertical shaded bars correspond to menses. The solid curve in the first panel shows the levels of a major estrogen metabolite, whereas the broken curve shows levels of a progesterone metabolite, both corrected for creatinine excretion to control for urinary diluteness. The day of ovulation was estimated by an algorithm that captures the rapid descent in the ratio of the two metabolites that accompanies luteinization of the ovarian follicle around the time of ovulation (Baird et al., 1991). The estimated days of ovulation are shown as vertical broken lines through each menstrual cycle. The pregnancy hormone, hCG, evinces the occurrence of an early loss followed by a clinical pregnancy.

specimens for only a few days in each cycle (Weinberg et al., 1992). If necessary, sample collection could be limited to the first 6 days of the menstrual cycle; this timing is adequate to detect most early losses, provided the laboratory assay is sufficiently sensitive and specific for hCG.

One concern raised in the context of studies of early pregnancy loss is that most assay-based algorithms for defining short-lived pregnancies have specificity less than 1.0. Imperfect specificity can seriously bias the findings, with false positives included as pregnancies in both the numerator and denominator. For example, if one group is subfertile, a higher proportion of apparent conceptions will end in early loss, even if there is no difference in risk of loss between groups. This difference arises because the subfertile group contributes a higher proportion of nonconception cycles, hence a greater opportunity for false positives. This "fertility bias" can be substantial unless the diagnostic specificity is very close to 1.0 (Weinberg et al., 1992). To protect against this bias, studies of early pregnancy loss should include a control group of women who are known to be invulnerable to pregnancy, such as women with tubal ligation. Urine specimens from this group should be interspersed with those from the main study, so that the criteria for diagnosing pregnancy are strict enough to have very high specificity (producing few or no false positives in the sterile group).

Urine can also be used to measure metabolites of the ovarian hormones, estrogen and progesterone, and the pituitary hormone, luteinizing hormone (LH). These hormones allow the time of ovulation to be estimated (Baird et al., 1995), and may also provide more subtle clues about the fertile potential of each menstrual cycle. Kits are now available that can permit a woman to identify the surge in LH that comes right before ovulation and can potentially obviate the need to collect daily specimens. If women record days with unprotected intercourse, the timing of intercourse in relation to ovulation can be taken into account in assessing the risk of pregnancy (Weinberg et al., 1994b; Zhou and Weinberg, 1996; Dunson and Weinberg, 2000).

PREGNANCY COMPLICATIONS

In trying to identify factors that adversely influence pregnancy, one must be especially careful about the direction and path of causality. As an example, if high consumption of coffee during pregnancy were associated with a particular complication, would this be compelling evidence for a deleterious effect of coffee? Or could it be that healthy pregnancies produce enough nausea to discourage coffee consumption? As another example, a pregnancy biomarker that predicts the occurrence of pre-eclampsia may be an early preclinical manifestation of pre-eclampsia that has little to do with its etiology. (Such a marker could still, of course, be of prognostic value.) In general, it is not enough to establish that the putative cause occurs before the diagnosis or before the adverse event under study.

One must also resist the temptation to adjust for intermediate variables, or for epiphenomena associated with the exposure under study. For example, smoking during pregnancy reduces birth weight, but low birth weight should not simply be controlled in an analysis of smoking in relation to perinatal mortality. We shall return to this issue later.

Preterm delivery is one of the most significant common complications, occurring in about 5% to 10% of pregnancies. This adverse outcome is usually defined as delivery before 37 completed weeks of gestation, when gestation is measured from the start of the last menstrual period. The most valid (and usually most costly) approach to studying preterm delivery is a prospective cohort study. Survival-analytic methods allow all pregnancies to be fully used in the analysis (see Part III of this book), where survival refers to the continuation of the pregnancy. Pregnancies should be left-censored by entering them at the time that a termination of the pregnancy would have been identified as an event in the study. One can then truncate the analysis at a prespecified definition of full-term gestation (e.g., 37 completed weeks), after which, by definition, no one is at risk. Interventions such as induction of labor and caesarian section should be treated as right-censoring events (events that terminate follow-up). Nevertheless, this censoring may distort the analysis if the interventions are in response to fetal distress (as is often the case), which may itself have otherwise increased the risk of spontaneous preterm delivery.

A related problem arises when specific pathologic mechanisms leading to prematurity are under study, for example, the premature rupture of membranes (PROM). If preterm deliveries without PROM are treated as independent censoring events, this implicitly assumes that the pregnancies ending in preterm delivery without rupture of the membranes would not have been at increased risk for PROM if the observed preterm delivery could have been prevented. This implicit assumption is not necessarily true.

Although prematurity is not a rare outcome, one can potentially improve study efficiency by sampling all preterm deliveries in some defined population of pregnancies and recording exposures experienced during these pregnancies and also in a random subcohort of pregnancies. This design would be straightforward, for example, in a health maintenance organization. Case-cohort methods of analysis are then needed to analyze the gestational survival of the pregnancy up to a cutoff at 37 weeks, in analogy with what has been proposed for studies of spontaneous abortion (Hertz-Picciotto et al., 1989). Such survival methods allow the investigator to model gestational-time-specific exposure effects.

Assessment of exposures specific to gestational time can be important if there are specific windows of embryologic and fetal vulnerability to adverse effects. Ascertaining only crudely whether an exposure was experienced sometime during pregnancy can lead to *de facto* exposure misclassification and bias (Hertz-Picciotto et al., 1996). One obvious problem is that pregnancies that last longer have a greater opportunity to have been exposed than pregnancies that end early. This bias can be avoided by treating exposure as time-dependent in a survival analysis, so that current hazard is not permitted to depend in any way on future exposures. A more detailed treatment of issues related to the study of pregnancy complications is provided by Olsen and Basso (2004).

BIRTH WEIGHT

A newborn's weight predicts its survival better than any other characteristic. The smallest babies not only have the highest mortality, they are at increased risk of long-term morbidity, including neurologic deficits and behavior problems (Illsley and Mitchell, 1984; Hack et al., 1994). Because birth weight is easily measured and routinely recorded for nearly every newborn, it has become a commonly used variable in perinatal research. Nonetheless, the epidemiologic use of birth weight as a surrogate for perinatal health presents some difficulties. Recent observations have heightened interest in birth weight by suggesting a role of prenatal experiences, as reflected in birth weight, in the development of susceptibility to diseases such as hypertension in later life (the "fetal origins of adult disease" hypothesis; (Barker, 1995)).

DICHOTOMIZED BIRTH WEIGHT

Birth weight is often dichotomized at 2,500 g, into babies of low birth weight (LBW), who have an elevated mortality and morbidity, and babies of higher weight, who are at lower risk. The prevalence of LBW varies widely across regions, ranging from 7% in Europe to 14% in Africa to 31% in middle south Asia (Control, 1984).

For many years, premature delivery was assumed to account for the high mortality of LBW babies. Indeed, prematurity and LBW were regarded as functionally equivalent; before 1961, the official World Health Organization (WHO) definition of prematurity was birth weight less than 2,500 g.

As better data on gestational age accumulated, however, it became clear that half or more of LBW babies are not premature according to their length of gestation (Chamberlain, 1975). The recognition that there are many term births among LBW infants was quickly followed by the observation that small term babies carry an excess risk of mortality. Prematurity could not explain their risk, so a new designation was created. Full-term babies that were small came to be regarded as "growth-retarded." A variant of the LBW dichotomy is to identify the smallest babies at each gestational age (usually based on tenth percentiles of a standard population). These babies are characterized as small for gestational age (SGA) or intrauterine growth-retarded (IUGR). One problem with a definition based on current percentiles is that the incidence rate for such a syndrome is fixed. Any change in incidence becomes logically impossible.

The term *growth retardation* implicitly attributes the smallness of IUGR babies to abnormal prenatal development. A short logical leap leads to the presumption that low weight per se is a meaningful pathology, analogous to high blood pressure. If smallness is harmful and perhaps preventable, then it becomes natural to look for public health interventions that produce bigger (hence "healthier") babies. Nevertheless, other evidence suggests that the causal pathway may not be so simple.

PARADOXES

Comparisons of LBW among populations can lead to paradoxes. First, an excess of LBW in a population does not necessarily mean that the population will have higher infant mortality. More girls are born LBW than boys, for example, but girls have better survival than boys. Second, when comparing LBW infants from two different populations, the LBW group with the lower mortality is often from the population with the higher overall mortality. For example, at each specific weight under 2,500 g, African American babies have lower mortality than white babies, even though overall mortality for African American babies is twice that for white babies (Wilcox and Russell, 1990). The same is true in comparisons of infants of mothers who smoke and mothers who don't smoke (Wilcox, 1993), twins compared to singletons (Buekens and Wilcox, 1993), and others (Skjaerven et al., 1988; Wilcox and Skjaerven, 1992). These paradoxes raise questions about the underlying relation between birth weight and survival.

In considering the causal pathway, it is obvious that low birth weight per se does not cause adverse outcomes, but that it serves as a biomarker for the truly causal factors. The question, therefore, is whether birth weight is a faithful correlate for some factor, such as impaired growth, that is on the causal pathway to disability and death. To pursue this question, we will examine more closely the relation of birth weight to survival.

WEIGHT-SPECIFIC MORTALITY

Figure 31–2 shows a typical pattern of neonatal mortality (i.e., death within the first month among live births) as a function of birth weight. Risk approaches 100% for the smallest babies and declines

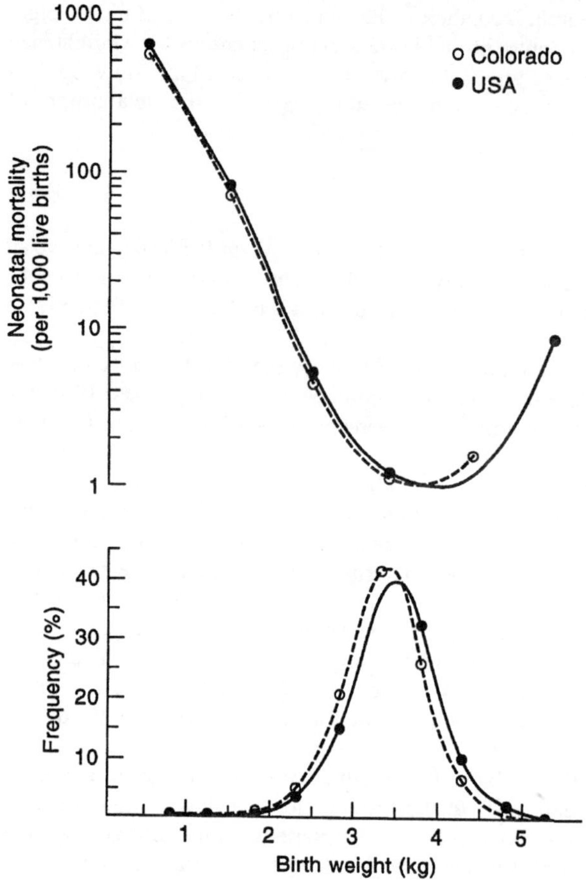

FIGURE 31–2 • Birth-weight-specific neonatal mortality and frequency distribution of birth weight for white singleton births, for Colorado and the United States, 1984. (Reproduced with permission from Wilcox, 1993. Birth weight and perinatal mortality: the effect of maternal smoking. *Am J Epidemiol.* 1993;137:1098–1104.)

to less than 1% in the mid-range of weights. Risk then rises again slightly for the largest weights. This pattern of weight-specific mortality is consistently seen in diverse populations. The pattern is not simply a reflection of preterm births at the lowest weights or postterm births at the highest weights; the same pattern is seen within each gestational-age stratum (Wilcox and Skjaerven, 1992).

If birth weight were the ideal biomarker for risk of perinatal mortality, then variations in birth weight would closely parallel changes in risk. An exposure that depressed fetal growth and lowered birth weights would predictably increase risk. We could estimate the likely effect of such an exposure by simply applying the weight-specific mortalities for the general population to the new distribution of birth weights.

In fact, when comparing groups of babies, the relation between birth weight and mortality does not behave according to this expected pattern. As the birth-weight distribution shifts to higher or lower weights, the corresponding mortality curve moves with it, shifting to the same extent. For example, in Colorado (where the average oxygen pressure is reduced because of high altitudes), babies have reduced birth weights compared with babies in the United States as a whole. At the same time, the corresponding mortality curve for these babies has shifted to the left to precisely the same extent (Fig. 31–2), so that the overall mortality of Colorado babies is unchanged (Wilcox, 1993). The matching lateral shifts in the distribution of birth weight and in the corresponding weight-specific mortality curve explain a seemingly paradoxical result: LBW is increased in Colorado, but mortality is not. The shift in the mortality curve is not what one would expect if birth weight were on the causal pathway or were a faithful surrogate for risk. Instead, the data suggest that birth weight is a factor that is susceptible to disturbance by exposures (here, gestation in Colorado) that do not affect risk, and that factors that shift the birth-weight distribution need not produce a corresponding effect on risk.

A more complicated but related phenomenon is seen with maternal smoking. Mothers who smoke have smaller babies, and their babies have higher neonatal mortality. Nonetheless, this higher mortality is not necessarily due, even in part, to smoking-induced smallness. Inspection of weight-specific mortality rates for babies of mothers who smoke shows that (as with the previous example) the mortality curve shifts laterally to the same extent as the birth-weight distribution. Superimposed on this shifted mortality curve is an upward shift, such that weight-specific mortality rates are increased across all birth weights. This comparison suggests that the increased perinatal mortality associated with smoking during pregnancy is not due to the lowering of birth weight but due to separate mechanisms. In fact, (Basso et al., 2006) have shown that one can reproduce the weight-specific mortality curve for full-term infants by a pure-confounding model: In this model, one rare factor produces a marked increase in mortality and independently a decrease in birth weight, while another rare factor produces an increase in mortality and independently an increase in birth weight.

Little may be accomplished by trying to increase birth weights to reduce neonatal mortality. We know of no example in which the weight-specific mortality rates stay fixed while the birth weight distribution as a whole shifts. This is not to say that exposures that affect birth weight should not be a concern. Exposures that decrease birth weights might also have morbid effects (e.g., subtle impairment of brain development) that are not as easy to detect as neonatal death.

RELATIVE BIRTH WEIGHT

The paradoxes associated with application of a rigid cutoff for LBW, together with the observed tendency of the mortality curve to realign itself to the location of the birth-weight distribution, has led to alternative approaches (Wilcox, 2001). One can measure relative weight in place of absolute weight by expressing the birth weight in standard deviations away from the population (or subpopulation) mean. A corresponding category of high-risk babies can then be defined according to some cutoff, such as 2 standard deviations below the mean (Rooth, 1980). This approach resembles the 10% criterion used to define small for gestational age (SGA) but allows for possible displacement of the birth-weight distribution by factors other than gestational age. Estimates of the standard deviation of birth weight are exaggerated to a degree by the presence of small (preterm) births in the lower tail of the distribution. Methods to avoid this exaggeration by basing the standard-deviation estimate on the predominant part of the distribution have been developed (Wilcox and Russell, 1983; Umbach and Wilcox, 1996).

BIRTH-WEIGHT SUMMARY

The fact that birth weight is highly predictive is not sufficient evidence that birth weight determines neonatal survival. As has been shown, the relation between the birth-weight distribution and weight-specific mortality reveals that factors that shift birth weight do not have readily predictable effects on mortality. As a result, the analysis of birth weight as a surrogate for mortality risk can be misleading. Furthermore, adjustment for birth weight in the analysis of other variables, as if it were a confounder, can actually produce confounding and distort results (Wilcox and Russell, 1983; Weinberg, 1993).

Birth weight has been a favored topic of study because of its accessibility, its precision, and its apparently close relation to newborn health. The assumption, however, that birth weight offers the reproductive epidemiologist a readily interpretable marker for newborn health is overly simplistic. Birth weight may be less relevant to our understanding of perinatal mortality and morbidity than, for example, preterm delivery.

PERINATAL MORTALITY

The transition from intrauterine to extrauterine life is dangerous, with the highest risk occurring during labor and the immediate postpartum period. This risk is commonly divided into two distinct outcomes: stillbirth and neonatal mortality. Neonatal mortality is a straightforward concept, defined as any death in the first 28 days after birth. Stillbirth mortality (late fetal death) is not so easily specified.

Stillbirth implies the death of a viable fetus before delivery. Because the "viability" of a fetus who has died can only be inferred, there is no standard definition in vital statistics (and thus in epidemiology). For many years, viability was defined as a pregnancy that has advanced to at least 28 completed weeks of gestation. Modern medical interventions have moved the lower boundary of viability downward, so that today it is not uncommon for babies to survive at 24 weeks and even earlier. As a consequence, the legal definition of stillbirth now varies widely across jurisdictions (e.g., 16, 20, 22, 24, 28 weeks), and sometimes includes a birth-weight criterion as well (e.g., 350, 400, 500, 1,000 g) (Gourbin and Masuy-Stroobant, 1995; Kowaleski, 1997).

There are other complications in the definition of stillbirth mortality. There is often little to distinguish a fetal death during labor from death shortly thereafter. Signs of life may be uncertain and left to the discretion of the birth attendant. Regional or cultural differences in defining a borderline death as stillbirth or neonatal death may therefore bias both outcomes. Gestational age itself is hard to determine, and population differences in the methods of determining gestational age (for example, last menstrual period dating versus early ultrasound examination) may affect the proportion of fetal deaths defined as stillbirth. For all these reasons, valid comparisons of stillbirth rates across populations require that similar definitions are being used in all groups. This point applies also to the analysis of perinatal mortality, which is the combination of stillbirth and neonatal mortality.

BIRTH-WEIGHT OR GESTATIONAL-AGE-SPECIFIC MORTALITY

Birth weight and gestational age are both powerful predictors of perinatal survival. As a consequence, there is an extensive literature on the analysis of perinatal mortality stratified or adjusted by these variables. Special problems arise, however, when stillbirth or neonatal mortality is stratified by birth weight and gestational age. Analysis of stillbirth mortality by birth weight is complicated by the fact that some fetal deaths might occur days before delivery. In these cases, there is presumably loss of weight between the death and the expulsion of the fetus, contributing to an association between low birth weight and stillbirth mortality on the basis of reverse causation. The extent of this problem in the observed high risk of late fetal death among small fetuses is not known. The conundrum could be avoided by limiting attention to those fetuses who died during labor. Unfortunately, such information is not routinely available in vital statistics, the routine source of stillbirth data for epidemiologic purposes.

Stratification of stillbirth mortality by gestational age is even more problematic. Such mortality has been routinely defined as the number of stillbirths divided by the total number of live and stillbirths at a given gestational age. Some have argued (Cheung, 2004; Platt, 2004) that the proper denominator should include all pregnancies that are continuing, because those fetuses were also at risk of fetal death at the given gestational age. Both approaches have limitations. In general, analyses of stillbirth mortality that stratify by birth weight or gestational age should be undertaken with close attention to the underlying biologic hypotheses being addressed (Wilcox and Weinberg, 2004).

BIRTH DEFECTS

In 1941, Gregg linked an outbreak of rubella to a rare eye defect in newborn infants (Gregg, 1941), which led to the discovery of the rubella syndrome and dethroned the medical dogma that the fetus is shielded by the placenta from adverse influences. In 1961, another dogma fell when the link between thalidomide and limb-reduction defects was recognized. This effect became a paradigm for the damage that could be done to a fetus by toxicants that are benign in other mammalian species and benign (or even therapeutic) to the mother (Brent, 1986). Perhaps most disturbing of all was the recognition in 1971 that diethylstilbestrol (DES) is a transplacental carcinogen, leading to a rare cancer in adulthood (Herbst et al., 1971). This finding demonstrated the possibility of harmful effects on the fetus that might not become apparent for decades.

Despite these discoveries and the resulting expansion of epidemiologic research related to birth defects, little is known about the causes of most defects. Methodologic difficulties persistently frustrate research in this area. Perhaps the single most important difficulty is estimating rates. True biologic incidence is impossible to determine because most birth defects originate in the earliest stages of pregnancy, when direct observation is virtually impossible. Many embryos with defects do not survive early pregnancy; the prevalence of the defect at birth is therefore a function not just of embryologic incidence but of intrauterine survival. Survival may be affected by the severity of the defect (with maternal mechanisms possibly leading to selective rejection of defective fetuses; (Warkany, 1978)), and by diagnostic screening leading to elective abortion. Elective abortion is a particularly likely source of bias for certain birth defects, because access to prenatal diagnosis (and the decision to use it) is not random. Thus, even perfect ascertainment at birth would produce rates subject to distortion by differential selection and survival, which may vary by exposure.

Ascertainment of defects at birth is itself problematic. Birth defects are highly heterogeneous in presentation, and not all are apparent at delivery. Many heart defects, for example, do not manifest themselves until after initial discharge from hospital, and some may go undiagnosed until well into adulthood. Mental retardation may not be apparent until long after birth, and more subtle abnormalities of neurologic development may never be recognized as prenatal in origin. The skill of the examiner and the thoroughness of examination can have a large effect on the apparent birth prevalence for a particular defect. With careful examination, major birth defects can be found among an estimated 3% of babies at birth and among another 3% later (Kalter and Warkany, 1983). Minor defects are at least as common. Population registries that depend on routine examination of newborns find overall prevalence in the range of 2 to 3%.

Most studies of birth defects fall into two general categories: descriptive studies based on population registries and case-control studies (which may be based on clinic or registry data). Although registries have not uncovered evidence of powerful new teratogens being introduced into the environment, registries are limited in their power to detect new teratogens with moderate effects, or that affect small subgroups of the population (Khoury and Holtzman, 1987).

Even the most common birth defects occur in only 1 to 4 per 1,000 babies, so that the rarity of the outcome renders the case-control approach particularly advantageous. The overriding methodologic question in case-control studies of birth defects has been whether a couple with a defective infant will be motivated (by guilt or concern) to report more or fewer adverse exposures than a couple with a normal infant (MacKenzie and Lippman, 1989; Werler et al., 1989; Swan et al., 1992; Rockenbauer et al., 2001), and whether the additional reporting is spurious or of greater accuracy than for other couples.

One controversial remedy for this potential recall bias is to use babies with other birth defects as controls. There is a practical advantage as well: Parents of babies with birth defects are easier to recruit than parents of normal infants. Controls with defects can often be taken conveniently from the same clinic or birth-defect registry as the cases. A problem with such controls is that—if they share etiologies with the cases (Khoury et al., 1992)—the effect measure can be biased toward the null.

Moreover, the available evidence suggests that recall bias is not necessarily an important problem in case-control studies of birth defects. A comparison of odds ratios using the two types of control groups provided no evidence that differential recall of exposure is an important concern in such studies (Khoury et al., 1994).

Case-control studies of birth defects can take advantage of short latencies for teratogenic effects. The relevant window of exposure for most defects is within the first trimester of pregnancy. Although this timing is within months of the identification of the defect in most cases, timing of exposure even within that interval of fetal development can be crucially important. Teratogens may have an effect only during a very brief stage of organogenesis. This precision of timing is difficult to establish with recall, which weakens the power of a study to detect an effect (Khoury et al., 1992). Associations could also be weakened by etiologic heterogeneity. Even well-defined defects have many possible causes; a single teratogen may cause only a fraction of the observed cases.

Amidst this uncertainty over etiology, we do know that there are specific genetic and environmental factors that play a role in most defects, presumably in interaction with each other. Concordance rates in monozygotic twins are elevated, as are recurrence risks in families that have already had a child with a birth defect (Lie et al., 1995; Basso et al., 1999). New methods of design and analysis can help elucidate effects of particular susceptibility genes.

GENETIC FACTORS IN REPRODUCTIVE EPIDEMIOLOGY

Because birth defects and pregnancy complications (and some diseases with early onset, such as autism and acute lymphoblastic leukemia) have their origins during prenatal life, the mother's genome can play a major role by influencing the prenatal environment (Mitchell, 1997). For example, the mother's genotype may impair her ability to metabolize toxicants during pregnancy. Thus, when exploring the genetic components of risk, one should consider both individuals and think of the affected unit as the maternal/fetal pair. If one studies only the baby's genotype, or only the mother's genotype, the potential for confounding is strong because of the high correlation between maternal and fetal genotypes (Mitchell, 2004). Thus, a carefully designed case-control study would include mother–child case pairs and mother–child control pairs.

An alternative design can be particularly useful when studying birth defects, pregnancy complications, and conditions with onset early in the child's life. In this design, affected offspring and their two parents (and possibly their four grandparents (Weinberg, 2003)) are genotyped. Alleles associated with risk can be identified because they will be found in affected offspring more often than Mendelian transmission would predict (see also Chapter 28). Geneticists have made use of this apparent distortion by comparing the total number of transmissions from heterozygous parents to affected offspring with a binomial (probability $\frac{1}{2}$) distribution, in a chi-squared procedure called the transmission disequilibrium test (TDT) (Spielman et al., 1993).

A family-based analysis is also possible. Consider a di-allelic locus, so that each person carries 0, 1, or 2 copies of the variant allele (it does not matter which allele is designated as the "variant"). Based on the trio of genotypes for the mother, father, and child, each family is categorized into one of 15 possible cells in a contingency table of family-based genetic outcomes. The resulting multinomial counts can be analyzed by stratified Poisson regression (Weinberg et al., 1998), which yields estimates of the two relative risk parameters associated with 2 copies or 1 copy, respectively, of the variant allele inherited by the affected offspring, treating the 0-copy offspring as the referent category. Despite the absence of controls, statistical power for this approach often exceeds that of the TDT (Weinberg et al., 1998), and is similar to that of a case-control study with the same number of cases and an equal-size control group (Lee, 2004). Thus, compared with a case-control design that studies both cases and their mothers, the case-parent approach provides about the same precision and power while requiring a smaller total number of genotyped individuals.

Methods based on parents also avoid worries about bias related to control selection, because the biologic parents are always inherently well-matched controls for genetic effects. On the other hand, because Mendelianism serves as the leveraging assumption for parent-based methods, for validity one must be able to assume not only Mendelian assortment for the gametes, but that survival of affected offspring to the point of study does not depend on genotype, conditional on the parents' genotypes.

To develop intuition for why the log-linear approach works, suppose that families with one child per couple are randomly sampled from families in which both parents are heterozygous. By Mendelian genetics, the offspring should have 0, 1, or 2 copies, with expected cell counts showing a ratio of 1:2:1. If instead we sample families in which the child has a particular birth defect, one can show that the expected counts will show a ratio of $1{:}2R_1{:}R_2$, where R_1 and R_2 are the relative risks associated with inheriting 1 or 2 copies of the variant allele. This pattern is multiplicative in the expected count, corresponding to a log-linear Poisson regression model (see Chapter 21), which means that maximum-likelihood estimates and confidence intervals can be obtained for the relative-risk parameters using widely available statistical packages.

What if there are maternally mediated genetic effects, through which the mother's phenotype during gestation affects her offspring? This kind of causal mechanism will produce asymmetry between the parents, in which mothers of affected offspring carry more copies of the susceptibility allele than do fathers. There would be no distortion in transmissions to affected offspring. A simple extension of the same Poisson model accommodates such maternally-mediated effects and allows them to be distinguished from direct effects due to the child's inherited genotype (Wilcox et al., 1998). Families in which the genotype for a parent is missing (e.g., due to nonparticipation or due to misidentified paternity) can also be fully used (Weinberg, 1999).

The case-parent approach has several practical and theoretical advantages over a case-control design. First, it requires only affected families, who are usually willing to be studied. This design also obviates selecting a comparable control group, always one of the most problematic aspects of case-control studies. Second, the case-parent approach is relatively robust against bias due to self-selection. Genetic "population stratification" (which occurs when subgroups tend to avoid reproducing with other subgroups and also differ in prevalence of the allele and the baseline risk of disease) is one of the potential sources of confounding avoided by the case-parents design, provided the analysis is conditional on parental genotypes. (Some investigators suggest that genetic stratification is not an important source of bias in diverse populations (Wacholder et al., 2002).) One can also extend the model to look at effects due to *imprinting,* which occurs when a copy of the variant allele can be expressed differently depending on whether it came from the mother or the father (Weinberg, 1999). Evidence is mounting, for example, that imprinting plays a role in autism (Nurmi et al., 2003). Finally, statistical missing-data methods can be used to make full use of the data from incomplete triads (Weinberg, 1999), even if the missing-data mechanism depends on the missing genotype (Allen et al., 2003; Chen, 2004).

Regarding the maternal/fetal pair as the unit at risk leads naturally to questions about the potential for synergistic effects of the fetal and maternal genotypes. The example of Rh-factor maternal–fetal incompatibility is well known: If the mother is Rh-negative (double null) and has previously been sensitized by an Rh-positive fetus, and the fetus of the current pregnancy is Rh-positive, the baby can suffer hemolytic disease of the newborn. The log-linear model has been extended to detect such interactive causal mechanisms (Sinsheimer et al., 2003). Incompatible maternal/fetal genotypes may also be related to risk of schizophrenia in the offspring (Palmer et al., 2002). Thus, the case-parent design offers the opportunity to study maternal effects, parent-of-origin effects, and fetal–maternal interactions that would be difficult to elucidate with a case-control design.

An extension of the log-linear model also allows the investigator to explore gene-by-environment interaction on the multiplicative scale (Umbach and Weinberg, 2000). Note, however, that the case-parent design does not permit the study of the "main" effects of exposures without adding population controls. Nonetheless, one can estimate the main effects of the fetal/maternal genotypes and assess departures from multiplicative joint effects between genotypes and categorical exposures using Poisson regression. Either the mother or the fetus/offspring, or both, may be exposed to the relevant factor.

Interactions between genotypes and continuous exposures, such as number of cigarettes smoked, can be studied in a closely related framework by looking for apparent "effects" of the offspring exposure on the patterns of allele transmission from parents to affected offspring (Kistner and Weinberg, 2004), assessed by polytomous logistic regression (see Chapter 20). Note that the design is retrospective, and the exposure obviously does not actually influence the transmission of alleles. Rather, the occurrence of the disease (our basis for sampling) potentially reflects the prior transmission of risk alleles and the co-occurrence of deleterious exposures, which may together have led to the condition and hence to sampling.

The case-parents design suffers from its inability to estimate exposure "main" effects, although it can be used to study multiplicative gene-by-environment interactions. A third alternative is a hybrid design, which exploits the best features of the case-parents approach and the population-based case-control approach. One recruits cases and their parents and also unrelated controls and their parents. The parents of controls are genotyped, but not the controls themselves, who provide only nongenetic information to the study (Weinberg and Umbach, 2005). Under the assumption that the disease is rare and that Mendelian transmission rates apply in the general population, this design permits efficient estimation of all risk-related parameters of interest under a multiplicative formulation.

Quantitative traits such as birth weight can also be studied in place of dichotomous outcomes by using the same polytomous logistic regression described for assessing gene-by-exposure interaction, but with the trait in place of the exposure. In such analysis, the outcome is the number of copies carried by the offspring, conditional on the parental genotypes, in relation to the value of the trait (Kistner and Weinberg, 2004; Laird and Lange, 2006). A convenient feature of this approach is that one need not assume Mendelian inheritance under the null, and thus one gains robustness against potential effects of the gene (and any genetic correlates) on gestational survival. The inference is based on whether the distribution of offspring genotypes, conditional on parental genotypes, varies across levels of the quantitative trait. Extensions also allow for the incorporation of trait data from multiple offspring from the same family (Kistner and Weinberg, 2004).

The availability of tools for genotyping will no doubt lead to still other options for the design of epidemiologic studies. As new biologic hypotheses are framed, the opportunities will expand for analysis of the interplay of genetic and environmental factors. This expanded research may have powerful implications for the way we understand not just birth defects but many other problems of reproduction, pregnancy, and development.

APPENDIX

Formally, the proportional probabilities model for analysis of retrospective (pregnancy-based or attempt-based) or prospective (cohort study-based) time-to-pregnancy data is based on outcomes at each woman-cycle of observation:

$$\ln\{\text{conception rate at cycle } i,\ \text{given } E, X_1, X_2, \ldots, X_P\} = c_i + \beta E + \beta_1 X_1 + \beta_2 X_2 + \beta_P X_P$$

where ln denotes the natural logarithm; the conception rate is the cycle-specific probability of pregnancy, given the couple is still at risk; E is the exposure of interest; and $X_1, X_2, \ldots, X_P$ denote P potential confounders. The parameter c_i denotes the baseline conception rate for the ith cycle; in effect, we establish a set of baseline stratum parameters to allow for the above-described decline in conception rate with attempt cycle. The fecundability ratio is estimated by exponentiating the estimated β based on this model. Confidence intervals can be obtained by exponentiating the upper and lower confidence limits based on the estimated coefficient β and its estimated standard error.

Because this is a generalized linear model (see Chapter 20), it can be fitted using standard software (GLIM, or SAS using the GENMOD procedure); however, one must force extra iterations to ensure that convergence has been achieved. One annoying feature of this model is that it can sometimes result in fitted probabilities that exceed 1.0 for individual couples, which occurs whenever their fitted linear predictor (the right-hand side of the above equation) exceeds 0. Although this feature is undesirable in a model and can interfere with estimation of parameters, such invalid excursions seem to be rare in practice, unless the model is overparameterized or there are covariate outliers.

Other models can be used. The discrete-time model proposed by Cox (Cox and Oakes, 1984) uses as the link function the log odds of the conception rate instead of its logarithm. Otherwise, the preceding formulation is unchanged. This alternative formulation is a logistic model and can be fitted using standard software, provided attempt cycle is entered as an unordered categorical (in SAS a *class*) variable. It is important, however, to be aware that when this Cox discrete-time model is used, the parameter being estimated by exponentiating β is now the fecundability-odds ratio, not the fecundability ratio. The fecundability ratio will always be closer to 1.0 than the fecundability-odds ratio, just as the risk ratio is closer than the odds ratio to 1.0. Because the outcome here is not rare, the two parameters may be quite different. The assumption that the fecundability ratio or, alternatively, the fecundability-odds ratio, is constant across time can be checked by examining in the respective model the coefficient for a product of the exposure and cycle time.

CHAPTER 32

Clinical Epidemiology

Noel S. Weiss

Studies of the Natural History of Illness 642
Studies of Diagnostic and Screening Tests 642
Studies of Therapy—Randomized Controlled Trials 646
Selection of Subjects 647
Selection of the Intervention Measure 648
Definition of Study Endpoints 649
Using Patients as Their Own Controls (Crossover Studies) 649
Studies of Therapy—Nonrandomized Studies 649
Selected Reading 651

Clinical epidemiology is the study of the variation in the outcome of illness and of the reasons for that variation. The overall strategy used in clinical epidemiology is exactly that used in other areas of epidemiology: observations of events in groups of individuals who share a particular characteristic, comparisons of rates of the events among groups, and then inferences regarding the basis for any differences seen. In clinical epidemiologic studies, the characteristic that defines the group can be a symptom, a sign, an illness, or a diagnostic procedure or treatment given for the symptom, sign, or illness.

The ways in which the observations in clinical epidemiology are structured are also similar to those of epidemiology per se. There are studies in which randomization is employed and others in which it is not. Among the nonrandomized studies, there may be comparisons of aggregated patient data across geographic areas or time periods, or there may be cohort, case-control, or cross-sectional studies of individual patients. Relative to epidemiologic studies, those in clinical epidemiology more often tend to involve randomization, because:

1. The "exposure," often a therapy, lends itself to randomization more than do the exposures under consideration in most epidemiologic studies (e.g., diet, tobacco or alcohol consumption, or characteristics of a person or his/her environment);
2. The illness outcomes considered in clinical epidemiologic studies—usually disease progression, complications, or mortality—are often relatively frequent within the patient groups being compared, which makes randomized studies more feasible; and
3. In clinical epidemiologic studies, there is a particularly great potential for confounding in the absence of randomization. In many nonrandomized studies of therapy in which an association has been found, it is uncertain whether it was the treatment or the type of patient to whom that treatment was administered that was related to the altered risk for disease progression, complications, or mortality.

STUDIES OF THE NATURAL HISTORY OF ILLNESS

Studies of the natural history of illness (or any abnormality that comes to the attention of a health care provider, including symptoms and signs of illness) measure health outcomes in ill persons who are not receiving a therapy that influences the presence or rate of these outcomes. Unless the natural history is adverse relative to the experience of unaffected persons, there would be little purpose in seeking to identify and treat the illness, symptom, or sign. For example, among infants with a fever of unknown cause, the decision to identify an infecting organism that may be responsible for the fever (e.g., via blood culture) or to treat the possible infection (e.g., with antibiotics) would be based in part on the knowledge of the frequency with which these febrile infants developed one or more important complications of the presumed infection (e.g., meningitis). As another example, among men with localized cancer of the prostate, the decision to treat (perhaps with local radiation or radical prostatectomy) would be influenced by the probability of death from prostate cancer in such individuals in the absence of therapy.

Data from cohort studies (see Chapter 7) are the major source of information on the natural history of a condition. For example, in Sweden during the late 1970s and early 1980s, men over 75 years of age with localized prostate cancer and younger men with highly differentiated localized tumors received no specific treatment for their tumor (Johansson et al., 1992). Their experiences were evaluated in a 10-year cohort study in which 19 of 223 such patients died of prostate cancer, corresponding to a relative survival (i.e., survival taking into account mortality from other causes) of about 87%.

Case-control studies (see Chapter 8) also can be used for studying natural history. For example, echocardiographic evaluations of persons under 45 years of age who had sustained an ischemic stroke and controls of similar age revealed a nearly identical prevalence of mitral valve prolapse in the two groups (Gilon et al., 1999). These results argue that stroke prophylaxis need not be preferentially recommended for persons with mitral valve prolapse. Case-control studies can play a role as well in the identification of subgroups of patients with a given illness who are at altered risk of the outcome under study. For example, Dornan et al. (1982) sought to characterize insulin-dependent diabetics who are resistant to the development of retinopathy. They compared persons with long-standing diabetes who had normal eyes with diabetic controls who had retinopathy, matched for duration and age at onset of diabetes, with regard to such characteristics as weight, blood pressure, and smoking habits.

STUDIES OF DIAGNOSTIC AND SCREENING TESTS

Diagnostic or screening tests are done to obtain information that can guide a health care provider's decision to initiate or continue a therapeutic intervention. Tests performed in persons with a symptom or sign of an illness are usually termed *diagnostic,* whereas those done in individuals with no such symptom or sign are referred to as *screening*. The underlying rationale as to when a test ought to be applied, however, is identical for these two types. That rationale requires a judgment that among patients to whom the test is administered, the costs of the illness, both monetary and physical, along with the cost of the test and the errors that arise when it does not classify patients accurately, will be exceeded by the costs of the illness (both monetary and physical) had the test not been done. A positive test result can lead to the introduction of therapy when it might not otherwise have been considered, such as prostatectomy following a positive test for serum prostate-specific antigen that leads to a diagnosis of cancer. Alternatively, a negative test can lead to the decision *not* to initiate therapy when it otherwise would have been given (see the example below).

To assess a test's validity, the results it provides can be compared either with a "true" measure of the physiologic, biochemical, or pathologic state the test is seeking to characterize or with the occurrence of disease progression or a disease complication that the test result seeks to predict. For example, arterial blood pressure as assessed via a sphygmomanometer can be compared either with readings obtained from direct intra-arterial pressure measurements or with the subsequent occurrence of stroke or other forms of cardiovascular disease. In clinical epidemiology, particular interest lies in the test's ability to predict progression or complications.

The following example will introduce the ways in which the validity of a test can be measured.

Although the majority of persons undergoing an acute myocardial infarction (MI) experience chest pain, most persons with chest pain have another basis for their symptoms. Because of the

TABLE 32–1

Validity of Emergency Room Criteria for Myocardial Infarction

Emergency Room Criteria for MI	MI Present Yes	MI Present No	Total
Positive	50	91	141
Negative	5	211	216
Total	55	302	357

potential lethality of a MI, however, physicians hospitalize many patients with chest pain for a period of time until they are reasonably certain that a MI has not occurred. In an attempt to avoid hospitalization for those patients with chest pain but not infarction, several investigators (Goldman et al., 1982) sought to develop clinical criteria to predict better the presence of MI. For all patients with chest pain who were seen in an emergency room over a period of several months; they obtained information on characteristics at the time the patient was first seen and on each patient's status 6 to 10 months later. To some extent, the presence of MI, determined during hospitalization or the follow-up period by electrocardiographic (ECG) changes, elevated serum levels of cardiac enzymes, or abnormalities on radionuclide testing, was predicted by an algorithm that considered ECG abnormalities present during the emergency room visit, the nature and duration of symptoms present at that time, and the patient's age. Persons classified as positive or negative according to the algorithm had experienced a MI as shown in Table 32–1.

The validity of the clinical criteria (the "test") could be described in terms of the degree to which persons with and without the condition under study (MI) are correctly categorized. So the percentage of persons with an infarction who tested positive by the clinical criteria—the "sensitivity" of the criteria—was 50/55 = 90.9%. The percentage of persons without an infarction who were correctly categorized as negative by the criteria—the "specificity"—was 211/302 = 69.9%.

Alternatively, the validity of the criteria could be expressed as the extent to which being categorized as positive or negative actually predicts the presence of MI. In this example, the percentage of persons who were deemed clinically positive and who were found to have an infarction—the predictive value of a positive test (PV+)—was 50/141 = 35.5%. The percentage who were clinically negative and who truly had no infarction—the predictive value of a negative test (PV−)—was 211/216 = 97.7%. These measures are summarized in Table 32–2.

Because the predictive values—the probabilities that a person who tests positive (or negative) has or will develop the disease or complication—provide the results that most directly apply to the decision to use or not use a given test, it is important to be able to estimate these even when the data have not been gathered in such a way as to calculate them directly. In the following example, data from a hypothetical case-control study of predictors of MI are presented, in which 33 cases and 33 noncases have been chosen for study. Table 32–3 shows what happens when the proportions of clinically positive and clinically negative patients among cases and noncases mirror those of the patients with chest pain in the emergency room [(50/55) ×33 = 30 cases and (91/302) ×33 = 10 noncases testing positive].

It would be incorrect to calculate PV+ as 30/40 or PV− as 23/26. The predictive values depend on the relative number of persons in the groups with and without infarction, and in this example, these numbers have been set arbitrarily (one control per one patient with infarction). The sensitivity and specificity of the screening criteria, however, can be accurately determined (each is calculated *within* the group of MI cases and noncases, respectively). If the frequency of the condition for which screening is being performed can be estimated, both predictive values can be estimated as well. The following formulas are used to do this.

$$PV+ = \frac{\Pr(D)}{\Pr(D) + \dfrac{1 - \Pr(D)}{LR+}} \qquad [32\text{–}1]$$

TABLE 32-2

Measures of the Validity of a Diagnostic or Screening Test

	Reference Criterion				Reference Criterion		
Test Result	Positive	Negative		Test Result	Infarction	No Infarction	
Positive	a	b	$a+b$	Positive	50	91	141
Negative	c	d	$c+d$	Negative	5	211	216
	$a+c$	$b+d$	n		55	302	357

Term	General	Example	Definition
Sensitivity	$a/(a+c)$	50/55 (90.9%)	Proportion of those with the condition who have a positive test
Specificity	$d/(b+d)$	211/302 (69.9%)	Proportion of those without the condition who have a negative test
PV+	$a/(a+b)$[a]	50/141 (35.5%)	Proportion of those with a positive test who have the condition
PV−	$d/(c+d)$[a]	211/216 (97.7%)	Proportion of those with a negative test who do not have the condition

[a] Meaningful only if $(a+b)/n$ represents the actual proportion of the positives in the relevant population.

where Pr(D) is the relative frequency of the condition for which testing is being performed and LR+, the likelihood ratio for a positive test, is

$$\frac{\text{sensitivity}}{1-\text{specificity}}$$

The second formula is

$$PV- = \frac{\Pr(1-D)}{\Pr(1-D) + (\Pr(D) \times LR-)} \quad [32\text{–}2]$$

where Pr(1 −D) is the relative frequency of patients who do *not* have the condition and LR−, the likelihood ratio for a negative test, is

$$\frac{1-\text{sensitivity}}{\text{specificity}}$$

TABLE 32-3

Results of a Hypothetical Case-Control Study of Testing for MI

	MI		
Test Result	Yes	No	Total
Positive	30	10	40
Negative	3	23	26

In the present example,

$$\Pr(D) = 55/357 = 0.1541, \Pr(1 - D) = 302/357 = 0.8459$$

From the case control data, we estimate

$$LR+ = \frac{30/33}{1 - (23/33)} = 3.0$$

$$LR- = \frac{1 - (30/33)}{23/33} = 0.1304$$

Thus,

$$PV+ = \frac{0.1541}{0.1541 + \dfrac{1 - 0.1541}{3.0}} = 0.353$$

and

$$PV- = \frac{0.8459}{0.8459 + (0.1541)(0.1304)} = 0.977$$

Except for rounding, these values are identical to those obtained from the complete patient group (Table 32–1).

The results of many forms of medical testing are available not only as a dichotomy—positive versus negative—but as a graded characteristic (e.g., a serum sodium concentration). For purposes of medical decision making, however, we generally consider the results of tests such as these in no more than several categories, even if that means lumping together persons whose test results are only broadly similar to one another. For instance, the algorithm used by Goldman et al. to predict the presence of an MI in persons with chest pain undoubtedly produced a wide range of scores, but the decision confronting the physician treating a patient with chest pain—to hospitalize that person or not to do so—encouraged combining scores to obtain a dichotomous result. Still, some of the measures of test accuracy presented earlier apply even if there are more than two possible results of the test. As an example, the results of the algorithm that characterized persons with chest pain conceivably could have been used to classify them into three groups: "strongly positive," "borderline positive," and "negative."

Suppose the presence of an MI in these persons were as shown in Table 32–4. Among persons who, based on their signs and symptoms, were "strongly positive," 46.3% had a myocardial infarction. The corresponding values for "borderline positive" and "negative" persons are 20.3% and 2.3%, respectively. Each of these predictive values can be compared not only to one another, but also to the probability of an MI being present without considering the results of the algorithm (55/357 = 15.4%). In a case-control design, an accurate estimate of these predictive values can be

TABLE 32–4

Hypothetical Performance of a Three-Level Test to Predict the Presence of MI

	MI		
Test Result	**Yes**	**No**	**Total**
Strongly positive	38 (46.3%)	44 (53.7%)	82
Borderline positive	12 (20.3%)	47 (79.7%)	59
Negative	5 (2.3%)	211 (97.7%)	216
	55 (15.4%)	302 (84.6%)	357

obtained by the use of likelihood ratios and an estimate of the true prevalence of the condition that the test seeks to identify (Weiss, 2006).

One or more measures of the validity of a test may be estimated erroneously if (a) in terms of severity, the patients with the condition (e.g., MI) for whom data are available are not typical of patients with the condition in the population for whom the test is intended, or (b) for diagnostic tests, if the proportions of study subjects who do and do not receive the test fail to reflect those of the patients in which the results are to be applied. These issues are discussed in greater detail elsewhere (Begg, 1987; Weiss, 2006).

The ability of a test to lead to improved illness outcomes in a given population is influenced by the frequency of the condition or abnormality being sought, the degree to which the test allows that condition or abnormality to be detected before it or its consequences would otherwise be evident, and the degree to which early treatment of the condition or abnormality is better than late (or no) treatment. For most tests, information regarding each of these is generated in separate studies. For example, the value of blood-pressure screening in reducing mortality from cardiovascular disease was determined by conducting three types of study:

1. Surveys of the prevalence of high blood pressure
2. Investigations of the relative increase in mortality from cardiovascular disease in persons with high blood pressure
3. Comparisons of treated and untreated hypertensives with respect to mortality from cardiovascular disease

A single study that attempts to determine whether all requirements are met (a "one-step" study; Weiss, 2006) is usually far less feasible than each of the component investigations. A one-step study would compare the rates of disease progression or disease complications between two groups of persons:

1. Those who received the test and then received treatment based on the test result
2. Persons who did not receive the test and thus whose treatment (or lack thereof) was not guided by the test result

These one-step studies attempt to assess in aggregate the effects of test accuracy and early-treatment efficacy. Typically, they need a large number of subjects because, as a rule, most individuals do not test positive or do not have the condition being sought. Nonetheless, studies of this sort are required when all (or nearly all) patients who are found to be positive on a certain test receive treatment as a result (thus precluding study type 3 above). This situation is common for cancer screening tests. For example, a woman who tests positive on a mammogram, or who is found to have a rectal tumor during a screening sigmoidoscopy, will not have treatment withheld from her; no comparison of treatment versus nontreatment of screen-detected breast or rectal cancer can be made.

One-step studies can employ any of the traditional designs. For example, the ability of screening for colorectal cancer to reduce mortality from that disease has been evaluated by randomized controlled trials (individuals randomly assigned to receive or not receive fecal occult blood testing), cohort studies (comparison of colorectal cancer mortality among persons who did and did not receive screening sigmoidoscopy), and case-control studies (a comparison of fatal cases of colorectal cancer and controls for a history of prior sigmoidoscopy). Ecologic studies also have the potential to assist in the evaluation of screening efficacy. For example, arguably the most convincing data that bear on the efficacy of cervical cancer screening come from a comparison of mortality from cervical cancer in those Nordic countries that did and those that did not introduce such screening on a wide scale (Day, 1984).

STUDIES OF THERAPY—RANDOMIZED CONTROLLED TRIALS

Randomized controlled trials of therapeutic interventions are ones in which (a) patients are assigned to one of two or more groups to be offered different therapeutic measures; (b) chance alone dictates whether a particular patient will be assigned to a particular group; and (c) patients in each group are monitored for the abatement of their illness, the occurrence of the event(s) that the therapy seeks to prevent, or the occurrence of untoward effects. Although randomized controlled trials have an important role to play in identifying adverse effects of therapy that are relatively common and occur relatively soon after therapy has been initiated, the primary role of these trials is to assess the efficacy of therapy. Randomized trials provide results that can be interpreted relatively easily, for the common concern in *non*randomized studies of treatment efficacy—that the various treatment groups had inherently unequal probabilities of doing well—is much less an issue when it is only chance that determines the membership of the groups.

Relative to studies of patient groups in which randomization has not taken place, randomized controlled trials are labor-intensive and generally entail a high cost per patient. This relatively high cost, in addition to the difficulties that can occur in encouraging patients and their physicians to participate actively in a study, prevents many randomized trials from enrolling a large number of participants. Often, such studies include a few dozen to a few hundred patients. Trials of this size can assess large differences between treatments but may have inadequate statistical precision to evaluate a true small or moderate influence of treatment. For this reason, persons planning a randomized trial often endeavor to incorporate one or more design features that will increase the trial's sensitivity (ability to detect a treatment effect). Such an increase may be possible by careful attention to the selection of subjects, the intervention measure, and the definition of study endpoints. In addition, a design in which patients serve as their own controls sometimes can lead to greater efficiency. Despite these methods to enhance efficiency, few randomized trials are large enough to evaluate rare adverse outcomes related to the treatment. As described later, such adverse outcomes are often discovered from spontaneous reporting systems or from nonrandomized studies conducted after therapies are widely adopted.

SELECTION OF SUBJECTS

A study conducted in England and Wales randomized 1,017 50- to 69-year-old female survivors of a first MI to receive estradiol valerate (2 mg/day) or a placebo for 2 years beginning at the time of hospital discharge (The Esprit team, 2002). Despite the investigators' efforts to restrict participation in the trial to women who would adhere to their assigned regimen—potential subjects were visited twice while in the hospital and provided with detailed information about the study—nonadherence after randomization was high. As of 3 months after discharge, only 74% of women were taking their assigned preparation, and as of 1 year only 59% were doing so. Because of this low level of adherence, the trial's finding of no difference in MI recurrence and cardiac death between women in the two treatment arms has two plausible interpretations: (a) There is no effect of estradiol valerate at this dose on these cardiac outcomes; versus (b) A true modest effect of the drug was underestimated because of the high proportion of participants who did not receive the interventions for an adequate duration.

In an effort to keep the effect of nonadherence to a minimum, many randomized controlled trials begin with a *run-in* phase in which all potential subjects are given a placebo or a control therapy. Their adherence with the regimen is determined, and only those with good adherence are entered into the randomized portion of the study. Measurement of adherence can take many forms (pill counts, biochemical tests, etc.). The goal, however, is to identify and eliminate, before the start of the study, patients who have a high likelihood of not adhering to the regimen offered, because nonadherence can greatly complicate proper analysis and interpretation of a randomized trial. Only the assigned (original) treatment category is randomized, and subjects switch to other treatments in a nonrandom fashion. Hence there is great potential for confounding in comparisons based only on actual (received) treatment.

There are several methods for dealing with this confounding problem, each with strengths and weaknesses. The most commonly used method is called *intent-to-treat* analysis, in which nonadherence is ignored and subjects are compared based on their assigned treatment category. The advantage of this method is that it eliminates the confounding described above. The drawback of an intent-to-treat analysis is that it will tend to underestimate the size of the effect that a treatment may have. Essentially, assigned treatment is a misclassified measure of received treatment and so cannot be expected to produce unbiased estimates of the effect of received treatment (see Chapter 9), i.e., of treatment "efficacy." To the extent that the level of nonadherence in the trial reflects that present in the target population—arguably, this is not a common occurrence—intent-to-treat estimates will be a good measure of "effectiveness," i.e., the effect of the intervention in all to whom it is offered.

Nonadherence in some randomized trials plausibly is not due to the study participants' perception of lack of treatment efficacy, nor to an untoward effect of the treatment. For example, among persons assigned to receive a given treatment there may be some who do not receive it at all. In such instances, steps can be taken to remove the bias that would otherwise be present in an intent-to-treat analysis. One approach involves monitoring the occurrence of outcome events in both adherers and nonadhererers, and then using these data to estimate the size of the difference in outcome occurrence among treatment adherers and their hypothetical counterparts in the control arm of the trial (Sommer and Zeger, 1991; Cuzick et al., 1997; Greenland, 2000b). These methods are discussed in Chapter 12 under the heading of instrumental variables. A related approach is discussed in Chapter 21 under the topic of g-estimation for problems of nonadherence.

Conventional analytic methods that are based on actual treatment rather than on the treatment assigned by the original randomization ("as treated" analysis) are subject to bias from factors that influence whether subjects in the study adhere with the treatment assigned by randomization. To reduce such bias, the investigator can adjust for confounding by controlling variables thought to affect both adherence (hence received treatment) and outcome. The problem with this approach is that (as in many nonexperimental studies) one can rarely if ever be confident that one has properly recorded and controlled a sufficient set of confounders.

Another approach is simply to eliminate nonadherers from the analysis ("per-protocol" analysis), which is subject to even more confounding than "as-treated" analysis. If adherence is affected by treatment and by uncontrolled risk factors for the outcome, then treatment will become associated with (and hence confounded by) those factors among the adherers (see Chapter 9). For instance, there are therapies that, if effective, are expected to produce demonstrable improvement in the patient's status before the full course of therapy is finished. It would be expected that patients who do not complete the full course will be disproportionately numerous in the group assigned to the therapy that is truly less effective. In such situations, the elimination of patients with an incomplete course of therapy from the analysis will diminish the estimated efficacy of the superior therapy. In other examples, elimination of nonadherers can inflate estimated efficacy.

Even when the treatment or the outcome does not influence adherence in such a direct way, the failure to take account of the originally assigned groups can lead to a biased result. An instructive example comes from a randomized trial in which, in an effort to reduce cardiac mortality, clofibrate (an agent that lowers the concentration of serum cholesterol) or a placebo was prescribed to patients who had sustained a MI (Coronary Drug Project Research Group, 1980). During the 5-year period of the study, adherence to the prescribed regimen was monitored in both treatment and placebo groups. Cumulative mortality was found not to differ between the two groups. About 15% of those who had adhered to the assigned treatment (adhered 80% or more of the time) subsequently died, regardless of which regimen had been prescribed. The mortality in persons who were less than 80% adherent was about 27%. If in the analysis the investigators had placed the nonadherent clofibrate patients into the placebo group, they would have found a spurious association of favorable outcomes with use of clofibrate.

Sometimes the nature of the treatment being evaluated does not lend itself to a run-in phase (e.g., a surgical procedure). In such studies, the randomization of patients should be as close as possible to the time of the actual administration of the therapy. Consider, for example, a randomized trial of "second-look" surgery in women with initially advanced ovarian cancer who were in clinical remission following surgery plus chemotherapy (Luesley et al., 1988). Interpretation of this trial was hindered by the relatively early randomization of women—it occurred before the response to the initial chemotherapy had been determined and before all patients had agreed to participate in the study—and led to a sizable fraction of women not receiving the treatment to which they had been randomized.

SELECTION OF THE INTERVENTION MEASURE

It is important to make the actual intervention selected for study as different as possible from whatever treatment will be received by control patients, within the range of what is believed to be possible and ethical for a particular condition. For example, in a randomized trial whose purpose is to measure the extent to which a low-saturated-fat diet can reduce the recurrence of MI, it would be desirable to seek a dietary modification that is a substantial one. It is easier for a randomized trial (or for any epidemiologic or clinical epidemiologic study) to document a large than a small association, and if the risk of MI recurrence does indeed vary monotonically with saturated-fat intake, the bigger the dietary difference is, the bigger the effect on risk.

DEFINITION OF STUDY ENDPOINTS

Some conditions that one is attempting to treat or prevent have measurable antecedents. For example, following treatment for cancer, a death from that cancer is usually preceded by tumor recurrence or metastasis. Death from ventricular arrhythmia following MI is often preceded by nonfatal episodes of ventricular arrhythmia. Neonatal death can be a consequence of prematurity. Because one of the factors limiting the power of a randomized study is the number of endpoints observed, and because these antecedent conditions often occur more commonly than do the endpoints themselves, the monitoring and analysis of these antecedents should increase the study's statistical efficiency.

We should be pleased to accept this increase in efficiency as long as the analysis of the occurrence of such an antecedent condition leads to the same conclusion as would a study of a larger number of subjects in which the endpoint itself was measured. It is necessary, however, to be highly judicious in the selection of such endpoints: In a number of instances, it has been learned that antecedent conditions that plausibly were highly related to a particular endpoint of interest turned out not to be so. For example, some agents that can reduce the *occurrence* of one form of cardiac arrhythmia, ventricular premature depolarizations, actually increase *mortality* from cardiac arrhythmia (Echt et al., 1991).

USING PATIENTS AS THEIR OWN CONTROLS (CROSSOVER STUDIES)

Studies of the efficacy of therapies intended to reduce the frequency or severity of chronic, recurrent problems, such as seizures, arthritic pain, or menopausal hot flashes, can lead to more precise estimates if the subject can serve as his or her own control (Hills and Armitage, 1979). By evaluating the same subject at different times in the presence and absence of the therapy under study, the variability *among* subjects in the frequency or severity of the problem will not blur true differences in efficacy. This goal can be achieved experimentally in a *crossover* design, in which patients receive different therapies during different periods of time. The particular therapy to be administered first is selected at random for each patient. The rates of outcome events (e.g., seizures) or levels of symptoms (e.g., joint pain) that are present during or at the end of the periods of time are compared within individual study subjects. Sufficient time is allowed between treatment periods to permit the effects of the intervention administered previously to dissipate. Thus, crossover studies are appropriate for evaluating the efficacy of therapeutic measures only when the effect fades rapidly after discontinuation.

It is also possible to conduct studies of individual patients over the course of several randomly chosen periods during which either a treatment or control intervention is provided. Such an "*N* of 1" study (Guyatt et al., 1986; McLeod et al., 1986) would contrast the aggregate experience of that patient (e.g., with respect to symptoms) during or immediately after treatment and control intervals, and would have the potential to determine what therapy is most successful in him or her.

STUDIES OF THERAPY—NONRANDOMIZED STUDIES

Many important unintended effects of therapy (side effects) neither are common nor occur within a short time (i.e., less than several weeks) following receipt of the therapy. As mentioned earlier, most randomized trials are not of the size or duration to evaluate such effects, so it is necessary to rely on other means if we are to learn of their existence. Adverse events that are reported to pharmaceutical manufacturers by patients who have used a particular product (and/or by their physicians) often serve as clues as to the presence of a negative unintended effect. If there are substantial numbers of reports pertaining to an otherwise quite uncommon condition—such as the hundreds of reports of hepatic injury in users of the diuretic ticrynofen that led to withdrawal of this drug from the market within 1 year of its introduction (Zimmerman et al., 1984)—formal pharmacoepidemiologic study of the question may not be necessary to form a judgment of a cause–effect relation. In other circumstances, a comparison of adverse events reported for different drugs with a similar indication and similar time of entry into the market, combined with sales data on the drugs, can be informative. For example, the nearly 100-fold higher frequency of reports of rhabdomyolysis in users of cerivastatin compared with atorvastatin, taking into account the estimated number of users of each drug, provided compelling evidence of a particular hazard associated with use of cerivastatin (Staffa et al., 2002).

Nonetheless, in most instances, formal nonrandomized studies are needed to document the safety of therapies. Fortunately, the factors that influence the need for or choice of therapy for a particular patient often are unrelated to that patient's risk of developing the unintended effect. For example, the patients who happened to receive cerivastatin rather than atorvastatin were probably not otherwise predisposed to rhabdomyolysis. Thus, many follow-up and case-control studies can provide a valid estimate of the relative frequency of unintended health outcomes in recipients of a given treatment. With the advent of computerized data on use of prescription medications and health events among persons enrolled in health insurance plans, it has become particularly feasible to assess potential unintended effects of medication use (Ray, 2003; Strom, 2000).

Only infrequently can nonrandomized studies provide a valid estimate of the efficacy of a treatment. In most situations, the measured differences between the experiences of patient groups receiving alternative therapies are primarily the result of underlying differences between the groups regarding the chances of progression or complications. In other words, patients are selected for different therapies based on clinical indications. If, as one would expect, these indications are also prognostic factors, the estimates of treatment efficacy become confounded by these factors. This phenomenon is often referred to as *confounding by indication* (Strom, 2000 MacMahon, 2003). To alleviate this problem, strategies to prevent and control confounding (such as restriction, matching, and stratification; see Chapters 11 and 15) must be deployed, although these strategies can work only to the extent that the relevant factors can be measured accurately.

A problem that can afflict all studies (whether of intended or unintended outcomes) is that patients receiving different therapies may be monitored differently (differential outcome ascertainment). This problem can result in spurious differences in outcomes, but it can be avoided if steps can be taken to ensure comparable monitoring of the various treatment groups. Even if the monitoring is identical across compared groups, however, the observed associations will be biased by incomplete ascertainment (a form of nondifferential outcome measurement; see Chapter 9), usually toward the null.

The above problems often cannot be completely addressed by design and analysis methods. Nonetheless, the study results may have some value if the size of the observed difference in outcome among the treatment groups substantially exceeds that which could be expected on the basis of inherent differences among the groups with respect to prognostic factors (e.g., illness severity) or bias due to outcome misclassification. Sensitivity analysis (see Chapter 19) may be needed in making such arguments, however.

To illustrate this point, consider the following two examples. The first provides a result that *cannot* be regarded as a valid estimate of therapeutic efficacy. Among 106 women with advanced ovarian cancer who underwent primary surgery followed by chemotherapy, 32 later underwent secondary cytoreductive operations (Berek et al., 1983). In 12 women, the cytoreduction was "optimal" (i.e., diameter of largest residual tumor mass <1.5 cm), and among them the median survival was 20 months. In the remaining 20 women, the procedure was "nonoptimal," and among them the median survival was 5 months. The authors' conclusion was that "resection of macroscopic disease that persists after completion of chemotherapy enhances survival." The conclusion is unduly optimistic: The better survival in the "optimal" group just as easily could have been the result of their inherently better prognosis as the influence of the surgery itself.

Contrast the preceding example with an evaluation of bone-marrow transplantation in 24 children who had a relapse after an initial course of chemotherapy for acute lymphoblastic leukemia (Johnson et al., 1981). At the end of a mean follow-up period of about 2 years, 11 of these children were alive, in contrast to only 2 of 21 children who had relapsed but received only additional chemotherapy. The children had not been randomly assigned to the two treatment groups; rather, those who had an HLA-identical donor available were offered marrow transplantation, whereas the others were not. Because there is no reason to believe that the availability of an HLA-identical donor correlates much, if at all, with survival in this disease, it seems very likely that the difference in survival is almost entirely the result of a difference in the efficacy of the two therapeutic approaches.

SELECTED READING

A number of books have been written that contain the words "clinical epidemiology" in their title, or that deal heavily with this topic, including Feinstein (1985), Fletcher and Fletcher, 2005, Hulley et al. (2001), Katz (2001), Kramer (1988), Sackett et al. (1991), and Weiss (2006). Probably as testimony to the relative youth of clinical epidemiology as an identified entity, these books differ considerably from one another not only in their emphasis but in their content.

CHAPTER 33

Meta-Analysis

Sander Greenland and Keith O'Rourke

Preliminaries 652
- The Nature of Meta-Analysis 652
- When Is Meta-Analysis Needed? 653
- Goals of Meta-Analysis 654
- Conducting a Sound and Credible Meta-Analysis 655

Initial Tasks of a Meta-Analysis 655
- Specifying the Study Variables 655
- Study Identification 656
- Quantification of Effects 657
- Regression Models 658

Statistical Reanalysis of Individual Studies 659
- Extraction of Estimates 659
- Adjustments Using External Estimates of Confounding 660
- Adjustment for Selection Bias and Misclassification 662
- Regression on Rates and Ratios 663
- Estimation from Reports Employing Only Broad Exposure Categories 666
- Estimation of Coefficients from Reports Presenting Only Mean Exposure Levels 666
- Reporting the Results 667

Statistical Methods for Meta-Analysis 668
- Basic Methods 668
- Meta-Regression Methods 673

Problems in Application of Methods 677
- Overconclusiveness 677
- Aggregation Bias 678
- Publication Bias 678
- Issues of Study Size 679
- Bias in Exclusion of Studies 679

Some Methods to Avoid 680
- Qualitative Tally (Vote Counting) 680
- Scatterplots of Test Statistics 681
- Standardized Coefficients, Correlations, and Effect Sizes 681
- Quality Scoring 681

Role and Limitations of Meta-Analysis 682

Conclusion 682

PRELIMINARIES

THE NATURE OF META-ANALYSIS

Meta-analysis refers to the analysis of multiple studies, including statistical techniques for merging and contrasting results across studies. Synonyms and related terms include research synthesis, cross-design synthesis, systematic review, systematic overview, pooling, and scientific audit. Some use meta-analysis to refer only to the quantitative aspects of the review. Whatever the term, these methods focus on contrasting and combining results from different studies, in the hopes of identifying patterns among study results, sources of disagreement among those results, or other interesting relationships that may come to light in the context of multiple studies. Such methods have been an integral part of educational, social science, policy, and medical research for decades (Louis et al., 1985; Yusuf et al., 1987; Sacks et al., 1987; L'Abbe et al., 1987; Mosteller and Chalmers, 1992), and books on meta-analysis in medical care have been available for some time (Eddy et al., 1992; Pettiti, 1994a; Chalmers and Altman, 1995; Mulrow and Cook, 1998; Glasziou et al., 2001, Egger et al., 2001).

Meta-analysis has not been as integral to epidemiology, in part because of objections (Shapiro, 1994) and in part because of less obvious pressing need. Social science and medical topics often involve hundreds of studies, from which policy researchers must often distill a few simple recommendations (Eddy et al., 1992; Pettiti, 1994a). As a result, there has been greater pressure to refine summarization techniques in those fields. In contrast, epidemiologic studies of specific topics have tended to be fewer, and the epidemiologic community appears to be more hospitable to tentative, limited inferences based on narrative reviews. Nonetheless, to neglect quantitative aspects of review would be akin to presenting a study and supplying only a narrative discussion of the raw data, with no attempt to group and compare subject outcomes.

Meta-analysis can be viewed as the transference of good analytic practice from the single-study to the multiple-study context. It begins with thorough and critical evaluation of the available data in a manner that is explicit and fully replicable by others. The need to identify, abstract, and analyze data from multiple studies parallels the need of single studies to identify eligible subjects, abstract their information, and analyze the resulting data by summarizing information across subjects.

There are, however, crucial differences between analyzing a single study and conducting a meta-analysis. In any credible single study, a single explicit protocol is applied to locating and recruiting subjects, and to data collection. Indeed, the homogeneity of the study protocol is presumed by standard statistical methods, such as those described in Part III of this book. In contrast, the opposite extreme holds in a meta-analysis. Studies are undertaken for various reasons, which may or may not be related to the question of interest to the meta-analyst. Different studies may employ vastly different protocols to collect, analyze, and report their data. The result is that the meta-analyst is faced with a collection of data with remarkable heterogeneity, sometimes so much that application of standard statistical methods is unjustifiable if not impossible. For example, in a review of the relation of socioeconomic status (SES) to childhood leukemia, Poole et al. (2006) found such large difference in SES definition and measurement that they could justify only qualitative contrasts among study results.

The meta-analytic situation is analogous to an individual study in which every subject is selected according to a different eligibility criterion, and had data obtained by a different method—some from face-to-face interview, some from mail-in questionnaire, some from records, with different forms used for each subject. Thus, one should not expect the analytic tasks to be as simple in a meta-analysis as in a single study, and one should expect the results to be affected by sources of uncertainty (such as between-study protocol differences) that are absent in single studies. These extra sources of uncertainty need to be explicitly acknowledged and addressed.

The diversity of study methods can be viewed as an opportunity for discovering the extent to which study context and methods influence study results—making the meta-analysis a study of studies and their results. In the SES and childhood-leukemia example, there was a clear divergence between early ecologic studies (which largely showed positive associations) and later case-control studies (which largely showed inverse associations). Even if no pattern emerges, documenting that the current literature supports no inference is valuable.

The present chapter provides an overview and illustration of basic principles and quantitative methods for reviewing typical epidemiologic literature. The examples concern nonexperimental studies of easily defined antecedent variables and discrete, nonrecurrent outcomes (although easily defined does not necessarily imply easily measured). We focus on situations in which most or all of the research results are available only in the form of journal articles, and therefore in which crucial details of certain studies are lacking. We will not address randomized-trial meta-analyses or overviews in which original data are accumulated and reanalyzed as a pooled dataset, although many of the same primary concerns and methods apply (Sutton et al., 2000; Senn, 2002; Whitehead, 2002).

WHEN IS META-ANALYSIS NEEDED?

Most researchers want to see individual studies placed in the context of previous studies, as evinced by the inclusion of a literature review section in almost all published research reports. Meta-analysis offers a more rigorous and coherent treatment of past research work than typical narrative reviews. Some commentators have even suggested that no randomized-trial result should be published without the inclusion of a meta-analysis in place of the narrative literature review section (O'Rourke and

Detsky, 1989). Similarly, because of the rapid growth of epidemiologic literature, the traditional narrative review may no longer be a reliable way to summarize research in certain areas.

Although we have no doubt that a well-conducted meta-analysis provides valuable information to put a new study in context and guide its design and interpretation, the thought and effort needed to conduct a reliable meta-analysis may be far too excessive to demand of authors of those studies. These authors will also have an intrinsic conflict of interest given their involvement in the new study that needs to be critically evaluated in the context of all other studies. This practical limitation has led some commentators to suggest that reports of single studies should be relieved of the tasks of formulating conclusions, and thus of reviewing the literature in detail. Instead, they suggest that single-study reports should focus on describing their methods and data in as much detail as feasible, to facilitate later meta-analyses of the topic (Greenland et al., 2004). Meta-analyses conducted separately from a single study reduce the risk that the meta-analysis will be heavily influenced by that study, and can be published as a separate article providing far more detail of the literature and the meta-analysis than could be put in combination with the single study's report.

Another issue is the idea that authors of a relevant study will have an intrinsic conflict of interest for meta-analysis, given that their study will need to be critically evaluated relative to other studies. Although authors involved in a relevant study may be the most qualified to undertake the meta-analysis, it has been recommended that their meta-analysis should acknowledge this possible conflict by indicating their authorship of studies considered for inclusion in the meta-analysis (Stelfox et al., 1998).

GOALS OF META-ANALYSIS

An important controversy concerns whether the primary objective of a meta-analysis should be the estimation of an average effect across studies (a synthetic goal) or the identification and estimation of differences among study-specific effects (an analytic goal) (Maclure, 1993). The synthetic approach is well established in the clinical-trial literature but has come under harsh criticism by various authors, especially in epidemiology (O'Rourke and Detsky, 1989; Greenland, 1994d, 1994e, 1994f; Shapiro, 1994; Thompson, 1994). Regardless of approach, a sound meta-analysis needs to assess each study's limitations as well as gaps in the entire literature being assessed.

A major problem with a purely synthetic meta-analysis is that it can give a false impression of consistency across study results, especially when the individual study results are too imprecise to reveal inconsistencies between studies. Thus there should be no compulsion to produce a combined estimate, especially when background information suggests that no such estimate could capture the diversity of study results. Instead, one should seek to identify systematic variation (heterogeneity) in study results. Averaging should be limited to those results that could be reasonably expected to be similar among the studies. As with many guidelines for meta-analysis, the same caution applies to analysis of individual studies. For example, in a single study it would be inappropriate to combine sex-specific estimates of effects of hormonally based cancer therapies.

No meta-analysis can compensate for the inherent limits of nonexperimental data for making inferences about causal effects. Even if one approaches a meta-analysis with a synthetic goal foremost in mind, it is nonetheless imperative to search for systematic variations in estimates across studies and study designs and to report any suggestive patterns (as always, regardless of whether they are "statistically significant"). The meta-analyst should remember that even if the variations across studies appear to be no more than random, it remains possible that all studies suffered similar systematic errors, or have net error in the same direction.

One should also bear in mind that the collection of all studies on a topic is haphazard, with some poorly done, others possibly misreported, and yet others not published at all. Each study should be viewed critically with an eye to contradictions as well as omissions. Sometimes data that are unfavorable to a research sponsor or a researcher's pet hypothesis are hidden (Berenson, 2005). In other cases, data may go unpublished or be hard to find simply because they were not of primary interest. For example, in many studies SES is collected secondarily as a potential confounder, and hence is reported only descriptively, if at all (Poole et al., 2006). Also, far too many studies report only "statistically significant" associations. As a consequence, critical nonsignificant results go unpublished, and the associations reported may be those from the most "significant" analysis, making them unrepresentative of all available data. This type of selection bias has been well documented in randomized clinical trials (Chan et al., 2004). Therefore, one of the goals of meta-analysis must be to evaluate the extent of such bias, a topic to which we will return under the heading of publication bias.

CONDUCTING A SOUND AND CREDIBLE META-ANALYSIS

Like any scientific study, an ideal meta-analysis would follow an explicit protocol that is fully replicable by others. This ideal can be hard to attain, but meeting certain conditions can enhance soundness (validity) and credibility (believability). Among these conditions we include the following:

1. A clearly defined set of research questions to address.
2. An explicit and detailed working protocol.
3. A replicable literature-search strategy.
4. Explicit study inclusion and exclusion criteria, with a rationale for each.
5. Nonoverlap of included studies (use of separate subjects in different included studies), or use of statistical methods that account for overlap.
6. Reanalysis of included studies as needed and feasible (which may involve requests for more information from study authors).
7. A listing or graphical display of individual study results or inputs, along with a listing of what is believed to be the most relevant clinical and methodologic differences between studies, so that the analyses can be easily replicated by others.
8. Explanatory analysis of differences among study results, with the aim of finding any systematic relations between study properties and study results. Study properties include biologic and clinical characteristics of the study population (e.g., studies of men vs. studies of women), as well as methodologic properties (e.g., study design, methods of measurement, susceptibility to measurement error, and manner and extent of confounder control).
9. Avoidance of invalid analytic methods, even if those methods are popular (such as those based on effect sizes or standardized coefficients).
10. A summary of limitations and shortcomings known to the meta-analysts, along with some indication (if not analysis) of how these problems may have affected the meta-analytic results.

Though not necessarily relevant to the validity of a meta-analysis, it can also be helpful to formulate suggestions for future research to help overcome the limitations and shortcomings identified in item 10, along with possibly promising research opportunities that may have become apparent.

The following sections discuss most of these considerations in detail. We will illustrate points with a relatively transparent meta-analysis of the association of coffee consumption with coronary heart disease (Greenland, 1993e). This illustration is now dated, but it is used here for simplicity and convenience, although the points made would apply to any newer analysis of this topic.

INITIAL TASKS OF A META-ANALYSIS

When determining the tasks needed in a meta-analysis, it is important to define clearly the main components. Poorly focused research questions can lead to poor decisions about what research to include and how to summarize it. There are several key components to a well-formulated question. A clearly defined question will be reasonably precise in specifying the exposures and outcomes under study, and the populations to which the meta-analysis will apply (e.g., children, fertile women, the elderly, etc.).

SPECIFYING THE STUDY VARIABLES

Outcome

The outcome "coronary heart disease" subsumes such heterogeneous endpoints as sudden cardiac death, myocardial infarction, coronary insufficiency, and angina pectoris. Furthermore, these subcategories represent neither mutually exclusive nor completely exhaustive subdivisions of the outcome. Coffee drinking might affect risk of one or some but not all of these subcategories, in which case its effect on the gross outcome of coronary heart disease would be a dilute echo of its primary effect. On the other hand, coffee effects might be similar across these categories, in which case maximum precision would be obtained by taking all coronary heart disease as the outcome. After considering these possibilities, the reviewer must decide whether to narrow the review to only one subcategory (say, acute myocardial infarction) and acknowledge the potential irrelevance of the findings for other subcategories (say, angina), or to perform a meta-analysis on several or all subcategories.

Exposure

Another item requiring precise specification is the antecedent variable or exposure under study. For example, many studies of diet and health in fact focus on nutrients (e.g., calcium and β-carotene) rather than on dietary factors (e.g., milk and vegetables). Each is a legitimate study topic, but which is chosen has profound implications for issues such as confounding and measurement error. Taking again the coffee–heart disease issue, one must decide whether to study an effect of caffeine or of coffee. A study of caffeine would demand consideration of type of coffee consumed (ordinary or decaffeinated), as well as tea and cola consumption.

Confounders

Having precisely specified the study exposure and outcome, one will be in a position to identify potential confounders. In identifying confounders, we note that just because a variable has a potential to confound does not mean that failure to control it leads to important bias. Nevertheless, some confounders may be generally recognized as so important that any report that fails to fully adjust for them will be immediately suspect. An example is cigarette smoking in the study of coffee and heart disease.

Intermediates

Although this issue is often neglected, it can be important to identify certain potential intermediates (variables along a possible causal pathway from exposure to outcome). Intermediate variables, if controlled in an analysis, bias effect estimates, typically, though not necessarily, toward the null (i.e., toward finding no effect); see Chapters 9 and 12. Despite these problems, in many topic areas, studies routinely report effect estimates adjusted for potential intermediates. For example, in the coffee–heart disease literature, serum cholesterol is often used for adjustment, despite the potential effects of coffee on serum lipids (Jacobsen and Thelle, 1987; Stensvold et al., 1989; Pietinen et al., 1990; Zock et al., 1990; Salvaggio et al., 1991).

Modifiers of the Effect Measure

Finally, one should also attempt to identify potentially important modifiers of the effect measure under study, especially qualitative effect modifiers, that is, variables for which the study factor has an effect within some but not all categories or has opposite effects across categories. Identification of quantitative effect-measure modifiers will depend on which effect measure is reported.

STUDY IDENTIFICATION

A difficult but crucial task is identifying studies that recorded the exposure and outcome of interest. A search of computerized databases (e.g., MEDLINE) may provide a reasonable start but is often insufficient because not all studies are entered in such databases. In particular, some studies may go unpublished, some may be published only as abstracts or in journals that are not included in the database, and others may obtain relevant data but do not publish those data. Of course, identifying all such data may be impossible, but one should search through each identified report to find references to as yet unidentified reports. One may also inquire among researchers in the topic area to see if they know of unpublished data on the topic.

A systematic relation between study results and chance of inclusion in the meta-analysis (whether through inappropriate exclusion criteria or failure to search thoroughly for studies) will be a source of bias in the meta-analysis. Such study-selection bias is the analogue of subject-selection bias in individual studies and is a major concern in some topic areas. A specific and common form of study-selection bias, described earlier, is *publication bias,* which is the systematic failure to publish or report certain types of results. There is evidence that publication bias is common in epidemiology (Min and Dickersin, 2005), and it will be discussed further in a later section. Restricting one's analysis to published articles may only aggravate this source of study-selection bias. The only safeguard against such biases is to diligently seek out unpublished results, as well as published ones, through methods such as direct inquiry among researchers in the area.

QUANTIFICATION OF EFFECTS

To quantify effects, one needs to specify how effects will be measured. A measure of effect quantifies the change in the occurrence of the study outcome that would result from shifting an entire target population of interest from one exposure level to another (see Chapter 4). The measures used in the overwhelming majority of epidemiologic reports are relative risks, which measure the proportionate change in incidence produced by moving from one exposure level to another. Thus, the relative risk for the effect on myocardial infarction incidence of drinking five cups of coffee per day versus none might be specified as the rate ratio, the proportionate increase in incidence rate produced by coffee drinking among drinkers of five cups per day in a specific cohort after 12 years of follow-up. This effect would ideally be consistently estimated by an adjusted rate ratio for the cohort, were it possible to adjust perfectly for all confounding, misclassification, and loss to follow-up. Of course, other effect measures may be of greater interest—for example, the risk difference is more closely related to models for biologic interaction and public health issues (see Chapter 5)—but few are as commonly reported or as easy to extract from published data as relative-risk estimates.

If the outcome under study is rare in all populations and subgroups under review, one can generally ignore the distinctions among the various measures of relative risk (e.g., risk ratios, rate ratios, and odds ratios). These distinctions can be important, however, when considering common outcomes, especially in case-control design and analysis; see Chapter 4 for more details.

The specification of the population and follow-up in the definition of effect is necessary because there is rarely any basis for believing the effect will be identical across different populations or follow-up periods. Nonetheless, the assumption that a particular effect measure is homogeneous across populations and follow-up periods is often implicit in informal reviews. Given that assumption, the objective of a meta-analysis can be concisely stated as, for example, to estimate the relative risk for the exposure effect on the outcome. Often, the homogeneity assumption is weakened slightly to allow the true (causal) logarithm of the relative risk to vary in a symmetric but random fashion across studies; under this random-effects assumption, the objective usually becomes to estimate the geometric mean relative risk. Occasionally, some measure of spread or variability of relative risks may be of equal or more interest.

Because many factors (both methodologic and biologic) that could affect relative risk estimates will vary across studies, the homogeneity assumption is at best a convenient fiction. Similarly, the variation in these factors will tend to be systematic, making a random distribution for effects a fiction, and any measure of average or spread of relative risks potentially misleading. Thus one should be prepared to question and discard these assumptions, especially if distributions of suspected effect-measure modifiers vary across the source populations of the studies. For example, one study of coffee and myocardial infarction was restricted to women aged 30 to 49 years (Rosenberg et al., 1980). The assumption that the effect estimated from this study equals that found in unrestricted studies (or in studies of men only) should be discarded if much variation in the effect across sex or age is expected or observed. Furthermore, if such variation exists, it is (by definition) systematic variation across sex and age, and therefore not a random effect.

Methodologic variation will also lead to systematic variation in the quantities estimated by different studies. For example, interview data is subject to measurement errors quite different from those of medical record data. Methodologic variation, however, entails variation in bias rather than the actual effect under study, and so is not effect-measure modification. Additionally, unlike actual treatment effect variation, methodologic variation is not of any intrinsic biologic interest for the underlying science or clinical application.

Although the homogeneity assumption can be statistically tested (as described later), the tests have little power in most epidemiologic settings (Greenland, 1983). Consequently, a "nonsignificant" P-value ($P > 0.05$) provides no justification for the assumption. This problem is sometimes partially addressed by requiring a higher cutoff (e.g., $P > 0.20$) before using the assumption.

A more thoughtful approach considers interval estimates for the magnitude of effect-measure variation, as well as contextual expectations (prior information) about whether the chosen effect measure is likely to vary much across studies.

REGRESSION MODELS

Relative risks are convenient to work with when the effects of dichotomous variables are being examined, such as seatbelt use in a study of crash injuries. Nonetheless, when the exposure of interest is a quantity, such as coffee consumption, it is best to take account of differing average exposure levels across the "exposed" categories in different studies (Hertz-Picciotto and Neutra, 1994; Greenland, 1995b). Regression analysis is the easiest way to do this. Chapters 20 and 21 review regression models and methods in general; here we focus on some aspects that are important to meta-analysis.

Specifying a model for effect measures is an important step in a meta-analysis (Greenland, 1987d; Rubin, 1990b). This step need not be highly technical but should be reasonably precise. Within a regression context, the effect measure is the coefficient (or coefficients) for exposure. Consider a follow-up study of coffee and myocardial infarction, with coffee use measured as average cups of coffee per day. Using a proportional-hazards model with coffee coefficient β, e^{β} is the rate ratio (proportionate change in the rate) incurred by a one-cup-a-day increase in coffee use; similarly, e^{β} from a logistic model is the odds ratio (proportionate change in the odds) incurred by a one-cup-a-day increase in coffee use (see Chapter 20). Of course, these causal interpretations presume that all important confounders have been adequately controlled, which may be true in some (but usually not all) studies; even when it is true, selection biases and measurement error will distort the resulting estimate.

In most epidemiologic situations (e.g., rare diseases), the logistic coefficient can be treated as an approximation to the Cox model coefficient (Green and Symons, 1983; Efron, 1988). In either formulation, the coefficient β of exposure in the model is the effect measure. Thus, one could state the primary objectives of a meta-analysis of relative risk as (1) to determine if the exposure coefficient β is nonzero in any of the study populations, and (2) to measure and explain variation in β across studies.

Both the Cox and logistic models are types of exponential (multiplicative) models. Absence of product terms in such models automatically implies a multiplicative relation between exposure and covariate effects, in the following sense: Given a baseline (reference) value x_0 for exposure, the disease rate at exposure level x_1 relative to the rate at exposure level x_0 will always be $\exp[\beta(x_1 - x_0)]$, no matter what the values of the covariates. This relation implies that in a report comparing only two levels of exposure, say, x_1 and x_0, and providing an adjusted estimate of relative risk, RR_a, an estimate b of the regression coefficient β is given by $(\ln RR_a)/(x_1 - x_0)$, where "ln" is the natural logarithm. For example, in a study of coffee consumption and myocardial infarction that compared only drinkers of five cups per day with nondrinkers and gave an adjusted rate-ratio estimate of 2.5, an estimate of the Cox regression coefficient would be $b = (\ln 2.5)/(5 - 0) = 0.18$.

Although exponential models are convenient to work with, the relations they imply may poorly represent the actual exposure and covariate effects. For example, multiplicative exposure–covariate effects are not always biologically realistic. The models also imply exponential dose–response relations between the regressor variables and the incidence measure, which are rarely plausible. For example, the Cox model given earlier for the effect of coffee on myocardial infarction implies that the infarction rate increases exponentially with coffee consumption (holding the other variables constant).

Ideally, the multiplicative-exponential model should be evaluated against various alternative models. If the model fails to hold, however, it can still be used as a device for estimating summary relative risks. Within the central range of the regressors (independent variable and covariates) under study, a fitted model can provide acceptably accurate estimates of relative risks if the latter are not too large, even if the model itself is moderately violated overall (Maldonado and Greenland, 1993b; Greenland and Maldonado, 1994). For example, suppose that the coffee effect on myocardial infarction risk is linear (risk $= \alpha + \beta x$) but that an exponential risk model $= \exp(\alpha + \beta x)$ is fitted to the data, and suppose that in the data substantial proportions of the subjects consume zero cups of coffee per day and five or more cups per day. Then, in typical datasets, $\exp(b5)$, the estimate of relative risk for five cups versus zero cups obtained from the exponential model, will not be far from the result that would have been obtained using the (correct) linear model. On the other hand, if few or no subjects drank 10 or more cups per day, there would usually be upward bias in the estimate $\exp(b10)$ of the relative risk for 10 cups versus zero cups obtained from the model.

STATISTICAL REANALYSIS OF INDIVIDUAL STUDIES

Ideally, one would obtain the raw data from every study that recorded the exposure and outcome of interest, transform these data sets into a common format, merge the datasets together, and analyze the merged data set in a *pooled analysis*. These tasks would require some guidelines. For example, one would have to include a variable that identified the study from which each subject came; this variable would allow one to analyze effect variation across studies. One might also have to devote much labor to producing a common format for data from different studies, especially given the very different and often extensive database problems across studies. For example, some variables (e.g., smoking habits) might not be recorded in some studies, and one would have to assign all subjects from those studies a missing-value code for the unrecorded variables. Nonetheless, statistical methods used for single studies could be applied to the merged data, as long as one handled the missing data properly and analyzed the study identifier as a potential modifying variable (examining products of the study indicators with the exposure variables). More involved methods may be required for continuous outcomes (Higgins et al., 2001).

Unfortunately, the preceding ideal is often unattainable in epidemiologic settings. Original study data may have been discarded, or investigators may refuse to supply their data. Even if they do supply what they believe was the finalized study data, later editing may have made it impossible to replicate closely their earlier published findings and establish any confidence in what they have supplied. Often personnel have changed and the original care taken to ensure data and analysis validity in the published study submission was not fully documented. If (as is more usual) unpublished data cannot be obtained, the meta-analysis has to rely on data available in circulated research reports (e.g., published articles). Because research reports usually present only data reductions and summary statistics rather than complete data, one must resort to rather crude methods for extracting or constructing summary estimates and their standard errors from each study.

EXTRACTION OF ESTIMATES

A large proportion of research reports neither present nor permit extraction of estimates other than of relative risks and multiplicative-exponential model coefficients. Consequently, the remainder of this chapter will treat the objective of the meta-analysis as estimation of either log relative risks or multiplicative-exponential model coefficients.

Extracting an estimate from a published report may involve no more than copying it out of the report, if the report gives the desired estimate and its standard-error estimate. Nonetheless, it is best to check the reported values against other pieces of information both in the text and in graphs. Inconsistencies occur, and may indicate errors in the reported estimates. Garcia-Berthou and Alcaraz (2004) found inconsistencies in over 10% of the computations reported in a sample of articles from *Nature* and the *British Medical Journal*.

If confidence limits are given instead of a standard error (SE), extra computation is required. Consider a relative risk estimate RR with a given 95% lower limit of $\underline{RR}$ and upper limit of $\overline{RR}$. If the confidence limits are proportionally symmetric about the ratio (i.e., if $\overline{RR}/RR = RR/\underline{RR}$), an estimate SE of the standard error is given by $SE = (\ln \overline{RR} - \ln \underline{RR})/3.92$, where $3.92 = 2 \cdot 1.96$ is twice the normal percentile for 95% limits (for 90% confidence limits, the divisor in this formula should be $2 \cdot 1.645 = 3.29$). For a coefficient estimate b and 95% confidence limits of $\overline{b}$ and $\underline{b}$, the estimated standard error would be $(\overline{b} - \underline{b})/3.92$. See Follmann et al. (1992) for a method applicable to analyses of continuous outcomes.

Often, a P-value for the null hypothesis is given instead of a standard error or confidence interval. If the given value is accurate enough (to at least two significant digits if $P > 0.1$ and one digit if $P < 0.1$), one can compute a "test-based" standard-error estimate from $SE = (\ln RR)/Z_p$ or $SE = b/Z_p$, where Z_p is the value of a standard-normal test statistic corresponding to the P-value (e.g., $Z_p = 1.96$ if $P = 0.05$, two-tailed test). Unfortunately, because many reports use few significant digits in presenting P-values, this method can be highly unstable for near-null results, and it breaks down completely if ln RR or b is zero. For example, given RR = 1.1, $P = 0.9$ (two-sided), one can only infer that the estimated RR is between 1.05 and 1.15 and that P is between 0.85 and 0.95, implying that Z_p is between 0.063 and 0.188; consequently, the original data could yield a standard error for b of anywhere from (ln 1.05)/0.188 = 0.26 to (ln 1.15)/0.063 = 2.22, compared with the test-based estimate of (ln 1.1)/0.126 = 0.76.

Another problem with the test-based method is that it gives a biased standard-error estimate when the point estimate is far from the null (Halperin, 1977). For odds ratios and logistic coefficients, this bias will be small in most applications; for other measures, however, such as standardized mortality ratios, the bias can be substantial (Greenland, 1984a). In any case, the applicability of the test-based method is limited by the fact that most reports do not precisely specify P-values unless P is between 0.01 and 0.10, and often not even then.

The remainder of this section presents quantitative methods for extracting estimates from reports with incomplete information. Most of these methods are quite rough and should be regarded as appropriate only when a report does not give sufficient information to allow use of more accurate statistical methods. Nevertheless, even these rough methods require certain minimum pieces of information, and some reports may have to be excluded from a meta-analysis on the basis of inadequate data presentation, or used only in a qualitative analysis of observed direction of association (as in Poole et al., 2006). In such cases, however, it may be possible to contact the authors for additional information. Contact may also be worthwhile if there is doubt about the accuracy of the following methods.

ADJUSTMENTS USING EXTERNAL ESTIMATES OF CONFOUNDING

One frequently finds published results that are partially or wholly unadjusted for known or suspected important confounders. Examples include the lack of adjustment for smoking in the published data of several studies of coffee and heart disease (Yano et al., 1977) and in other reports on the same topic in which smoking adjustment involved only very broad categories (Paul et al., 1968; Jick et al., 1973). In these situations we must estimate the residual confounding left by this lack of confounder control. Such estimation must necessarily be based on those studies of the same outcome that provided data on the effects of the putative confounder. In practice, this adjustment usually requires that one use estimates of confounding derived from data external to the study under review, thus greatly adding to the uncertainty of the results (see Chapter 19).

Factorization of the Relative Risk

One approach to external adjustment is to write the unadjusted (or partially adjusted) relative risk RR_u from the study under review as a product of two terms: $RR_u = RR_a U$, where RR_a is what the relative risk would be after full adjustment for the putative confounder or confounders and U is the multiplicative bias produced by having failed to fully control for the factor (Bross, 1967). Given U, a fully adjusted estimate can be derived from the unadjusted estimate via the equation $RR_a = RR_u/U$.

The problem confronting the reviewer is how to get an acceptable estimate of the bias factor U. Chapter 19 described how one could estimate U from estimates of confounder prevalence and the strength of confounder association with the study exposure and disease, and more generally estimate a distribution for U from prior information about these quantities. Another, simpler approach assumes that one has external data that provide estimates of RR_u and RR_a; one can then estimate U via the equation $U = RR_u/RR_a$. This estimate will be valid only to the extent that the confounding effect (U) of the covariate in question is similar in both the external data and the study under review. Even if it is valid, the estimate of U will itself be subject to statistical error, which in some cases can be estimated and incorporated into the final adjustment (Greenland and Mickey, 1988).

Consider the study by Jick et al. (1973) of coffee and discharge diagnosis of myocardial infarction: An adjusted odds ratio of 2.2 was given for the effect of drinking six or more cups per day versus none, but smoking was treated as the trichotomy ex-smoker/current smoker/other. This treatment raises the possibility that residual confounding by smoking remains because of failure to adjust for the amount smoked by current and former smokers. No comparable published data exist that allow estimation of the confounding effect of amount smoked in the study by Jick et al. Thus, an estimate of this effect will be derived from the study by Rosenberg et al. (1980) on coffee and hospital admission for first myocardial infarction.

From the data in Table 3 of Rosenberg et al. (1980), one can calculate an odds ratio of $RR_u = 1.7$ for the effect of drinking five or more cups per day versus none, adjusted for smoking in the same trichotomy used by Jick et al. (1973). When the adjustment is based on the full smoking detail given in the table (nonsmoker, ex-smoker, smokers of 1 to 14, 15 to 24, 25 to 34, 35 to 44, or 45 or more cigarettes per day), the odds ratio drops to $RR_a = 1.4$. Thus, for the Rosenberg et al. data, the estimate of the confounding produced by controlling smoking only as a trichotomy is $U = 1.7/1.4 = 1.2$. For the Jick et al. study, $RR_u = 2.2$, which may be divided by the external estimate of U, 1.2, to obtain the externally adjusted estimate for the Jick et al. study, $RR_a = 2.2/1.2 = 1.8$.

RR_a is an estimate of what would have been obtained from the Jick et al. study had smoking been controlled in the same detail as in the Rosenberg et al. study. It will be accurate if the joint distributions of coffee, cigarettes, and infarction are similar in both studies. Both studies used hospitalized subjects from the northeastern United States, but the subjects of Jick et al. were 40- to 69-year-old whites and mostly male, whereas the subjects of Rosenberg et al. were 30- to 49-year-old females and 88% white. Furthermore, the exposure and outcome variables are not identical in the two studies: In the Jick et al. study, the exposure is six or more cups per day of any coffee, and the outcome is hospital discharge after hospitalization for myocardial infarction, whereas in the Rosenberg et al. study, the exposure is five or more cups per day of caffeine-containing coffee, and the outcome is hospital admission for myocardial infarction.

As shown in Chapter 19, U depends on the prevalence of the confounder and the associations of the confounder with the study factor and the outcome. In the preceding example, there is no basis for believing that the coffee–smoking association was the same in the two studies, given the associations of coffee use and smoking with age and sex. Thus, the externally adjusted estimate of 1.8 may be considerably overadjusted or underadjusted for smoking, and would have to be regarded as inferior to an estimate that was fully adjusted for smoking and depended only on more complete smoking data in the original Jick et al. study, were it available.

Coefficient Adjustment

To translate the preceding adjustment into an adjustment for a Cox or logistic regression coefficient, let x be the exposure, b_u the unadjusted (or partially adjusted) x coefficient estimate, and b_a the fully adjusted estimate from a study or set of studies. The estimated confounding in estimating the effect of one unit of x is then $U = RR_u/RR_a = \exp(b_u)/\exp(b_a) = \exp(b_u - b_a)$, where RR_a and RR_u now represent the estimated increase in the rate produced by one unit of x. Taking logs, we see that $\ln(U) = b_u - b_a$. Thus, to externally adjust an estimate from a study under review, one must obtain an estimate of $\ln(U)$ from another study (or studies) and subtract this estimate from the coefficient estimate being adjusted.

Continuing the preceding example, an estimate of the logistic regression coefficient for coffee (in cups per day) in the Jick et al. (1973) study is 0.110. This estimate is adjusted for numerous confounders but is adjusted for smoking using only the trichotomy described earlier. The coefficient estimate computed from Table 3 of Rosenberg et al. (1980) is 0.073 after adjustment for smoking in the trichotomy used by Jick et al., but it decreases to 0.046 when adjustment for smoking includes categories of cigarettes per day. Thus, in the Rosenberg et al. study, $\ln(U) = 0.073 - 0.046 = 0.027$. This correction factor applied to the Jick et al. study yields an externally adjusted coefficient of $0.110 - 0.027 = 0.083$. All the caveats discussed for the externally adjusted odds ratio apply to this coefficient estimate as well.

Standard Error of the Externally Adjusted Estimate

Let V_U be an estimate of the variance of $\ln(U)$, and SE the estimated standard error for the unadjusted estimate $\ln RR_u$ or b_u from the study under review. An estimate of the standard error of the externally adjusted estimate $\ln(RR_u/U)$ or $b_u - \ln(U)$ is then $(V_U + SE^2)^{1/2}$. Suppose that RR_c is the crude relative-risk estimate from external data, RR_a is a common relative-risk estimate from the same data (e.g., a Mantel-Haenszel odds ratio or a logistic regression–based odds ratio), $U = RR_c/RR_a$, and V_c and V_a are variance estimates for $\ln RR_c$ and $\ln RR_a$. Then V_U may be estimated by $V_a - V_c$, provided that this quantity is positive (Greenland and Mickey, 1988).

Unfortunately, if one of V_a or V_c is unavailable (as in the examples given here), one will have to employ the crude SE as the standard error of the externally adjusted estimate, and the resulting confidence interval will understate the uncertainty one should have about the final estimate. Nonetheless, there will usually be much more uncertainty about the difference in confounding factors U between the two studies (the one supplying the estimate of U and the one being adjusted), and that uncertainty will be much larger than indicated by the variance estimate V_U.

Bounds for Confounding

As discussed in Chapter 19, one can conduct a sensitivity analysis (seeing how U varies over plausible values for its components) or a Bayesian analysis (averaging results over plausible values for the U components) to take account of this uncertainty. One simple sensitivity analysis places bounds on confounding based on plausible values for the associations that determine the confounding. Consider bounds for the magnitude of confounding in studies involving a dichotomous exposure and a dichotomous confounder. For case-control studies, the bounds are a function of the odds ratios for the associations of the confounder with the exposure and the disease (see Chapter 19). In Rosenberg et al. (1980), the association of current smoking versus nonsmoking seen among nondrinkers of caffeine-containing coffee is around an odds ratio of 3, and the association of current smoking with drinking caffeine-containing coffee among the controls is around an odds ratio of 2. From Table 1 of Yanagawa (1984), a dichotomous confounder with an effect corresponding to an odds ratio of 3 and an association with exposure corresponding to an odds ratio of 2 produce at most a 20% inflation in the odds ratio relating exposure to outcome. This result suggests that the confounding factor U due to current smoking versus nonsmoking must be less than 1.2. Nonetheless, this calculation does not address additional confounding by amount smoked.

Unfortunately, the utility of such confounding bounds is limited. First, for small effects (relative risks less than 2), even a small amount of confounding can be critical; second, in order to compute the bounds, one must know the confounder–exposure association in the source population and the confounder–outcome association conditional on exposure; third, the extent of confounding produced by several variables or a single variable with more than two levels can greatly exceed the bounds computed when treating the exposure variable as a single dichotomy. The data of Rosenberg et al. (1980) provide an example: The crude odds ratio comparing five or more cups per day versus none is 2.0, whereas after logistic-regression adjustment for multiple variables (including multiple smoking levels) it decreases to 1.4. In contrast, the 20% upper bound on confounding based on treating the confounder as a single dichotomy is $1.2(1.4) = 1.7$. Thus, the amount of confounding appears to be much greater than that indicated by the computations for a dichotomous confounder. Note that there is no limit on the amount of confounding that can be produced by a single dichotomous confounder (Greenland, 2003c). Rather, the discrepancy occurs because dichotomization of a confounder with multiple levels can make the degree of confounding appear much less than it actually is.

ADJUSTMENT FOR SELECTION BIAS AND MISCLASSIFICATION

Selection Bias

In rare situations, one can estimate exposure-specific selection probabilities and correct for selection bias from available data (Chapter 19). Occasionally, one may be able to reduce bias in a study by applying more strict exclusion criteria to the subjects and then reanalyzing the study using only the subjects that meet the new criteria. For example, it has been observed that persons who are hospitalized for chronic conditions exhibit lower coffee consumption than either persons hospitalized for acute conditions or persons in the general population (Rosenberg et al., 1981; Silverman et al., 1983). On this basis, one might wish to reanalyze hospital-based case-control studies of coffee effects after excluding controls hospitalized for chronic conditions.

In most situations, there will be sufficient information to reanalyze only the crude data, but in such cases one can parallel external adjustment for confounding. Given a crude log relative-risk (or coefficient) estimate b_c, an uncorrected adjusted estimate b_a, and a corrected crude estimate b_{cc} (e.g., the crude computed after restrictions), one can use $U_c = b_c - b_{cc}$ as a correction factor to obtain a corrected adjusted estimate $b_a - U_c$. The assumption underlying this method is that the selection bias in the crude estimate b_c and the adjusted estimate b_a are the same.

The first Boston Collaborative Drug Surveillance Program study (1972) and the Jick et al. study (1973) of coffee and myocardial infarction were criticized for their use of general hospital control groups. Such control groups, it was argued, would underrepresent coffee consumption in the source population because of reduced coffee consumption among controls with digestive disorders. Rosenberg et al. (1981) and Silverman et al. (1983) offered evidence in support of this hypothesis, showing lower coffee consumption among patients hospitalized for chronic conditions than among patients hospitalized for acute conditions (e.g., fractures). Jick (1981) responded to these criticisms by publishing a comparison of coffee consumption among controls with chronic conditions and those with acute conditions in the Jick et al. study (1973). The data in Jick (1981, Table 1) exhibit an average rate of drinking one to five cups per day that is higher among the acute controls: The (exposure) odds of drinking one to five cups versus none is 3.65 among the acute controls versus 2.61 among all the controls. For six or more cups per day versus none, these figures become 0.44 and 0.45, respectively. The crude logistic coefficient when only the acute controls are used is 0.104, as opposed to 0.108 when all controls are used, indicating a net upward bias of 0.004 when all controls are used. This quantity can be subtracted as a selection-bias correction from the coefficients in the Boston Collaborative Drug Surveillance Program study and the Jick et al. study. When this correction is added to the smoking correction factor of -0.027 estimated in example 2, the total correction becomes -0.031, yielding $0.11 - 0.031 = 0.079$ for Jick et al. in Table 2. The small value of the selection-bias correction is actually in accord with the findings of Rosenberg et al. (1981), because the differences in coffee consumption between acute and chronic controls in the latter report were also not large enough to alter importantly the Jick et al. results.

In theory, the selection-bias correction U can be estimated from other studies, but if the parameters determining bias (here, the selection probabilities and their associations with the study factors) vary across studies, external correction could increase bias. Nevertheless, external estimates may still serve as a starting point for a sensitivity analysis of selection bias, in which one experiments with various plausible values for the selection probabilities to assess the likely effect of bias (Chapter 19).

Misclassification

Given estimates of the classification rates of key measures used in a study and a detailed tabulation of the original data, one can apply correction formulas for misclassification to the tabulation and obtain corrected effect estimates from the resulting corrected tabulations (Chapter 19). If this correction cannot be done, one may of course resort to more informal speculation about the direction and magnitude of the bias. Such speculation may be based on a sensitivity analysis, in which one experiments with plausible values for the data tabulations and classification rates in order to assess the likely effect of misclassification of exposure, disease, or confounders; again, see Chapter 19 for details. Note that confounder misclassification can be as important as exposure and disease misclassification, because misclassification of confounders will introduce confounding into adjusted estimates (Greenland, 1980; see Chapter 9).

REGRESSION ON RATES AND RATIOS

Results concerning an ordered exposure variable are often presented in terms of exposure-level-specific rates or ratios, and these ratios are usually computed without taking account of the ordering of exposure levels. It is often possible to estimate an exposure coefficient from such presentations using approximate inverse-variance weighted methods. The relevant criterion for application of these methods is that the study-specific estimates (log-rate, logit-risk, or log-ratio estimates) are approximately normally distributed. Simulation studies (Howe, 1983; Walker, 1985) indicate that such a criterion will be approximated if the expectations of the counts contributing to the rates or ratios are 4 or greater. Analysis of studies too small to meet such a criterion will be discussed later.

Rates and Risks

If crude or adjusted incidence rates or proportions and their estimated standard errors are given, the coefficient for exposure in an exponential or logistic model may be estimated by weighted linear regression of log rate or logit risk on exposure level. For log person-time rates, the appropriate weights are $(R/\text{SE})^2$, where R is the exposure-specific rate and SE is its standard error on the original (untransformed) scale. For the logit of a proportion, $\ln[R/(1-R)]$, the appropriate weights are $[R(1-R)/\text{SE}]^2$, where R is the exposure-specific proportion (risk). If 95% confidence limits are given instead of standard errors and the limits are arithmetically symmetric about the rates, that is, if $\overline{R}-R = R-\underline{R}$, the standard errors may be estimated as $\text{SE} = (\overline{R}-\underline{R})/3.92$, where $\overline{R}$ and $\underline{R}$ are the upper and lower confidence limits. If 95% confidence limits are given and the limits appear proportionally symmetric about the rates, that is, if $\overline{R}/R = R/\underline{R}$, the standard errors for the rates may be estimated as $\text{SE} = R[\ln(\overline{R}/\underline{R})/3.92]$.

Often, no standard error or confidence interval for the rates is given. If, however, the report gives the size of the denominator for the rate in each exposure group, *ad hoc* approximate standard errors can be computed in the following manner:

1. If N is the amount of person-time contributing to person-time rate R in a group, an *ad hoc* standard error for R is $(R/N)^{1/2}$, yielding a weight of RN for $\ln(R)$.
2. If N and R instead represent the number of persons and proportion with the outcome in a group, an *ad hoc* standard error for R is $[R(1-R)/N]^{1/2}$, yielding a weight of $R(1-R)N$ for logit(R).

These estimates are appropriate if the rates under consideration are crude (unadjusted) rates; otherwise, they may incorporate considerable absolute bias. Because only relative weighting is important for point estimation, no error in the coefficient estimate will arise even if there are biases in the weights, as long as these biases are proportional across exposure levels. Even if the biases are not proportional, they must be large in order to produce large error in the coefficient estimate. Biases in the estimated weights may, however, produce bias in the standard error of the coefficient as computed by the regression program, even if the bias is uniform across exposure groups.

When computing the weighted regression estimates discussed here, the coefficient standard error supplied by standard linear least-squares regression programs will not be valid (Greenland and Engleman, 1988). For univariate regressions, a valid large-sample standard-error estimate may be computed as the inverse square root of the weighted sum of squared deviations of the regressor from its weighted mean. This approach is illustrated next.

The following data on coffee consumption and myocardial infarction incidence are derived from Table 1 of Yano et al. (1977):

Cups of Coffee per Day	Coffee Code	Persons (N)	Directly Age-Standardized Incidence (per 1,000)
0	0.0	1,235	14.5
1–2	1.8	2,484	17.2
3–4	3.4	2,068	19.7
5+	7.0	1,918	16.9

The *ad hoc* standard-error estimate for the zero-cup incidence of $14.5/1{,}000 = 0.0145$ is $[0.0145(1-0.0145)/1{,}235]^{1/2} = 0.00340$, yielding a weight of $0.0145(1-0.0145)1{,}235 = 17.6$; the weights for the remaining incidences are 42.0, 39.9, and 31.9, respectively.

The logit of the zero-cup incidence is $\ln[0.145/(1-0.0145)] = -4.22$; the logits of the remaining incidences are -4.05, -3.91, and -4.06, respectively. Use of these weights for a linear regression of the logits on coffee consumption (coding 1 to 2 cups as 1.8, 3 to 4 cups as 3.4, and 5+ cups as 7, a coding scheme based on the histogram of coffee consumption given in Table 1 of Yano et al.) yields a coefficient estimate of 0.012. The sum of the weights is 131.4; the weighted mean coffee consumption is $[17.6(0.0) + 42.0(1.8) + 39.9(3.4) + 31.9(7.0)]/131.4 = 3.31$; and the weighted sum of squared deviations from this mean is $[17.6(0.0-3.31)^2 + \ldots + 31.9(7.0-3.31)^2] = 723$. This sum yields an estimated standard error for the coffee coefficient of $1/723^{1/2} = 0.0372$.

Standardized Morbidity Ratios Derived Using an External Reference Population

A standardized morbidity ratio (SMR), or observed/expected ratio, is often constructed by computing the expected values based on some external reference population. These external reference rates are usually assumed to be known without error, such as general U.S. population rates. In such instances, an estimate of the exposure coefficient in an exponential regression may be obtained from a weighted linear regression of ln(SMR) on exposure. The appropriate weighting for such a regression is $1/SE^2$, where SE is the standard error of ln(SMR). If proportionally symmetric 95% confidence intervals are given for each SMR, the standard error for ln(SMR) may be estimated as $SE = \ln(\overline{SMR}/\underline{SMR})/3.92$, where $\overline{SMR}$ and $\underline{SMR}$ are the upper and lower confidence limits. If the report gives no standard error or confidence interval but gives A, the number of cases observed in each exposure group, $1/A$ will estimate the squared standard error of ln(SMR), and so A may be taken as the regression weight.

Suppose now that the report does not give standard errors or confidence intervals for SMR or ln(SMR), or the number of cases in each exposure group. If the report gives A_+, the total number of cases of the outcome under study, and for each exposure group gives N, the number of person-years or persons in the group, one can compute a crude "null" weight for each ln(SMR) as NA_+/N_+, where N_+ is the total of the N across groups.

As an example, the initial Framingham report on coffee and heart disease (Dawber et al., 1974) did not provide the total number of cases in each exposure or outcome category. Although the coffee-specific numbers of cases were no longer available, Dr. Paul Sorlie of the National Heart, Lung, and Blood Institute kindly provided an estimate of the total number of myocardial infarction cases. This estimated total number of cases, $A_+ = 138$, and the total number of men starting follow-up, $N_+ = 1{,}992$, were then used to construct crude estimates of the total number of cases expected in each coffee-consumption category under the null hypothesis of no association between coffee and myocardial infarction. For example, the number of drinkers of two cups of coffee per day out of the total starting follow-up was 486 (Dawber et al., 1974, Table 4); the crude null expected number of infarction cases among drinkers of two cups per day is thus $138(486)/1{,}992 = 33.7$, which is taken as the weight for the ln(SMR) for myocardial infarction among drinkers of two cups per day.

An "indirectly adjusted" rate is often defined as the exposure-specific SMR multiplied by the overall crude rate in the reference population (Porta, 2008). Therefore, the aforementioned SMR techniques (and weights) may also be applied with the indirectly adjusted rate replacing SMR. Note that $\ln(SMR) = \ln(R_j) - \ln(R_+)$, where R_j is the exposure-specific indirectly adjusted rate and R_+ is the overall crude rate in the reference population. As a consequence, the coefficients from a regression using indirectly adjusted rates are the same as from SMR regression; only the intercept is changed.

Strictly speaking, comparisons of standardized morbidity ratios (and thus indirectly adjusted rates) with one another are invalid unless all stratum-specific study population rates are a constant multiple of the specific reference population rates (Breslow et al., 1983). Thus, regressions using ln(SMR) as the outcome will be biased unless the latter condition holds. The extent of this bias will be small, however, unless large departures from multiplicativity are present (Breslow et al., 1983).

Ratios Derived Using an Internal Reference Group

When a report presents results in terms of relative-risk estimates that are computed using an internal exposure group as referent, one can perform a weighted linear regression of the log relative risk on exposure. Because the log relative risk for the reference level is necessarily 0 (corresponding to a relative risk of 1), the computations employ only the nonreference exposure groups, and the fitted line must be forced to pass through 0 when the exposure is at the reference level. The latter is easily accomplished with most regression programs by recoding (if necessary) the exposure values so that the reference level is 0 and specifying "no intercept" or "intercept = 0" in the program.

Because the numbers in the reference group are subject to statistical error and are employed in all the log relative-risk estimates, the estimates derived from these numbers will have nonzero covariances. The optimal weighting scheme would take account of these covariances (and would require matrix inversion for derivation), but in most cases the data are not presented in sufficient detail to allow computation of these covariances. If they were, one could merely reanalyze the whole data set by using a nonlinear regression program. The regression may still be performed (with possible bias and loss in efficiency) by weighting each log relative-risk estimate by $1/SE^2$ (where SE is its estimated standard error) and ignoring the covariances among the estimates. Alternatively, one may estimate the covariances using a procedure given by Greenland and Longnecker (1992); see Orsini et al. (2006) for a Stata program to do this.

ESTIMATION FROM REPORTS EMPLOYING ONLY BROAD EXPOSURE CATEGORIES

Many reports treat continuous exposures in a categorical fashion and provide relative-risk estimates only for broad categories of exposure. For example, the study of coffee and myocardial infarction by Klatsky et al. (1973) recorded and analyzed coffee consumption as "six or fewer cups per day/over six cups per day." In such cases, it is necessary to assign numeric values (codes) to the categories before estimating the exposure coefficient from the study. When the categories are broad, results may be sensitive to the method of assignment (Greenland, 1995b, 1995c).

One needs to know the distributions of exposure within categories to make a good assignment, especially when attempting to estimate a nonlinear regression coefficient (as in Cox and logistic models) (Greenland, 1995b, 1995c). If these distributions are unknown, a common method is to assign category midpoints to categories; unfortunately, this method gives no answer for open-ended categories (e.g., "over six cups per day"). An alternative is to assume a distributional shape for exposure (e.g., normality); one can then calculate category means from the category boundaries (Chene and Thompson, 1996).

Suppose now that one has a detailed frequency distribution for exposure, preferably from the data in question but, if not, then from a study of a population with a similar exposure distribution. One may then use this distribution to estimate category means. Consider the distribution of coffee consumption among men in the original Framingham cohort (Dawber et al., 1974; Table 4):

Cups/day	0	1	2	3	4	5	6	7+
Men (N)	170	363	486	381	220	141	102	129

From these data, we see that the mean coffee consumption among drinkers of zero to six cups per day was about 2.5 in the Framingham study. We may use this value as an external estimate of the mean consumption among drinkers of zero to six cups per day in the Klatsky et al. study (1973). This estimate assumes that the distributions in the two studies had similar means among drinkers of zero to six cups per day.

Suppose now that we estimate the mean consumptions in the Klatsky et al. study to be 2.5 in the category zero to six cups and 8.5 in the category 7+ cups. The Mantel-Haenszel odds ratio for seven or more cups versus six or fewer cups was 0.77 in the study (the estimate was computed from the "risk" controls and percentages given in Table 2 of Klatsky et al.). This odds ratio is an estimate of the effect of 8.5 cups versus 2.5 cups per day. We thus solve the equation $\exp[b(8.5 - 2.5)] = 0.77$ to obtain the coefficient estimate $b = \ln(0.77)/(8.5 - 2.5) = -0.044$.

An indication of the sensitivity of the results to the assignments is given by noting that if one had assigned 3 (the category midpoint) to six or fewer cups and 7 to seven or more cups, the coefficient estimate would have been $b = \ln(0.77)/(7 - 3) = -0.065$, or 50% greater. This sensitivity points out the need to use the best information available in making assignments. Note that means are not necessarily the "best" assignment values: Even if one had the true category means, the resulting estimate could still be biased by the categorization (Greenland, 1995c).

ESTIMATION OF COEFFICIENTS FROM REPORTS PRESENTING ONLY MEAN EXPOSURE LEVELS

Before 1980, many reports presented results for continuous exposures in terms of mean exposure levels among cases and noncases, rather than in modern terms of relative-risk estimates or relative-risk functions; such reports still occasionally appear. If such a report supplies a cross-classification of the data by exposure levels and outcome status, crude relative-risk and coefficient estimates can be computed from this cross-classification. If no such cross-classification is reported but standard errors for the means are given, crude logistic coefficient estimates can be constructed by the linear discriminant-function method (Cornfield, 1962). See Greenland (1987d) and Chene and Thompson (1996) for further details and an illustration of this method.

REPORTING THE RESULTS

It is important that a meta-analyst presents the basic details of each study supplying data on the topic under study. This requirement can be met in a table that provides essentials such as the primary author, year, design, crude data, and derived summary estimates of each study, as in Table 33–1. The inclusion of the individual study results allows readers to check the summaries used against what was given in the original reports, and to check meta-analytic results against their own impression

TABLE 33–1

Summary of Reanalyses for Cohort Studies of Coffee and Myocardial Infarction or Coronary Death up to 1992

Study	Outcome	Cases (n)	% ≥ n Cups[a]	Coeff[b]	Standard Error[b]	Weight	Rate Ratio, 5 Cups/d	Follow-up (y)
Klatsky et al. (1973)[c]	M	464	22 ≥ 7	−44	29	1,171	0.80	6
Dawber et al. (1974)	M	322	15 ≥ 5	−39[d]	40	625	0.82	12
Wilhelmsen[e] et al. (1977)	M	60	50 ≥ 5	109	153	43	1.72	12
Heyden et al. (1978)	D	36	13 ≥ 5	−44[d]	76	5	0.80	4.5
Murray et al. (1981)	D	721	31 ≥ 5	−4	19	2,921	0.98	11.5
La Croix et al. (1986)	C	37	13 ≥ 5	86	58	294	1.54	25
Jacobsen et al.[e] (1986)	D	941	37 ≥ 5	−3	19	2,887	0.99	11.5
Yano et al. (1987)	C	730	25 ≥ 5	49	36	766	1.28	15
LeGrady et al. (1987)	D	232	53 ≥ 4	82	27	1,351	1.51	19
Klatsky et al. (1990)	M	724	17 ≥ 4	68	19	2,746	1.40	5
Grobbee et al. (1990)	DM	221	20 ≥ 4	4	30	1,076	1.02	2
Tverdal et al.[e] (1990)	D	184	57 ≥ 5	86	35	825	1.54	6.4
Rosengren and Wilhelmsen[e] (1991)	DM	399	44 ≥ 5	31	26	1,504	1.17	7.1
Lindsted et al. (1992)	D	NG	10 ≥ 3	86	21	2,166	1.53	26

C, coronary disease incidence; D, coronary death; DM, coronary death or myocardial infarction; M, myocardial infarction (La Croix et al., 1986, included angina); NG, quantity not given in study report.

[a] Percentage of cohort drinking at least given number of cups per day; for example, 22 ≥ 5 indicates 22% of subjects reported drinking five or more cups per day.

[b] Times 1,000, rounded to nearest thousandth. Coefficients represent estimated increments in log rate or logit risk per cup of coffee per day.

[c] Case-control within cohort (nested case-control) study.

[d] "Corrected" coefficient: uncorrected coefficient plus external adjustment.

[e] Scandinavian study.

or analysis of the table. Reanalysis by others can be especially important in literature overviews, as meta-analyses can be done many ways and need not resolve conflicts and controversies. A prominent example of a failed replication of a published meta-analysis involved mammographic screening for breast cancer, in which a reanalysis attributed all the negative conclusions of the original meta-analysis to errors in the latter (Freedman et al., 2004).

STATISTICAL METHODS FOR META-ANALYSIS

The fundamental meta-analytic approach emphasized here is based on weighted regression, which treats each study result b (where b is either a log relative risk or coefficient estimate) as the dependent variable with an accompanying weight. If sufficient data from each study are available, a likelihood-based approach can be used, but the weighted approach is simpler to understand and to apply, and the required computations can be carried out more easily (Chapter 8.4 of Cox, 2006). Furthermore, if the study likelihoods are approximately normal—which will be the situation when all the studies have adequate size—the results of the two approaches will be close.

The conventional statistical component of a study weight, w, is the inverse variance or precision of the result, computed from the estimated standard error, SE, as $1/\text{SE}^2$. This quantity need not (and arguably should not) be the only component of the weight; for example, discarded studies are studies with zero weight, regardless of the value of $1/\text{SE}^2$. There can sometimes be good reason for downweighting but not discarding a study, as when the uncertainty of a result is not entirely reflected by the computed standard-error estimate (Cox, 1982). This added uncertainty can be especially large when there are uncontrolled sources of potential bias. For example, after external adjustment, one could legitimately argue that the weight of the corrected coefficient should be less than that computed from the standard error of the original unadjusted estimate, because the original standard error reflects neither the error in estimating the correction term nor the bias from applying the correction to a new, noncomparable study setting. Decisions to discard or downweight studies based on unquantified problems (e.g., questions of case identification) need careful explanation in the report, however, and should best be made before the statistical meta-analysis, lest they be influenced by the results of the latter.

It can be problematic to determine the appropriate degree of downweighting. Although suspect results or extreme "outliers" among the results can often be identified, one usually cannot quantify all the error beyond that reflected in the original standard-error estimate. Furthermore, downweighting cannot rectify problems that tend toward a particular direction, such as biases from simple forms of classification error. These problems can be dealt with to some extent via sensitivity and influence analysis, as discussed in Chapter 19 and at the end of this section, respectively. An alternative to downweighting that does account for directional problems is bias analysis using prior distributions for study-specific bias parameters in the meta-analysis (Eddy et al., 1992; Greenland, 2003c, 2005b; Chapter 19).

BASIC METHODS

Descriptive and Graphical Analyses

In addition to study description (e.g., number of cases and noncases), a review should present a table of the results of the study reanalyses, showing at least the point estimate, net correction, and standard error or confidence interval from each study. Such tables can make it easy to detect patterns in the results as well as facilitate reanalysis of the meta-analysis by third parties. When there are many studies, a graphical picture can be provided by a weighted histogram of the study results (Greenland, 1987d) or by a plot of the study-specific confidence intervals (Walker et al., 1988) or other study-specific summaries.

Tables 33–1 and 33–2 present the results of reanalyses of studies of coffee consumption and myocardial infarction or sudden coronary death published up to 1992, and one unpublished study by Ulrik Gerdes from the same period; it omits one small case-control study of 64 myocardial infarction patients (Mann and Thorogood, 1975). Details of the studies and their selection are omitted here; see Greenland (1993e) for further information, as well as a discussion of the studies through 1992 as they pertain to possible effects of coffee on heart disease. Studies of this topic continue to be

TABLE 33–2

Summary of Reanalyses for Case-Control Studies of Coffee and Myocardial Infarction or Coronary Death up to 1992

Study	Outcome	Cases (*n*)	% ≥ *n* Cups[a]	Coeff[b]	Standard Error[b]	Weight	Rate Ratio, 5 cups/d
Boston Collaborative (1972)	M	276	9 ≥ 6	66	36	772	1.39
Jick et al. (1973)	M	440	11 ≥ 6	79	24	1,736	1.48
Hennekens et al. (1976)	D	649	NG	30	43	538	1.16
Wilhelmsen et al.[c] (1977)	M	230	50 ≥ 5	62	23	1,890	1.36
Rosenberg et al. (1987)	M	491	22 ≥ 5	70	22	2,141	1.42
Rosenberg et al. (1988)	M	1541	28 ≥ 5	74	15	4,526	1.45
La Vecchia et al. (1989)	M	262	23 ≥ 4	120	46	465	1.82
Gerdes[c] (1992)	M	57	61 ≥ 5	31	52	367	1.17

D, coronary death; M, myocardial infarction.
[a] Percentage of controls drinking at least given number of cups per day; for example, 22 ≥ 5 indicates 22% of subjects reported drinking five or more cups per day.
[b] Times 1,000, rounded to nearest thousandth. Coefficients represent estimated increments in log rate or logit risk per cup of coffee per day.
[c] Scandinavian study.

published and continue to exhibit somewhat conflicting results (e.g., Klag et al., 1994; Palmer et al., 1995; Willett et al., 1996; and Stensvold et al., 1996).

The studies in Tables 33–1 and 33–2 were reanalyzed as necessary by the methods described earlier. Net correction values represent estimated corrections to the original coefficients, primarily for incomplete smoking adjustment. Because of space limitations, the derivations of all the quantities in the tables are not given here; the earlier examples provide representative illustrations. The findings of this meta-analysis are insensitive to the exact values of these quantities.

One can construct and compare separate tables, histograms, and plots for different subgroups of studies (e.g., case-control vs. cohort studies). If the studies have associated quantitative characteristics (e.g., year of conduct), their point and interval estimates can be plotted against these characteristics. Bimodal (or multimodal) distributions are indicative of two (or multiple) distinct sets of studies with different expectations for their effect estimates; one may be able to identify a factor associated with proximity to a particular mode. Similarly, outlier studies may be identified in a histogram or graph, and one may be able to identify some characteristics unique to the outlier as possible explanations of the results.

One may sometimes be alerted to bias in the identification of studies by the shape of the histogram of study results (Light and Pillemer, 1984). For example, if a review is based solely on published reports and there is a bias against publishing studies that report no effect, the histogram of results from published reports will be depressed in the region of zero effect. As a consequence, if the study exposure has no effect, the histogram will likely show a bimodal distribution with clusters of positive and negative estimates; if the study exposure has an effect, the histogram will likely show a distribution skewed away from 0. In either case, one should expect to see the pattern most strongly among studies with smaller weight, such as small studies, because small studies are more likely to go unpublished (Dickersin, 1990).

Another graphical method of identifying possible divergence in study results is the funnel display (Light and Pillemer, 1984), in which results are plotted against a measure of precision, such as sample size or weight. If all studies are estimating a similar value for the effect, the spread of results should become narrow as precision increases, forming a funnel-like shape if enough studies are plotted. As with histograms, such displays may also signal the existence of a bias in the identification of studies via gaps in the display. For example, underrepresentation of studies reporting no effect will result in a gap or sparsity of the display in the region around zero effect and low precision. Unfortunately, large numbers of studies are needed to distinguish actual from imagined patterns (Dickersin and Berlin, 1992; Greenland, 1994d). A test for publication bias in a funnel display is given by Begg and Mazumdar (1994); unfortunately this test has very low power in typical settings. Model-based methods for sensitivity analysis of certain types of publication bias have also been proposed (Copas, 1999; Shi and Copas, 2002).

One can graphically summarize studies by plotting the point estimates and confidence intervals. Some care is needed in the scaling of such a plot. The relative-risk scale has the disadvantage of making a confidence interval from, say, 0.2 to 1.0 appear much more precise than a confidence interval from 1.0 to 5.0, even though both intervals would arise from the same degree of imprecision (statistical variability) on the log scale. This problem can be avoided by plotting the relative risks on a logarithmic scale (Rifat, 1990). (Note that logistic and Cox model coefficients correspond to log relative-risk estimates, and so require no transformation before plotting.) See Chapter 17 for further discussion of plot scaling. Walker et al. (1988) have studied the statistical properties of certain summaries derived by plotting relative-risk confidence intervals.

Weighted Averages

A weighted mean (or pooled summary) $\bar{b}$ of the study results is a weighted sum of the results, $\sum wb$, divided by the sum of the weights, $\sum w$. Table 33–3 gives $\bar{b}$, separately calculated using precision (inverse-variance) weights $w = 1/\text{SE}^2$ for the cohort studies and case-control studies. It also provides the conversion of each $\bar{b}$ into a rate-ratio estimate for the effect of five cups per day versus none via the formula $\exp[\bar{b}(5-0)]$.

The appropriateness of the precision-weighted mean as a meta-analytic summary of the effect under study depends on a very stringent homogeneity assumption. This assumption states that the studies are estimating the same value for the effect; that is, after considering the extent of real effect and bias in each study, the studies should on average yield the same value, so that differences between the estimates are due entirely to random error. Under this assumption, the precision-weighted mean is an appropriate estimate of the (common) value being estimated by the studies, and an estimate s of the standard error of this mean is the inverse of the square root of the sum of the weights, $s = 1/(\sum w)^{1/2}$. Approximate 95% confidence limits for the assumed common value are given by $\exp(\bar{b} \pm 1.96s)$. A test statistic for whether the assumed common value is 0 is given by $Z = \bar{b}/s$, which has an approximate standard normal distribution if the assumed common value is 0.

TABLE 33–3

Summary Statistics for Meta-Analysis

		All Cohort		Cohort	
	Case-Control	Fixed[a]	Random	Later (≥ 1986)	Earlier (≤ 1981)
Average coefficient ($\bar{b}$)[b]	70.20	31.40	32.50	48.50	−17.40
Standard error (SE) of ($\bar{b}$)[b]	9.00	7.40	13.30	8.60	14.50
Rate ratio (RR) for 5 cups/d[c]	1.42	1.17	1.18	1.27	0.92
95% Confidence limits for RR	1.30, 1.55	1.09, 1.26	1.03, 1.34	1.17, 1.39	0.80, 1.06
Z-statistic ($\bar{b}$/SE)	7.83	4.26	2.46	5.65	−1.20
Homogeneity chi-squared	2.93	35.10		17.40	2.34
Degrees of freedom	7	13		8	4
Homogeneity P-value	0.89	0.0008		0.03	0.67

All computations are based on the corrected coefficients. "Fixed" refers to fixed-effects mean; "random" to random-effects mean.
[a] Valid only under homogeneity hypothesis.
[b] Times 1,000; $\bar{b}$ is weighted-average coefficient using inverse-variance weights; SE is square root of inverse sum of weights.
[c] Estimated weighted geometric mean rate ratio $\exp(5\bar{b})$.

Table 33–3 also provides these statistics separately for the case-control and cohort studies in Tables 33–1 and 33–2.

If tabular data are available from each study, one may be able to construct summary estimates of a common effect via Mantel-Haenszel or maximum-likelihood methods (see Chapter 15). Although based on the same homogeneity assumption as the precision-weighted mean b, these estimates have better statistical properties than $\bar{b}$ when several of the studies are very small. Unfortunately, many reports do not provide enough information to allow them to contribute directly to a summary based on these methods.

Homogeneity Assumptions versus Reality

As many authors have stressed, analysis of heterogeneity can be the most important function of meta-analysis, often more important than computing a fictional common or "average" effect (Pearson, 1904; Light and Pillemer, 1984; Greenland, 1987d, 1994d; L'Abbe et al., 1987; Bailey, 1987; Rubin 1990b, 1992; Dickersin and Berlin, 1992; Hertz-Picciotto and Neutra, 1994; Thompson, 1994; Pettiti, 1994b; Berlin, 1995). Finding or confirming systematic variation in study results, along with exploring such variation, can be particularly valuable in planning further studies, because one might want to concentrate resources on populations in which effects are strongest and to identify study designs that give the most accurate results for the problem at hand.

There is ordinarily no basis for assuming that the true relative risk or coefficient is constant across study populations. In fact, many situations imply heterogeneity instead; for example, simple variation in background rates can produce large variation in the rate ratio, if the exposure effect is to add a constant amount to the background rate (see Chapters 4 and 15). Thus, whereas the pooled statistics given thus far may be useful for detecting the existence of an effect, it will always be more accurate to picture the effect as a function of other variables rather than as a single number (Greenland, 1987d; Rubin, 1992). The typical range of this function may be a useful summary but cannot in general be estimated accurately. Unfortunately, the standard error and confidence limits given earlier for the common effect will not adequately reflect the variability and range of effects if important heterogeneity is present.

Even if the effect of a single well-defined exposure is assumed constant across every study population, there will still be little reason to assume that the estimates will not vary systematically across studies, because some bias is usually present in nonexperimental studies and this bias will vary across studies. In addition, the exposure being studied will usually vary somewhat across studies, and this will contribute to variation in effect. For example, some studies of coffee and myocardial infarction measured coffee consumption at a baseline examination, whereas other studies measured coffee consumption immediately before the outcome event. This is not just a difference in measurement, but a difference in the actual exposure being measured. Despite such differences, both types of study address the same general issue of whether coffee consumption affects infarction risk and so would be included in the same review.

To summarize, one should regard any homogeneity assumption as extremely unlikely to be satisfied, given the differences in covariates, bias, and exposure variables among the studies. The question at issue in employing the assumption is whether the existing heterogeneity is small enough relative to other sources of variation to be reasonably ignored. A statistical test of homogeneity can serve as a warning light with high specificity but low sensitivity: Small P-values indicate that the heterogeneity should not be ignored, but large P-values do not indicate that it can be safely ignored. The same warning applies to tests of publication bias, and for that matter, to all statistical tests; see Chapter 10.

Basic Statistical Analysis of Heterogeneity

The most elementary form of heterogeneity analysis involves pairwise comparisons of studies. Given a pair of studies, the difference between their results has a standard error equal to the square root of the sum of the squared standard errors of the two results. This standard error of the difference can be used to construct confidence limits and a test statistic for the difference between the two studies.

In Table 33–2, the difference in the coefficient estimates from the Jick et al. (1973) and Hennekens et al. (1976) studies is $0.079 - 0.031 = 0.048$; this has a standard-error estimate of $(0.024^2 + 0.043^2)^{1/2} = 0.049$. The point estimate for the ratio of the estimated effects of x = five cups per day from the two studies is then $\exp[0.048(5)] = 1.3$, with 95% confidence limits of $\exp\{[0.048 \pm$

$1.96(0.049)]5\} = 0.79, 2.1$. The Z-statistic is $0.048/0.049 = 0.98$, which yields $P = 0.3$. This type of finding, essentially indeterminate with respect to homogeneity, is probably the most common outcome of single-study comparisons. More helpful results can often be obtained by grouping of studies or by meta-regression, as discussed below.

For multiple studies, a statistical test of the homogeneity assumption is given by $X_h^2 = \sum w(b - \bar{b})^2$, which, if the studies are estimating the same value for the effect, has a chi-squared distribution with degrees of freedom one less than the number of studies. When only two studies are being tested, X_h^2 is just the square of the Z-statistic for comparing two studies. For all the studies in Tables 33–1 and 33–2, $X_h^2 = 49$ on 21 degrees of freedom ($P = 0.0005$). Table 33–3 gives X_h^2 and the corresponding degrees of freedom and P value for the cohort and case-control studies considered separately. The P value from all studies is very small, in part because of the disparity between the cohort and case-control results and in part because of the heterogeneity among the cohort-study results.

Because a large P-value should not be taken as justifying the homogeneity assumption, one should always refer to the tabular and visual displays to see if the spread of results appears consistent with the notion of only random differences among the studies. A graphical check of statistical variation in the results can be obtained by placing the Z-scores, $(b - \bar{b})/\text{SE}$, in a histogram; under the hypothesis of only random differences among the studies, this histogram should have an approximately normal shape. Large absolute Z-scores can signal important departures of individual studies from the average result.

The homogeneity assumption can be further assessed by partitioning the studies along characteristics likely to be associated with heterogeneity. For instance, suppose that the studies are partitioned into K groups numbered 1 to K (e.g., two groups: group 1 consisting of the cohort studies and group 2 consisting of the case-control studies), within which the homogeneity assumption is thought to hold approximately. Let $\bar{b}_k$ be the precision-weighted mean result within group k, w_k the sum of weights from group k, and $s_k = 1/w_k^{1/2}$ the estimated standard error of $\bar{b}_k$. The estimated difference between the quantities being estimated in groups i and j is $\bar{d}_{ij} = \bar{b}_i - \bar{b}_j$ under the assumption of within-group homogeneity, this has a standard-error estimate $s_d = (1/w_i + 1/w_j)^{1/2}$. If x represents an exposure difference of interest, then $\exp(\bar{d}_{ij}x)$ is a point estimate of the ratio of the relative risks from the two groups, and $\exp[(\bar{d}_{ij} \pm 1.96s_d)x]$ is a 95% confidence interval for this ratio; a Z-statistic for the hypothesis of no difference between the groups is $Z_g = \bar{d}_{ij}/s_d$.

The difference between the case-control and cohort results in Tables 33–1 and 33–2 is $\bar{d}_{21} = \bar{b}_2 - \bar{b}_1 = (0.070 - 0.031) = 0.039$, with standard-error estimate $s_d = (1/18{,}380 + 1/12{,}435)^{1/2} = 0.012$. The point estimate and 95% confidence limits, respectively, for the ratio of the case-control and cohort estimated effects of x = five cups per day are then $\exp[0.039(5)] = 1.2$ and $\exp([0.039 \pm 1.96(0.012)]5) = 1.1, 1.4$. The Z-statistic is $0.039/0.012 = 3.3$, yielding $P = 0.001$. These results indicate that the case-control studies have tended to estimate a larger value for the coffee effect than the cohort studies. Nevertheless, the confidence interval is too narrow because of the severe heterogeneity among the cohort studies, which results in $s_d = 0.012$ being an underestimate.

A global test statistic for any difference among groups is given by $X_g^2 = \sum w_k(\bar{b}_k - \bar{b})^2$, where $\bar{b}$ is the precision-weighted mean of all the studies. If all the studies are estimating a common value, X_g^2 will have a chi-squared distribution with degrees of freedom equal to one less than the number of groups. Note that $\bar{b}$ can be computed directly from the $\bar{b}_k$ via the formula $\bar{b} = \sum w_k \bar{b}_k / \sum w_k$, where the sums are over k; the standard-error estimate for $\bar{b}$ is $s = 1/(\sum w_k)^{1/2}$. From Table 33–3, $X_g^2 = 18{,}380(0.031 - 0.047)^2 + 12{,}435(0.070 - 0.047)^2 = 11$, with one degree of freedom, which yields $P = 0.001$. To within rounding error, X_g^2 is the square of $Z_g = 3.3$ from the last example, and $\bar{b} = 0.047 = [18{,}380(0.031) + 12{,}435(0.070)]/(18{,}380 + 12{,}435)$.

If there is important within-group heterogeneity (i.e., heterogeneity unaccounted for by the grouping variable), s_d will tend to underestimate the true standard error of $\bar{d}_{ij}$; as a consequence, the confidence interval and test based on s_d will not be valid. One may test for within-group heterogeneity by computing the residual-heterogeneity chi-squared $X_r^2 = X_h^2 - X_g^2$. The degrees of freedom for X_r^2 is equal to the difference between the number of studies and the number of groups. For the studies in Tables 33–1 and 33–2, $X_r^2 = 49 - 11 = 38$ on $22 - 2 = 20$ degrees of freedom, $P = 0.001$, strongly indicative of heterogeneity within the case-control or cohort groups. As may be apparent from Tables 33–1 and 33–2, this result is attributable to severe heterogeneity among the cohort studies, especially between the earlier (pre-1982) and later (post-1985) cohort studies. There is no more heterogeneity among the case-control studies than one would expect from sampling variation.

META-REGRESSION METHODS

If more than two groups of studies have been formed and the characteristic used for grouping is ordered, greater power to identify sources of heterogeneity may be obtained by regressing study results on the characteristic. Such *meta-regression* or *effect-size modeling* also allows simultaneous examination of multiple characteristics.

With meta-regression, it is not necessary or even desirable to group the studies. Instead, the individual study results can be entered directly in the analysis. For example, suppose that for each cohort study one has the follow-up time t, in addition to a coefficient estimate b and a weight w. Consider a simple linear model for the dependence of the study-specific expected coefficient on time t: $E(b|t) = \mu + \theta t$. The parameters in this model can be estimated using any standard linear-regression program that allows the use of weights. Each study becomes a "subject" (observed unit) in the input data file. In this meta-analysis file, the coefficient estimate b is the outcome or dependent variable for each study, and the follow-up time t is the independent variable. The coefficient estimate $\hat{\theta}$ given by the program then serves as an estimate of the "meta-coefficient" θ in the linear model for $E(b|t)$. If x is an exposure difference of interest and b represents change in log rate or logit risk per unit change in exposure, $\exp(\hat{\theta}\Delta tx)$ is an estimate of the ratio of the relative risk being estimated by studies with a follow-up time of $t + \Delta t$ to the relative risk estimated by studies with a follow-up time of t.

Two useful quantities produced by a meta-regression are the residual degrees of freedom and the residual sum of squares. The residual degrees of freedom df is the number of studies used in the regression minus the number of parameters in the model (intercept and meta-coefficients). In a regression of the cohort-study estimates in Table 33–1 on follow-up time, df would be 12:14 studies minus two parameters, μ and θ. The weighted residual sum of squares, RSS, from the meta-regression is the weighted sum of the squared residuals,

$$\text{RSS} = \sum w_k(b_k - \hat{b}_k)^2$$

where $\hat{b}_k$ is the fitted (predicted) value of the coefficient in study k and the sum is over all the studies in the regression. In a regression of estimates on follow-up times, $\hat{b}_k = \hat{\mu} + \hat{\theta} t_k$, where t_k is the follow-up time for study k. Some regression programs provide a residual mean square (RMS) instead of a residual sum of squares, which varies somewhat in its definition (Greenland and Engelman, 1988) but is usually RSS/df.

The residual sum of squares may be used as a chi-squared statistic (with df degrees-of-freedom) for the fit of the preceding model. Large values of the residual sum of squares may arise if $E(b|t)$ depends on t in a nonlinear fashion or if $E(b|t)$ is heterogeneous within levels of t. Although a small P-value from this statistic indicates that the model is insufficient to account for the observed variation in the study results, a large P-value should not be interpreted to mean that the model adequately explains all of this variation.

Under the assumption that the regression model is correct, $\hat{\theta}$ has an approximate standard-error estimate of $\hat{\sigma} = s_\theta/(\text{RMS})^{1/2}$, where s_θ is the standard error of $\hat{\theta}$ given by the program and RMS is the residual mean square given by the program (Wallenstein and Bodian, 1987). From these quantities, approximate 95% confidence intervals can be constructed as $\hat{\theta} \pm 1.96\hat{\sigma}$, and an approximate Z (standard normal)-statistic can be constructed as $\hat{\theta}/\hat{\sigma}$. If, however, the regression model is inadequate (as would be indicated by a large value for RSS), $\hat{\sigma}$ will tend to underestimate the standard error of $\hat{\theta}$, and the interval and P-value based on $\hat{\sigma}$ will not be valid. In such cases, one should seek other regression variables that explain the residual variation.

The regression approach can be used to compare results of a study or a group of studies with the remaining studies by adding to the meta-regression an indicator variable for the study or group of studies. The estimated meta-coefficient of this variable is an estimate of the difference between the value estimated by that study or group and the value estimated by the remaining studies; the standard error of the meta-coefficient equals the estimated standard error of this difference.

To compare case-control with cohort results in Table 33–1, one could perform a meta-regression of study results on an indicator variable coded 1 = cohort, 0 = case-control. The estimated coefficient for this variable, $\hat{\theta}$, would be the difference, −0.039, between the average fixed-effects coefficients of the cohort and the case-control studies. The estimated standard error of the coefficient, $\hat{\sigma}$, would equal the estimated standard error of this difference, $s_d = 0.012$, as calculated earlier.

Indicators can simultaneously be added for several groups of studies; the meta-coefficients of these indicators represent differences between group average coefficients and the average coefficients for the studies not coded into a group. Heterogeneity across several characteristics can also be simultaneously analyzed by employing weighted multiple regression of results on the characteristics. Such analyses may reveal and adjust for confounding among the characteristics.

As can be seen in Tables 33–1 and 33–3, among the cohort studies, publication year is strongly associated with the magnitude of relative-risk estimate. Because this association is difficult to explain, it is of special interest to see whether it is reduced by adjustment for other factors. To this end, the cohort study coefficients b were regressed simultaneously on study location (1 = Scandinavian; 0 = other), length of follow-up, and publication year, using a standard multiple regression program. The fit of the model with only these variables was excellent (RSS = 9.7 on $14 - 4 = 10$ df, $P = 0.47$). Table 33–4 summarizes the model results. The P values for fit and for publication year cannot be regarded as valid because the data led to the recognition and inclusion of publication year. Nevertheless, the results do suggest that much of the heterogeneity seen in the earlier examples cannot be "explained" (in the statistical sense) by differences in study location or follow-up time.

Regression methods are not limited to examining simple linear dependencies. For example, one can transform the dependent variable b or the regressors before doing the meta-regression by using $\ln(t)$ in the previous formulas; or one can add terms to the meta-regression such as a quadratic term t^2. In fact, the full range of regression models and methods (Chapters 20 and 21) may be employed in meta-analysis, with limitations arising chiefly from lack of data. For example, the dependency of relative risks on background (unexposed) risks cannot be examined among case-control studies, because the latter usually do not provide information on background risks.

Greenland and Longnecker (1992) discuss methods for dose–response meta-analysis when category-specific relative-risk estimates are available from a number of studies. They focus on evaluation of quadratic components of trend. A more general approach involves the use of scatter-plot smoothers (Hastie and Tibshirani, 1990; Hastie et al., 2001), which impose no shape restriction on the dose–response curve other than smoothness (see Chapters 17 and 21). Currently, the chief drawback of such analyses is the need for special software for implementation. See Greenland

TABLE 33–4

Results of Multiple-Linear Regression Analysis of Cohort-Study Coefficients

	Location[a]	Follow-up (y)	Publication Year (minus 1973)
Meta-coefficient ($\hat{\theta}$)[b]	−26.8	1.08	6.41
Standard error ($\hat{\sigma}$)[b]	17.0	1.04	1.39
Estimated ratio of rate ratios[c]	0.87	1.10	1.67
95% Confidence limits	0.74, 1.03	0.92, 1.33	1.34, 2.08
Z-statistic ($\hat{\theta}/\hat{\sigma}$)	−1.58	1.04	4.60
P-Value from Z	0.12	0.30	<0.0001

Residual chi-squared = 9.7 on 10 df, $P = 0.47$.

[a] 1, if Scandinavia; 0, otherwise.

[b] Times 1,000.

[c] Estimated *ratio* of rate ratios for the effect of five cups a day of coffee. Compares Scandinavian versus non-Scandinavian studies for location, 20 years versus 2 years for follow-up, and 1990 versus 1974 for publication year; computed as $\exp[\hat{\theta}(5)]$ for location, $\exp[\hat{\theta}(18)5]$ for follow-up, and $\exp[\hat{\theta}(16)5]$ for publication year.

(1994d) for an example of a smoother applied to the coffee–coronary heart disease studies in Table 33–1.

Sensitivity and Influence Analysis

Given the regression format, regression diagnostic procedures (e.g., residual analysis) can be used to improve the meta-analysis. Two methods of particular utility are sensitivity analysis and influence analysis.

As discussed in Chapter 19, sensitivity analysis examines how inferences change with variations in or violations of assumptions, corrections, and models. For example, one may have externally controlled for cigarette smoking in all studies that failed to control for smoking by subtracting a bias-correction factor from the unadjusted coefficients in those studies. The sensitivity of inferences to the assumptions about the bias produced by failure to control for smoking can be checked by repeating the meta-analysis using other plausible values of the bias, or by varying the correction across studies. If such reanalysis produces little change in the confidence interval, one can say that the limits appear to be insensitive to assumptions about confounding by smoking. On the other hand, one may find that the interval appears to be deceptively precise relative to the variation that can be produced by varying assumptions, and thus choose to base the meta-analysis only on those studies that present results adjusted for smoking. In the present example, the disparity between the case-control and cohort results is not much changed by dropping the correction factors or inflating them by 50%; in other words, the observation of a disparity is fairly insensitive to the correction factors. Likewise, the disparity is fairly insensitive to the values of the standard-error estimates.

In influence analysis, the extent to which inferences depend on a particular study or group of studies is examined; this can be accomplished by varying the weight of that study or group. Thus, in looking at the influence of a study, one could repeat the meta-analysis without the study, or perhaps with half its usual weight. In looking at the influence of a group of studies, say, all case-control studies, one can again repeat the meta-analysis without them, or give them a smaller weight. If change in weight of a study produces little change in an inference, inclusion of the study cannot produce a serious problem, even if unquantified biases exist in the study. On the other hand, if an inference hinges on a single study or group of studies, one should refrain from making that inference. In the present example, the disparity between the case-control and cohort results is not much changed by dropping any one study; in other words, the observation of a disparity was not unduly influenced by any one study.

Random-Effects Models

The models used earlier are fixed-effects models, in that within groups or levels of the regressors, each study is assumed to be estimating the same value for β, the exposure coefficient. This is essentially a within-group homogeneity assumption, and as such cannot be realistic. If a large amount of unexplained heterogeneity remains after fixed-effect regression modeling (e.g., as indicated by failure to find a good-fitting and sensible fixed-effects model), one should consider turning to random-effects models, in which the meta-regression model is augmented by the addition of a term representing unexplained sources of between-study heterogeneity (DerSimonian and Laird, 1986; Stijnen and van Houwelingen, 1990; Berlin et al., 1993).

As an example, the earlier model for the dependence of the expected study coefficient on follow-up time could become

$$E(b|t) = \mu + \theta t + \varepsilon$$

where ε is a normal (Gaussian) random variable with mean 0 and unknown variance τ^2; ε is assumed to be independent with identical variance across studies. Here, ε represents the component of between-study variation (modification) of the coffee log risk ratio that is unaccounted for by linear effects θt of follow-up time. In the context of meta-analysis, a random effect such as ε is more accurately viewed as random-effect modification, random bias, or some combination of the two.

The assumption that both modification (heterogeneity) and bias are randomly distributed across the studies is a strong one, and (as with the fixed-effects model) the model does not account for systematic variation in effects or bias across studies. Nonetheless, the fixed-effects analysis is essentially a special case of the random-effects analysis, with the added assumption that $\tau^2 = 0$ (or, equivalently, that all the ε are 0), which is the homogeneity assumption within levels of the regressor t; it is thus based on the same strong assumptions, and more.

Random-effects meta-regression requires an iterative procedure in which the study weights w are updated at each cycle. In addition, one must make corrections to the estimated standard errors to take account of uncertainty about the residual variance τ^2. See, for example, Stijnen and van Houwelingen (1990) for details.

The random-effects extension usually does little to change the point estimates from meta-regression but can considerably widen the confidence intervals (Dickersin and Berlin, 1992). Nonetheless, it is possible for the random-effects coefficient to move far enough away from the null (e.g., as a result of publication bias) so that the exposure or treatment P-value becomes smaller than in the fixed-effects analysis (Poole and Greenland, 1999). An indication of whether a random-effects approach will appreciably widen the interval can be obtained by examining the quantity $(\text{RSS/df})^{1/2}$ from the final fixed-effects regression model. This quantity indicates roughly the degree to which confidence intervals would be expanded by adding a random effect to the final model. For example, averaging over all cohort studies in Table 33–1, we see in Table 33–3 that the fixed-effects estimate for the effect of five cups a day versus none is 1.17, with 95% confidence limits of $1.17 \exp[\pm 1.96(0.00738)5] = 1.09, 1.26$. These estimates assume the model $E(b) = \mu$. Under this model, however, $(\text{RSS/df})^{1/2} = (35.1/13)^{1/2} = 1.64$, which suggests that using the random-effects model $E(b) = \mu + \varepsilon$ instead would produce 95% confidence limits of $1.17 \exp[\pm 1.96(1.64)(0.00738)5] = 1.04, 1.32$. The actual estimate and limits under this random-effects model are 1.18 and 1.03, 1.34. On the other hand, for the regression in Table 33–4, $(\text{RSS/df})^{1/2} = (9.7/10)^{1/2} = 0.98$, indicating that the normal confidence intervals from the fixed-effects and random-effects models would be nearly identical (as indeed they are).

Several cautions should be borne in mind when considering random-effects models for meta-analysis.

1. In situations in which addition of a random effect to the model yields important changes in inferences, the degree of heterogeneity present will often (if not usually) be so large as to nullify the value of the summary estimates (with or without the random effects). Such a situation is indicative of the need to explore further sources of conflict among the study results (Greenland, 1994d).
2. Specific distributional forms for the random effects have no empirical, epidemiologic, or biologic justification in typical applications. Therefore, use of methods that specify the random-effects distribution should be accompanied by checks on the assumed distributional form, such as a histogram of the residuals (which would be the $b_k - \hat{\mu} - \hat{\theta} t$ in the preceding example). As always, these checks are one-directional in logic: Although they may detect problems, failure to detect a problem does not mean that the assumption is correct.
3. The summary estimate obtained from a random-effects model has no population-specific interpretation; it instead represents the mean of a distribution that generates effects. Unlike a standardized rate ratio, it does not correspond to an average effect in an actual population.
4. Random-effects summaries give proportionally greater weight to small studies than do fixed-effects summaries: The random-effects weight is $1/(\text{SE}^2 + \hat{\tau}^2)$, which varies less across studies than the fixed-effects weight $1/\text{SE}^2$. As a consequence, random-effects summaries will be more affected by biases that more strongly affect small studies, such as publication bias (Thompson and Pocock, 1991; Poole and Greenland, 1999; O'Rourke, 2001).
5. Unlike fixed-effects statistics, standard normal-theory random-effects tests and confidence limits depend on having a "large" number of studies. To address possible deficiencies in this regard, one may use a t-multiplier instead of a normal multiplier when constructing P-values and confidence intervals (Follmann and Proschan, 1999). Thus, for a random-effects regression paralleling that of Table 33–4, one would use a t-distribution with 10 degrees of freedom, which has a 97.5th percentile of 2.23, rather than the normal percentile of 1.96.

We emphasize that a random-effects model replaces a doubtful homogeneity assumption (that $\varepsilon = 0$ for all studies) with a fictitious random distribution of effects (allowing ε to vary across studies, but only in a purely random fashion). The advantage purchased by this generalization is that the standard errors and confidence limits can more accurately reflect uncertainty about unaccounted-for sources of variation in study results (e.g., measurement variation) than can estimates from fixed-effects models. Drawbacks are that some simplicity of interpretation is lost and that more weight is given to small studies.

When residual heterogeneity is small relative to study-specific variance (so that, say, residual sum of squares ends up smaller than its degrees of freedom), similar conclusions should result from either a fixed-effects or a random-effects approach. Nonetheless, a much smaller than expected variance may signal serious problems, for example, computational errors; multiple publication of the same group of patients being entered as separate studies in the analysis; or "conformity bias," a form of publication bias wherein authors preferentially publish analyses that give estimates similar to those already published.

A more general approach for multiple meta-regression that includes the fixed- and random-effects models as special cases is provided by random-coefficient or mixed models, which are also known as mixed-effects, empirical-Bayes, hierarchical, or multilevel models (see Chapter 21; Raudenbush and Bryk, 1985; Stram, 1996; Greenland and O'Rourke, 2001; Skrondal and Rabe-Hesketh, 2004). In these models the multiple meta-coefficients are given a distribution instead of being treated as fixed. In the simplest applications of these models, the estimated meta-coefficients of the study characteristics are shifted toward 0 (their null value) by an amount that is directly dependent on their estimated variances. The resulting "shrunken" meta-coefficient estimates have smaller variances and smaller mean-squared error than the original estimates. See the section on hierarchical regression in Chapter 21 and the references therein for further discussion of these methods.

PROBLEMS IN APPLICATION OF METHODS

OVERCONCLUSIVENESS

Like large epidemiologic studies, meta-analyses run the risk of appearing to give results that are more precise and conclusive than are warranted (Egger et al., 1998). The large number of subjects contributing to a meta-analysis will often lead to very narrow confidence intervals for the effect estimate. It is thus crucial to remember that these intervals take no account of average bias across studies, and take account of between-study variation in effect or bias only under restrictive assumptions. When uncertainties about bias sources are included, interval estimates will expand dramatically (Greenland, 2005b; see Chapter 19).

Consider again the coffee–myocardial infarction example. Suppose that no cohort study had been done and that only the case-control results in Table 33–2 were available for analysis. The meta-analysis would then supply only the first column in Table 33–3, which makes it appear that five cups per day of coffee consumption probably increases the myocardial infarction rate by 30% to 55%. Without the cohort data, these results might be misinterpreted in just this fashion. Instead, the appearance of precise results implies only that random error alone is no longer the major source of uncertainty. One must then shift one's focus to bias considerations and emphasize that the ordinary statistics do not address these considerations. In this example, one would have to emphasize that the confidence intervals do not account for possible recall bias, selection bias, or residual confounding (e.g., due to inadequate control of lifestyle factors) in the case-control results.

If one instead focused only on the cohort studies, one would be alerted to the fact that biases are probably operating, because of the gross conflict among those studies. Again, however, one must resist the temptation to overinterpret statistical summaries, such as the random-effects summary from the cohort studies, because these summaries blend together study results without regard to possible unmeasured differences in validity among the studies. For example, the analyses in Tables 33–2 and 33–4 did not account for differences in measurement accuracy among the cohort studies.

The major point is that failure to properly and fully emphasize the nonrandom sources of uncertainty in a meta-analysis may encourage and even support faulty conclusions and bad policy decisions; examples are provided by disturbing conflicts between observational and randomized trial evidence (Lawlor et al., 2004a, 2004b; Pettiti, 2004). One approach to avoiding this type of problem is to apply methods of uncertainty (bias) analysis to the meta-analysis (Eddy et al., 1992; Greenland, 2005b; see Chapter 19).

AGGREGATION BIAS

The previously described methods of regressing study results on study characteristics are ecologic regression methods (i.e., regressing area or group outcome rates on group exposure means or rates). It is well known that ecologic regression methods can yield misleading results, in that the relation between group rates or means may not resemble the relation between individual values of exposure and outcome (Chapter 25). This phenomenon is known as aggregation bias or ecologic bias. Such problems can arise in meta-analysis and need to be considered when interpreting meta-analytic results. Further bias can arise from regressing adjusted study results on unadjusted average values for covariates (Rosenbaum and Rubin, 1984). Such bias is a potential problem unless the covariates under study are not associated with the adjustment factors.

PUBLICATION BIAS

Meta-analytic corrections for publication bias are generally insufficient for bias removal; nevertheless, as discussed previously, some meta-analytic methods are useful for detecting and analyzing such biases (Light and Pillemer, 1984; Dear and Begg, 1992; Begg and Mazumdar, 1994; Copas, 1999; Copas and Jackson, 2004; Copas and Shi, 2000a, 2000b, 2004; Shi and Copas, 2002).

Several sources of publication bias have provoked serious concern. The classic source may be termed *significance bias,* the tendency of investigators to preferentially report (and in some cases, of editors to preferentially accept) associations that are "statistically significant" at the 0.05 level ($P < 0.05$). Such associations tend to be farther from the null than nonsignificant associations; consequently, if significant associations are preferentially published, the average published result will be farther from the null than the average result overall. Thus, significance bias is a bias away from the null. There is empirical evidence that significance bias is severe in some health science literature (Dickersin, 1990; Min and Dickersin, 2005). It is not a problem in all situations, however: In some topic areas, any finding from a sound study may be of great interest, especially when the association under study is controversial.

Significance bias results in *size bias,* the preferential submission and acceptance of larger studies, because the latter have more power (i.e., have a higher probability of significance if an association is present). Size bias also occurs directly—for example, when editors preferentially accept larger "null" studies on the grounds that those rule out important effects. If there are many small studies and few large ones, this bias against smaller studies can result in a substantial portion of the totality of relevant data being unavailable or difficult to locate.

Another form of publication bias may be termed *suppression bias,* in which certain types of results are intentionally not submitted (suppressed) because they do not conform to the desires of research sponsors. This concern has been raised in areas (such as occupational, environmental, and pharmaceutical epidemiology) in which private industry funds a major portion of research. Some research contracts allow the sponsor to veto publication, a veto presumably exercised when the results (for example) show an association of the sponsor's products or pollutants with adverse health events. Even when veto power is not present, some research groups may be dependent enough on funding from the industry, government, or other funding agencies to suppress reporting of adverse results or exaggerate evidence for promising results, in order to ensure continued funding. Other research, conducted directly by industry, is likely to be published selectively. This selectivity has been common in the pharmaceutical industry (Berenson, 2005), and is a source of bias toward the null in the published literature on adverse side effects.

As with selection bias in single studies, study-selection biases such as publication bias tend to be difficult if not impossible to remedy. Methods that estimate the number of undetected null studies needed to "refute" a non-null meta-analytic result can be misleading. Such methods overlook the fact that failure to include null studies cannot bias a pooled estimate if the parameter being estimated by all studies is null, for in the latter case one should expect equal numbers of negative (inverse) associations and positive associations. Similarly, one should expect a non-null pooled estimate to remain non-null no matter how many null studies are added (although of course it will become attenuated, possibly becoming almost null). Thus, failure to locate all null studies by itself cannot easily explain a non-null summary estimate. Among other explanations to consider is systematic failure to publish studies with results in a particular direction. Such directional publication bias can warp a null reality into a predominantly non-null literature or vice versa, and even make the literature tend to the direction opposite reality (Jackson, 2006).

Because small studies tend to display more publication bias, some authors have attempted to avoid or minimize the problem by excluding studies below a certain size. The strategy would make an important difference only when the excluded studies contain (in aggregate) a large portion of the observed data. One problem with the strategy is that the exact size limit for inclusion is arbitrary. Another is that, in some fields, all or almost all studies are small, so that the strategy would exclude most observations on the topic. Yet another problem is the possibility that the small studies might be the more valid of those available; for example, if the large studies are from administrative data bases while the small studies generate their own data through record abstraction and medical exams, the latter might have less bias from measurement error (Harbord et al., 2006).

An alternative to exclusion based on size is to include all studies but check for publication bias using the methods discussed earlier, such as funnel plots. For further discussion of publication bias, see Begg and Berlin (1988), Dickersin (1990), Copas and Shi (2000a), and Phillips (2004).

ISSUES OF STUDY SIZE

The weighted-averaging and regression methods presented above assume that each study is large enough to yield an effect estimate with an approximately normal distribution. As mentioned earlier, simulations indicate that, for log relative risks, studies with expected cell sizes as small as four can be large enough for practical purposes.

Normality of log relative-risk estimates computed by Mantel-Haenszel or conditional-likelihood methods depends on special summations across strata rather than on cell sizes. Simulation studies indicate that the relevant sums need not be very large when the true relative risk is not large; for example, if the true odds ratio is between 0.3 and 3.3, as few as 25 cases in a 1:4 matched case-control study can be sufficient for approximate normality of the Mantel-Haenszel log odds ratio (Robins et al., 1986c).

For studies so small that it is unreasonable to assume normality of the estimate, precise specification of the proper statistical weight for the study will be unimportant if the study contributes little to the total weight. Nevertheless, when a large proportion of the total weight comes from very small studies, the heterogeneity and regression statistics described earlier may no longer follow their large-sample (normal or chi-squared) distributions. In such cases, one will need study-specific cell counts and have to employ sparse-data or exact methods (see Chapters 15 and 21) to analyze the combined data, using "study" as a stratifying variable. Similarly, to contrast properly results from a small study with results from other studies, sparse-data or exact methods may be required.

BIAS IN EXCLUSION OF STUDIES

Exclusion of studies is a controversial practice. Some authors exclude unpublished studies from meta-analyses on the grounds that such studies tend to be of lower quality and that only a biased sample of such studies can be located. On the other hand, it can be argued that exclusion of unpublished studies aggravates publication bias. Other authors exclude studies based on methodologic features or low quality scores. It can be argued that such exclusions can lead to selection based on prejudice against certain methods (e.g., case-control studies) and mere speculations about bias. By controlling for quality items in the analysis, one can test these bias hypotheses rather than rely on exclusions, and efficiently estimate the relation of quality items to the estimated effect of exposure on outcome.

Three uncontroversial observations can be made: First, any weighting or decision to exclude a study should not be based on the results of the study, such as the point or interval estimates, lest it bias the meta-analysis (Yates and Cochran, 1938; Sacks et al., 1987). Second, even if one wants to include all studies, some studies may have to be excluded because the presentation of results is too uninformative to allow extraction of a credible effect estimate or weight. In such a case, an analysis constrained to qualitative results (e.g., direction) may allow the inclusion of more studies, and can be compared with a more quantitative but restrictive analysis. Third, all exclusions and reasons for them should be noted in the review.

SOME METHODS TO AVOID

QUALITATIVE TALLY (VOTE COUNTING)

In many traditional, qualitative reviews, one can find the explicit or implicit use of a qualitative tally or vote count. Consider a hypothetical literature summary stating, "of 17 studies to date, five have found a positive association, 11 have found no association, and one has found a negative association; thus, the preponderance of evidence favors no association." Such a tally can be extremely misleading, even if every single study is methodologically flawless, every study is included, and all the studies are comparable in every relevant aspect (Light and Pillemer, 1984). For example, the 11 studies counted as finding no association may have tended on the average toward a positive (if "nonsignificant") association, the single negative association may have been weak, and the five positive results may have ranged from weak to very strong—so that the average association across the studies might have been unequivocally positive. Mere lack of power might cause most or all of the study results to be erroneously reported as null (Hedges and Olkin, 1980).

Taking "nonsignificant" results as evidence for the null is a common fallacy involving the improper use of significance testing (Chapter 10). As usual, the best way to avoid such misinterpretations is to base interpretation on estimates, rather than on tests and tallies. Because of its lack of power, a tally can also miss important sources of heterogeneity. More serious still, a quick tally completely obscures the role of bias. In the preceding example, perhaps the positive studies were the least biased ones, or perhaps all the studies were positively biased, and the true association is negative. Thus, unless no further analysis is feasible, a qualitative tally should not serve as anything more than a provocative introduction to a more detailed and thoughtful analysis.

In cases in which the available data are so crude that a qualitative tally is the only feasible analysis, it is sometimes recommended that one use a binomial test of the proportion π of studies that are "positive" according to some criterion. Such tests can be done using the methods given in Chapter 13. If the criterion for positivity is merely that the observed association is in the positive direction (regardless of its size or P-value), half the studies would be expected to be positive under the null hypothesis of no effect or bias; this test of $\pi = 1/2$ is traditionally called a *sign test*. If the criterion for positivity is that the association is in the positive direction and also significant at the 0.05 level ($P < 0.05$) by a two-sided test, the null value of π would be $0.05/2 = 0.025$. Regardless of the criterion, if H is the number of "positive" studies and K is the total number of studies, the score statistic to test that $\pi = p$ is $\chi_{\text{score}} = (H - Kp)/[Kp(1 - p)]^{1/2}$. One can use the same method to test the proportion of studies that are "negative" according to some criterion; H then becomes the number of studies negative by chosen criterion.

Under the criterion that "positive" means a positive association significant at the two-sided 0.05 level, finding $H = 5$ of $K = 17$ studies to be positive would result in a score statistic for $\pi = 0.025$ of

$$\chi_{\text{score}} = [5 - 17(0.025)]/[17(0.025)(0.975)]^{1/2} = 7.1$$

From a normal table the value of 7.1 yields a "vote count" $P < 0.0001$, indicating that there are far more positive studies than one should expect under the null. Note that many researchers would misinterpret having "only" 5 of 17 studies significant and positive to mean that the preponderance of evidence favors the null; the test shows how mistaken this judgment is. Under the null hypothesis we should expect only 1 in 20 to be "significant" at the 0.05 level in either direction, and only 1 in 40 to be significant and positive. Thus, seeing 5 out of 17 studies significant and positive would be extremely unusual if there were no effect or bias in any of the studies.

Although the previous lesson is valuable, we still emphasize that the binomial test lacks power because it dichotomizes the continuum of information contained in the study-specific P-values. A much more powerful qualitative test of the null can be constructed by combining the P-values from the individual studies. There are various ways to define and combine P-values (P_k) from the individual studies, depending on the alternative hypothesis against which one wishes to maximize power. For an alternative in one direction (e.g., "studies tend to report positive associations more than expected by chance alone"), a one-sided P-value in the stated direction would be computed from each study and then combined. On the other hand, if the alternative were nondirectional (e.g., "studies tend to report associations more than expected by chance alone"), two-sided P-values would be computed and combined. Perhaps the best known method for combining P-values uses $-2\sum_k \ln(P_k)$, which has approximately a chi-squared distribution with $2K$ degrees of freedom under the null hypothesis that there is no association in any study (Fisher, 1932, p. 99; Cox and Hinkley, 1974, p. 80).

SCATTERPLOTS OF TEST STATISTICS

Cox and Hinkley (1974) warn against the practice of plotting test statistics (e.g., chi-squared or Z-values) versus explanatory variables, because the magnitude of the test statistics depends on study size and so cannot be taken as a measure of association or "distance" from the null value. Identical objections apply to scatterplots of P-values. This objection does not apply to simple histograms of test statistics or P-values; these have known distributions under the null hypothesis and can be examined for departures from those distributions (Cox and Hinkley, 1974).

STANDARDIZED COEFFICIENTS, CORRELATIONS, AND EFFECT SIZES

Detailed arguments have been given against the use of so-called standardized coefficients, correlations, variance explained, and related measures based on the use of standard-deviation units (Greenland et al., 1986, 1991). A key problem with such measures is that the so-called standard unit used to construct them actually varies across studies, rendering them noncomparable and useless for meta-analysis. Unfortunately, a fair portion of the meta-analysis literature in the social sciences has focused on an index of this sort, the *effect size,* defined as the difference in mean outcomes of the exposed (treated) and unexposed (control) groups, divided by the standard deviation of the outcome in the unexposed group; some authors divide by the pooled standard deviation.

It has been claimed that "expressing the effect sizes in standard deviation limits makes it possible to compare outcomes across different studies" (Light and Pillemer, 1984, p. 56). In fact, the opposite is the case: By expressing effects in standard-deviation units, one can make studies with identical results spuriously appear to yield different results; one can even reverse the order of strength of results (Greenland et al., 1986). These are severe distortions, and they imply that use of standardized coefficients, correlations, variance explained, and effect size (as defined in the meta-analytic literature) should be avoided (Greenland et al., 1991). Effect estimates should be expressed in a substantively meaningful unit that is uniform across studies, not in standard-deviation units. If this cannot be done credibly, one can limit statistical analysis to examining only the direction of association (Poole et al., 2006).

QUALITY SCORING

A very common practice is to weight studies or regress studies on a "quality score," usually based on some subjective assignment of points based on features of the studies. For example, one might score the studies in Table 33–1 by giving 10 quality points for a cohort design, 8 points for a nested case-control design, and 4 points for a population-based case-control design. The studies could then receive 2, 3, or 4 points if they controlled for smoking as a dichotomy, trichotomy, or in four or more categories. One would then use this score in the weighting (e.g., study weight = score/SE^2) or regress study estimates on the score.

Unfortunately, quality scoring submerges important information by combining disparate study features into a single score (Greenland, 1994d, 1994e; Greenland and O'Rourke, 2001). It also introduces an unnecessary and somewhat arbitrary subjective element into the analysis via the scoring scheme. Quality scoring can and should be replaced by direct categorical and regression analyses of the effect of each quality item (e.g., study design), as illustrated earlier (Greenland, 1994d, 1994e, 1994f). Such item-specific analyses let the data, rather than the investigator, indicate the importance of each item in determining the estimated effect. It is possible to reconstruct quality scores to reflect prior expectations about heterogeneity and use the resulting scores in a hierarchical meta-regression (Greenland and O'Rourke, 2001), but such usage also includes the contributing quality items as separate factors in the regression.

ROLE AND LIMITATIONS OF META-ANALYSIS

Meta-analytic and narrative (qualitative) aspects of research review can and should be complementary. A review is like a report of a single study, in that both quantitative and narrative elements will be necessary to convey a balanced picture of the material (Light and Pillemer, 1984). A purely statistical analysis cannot convey all the caveats or address all the shortcomings of the material, nor can it convey explanations of results in terms of biology and bias, whereas a purely qualitative analysis will lack precision and can easily miss small (but important) associations or subtle patterns in the material. Thus, where possible, a review should attempt some sort of meta-analysis and give explicit reasons for limiting attempts, just as an epidemiologic report should provide at least descriptive statistics.

In recognizing the necessity of meta-analysis, one should also be aware of its limitations. In particular, causal explanation of similarities and differences among study results noted in meta-analysis is a qualitative aspect of the review and thus outside the realm of ordinary statistical meta-analysis. This limitation is entirely analogous to the fact that causal explanation of associations noted in statistical analysis of basic data is beyond the scope of ordinary statistics. In either case, the statistics serve as fallible pattern-recognition devices; explanation of the origin of observed patterns is beyond the scope of these devices.

Meta-analytic methods do not provide a means for directly evaluating the bias of the individual studies considered in a review. As illustrated earlier, *ad hoc* corrections may be performed in an attempt to account for quantifiable biases, and one can analyze the effect of features that are thought to affect bias. It is also possible to employ more elaborate bias models for the analysis, along with formal prior distributions for the bias components (Greenland, 2005b; Chapter 19). Nevertheless, many problems will remain unquantified, and these problems will contribute to the observed patterns among study results. Again, explanation of the observed heterogeneity in terms of such unquantified problems (e.g., use of different case definitions, use of different sources of controls) will depend on the amount of detail in the reports and the skill of the reviewer, and is beyond the scope of meta-analytic methods.

CONCLUSION

This chapter has provided an exposition of basic considerations and quantitative methods for literature review, including methods that are useful in constructing statistical summaries and comparisons of studies. These methods cannot address unquantified problems that affect study results. Nevertheless, the methods provide a means of quantitatively comparing and (in some instances) summarizing study results, thus aiding in assessment of a literature.

Most meta-analyses will require from each study both a point estimate of effect and an estimate of its standard error. The actual study data would arguably be preferable, if correctly coded and documented adequately. Therefore, in the interest of facilitating reviews, authors, referees, and editors should consider making the study data available with the least restrictions on availability as is ethically possible (some funding agencies may even require funding recipients to make data available). At the very least, published abstracts and reports should provide both the point estimate for an association and its standard error or confidence limits (from which an accurate standard-error estimate can easily be recovered). A point estimate with a P-value may not provide an accurate standard error, and so should not be considered sufficient for reporting purposes.

References

Abadie A, Imbens GW. On the failure of the bootstrap for matching estimators. NBER Working Paper No. T0325, June 2006. Available at: http://ssrn.com/abstract=912426.

Abarca JF, Casiccia CC, Zamorano FD. Increase in sunburns and photosensitivity disorders at the edge of the Antarctic ozone hole, southern Chile, 1986–2000. *J Am Acad Dermatol* 2002;46:193–199.

Abbey H. An examination of the Reed-Frost theory of epidemics. *Hum Biol* 1952;24:201–233.

Adams P, Hurd MD, McFadden D, Merrill A, Ribeiro T. Healthy, wealthy, and wise? Tests for direct causal paths between health and socioeconomic status. *J Econometrics* 2003;112:3–56.

Adelstein AM, Staszewski J, Muir CS. Cancer mortality in 1970–1972 among Polish-born migrants to England and Wales. *Br J Cancer* 1979;40:464–475.

Agresti AA. *Categorical data analysis*, 2nd ed. New York: Wiley, 2002.

Ahluwalia IB, Mack KA, Murphy W, Mokdad AH, Bales VS. State-specific prevalence of selected chronic disease-related characteristics-Behavioral Risk Factor Surveillance System, 2001. In: *Surveillance summaries*, August 22, 2003. *MMWR Morb Mortal Wkly Rep* 2003;52(No. SS-8):1–84.

Alavanja MC, Brown CC, Swanson C, Brownson RC. Saturated fat intake and lung cancer risk among nonsmoking women in Missouri. *J Natl Cancer Inst* 1993;85:1906–1916.

Alberti C, Métivier F, Landais P, Thervet E, Legendre C, Chevret S. Improving estimates of event incidence over time in populations exposed to other events: application to three large databases. *J Clin Epidemiol* 2003;56:536–545.

Alho JM. On prevalence, incidence and duration in stable populations. *Biometrics* 1992;48:578–592.

Anderson JA. Separate-sample logistic discrimination. *Biometrika* 1992;59:19–35.

Allison PD. *Missing data*. Thousand Oaks: Sage, 2001.

Altman DG, Bland JM. Absence of evidence is not evidence of absence. *Br Med J* 1995;311:485.

Altman DG, Machin D, Bryant TN, Gardner MJ, eds. *Statistics with confidence*, 2nd ed. London: BMJ Books, 2000.

Ananth CV, Kleinbaum DG. Regression models for ordinal responses: a review of methods and applications. *Int J Epidemiol* 1997;26:1323–1333.

Ananth CV, Balasubramanian B, Demissie K, Kinzler WL. Small-for-gestational-age births in the United States. An age-period-cohort analysis. *Epidemiology* 2004;15:28–35.

Anderson JA. Separate sample logistic disrimination. *Biometrika* 1972;59:19–35.

Anderson JR, Bernstein L, Pike MC. Approximate confidence intervals for probabilities of survival and quantiles in life-table analysis. *Biometrics* 1982;38:407–416.

Anderson TW, Le Riche WH. Cold weather and myocardial infarction. *Lancet* 1970;1:291–296.

Angrist JD, Imbens GW, Rubin DB. Identification of causal effects using instrumental variables (with comments). *J Am Stat Assoc* 1996;91:444–472.

Angrist JD, Krueger AB. Instrumental variables and the search for identification: from supply and demand to natural experiments. *J Econ Perspect* 2001;15:69–85.

Anscombe FJ. The summarizing of clinical experiments by significance levels. *Stat Med* 1990;9:703–708.

Antunes CM, Strolley PD, Rosenshein NB, Davies JL, Tonascia JA, Brown C, Burnett L, Rutledge A, Pokempner M, Garcia R. Endometrial cancer and estrogen use: report of a large case-control study. *N Engl J Med* 1979;300:9–13.

Aoki K, Hayakawa N, Kurihara M Suzuki S. Death rates for malignant neoplasms for selected sites by sex and five-year age group in 33 countries, 1953–1957 to 1983–1987. In: *International Union Against Cancer,* Nagoya, Japan: University of Nagoya Cooperative Press, 1992.

ARIC Investigators. The Atherosclerosis Risk in Communities (ARIC) Study: design and objectives. *Am J Epidemiol* 1989;129:687–702.

Armitage P. The search for optimality in clinical trials. *Int Stat Rev* 1985;53:1–13.

Armitage P, McPherson CK, Rowe BC. Repeated significance tests on accumulating data. *J R Stat Soc Ser A* 1969;132:235–244.

Armstrong B, Doll R. Environmental factors and cancer incidence and mortality in different countries, with special reference to dietary practices. *Int J Cancer* 1975;15:617–631.

Armstrong BK. Stratospheric ozone and health. *Int J Epidemiol* 1994;23:873–885.

Armstrong BK, White E, Saracci R. *Principles of exposure measurement in epidemiology. Monographs in epidemiology and biostatistics, vol 21.* New York: Oxford University Press, 1992.

Arrighi HM. U.S. asthma mortality: 1941 to 1989. *Ann Allergy Asthma Immunol* 1995;74:321–326.

Ascherio A, Stampfer MJ, Colditz GA, Rimm EB, Litin L, Willett WC. Correlations of vitamin A and E intakes with the plasma concentrations of carotenoids and tocopherols among American men and women. *J Nutr* 1992;122:1792–1801.

Aselton P, Jick H, Chentow SJ, Perera DR, Hunter JR, Rothman KJ. Pyloric stenosis and maternal Bendectin exposure. *Am J Epidemiol* 1984;120:251–256.

Ast DB. Dental public health. In: Sartwell PE, ed. *Preventive medicine and public health,* 9th ed. New York: Meredith, 1965.

Ast DB, Smith DJ, Wachs B, Cantwell KT. Newburgh-Kingston caries-fluorine study. XIV. Combined clinical and roentgenographic dental findings after ten years of fluoride experience. *J Am Dent Assoc* 1956;52:314–325.

Atkins L, Jarrett D. The significance of "significance tests." In: Irvine J, Miles I, Evans J, eds. *Demystifying social statistics.* London: Pluto Press, 1979.

Austin H, Flanders WD, Rothman KJ. Bias arising in case-control studies from selection of controls from overlapping groups. *Int J Epidemiol* 1989;18:713–716.

Austin PC, Brunner LJ. Inflation of the type I error rate when a continuous confounding variable is categorized in logistic regression analyses. *Stat Med* 2004;23:1159–1178.

Austin PC, Grootendorst P, Lise-Normand ST, Anderson, GM. Conditioning on the propensity score can result in biased estimation of common measures of treatment effect. *Stat Med* 2007;26:754–768.

Avins AL. Can unequal be more fair? Ethics, subject allocation, and randomized clinical trials. *J Med Ethics* 1998;24:401–408.

Axelson O, Steenland K. Indirect methods of assessing the effect of tobacco use in occupational studies. *Am J Ind Med* 1988;13:105–118.

Aymard M, Valette M, Lina B, Thouvenot D. Surveillance and the impact of influenza in Europe. *Vaccine* 1999;17:S30–S41.

Backlund D, Sorlie PD, Johnson NJ. The shape of the relationship between income and mortality in the United States: evidence from the National Longitudinal Mortality Study. *Ann Epidemiol* 1996;6:12–23.

Bailey KR. Inter-study differences: how should they influence the interpretation and analysis of results? *Stat Med* 1987;6:351–360.

Baird DD, Wilcox AJ. Cigarette smoking associated with delayed conception. *JAMA* 1985;253:2979–2983.

Baird DD, Wilcox AJ, Weinberg CR. Use of time to pregnancy to study environmental exposures. *Am J Epidemiol* 1986;124:470–480.

Baird DD, Weinberg CR, Rowland AS. Reporting errors in time-to-pregnancy data collected with a short questionnaire: impact on power and estimation of fecundability ratios. *Am J Epidemiol* 1991a;133:1282–1290.

Baird DD, Weinberg CR, Wilcox AJ, McConnaughey DR, Musey PI, Collins DC. Hormonal profiles of natural conception cycles ending in early, unrecognized pregnancy loss. *J Clin Endocrinol Metab* 1991b;72: 793–800.

Baird DD, Weinberg CR, Wilcox AJ, McConnaughey DR, Musey PI. Using the ratio of urinary oestrogen and progesterone metabolites to estimate day of ovulation. *Stat Med* 1991c;10:255–266.

Baird DD, Weinberg CR, Schwingl P, Wilcox AJ. Selection bias associated with contraceptive practice in time-to-pregnancy studies. In: Campbell KL, Wood JW, eds. *Human reproductive ecology: interactions of environment, fertility, and behavior.* New York: New York Academy of Sciences, 1994:156–164.

Baird DD, McConnaughey DR, Weinberg CR, Musey PI, Collins DC, Kesner JS, Knecht EA, Wilcox AJ. Application of a method for estimating day of ovulation using urinary estrogen and progesterone metabolites. *Epidemiology* 1995;6:547–550.

Baker G. *An essay concerning the cause of the endemial colic of Devonshire.* Read in the Theatre of the College of Physicians in London, June 29, 1767. London: J Hughs near Lincoln's-Inn-Fields, 1767.

Bancroft TW, Han CP. Inference based on conditional specification. *Int Stat Rev* 1977;45:117–128.

Bandt CL, Boen JR. A prevalent misconception about sample size, statistical significance, and clinical importance. *J Periodontol* 1972;43:181–183.

Bang H, Robins JM. Doubly robust estimation in missing data and causal inference models. *Biometrics* 2005;61:962–972.

Bannerjee S, Carlin BP, Gelfand AE. *Hierarchical modeling and analysis for spatial data.* Boca Raton: CRC Press, 2004.

Barker DJ. Fetal growth and adult disease. *Br J Obstet Gynaecol* 1992;99:275–276.

Barnett E, Armstrong DL, Casper ML. Evidence of increasing coronary heart disease mortality among black men of lower social class. *Ann Epidemiol* 1999;9:464–471.

Baum FE, Ziersch AM. Social capital. *J Epidemiol Community Health* 2003;57:320–323.

Barron BA. The effects of misclassification on the estimation of relative risk. *Biometrics* 1977;33:414–418.

Basso O, Christensen K, Olsen J. Higher risk of pre-eclampsia after change of partner. An effect of longer interpregnancy intervals? *Epidemiology* 2001;12:624–629.

Batterham AM, Hopkins WG. Making meaningful inferences about magnitudes. *Int J Sports Physiol Perform* 2006;1:50–57.

Bayer R, Fairchild AL. Surveillance and privacy. *Science* 2000;290:1898–1899.

Bayes T. An essay towards solving a problem in the doctrine of chances. *Philos Trans R Soc Lond* 1764;53:370–418.

Beaglehole R, Magnus P. The search for new risk factors for coronary heart disease: occupational therapy for epidemiologists. *Int J Epidemiol* 2002;31:1117–1122.

Beaton GH, Milner J, Corey P, McGuire V, Cousins M, Stewart E, de Ramos M, Hewitt D, Grambsch PV, Kassim N, Little JA. Sources of variance in 24-hour dietary recall data: implications for nutrition study design and interpretation. *Am J Clin Nutr* 1979;32:2546–2549.

Beck LR, Rodriguez MH, Dister SW, Rodriguez AD, Rejmankova E, Ulloa A, Meza RA, Roberts DR, Paris DF, Spanner MA, Washino RK, Hacker C, Legters LJ. Remote sensing as a landscape epidemiologic tool to identify villages at high risk for malaria transmission. *Am J Trop Med* 1994;51:271–280.

Bedrick EJ, Christensen R, Johnson W. A new perspective on generalized linear models. *J Am Stat Assoc* 1996;91:1450–1460.

Beebe GW. Reflections on the work of the Atomic Bomb Casualty Commission in Japan. *Epidemiol Rev* 1979;1:184–210.

Begg CB. Biases in the assessment of diagnostic tests. *Stat Med* 1987;6:411–419.

Begg CB, Berlin JA. Publication bias: a problem in interpreting medical data. *J R Stat Soc Ser A* 1988;151:419–463.

Begg CB, Mazumdar M. Operating characteristics of a rank correlation test for publication bias. *Biometrics* 1994; 50:1088–1101.

Begg CB, Zhang ZF. Statistical analysis of molecular epidemiology studies employing case-series. *Cancer Epidemiol Biomarkers Prev* 1994;3:173–175.

Bell EM, Hertz-Picciotto I, Beaumont JJ. A case-control study of pesticides and fetal death due to congenital anomalies. *Epidemiology* 2001a;12:148–156.

Bell EM, Hertz-Picciotto I, Beaumont JJ. Pesticides and fetal death due to congenital anomalies: implications of an erratum. Erratum in: *Epidemiology* 2001b;12:596.

Bell EM, Hertz-Picciotto I, Beaumont JJ. Case-cohort analysis of agricultural pesticide applications near maternal residence and selected causes of fetal death. *Am J Epidemiol* 2001c;154:702–710.

Bellinger DC. Perspectives on incorporating human neurobehavioral end points in risk assessments. *Risk Anal* 2003;23:163–174.

Bellinger DC. Assessing environmental neurotoxicant exposures and child neurobehavior: confounded by confounding? *Epidemiology* 2004a;15:383–384.

Bellinger DC. What is an adverse effect? A possible resolution of clinical and epidemiological perspectives on neurobehavioral toxicity. *Environ Res* 2004b;95:394–405.

Bellinger D, Leviton A, Allred E, Rabinowitz M. Pre- and postnatal lead exposure and behavior problems in school-aged children. *Environ Res* 1994a;66:12–30.

Bellinger D, Hu H, Titlebaum L, Needleman HL. Attentional correlates of dentin and bone lead levels in adolescents. *Arch Environ Health* 1994b;49:98–105.

Belsley DA, Kuh E, Welsch RE. *Regression diagnostics: identifying influential data and sources of collinearity*. New York: Wiley, 2004.

Benichou J, Gail MH. Estimates of absolute cause-specific risks in cohort studies. *Biometrics* 1990a;46:813–826.

Benichou J, Gail MH. Variance calculations and confidence intervals for estimates of the attributable risk based on logistic models. *Biometrics* 1990b;46:991–1003.

Benichou J, Wacholder S. A comparison of three approaches to estimate exposure-specific incidence rates from population-based case-control data. *Stat Med* 1994;13:651–661.

Beral V, Chilvers C, Fraser P. On the estimation of relative risk from vital statistical data. *J Epidemiol Community Health* 1979;33:159–162.

Berek JS, Hacker NF, Lagasse LD, Nieberg RK, Elashoff RM. Survival of patients following secondary cytoreductive surgery in ovarian cancer. *Obstet Gynecol* 1983;61:189–193.

Berenson A. Despite vow, drug makers still withhold data. *New York Times*, May 31 2005.

Berger JO. The case for objective Bayesian analysis. *Int Soc Bayesian Analysis* 2004;1:1–17.

Berger JO, Berry DA. Statistical analysis and the illusion of objectivity. *Am Scientist* 1988;76:159–165.

Berger JO, Delampady M. Testing precise hypotheses (with discussion). *Stat Sci* 1987;2:317–352.

Berger JO, Sellke T. Testing a point null hypothesis: the irreconcilability of p values and evidence (with discussion). *J Am Stat Assoc* 1987;82:112–139.

Berger JO, Wolpert RL. *The likelihood principle,* 2nd ed. Hayward, CA: Institute of Mathematical Statistics, 1988.

Bergfeldt K, Rydh B, Granath F, Grönberg H, Thalib L, Adami HO, Hall P. Risk of ovarian cancer in breast-cancer patients with a family history of breast or ovarian cancer: a population-based cohort study. *Lancet* 2002;360:891–894.

Berk RA. *Regression analysis: a constructive critique*. Newbury Park, CA: Sage, 2004.

Berk RA, Western B, Weiss RE. Statistical inference for apparent populations. *Sociol Methodol* 1995;25:421–458.

Berkman LF. Assessing the physical health effects of social networks and social support. *Annu Rev Public Health* 1984;5:413–432.

Berkson J. Some difficulties of interpretation encountered in the application of the chi-square test. *J Am Stat Assoc* 1938;33:526–536.

Berkson J. Tests of significance considered as evidence. *J Am Statist Assoc* 1942;37:325–335. Reprinted in *Int J Epidemiol* 2003;32:687–691.

Berkson J. Limitations of the application of fourfold table analysis to hospital data. *Biomet Bull* 1946;2:47–53.

Berkson J. Smoking and lung cancer: some observations on two recent reports. *J Am Stat Assoc* 1958;53:28–38.

Berlin JA. Benefits of heterogeneity in meta-analysis of data from epidemiologic studies. *Am J Epidemiol* 1995;142:383–387.

Berlin JA, Longnecker MP, Greenland S. Meta-analysis of epidemiologic dose-response data. *Epidemiology* 1993;4:218–228.

Berman LE, Porter K, Binzer G, McQuillan G, Ostchega Y, Dupree N, Slobasky R. Use of information technology to support collection and reporting of data in the National Health and Nutrition Examination Survey. Presented at the International Conference on Improving Surveys, August 25–28, 2002, University of Copenhagen, Denmark.

Berry DA. A case for Bayesianism in clinical trials. *Stat Med* 1993;12:1377–1393.

Berry DA. Teaching elementary Bayesian statistics with real applications in science (with discussion). *Am Stat* 1997;51:241–271.

Berry G, Armitage P. Mid-P confidence intervals: a brief review. *Statistician* 1995;44:417–423.

Berry G, Liddell FDK. The interaction of asbestos and smoking in lung cancer: a modified measure of effect. *Ann Occup Hyg* 2004;48:459–462.

Besag J. Discussion. *J R Stat Soc Ser A* 1989;(Part 3):367–368.

Besag J, Newell J. The detection of clusters in rare diseases. *J R Stat Soc Ser A* 1991;154:143–155.

Beskow LM, Burke W, Merz JF, Barr PA, Terry S, Penchaszadeh VB, Gostin LO, Gwinn M, Khoury MJ. Informed consent for population-based research involving genetics. *JAMA* 2001;286:2315–2321.

Best N, Cockings S, Bennett J, Wakefield J, Elliott P. Ecological regression analyses of environmental benzene exposure and childhood leukemia: sensitivity to data inaccuracies, geographical scale and ecological bias. *J R Stat Soc A* 2001;164(Part 1):155–174.

Beyea J, Greenland S. The importance of specifying the underlying biologic model in estimating the probability of causation. *Health Physics*, 1999;76:269–274.

Biemer PP, Groves RM, Lyberg LE, Mathiowetz NA, Sudman S, eds. *Measurement errors in surveys.* New York: Wiley, 1991.

Bigler J, Whitton J, Lampe JW, Fosdick L, Bostick RM, Potter JD. CYP2C9 and UGTIA6 genotypes modulate the protective effect of aspirin on colon adenoma risk. *Cancer Res* 2001;61:3566–3569.

Bingenheimer JB, Raudenbush SW. Statistical and substantive inferences in public health: issues in the application of multilevel models. *Ann Rev Public Health* 2004;25:53–77.

Bingham SA, Cummings JH. Urine nitrogen as an independent validatory measure of dietary intake: a study of nitrogen balance in individuals consuming their normal diet. *Am J Clin Nutr* 1985;42:1276–1289.

Birkett NJ. Effect of nondifferential misclassification of estimates of odds ratios with multiple levels of exposure. *Am J Epidemiol* 1992;136:356–362.

Birnbaum A. A unified theory of estimation, I. *Ann Math Stat* 1961;32:112–135.

Birnbaum A. Median unbiased estimators. *Bull Math Stat* 1964;11:25–34.

Birnbaum LS, Fenton SE. Cancer and developmental exposure to endocrine disruptors (review). *Environ Health Perspect* 2003;111:389–394.

Birnbaum LS, Tuomisto J. Non-carcinogenic effects of TCDD in animals (review). *Food Addit Contam* 2000;17:275–288.

Bishop YMM, Fienberg SE, Holland PW. *Discrete multivariate analysis: theory and practice.* Cambridge, MA: MIT Press, 1975.

Bithell JF, Stone RA. On statistical methods for analysing the geographical distribution of cancer cases near nuclear installations. *J Epidemiol Community Health* 1989;43:79–85.

Blackwelder WC. Equivalence trials. In: Armitage P, Colton T, eds. *Encyclopedia of biostatistics.* New York, NY: John Wiley and Sons, Inc, 1998.

Blakely TA. Commentary: estimating direct and indirect effects—fallible in theory, but in the real world? *Int J Epidemiol* 2002;31:166–167.

Blank RM, Dabady M, Citro CF, eds. *Measuring racial discrimination.* Washington, D.C.: National Academy Press, 2003.

Blaser MJ, Newman LS. A review of human salmonellosis: I. infective dose. *Rev Infect Dis* 1982;4:1096–1106.

Block G, Hartman AM, Dresser CM, Carroll MD, Gannon J, Gardner L. A data-based approach to diet questionnaire design and testing. *Am J Epidemiol* 1986;3:453–469.

Blot WJ, Day NE. Synergism and interaction: are they equivalent? (letter). *Am J Epidemiol* 1979;110:99–100.

Blot WJ, Fraumeni JF Jr. Geographic patterns of lung cancer: industrial correlations. *Am J Epidemiol* 1976;103:539-550.

Blot WJ, Fraumeni JF Jr. Geographic patterns of oral cancer in the United States: etiologic implications. *J Chronic Dis* 1977;30:745–757.

Bodnar LM, Tang G, Ness RB, Harger G, Roberts JM. Periconceptional multivitamin use reduces the risk of preeclampsia. *Am J Epidemiol* 2006;164:470–477.

Bogle M, Stuff J, Davis L, Forrester I, Strickland E, Casey PH, Ryan D, Champagne C, McGee B, Mellad K, Neal E, Zaghloul S, Yadrick K, Horton J. Validity of a telephone-administered 24-hour dietary recall in telephone and non-telephone households in the rural Lower Mississippi Delta region. *J Am Diet Assoc* 2001;101:216–222.

Boice JD, Monson RR. Breast cancer in women after repeated fluoroscopic examinations of the chest. *J Natl Cancer Inst* 1977;59:823–832.

Boice JD Jr. Follow-up methods to trace women treated for pulmonary tuberculosis, 1930–1954. *Am J Epidemiol* 1978;107:127–139.

Bolumar R, Olsen J, Boldsen J. Smoking reduces fecundity: a European multicenter study on infertility and subfecundity. *Am J Epidemiol* 1996;143:578–587.

Bonen DK, Cho JH. The genetics of inflammatory bowel disease. *Gastroenterology* 2003;124:521–536.

Boring EG. Mathematical versus statistical importance. *Psychol Bull* 1919;16:335–338.

Borja-Aburto VH, Loomis DP, Bangdiwala SI, Shy CM, Rascon-Pacheco RA. Ozone, suspended particulates, and daily mortality in Mexico City. *Am J Epidemiol* 1997;145:258–268.

Boshuizen H, Greenland S. Average age at first occurrence as an alternative occurrence parameter in epidemiology. *Int J Epidemiol* 1997;26:867–872.

Boston Collaborative Drug Surveillance Program. Coffee drinking and acute myocardial infarction. *Lancet* 1972;2:1278–1281.

Botto LD, Khoury MJ. Commentary: facing the challenge of gene-environment interaction: the two-by-four table and beyond. *Am J Epidemiol.* 2001;153:1016–1020.

Botto LD, Khoury MJ. Facing the challenge of complex genotypes and gene-environment interaction: the basic epidemiologic units in case-control and case-only designs. In: Khoury MJ, Little J, Burke W, eds. *Human genome epidemiology: a scientific foundation for using genetic information to improve health and prevent disease*. New York: Oxford University Press, 2004:111–126.

Boucot KR, Dillon ES, Cooper DA, Meier P, Richardson R. Tuberculosis among diabetics: the Philadelphia survey. *Am Rev Tuberc* 1952;65:1–50.

Bowles S, Gintis H, Osborne M, eds. *Unequal chances: family background and economic success*. Princeton, NJ: Princeton University Press, 2004.

Box G, Jenkins G. *Time series analysis, forecasting and control.* San Francisco: Holden Day, 1976.

Box GEP. Sampling and Bayes inference in scientific modeling and robustness. *J R Stat Soc Ser A* 1980;143:383–430.

Boyd LH Jr, Iversen GR. *Contextual analysis: concepts and statistical techniques.* Belmont, CA: Wadsworth, 1979.

Bradburn NM, Sudman S, Wansink B. *Asking questions: the definitive guide to questionnaire design-for market research, political polls, and social and health questionnaires*, rev ed. New York: Jossey-Bass, 2004.

Brambilla D, McKinlay S. A prospective study of factors affecting age at menopause. *J Clin Epidemiol* 1989;42:1031–1039.

Brammer TL, Murray EL, Fukuda K, Hall HE, Klimov A, Cox NJ. Surveillance for influenza—United States, 1997–1998, 1988–1999, and 1999–2000 seasons. MMWR Morb Mortal Wkly Rep 2002:51(No. SS-7):1–10.

Brandwein AC, Strawderman WE. Stein estimation: the spherically symmetric case. *Stat Sci* 1990;5:356–369.

Brant SR, Picco MF, Achkar JP, Bayless TM, Kane SV, Brzezinski A, Nouvet FJ, Bonen D, Karban A, Dassopoulos T, Karaliukas R, Beaty TH, Hanauer SB, Duerr RH, Cho JH. Defining complex contributions of NOD2/CARD15 gene mutations, age at onset, and tobacco use on Crohn's disease phenotypes. *Inflamm Bowel Dis* 2003;9:281–289.

Brenner H. Bias due to non-differential misclassification of polytomous confounders. *J Clin Epidemiol* 1993;46:57–63.

Brenner H. Correcting for exposure misclassification using an alloyed gold standard. *Epidemiology* 1996;7:406–410.

Brenner H, Gefeller O. Use of positive predictive value to correct for disease misclassification in epidemiologic studies. *Am J Epidemiol* 1993;138:1007–1015.

Brenner H, Savitz DA. The effects of sensitivity and specificity of case selection on validity, sample size, precision, and power in hospital-based case-control studies. *Am J Epidemiol* 1990;132:181–192.

Brenner H, Greenland S, Savitz DA. The effects of nondifferential confounder misclassification in ecologic studies. *Epidemiology* 1992a;3:456–459.

Brenner H, Savitz DA, Jöckel KH, Greenland S. Effects of nondifferential exposure misclassification in ecologic studies. *Am J Epidemiol* 1992b;135:85–95.

Brenner H, Gefeller O, Greenland S. Risk and rate advancement periods as measures of exposure impact on the occurrence of chronic diseases. *Epidemiology* 1993;4:229–236.

Brenner H, Blettner M. Controlling for continuous confounders in epidemiological research. *Epidemiology* 1997;8:429–434.

Brenner H. A potential pitfall in control of covariates in epidemiologic studies. *Epidemiology* 1998;9:68–71.

Breslow L. Musing on sixty years in public health. *Annu Rev Pub Health* 1998;19:1–15.

Breslow NE. Odds ratio estimators when the data are sparse. *Biometrika* 1981;68:73–84.

Breslow NE. Extra-Poisson variation in log-linear models. *Appl Stat* 1984;33:38–44.

Breslow NE, Cain KC. Logistic regression for two-stage case-control data. *Biometrika* 1988;75:11–20.

Breslow NE, Clayton DG. Approximate inference in generalized linear mixed models. *J Am Stat Assoc* 1993;88:9–25.

Breslow NE, Day NE. *Statistical methods in cancer research. Vol I: the analysis of case-control data.* Lyon: IARC, 1980.

Breslow NE, Day NE. *Statistical methods in cancer research. Vol II: the design and analysis of cohort studies.* Lyon: IARC, 1987.

Breslow NE, Holubkov R. Maximum likelihood estimation of logistic regression parameters under two-phase, outcome dependent sampling. *J R Stat Soc Ser B* 1997a;59:447–461.

Breslow NE, Holubkov R. Weighted likelihood, pseudo-likelihood and maximum likelihood methods for logistic regression analysis of two-stage data. *Stat Med* 1997b;16:103–116.

Breslow NE, Liang KY. The variance of the Mantel-Haenszel estimator. *Biometrics* 1982;38:943–952.

Breslow NE, Lubin JH, Marek P, Langholz, B. Multiplicative models and cohort analysis. *J Am Stat Assoc* 1983;78:1–12.

Brick JM, Judkins D, Montaquila J, Morganstein D. Two-phase list-assisted RDD sampling. *J Off Stat* 2002;18:203–216.

Brinton LA, Blot WJ, Stone BJ, Fraumeni JF Jr. A death certificate analysis of nasal cancer among furniture workers in North Carolina. *Cancer Res* 1977;37:3473–3474.

Brody H, Rip MR, Vinten-Johansen P, Paneth N, Rachman S. Map-making and myth-making in Broad Street: the London cholera epidemic, 1854. *Lancet* 2000;356;64–68.

Brogan DJ, Denniston MM, Liff JM, Flagg EW, Coates RJ, Brinton LA. Comparison of telephone sampling and area sampling: response rates and within-household coverage. *Am J Epidemiol* 2001;153:1119–1127.

Brookhart MA, Schneeweiss S, Rothman KJ, Glynn RJ, Avorn J, Stürmer T. Variable selection for propensity score models. *Am J Epidemiol* 2006;163:1149–1156.

Brookmeyer R, Gail MH. *AIDS epidemiology: A quantitative approach*, Oxford University Press, 1994.

Brookmeyer R, Liang KY, Linet M. Matched case-control designs and overmatched analyses. *Am J Epidemiol* 1986;124:693–701.

Bross I. Misclassification in 2 × 2 tables. *Biometrics* 1954;10:478–486.

Bross IDJ. Spurious effects from an extraneous variable. *J Chronic Dis* 1966;19:637–647.

Bross IDJ. Pertinency of an extraneous variable. *J Chronic Dis* 1967;20:487–495.

Brown AS, Begg MD, Gravenstein S, Schaefer CA, Wyatt RJ, Bresnahan M, Babulas VP, Susser ES. Serologic evidence of prenatal influenza in the etiology of schizophrenia. *Arch Gen Psychiatry* 2004;61:774–780.

Brown PJ, Vannucci M, Fearn, T. Bayes model averaging with selection of regressors. *J R Stat Soc Ser B* 2002;64:519–536.

Brumback BA, Berg A. On effect-measure modification: Relations among changes in the relative risk, odds ratio, and risk difference. *Stat Med* 2008; in press.

Brumback BA, Greenland S, Redman M, Kiviat N, Diehr P. The intensity-score approach to adjusting for confounding. *Biometrics* 2003;59:274–285.

Brumback BA, Hernan MA, Haneuse S, Robins JM. Sensitivity analyses for unmeasured confounding assuming a marginal structural model for repeated measures. *Stat Med* 2004;23:749–767.

Brunekreef B, Noy D, Clausing P. Variability of exposure measurements in environmental epidemiology. *Am J Epidemiol* 1987;125:892–898.

Bruzzi P, Green SB, Byar DP, Brinton LA, Schairer C. Estimating the population attributable risk for multiple risk factors using case-control data. *Am J Epidemiol* 1985;122:904–914.

Bryk AS, Raudenbush SW. *Hierarchical linear models: applications and data analysis methods.* Thousand Oaks, CA: Sage, 1992.

Buehler JW, Berkelman RL. Surveillance. In: Holland WW, Detels R, Know G, eds. *Oxford textbook of public health,* 2nd ed. *Volume 2: methods of public health.* Oxford: Oxford University Press, 1991:161–176.

Buehler JW, Devine OJ, Berkelman RL, Chevarley FM. Impact of the human immunodeficiency virus epidemic on mortality trends in young men, United States. *Am J Public Health* 1990;80:1808–1086.

Buehler JW, Prager K, Hogue CJR. The role of linked birth and infant death certificates in maternal and child health epidemiology in the United States. *Am J Preventive Med* 2000;19(1S):3–11.

Buehler JW, Berkelman RL, Hartley DM, Peters CJ. Syndromic surveillance and bioterrorism-related epidemics. *Emerging Infect Dis J* 2003;9:1197–1204.

Buekens P, Wilcox A. Why do small twins have a lower mortality rate than small singletons? *Am J Obstet Gynecol* 1993;168:937–941.

Buell P. Changing incidence of breast cancer in Japanese-American women. *J Natl Cancer Inst* 1973;51:1479–1483.

Buhmann B, Rainwater L, Schmaus G, Smeeding, T. Equivalence scales, well-being, inequality and poverty: sensitivity estimates across ten countries using the Luxembourg Income Study database. *Rev Income Wealth* 1988;34:115–142.

Bull GM, Morton J. Relationships of temperature with death rates from all causes and from certain respiratory and arteriosclerotic diseases in different age groups. *Age Ageing* 1975;4:232–246.

Bunker JP, Forrest WH, Mosteller F, Vandam LD, eds. *The National Halothane Study. Report of the Subcommittee on the National Halothane Study of the Committee on Anesthesia.* Division of Medical Sciences, National Academy of Sciences-National Research Council. U.S. Government Printing Office: Washington, DC, 1969, Part IV.

Burke BS. The dietary history as a tool in research. *J Am Diet Assoc* 1947;23:1041–1046.

Burke W, Atkins D, Gwinn M, Guttmacher A, Haddow J, Lau J, Palomaki G, Press N, Richards CS, Wideroff L, Wiesner GL. Genetic test evaluation: information needs of clinicians, policy makers, and the public. *Am J Epidemiol.* 2002;156:311–318.

Burke W. Genomics as a probe for disease biology. *N Engl J Med* 2003;349:969–974.

Butler LM, Sinha R, Millikan RC, Martin CF, Newman B, Gammon MD, Ammerman AS, Sandler RS. Heterocyclic amines, meat intake, and association with colon cancer in a population-based study. *Am J Epidemiol* 2003;157:434–445.

Byar DP, Simon RM, Friedewald WT, Schlesselman JJ, DeMets DL, Ellenberg JH, Gail MH, Ware JH. Randomized clinical trials: perspectives on some recent ideas. *N Engl J Med* 1976;295:74–80.

Byers T, Marshall J, Anthony E, Fiedler R, Zielezny M. The reliability of dietary history from the distant past. *Am J Epidemiol* 1987;125:999–1011.

Byers TE, Rosenthal RI, Marshall JR, Rzepka TF, Cummings KM, Graham S. Dietary history from the distant past: a methodological study. *Nutr Cancer* 1983;5:69–77.

Byers TE, Graham S, Haughey BP, Marshall JR, Swanson MK. Diet and lung cancer risk: findings from the Western New York Diet Study. *Am J Epidemiol* 1987;125:351–363.

Cain KC, Breslow NE. Logistic regression analysis and efficient design for two-stage studies. *Am J Epidemiol* 1988;128:1198–1206.

Caldwell GG, Kelley DB, Heath CW Jr. Leukemia among participants in military maneuvers at a nuclear bomb test: a preliminary report. *JAMA* 1980;244:1575–1578.

California Department of Developmental Services. Autism Spectrum Disorders: Changes in the California Caseload, an Update: 1999-2002. California Health and Human Services Agency, State of California, 2003. available at URL www.dds.ca.gov (accessed December, 2007).

Callebaut W, ed. *Taking the naturalistic turn, or how real philosophy of science is done.* Chicago: University of Chicago Press, 1993.

Cannistra SA. The ethics of early stopping rules: who is protecting whom? *J Clin Oncol* 2004;22:1542–1545.

Carlin B, Louis TA. *Bayes and Empirical-Bayes methods of data analysis*, 2nd ed. New York: Chapman and Hall. 2000.

Carlin BP, Sargent DJ. Robust Bayesian approaches for clinical trial monitoring. *Stat Med* 1996;15:1093–1106.

Carpenter J, Bithell J. Bootstrap confidence intervals: when, which, and what? *Stat Med* 2000;19:1141–1164.

Carriere KC, Roos LL. Comparing standardized rates of events. *Am J Epidemiol* 1994;140:472–482.

Carroll RJ, Ruppert D, Stefanski LA, Crainiceanu C. *Measurement error in nonlinear models.* Boca Raton, FL: Chapman and Hall, 2006.

CARTaGENE project. Website accessed May, 2004 at http://www.cartagene.qc.ca/en/index.htm.

Cartwright RA, Glashan RW, Rogers HJ, Ahmad RA, Barham-Hall D, Higgins E, Kahn MA. Role of *N*-acetyl transferase phenotypes in bladder carcinogenesis: a pharmacogenetic epidemiological approach to bladder cancer. *Lancet* 1982;2:842–846.

Casady R, Leplowski J. Stratified telephone survey designs. *Surv Methodol* 1993;19:103–113.

Casella G, Berger RL. Reconciling Bayesian and frequentist evidence in the one-sided testing problem. *J Am Stat Assoc* 1987;82:106–111.

Casper M, Wing S, Strogatz D, Davis CE, Tyroler HA. Antihypertensive treatment and U.S. trends in smoking mortality, 1962 to 1980. *Am J Public Health* 1992;82:1600–1606.

Catalano R, Serxner S. Time series designs of potential interest to epidemiologists. *Am J Epidemiol* 1987;126:724–731.

Cederlof R, Doll R, Fowler B, Friberg L, Nelson N, Vouk V, eds. Air pollution and cancer: risk assessment of methodology and epidemiological evidence: report of a task group. *Environ Health Perspect* 1978;22.

Caughy MO, O'Campo PJ, Patterson J. A brief observational measure for urban neighborhoods. Health and Place 2001;7:225–236.

Celentano DD, Nelson KE, Lyles CM, Beyrer C, Eiumtrakul S, Go VF, Kuntolbutra S, Khamboonruang C. Decreasing incidence of HIV and sexually transmitted diseases in young Thai men: evidence for success of the HIV/AIDS control and prevention program. *AIDS* 1998;12:F29–36.

Centers for Disease Control. Guidelines for investigating clusters of health events. *MMWR Morb Mortal Wkly Rep* 1990b;39:1–23.

Centers for Disease Control. Reduced incidence of menstrual toxic-shock syndrome-United States, 1980–1990. *MMWR Morb Mortal Wkly Rep* 1990d;39:421–424.

Centers for Disease Control and Prevention. Summary of notifiable diseases, United States, 1996. *MMWR Morb Mortal Wkly Rep* 1996;45:43.

Centers for Disease Control and Prevention. Case definitions for infectious conditions under public health surveillance. *MMWR Morb Mortal Wkly Rep* 1997;46(No.RR-10):1–55.

Centers for Disease Control and Prevention. Diabetes Surveillance System, 1999 Surveillance Report, Appendix: Data Sources and Limitations, 1999a. [Accessed June 2004]. Available at URL: http://www.cdc.gov/diabetes/statistics/survl99/chap1/appendix.htm.

Centers for Disease Control and Prevention. Guidelines for national human immunodeficiency virus case surveillance, including monitoring for human immunodeficiency virus infection and acquired immunodeficiency syndrome. *MMWR Morb Mortal Wkly Rep* 1999b;48(No. RR-13):11–17.

Centers for Disease Control and Prevention. Updated guidelines for evaluating public health surveillance systems: recommendations from the guidelines working group. *MMWR Morb Mortal Wkly Rep* 2001;50(No. RR-13):14–24.

Centers for Disease Control and Prevention. Informed consent template for population-based research involving genetics. 2001a. Accessed June 2004 at http://www.cdc.gov/genomics/oldWeb01_16_04/info/reports/policy/consent.htm

Centers for Disease Control and Prevention. Supplemental brochure for population-based research involving genetics. 2001b. Accessed June 2004 at http://www.cdc.gov/genomics/oldWeb01_16_04/info/reports/policy/brochure.htm.

Centers for Disease Control and Prevention. State-specific prevalence of current cigarette smoking among adults - United States, 2002. *MMWR Morb Mortal Wkly Rep* 2004;52:1277–1280.

Centers for Disease Control and Prevention. Second national report on human exposures to environmental chemicals. 2003. Accessed online at http://www.cdc.gov/exposurereport/2nd/pdf/secondner.pdf.

Centers for Disease Control and Prevention. HIPAA Privacy Rule and public health: guidance from CDC and the U.S. Department of Health and Human Services. *MMWR Morb Mortal Wkly Rep* 2003a;52(Supl):1–20.

Centers for Disease Control and Prevention. *CDC/ATSDR Policy on Releasing and Sharing Data. Manual GUIDE: General Administration, CDC-102*, Office of the Director, Office of Science Policy and Technology Transfer, Date of Issue: 04/16/2003b [Accessed June 2004] Available at URL: http://www.cdc.gov/od/ads/pol-385.htm.

Centers for Disease Control and Prevention. Summary of notifiable diseases-United States, 2002. *MMWR Morb Mortal Wkly Rep* 2002;51(No. 53):1–5.

Centers for Disease Control and Prevention. Framework for evaluating public health surveillance systems for early detection of outbreaks; recommendations from the CDC Working Group. *MMWR Morb Mortal Wkly Rep* 2004b;53(No. RR-5):1–11.

Centerwall BS. Exposure to television as a risk factor for violence. *Am J Epidemiol* 1989;129:643–652.

Cepeda MS, Boston R, Farrar JT, Strom BL. Comparison of logistic regression versus propensity score when the number of events is low and there are multiple confounders. *Am J Epidemiol* 2003;158:280–287.

Chalmers I, Altman DG, eds. *Systematic reviews*. London: BMJ Publishing, 1995.

Chamberlain R. *British births 1970*. London: Heinemann Medical Books, 1975.

Chambers RL, Steel DG. Simple methods for ecological inference in 2 × 2 tables. *J R Stat Soc Ser A* 2001;164(Part 1): 175–192.

Chan AW, Hrobjartsson A, Haahr MT, Gotzsche PC, Altman DG. Empirical evidence for selective reporting of outcomes in randomized trials: comparison of protocols to published articles. *JAMA* 2004;291:2457–2465.

Chatfield C. *Time-series forecasting*. Boca Raton: Chapman & Hall/CRC, 2001.

Chavance M, Dellatolas G, Lellouch J. Correlated nondifferential misclassification of disease and exposure. *Int J Epidemiol* 1992;21:537–546.

Checkoway H, Pearce N, Kriebel D. *Research methods in occupational epidemiology*, 2nd ed. New York: Oxford University Press, 2004.

Checkoway H, Pearce N, Hickey JLS, Dement JM. Latency analysis in occupational epidemiology. *Arch Environ Health* 1990;45:95–100.

Chen J, Campbell CT, Junyao L, Peto R. *Diet, lifestyle, and mortality: a study of the characteristics of 65 Chinese counties*. Oxford: Oxford University Press, 1990.

Chen J, Giovannucci E, Kelsey K, Rimm EB, Stampfer MJ, Colditz GA, Spiegelman D, Willett WC, Hunter DJ. A methylenetetrahydrofolate reductase polymorphism and the risk of colorectal cancer. *Cancer Res* 1996;56:4862–4864.

Chen YC, Yu ML, Rogan WJ, Gladen BC, Hsu CC. A 6-year follow-up of behavior and activity disorders in the Taiwan Yu-cheng children. *Am J Public Health* 1994;84:415–421.

Chene G, Thompson SG. Methods for summarizing the risk associations of quantitative variables in a consistent form. *Am J Epidemiol* 1996;144:610–621.

Cho SI, Goldman MB, Ryan LM, Chen C, Damokosh AI, Christiani DC, Lasley BL, O'Connor JF, Wilcox AJ, Xu X. Reliability of serial urine hCG as a biomarker to detect early pregnancy loss. *Hum Reprod* 2002;17:1060–1066.

Cho WKT. Iff the assumption fits . . .: a comment on the King ecological inference solution. Polit Anal 1998;7:143–163.

Chowdhury AM. Arsenic crisis in Bangladesh. *Sci Am* 2004;291:86–91.

Christian P, Khatry SK, Katz J, Pradhan EK, LeClerq SC, Shrestha SR, Adhikari RK, Sommer A, West KP Jr. Effects of alternative maternal micronutrient supplements on low birth weight in rural Nepal: double blind randomised community trial. *Br Med J* 2003;326:1–6.

Chu H, Wang Z, Cole SR, Greenland S. Illustration of a graphical and a Bayesian approach to sensitivity analysis of misclassification. *Ann Epidemiol* 2006;16:834–841.

Church A. Estimating the effect of incentives on mail survey response rates: a meta-analysis. *Public Opin Q* 1993;57:62–79.

Church TR, Yeazel MW, Jones RM, Kochevar LK, Watt GD, Mongin SJ, Cordes JE, Engelhard D. A randomized trial of direct mailing of fecal occult blood tests to increase colorectal cancer screening. *J Natl Cancer Inst* 2004;96:770–780.

Cifuentes L, Borja-Aburto VH, Gouveia N, Thurston G, Davis DL. Climate change. Hidden health benefits of greenhouse gas mitigation. *Science* 2001;293:1257–1259.

Citro CF, Michael RT, eds. *Measuring poverty: a new approach.* Washington, D.C., National Academy Press, 1995.

Clark HH, Schober MF. Asking questions and influencing answers. In: Tanur JM, ed. *Questions about questions: inquiries into the cognitive bases of surveys.* New York: Sage Foundation, 1992.

Clayton D, Hills M. *Statistical models in epidemiology.* New York: Oxford University Press, 1993.

Clayton D, Kaldor J. Empirical Bayes estimates of age-standardized relative risks for use in disease mapping. *Biometrics* 1987;43:671–681.

Clayton DG, Bernardinelli L, Montomoli C. Spatial correlation in ecological analysis. *Int J Epidemiol* 1993;22:1193–1202.

Clumeck N, Taelman H, Hermans P, Piot P, Schoumacher M, De Wit S. A cluster of HIV infection among heterosexual people without apparent risk factors. *N Engl J Med* 1989;321:1460–1462.

Coates RJ, Eley JW, Block G, Gunter EW, Sowell AL, Grossman C, Greenberg RS. An evaluation of a food frequency questionnaire for assessing dietary intake of specific carotenoids and vitamin E among low-income black women. *Am J Epidemiol* 1991;134:658–671.

Cochran WG. Some methods for strengthening common chi-square tests. *Biometrics* 1954;10:417–451.

Cochran WG. The effectiveness of adjustment by subclassification in removing bias in observational studies. *Biometrics* 1968;24:295–313.

Cohen J. The earth is round ($p < 0.05$). *Am Psychol* 1994;47:997–1003.

Cohen NL, Laus MJ, Ferris AM et al. *The contributions of portion data to estimating nutrient intake by food frequency.* Amherst, MA: Mars Agricultural Experiment Station, University of Massachusetts, 1990. Research Bulletin No 730/ Dec 1990.

Cohn DL, O'Brien RJ, and the writing group for the ATS/CDC statement committee on latent tuberculosis infection. Targeted tuberculin testing and treatment of latent tuberculosis infection. *Am J Respir Crit Care Med* 2000; 161:S221–S247.

Colborn T. *Our stolen future.* Dutton: New York, 1996.

Cole P. The evolving case-control study. *J Chronic Dis* 1979;32:15–27.

Cole SR, Ananth CV. Regression models for unconstrained, partially or fully constrained continuation odds ratios. *Int J Epidemiol* 2001;30:1379–1382.

Cole SR, Hernán MA. Fallibility in estimating direct effects. *Int J Epidemiol* 2002;31:163–165.

Cole SR, Chu H. Effect of acyclovir on herpetic ocular recurrence using a structural nested model. *Contemp Clin Trials* 2005;26:300–310.

Cole SR, Hernán MA, Robins JM, Anastos K, Chmiel J, Detels R, Ervin C, Feldman J, Greenblatt R, Kingsley L, Lai S, Young M, Cohen M, Muñoz A. Effect of highly antiretroviral therapy on time to acquired immunodeficiency syndrome or death using marginal structural models. *Am J Epidemiol* 2003;158:687–694.

Cole SR, Chu H, Greenland S. Multiple-imputation for measurement error correction (with comment). *Int J Epidemiol* 2006;35:1074–1082.

Collins FS, Guttmacher AE. Welcome to the genomics era. *New Engl J Med* 2003;349:996–998.

Collins FS, Morgan M, Patrinos A. The human genome project: lessons from large scale biology. *Science* 2003; 300:286–290.

Cologne JB, Sharp GB, Neriishi K, Verkasalo PK, Land CE, Nakachi K. Improving the efficiency of nested case-control studies of interaction by selecting controls using counter matching on exposure. *Int J Epidemiol* 2004;33:485–449.

Colt JS, Zahm SH, Camann DE, Hartge P. Comparison of pesticides and other compounds in carpet dust samples collected from used vacuum cleaner bags and from the high-volume surface sampler. *Environ Health Perspect* 1998;106:721–724.

Cone LA, Woodard DR, Schlievert PM, Tomory GS. Clinical and bacteriologic observations of a toxic shock-like syndrome due to *Streptococcus pyogenes*. *N Engl J Med* 1987;317:146–149.

Connor MJ, Gillings D. An empiric study of ecological inference. *Am J Public Health* 1984;74:555–559.

Cook EF, Goldman L. Performance of tests of significance based on stratification by a multivariate confounder score or by propensity score. *J Clin Epidemiol* 1989;42:317–324.

Cook TD, Campbell OT. *Quasi-experimentation*. Chicago: Rand McNally, 1979.

Copas JB. Regression, prediction, and shrinkage. *J R Stat Soc Ser B* 1983;45:311–354.

Copas JB. What works? Selectivity models and meta-analysis. *J R Stat Soc Ser B* 1999;162:95–109.

Copas JB, Shi JQ. Meta analysis, funnel plots and sensitivity analysis. *Biostatistics*, 2000a;1:247–262.

Copas JB, Shi JQ. A sensitivity analysis for publication bias in systematic reviews. *Stat Methods Med Res* 2000b;10:251–265.

Copas JB, Shi JQ. Meta-analysis for trend estimation. *Stat Med* 2004;23:3–19.

Copas JB, Jackson D. A bound for publication bias based on the fraction of unpublished studies. *Biometrics* 2004;60:146–153.

Copeland KT, Checkoway H, Holbrook RH, McMichael AJ. Bias due to misclassification in the estimate of relative risk. *Am J Epidemiol* 1977;105:488–495.

Corley DA, Levin TR, Habel LA, Weiss NS, Buffler PA. Surveillance and survival in Barrett's adenocarcinomas: a population-based study. *Gastroenterology* 2002;122:633–640.

Corman LC. The relation between nutrition, infection, and immunity. *Med Clin North Am* 1985;69:519–531.

Cornfield J. A method of estimating comparative rates from clinical data: application to cancer of the lung, breast and cervix. *J Natl Cancer Inst* 1951;11:1269–1275.

Cornfield J. Joint dependence of risk of coronary heart disease on serum cholesterol and systolic blood pressure: a discriminant function analysis. *Fed Proc* 1962;21:58–61.

Cornfield J. Recent methodological contributions to clinical trials. *Am J Epidemiol* 1976;104:408–424.

Cornfield J, Haenszel WH, Hammond EC, Lilienfeld AM, Shimkin MB, Wynder EL. Smoking and lung cancer: recent evidence and a discussion of some questions. *J Natl Cancer Inst* 1959;22:173–203.

Coronary Drug Project Research Group. Influence of adherence to treatment and response of cholesterol on mortality in the Coronary Drug Project. *N Engl J Med* 1980;303:1038–1041.

Corti MC, Guralnik JM, Ferrucci L, Izmirlian G, Leveille SG, Pahor M, Cohen HJ, Pieper C, Havlik RJ. Evidence for a Black-White crossover in all-cause and coronary heart disease mortality in an older population: The North Carolina EPESE. *Am J Public Health* 1999;89:308–314.

Costello EJ, Compton SN, Keeler G, Angold A. Relationships between poverty and psychopathology: a natural experiment. *JAMA* 2003;290:2023–2029.

Cowell FA. *Measuring inequality*. 2nd ed. Prentice Hall: London, 1995.

Cox DR. Regression models and life tables (with discussions). *JR Stat Soc B* 1972;34:187–220.

Cox DR. Combination of data. In: Kotz S, Johnson NL, eds. *Encyclopedia of statistical sciences*, 2nd ed. New York: Wiley, 1986:45–53.

Cox DR. *Principles of statistical inference*. Cambridge: Cambridge University Press, 2006.

Cox DR, Hinkley DV. *Theoretical statistics*. New York: Chapman and Hall, 1974.

Cox DR, Oakes D. *Analysis of survival data*. New York: Chapman and Hall, 1984.

Cox DR, Wermuth N. A comment on the coefficient of determination for binary responses. *Am Statist* 1992;46: 1–4.

Crawford MD, Gardner MJ, Morris JN. Changes in water hardness and local death-rates. *Lancet* 1971;2:327–329.

Cressie N. Regional mapping of incidence rates using spatial Bayesian models. *Med Care* 1993;31(suppl): YS60–YS65.

Cressie NAC. *Statistics for spatial data*. New York: Wiley, 1991.

Criqui MH, Austin M, Barrett-Connor E. The effect of non-response on risk ratios in a cardiovascular disease study. *J Chronic Dis* 1979;32:633–638.

Cromley EK. GIS and disease. *Ann Rev Public Health* 2003;24:7–24.

Cromley EK, McLafferty SL. *GIS and public health*. The Guilford Press: New York, 2002.

Crouch EAC, Lester RL, Lash TL, Armstrong SA, Green LC. Health risk assessments prepared per the risk assessment reforms under consideration in the U.S. Congress. *Human and Ecological Risk Assessment* 1997;3:713–785.

Croucher PJ, Mascheretti S, Hampe J, Huse K, Frenzel H, Stoll M, Lu T, Nikolaus S, Yang SK, Krawczak M, Kim WH, Schreiber S. Haplotype structure and association to Crohn's disease of CARD15 mutations in two ethnically divergent populations. *Eur J Hum Genet* 2003;11:6–16.

Croyle RT, Loftus EE. Improving episodic memory performance of survey respondents. In: Tanur JM, ed. *Questions about questions: inquiries into the cognitive bases of surveys*. New York: Sage Foundation, 1992.

Cummings SR, Block G, McHenry K, Baron RB. Evaluation of two food frequency methods of measuring dietary calcium intake. *Am J Epidemiol* 1987;126:796–802.

Curd M, Cover JA eds. *Philosophy of science*, Section 3: The Duhem-Quine Thesis and Underdetermination, W.W. Norton & Company, 1998.

Curfman GD, Morissey S, Drazen JM. Expression of concern reaffirmed. *N Eng J Med* 2006;354:1193.

Curriero FC, Patz JA, Rose JB , Lele S. The association between extreme precipitation and waterborne disease outbreaks in the United States, 1948–1994. *Am J Public Health* 2001;91:1194–1199.

Cuzick J, Edwards R, Segnan N. Adjusting for non-compliance and contamination in randomized clinical trials. *Stat Med* 1997;16:1017–1029.

Cytel Corporation. Statexact 7. 2006.

Dales LD, Ury HK. An improper use of statistical significance testing in studying covariables. *Int J Epidemiol* 1978; 4:373–375.

Dalen P. Month of birth and schizophrenia. *Acta Psychiatr Scand Suppl* 1968;203:55–60.

Daly MB, Offit K, Li F, Glendon G, Yaker A, West D, Koenig B, McCredie M, Venne V, Nayfield S, Seminara D. Participation in the cooperative family registry for breast and ovarian cancer studies: issues of informed consent. *J Natl Cancer Inst* 2000;92:452–456.

Darby S, Deo H, Doll R, Whitley E. A parallel analysis of individual and ecological data on residential radon and lung cancer in south-west England. *J R Stat Soc Ser A* 2001;164(Part 1):193–203.

Darby SC, Doll R. Fallout, radiation doses near Dounreay, and childhood leukaemia. *Br Med J* 1987;294:603–607.

Darity WA. Employment discrimination, segregation, and health. *Am J Public Health* 2003;93:226–231.

Darroch J. Biologic synergism and parallelism. *Am J Epidemiol* 1997;145:661–668.

Darroch JN, Borkent M. Synergism, attributable risks and interaction for two binary exposure factors. *Biometrika* 1994;81:259–270.

Dashwood R. Use of transgenic and mutant animal models in the study of heterocyclic amine-induced mutagenesis and carcinogenesis. *J Biochem Mol Biol* 2003;36:35–42.

Davey Smith G. Classics in epidemiology: Should they get it right? *Int J Epidemiol* 2004;33:441–442.

Davey Smith G. Specificity as a criterion for causation: a premature burial? *Int J Epidemiol* 2002;31:710.

Davis JP, Chesney PJ, Wand PJ, Laventure M, Vergeront JM. Toxic shock syndrome, epidemiologic features, recurrence, risk factors, and prevention. *N Engl J Med* 1980;303:1429–1435.

Davis L, Wellman H, Punnett L. Surveillance of work-related carpal tunnel syndrome in Massachusetts, 1992–1997: A report from the Massachusetts Sentinel Event Notification System for Occupational Risks (SENSOR). *Am J Industrial Medicine* 2001;39:58–71.

Davison AC, Hinkley DV. *Bootstrap methods and their application*. New York: Cambridge, 1997.

Dawber T, Kannel W, Pearson G, Shurtleff D. Assessment of diet in the Framingham study, methodology and preliminary observations. *Health News* 1961;38:4–6.

Dawber TR, Kannel WB, Gordon T. Coffee and cardiovascular disease. *N Engl J Med* 1974;291:871–874.

Dawber TR, Moore FE, Mann GV II. Coronary heart disease in the Framingham study. *Am J Public Health* 1957;47:4–24.

Day NE. Effect of cervical cancer screening in Scandinavia. *Obstet Gynecol* 1984;63:714–718.

De Boor C. *A practical guide to splines*. New York: Springer, 2001.

de la Burde B, Choate MS. Early asymptomatic lead exposure and development at school age. *J Pediatr* 1975;87:638–642.

de Solla SR, Bishop CA, Van der Kraak G, Brooks RJ. Impact of organochlorine contamination on levels of sex hormones and external morphology of common snapping turtles (Chelydra serpentina serpentina) in Ontario, Canada. *Environ Health Perspect* 1998;106:253–260.

De Roos AJ, Poole C, Teschke K, Olshan AF. An application of hierarchical regression in the investigation of multiple paternal occupational exposures and neuroblastoma in offspring. *Am J Ind Med* 2001;39:477–486.

De Stefani E, Deneo-Pellegrini H, Mendilaharsu M, Carzoglio JC, Ronco A. Dietary fat and lung cancer: a case-control study in Uruguay. *Cancer Causes Control* 1997;8:913–921.

Dear KBG, Begg CB. An approach for assessing publication bias prior to performing a meta-analysis. *Stat Sci* 1992;7:237–245.

Deely JE, Lindley DV. Bayes empirical Bayes. *J Am Stat Assoc* 1981;76:833–841.

DeFinetti B. Foresight: its logical laws, its subjective sources In: Kyburg HE, Smokier HE, eds. *Studies in subjective probability.* New York, Wiley, 1964. (Original publication in Italian, 1937.).

DeFinetti B. *The theory of probability. Vol. 1.* New York: Wiley, 1974.

DeLong GR. Effects of nutrition on brain development in humans. *Am J Clin Nutr* 1993;57(suppl):286S–2905.

DerSimonian R, Laird N. Meta-analysis in clinical trials. *Control Clin Trials* 1986;7:177–188.

Detre KM, Shaw L. Long-term changes of serum cholesterol with cholesterol-altering drugs in patients with coronary heart disease. *Circulation* 1974;50:998–1005.

Deubner DC, Wilkinson WE, Helms MJ, Tyroler HA, Hames CG. Logistic model estimation of death attributable to risk factors for cardiovascular disease in Evans County, Georgia. *Am J Epidemiol* 1980;112:135–143.

Devesa SS, Pollack ES, Young JL. Assessing the validity of observed cancer incidence trends. *Am J Epidemiol* 1984;119:274–291.

Devesa SS, Donaldson J, Fears T. Graphical presentation of trends in rates. *Am J Epidemiol* 1995;141:300–304.

Devine O. Exploring temporal and spatial patterns in public health surveillance data. In: Brookmeyer R, Stroup DF, eds. *Monitoring the health of populations: statistical principles and methods for public health surveillance*. Oxford: Oxford University Press, 2004:71–98.

Devine OJ, Louis TA, Halloran ME. Empirical Bayes methods for stabilizing incidence rates before mapping. *Epidemiology* 1994;5:622–630.

Dickersin K. The existence of publication bias and risk factors for its occurrence. *JAMA* 1990;263:1385–1389.

Dickersin K, Berlin JA. Meta-analysis: state-of-the-science. *Epidemiol Rev* 1992;14:154–176.

Diez Roux AV. Bringing context back into epidemiology: variables and fallacies in multilevel analysis. *Am J Public Health* 1998;88:216–222.

Diez Roux AV. Estimating neighborhood health effects: the challenge of causal inference in a complex world. *Soc Sci & Med* 2004;58:1953–1960.

Diffey B. Climate change, ozone depletion and the impact on ultraviolet exposure of human skin. *Phys Med Biol* 2004;49(1):R1–11.

DiGaetano R, Waksberg J. Commentary: trade-offs in the development of a sample design for case-control studies. *Am J Epidemiol* 2002;155:771–775.

Diggle PJ, Heagerty P, Liang K-Y, Zeger SL. *Analysis of longitudinal data*, 2nd ed. New York: Oxford, 2002.

Dixon WD, Massey FJ. *Introduction to statistical analysis,* 3rd ed. New York: McGraw-Hill, 1969.

Dobson AJ. *An Introduction to generalized linear models*, 2nd ed. Chapman and Hall/CRC: London, 2001.
Dogan M, Rokkan S. Introduction. In: Dogan M, Rokkan S, eds. *Social ecology.* Cambridge, MA: MIT Press, 1969:1–15.
Doll R, Hill AB. A study of the aetiology of carcinoma of the lung. *Br Med J* 1952;2:1271–1286.
Doll R, Hill AB. Mortality of British doctors in relation to smoking; observations on coronary thrombosis. In: Haenszel W, ed. *Epidemiological approaches to the study of cancer and other chronic diseases*. Monogr Natl Cancer Inst 1966;19:205–268.
Doll R, Peto R. *The causes of cancer.* New York: Oxford University Press, 1981.
Dong SM, Traverso G, Johnson C, Geng L, Favis R, Boynton K, Hibi K, Goodman SN, D'Allessio M, Paty P, Hamilton SR, Sidransky D, Barany F, Levin B, Shuber A, Kinzler KW, Vogelstein B, Jen J. Detecting colorectal cancer in stool with the use of multiple genetic targets. *J Natl Cancer Inst* 2001;93:858–865.
Doody MM, Hayes HM, Bilgrad R. Comparability of National Death Index Plus and standard procedures for determining causes of death in epidemiologic studies. *Ann Epidemiol* 2001;11:46–50.
Doody MM, Sigurdson AS, Kampa D, Chimes K, Alexander BH, Ron E, Tarone RE, Linet MS. Randomized trial of financial incentives and delivery methods for improving response to a mailed questionnaire. *Am J Epidemiol* 2003;157:643–651.
Dorman SE, Holland SM. Mutation in the signal-transducing chain of the interferon-gamma receptor and susceptibility to mycobacterial infection. *J Clin Invest* 1998;101:2364–2369.
Dornan T, Mann JI, Turner R. Factors protective against retinopathy in insulin-dependent diabetics free of retinopathy for 30 years. *Br Med J* 1982;285:1073–1077.
Dosemeci M, Wacholder S, Lubin J. Does nondifferential misclassification of exposure always bias a true effect toward the null value? *Am J Epidemiol* 1990;132:746–749.
Dosemeci M, Hoover RN, Blair A, Figgs LW, Devesa S, Grauman D, Fraumeni JF Jr. Farming and prostate cancer among African Americans in the southeastern United States. *J Natl Cancer Institute* 1994;86:1718–1719.
Drake C. Effects of misspecification of the propensity score on estimators of treatment effect. *Biometrics* 1993;49:1231–1236.
Drake C, Fisher L. Prognostic models and the propensity score. *Int J Epidemiol* 1995;24:183–187.
Draper D. Assessment and propagation of model uncertainty. *J R Stat Soc Ser B*. 1995;57:45–97.
Draper NR, Guttman I, Lapczak L. Actual rejection levels in a certain stepwise test. *Communications in Statistics* 1979;A8:99–105.
Dreger AD. Ambiguous sex - or ambivalent medicine? Ethical issues in the treatment of intersexuality. *Hastings Cent Rep* 1998;28:24–35.
Drews CD, Flanders WD. Use of two data sources to estimate odds ratios in case-control studies. *Epidemiology* 1993;4:327–335.
Drews CD, Greenland S. The impact of differential recall on the results of case-control studies. *Int J Epidemiol* 1990;19:1107–1112.
Duhem P. *La théorie physique son objet et sa structure* (The aim and structure of physical theory). 1906. Translated from the French by Philip P. Wiener. Princeton: Princeton University Press, 1954.
DuMouchel W. Bayesian data mining in large frequency tables, with an application to the FDA spontaneous Reporting System (with discussion). *Am Stat* 1999;53:177–190.
Duncan OD. *Introduction to structural equation models.* New York: Academic Press, 1975.
Duncan OD, Cuzzort RP, Duncan B. *Statistical geography: problems in analyzing areal data.* Westport, CT: Greenwood Press, 1961:64–67.
Duncan OD, Davis B. An alternative to ecological correlation. *Am Sociol Rev* 1953;18:665–666.
Dunn KM, Jordan K, Lacey RJ, Shapley M, Jinks C. Patterns of consent in epidemiologic research: evidence from over 25,000 responders. *Am J Epidemiol* 2004;159:1087–1094.
Dunson D. Practical advantages of Bayesian analysis of epidemiologic data. *Am J Epidemiol* 2001;153:1222–1226.
Durack DT, Lukes AS, Bright DK. New criteria for the diagnosis of infective endocarditis. *Am J Med* 1994;96:2300–2309.
Durkheim E. *Suicide: a study in sociology.* New York: Free Press, 1951:153–154.
Dykes MHM, Meier P. Ascorbic acid and the common cold: evaluation of its efficacy and toxicity. *JAMA* 1975; 231:1073–1079.
Easton DF, Peto J, Babiker AG. Floating absolute risk: an alternative to relative risk in survival and case-control analysis avoiding an arbitrary reference group. *Stat Med* 1991;10:1025–1035.
Echt DS, Liebson PR, Mitchell LB, Peters RW, Obias-Manno D, Barker AH, Arensberg D, Baker A, Friedman L, Greene HL, and the CAST Investigators. Mortality and morbidity in patients receiving encainide, flecainide, or placebo. *N Engl J Med* 1991;324:781–788.
Eddy DM, Hasselblad V, Schachter R. *Meta-analysis by the confidence profile method.* New York: Academic Press. 1992.
Edwards AWF. *Likelihood*, 2nd ed. Baltimore: Johns Hopkins University Press. 1992.
Edwards JH. The recognition and estimation of cyclical trends. *Ann Hum Genet* 1961;25:83–86.
Efron B. Logistic regression, survival analysis, and the Kaplan-Meier curve. *J Am Stat Assoc* 1988;83:414–425.
Efron B. The estimation of prediction error: covariance penalties and cross-validation. *J Am Stat Assoc* 2004;99:619–642.
Efron B. Bayesians, frequentists, and scientists. *J Am Stat Assoc* 2005;100:1–5.
Efron B, Morris C. Stein's estimation rule and its competitors-an empirical Bayes approach. *J Am Stat Assoc* 1973;68:117–130.
Efron B, Morris CN. Data analysis using Stein's estimator and its generalizations. *J Am Stat Assoc* 1975;70:311–319.

Efron B, Morris C. Stein's paradox in statistics. *Sci Am* 1977;236:119–127.
Efron B, Tibshirani RJ. *An introduction to the bootstrap.* New York: Chapman and Hall, 1994.
Egger M, Davey Smith G, Altman D. *Systematic reviews in health care. Meta-analysis in context.* London: BMJ Publishing Group, 2001.
Egger M, Schneider M, Davey Smith G. Spurious precision? Meta-analysis of observational studies. *Br Med J* 1998;316:140–144.
Eisenberger MA, Blumenstein BA, Crawford ED, Miller G, McLeod DG, Loehrer PJ, Wilding G, Sears K, Culkin DJ, Thompson IM Jr, Bueschen AJ, Lowe BA. Bilateral orchiectomy with or without flutamide for metastatic prostate cancer. *N Engl J Med* 1998;339:1036–1042.
Elandt-Johnson RC. Definition of rates: some remarks on their use and misuse. *Am J Epidemiol* 1975;102:267–271.
Elias MF, Sullivan LM, D'Agostino RB, Elias PK, Beiser A, Au R, Seshadri S, DeCarli C, Wolf PA. Framingham stroke risk profile and lowered cognitive performance. *Stroke* 2004;35:404–409.
Elias P, McKnight A, Davies R, Kinshott, G. *Occupational change: revision of the standard occupational classification.* Coventry: Institute of Employment Research, University of Warwick, 2000.
Elliott P, Kleinschmidt I, Westlake AJ. Use of routine data in studies of point sources of environmental pollution. In: Elliott P, Cuzick J, English D, Stern R, eds. *Geographical and environmental epidemiology: methods for small-area studies.* New York: Oxford University Press, 1992:106–114.
Elliott P, Wakefield JC, Best NG, Briggs DJ, eds. *Spatial epidemiology: methods and applications.* New York: Oxford, 2000.
Elo IT, Preston SH. Educational differentials in mortality: United States, 1979–1985. *Social Science & Medicine* 1996;42:47–57.
Elson CO. Genes, microbes, and T cells-new therapeutic targets in Crohn's disease. *New Engl J Med* 2002;346:614–616.
Espeland M, Hui SL. A general approach to analyzing epidemiologic data that contain misclassification errors. *Biometrics* 1987:43:1001–1012.
Estonian Genome Project. Website accessed May, 2004 http://www.geenivaramu.ee/index.php?show=main&lang=eng.
Evans GW, Kantrowitz E. Socioeconomic status and health: the potential role of environmental risk exposure. *Annu Rev Public Health* 2002;23:303–331.
Evans L, Frick MC. Helmet effectiveness of preventing motorcycle driver and passenger fatalities. *Accid Anal Prev* 1988;20:447–458.
Evans SJW, Mills P, Dawson J. The end of the P-value? *Br Heart J* 1988;60:177–180.
Evans SJW, Waller PC, Davis S. Use of proportional reporting ratios (PRRs) for signal generation from spontaneous adverse drug reaction reports. *Pharmacoepidemiol Drug Saf* 2001;10:483–486.
Eylenbosch WJ, Noah ND. Historical aspects. In: Eylenbosch WJ, Noah ND, eds. *Surveillance in health and disease.* Oxford: Oxford University Press, 1988:1–8.
Fairchild AL, Bayer R. Ethics and the conduct of public health surveillance. *Science* 2004;303:631–632.
Fan J, Gijbels I. *Local polynomial modeling and its applications.* New York: Chapman and Hall, 1996.
Fananas L, Marti-Tusquets JL, Bertranpetit J. Seasonality of birth in schizophrenia. An insufficient stratification of control population? *Soc Psychiatry Psychiatr Epidemiol* 1989;24:266–270.
Faraway JJ. On the cost of data analysis. *Journal of Computational and Graphical Statistics* 1992;1:213–219.
Farewell VT. Some results on the estimation of logistic models based on retrospective data. *Biometrika* 1979;66:27–32.
Fauci AS. Host factors and the pathogenesis of HIV-induced disease. *Nature* 1996;384:529–534.
Federal Committee on Statistical Methodology. Report on statistical disclosure methodology [statistical working paper 22]. Washington: Office of Management and Budget, Office of Information and Regulatory Affairs, Statistical Policy Office; May 1994:66–67 [Accessed June 2004] Available at: URL: http:/www.fesm.gov/working-papers/wp22.html.
Feigl P, Zelen M. Estimation of exponential survival probabilities with concomitant information. *Biometrics* 1965;21:826–838.
Feinleib M, Leaverton PE. Ecological fallacies in epidemiology. In: Leaverton PE, Masse L, eds. *Health information systems.* New York: Praeger, 1984:33–61.
Feinstein AR. *Clinical epidemiology: the architecture of clinical research.* Philadelphia: WB Saunders, 1985.
Feinstein AR. Clinical biostatistics. XX. The epidemiologic trohoc, the ablative risk ratio, and "retrospective" research. *Clin Pharmacol Ther* 1973;14:291–307.
Felarca LC, Wardell DM, Rowles B. Vaginal spermicides and congenital disorders. *JAMA* 1981;246:2677–2678.
Felton JS, Knize MG, Bennett LM, Malfatti MA, Colvin ME, Kulp KS. Impact of environmental exposures on the mutagenicity/carcinogenicity of heterocyclic amines. *Toxicology* 2004;198:135–145.
Fennelly KP, Martyny JW, Fulton KE, Orme IM, Cave DM, Heifets LB. Cough-generated aerosols of Mycobacterium tuberculosis: a new method to study infectiousness. *Am J Respir Crit Care Med* 2004;169:604–609.
Ferlay J, Bray F, Pisani P, Parkin DM. *GLOBOCAN 2000: Cancer Incidence, Mortality and Prevalence Worldwide.* Version 1.0. Lyon: IARC Press, 2001.
Fewell Z, Smith GD, Sterne JAC. The impact of residual and unmeasured confounding in epidemiologic studies (with comment). *Am J Epidemiol* 2007;166:646–661.
Feyerabend P. *Against method.* New York: New Left Books, (3rd ed. 1993, New York: Verso) 1975.
Fine PE. A commentary on the mechanical analogue to the Reed-Frost epidemic model. *Am J Epidemiol* 1977;106:87–100.
Fine PE. Variation in protection by BCG: implications of and for heterologous immunity. *Lancet* 1995;346:1339–1345.
Fine PE, Zell ER. Outbreaks in highly vaccinated populations: implications for studies of vaccine performance. *Am J Epidemiol* 1994;139:77–90.

Firebaugh G. A rule for inferring individual-level relationships from aggregate data. *Am Sociol Rev* 1978;43:557–572.
Firket M. Sur les causes des accidents survenus dans la vallée de la Meuse, lors des brouillards de décembre 1930. *Bull Acad R Med Belg* 1931;11:683–739.
Fisher B, Costantino JP, Wickerham DL, Redmond CK, Kavanah M, Cronin WM, Vogel V, Robidoux A, Dimitrov N, Atkins J, Daly M, Wieand S, Tan-Chiu E, Ford L, Wolmark N. Tamoxifen for prevention of breast cancer: report of the National Surgical Adjuvant Breast and Bowel Project P-1 Study. *J Natl Cancer Inst* 1998;90:1371–1388.
Fisher GM. The development and history of the poverty thresholds. *Soc Secur Bull* 1992;55:3–14.
Fisher RA. *Statistical methods for research workers*, 4th ed. London: 1932.
Fisher RA. The logic of inductive inference. *J R Stat Soc Ser A* 1935;98:39–54.
Fisher RA. Note on Dr. Berkson's criticism of tests of significance. *J Am Statist Assoc* 1943;38:103–104. Reprinted in *Int J Epidemiol* 2003;32:692.
Fisher RP, Quigley KL. Applying cognitive theory in public health investigations: enhancing food recall with the cognitive interview. In: Tanur JM, ed. *Questions about questions: inquiries into the cognitive bases of surveys*. New York: Sage Foundation, 1992.
Flack VF, Chang PC. Frequency of selecting noise variables in subset regression analysis: a simulation study. *Am Statist* 1987;41:84–86.
Flanders WD, Austin H. Possibility of selection bias in matched case-control studies using friend controls. *Am J Epidemiol* 1986;124:150–153.
Flanders WD, Greenland S. Analytic methods for two-stage case-control studies and other stratified designs. *Stat Med* 1991;10:729–747.
Flanders WD, Khoury MJ. Indirect assessment of confounding: graphic description and limits on effect of adjusting for covariates. *Epidemiology* 1990;1:199–246.
Flanders WD, Khoury MJ. Analysis of case-parental control studies. *Am J Epidemiol* 1996;144:696–703.
Flanders WD, Rhodes PH. Large-sample confidence intervals for regression standardized risks, risk ratios, and risk differences. *J Chronic Dis* 1987;40:697–704.
Flanders WD, DerSimonian R, Rhodes P. Estimation of risk ratios in case-base studies with competing risks. *Stat Med* 1990;9:423–435.
Flanders WD, Lin L, Pirkle JL, Caudill SP. Assessing the direction of causality in cross-sectional studies. *Am J Epidemiol* 1992;135:926–935.
Flanders WD, Sun F, Yang Q. New estimator of the genotype risk ratio for use in case-parental control studies. *Am J Epidemiol* 2001;154:259–263.
Flegal KM, Keyl PM, Nieto FJ. Differential misclassification arising from nondifferential errors in exposure measurement. *Am J Epidemiol* 1991;134:1233–1244.
Fleming DM, van der Velden J, Paget WJ. The evolution of influenza surveillance in Europe and prospects for the next 10 years. *Vaccine* 2003;21:1749–1753.
Fletcher RH, Fletcher SW. *Clinical epidemiology: the essentials,* 4th ed. Lippincott Williams & Wilkins, New York, 2005.
Folks JF. *Ideas of statistics*. New York: Wiley, 1981.
Follmann DA, Elliott P, Suh I, Cutler J. Variance imputation for overviews of clinical trials with continuous response. *J Clin Epidemiol* 1992;45:769–773.
Follmann DA, Proschan MA. Valid Inference in Random Effects Meta-Analysis. *Biometrics* 1999;55:732–737.
Folstein MF, Folstein SE, McHugh PR. "Mini-mental state." A practical method for grading the cognitive state of patients for the clinician. *J Psychiatr Res*, 1975;12:189–198.
Forsdahl A. Living conditions in childhood and subsequent development of risk factors for arteriosclerotic heart disease. The cardiovascular survey in Finnmark 1974–75. *J Epidemiol Community Health* 1978;32:34–37.
Foster SO, Ward NA, Joarder AK, Arnt N, Tarantola D, Rahman M, Hughes K. Smallpox surveillance in Bangladesh: I-development of surveillance containment strategy. *Int J Epidemiol* 1980;9:329–334.
Fox AJ, Collier PF. Low mortality rates in industrial cohort studies due to selection for work and survival in the industry. *Br J Prev Soc Med* 1976;30:225–230.
Fox CS, Cupples LA, Chazaro I, Polak JF, Wolf PA, D'Agostino RB. Genomewide linkage analysis for internal carotid artery intimal medial thickness: Evidence for linkage to chromosome 12. *Am J Hum Genet* 2004;74:253–261.
Fox MP, Lash TL, Greenland S. A method to automate probabilistic sensitivity analyses of misclassified binary variables. *Int J Epidemiol* 2005;34:1370–1376.
Francis TF, Korns RF, Voight RB, Boisen M, Hemphill FM, Napier JA, Tolchinsky E. An evaluation of the 1954 poliomyelitis vaccine trials. *Am J Public Health* 1955;45(suppl):1–63.
Francis T, Napier JA, Voight BS, Hemphill FM, Wenner HA, Korns RF, Boisen M, Tolchinsky E, Diamond EL. *Evaluation of the 1954 field trial of poliomyelitis vaccine: final report.* Ann Arbor, MI: Poliomyelitis Vaccine Evaluation Center, University of Michigan, 1957.
Freedman DA. A note on screening regression equations. *Am Statist* 1983;37:152–155.
Freedman DA. Statistics and the scientific method. In: Mason W, Feinberg SE, eds. *Cohort analysis and social research*. New York: Springer-Verlag, 1985:345–390.
Freedman DA. As others see us: a case study in path analysis (with discussion). *J Educ Stat* 1987;12:101–223.
Freedman DA, Zeisel H. Cancer and risk assessment: From mouse to man. *Stat Sci* 1988;3:1–28.
Freedman DA, Humphreys P. Are there algorithms that discover causal structure? *Synthese* 1999;121:29–54.
Freedman DA, Klein SP, Ostland M, Roberts MR. Review of *A Solution to the Ecological Inference Problem* (by G. King). *J Am Stat Assoc* 1998;93:1518–1522.
Freedman DA, Navidi W, Peters SC. On the impact of variable selection in fitting regression equations. In: Dijlestra TK, ed. *On model uncertainty and its statistical implications*. Berlin: Springer-Verlag, 1988:1–16.

Freedman DA, Ostland M, Roberts MR, Klein SP. Reply to G. King. *J Am Stat Assoc* 1999;94:355–357.

Freedman DA, Petitti DB, Robins JM. On the efficacy of screening for breast cancer (with discussion). *Int J Epidemiol* 2004;33:43–73.

Freedman DA, Pisani R, Purves R. *Statistics,* 4th ed. New York: Norton, 2007.

Freedman LS, Fainberg V, Kipnis V, Midthune D, Carroll RJ. A new method for dealing with measurement error in explanatory variables of regression models. *Biometrics* 2004;60:172–181.

Freeman J, Hutchison GB. Prevalence, incidence and duration. *Am J Epidemiol* 1980;112:707–723.

Freiman JA, Chalmers TC, Smith H Jr, Kuebler RR. The importance of beta, the Type II error and sample size in the design and interpretation of the randomized control trial: survey of 71 "negative" trials. *N Engl J Med* 1978;299: 690–694.

Friedenreich CM, Howe GR, Miller AB. An investigation of recall bias in the reporting of past food intake among breast cancer cases and controls. *Ann Epidemiol* 1991;1:439–453.

Frost WH. The age selection of mortality from tuberculosis in successive decades. *Am J Hyg* 1939;30:91–96.

Gail MH, Simon R. Testing for qualitative interactions between treatment effects and patient subsets. *Biometrics* 1985;41:361–372.

Gail MH, Wacholder S, Lubin JH. Indirect corrections for confounding under multiplicative and additive risk models. *Am J Ind Med* 1988;13:119–130.

Gail MH, You WC, Chang YS, Zhang L, Blot WJ, Brown LM, Groves FD, Heinrich JP, Hu J, Jin ML, Li JY, Liu WD, Ma JL, Mark SD, Rabkin CS, Fraumeni JF Jr, Xu GW. Factorial trial of three interventions to reduce the progression of precancerous gastric lesions in Shandong, China: design issues and initial data. *Control Clin Trials* 1998;19:352–369.

Garcia-Berthou E, Alcaraz C. Incongruence between test statistics and P values in medical papers. *BMC Med Res Methodol* 2004;4:13.

Gardner MA, Altman DG. Confidence intervals rather than P values: estimation rather than hypothesis testing. *Br Med J* 1986;292:746–750.

Gart JJ, Tarone RE. The relation between score tests and approximate UMPU tests in exponential models common in biometry. *Biometrics* 1983;39:781–786.

Gelman A, Carlin JB, Stern HS, Rubin DB. *Bayesian data analysis*, 2nd ed. New York: Chapman and Hall/CRC. 2003.

Gelman A, Park DK, Ansolabehere S, Price PN, Minnite LC. Models, assumptions and model checking in ecological regressions. *J R Stat Soc Ser A* 2001;164(Part 1):101–118.

Gelman A, Price PN, All maps of parameter estimates are misleading, *Stat Med* 1999,18:3221–3234.

GenomEUtwin project. Website at http://www.genomeutwin.org/ accessed May, 2004.

George SL, Freidlin B, Korn EL. Strength of accumulating evidence and data monitoring committee decision making. *Stat Med* 2004;23:2659–2672.

Germolec DR, Yang RS, Ackermann MF, Rosenthal GJ, Boorman GA, Blair P, Luster MI. Toxicology studies of a chemical mixture of 25 groundwater contaminants. II. Immunosuppression in B6C3F1 mice. *Fundam Appl Toxicol* 1989;13:377–378.

Geweke J. Simulation methods for model criticism and robustness analysis. In: Bernardo JM, Berger JO, Dawid AP, Smith AFM. *Bayesian statistics 6*. New York: Oxford University Press, 1998.

Giere, R. *Science without laws*. Chicago: University of Chicago Press, 1999.

Gigerenzer G. Mindless statistics. *Journal of Socioeconomics* 2004; 33:567–606.

Gillet Y, Issartel B, Vanhems P, Fournet JC, Lina G, Bes M, Vandenesch F, Piémont Y, Brousse N, Floret D, Etienne J. Association between *Staphylococcus aureus* strains carrying gene for Panton-Valentine leukocidin and highly lethal necrotising pneumonia in young immunocompetent patients. *Lancet* 2002;359:753–759.

Gillman D. Decision criteria for using automated coding in survey processing. Proceedings of the Survey Research Methods Section of the American Statistical Association, 2002:1168–1173.

Gilon D, Buonanno FS, Joffe MM, Leavitt M, Marshall JE, Kistler JP, Levine RA. Lack of evidence of an association between mitral-valve prolapse and stroke in young patients. *N Engl J Med* 1999;341:8–13.

Gilovich T. *How we know what isn't so*. Free Press, 1993.

Gilovich T, Griffin D, Kahneman D. *Heuristics and biases: the psychology of intuitive judgment*. New York: Cambridge University Press; 2002.

Gilpin E, Pierce JP. Measuring smoking cessation: problems with recall in the 1990 California tobacco survey. *Cancer Epidemiol Biomarkers Prev* 1994;3:613–617.

Giovannucci E, Stampfer MJ, Colditz GA, Manson JE, Rosner BA, Longnecker M, Speizer FE, Willett WC. A comparison of prospective and retrospective assessments of diet in the study of breast cancer. *Am J Epidemiol* 1993; 137:502–511.

Gladen BC. On the role of "habitual aborters" in the analysis of spontaneous abortion. *Stat Med* 1986;5:557–564.

Gladen BC, Rogan WJ. On graphing rate ratios. *Am J Epidemiol* 1983;118:905–908.

Glanz K, Lewis FM, Rimer BK, eds. *Health behavior and health education*. 3rd ed. San Francisco: Jossey-Bass Publishers, 2002.

Glass RI, Svennerholm AM, Stoll BJ, Khan MR, Hossain KM, Huq MI, Holmgren J. Protection against cholera in breast-fed children by antibiotics in breast milk. *N Engl J Med* 1983;308:1389–1392.

Glasziou P, Irwig L, Bain C, Colditz G. *Systematic reviews in health care: a practical guide*. Cambridge University Press, 2001.

Glenn ND. *Cohort analysis*. Thousand Oaks, CA: Sage Foundation, 1977. Series/no 07-005.

Glymour C, Spirtes P, Richardson T. On the possibility of inferring causation from association without background knowledge. In: Glymour C, Cooper G, eds. *Computation, causation, and discovery*. Menlo Park, CA and Cambridge, MA: AAAI Press/ The MIT Press. 1999:323–331.

Glymour MM, Weuve J, Berkman LF, Kawachi I, Robins JM. When is baseline adjustment useful in analyses of change? An example with education and cognitive change. *Am J Epidemiol* 2005;162:267–278.

Glymour MM. Natural experiments and instrumental variables analyses in social epidemiology. In: Oakes JM, Kaufman JS, eds. *Methods in social epidemiology*. San Francisco: Jossey-Bass, 2006a.

Glymour MM. Using causal diagrams to understand common problems in social epidemiology. In: Oakes JM, Kaufman JS, eds. *Methods in social epidemiology*. San Francisco: Jossey-Bass, 2006b.

Goetghebeur E, van Houwelingen H, eds. Analyzing non-compliance in clinical trials (special issue). *Stat Med* 1998;17:247–393.

Goldbohm RA, van den Brandt PA, Brants HA, van't Veer P, Al M, Sturmans F, Hermus RJ. Validation of a dietary questionnaire used in a large prospective cohort study on diet and cancer. *Eur J Clin Nutr* 1994;48:253–265.

Goldman L, Weinberg M, Weisberg M, Olshen R, Cook EF, Sargent RK, Lamas GA, Dennis C, Wilson C, Deckelbaum L, Fineberg H, Stiratelli R. A computer-derived protocol to aid in the diagnosis of emergency room patients with acute chest pain. *N Engl J Med* 1982;307:588–596.

Goldstein H. Age, period and cohort effects-a confounded confusion. *Bias* 1979;6:19–24.

Goldstein H. *Multilevel statistical models*, 3rd ed. London: Arnold, 2003.

Goldstein H, Browne W, Rasbash J. Multilevel modelling of medical data. *Stat Med* 2002;21:3291–3315.

Goldstein M. Subjective Bayesian analysis: Principles and practice. *Bayesian Analysis*, to appear (preprint at http://www.stat.cmu.edu/bayesworkshop/2005/panel.html). 2006.

Good IJ. *The Estimation of probabilities*. Boston: MIT Press, 1965.

Good IJ. *Good thinking*. Minneapolis, MN: University of Minnesota Press, 1983.

Good IJ. Hierarchical Bayesian and empirical Bayesian methods (letter). *Am Stat* 1987;41:92.

Goodman LA. Some alternatives to ecological correlation. *Am J Social* 1959;64:610–625.

Goodman MT, Kolonel LN, Yoshizawa CN, Hankin JH. The effect of dietary cholesterol and fat on the risk of lung cancer in Hawaii. *Am J Epidemiol* 1988;128:1241–1255.

Goodman SN. A comment on replication, p-values and evidence. *Stat Med* 1992;11:875–879.

Goodman SN. P Values, hypothesis tests, and likelihood: implications for epidemiology of a neglected historical debate. *Am J Epidemiol* 1993;137:485–496.

Goodman SN, Berlin J. The use of predicted confidence intervals when planning experiments and the misuse of power when interpreting results. *Ann Intern Med* 1994;121:200–206.

Goodman SN, Royall R. Evidence and scientific research. *Am J Public Health* 1988;78:1568–1574.

Goodwin PJ, Boyd NF. Critical appraisal of the evidence that dietary fat intake is related to breast cancer risk in humans. *J Natl Cancer Inst* 1987;79:473–485.

Gooley TA, Leisenring W, Crowley J, Storer BE. Estimation of failure probabilities in the presence of competing risks: new representations of old estimators. *Stat Med* 1999;18:695–706.

Gordis L. Should dead cases be matched to dead controls? *Am J Epidemiol* 1982;115:1–5.

Gordon T, Kagan A, Garcia-Palmieri M, Kannel WB, Zukel WJ, Tillotson J, Sorlie P, Hjortland M. Diet and its relationship to coronary heart disease and death in three populations. *Circulation* 1981;63:500–515.

Gostin LO, Bayer R, Fairchild AL. Ethical and legal challenges posed by severe acute respiratory syndrome. *JAMA* 2003;290:3229–3237.

Gover M. Mortality during periods of excessive temperature. *Public Health Rep* 1938;53:1122–1143.

Goyer RA. Nutrition and metal toxicity. *Am J Clin Nutr* 1995;61(suppl):646S–650S.

Graham P. Bayesian inference for a generalized population attributable fraction. *Stat Med* 2000;19:937–956.

Graham S, Dayal H, Swanson M, Mittelman A, Wilkinson G. Diet in the epidemiology of cancer of the colon and rectum. *J Natl Cancer Inst* 1978;61:709–714.

Gramenzi A, Gentile A, Fasoli M, Negri E, Parazzini F, La Vecchia C. Association between certain foods and risk of acute myocardial infarction. *Br Med J* 1990;300:771–773.

Gravelle H. How much of the relation between population mortality and unequal distribution of income is a statistical artifact? *Br Med J* 1998;316:382–385.

Green MS, Symons MJ. A comparison of the logistic risk function and the proportional hazards model in prospective epidemiologic studies. *J Chronic Dis* 1983;36:715–724.

Greene WH. *Econometric analysis*, 5th ed. Prentice Hall: Upper Saddle River, NJ, 2003.

Greenland S. Response and follow-up bias in cohort studies. *Am J Epidemiol* 1977;106:184–187.

Greenland S. The effect of misclassification in the presence of covariates. *Am J Epidemiol* 1980;112:564–569.

Greenland S. Multivariate estimation of exposure-specific incidence from case-control studies. *J Chronic Dis* 1981;34:445–453.

Greenland S. The effect of misclassification in matched-pair case-control studies. *Am J Epidemiol* 1982a;116:402–406.

Greenland S. Interpretation and estimation of summary ratios under heterogeneity. *Stat Med* 1982b;1:217–227.

Greenland S. Tests for interaction in epidemiologic studies: a review and a study of power. *Stat Med* 1983;2:243–251.

Greenland S. A counterexample to the test-based principle of setting confidence limits. *Am J Epidemiol* 1984a;120:4–7.

Greenland S. Bias in methods for deriving standardized morbidity ratios and attributable fraction estimates. *Stat Med* 1984b;3:131–141.

Greenland S. Control-initiated case-control studies. *Int J Epidemiol* 1985a;14:130–134.

Greenland S. Power, sample size, and smallest detectable effect determination for multivariate studies. *Stat Med* 1985b;4:117–127.

Greenland S. Partial and marginal matching in case-control studies. In: Moolgavkar SH, Prentice RL, eds. *Modern statistical methods in chronic disease epidemiology*. New York: Wiley, 1986a;35–49.

Greenland S. Estimating variances of standardized estimators in case-control studies and sparse data. *J Chronic Dis* 1986b;39:473–477.

Greenland S. Adjustment of risk ratios in case-base studies (hybrid epidemiologic designs). *Stat Med* 1986c;5:579–584.
Greenland S. Interpretation and choice of effect measures in epidemiologic analysis. *Am J Epidemiol* 1987a;125:761–768.
Greenland S. Estimation of exposure-specific rates from sparse case-control data. *J Chronic Dis* 1987b;40:1087–1094.
Greenland S. Variance estimators for attributable fraction estimates consistent in both large strata and sparse data. *Stat Med* 1987c;6:701–708.
Greenland S. Quantitative methods in the review of epidemiologic literature. *Epidemiol Rev* 1987d;9:1–30.
Greenland S. Bias in indirectly adjusted comparisons due to taking the total study population as the reference group. *Stat Med* 1987e;6:193–195.
Greenland S. On sample-size and power calculations for studies using confidence intervals. *Am J Epidemiol* 1988a; 128:231–237.
Greenland S. Variance estimation for epidemiologic effect estimates under misclassification. *Stat Med* 1988b;7:745–757.
Greenland S. Statistical uncertainty due to misclassification: implications for validation substudies. *J Clin Epidemiol* 1988b;41:1167–1174.
Greenland S. Comment: cautions in the use of preliminary test estimators. *Stat Med* 1989a;8:669–673.
Greenland S. Modeling and variable selection in epidemiologic analysis. *Am J Public Health* 1989b;79:340–349.
Greenland S. Randomization, statistics, and causal inference. *Epidemiology* 1990;1:421–429.
Greenland, S. Reducing mean squared error in the analysis of stratified epidemiologic studies. *Biometrics* 1991;47:773–775.
Greenland S. A mathematical analysis of the "epidemiologic necropsy." *Ann Epidemiol* 1991a;1:551–558.
Greenland S. On the logical justification of conditional tests for two-by-two contingency tables. *Am Statist* 1991b; 45:248–251.
Greenland S. Estimating standardized parameters from generalized linear models. *Stat Med* 1991c;10:1069–1074.
Greenland S. A semi-Bayes approach to the analysis of correlated multiple associations, with an application to an occupational cancer-mortality study. *Stat Med* 1992a;11:219–230.
Greenland S. Divergent biases in ecologic and individual-level studies. *Stat Med* 1992b;11:1209–1223.
Greenland S. Basic problems in interaction assessment. *Environ Health Perspect* 1993a;101(suppl 4):59–66.
Greenland S. Methods for epidemiologic analyses of multiple exposures: a review and comparative study of maximum-likelihood, preliminary testing, and empirical-Bayes regression. *Stat Med* 1993b;12:717–736.
Greenland S. Summarization, smoothing, and inference. *Scand J Soc Med* 1993c;21:227–232.
Greenland S. Additive risk versus additive relative-risk models. *Epidemiology* 1993d;4:32–36.
Greenland S. A meta-analysis of coffee, myocardial infarction, and sudden coronary death. *Epidemiology* 1993e;4:366–374.
Greenland S. Alternative models for ordinal logistic regression. *Stat Med* 1994a;13:1665–1677.
Greenland S. Modeling risk ratios from matched cohort data: an estimating equation approach. *Appl Stat* 1994b;43:223–232.
Greenland S. Hierarchical regression for epidemiologic analyses of multiple exposures. *Environ Health Perspect* 1994c;102(suppl 8):33–39.
Greenland S. A critical look at some popular meta-analytic methods. *Am J Epidemiol* 1994d;140:290–296.
Greenland S. Quality scores are useless and potentially misleading. *Am J Epidemiol* 1994e;140:300–301.
Greenland S. Can meta-analysis be salvaged? *Am J Epidemiol* 1994f;140:783–787.
Greenland S. Dose-response and trend analysis: alternatives to category-indicator regression. *Epidemiology* 1995a;6:356–365.
Greenland S. Avoiding power loss associated with categorization and ordinal scores in dose-response and trend analysis. *Epidemiology* 1995b;6:450–454.
Greenland S. Problems in the average-risk interpretation of categorical dose-response analysis. *Epidemiology* 1995c; 6:563–565.
Greenland S. Absence of confounding does not correspond to collapsibility of the rate ratio or rate difference. *Epidemiology* 1996a;7:498–501.
Greenland S. Confounding and exposure trends in case-crossover and case-time-control designs. *Epidemiology* 1996b; 7:231–239.
Greenland S. Basic methods for sensitivity analysis of bias. *Int J Epidemiol* 1996c;25:1107–1116.
Greenland S. Historical HIV incidence modeling in regional subgroups: use of flexible discrete models with penalized splines based on prior curves. *Stat Med* 1996d;15:513–525.
Greenland S. A lower bound for the correlation of exponentiated bivariate normal pairs. *Am Statist* 1996e;50:163–164.
Greenland S. Re: "Estimating relative risk functions in case-control studies using a nonparametric logistic regression". *Am J Epidemiol* 1997a;146:883–884.
Greenland S. Second-stage least squares versus penalized quasi-likelihood for fitting hierarchical models in epidemiologic analyses. *Stat Med* 1997b;16:515–526.
Greenland S. Induction versus Popper: substance versus semantics. *Int J Epidemiol* 1998a;27:543–548.
Greenland S. Probability logic and probabilistic induction. *Epidemiology* 1998b;9:322–332.
Greenland S. The sensitivity of a sensitivity analysis (invited paper). In: *1997 Proceedings of the Biometrics Section*, Alexandria, VA. American Statistical Association, 1998c:19–21.
Greenland S. The relation of the probability of causation to the relative risk and the doubling dose: A methodologic error that has become a social problem. *Am J Public Health* 1999a;89:1166–1169.
Greenland S. A unified approach to the analysis of case-distribution (case-only) studies. *Stat Med* 1999c;8:1–15.

Greenland S. Multilevel modeling and model averaging. *Scand J Work Environ Health* 1999b;25 (suppl 4):43–48.
Greenland S. Causal analysis in the health sciences. *J Am Stat Assoc*, 2000a;95:286–289. Reprinted in: Raftery AE, Tanner MA, Wells MT. *Statistics in the 21st Century*. New York: Chapman and Hall/CRC, 2001:12–19.
Greenland S. An introduction to instrumental variables for epidemiologists. *Int J Epidemiol* 2000b;29:722–729. (Erratum: 2000;29:1102).
Greenland S. When should epidemiologic regressions use random coefficients? *Biometrics* 2000c;56:915–921.
Greenland S. Principles of multilevel modelling. *Int J Epidemiol* 2000d;29:158–167.
Greenland S. Small-sample bias and corrections for conditional maximum-likelihood odds-ratio estimators. *Biostatistics* 2000e;1:113–122.
Greenland S. Ecologic versus individual-level sources of confounding in ecologic estimates of contextual health effects. *Int J Epidemiol* 2001a;30:1343–1350.
Greenland S. Putting background information about relative risks into conjugate priors. *Biometrics* 2001b;57:663–670.
Greenland S. Sensitivity analysis, Monte-Carlo risk analysis, and Bayesian uncertainty assessment. *Risk Anal* 2001c;21:579–583.
Greenland S. Attributable fractions: Bias from broad definition of exposure. *Epidemiology* 2001d;12:518–520.
Greenland S. Estimating population attributable fractions from fitted incidence ratios and exposure survey data, with an application to electromagnetic fields and childhood leukemia. *Biometrics* 2001e;57:182–188.
Greenland S. Causality theory for policy uses of epidemiologic measures. Ch. 6.2 in: Murray CJL, Salomon JA, Mathers CD, Lopez AD, eds. *Summary Measures of Population Health*. Cambridge, MA: Harvard University Press/WHO, 2002a:291–302.
Greenland S. A review of multilevel theory for ecologic analyses. *Stat Med* 2002b;21:389–395.
Greenland S. Quantifying biases in causal models: Classical confounding vs collider-stratification bias. *Epidemiology* 2003a;14:300–306.
Greenland S. Generalized conjugate priors for Bayesian analysis of risk and survival regressions. *Biometrics* 2003b;59:92–99.
Greenland S. The impact of prior distributions for uncontrolled confounding and response bias: A case study of the relation of wire codes and magnetic fields to childhood leukemia. *J Am Stat Assoc* 2003c;98:47–54.
Greenland S. An overview of methods for causal inference from observational studies. In: Gelman A, Meng XL, eds. *Applied Bayesian modeling and causal inference from an incomplete-data perspective*. New York: Wiley, 2004a.
Greenland S. Ecologic inference problems in studies based on surveillance data. Ch. 12 in: Stroup DF Brookmeyer R, eds. *Monitoring the health of populations: statistical principles and methods for public health surveillance*. New York: Oxford University Press, 315–340. 2004b.
Greenland S. Interval estimation by simulation as an alternative to and extension of confidence intervals. *Int J Epidemiol* 2004c;33:1389–1397.
Greenland S. Model-based estimation of relative risks and other epidemiologic measures in studies of common outcomes and in case-control studies. *Am J Epidemiol* 2004d;160:301–305.
Greenland S. Epidemiologic measures and policy formulation: Lessons from potential outcomes (with discussion). *Emerg Themes Epidemiol* 2005a;2:1–4.
Greenland S. Multiple-bias modeling for analysis of observational data (with discussion). *J R Stat Soc Ser A* 2005b;168:267–308.
Greenland S. Bayesian perspectives for epidemiologic research. I. Foundations and basic methods (with comment and reply). *Int J Epidemiol* 2006a;35:765–778.
Greenland S. Smoothing observational data: a philosophy and implementation for the health sciences. *Int Stat Rev* 2006b;74:31–46.
Greenland S. Bayesian methods for epidemiologic research. II. Regression analysis. *Int J Epidemiol* 2007a;36:195–202.
Greenland S. Prior data for non-normal priors. *Stat Med* 2007b;26:3578–3590.
Greenland S. Maximum-likelihood and closed-form estimators of epidemiologic measures under misclassification. *J Stat Plan Inference* 2007c;138:528–538.
Greenland S. Variable selection and shrinkage in the control of multiple confounders (invited commentary). *Am J Epidemiol* 2008;167:in press.
Greenland S, Brenner H. Correcting for non-differential misclassification in ecologic analyses. *Appl Stat* 1993;42:117–126.
Greenland S, Brumback BA. An overview of relations among causal modeling methods. *Int J Epidemiol* 2002;31:1030–1037.
Greenland S, Christensen R. Data augmentation for Bayesian and semi-Bayes analyses of conditional-logistic and proportional-hazards regression. *Stat Med* 2001;20:2421–2428.
Greenland S, Drescher K. Maximum likelihood estimation of attributable fractions from logistic models. *Biometrics* 1993;49:865–872.
Greenland S, Engelman L. Re: "Inferences on odds ratios, relative risks, and risk differences based on standard regression programs." *Am J Epidemiol* 1988;128:145.
Greenland S, Finkle WD. A critical look at methods for handling missing covariates in epidemiologic regression analyses. *Am J Epidemiol* 1995;142:1255–1264.
Greenland S, Finkle WD. A case-control study of prosthetic implants and selected chronic diseases. *Ann Epidemiol* 1996;6:530–540.
Greenland S, Finkle WD. A retrospective cohort study of implanted medical devices and selected chronic diseases in Medicare claims data. *Ann Epidemiol* 2000;10:205–213.

Greenland S, Gustafson P. Adjustment for independent nondifferential misclassification does not increase certainty that an observed association is in the correct direction. *Am J Epidemiol* 2006;164:63–68.
Greenland S, Holland PW. Estimating standardized risk differences from odds ratios. *Biometrics* 1991;47:319–322.
Greenland S, Kheifets L. Leukemia attributable to residential magnetic fields: Results from analyses allowing for study biases. *Risk Anal* 2006;26:471–482.
Greenland S, Kleinbaum DG. Correcting for misclassification in two-way tables and matched-pair studies. *Int J Epidemiol* 1983;12:93–97.
Greenland S, Longnecker MP. Methods for trend estimation from summarized dose-response data, with applications to meta-analysis. *Am J Epidemiol* 1992;135:1301–1309.
Greenland S, Maldonado G. The interpretation of multiplicative model parameters as standardized parameters. *Stat Med* 1994;13:989–999.
Greenland S, Mickey RM. Closed-form and dually consistent methods for 2×2×K and I×J×K tables. *Appl Stat* 1988; 37:335–343.
Greenland S, Morgenstern H. Ecological bias, confounding, and effect modification. *Int J Epidemiol* 1989;18:269–274.
Greenland S, Morgenstern H. Matching and efficiency in cohort studies. *Am J Epidemiol* 1990;131:151–159.
Greenland S, Morgenstern H. Confounding in heath research. *Annu Rev Pub Health* 2001;22:189–212.
Greenland S, Neutra RR. Control of confounding in the assessment of medical technology. *Int J Epidemiol* 1980;9:361–367.
Greenland S, Neutra R. An analysis of detection bias and proposed corrections in the study of estrogens and endometrial cancer. *J Chronic Dis* 1981;34:433–438.
Greenland S, O'Rourke K. On the bias produced by quality scores in meta-analysis, and a hierarchical view of proposed solutions. *Biostatistics* 2001;2:463–471.
Greenland S, Pearl J. Causal diagrams. In: Boslaugh S ed. *Encyclopedia of epidemiology*. Thousand Oaks, CA: Sage Publications, 2008:149–156.
Greenland S, Poole C. Invariants and noninvariants in the concept of interdependent effects. *Scand J Work Environ Health* 1988;14:125–129.
Greenland S, Poole C. Empirical Bayes and semi-Bayes approaches to occupational and environmental hazard surveillance. *Arch Environ Health* 1994;49:9–16.
Greenland S, Poole C. Interpretation and analysis of differential exposure variability and zero-dose categories for continuous exposures. *Epidemiology* 1995;6:326–328.
Greenland S, Robins JM. Confounding and misclassification. *Am J Epidemiol* 1985a;122:495–506.
Greenland S, Robins JM. Estimation of a common effect parameter from sparse follow-up data. *Biometrics* 1985b;41:55–68.
Greenland S, Robins JM. Identifiability, exchangeability and epidemiological confounding. *Int J Epidemiol* 1986;15:413–419.
Greenland S, Robins J. Conceptual problems in the definition and interpretation of attributable fractions. *Am J Epidemiol* 1988;128:1185–1197.
Greenland S, Robins JM. Empirical-Bayes adjustments for multiple comparisons are sometimes useful. *Epidemiology* 1991;2:244–251.
Greenland S, Robins J. Invited commentary: ecologic studies-biases, misconceptions, and counterexamples. *Am J Epidemiol* 1994;139:747–760.
Greenland S, Robins JM. Epidemiology, justice, and the probability of causation. *Jurimetrics* 2000;40:321–340.
Greenland S, Thomas DC. On the need for the rare disease assumption in case-control studies. *Am J Epidemiol* 1982; 116:547–553.
Greenland S, Schlesselman JJ, Criqui MH. The fallacy of employing standardized regression coefficients and correlations as measures of effect. *Am J Epidemiol* 1986;123:203–208.
Greenland S, Maclure M, Schlesselman JJ, Poole C, Morgenstern H. Standardized regression coefficients: a further critique and review of some alternatives. *Epidemiology* 1991;2:387–392.
Greenland S, Salvan A, Wegman DH, Hallock MF, Smith TJ. A case-control study of cancer mortality at a transformer-assembly facility. *Int Arch Occup Environ Health* 1994;66:49–54.
Greenland S, Pearl J, Robins JM. Causal diagrams for epidemiologic research. *Epidemiology* 1999a;10:37–48.
Greenland S, Robins JM, Pearl J. Confounding and collapsibility in causal inference. *Statistical Science* 1999b;14:29–46.
Greenland S, Michels KB, Robins JM, Poole C, Willett WC. Presenting statistical uncertainty in trends and dose-response relations. *Am J Epidemiol* 1999c;149:077–1086.
Greenland S, Schwartzbaum JA, Finkle WD. Problems from small samples and sparse data in conditional logistic regression analysis. *Am J Epidemiol* 2000a;151:531–539.
Greenland S, Sheppard AR, Kaune WT, Poole C, Kelsh MA. A pooled analysis of magnetic fields, wire codes, and childhood leukemia. *Epidemiology* 2000b;11:624–634.
Greenland S, Gago-Domiguez M, Castellao JE. The value of risk-factor ("black-box") epidemiology (with discussion). *Epidemiology* 2004;15:519–535.
Greenland S, Lanes SF, Jara M. Estimating efficacy from randomized trials with discontinuations: The need for intent-to-treat design and g-estimation. *Clinical Trials* 2008:5, in press.
Gregg N. Congenital cataract following German measles in the mother. *Trans Ophthalmol Soc Aust* 1941;3:35–46.
Griem ML, Kleinerman RA, Boice JD Jr, Stovall M, Shefner D, Lubin JH. Cancer following radiotherapy for peptic ulcer. *J Natl Cancer Inst* 1994;86:842–849.
Grobbee DE, Rimm EB, Giovannucci E, Colditz G, Stampfer M, Willett W. Coffee, caffeine, and cardiovascular disease in men. *N Eng J Med* 1990;323:1026–1032.

Groves RM. *Survey errors and survey costs.* New York: Wiley, 1989.

Groves RM, Fowler FJ, Couper MP, Lepkowski ES, Tourangeau R. Nonresponse in sample surveys. Chapter 6 in *Survey methodology*. New York: John Wiley, 2004, 169–200.

Gruchow HW, Rimm AA, Hoffman RG. Alcohol consumption and ischemic heart disease mortality: are time-series correlations meaningful? *Am J Epidemiol* 1983;118:641–650.

Guillette LJ Jr, Woodward AR, Crain DA, Pickford DB, Rooney AA, Percival HF. Plasma steroid concentrations and male phallus size in juvenile alligators from seven Florida lakes. *Gen Comp Endocrinol* 1999;116:356–372.

Gullen WH, Berman JE, Johnson EA. Effects of misclassification in epidemiologic studies. *Public Health Rep* 1968; 53:1956–1965.

Gustafson P. *Measurement error and misclassification in statistics and epidemiology*. Boca Raton, FL: Chapman and Hall, 2003.

Gustafson P. On model expansion, model contraction, identifiability, and prior information (with discussion). *Stat Sci* 2005;20:111–140.

Gustafson P, Greenland S. Curious phenomena in Bayesian adjustment for exposure misclassification. *Stat Med* 2006a;25:87–103.

Gustafson P, Greenland S. The performance of random coefficient regression in accounting for residual confounding. *Biometrics* 2006b;62:760–768.

Gutensohn N, Li FP, Johnson RE, Cole P. Hodgkin's disease, tonsillectomy and family size. *N Engl J Med* 1975;292:22–25.

Guthrie KA, Sheppard L. Overcoming biases and misconceptions in ecological studies. *J R Stat Soc Ser* A 2001; 164(Part 1): 141–154.

Guttmacher AE, Collins FS. Genomic medicine–a primer. *New Engl J Med* 2002;347:1512–1520.

Guyatt G, Sackett D, Taylor DW, Chong J, Roberts R, Pugsley S. Determining optimal therapy—randomized trials in individual patients. *N Engl J Med* 1986;314:889–892.

Haack S. Defending Science – Within Reason. Between Scientism and Cynicism. Prometheus Books, Amherst, N.Y., 2003.

Haan M, Kaplan G, Camacho C. Poverty and health: prospective evidence from the Alameda County study. *Am J Epidemiol* 1987;125:989–998.

Hack M, Taylor HG, Klein N, Eiben R, Schatschneider C, Mercuri-Minich N. School-age outcomes in children with birth weights under 750 g. *N Engl J Med* 1994;331:753–759.

Haddow JE, Palomoaki GE. ACCE: a model for evaluating data on emerging genetic tests. In: Khoury MJ, Little J, Burke W, eds. *Human genome epidemiology: a scientific foundation for using genetic information to improve health and prevent disease*. Oxford University Press, New York, 2004;217–233.

Hadler SC, Webster HM, Erben JJ, Swanson JE, Maynard JE. Hepatitis A in day-care centers. A community-wide assessment. *N Engl J Med* 1980;302:1222–1227.

Haenszel W, Kurihara M, Segi M, Lee RK. Stomach cancer among Japanese in Hawaii. *J Natl Cancer Inst* 1972;49:969–988.

Hahn LW, Ritchie MD, Moore JH. Multifactor dimensionality reduction software for detecting gene-gene and gene-environment interactions. *Bioinformatics* 2003;19:376–382.

Haines A, McMichael AJ, Epstein PR. Environment and health: 2. Global climate change and health. *Can Med Assoc J* 2000;163:729–734.

Hakonarson H, Gulcher JR, Stefansson K. deCODE genetics, Inc. *Pharmacogenomics* 2003;4:209–215.

Hall P. *The bootstrap and edgeworth expansions*. Springer: New York, 1992.

Hall P, Adami HO, Trichopoulos D, Pedersen NL, Lagiou P, Ekbom A, Ingvar M, Lundell M, Granath F. Effect of low doses of ionising radiation in infancy on cognitive function in adulthood: Swedish population based cohort study. *Br Med J* 2004;328:19.

Halloran ME. Concepts of transmission and dynamics. In: Thomas JC, Weber DJ, eds. *Epidemiologic methods for the study of infectious diseases*. Oxford University Press, Oxford, 2003;56–85.

Halperin M. Re: "Estimability and estimation in case-control studies" (letter). *Am J Epidemiol* 1977;105:496–498.

Halstead SB, O'Rourke EJ. Dengue viruses and mononuclear phagocytes. I. Infection enhancement by non-neutralizing antibody. *J Exp Med* 1977;146:201–217.

Hampe J, Grebe J, Nikolaus S, Solberg C, Croucher PJ, Mascheretti S, Jahnsen J, Moum B, Klump B, Krawczak M, Mirza MM, Foelsch UR, Vatn M, Schreiber S. Association of NOD2 (CARD 15) genotype with clinical course of Crohn's disease: a cohort study. *Lancet* 2002;359:1661–1665.

Hanahan D, Weinberg R. The hallmarks of cancer. *Cell* 2000;100:57–70.

Hankin JH, Nomura AM, Lee J, Hirohata T, Kolonel LN. Reproducibility of a dietary history questionnaire in a case-control study of breast cancer. *Am J Clin Nutr* 1983;37:981–985.

Hardin J, Hilbe J. *Generalized linear models and extensions*, 2nd ed. New York: Chapman and Hall/CRC Press, 2007.

Hare E, Price J, Slater E. Mental disorder and season of birth: a national sample compared with the general population. *Br J Psychiatry* 1974;124:81–86.

Harlow SD, Ephross S. Epidemiology of menstruation and its relevance to women's health. *Epidemiol Rev* 1995; 17:265–286.

Harlow SD, Zeger SL. An application of longitudinal methods to the analysis of menstrual diary data. *J Clin Epidemiol* 1991;44:1015–1025.

Harrell F. *Regression modeling strategies*. Springer: New York, 2001.

Hartge P, Brinton LA, Rosenthal JF, Cahill JI, Hoover RN, Waksberg J. Random digit dialing in selecting a population-based control group. *Am J Epidemiol* 1984;120:825–833.

Hastie T, Tibshirani R. *Generalized additive models*. New York: Chapman and Hall, 1990.

Hastie T, Tibshirani R, Friedman J. *The elements of statistical learning: data mining, inference, and prediction*. New York: Springer, 2001.
Hatch M, Susser M. Background gamma radiation and childhood cancers within ten miles of a U.S. nuclear plant. *Int J Epidemiol* 1990;19:546–552.
Hauer E. The harm done by tests of significance. *Accid Anal Prev* 2003;36:495–500.
Hauser R, Calafat AM. Phthalates and human health. *Occup Environ Med* 2005;62:806–818.
Hauser RM, Warren JR. Socioeconomic indexes for occupations: a review, update, and critique. *Sociological Methodology* 1997;27:177–298.
Hausmann JA, Taylor WE. Panel data and unobservable individual effects. *Econometrica* 1981;49:1377–1398.
Heady JA. Diets of bank clerks: development of a method of classifying the diets of individuals for use in epidemiologic studies. *J R Stat Soc Ser A* 1961;124:336–361.
Hearst N, Newman T, Hulley S. Delayed effects of the military draft on mortality: a randomized natural experiment. *N Engl J Med* 1986;314:620–624.
Hebert JR, Miller DR. Methodologic considerations for investigating the diet-cancer link. *Am J Clin Nutr* 1988;47: 1068–1077.
Heckman J. Detecting discrimination. *J Econ Perspect* 1998;12:101–116.
Hedges LV, Olkin I. Vote counting methods in research synthesis. *Psychol Bull* 1980;88:359–369.
Heiat A, Gross CP, Krumholz HM. Representation of the elderly, women, and minorities in heart failure clinical trials. *Arch Int Med* 2002;162:1682–1688.
Helfenstein U. The use of transfer function models, intervention analysis and related time series methods in epidemiology. *Int J Epidemiol* 1991;20:808–815.
Hennekens CH, Buring JE. *Epidemiology in medicine*. Boston/Toronto, Little, Brown and Company, 1987.
Hennekens CH, Drolette ME, Jesse MJ, Davies JE, Hutchison GB. Coffee drinking and death due to coronary heart disease. *N Eng J Med* 1976;294:633–636.
Herbst A, Ulfelder H, Poskanzer D. Adenocarcinoma of the vagina: association of maternal stilbestrol therapy with tumor appearance in young women. *N Eng J Med* 1971;284:878–881.
Hernán MA. Hypothetical interventions to define causal effects—afterthought or prerequisite? *Am J Epidemiol* 2005;162:618–620.
Hernán MA, Robins JM. Instruments for causal inference—An epidemiologist's dream? *Epidemiology* 2006;17: 360–372.
Hernán MA, Hernandez-Diaz S, Werler MM, Mitchell AA. Causal knowledge as a prerequisite for confounding evaluation: An application to birth defects epidemiology. *Am J Epidemiol* 2002;155:176–184.
Hernán MA, Brumback B, Robins JM. Marginal structural models to estimate the causal effect of zidovudine on the survival of HIV-positive men. *Epidemiology* 2000;11:561–570.
Hernán MA, Brumback BA, Robins JM. Marginal structural models to estimate the joint causal effect of nonrandomized treatments. *J Am Stat Assoc* 2001;96:440–448.
Hernán M A, Hernandez-Diaz S, Robins JM. A structural approach to selection bias. *Epidemiology* 2004;15:615–625.
Hernandez-Avila M, Master C, Hunter DJ, Buring J, Phillips, J, Willett WC, Hennekens CH. Influence of additional portion size data on the validity of a semi-quantitative food frequency questionnaire. *Am J Epidemiol* 1988;128:891.
Hertz-Picciotto I. Epidemiology and quantitative risk assessment: a bridge from science to policy. *Am J Public Health* 1995;4:484–491.
Hertz-Picciotto I. Towards a coordinated system for surveillance of environmental health hazards (Commentary). Am *J Public Health* 1996;86:638–641.
Hertz-Picciotto I, Berhane KT, Bleecker ML, Engstrom PF, Fenske RA, Gasiewicz TA, Guidotti TL, Koller LD, Stegeman JJ, Strogatz DS [Committee to review the health effects in Vietnam Veterans of exposure to herbicides (Fourth Biennial Update)], *Veterans and Agent Orange, Update 2002*. Institute of Medicine (IOM), Washington, DC. National Academy Press, 2003.
Hertz-Picciotto I, Berhane KT, Bleecker ML, Engstrom PF, Fenske RA, Gasiewicz TA, Guidotti TL, Koller LD, Stegeman JJ, Strogatz DS [Committee to review the health effects in Vietnam Veterans of exposure to herbicides (Fourth Biennial Update)], *Veterans and Agent Orange, Length of Presumptive Period for Association Between Exposure and Respiratory Cancer.* Institute of Medicine (IOM), Washington, DC. National Academy Press, 2004.
Hertz-Picciotto I, Hu S-W. Contribution of cadmium in cigarettes to lung cancer: an evaluation of risk assessment methodologies. *Arch Environ Health* 1994:49:297–302.
Hertz-Picciotto I, Neutra RR. Resolving discrepancies among studies: the influence of dose on effect size. *Epidemiology* 1994:5:156–163.
Hertz-Picciotto I, Swan SH, Neutra RR, Samuels SJ. Spontaneous abortions in relation to consumption of tap water: an application of methods from survival analysis to a pregnancy follow-up study. *Am J Epidemiol* 1989;130:79–93.
Hertz-Picciotto I, Smith AH, Holtzman D, Lipsett M, Alexeeff G. Synergism between occupational arsenic exposure and smoking in the induction of lung cancer. *Epidemiology* 1992;3:23–31.
Hertz-Picciotto I, Pastore L, Beaumont J. Timing and patterns of exposures during pregnancy and their implications for study methods. *Am J Epidemiol* 1996;143:597–607.
Hessol NA, Koblin BA, van Griensven GJ, Bacchetti P, Liu JY, Stevens CE, Coutinho RA, Buchbinder SP, Katz MH. Progression of human immunodeficiency virus type 1 (HIV-1) infection among homosexual men in hepatitis B vaccine trial cohorts in Amsterdam, New York City, and San Francisco, 1978–1991. *Am J Epidemiol* 1994;139:1077–1087.
Heyden S, Tyroler HA, Heiss G, Hames CG, Bartel A. Coffee consumption and total mortality. *Arch Intern Med* 1978;138:1472–1475.
Heyman DL, Rodier G. Global surveillance, national surveillance, and SARS. *Emerging Infect Dis J* 2004;10:173–175.

Higgins JPT, Spiegelhalter DJ. Being skeptical about meta-analyses: a Bayesian perspective on magnesium trials in myocardial infarction. *Int J Epidemiol* 2002;31:96–104.

Higgins JP, Whitehead A, Turner RM, Omar RZ, Thompson SG. Meta-analysis of continuous outcome data from individual patients. *Stat Med* 2001;20:2219–2241.

Higginson J. Population studies in cancer. *Acta Unio Int Contra Cancrum* 1960;16:1667–1670.

Higginson J. Proportion of cancer due to occupation. *Prev Med* 1980;9:180–188.

Hilden J, Modvig J, Damsgaard MT, Schmidt L. Estimation of the spontaneous abortion risk in the presence of induced abortions. *Stat Med* 1991;10:285–297.

Hill AB. The environment and disease: association or causation? *Proc R Soc Med* 1965;58:295–300.

Hill J, McCulloch RE. Bayesian nonparametric modeling for causal inference. *J Am Stat Assoc* 2008; in press.

Hill J, Reiter JP. Interval estimation for treatment effects using propensity score matching. *Stat Med* 2006;25:2230–2256.

Hiller JE, McMichael AJ. Ecological studies. In: Margetts BM, Nelson M, eds. *Design concepts in nutritional epidemiology.* Oxford: Oxford University Press, 1991:323–353.

Hills M, Armitage P. The two-period cross-over clinical trial. *Br J Clin Pharmacol* 1979;8:7–20.

Hirano K, Imbens GW, Ridder G. Efficient estimation of average treatment effects using the estimated propensity score. *Econometrica* 2003;71:1161–1189.

Hirji K. *Exact analysis of discrete data*. Boca Raton, FL: CRC Press/Chapman and Hall, 2006.

Hodges JG, Gostion LO, Jacobson PD. Legal issues concerning electronic health information: privacy, quality, and liability. *JAMA* 1999;282:1466–1471.

Hoening JM, Heisey DM. The abuse of power: The pervasive fallacy of power calculations for data analysis. *Am Stat* 2001;55:19–24.

Hoffman FO, Hammonds JS. Propagation of uncertainty in risk assessments. *Risk Anal* 1994;14:707–712.

Hoffman JP. *Generalized linear models*. Boston: Allyn and Bacon, 2003.

Hoffman K, Heidemann C, Weikert C, Schulze MB, Boeing H. Estimating the proportion of disease due to classes of sufficient causes. *Am J Epidemiol* 2006;163:76–83.

Hogan MD, Kupper LL, Most BM, Haseman JK. Alternative to Rothman's approach for assessing synergism (or antagonism) in cohort studies. *Am J Epidemiol* 1978;108:60–67.

Hogben L. *Nature and nurture.* London: Williams and Norgate, 1933.

Hogben L. Statistical theory. Allen and Unwin, London, U.K., 1957.

Hoh J, Ott J. Mathematical multi-locus approaches to localizing complex human trait genes. *Nat Rev Genet* 2003;4:701–709.

Holford TR. Understanding the effects of age, period, and cohort on incidence and mortality rates. *Annu Rev Public Health* 1991;12:425–457.

Holland PW. Statistics and causal inference. *J Am Stat Assoc* 1986;81:945–960.

Holland PW. The false linking of race and causality: lessons from standardized testing. *Race and Society* 2001;4:219–233.

Holland SM, Dorman SE, Kwon A, Pitha-Rowe IF, Frucht DM, Gerstberger SM, Noel GJ, Vesterhus P, Brown MR, Fleisher TA. Abnormal regulation of interferon-gamma, interleukin-12, and tumor necrosis factor-alpha in human interferon-gamma receptor 1 deficiency. *J Infect Dis* 1998;178:1095–1104.

Holman CDJ, Arnold-Reed DE, de Klerk N, McComb C, English DR. A psychometric experiment in causal inference to estimate evidential weights used by epidemiologists. *Epidemiology* 2001;12:246–250.

Holmberg SD, Osterholm MT, Senger KA, Cohen ML. Drug-resistant salmonella from animals fed antimicrobials. *N Engl J Med* 1984;311:617–622.

Hook EB, Regal RR. Accuracy of alternative approaches to capture-recapture estimates of disease frequency: internal validity analysis of data from five sources. *Am J Epidemiol* 2000;152:771–779.

Hoover R, Mason TJ, McKay F, Fraumeni JF Jr. Cancer by county: new resource for etiologic clues. *Science* 1975;189:1005–1007.

Hopkins DR. Public health surveillance: where are we? where are we going? *MMWR Morb Mortal Wkly Rep* 1992;41(suppl):5–9.

Hopper JL. Commentary: Case-control-family designs: a paradigm for future epidemiology research? *Int J Epidemiol* 2003;32:48–50.

Hornick RB, Greisman SE, Woodward TE, DuPont HL, Dawkins AT, Snyder MJ. Typhoid fever: pathogenesis and immunologic control. *N Engl J Med* 1970;283:686–691.

Hornsby PP, Wilcox AJ, Weinberg CR, Herbst AL. Effects on the menstrual cycle of *in utero* exposure to diethylstilbestrol. *Am J Obstet Gynecol* 1994;170:709–715.

Horsburgh CR Jr. Priorities for the treatment of latent tuberculosis infection in the United States. *N Engl J Med* 2004;350:2060–2067.

Horvitz DG, Thompson DJ. A generalization of sampling without replacement from a finite population. *J Am Stat Assoc* 1952;47:663–685.

Horwitz RI, Feinstein AR. Alternative analytic methods for case-control studies of estrogens and endometrial cancer. *N Engl J Med* 1978;299:1089–1094.

Hosmer D, Lemeshow S. Confidence interval estimation of interaction. *Epidemiology* 1992;3:452–456.

Hosmer D, Lemeshow S. *Applied survival analysis*. New York: Wiley, 1999.

Hosmer D, Lemeshow S. *Applied logistic regression*, 2nd ed. New York: Wiley, 2000.

Hosmer DW, Hosmer T, Le Cessie S, Lemeshow S. A comparison of goodness-of-fit tests for the logistic regression model. *Stat Med* 1997;16:965–980.

Houlston R, Tomlinson I. Polymorphisms and colorectal tumor risk. *Gastroenterology* 2001;121:282–301.

Howard G, Goff DC. A call for caution in the interpretation of the observed smaller relative importance of risk factors in the elderly. *Ann Epidemiol* 1998;8:411–414.

Howe GR. Confidence interval estimation for the ratio of simple and standardized rates in cohort studies. *Biometrics* 1983;39:325–331.

Howe GM. Historical evolution of disease mapping in general and specifically of cancer mapping. *Recent Results Cancer Res* 1989;114:1–21. [Also appears in *Cancer mapping.* P Boyle, CS Muir, E Grundmann, eds. Springer-Verlag, New York.]

Howe GR, Choi BCK. Methodological issues in case-control studies: validity and power of various design/analysis strategies. *Int J Epidemiol* 1983;12:238–245.

Howe GR, Hirohata T, Hislop TG, Iscovich JM, Yuan J, Katsouyanni K, Lubin F, Marubini E, Modan B, Rohan T, Toniolo P, Shunzhang Y. Dietary factors and risk of breast cancer: combined analysis of 12 case-control studies. *J Natl Cancer Inst* 1990;82:561–569.

Howson C, Urbach P. *Scientific reasoning: the Bayesian approach,* 2nd ed. LaSalle, IL: Open Court, 1993.

Hu FB, Stampfer MJ, Rimm E, Ascherio A, Rosner BA, Spiegelman D, Willett WC. Dietary fat and coronary heart disease: a comparison of approaches for adjusting total energy intake and modeling repeated dietary measurements. *Am J Epidemiol* 1999;149:531–540.

Hu FB, Willett WC. Optimal diets for prevention of coronary heart disease. *JAMA* 2002;288:2569–2578.

Hugot JP, Laurent-Puig P, Gower-Rousseau C, Olson JM, Lee JC, Beaugerie L, Naom I, Dupas JL, Van Gossum A, Orholm M, Bonaiti-Pellie C, Weissenbach J, Mathew CG, Lennard-Jones JE, Cortot A, Colombel JF, Thomas G. Mapping of a susceptibility locus for Crohn disease on chromosome 16. *Nature* 1996;379:821–823.

Hugot JP, Chamaillard M, Zouali H, Lesage S, Cézard JP, Belaiche J, Almer S, Tysk C, O'Morain CA, Gassull M, Binder V, Finkel Y, Cortot A, Modigliani R, Laurent-Puig P, Gower-Rousseau C, Macry J, Colombel JF, Sahbatou M, Thomas G. Association of NOD2 leucine-rich repeat variants with susceptibility to Crohn disease. *Nature* 2001;411:599–603.

Hugot JP, Alberti C, Berrebi D, Bingen E, Cézard JP. Crohn's disease: the cold chain hypothesis. *Lancet* 2003;362: 2012–2015.

Hulka BS, Margolin BH. Methodological issues in epidemiologic studies using biologic markers. *Am J Epidemiol* 1992;135:200–209.

Hulley SB, Cummings SR, Browner WS, Grady D, Hearst N, Newman TB. *Designing clinical research*, 2nd ed. Lippincott Williams & Wilkins: Philadelphia, 2001.

Humble CG, Samet JM, Skipper BE. Use of quantified and frequency indices of vitamin A intake in a case-control study of lung cancer. *Int J Epidemiol* 1987;16:341–346.

Hume D. *A treatise of human nature.* Oxford: Oxford University Press, 1888; 2nd ed, 1978. (Original publication, 1739.)

Humphreys K, Carr-Hill R. Area variations in health outcomes: artefact or ecology. *Int J Epidemiol* 1991;20:251–258.

Hunter D. Biochemical Indicators of Dietary Intake. In: Willett W, ed. *Nutritional epidemiology*, 2nd ed. New York: Oxford University Press, 1998:174–243.

Hunter DJ, Rimm EB, Sacks FM, Stampfer MJ, Colditz GA, Litin LB, Willett WC. Comparison of measures of fatty acid intake by subcutaneous fat aspirate, food frequency questionnaire, and diet records in a free-living population of U.S. men. *Am J Epidemiol* 1992;135:418–427.

Hunter DJ, Spiegelman D, Adami HO, Beeson L, van den Brandt PA, Folsom AR, Fraser GE, Goldbohm RA, Graham S, Howe GR, Kushi LH, Marshall JR, McDermott A, Miller AB, Speizer FE, Wolk A, Yaun SS, Willett W. Cohort studies of fat intake and the risk of breast cancer—a pooled analysis. *N Eng J Med* 1996;334:356–361.

Hurvich CM, Tsai CL. The impact of model selection on inference in linear regression. *Am Statist* 1990;44:214–217.

Hurwitz ES, Schonberger LB, Nelson DB, Holman RC. Guillain-Barre syndrome and the 1978–1979 influenza vaccine. *N Eng J Med* 1981;304:1557–1561.

Hutchison GB, Rothman KJ. Correcting a bias? *N Engl J Med* 1978;299:1129–1130.

Hutwagner L, Thompson W, Seeman GM, Treadwell T. The Bioterrorism Preparedness and Response Early Aberration Reporting System (EARS). *J Urban Health: Bulletin of the New York Academy of Medicine* 2003;80(Suppl 1): i89–i96.

Ibrahim MA, Spitzer WO. The case-control study: the problem and the prospect. *J Chronic Dis* 1979;32:139–144.

Iceland J, Weinberg DH, Steinmetz E. U.S. Census Bureau, Series CENSR-3. Racial and Ethnic Residential Segregation in the United States: 1980–2000, U.S. Government Printing Office, Washington, DC, 2002.

Illsley R, Mitchell RG. *Low birth weight: a medical, psychological, and social study.* New York: Wiley, 1984.

Inskip PD, Monson RR, Wagoner JK, Stovall M, Davis FG, Kleinerman RA, Boice JD Jr. Cancer mortality following radium treatment for uterine bleeding. *Radiat Res* 1990;123:331–344.

Institute of Medicine. *The future of public health.* Washington, DC: National Academy Press, 1988.

Iversen GR. *Contextual analysis.* Thousand Oaks, CA: Sage Foundation, 1991.

Izurieta HS, Thompson WW, Kramarz P, Shay DK, Davis RL, DeStefano F, Black S, Shinefield H, Fukuda K. Influenza and the rates of hospitalization for respiratory disease among infants and young children. *N Engl J Med* 2000;342:232–239.

Jackson D. The implications of publication bias for meta-analysis' other parameter. *Stat Med* 2006;25:2911–2921.

Jacobsen BK, Bjelke E, Kvale G, Heuch I. Coffee drinking, mortality, and cancer incidence: results from a Norwegian prospective study. *J Natl Cancer Inst* 1986;76:823–831.

Jacobsen BK, Thelle DS. Coffee, cholesterol, and colon cancer: is there a link? *Br Med J* 1987;294:4–5.

Jacobsen R, Von Euler M, Osler M, Lynge E, Keiding N. Women's death in Scandinavia—what makes Denmark different? *Eur J Epidemiol* 2004;19:117–121.

Jacques PF, Sulsky SI, Sadowski JA, Phillips JC, Rush D, Willett WC. Comparison of micronutrient intake measured by a dietary questionnaire and biochemical indicators of micronutrient status. *Am J Clin Nutr* 1993;57:182–189.

Jaffe HW, Bregman DJ, Selik RM. Acquired immune deficiency syndrome in the United States: the first 1,000 cases. *J Infectious Diseases* 1983;148:339–345.
Jakes RW, Day NE, Luben R, Welch A, Bingham S, Mitchell J, Hennings S, Rennie K, Wareham NJ. Adjusting for energy intake–what measure to use in nutritional epidemiological studies? *Int J Epidemiol* 2004;33:1382–1386.
James RA, Hertz-Picciotto I, Willman E, Keller JA, Charles MJ. Determinants of serum polychlorinated biphenyls and organochlorine pesticides measured in women from the child health and development study cohort, 1963–1967. *Environ Health Perspect* 2002;110:617–624.
Janes GR, Hutwagner L, Cates W, Stroup DF, Williamson GD. Descriptive epidemiology: analyzing and interpreting surveillance data. In: Teutsch SM, Churchill RE, eds. *Principles and practice of public health surveillance*, 2nd ed. Oxford: Oxford University Press, 2000:112–167.
Janes H, Sheppard L, Lumley T. Overlap bias in the case-crossover design, with application to air pollution exposures. *Stat Med* 2004;24:285–300.
Janes H, Sheppard L, Lumley T. Case-crossover analyses of air pollution exposure data: referent selection strategies and their implications for bias. *Epidemiology* 2005;16:717–726.
Jarvis MJ, Feyerabend C, Bryant A, Hedges B, Primatesta P. Passive smoking in the home: plasma cotinine concentrations in non-smokers with smoking partners. *Tobacco Control* 2001;10:368–374.
Jaynes ET, Bretthorst GL. *Probability theory: the logic of science*. New York: Cambridge University Press, 2003.
Jewell N. *Statistics for epidemiology*. Boca Raton, Chapman and Hall/CRC, 2004.
Jick H. Re: Coffee and myocardial infarction (letter). *Am J Epidemiol* 1981;113:103–104.
Jick H, Miettinen OS, Neff RK, Shapiro S, Heinonen OP, Slone D. Coffee and myocardial infarction. *N Engl J Med* 1973;289:63–67.
Jick H, Watkins RN, Hunter JR, Dinan BJ, Madsen S, Rothman KJ, Walker AM. Replacement estrogens and endometrial cancer. *N Engl J Med* 1979;300:218–222.
Jick H, Walker AM, Rothman KJ, Hunter JR, Holmes LB, Watkins RN, D'Ewart DC, Danford A, Madsen S. Vaginal spermicides and congenital disorders. *JAMA* 1981a;245:1329–1332.
Jick H, Walker AM, Rothman KJ, Hunter JR, Holmes LB, Watkins RN, D'Ewart DC, Danford A, Madsen S. Re: "Vaginal spermicides and congenital disorders" (letter). *JAMA* 1981b;246:2677–2678.
Joffe M. Biases in research on reproduction and women's work. *Int J Epidemiol* 1985:14:118–123.
Joffe M, Villard L, Li Z, Plowman R, Vessey M. Long-term recall of time-to-pregnancy. *Fertil Steril* 1993;60:99–104.
Joffe MM, Greenland S. Estimation of standardized parameters from categorical regression models. *Stat Med* 1995;14:2131–2141.
Johansson JE, Adami HO, Andersson SO, Bergström R, Holmberg L, Krusemo UB. High 10-year survival rate in patients with early, untreated prostatic cancer. *JAMA* 1992;267:2191–2196.
Johnson FL, Thomas ED, Clark BS, Chard RL, Hartmann JR, Storb R. A comparison of marrow transplantation with chemotherapy for children with acute lymphoblastic leukemia in second or subsequent remission. *N Engl J Med* 1981;305:846–851.
Johnston SC. Combining ecological and individual variables to reduce confounding by indication: subarachnoid hemorrhage treatment. *J Clin Epidemiol* 2000;53:1236–1241.
Jones MC. Families of distributions arising from distributions of order statistics. *Test* 2004;13:1–44.
Jurek AM, Greenland S, Maldonado GM, Church TR. Proper interpretation of nondifferential misclassification effects: expectations versus observations. *Int J Epidemiol* 2005;34:680–687.
Jurek AM, Maldonado GM, Greenland, S, Church TR. Exposure measurement error is frequently ignored when interpreting epidemiologic study results. *Eur J Epidemiol* 2006;21;871–876.
Kabagambe EK, Baylin A, Allan DA, Siles X, Spiegelman D, Campos H. Application of the method of triads to evaluate the performance of food frequency questionnaires and biomarkers as indicators of long-term dietary intake. *Am J Epidemiol* 2001;154:1126–1135.
Kahneman D, Slovic P, Tversky A. *Judgment under uncertainty: heuristics and biases.* New York: Cambridge University Press, 1982.
Kalbfleisch JD, Prentice RL. *The statistical analysis of failure-time data*, 2nd ed. New York: Wiley, 2002.
Kalish LA. Matching on a non-risk factor in the design of case-control studies does not always result in an efficiency loss. *Am J Epidemiol* 1986;123:551–554.
Kalish LA. Reducing mean squared error in the analysis of pair-matched case-control studies. *Biometrics* 1990;46:493–499.
Kalter H, Warkany J. Congenital malformations: etiologic factors and their role in prevention. *N Eng J Med* 1983;308:424–431.
Kang JDY, Shafer JL. Demystifying double robustness: a comparison of alternative strategies for estimating a population mean from incomplete data. *Stat Sci* 2008; in press.
Kannel WB, Abbott RD. Incidence and prognosis of unrecognized myocardial infarction: an update on the Framingham study. *N Engl J Med* 1984;311:1144–1147.
Kannel WB, Dawber TR. Coffee and coronary disease. *N Engl J Med* 1973;289:100–101.
Kannel WB, Dawber TR, Kagan A, Revotskie N, Stokes JI. Factors of risk in the development of coronary heart disease-six year follow-up experience: the Framingham study. *Ann Intern Med* 1961;55:33–50.
Kannel WB, Wolf PA, Verter JI, McNamara PM. Epidemiologic assessment of the role of blood pressure in stroke: the Framingham study. *JAMA* 1970;214:301–310.
Karlowski TR, Chalmers TC, Frenkel LD, Kapikian AZ, Lewis TL, Lynch JM. Ascorbic acid for the common cold: a prophylactic and therapeutic trial. *JAMA* 1975;231:1038–1042.
Karon JM, Devine OJ, Morgan WM. Predicting AIDS incidence by extrapolating from recent trends. In: Castillo-Chavez C, ed. *Mathematical and statistical approaches to AIDS epidemiology.* Berlin: Springer-Verlag, 1989: 58–88. Lecture Notes in Biomathematics, Vol 83.

Karvetti RL, Knuts LR. Validity of the 24-hour recall. *J Am Diet Assoc* 1985;85:1437–1442.
Katz DL. Clinical epidemiology and evidence-based medicine. *Fundamental principles of clinical reasoning and research*. Sage Publications, Thousand Oaks, 2001.
Kaufman JS. How inconsistencies in racial classification demystify the race construct in public health statistics. *Epidemiology* 1999;10:101–103.
Kaufman JS, Cooper RS. Seeking causal explanations in social epidemiology. *Am J Epidemiol* 1999;150:113–120.
Kaufman JS, Cooper RS. Commentary: considerations for use of racial/ethnic classification in etiologic research. *Am J Epidemiol* 2001;154:291–298.
Kaufman JS, Kaufman S. Assessment of structured socioeconomic effects on health. *Epidemiology* 2001;12:157–167.
Kaufman JS, Poole C. Looking back on causal thinking in the health sciences. *Annu Rev Public Health* 2000;21:101–119.
Kaufman JS, Cooper RS, McGee DL. Socioeconomic status and health in blacks and whites: the problem of residual confounding and the resiliency of race. *Epidemiology* 1997;8:621–628.
Kaufman JS, Kaufman S, Poole C. Causal inference from randomized trials in social epidemiology. *Soc Sci Med* 2003;57:2397–2409.
Kaufman JS, MacLehose RF, Kaufman S. A further critique of the analytic strategy of adjusting for covariates to identify biologic mediation. *Epidemiol Perspect Innov* 2004;1:4 doi:10.1186/1742-5573-1-4
Kaufman S, Kaufman JS, MacLehose RF, Greenland S, Poole C. Improved estimation of controlled direct effects in the presence of unmeasured confounding by intermediate variables. *Stat Med* 2005;24:1683–1702.
Kawachi I, Berkman LF, eds. *Neighborhoods and Health*. Oxford University Press: Oxford, UK, 2003.
Keiding N. Age-specific incidence and prevalence: a statistical perspective. *JR Stat Soc A* 1991;154:371–412.
Keiding N, Vaeth M. Calculating expected mortality. *Stat Med* 1986;5:327–334.
Keku T, Millikan R, Worley K, Winkel S, Eaton A, Biscocho L, Martin C, Sandler R. 5,10-methylenetetrahydrofolate reductase codon 677 and 1298 polymorphisms and colon cancer in African Americans and whites. *Cancer Epidemiol Biomarkers Prev* 2002;11:1611–1621.
Kelsey JL, Whittemore AS, Evans AS, Thompson WD. *Methods in observational epidemiology*, 2nd ed. New York: Oxford University Press, 1996.
Kennedy P. *A guide to econometrics*. Cambridge, Massachusetts, The MIT Press, 1998.
Ketterer B. Dietary isothiocyanates as confounding factors in the molecular epidemiology of colon cancer. *Cancer Epidemiol Biomark Prev* 1998;7:645–646.
Keys A, Kihlberg JK. The effect of misclassification on the estimated relative prevalence of a characteristic. *Am J Public Health* 1963;53:1656–1665.
Khoury MJ. Genetic epidemiology. In Rothman KJ, Greenland S (eds). *Modern epidemiology*, 2nd ed. Lippincott-Raven Publishers: Philadelphia, PA, 1998:609–621.
Khoury MJ, Flanders WD. Nontraditional epidemiologic approaches in the analysis of gene-environment interactions: case-control studies with no controls! *Am J Epidemiol* 1996;144:207–213.
Khoury MJ, Holtzman NA. On the ability of birth defects monitoring to detect new teratogens. *Am J Epidemiol* 1987;126:136–143.
Khoury MJ, Flanders WD, Greenland S, Adams MJ. On the measurement of susceptibility in epidemiologic studies. *Am J Epidemiol* 1989a;129:183–190.
Khoury MJ, Flanders WD, James LM, Erickson JD. Human teratogens, prenatal mortality, and selection bias. *Am J Epidemiol* 1989b;130:361–370.
Khoury MJ, James L, Flanders W, Erickson J. Interpretation of recurring weak associations obtained from epidemiologic studies of suspected human teratogens. *Teratology* 1992;46:69–77.
Khoury MJ, Beaty TH, Cohen BH. *Fundamentals of genetic epidemiology*. New York: Oxford University Press, 1993.
Khoury M, James L, Erickson J. On the use of affected controls to address recall bias in case-control studies of birth defects. *Teratology* 1994;49:273–281.
Khoury MJ, Little J, Burke W. *Human genome epidemiology: a scientific foundation for using genetic information to improve health and prevent disease*. Oxford University Press: New York, 2004a.
Khoury MJ, Millikan R, Little J, Gwinn M. The emergence of epidemiology in the genomics age. *Int J Epidemiol* 2004b;33:936–944.
Kiechle FL, Holland-Staley CA. Genomics, transcriptomics, proteomics, and numbers. *Arch Pathol Lab Med* 2003;127:1089–1097.
Kim AI, Saab S. Treatment of hepatitis C. *Am J Med* 2005;118:808–815.
Kim HS, Newcomb PA, Ulrich CM, Keener CL, Bigler J, Farin FM, Bostick RM, Potter JD. Vitamin D receptor polymorphism and the risk of colorectal adenomas: evidence of interaction with dietary vitamin D and calcium. *Cancer Epidemiol Biomarkers Prev* 2001;10:869–873.
King G. *A solution to the ecological inference problem: reconstructing individual behavior from aggregate data*. Princeton, NJ: Princeton University Press, 1997.
King G. The future of ecological inference research: a comment on Freedman et al. *J Am Stat Assoc* 1999;94:352–355.
King G, Keohane RO, Verba S. *Designing Social Inquiry: Scientific Inference in Qualitative Research*. Princeton: Princeton University Press, 1994.
King G, Zeng L. When Can History be Our Guide? The Pitfalls of Counterfactual Inference. *Int Stud Q* 2007;51:183–210.
King G, Zeng L. Estimating risk and rate levels, ratios and differences in case-control studies. *Stat Med* 2002;21:1409–1427.
King H, Sinha A. Gene expression profile analysis by DNA microarrays: Promise and Pitfalls. *JAMA* 2001;286:2280–2288.
King H, Aubert RE, Herman WH. Global burden of diabetes, 1995–2025. *Diabetes Care* 1998;21:1414–1431.

Kington RS, Smith JP. Socioeconomic status and racial and ethnic differences in functional status associated with chronic diseases. *Am J Public Health* 1997;87:805–810.

Kinlen LJ. Fat and cancer. *Br Med J* 1983;286:1081–1082.

Kirkland JL. The biochemistry of mammalian senescence. *Clin Biochem* 1992;25:61–75.

Kitagawa EM. Components of a difference between two rates. *J Am Stat Assoc* 1955;50:1168–1194.

Kitler ME, Gavinio P, Lavanchy D. Influenza and the work of the World Health Organization. *Vaccine* 2002;20:S5–S14.

Klag MJ, Mead LA, LaCroix AZ, Wang NY, Coresh J, Liang KY, Pearson TA, Levine DM. Coffee intake and coronary heart disease. *Ann Epidemiol* 1994;4:425–433.

Klatsky AL, Friedman GD, Siegelaub AB. Coffee drinking prior to acute myocardial infarction. *JAMA* 1973;226:540–543.

Klatsky AL, Friedman GD, Armstrong MA. Coffee use prior to myocardial infarction restudied: heavier intake may increase risk. *Am J Epidemiol* 1990;132:479–488.

Kleinbaum DG, Kupper LL, Morgenstern H. *Epidemiologic research: principles and quantitative methods.* New York: Van Nostrand Reinhold, 1982 (1984 reprinting).

Klemetti A, Saxen L. Prospective versus retrospective approach in the search for environmental causes of malformations. *Am J Public Health* 1967;57:2071–2075.

Kliewer EV. Influence of migrants on regional variations of stomach and colon cancer mortality in the Western United States. *Int J Epidemiol* 1992;21:442–449.

Kliks SC, Nisalak A, Brandt WE, Wahl L, Burke DS. Antibody-dependent enhancement of dengue virus growth in human monocytes as a risk factor for dengue hemorrhagic fever. *Am J Trop Med Hyg* 1989;40:444–451.

Klinenberg E. *Heat Wave: A Social Autopsy of Disaster in Chicago.* The University of Chicago Press, Chicago, IL, 2002.

Knowler WC, Williams RC, Pettitt DJ, Steinberg AG. Gm3,5,13,14 and type 2 diabetes mellitus: an association in American Indians with genetic admixture. *Am J Hum Genet* 1988;43:520–526.

Koepsell TD, Weiss NS. *Epidemiologic Methods: Studying the Occurrence of Illness.* Oxford University Press, New York, New York, 2003.

Kolata G. Heart study produces a surprise result. *Science* 1982;218:31–32.

Koopman JS. Causal models and sources of interaction. *Am J Epidemiol* 1977;106:439–444.

Koopman JS. Interaction between discrete causes. *Am J Epidemiol* 1981;113:716–724.

Koopman JS, Longini IM Jr. The ecological effects of individual exposures and nonlinear disease dynamics in populations. *Am J Public Health* 1994;84:836–842.

Koopman JS, Lynch JW. Individual causal models and population system models in epidemiology. *Am J Public Health* 1999;89:1170–1174.

Koopman JS, Weed DL. Epigenesis theory. *Am J Epidemiol* 1990;132:366–390.

Korb K, Wallace C. In search of the philosopher's stone: remarks on Humphreys and Freedman's critique of casual discovery. *Br J Philos Sci* 1997;48:543–554.

Kovats RS, Haines A, Stanwell-Smith R, Martens P, Menne B, Bertollini R. Climate change and human health in Europe. *Brit Med J* 1999;318:1682–1685.

Krailo MD, Pike MC. Estimation of the distribution of age at natural menopause from prevalence data. *Am J Epidemiol* 1983;117:356–361.

Kramer MS. *Clinical epidemiology and biostatistics.* Berlin: Springer-Verlag, 1988.

Kraus AS. Comparison of a group with disease and a control group from the same families, in search of possible etiologic factors. *Am J Public Health* 1960;50:303–311.

Kreft I, de Leeuw J. *Introducing multilevel modeling.* London: Sage, 1998.

Krieger N. Epidemiology and the web of causation: has anyone seen the spider? *Soc Sci Med* 1994;39:887–903.

Krieger N, Fee E. Social class: the missing link in U.S. health data. *Int J Health Serv* 1994;24:25–44.

Krieger N. Embodying inequality: a review of concepts, measures, and methods for studying health consequences of discrimination. *Int J Health Serv* 1999;29:295–352.

Krieger N. Genders, sexes, and health: what are the connections—and why does it matter? *Int J Epidemiol* 2003;32:652–657.

Krieger N, Rowley DL, Herman AA, Avery B, Phillips MT. Racism, sexism and social class: implications for studies of health, disease, and well-being. *Am J Prev Med* 1993;9(suppl):82–122.

Krieger N, Williams DR, Moss NE. Measuring social class in U.S. public health research: concepts, methodologies, and guidelines. *Annu Rev Public Health* 1997;18:341–378.

Kristensen P. Bias from nondifferential but dependent misclassification of exposure and outcome. *Epidemiology* 1992;3:210–215.

Krupinski J, Stoller A, King D. Season of birth in schizophrenia: an Australian study. *Aust N Z J Psychiatry* 1976;10:311–314.

Kuh D, Ben Shlomo Y, eds. *A life course approach to chronic disease epidemiology*, 2nd ed. Oxford: Oxford University Press, 2004.

Kuhn TS. Reflections on my critics. In: Lakatos I, Musgrave A, eds. *Criticism and the growth of knowledge.* Cambridge: Cambridge University Press, 1970.

Kuhn TS. *The structure of scientific revolutions,* 2nd ed. Chicago: University of Chicago Press, 1962.

Kulldorff M. A spatial scan statistic. *Communications in statistics: theory and methods* 1997;26:1481–1496.

Künzli N, Tager IB. The semi-individual study of air pollution epidemiology: a valid design as compared to ecologic studies. *Environ Health Perspect* 1997;105:1078–1083.

Künzli N, Kaiser R, Medina S, Studnicka M, Chanel O, Filliger P, Herry M, Horak F Jr, Puybonnieux-Texier V, Quenel P, Schneider J, Seethaler R, Vergnaud JC, Sommer H. Public-health impact of outdoor and traffic-related air pollution: a European assessment. *Lancet* 2000;356:795–801.

Künzli N, Medina S, Kaiser R, Quenel P, Horak F Jr, Studnicka M. Assessment of deaths attributable to air pollution: should we use risk estimates based on time series or on cohort studies? *Am J Epidemiol* 2001;153:1050–1055.

Kupper LL. Effects of the use of unreliable surrogate variables on the validity of epidemiologic research studies. *Am J Epidemiol* 1984;20:634–638.

Kupper LL, Hogan MD. Interaction in epidemiologic studies. *Am J Epidemiol* 1978;106:447–453.

Kupper LL, McMichael AJ, Spirtas R. A hybrid epidemiologic design useful in estimating relative risk. *J Am Stat Assoc* 1975;70:524–528.

Kupper LL, Karon JM, Kleinbaum DG, Morgenstern H, Lewis DK. Matching in epidemiologic studies: validity and efficiency considerations. *Biometrics* 1981;37:271–292.

Kuratsune M, Yoshimura T, Matsuzaka J, Yamaguchi A. Epidemiologic study on Yusho, a poisoning caused by ingestion of rice oil contaminated with a commercial brand of polychlorinated biphenyls. *Environ Health Perspect* 1972;1:119–128.

Kurth T, Walker AM, Glynn RJ, Chan KA, Gaziano JM, Berger K, Robins JM. Results of multivariable logistic regression, propensity matching, propensity adjustment, and propensity-based weighting under conditions of nonuniform effect. *Am J Epidemiol* 2006;163:262–270.

Kurzawski G, Suchy J, Kadny J, Grabowska E, Mierzejewski M, Jakubowska A, Debniak T, Cybulski C, Kowalska E, Szych Z, Domagaa W, Scott RJ, LubiÒski J. The NOD2 3020insC mutation and the risk of colorectal cancer. *Cancer Res* 2004;64:1604–1606.

Kuss O. On the estimation of the stereotype regression model. *Comput Stat Data Anal* 2006;50:1877–1890.

L'Abbe KA, Detsky AS, O'Rourke K. Meta-analysis in clinical research. *Ann Intern Med* 1987;107:224–233.

LaCroix AZ, Mead LA, Liang KY, Thomas CB, Pearson TA. Coffee consumption and the incidence of coronary heart disease. *N Engl J Med* 1986;315:977–982.

Lafferty WE, Hopkins SG, Honey J, Harwell JD, Shoemaker PC, Kobayashi JM. Hospital discharges for people with AIDS in Washington state: utilization of a statewide hospital discharge data base. *Am J Public Health* 1988;78:949–952.

Lagakos SW. Effects of mismodeling and mismeasuring explanatory variables on tests of their association with a response variable. *Stat Med* 1988;7:257–274.

Lakatos I. Falsification and the methodology of scientific research programmes. In: Lakatos I, Musgrave A, eds. *Criticism and the growth of knowledge.* Cambridge: Cambridge University Press, 1970.

Lake SL, Laird NM. Tests of gene-environment interaction for case-parent triads with general environmental exposures. *Ann Hum Genet* 2004;68:55–64.

Lancaster HO. The combination of probabilities arising from data in discrete distributions. *Biometrika* 1949;36:370–382.

Lancaster HO. Significance tests in discrete distributions. *J Am Stat Assoc* 1961;56:223–234.

Lancaster PAL. Congenital malformations after in-vitro fertilization. *Lancet* 1987;2:1392–1393.

Lane PW, Nelder JA. Analysis of covariance and standardization as instances of prediction. *Biometrics* 1982;38:613–621.

Lanes SF, Rothman KJ. Tampon absorbency, composition, and oxygen content and risk of toxic shock syndrome. *J Clin Epidemiol* 1990;43:1379–1385.

Lanes SF, Poole C. "Truth in packaging?" The unwrapping of epidemiologic research. *J Occup Med* 1984;26:571–574.

Langbein LI, Lichtman AJ. *Ecological inference.* Thousand Oaks, CA: Sage Foundation, 1978. Series/no 07-010.

Langholz B, Clayton D. Sampling strategies in nested case-control studies. *Environ Health Perspect* 1994;102(suppl 8):47–51.

Langman MJS. Towards estimation and confidence intervals. *Br Med J* 1986;292;716.

Langmuir AD. The surveillance of communicable diseases of national importance. *N Engl J Med* 1963;268:182–192.

Lash TL, Heuristic thinking and inference from observational epidemiology. *Epidemiology* 2007;18:67–72.

Lash TL, Fink AK. Semi-automated sensitivity analysis to assess systematic errors in observational epidemiologic data. *Epidemiology* 2003a;14:451–458.

Lash TL, Fink AK. Re: "Neighborhood environment and loss of physical function in older adults: evidence from the Alameda County Study" (letter). *Am J Epidemiol.* 2003b;157:472–473.

Lash TL, Fink AK. A null association between pregnancy termination and breast cancer in a registry-based study of parous women. *Int J Cancer* 2004;110:443–448.

Lash TL, Silliman RA. A sensitivity analysis to separate bias due to confounding from bias due to predicting misclassification by a variable that does both. *Epidemiology* 2000;11:544–549.

Laurence KM, James N, Miller MH, Tennant GB, Campbell H. Double-blind randomised controlled trial of folate treatment before conception to prevent recurrence of neural-tube defects. *Br Med J* 1981;282:1509–1511.

Lauritzen SL, Richardson TS. Chain graph models and their causal interpretations. *J R Stat Soc Ser B* 2002;64:321–348.

Laursen M, Bille C, Olesen AW, Hjelmborg J, Skytthe A, Christensen K. Genetic influence on prolonged gestation: a population-based Danish twin study. *Am J Obstet Gynecol* 2004;190:489–494.

Lave LB, Seskin EP. Air pollution and human health. *Science* 1970;169:723–733.

La Vecchia C, Gentile A, Negri E, Parazzini F, Franceschi S. Coffee consumption and myocardial infarction in women. *Am J Epidemiol* 1989;130:481–485.

LaVeist TA, Wallace JM Jr. Health risk and inequitable distribution of liquor stores in African American neighborhood. *Soc Sci Med* 2000;51:613–617.

Lawlor DA, Davey Smith G, Bruckdorfer KR, Kundu D. Ebrahim S. Those confounded vitamins: what can we learn from the differences between observational versus randomized trial evidence? *Lancet* 2004a;363:1724–1727.

Lawlor DA, Davey Smith G, Ebrahim S. The hormone replacement-coronary heart disease conundrum: is this the death of observational epidemiology? *Int J Epidemiol* 2004b;33:464–467.

Lawson AB. *Statistical methods in spatial epidemiology.* Chichester: Wiley, 2001.

Leamer EE. False models and post-data model construction. *J Am Stat Assoc* 1974;69:122–131.

Leamer EE. Sensitivity analyses would help. *Am Econ Rev* 1985;75:308–313.

Leamer EE. *Specification searches.* New York: Wiley, 1978.

Lebret E. Models of human exposure based on environmental monitoring. *Sci Total Environ* 1995;168:179–185.

Le Cessie S, van Houwelingen HC. Ridge estimators in logistic regression. *Appl Stat* 1992;41:191–201.

Ledrans M, Pirard P, Tillaut H, Lee JAH. Melanoma and exposure to sunlight. *Epidemiol Rev* 1982;4:110–136.

Lee JAH, Petersen GR, Stevens RG, Vesanen K. The influence of age, year of birth, and date on mortality from malignant melanoma in the populations of England and Wales, Canada, and the white population of the United States. *Am J Epidemiol* 1979;110:734–739.

Lee WC. Case-control association studies with matching and genomic controlling. *Genet Epidemiol* 2004;27:1–13.

LeGrady D, Dyer AR, Shekelle RB, Stamler J, Liu K, Paul O, Lepper M, Shryock AM. Coffee consumption and mortality in the Chicago Western Electric Company Study. *Am J Epidemiol* 1987;126:803–812.

Lehmann EL. *Testing statistical hypotheses,* 2nd ed. New York: Wiley, 1986.

Le Marchand L, Seifried A, Lum-Jones A, Donlon T, Wilkens LR. Association of the cyclin D1 A870G polymorphism with advanced colorectal cancer. *JAMA*. 2003;290:2843–2848.

Leonard T, Hsu JSJ. *Bayesian Methods*. Cambridge: Cambridge University Press, 1999.

Leren P. The effect of plasma cholesterol lowering diet in male survivors of myocardial infarction. *Acta Med Scand Suppl* 1966;466:5–92.

Lesaffre E, Rizopoulos D, Tsonaka R. The logistic transform for bounded outcome scores. *Biostatistics* 2006;7:72–85.

Lesage S, Zouali H, Cézard JP, Colombel JF, Belaiche J, Almer S, Tysk C, O'Morain C, Gassull M, Binder V, Finkel Y, Modigliani R, Gower-Rousseau C, Macry J, Merlin F, Chamaillard M, Jannot AS, Thomas G, Hugot JP; EPWG-IBD Group; EPIMAD Group; GETAID Group. CARD15/NOD2 mutational analysis and genotype-phenotype correlation in 612 patients with inflammatory bowel disease. *Am J Hum Genet* 2002;70:845–857.

Leventhal T, Brooks-Gunn J. Moving to Opportunity: an experimental study of neighborhood effects on mental health. *Am J Public Health* 2003;93:1576–1582.

Levin ML. The occurrence of lung cancer in man. *Acta Unio Int Contra Cancrum* 1953;9:531–541.

Levy D, Lumley T, Sheppard L, Kaufman J, Checkoway H. referent selection in case-crossover analyses of acute health effects of air pollution. *Epidemiology* 2001;12:186–192.

Lewis D, Causation *J. Philos* 1973;70:556–567. (Reprinted with postscript in: Lewis D. *Philosophical papers.* New York: Oxford University Press, 1986.)

Lewis DK. A subjectivist's guide to objective chance. In: Jeffrey, R.C. (ed.): *Studies in inductive logic and probability.* Berkeley: University of California Press, 1981:263–293.

Li JY, Taylor PR, Li GY, Blot WJ, Yu Y, Ershow AG, Sun YH, Yang CS, Yang Q, Tangrea JA. Intervention studies in Linxian, China: an update. *J Nutr Growth Cancer* 1986;3:199–206.

Liang KY. Extended Mantel-Haenszel estimating equations for multivariate logistic regression models. *Biometrics* 1987;43:289–299.

Liang KY, Zeger SL. Longitudinal Data Analysis Using Generalized Linear Models *Biometrika* 1986;73:13–22.

Liberatos P, Link BG, Kelsey JL. The measurement of social class in epidemiology. *Epidemiol Rev* 1988;10:87–121.

Light RJ, Pillemer DB. *Summing up: the science of reviewing research.* Cambridge, MA: Harvard University Press, 1984.

Lin DY, Psaty BM, Kronmal RA. Assessing the sensitivity of regression results to unmeasured confounders in observational studies. *Biometrics* 1998;54:948–963.

Lin HJ, Lakkides KM, Keku TO, Reddy ST, Louie AD, Kau IH, Zhou H, Gim JS, Ma HL, Matthies CF, Dai A, Huang HF, Materi AM, Lin JH, Frankl HD, Lee ER, Hardy SI, Herschman HR, Henderson BE, Kolonel LN, Le Marchand L, Garavito RM, Sandler RS, Haile RW, Smith WL. Prostaglandin H Synthase 2 variant (Val511Ala) in African Americans may reduce the risk for colorectal neoplasia. *Cancer Epidemiol Biomarkers Prev* 2002;11:1305–1315.

Lindegren ML and the CDC NHANES working group. National Health and Nutrition Survey (NHANES) III DNA Bank: Gene Variants Important to Public Health. CDC report on genomics and population health, United States, 2003. Accessed online at http://www.cdc.gov/genomics/activities/ogdp/2003/chap01.htm.

Lindley DV. The Bayesian analysis of contingency tables. *Annals of Mathematical Statistics* 1964;35:1622–1643.

Lindley DV. *Introduction to probability and statistics from a Bayesian viewpoint.* Cambridge: Cambridge University Press. 1965.

Lindley DV. *Making decisions,* 2nd ed. New York: Wiley, 1985.

Lindsay SW, Martens WJM. Malaria in the African highlands: past, present and future. *Bull World Health Org* 1998;76:33–45.

Lindsted KD, Kuzma JW, Anderson JL. Coffee consumption and cause-specific mortality: association with age at death and compression of mortality. *J Clin Epidemiol* 1992;45:733–742.

Linet MS, Harlow SD, McLaughlin JK, Link BG, Phelan J. Social conditions as fundamental causes of disease. *J Health Soc Behav* 1995;(special no.):80–94.

Little RJA. On testing equality of two independent binomial proportions. *Am Statist* 1989;43:283–288.

Little RJA, Rubin DB. *Statistical analysis with missing data*, 2nd ed. New York: Wiley. 2002.

Liu K, Stamler J, Dyer A, McKeever J, McKeever P. Statistical methods to assess and minimize the role of intra-individual variability in obscuring the relationship between dietary lipids and serum cholesterol. *J Chronic Dis* 1978;31:399–418.

Liu X, Fallin MD, Linda Kao WH. Genetic dissection methods: designs used for tests of gene-environment interaction. *Curr Opinion Genet Devel* 2004;14:241–245.

Lloyd SA. Stratospheric ozone depletion. *Lancet* 1993;342:1156–1158.

Loftus EF, Smith KD, Klinger MR, Fiedler J. Memory and mismemory for health events. In: Tanur JM, ed. *Questions about questions: inquiries into the cognitive bases of surveys.* New York: Sage Foundation, 1992.

Loftus EV Jr. Clinical epidemiology of inflammatory bowel disease: incidence, prevalence, and environmental influences. *Gastroenterology* 2004;126:1504–1517.

Logan WPD. Mortality in the London fog incident, 1952. *Lancet* 1953;1:336–338.

London SJ, Sacks FM, Caesar J, Stampfer MJ, Siguel E, Willett WC. Fatty acid composition of subcutaneous adipose tissue and diet in post-menopausal U.S. women. *Am J Clin Nutr* 1991;54:340–345.

Longini IM, Koopman JS, Haber M, Cotsonis GA. Statistical Inference for infectious diseases. Risk-specific household and community transmission parameters. *Am J Epidemiol* 1988;128:845–859.

Longnecker MP, Daniels JL. Environmental contaminants as etiologic factors for diabetes. *Environ Health Perspect* 2001;109(Suppl 6):871–876.

Longnecker MP, Rogan WJ, Lucier G. The human health effects of DDT (dichlorodiphenyltrichloroethane) and PCBs (polychlorinated biphenyls) and an overview of organochlorines in public health. *Annu Rev Public Health* 1997;18:211–244.

Longnecker MP, Stram DO, Taylor PR, Levander OA, Howe M, Veillon C, McAdam PA, Patterson KY, Holden JM, Morris JS, Swanson CA, Willett WC. Use of selenium concentration in whole blood, serum, toenails, or urine as a surrogate measure of selenium intake. *Epidemiology* 1996;7:384–390.

Loring M, Powell B. Gender, race and DSM-III: a study of the objectivity of psychiatric diagnostic behavior. *J Health Soc Behav* 1988;29:1–22.

Louis TA, Fineberg HV, Mosteller F. Findings for public health from meta-analysis. *Annu Rev Public Health* 1985;6:1–20.

Lowy FD. Staphylococcus aureus infections. *N Engl J Med* 1998;339:520–532.

Lubin JH, Caporaso NE. Cigarette smoking and lung cancer: modeling total exposure and intensity. *Cancer Epidemiol Biomarkers Prev* 2006;15:517–523.

Lubin JH, Gail MH. Biased selection of controls for case-control analyses of cohort studies. *Biometrics* 1984;40:63–75.

Lubin JH, Hartge P. Excluding controls: misapplications in case-control studies. *Am J Epidemiol* 1984;120:791–793.

Lubin JH, Samet JM, Weinberg CR. Design issues in epidemiologic studies of indoor exposure to radon and risk of lung cancer. *Health Phys* 1990;59:807–817.

Luesley D, Lawton F, Blackledge G, Hilton C, Kelly K, Rollason T, Wade-Evans T, Jordan J, Fielding J, Latief T, et al. Failure of second-look laparotomy to influence survival in epithelial ovarian cancer. *Lancet* 1988;2:599–603.

Lumley T, Levy D. Bias in the case-crossover design: implications for studies of air pollution. *Environmetrics* 2000;11:689–704.

Lunceford JK, Davidian M. Stratification and weighting via the propensity score in estimation of causal treatment effects: A comparative study. *Stat Med* 2004;23:2937–2960.

Luneberg WV. The legal context of environmental protection in the United States. In: Talbott EO, Craun GF, eds. *Introduction to environmental epidemiology.* New York: CRC Lewis Publishers, 1995:1–21.

Luzzi GA, Merry AH, Newbold CI, Marsh K, Pasvol G, Weatherall DJ. Surface antigen expression on *Plasmodium falciparum*-infected erythrocytes is modified in alpha- and beta-thalassemia. *J Exp Med* 1991;173:785–791.

Lyles RH. A note on estimating crude odds ratios in case-control studies with differentially misclassified exposure. *Biometrics* 2002;58:1034–1037.

Lyles RH, Allen AS. Estimating crude or common odds ratios in case-control studies with informatively missing exposure data. *Am J Epidemiol* 2002;155:274–278.

Lynch H, de la Chapelle A. Hereditary colon cancer. *N Engl J Med* 2003;348:919–932.

Lynch J, Smith GD, Harper S, Hillemeier M, Ross N, Kaplan GA, Wolfson M. Is income inequality a determinant of population health? Part 1. A systematic review. *Milbank Q* 2004;82:5–99.

Lynch JW, Kaplan G. Socioeconomic position. In: Berkman LF, Kawachi I, eds. *Social epidemiology*. New York: Oxford University Press, 2000:13–35.

Lyon JL, Mahoney AW, West DW, Gardner JW, Smith KR, Sorenson AW, Stanish W. Energy intake: its relation to colon cancer risk. *J Natl Cancer Inst* 1987;78:853–861.

Lyons RA, Sibert J, McCabe. Injury surveillance programmes, ethics, and the Data Protection Act: sharing data to prevent injuries. *British Med J* 1999;319:372–373.

Ma X, Buffler PA, Layefsky M, Does MB, Reynolds P. Control selection strategies in case-control studies of childhood diseases. *Am J Epidemiol* 2004;159:915–921.

Macintyre K, Sosler S, Letipila F, Lochigan M, Hassig S, Omar SA, Githure J. A new tool for malaria prevention?: Results of a trial of permethrin-impregnated bedsheets (shukas) in an area of unstable transmission. *Int J Epidemiol* 2003;32:157–160.

Mack TM, Pike MC, Henderson BE, Pfeffer RI, Gerkins VR, Arthur M, Brown SE. Estrogens and endometrial cancer in a retirement community. *N Engl J Med* 1976;294:1262–1267.

MacKay AM, Rothman KJ. The incidence and severity of burn injuries following Project Burn Prevention. *Am J Public Health* 1982;72:248–252.

MacKenzie S, Lippman A. An investigation of report bias in a case-control study of pregnancy outcome. *Am J Epidemiol* 1989;129:65–75.

Mackie JL. Causes and conditions. *Am Philo Q* 1965;2:245–255. Reprinted in Sosa E, Tooley M, eds. *Causation*. New York: Oxford, 1993, 33–55.

MacLaughlin DS. A data validation program nucleus. *Comput Prog Biomed* 1980;11:43–47.

Maclehose RL, Kaufman S, Kaufman JS, Poole C. Bounding causal effects under uncontrolled confounding using counterfactuals. *Epidemiology* 2005;16:548–555.

Maclure M. Popperian refutation in epidemiology. *Am J Epidemiol* 1985;121:343–350.

Maclure M. The case-crossover design: a method for studying transient effects on the risk of acute events. *Am J Epidemiol* 1991;133:144–153.

Maclure M. Demonstration of deductive meta-analysis: ethanol intake and risk of myocardial infarction. *Epidemiol Rev* 1993;15:328–351.

Maclure M, Greenland S. Tests for trend and dose-response: misinterpretations and alternatives. *Am J Epidemiol* 1992;135:96–104.

MacMahon AD. Approaches to combat confounding by indication in observational studies of intended drug effects. *Pharmacoepidemiol Drug Saf* 2003;12:551–558.

MacMahon B. Strengths and limitations of epidemiology. In: National Academy of Sciences, The National Research Council. Washington, DC: National Academy of Sciences, 1979.

MacMahon B, Pugh TF. Causes and entities of disease. In: Clark DW, MacMahon B, eds. *Preventive medicine*. Boston: Little, Brown, 1967.

MacMahon B, Pugh TF. *Epidemiology: principles and methods*. Boston: Little, Brown, 1970:137–198, 175–184.

MacMahon B, Trichopoulos D. *Epidemiology: principles and methods*, 2nd ed. Philadelphia: Lippincott Williams & Wilkins, 1996.

MacQueen KM, Buehler JW. Ethical Issues in HIV, STD, and TB public health practice and research: results of a workshop. *Am J Public Health* 2004;94:928–931.

Madden JP, Goodman SJ, Guthrie HA. Validity of the 24-hour recall: analysis of data obtained from elderly subjects. *J Am Diet Assoc* 1976;68:143–147.

Magee B. *Philosophy and the real world: an introduction to Karl Popper.* La Salle, IL: Open Court, 1985.

Magnus P, Beaglehole R. The real contribution of the major risk factors to the coronary epidemics: Time to end the "Only-50%" myth. *Arch Intern Med* 2001;161:2657–2660.

Mahaffey KR, Annest JL, Roberts J, Murphy RS. National estimates of blood lead levels: United States, 1976–1980: association with selected demographic and socioeconomic factors. *N Engl J Med* 1982;307:573–579.

Maldonado G, Greenland S. Interpreting model coefficients when the true model form is unknown. *Epidemiology* 1993a;4:310–318.

Maldonado G, Greenland S. Simulation study of confounder-selection strategies. *Am J Epidemiol* 1993b;138:923–936.

Maldonado G, Greenland S. A comparison of the performance of model-based confidence intervals when the correct model form is unknown: coverage of asymptotic means. *Epidemiology* 1994;5:171–182.

Maldonado G, Greenland S. Estimating causal effects (with discussion). *Int J Epidemiol* 2002;31:421–438.

Maldonado G, Delzell E, Tyl S, Sever L. Occupational exposure to glycol ethers and human congenital malformations. *Int Arch Occup Environ Health* 2003;76:405–423.

Malkin JD, Broder MS, Keeler E. Do longer postpartum stays reduce newborn readmissions? Analysis using instrumental variables. *Health Serv Res* 2000;35:1071–1091.

Mann JI, Thorogood M. Coffee drinking and myocardial infarction. *Lancet* 1975;2:1215.

Mann JM, Gostin L, Gruskin S, Brennan T, Lazzarini Z, Fineberg H. Health and human rights. In: Mann JM, Gruskin S, Grodin MA, Annas GJ, eds. *Health and human rights: a reader*. New York: Routledge, 1999:7–20.

Manolio T. Novel risk markers and clinical practice. *N Engl J Med* 2003;349:1587–1589.

Manousos O, Day NE, Trichopoulos D. Diet and colorectal cancer: a case-control study in Greece. *Int J Cancer* 1983;32:1–5.

Mansson R, Joffe MM, Sun W, Hennessy S. On the estimation and use of propensity scores in case-control and case-cohort studies. *Am J Epidemiol* 2007;166:332–339.

Mantel N. Chi-square tests with one degree of freedom: extensions of the Mantel-Haenszel procedure. *J Am Stat Assoc* 1963;58:690–700.

Mantel N. Synthetic retrospective studies and related topics. *Biometrics* 1973;29:479–486.

Mantel N, Hankey BF. The odds ratios of a 2×2 table. *Am Stat* 1975;29:143–145.

Mantel N, Fleiss JL. Minimum expected cell size requirements for the Mantel-Haenszel one-degree-of-freedom test and a related rapid procedure. *Am J Epidemiol* 1980;112:129–134.

Mantel N, Haenszel WH. Statistical aspects of the analysis of data from retrospective studies of disease. *J Natl Cancer Inst* 1959;22:719–748.

Manton KG, Stallard E. *Chronic disease modelling*. London: Griffin, 1988.

Mariadason JM, Arango D, Shi Q, Wilson AJ, Corner GA, Nicholas C, Aranes MJ, Lesser M, Schwartz EL, Augenlicht LH. Gene expression profiling-based prediction of response of colon carcinoma cells to 5-fluorouracil and camptothecin. *Cancer Res* 2003;63:8791–8812.

Mark SD, Robins JM. Estimating the causal effect of smoking cessation in the presence of confounding factors using a rank preserving structural failure time model. *Stat Med* 1993a;12:1605–1628.

Mark SD, Robins JM. A method for the analysis of randomized trials with compliance information: an application to the Multiple Risk Factor Intervention Trial. *Control Clin Trials* 1993b;14:79–97.

Marmot M. Coronary heart disease: rise and fall of a modern epidemic. In: Marmot M, Elliott P, eds. *Coronary heart disease epidemiology: from aetiology to public health.* New York: Oxford University Press, 1992:3–19.

Marmot MG, Wilkinson RG, eds. Social Determinants of Health Oxford University Pres, Oxford UK, 1999.

Marmot MG, Smith GD, Stansfeld S, Patel C, North F, Head J, White I, Brunner E, Feeney A. Health inequalities among British civil servants: The Whitehall II study. *Lancet* 1991;8:1387–1393.

Marr JW. Individual dietary surveys: purposes and methods. *World Rev Nutr Diet* 1971;13:105–164.

Marshall JR, Hastrup JL. Mismeasurement and the resonance of strong confounders: uncorrelated errors. *Am J Epidemiol* 1996;143:1069–1078.

Marshall JR, Hastrup JL, Ross JS. Mismeasurement and the resonance of strong confounders: correlated errors. *Am J Epidemiol* 1999;150:88–96.

Marshall RJ. Validation study methods for estimating exposure proportions and odds ratios with misclassified data. *J Clin Epidemiol* 1990;43:941–947.

Marshall SW. Commentary on making meaningful inferences about magnitudes. *Sportscience* 2006;9:43–44.

Marshall SW, Mueller FO, Kirby DP, Yang J. Evaluation of safety balls and faceguards for prevention of injuries in youth baseball. *JAMA* 2003;289:568–574.

Martens WJM. Health impacts of climate change and ozone depletion: an ecoepidemiologic modeling approach. *Env Health Persp* 1998;106:241–251.

Martens EP, Pestman WR, de Boer A, Belitser SV, Klungel OH. Instrumental variables application and limitations. *Epidemiology* 2006;17:260–267.

Martin DO, Austin H. Exact estimates for a rate ratio. *Epidemiology* 1996;7:29–33.

Martinez ME, O'Brien TG, Fultz KE, Babbar N, Yerushalmi H, Qu N, Guo Y, Boorman D, Einspahr J, Alberts DS, Gerner EW. Pronounced reduction in adenoma recurrence associated with aspirin use and a polymorphism in the ornithine decarboxylase gene. *Proc Natl Acad Sci* 2003;100:7859–7864.

Marx J. A parent's sex may affect gene expression. *Science* 1988;239:352–353.

Mascheretti S, Hampe J, Croucher PJ, Nikolaus S, Andus T, Schubert S, Olson A, Bao W, Fölsch UR, Schreiber S. Response to infliximab treatment in Crohn's disease is not associated with mutations in the CARD15 (NOD2) gene: an analysis in 534 patients from two multicenter, prospective GCP-level trials. *Pharmacogenetics* 2002;12:509–515.

Mason KO, Mason W, Winsborough HH, Poole WK. Some methodological issues in the cohort analysis of archival data. *Am Sociol Rev* 1973;38:242–258.

Mason TJ, McKay FW, Hoover R, Blot W. *Atlas of cancer mortality for U.S. counties 1950–1969.* Washington, DC: U.S. Government Printing Office, 1975:36–37. DHEW Publ No (NIH) 75-780.

Mason TJ, McKay FW, Hoover R, Blot WJ, Fraumeni JF Jr. *Atlas of cancer mortality among U.S. nonwhites 1950–1969.* Washington, DC: U.S. Government Printing Office, 1976. DHEW Publ No (NIH) 76-1204.

Mason WM, Wong GY, Entwisle B. Contextual analysis through the multilevel linear model. In: Leinhardt S., ed. *Sociological Methodology* 83/84. San Francisco: Jossey-Bass, 1983:72–103.

Massey DS, Denton NA. The dimensions of residential segregation. *Social Forces* 1988;67:281–315.

Matthews RAJ. Methods for assessing the credibility of clinical trial outcomes. *Drug Inf J* 2001;35:1469–1478.

Mazumder DN, Das Gupta J, Santra A, Pal A, Ghose A, Sarkar S. Chronic arsenic toxicity in west Bengal–the worst calamity in the world. *J Indian Med Assoc* 1998;96:4–7,18.

Mayo DG, Cox DR. Frequentist statistics as a theory of inductive inference. In: Rojo J (ed.). 2nd Lehmann Symposium - Optimality. IMS Lecture Notes - Monographs Series 2006:1–28.

McCandless LC, Gustafson P, Levy AR. Bayesian sensitivity analysis for unmeasured confounders in observational studies. *Stat Med* 2007;26:2331–2347.

McClellan WM, Frankenfield DL, Frederick PR, Helgerson SD, Wish JB, Sugarman JR. Improving the care of ESRD patients: a success story. *Health Care Financing Review* 2003;24:89–100.

McCue KF. The statistical foundations of the EI method. *Am Statistician* 2001;55:106–110.

McCullagh P. Quasi-likelihood and estimating functions. In: Hinkley DV, Reid N, Snell EJ, eds. *Statistical theory and modeling.* London: Chapman and Hall, 1991. Chapter 11.

McCullagh P, Nelder JA. *Generalized linear models,* 2nd ed. New York: Chapman and Hall, 1989.

McCulloch CE, Searle SR. *Generalized, linear and mixed models.* New York: Wiley, 2001.

McDonough P, Duncan GJ, Williams D, House J. Income dynamics and adult mortality in the United States, 1972 through 1989. *Am J Public Health* 1997;87:1476–1483.

McDowall D, McCleary R, Meidinger EE, Hay RA Jr. *Interrupted time series analysis.* Beverly Hills, CA: Sage Foundation, 1980.

McDowall M. Adjusting proportional mortality ratios for the influence of extraneous causes of death. *Stat Med* 1983;2:467–475.

McGeehin MA, Qualters JR, Niskar AS. National environmental public health tracking program: bridging the information gap. *Environ Health Perspect* 2004;112:1409–1413.

McKee PA, Castelli WP, McNamara PM, Kannel WB. The natural history of congestive heart failure: the Framingham study. *N Engl J Med* 1971;285:1441–1446.

McKeown-Eyssen GE, Bright-See E. Dietary factors in colon cancer: international relationships: an update. *Nutr Cancer* 1985;7:251–253.

McKim VR, Turner SP. *Causality in crisis: statistical methods for causal knowledge in the social sciences.* Notre Dame, Ind.: University of Notre Dame Press, 1997.

McLaughlin JK, Blot WJ, Mehl ES, Mandel JS. Problems in the use of dead controls in case-control studies. I. General results. *Am J Epidemiol* 1985;121:131–139.

McLeod RS, Taylor DW, Cohen Z, Cullen JB. Single patient randomized controlled trial. Use in determining optimum treatment for patient with inflammation of Kock continent ileostomy reservoir. *Lancet* 1986;1:726–728.

McMichael AJ. Standardized mortality ratios and the "healthy worker effect:" scratching beneath the surface. *J Occup Med* 1976;18:165–168.

McMichael AJ. The health of persons, populations, and planets: epidemiology comes full circle. *Epidemiology* 1995;6:633–636.

McMichael AJ. The urban environment and health in a world of increasing globalization: issues for developing countries. *Bull World Health Organ* 2000;78:1117–1126.

McMichael AJ. Health consequences of global climate change. *J R Soc Med* 2001;94:111–114.

McMichael AJ, Giles GG. Cancer in migrants to Australia: extending the descriptive epidemiological data. *Cancer Res* 1988;48:751–756.

McMichael AJ, Patz J, Kovats RS. Impacts of global environmental change on future health and health care in tropical countries. *Brit Med Bull* 1998;54:475–488.

McNeilly MD, Anderson NB, Armstead CA, Clark R, Corbett M, Robinson EL, Pieper CF, Lepisto EM. The perceived racism scale: a multidimensional assessment of the experience of white racism among African Americans. *Ethn Dis* 1996;6:154–166.

McNemar Q. Note on the sampling of the difference between corrected proportions or percentages. *Psychometrika* 1947;12:153–157.

Meadows M. A look at the 2003–2004 flu season. *FDA Consumer* 2004:38:9–11.

Medawar PB. *Advice to a young scientist.* New York: Basic Books, 1979.

Melbye M, Wohlfahrt J, Olsen JH, Frisch M, Westergaard T, Helweg-Larsen K, Andersen PK. Induced abortion and the risk of breast cancer. *N Engl J Med* 1997;336:81–85.

Melnick JL, Ledinko N. Social serology; antibody levels in a normal young population during an epidemic of poliomyelitis. *Am J Hyg* 1951;54:354–382.

Meslin E, Thomson EJ, Boyer J. The ethical, legal, and social implications research program at the National Human Genome Research Institute. *Kennedy Inst Ethics J* 1997;7:291–298.

Mertz W. Foods and nutrients. *J Am Diet Assoc* 1984;84:769–770.

Meydrech EF, Kupper LL. Cost considerations and sample size requirements in cohort and case-control studies. *Am J Epidemiol* 1978;107:201–205.

Michels KB, Greenland S, Rosner BA. Does body mass index adequately capture the relation of body composition and body size to health outcomes? *Am J Epidemiol* 1998;147:167–172.

Mickey RM, Greenland S. The impact of confounder selection criteria on effect estimation. *Am J Epidemiol* 1989;129:125–137.

Mickle JE, Cutting GR. Genotype-phenotype relationships in cystic fibrosis. *Med Clin North Am* 2000;84:597–607.

Miech RA, Hauser RM. Socioeconomic status and health at midlife. A comparison of educational attainment with occupation-based indicators. *Ann Epidemiol* 2001;11:75–84.

Miettinen OS. Individual matching with multiple controls in the case of all-or-none responses. *Biometrics* 1969; 25:339–355.

Miettinen OS. Standardization of risk ratios. *Am J Epidemiol* 1972;96:383–388.

Miettinen OS. Comment. *J Am Stat Assoc* 1974a;69:380–382.

Miettinen OS. Proportion of disease caused or prevented by a given exposure, trait, or intervention. *Am J Epidemiol* 1974b;99:325–332.

Miettinen OS. Estimability and estimation in case-referent studies. *Am J Epidemiol* 1976a;103:226–235.

Miettinen OS. Stratification by a multivariate confounder score. *Am J Epidemiol* 1976b;104:609–620.

Miettinen OS. Design options in epidemiologic research: an update. *Scand J Work Environ Health* 1982a;8(suppl 1):7–14.

Miettinen OS. Causal and preventive interdependence: elementary principles. *Scand J Work Environ Health* 1982b;8: 159–168.

Miettinen OS. The "case-control" study: valid selection of subjects. *J Chron Dis* 1985a;38:543–548.

Miettinen OS. *Theoretical epidemiology.* New York: Wiley, 1985b.

Miettinen OS, Cook EF. Confounding: essence and detection. *Am J Epidemiol* 1981,114.593–603.

Miettinen OS, Wang J-D. An alternative to the proportionate mortality ratio. *Am J Epidemiol* 198I;114:144–148.

Mill JSA. *System of logic, ratiocinative and inductive*, 5th ed. London: Parker, Son and Bowin, 1862. (Cited in: Clark DW, MacMahon B, eds. *Preventive and community medicine,* 2nd ed. Boston: Little, Brown, 1981. Chapter 2.)

Min Y-I, Dickersin K. Rate of full publication and time to full publication of observational studies. *Am J Epidemiol* 2005;161(suppl):abstract 301.

Mirza MM, Fisher SA, King K, Cuthbert AP, Hampe J, Sanderson J, Mansfield J, Donaldson P, Macpherson AJ, Forbes A, Schreiber S, Lewis CM, Mathew CG. Genetic evidence for interaction of the 5q31 cytokine locus and the CARD15 gene in Crohn disease. *Am J Hum Genet* 2003;72:1018–1022.

Mitchell RS. Mortality and relapse of uncomplicated advanced tuberculosis before chemotherapy: 1,504 consecutive admissions followed for fifteen to twenty-five years. *Am Rev Tuberc* 1955;72:487–501.

Mittleman MA, Maclure M, Tofler GH, Sherwood JB, Goldberg RJ, Muller JE. Triggering of acute myocardial infarction by heavy physical exertion. *N Engl J Med* 1993;329:1677–1683.

Mittleman MA, Maclure M, Robins JM. Control sampling strategies for case-crossover studies: an assessment of relative efficiency. *Am J Epidemiol* 1995;142:91–98.

Mobius Research. Tackling declining response rates in Asia. Frequencies Newsletter. Available at www.Mobius-research.com/newsletter, 2003 (accessed 12/8/04).

Mohr DL, Blot WJ, Tousey PM, Van Doren ML, Wolfe KW. Southern cooking and lung cancer. *Nutr Cancer* 1999; 35:34–43.

Mohtashemi M, Levins R. Qualitative analysis of the all-cause Black-White mortality crossover. *Bull Math Biol* 2002; 64:147–173.

Mollie A, Richardson S. Empirical Bayes estimation of cancer mortality rates using spatial models. *Stat Med* 1991; 10:95–112.

Montaquila J, Mohadjer L, Khare M. The enhanced sample design of the future National Health and Nutrition Examination Survey (NHANES). *Proceedings of the Survey Research Methods Section of the American Statistical Association*, 1998:662–667.

Moolgavkar SH. Carcinogenesis modeling: from molecular biology to epidemiology. *Annu Rev Public Health* 1986; 7:151–169.

Moolgavkar SH. Commentary: Fifty years of the multistage model: remarks on a landmark paper. *Int J Epidemiol* 2004; 33:1182–1183.

Moolgavkar SH, Venzon DJ. General relative risk regression models for epidemiologic studies. *Am J Epidemiol* 1987; 126:949–961.

Morgan RW, Jain M, Miller AB, Choi NW, Matthews V, Munan L, Burch JD, Feather J, Howe GR, Kelly A. A comparison of dietary methods in epidemiologic studies. *Am J Epidemiol* 1978;107:488–498.

Morgenstern H. Uses of ecologic analysis in epidemiologic research. *Am J Public Health* 1982;72:1336–1344.

Morgenstern H, Bursic ES. A method for using epidemiologic data to estimate the potential impact of an intervention on the health status of a target population. *J Community Health* 1982;7:292–309.
Morgenstern H, Greenland S. Graphing ratio measures of effect. *J Clin Epidemiol* 1990;43:539–542.
Morgenstern H, Thomas DC. Principles of study design in environmental epidemiology. *Environ Health Perspect* 1993;101(suppl 4):23–38.
Morgenstern H, Winn DM. A method for determining the sampling ratio in epidemiologic studies. *Stat Med* 1983; 2:387–396.
Morris CN. Parametric empirical Bayes: theory and applications (with discussion). *J Am Stat Assoc* 1983:78:47–65.
Morris IN, Marr JW, Clayton DG. Diet and heart: a postscript. *Br Med J* 1977;2:1307–1314.
Morris M. *Network epidemiology: a handbook for survey design and data collection.* Oxford University Press: New York, 2004.
Morrison AS. Sequential pathogenic components of rates. *Am J Epidemiol* 1979;109:709–718.
Morrison AS, Buring JE, Verhoek WG, Aoki K, Leck I, Ohno Y, Obata K. Coffee drinking and cancer of the lower urinary tract. *J Natl Cancer Inst* 1982;68:91–94.
Morrison DE, Henkel RE, eds. *The significance test controversy.* Chicago: Aldine, 1970.
Mosteller F, Tukey JW. *Data analysis and regression.* Reading, MA: Addison-Wesley, 1977.
Mosteller F, Chalmers TC. Some progress and problems in meta-analysis of clinical trials. *Stat Sci* 1992;7:227–236.
Moulton LH, Foxman B, Wolfe RA, Port FK. Potential pitfalls in interpreting maps of stabilized rates. *Epidemiology* 1994;5:297–301.
Mulrow C, Cook D. Systematic Reviews. Synthesis of best evidence for health care decisions. Philadelphia: American College of Physicians, 1998.
Multiple Risk Factor Intervention Trial Research Group. Risk factor changes and mortality results. *JAMA* 1982; 248:1465–1477.
Murphy SA, Bentley GR, O'Hanesian MA. An analysis for menstrual data with time-varying covariates. *Stat Med* 1995; 14:1843–1857.
Murray CJL, Salomon JA, Mathers CD, Lopez, AD (eds.). *Summary Measures of Population Health.* Cambridge, MA: Harvard University Press/WHO; 2002.
Murray SS, Bjelke E, Gibson RW, Schuman LM. Coffee consumption and mortality from ischemic heart disease and other causes: results from the Lutheran Brotherhood Study. *Am J Epidemiol* 1981;113:661–667.
Murthy VH, Krumholz HM, Gross CP. Participation in cancer clinical trials - Race, sex, and age-based disparities. *JAMA* 2004;291:2720–2726.
Must A, Willett WC, Dietz WH. Remote recall of childhood height, weight, and body build by elderly subjects. *Am J Epidemiol* 1993;138:56–64.
Nash S, Tilley BC, Kurland LT, Gundersen J, Barnes AB, Labarthe D, Donohew PS, Kovacs L. Identifying and tracing a population at risk: the DESAD project experience. *Am J Public Health* 1983;73:253–259.
Nathanson N, Martin JR. The epidemiology of poliomyelitis: enigmas surrounding its appearance, epidemicity, and disappearance. *Am J Epidemiol* 1979;110:672–692.
National Cancer Institute. Current research: major areas of emphasis - consortia—cohorts. http://epi.grants.cancer.gov/consortia/cohort.html (accessed July 8, 2004).
National Center for Health Statistics. National Health and Nutrition Survey. Accessed August 2007. Available at URL: http://www.cdc.gov/nchs/nhanes.htm.
National Center for Health Statistics. Surveys and Data Collection Systems. Accessed August 2007. Available at URL: http://www.cdc.gov/nchs/express.htm.
National Heart, Lung, and Blood Institute. The Framingham Heart Study: 50 years of research success. Website accessed May, 2004 http://www.nhlbi.nih.gov/about/framingham/.
National Institutes of Health. National Children Study website accessed May, 2004 at http://www. nationalchildrensstudy.gov/.
National Library of Medicine. OMIM #266600. Website. Accessed June 2004 at http://www.ncbi.nlm.nih.gov/entrez/dispomim.cgi?id=266600.
National Research Council, National Academy of Sciences. *Risk assessment in the federal government: managing the process.* Washington, DC: National Academy Press, 1983.
National Research Council, Committee on Risk Assessment of Hazardous Pollutants. *Science and Judgment in Risk Assessment.* Washington: National Academy Press, 1994.
Navidi W, Thomas D, Stram D, Peters J. Design and analysis of multilevel analytic studies with applications to a study of air pollution. *Environ Health Perspect* 1994;102(suppl 8):25–32.
Navidi W, Weinhandl E. Risk set sampling for case-crossover designs. *Epidemiology* 2002;13:100–105.
Needleman HL, Gunnoe C, Leviton A, Reed R, Peresie H, Maher C, Barrett P. Deficits in psychologic and classroom performance of children with elevated dentine lead levels. *N Engl J Med* 1979;300:689–695.
Needleman HL, Shell A, Bellinger D, Leviton A, Allred EN. The long-term effects of exposure to low doses of lead in childhood: an 11-year follow-up report. *N Engl J Med* 1990;322:83–88.
Negoro K, McGovern DP, Kinouchi Y, Takahashi S, Lench NJ, Shimosegawa T, Carey A, Cardon LR, Jewell DP, van Heel DA. Analysis of the IBD5 locus and potential gene-gene interactions in Crohn's disease. *Gut* 2003;52:541–546.
Nelson MR, Kardia SL, Ferrell RE, Sing CF. A combinatorial partitioning method to identify multilocus genotypic partitions that predict quantitative trait variation. *Genome Res* 2001;11:458–470.
Newell DJ. Errors in interpretation of errors in epidemiology. *Am J Public Health* 1962;52:1925–1928.
Newhouse J, McClellan M. The use of instrumental variables. *Annu Rev Public Health* 1998;19:17–34.
Newman SC. *Biostatistical methods in epidemiology.* Wiley: New York, 2001.

Newman B, Silverberg MS, Gu X, Zhang Q, Lazaro A, Steinhart AH, Greenberg GR, Griffiths AM, McLeod RS, Cohen Z, Fernández-Viña M, Amos CI, Siminovitch K. CARD15 and HLA DRB1 alleles influence susceptibility and disease localization in Crohn's disease. *Am J Gastroenterol* 2004;99:306–315.

Newman SC. Odds ratio estimation in a steady-state population. *J Clin Epidemiol* 1988;41:59–65.

Newport MJ, Huxley CM, Huston S, Hawrylowicz CM, Oostra BA, Williamson R, Levin M. A mutation in the interferon-gamma-receptor gene and susceptibility to mycobacterial infection. *N Engl J Med* 1996;335:1941–1949.

Nicholson JK, Connelly J, Lindon JC, Holmes E. Metabonomics: a platform for studying drug toxicity and gene function. *Nat Rev Drug Discov* 2002;1:153–161.

Nicoll A, Gill ON, Peckham CS, Ades AE, Parry J, Mortimer P, Goldberg D, Noone A, Bennett D, Catchpole M. The public health applications of unlinked anonymous seroprevalence monitoring for HIV in the United Kingdom. *Int J Epidemiology* 2000;29:1–10.

Nieuwenhuijsen MJ, ed. *Exposure assessment in occupational and environmental epidemiology*. Oxford: Oxford University Press, 2003.

Nuckols JR, Ward MH, Jarup L. Using geographic information systems for exposure assessment in environmental epidemiology studies. *Environ Health Perspect* 2004;112:1007–1015.

Nurminen M. Asymptotic efficiency of general noniterative estimators of common relative risk. *Biometrika* 1981;68:525–530.

Nurminen M, Mutanen P. Exact Bayesian analysis of two proportions. *Scand J Stat* 1987;14:67–77.

Oakes JM. The (mis)estimation of neighborhood effects: causal inference for a practicable social epidemiology. *Soc Sci Med* 2004;58:1929–1952.

Oakes M. *Statistical inference.* Chestnut Hill, MA: ERI, 1990.

Oakes JM, Kaufman JS, eds. *Methods in Social Epidemiology*. Jossey-Bass: San Francisco, 2006.

Oakes JM, Rossi PH. The measurement of SES in health research: current practice and steps toward a new approach. *Soc Sci Med* 2003;56:769–784.

Oakley G Jr. Spermicides and birth defects. *JAMA* 1982;247:2405.

O'Campo P, Xue X, Wang MC, Caughy M. Neighborhood risk factors for low birthweight in Baltimore: a multilevel analysis. *Am J Public Health* 1997;87:1113–1118.

O'Campo P. Advancing theory and methods for multilevel models of residential neighborhoods and health. *Am J Epidemiol* 2003;157:9–13.

Office of Management and Budget. Directive Number 15: Race and Ethnic Standards for Federal Statistics and Administrative Reporting. Washington, DC: Off. Fed. Stat. Policy Standards, US Dep. Comm., 1977.

Office of Management and Budget. Revisions to the standards for classification of Federal data on race and ethnicity. *Fed Regist* 1997;62:58781–58790.

Ogura Y, Inohara N, Benito A, Chen FF, Yamaoka S, Nunez G. Nod2, a Nod1/Apaf-1 family member that is restricted to monocytes and activates NF-kappaB. *J Biol Chem* 2001a;276.4812–4818.

Ogura Y, Bonen DK, Inohara N, Nicolae DL, Chen FF, Ramos R, Britton H, Moran T, Karaliuskas R, Duerr RH, Achkar JP, Brant SR, Bayless TM, Kirschner BS, Hanauer SB, Nuñez G, Cho JH. A frameshift mutation in NOD2 associated with susceptibility to Crohn disease. *Nature* 2001b;411:603–606.

Oleinick A, Mantel N. Family studies in systemic Lupus erythematosis, II. *J Chronic Dis* 1970;22:617–625.

Oliver ML, Shapiro T. *Black wealth/white wealth: new perspective on racial inequality*. Routledge: New York, 1995.

Omar RZ, Thompson SG. Analysis of a cluster randomized trial with binary outcome data using a multi-level model. *Stat Med* 2000;19:2675–2688.

Openshaw S, Taylor PH. The modifiable area unit problem. In: Wrigley N, Bennett RJ, eds. *Quantitative geography: a British view*. London: Routledge & Kegan Paul, 1981: Chapter 9.

Opsahl R, Riddervold HO, Wessel-Aas T. Pulmonary tuberculosis in mitral stenosis and diabetes mellitus. *Acta Tuberc Scand* 1961;40:291–269.

O'Rourke K. Meta-analysis: Conceptual issues of addressing apparent failure of individual study replication or "inexplicable" heterogeneity. Ahmed SE, Reid N, eds. *Empirical Bayes and likelihood inference*. New York: Springer. 2001.

O'Rourke K, Detsky AS. Meta-analysis in medical research: strong encouragement for higher quality in individual research efforts. *J Clin Epidemiol* 1989;42:1021–1024.

Orsini N, Bellocco R, Greenland S. Generalized least squares for trend estimation of summarized dose-response data. *The Stata Journal* 2006;6:40–57.

Orzechowski S, Sepielli P. Household wealth and asset ownership: 1998 and 2000. Household economic studies. Current population reports. US Census Bureau, May 2003:70–88.

Oscarsson PN, Silwer H. Incidence of pulmonary tuberculosis among diabetics. *Acta Med Scand* 1958;161(Suppl 335):23–48.

Ostrom CW Jr. *Time series analysis: regression techniques,* 2nd ed. Newbury Park, CA: Sage Foundation, 1990.

Ouellet BL, Roemeder J-M, Lance J-M. Premature mortality attributable to smoking and hazardous drinking in Canada. *Am J Epidemiol* 1979;109:451–463.

Packard RM. *White plague, black labor: the political economy of health and diseases in South Africa.* Berkeley: University of California Press, 1989.

Paffenbarger RS, Hale WE. Work activity and coronary heart mortality. *N Engl J Med* 1975;292:545–550.

Pai JK, Pischon T, Ma J, Manson JE, Hankinson SE, Joshipura K, Curhan GC, Rifai N, Cannuscio CC, Stampfer MJ, Rimm EB. Inflammatory markers and the risk of coronary heart disease in men and women. *N Engl J Med* 2004;351:2599–2610.

Palmer JR, Rosenberg L, Rao S, Shapiro S. Coffee consumption and myocardial infarction in women. *Am J Epidemiol* 1995;141:724–731.

Pantell RH, Newman TB, Bernzweig J, Bergman DA, Takayama JI, Segal M, Finch SA, Wasserman RC. Management and outcomes of care of fever in early infancy. *JAMA* 2004;291:1203–1212.

Patz JA, McGeehin MA, Bernard SM, Ebi KL, Epstein PR, Grambsch A, Gubler DJ, Reiter P, Romieu I, Rose JB, Samet JM, Trtanj J. The potential health impacts of climate variability and change for the United States: Executive summary of the report of the health sector of the US National Assessment. *Environ Health Persp* 2000;108:(4)367–376.

Paul O, MacMillan A, McKean H, Park H. Sucrose intake and coronary heart disease. *Lancet* 1968;2:1049–1051.

Pearce N. Traditional epidemiology, modern epidemiology, and public health. *Am J Public Health* 1996;86:678–683.

Pearce N, Checkoway H, Dement J. Exponential models for analysis of time-related factors, illustrated with asbestos textile worker mortality data. *J Occup Med* 1988;30:517–522.

Pearce N, Merletti F. Complexity, simplicity, and epidemiology. *Int J Epidemiol* 2006;35:515–519.

Pearl J. *Probabilistic reasoning in intelligent systems*. Morgan Kaufmann, San Mateo, CA. 1988.

Pearl J. Causal diagrams for empirical research. *Biometrika* 1995;82:669–710.

Pearl J. *Causality*. New York: Cambridge University Press. 2000.

Pearl J. *Causality: models, reasoning and inference*. Cambridge, UK: Cambridge University Press, 2000.

Pearl J, Dechter R. *Identifying independencies in causal graphs with feedback*. 12th Conference on Uncertainty in Artificial Intelligence, San Francisco: Morgan Kaufman. 1996.

Pearl J, Robins JM. Probabilistic evaluation of sequential plans from causal models with hidden variables. In: *Uncertainty in artificial intelligence*. San Francisco: Morgan Kaufmann, 1995:444–453.

Pearson K. Report on certain enteric fever inoculation statistics. *Br Med J* 1904:3:1243–1246.

Pedace R, Bates N. Using administrative records to assess earnings reporting error in the Survey of Income and Program Participation. *J Econ Soc Meas* 2001;26:173–192.

Peduzzi P, Concato J, Kemper E, Holford TR, Feinstein AR. A simulation study of the number of events per variable in logistic regression analysis. *J Clin Epidemiol* 1996;49:1373–1379.

Peel DJ, Ziogas A, Fox EA, Gildea M, Laham B, Clements E, Kolodner RD, Anton-Culver H. Characterization of hereditary nonpolyposis colorectal cancer families from a population-based series of cases. *J Natl Cancer Inst* 2000;92:1517–1522.

Peltekova VD, Wintle RF, Rubin LA, Amos CI, Huang Q, Gu X, Newman B, Van Oene M, Cescon D, Greenberg G, Griffiths AM, St George-Hyslop PH, Siminovitch KA. Functional variants of OCTN cation transporter genes are associated with Crohn disease. *Nat Genet* 2004;36:471–475.

Peng RD, Dominici F, Zeger SL. Reproducible epidemiologic research. *Am J Epidemiol* 2006;163:783–789.

Pepe MS, Mori M. Kaplan-Meier, marginal or conditional probability curves in summarizing competing risks failure-time data? *Stat Med* 1993;12:737–751.

Perera F, Hemminki K, Jedrychowski W, Whyatt R, Campbell U, Hsu Y, Santella R, Albertini R, O'Neill JP. *In utero* DNA damage from environmental pollution is associated with somatic gene mutation in newborns. *Cancer Epidemiol Biomarkers Prev* 2002;11:1134–1137.

Peterson B, Harrell F. Partial proportional odss models for ordered response variables. *Appl Stat* 1990;39:205–217.

Petersen ML, van der Laan MJ. Direct effect models. *Biometrika* 2008; in press.

Petersen ML, Sinisi SE, van der Laan MJ. Estimation of direct causal effects. *Epidemiology* 2006;17:276–284.

Peto R. The preventability of cancer. In: Vessey MP, Gray M (eds). *Cancer risks and prevention*. Oxford: Oxford University Press,1985;1–14.

Peto R, Pike MC, Armitage P, Breslow NE, Cox DR, Howard SV, Mantel N, McPherson K, Peto J, Smith PG. Design and analysis of randomized clinical trials requiring prolonged observation of each patient. I. Introduction and design. *Br J Cancer* 1976;34:585–612.

Peto R, Doll R, Buckley JD, Sporn MD. Can dietary beta-carotene materially reduce human cancer rates? *Nature* 1981;290:201–208.

Pettiti DB. *Meta-analysis, decision analysis, and cost-effectiveness analysis in medicine*. New York: Oxford University Press, 1994a.

Pettiti DB. Of babies and bathwater. *Am J Epidemiol* 1994b;140:779–782.

Pettiti DB. Commentary: Hormone replacement therapy and coronary heart disease: four lessons. *Int J Epidemiol* 2004;33:461–463.

Pew Environmental Health Commission. http://healthyamericans.org/docs/print.php?DocID=77 2000.

Phillips CV. Quantifying and reporting uncertainty from systematic errors. *Epidemiology* 2003;14:459–466.

Phillips CV. Publication bias in situ. *BMC Med Res Methodol* 2004;4:20. http://www.biomedcentral.com/1471–2288/4/20. Accessed January 29, 2008.

Phillips CV, Goodman KJ. The missed lessons of Sir Austin Bradford Hill. *Epidemiol Perspect Innov* 2004;1:3. doi:10.1186/1742-5573-1-3

Phillips RL, Garfinkel L, Kuzma JW, Beeson WL, Lotz T, Brin B. Mortality among California Seventh-Day Adventists for selected cancer sites. *J Natl Cancer Inst* 1980;65:1097–1107.

Physicians' Health Study. Publications, http://phs.bwh.harvard.edu/pubs.htm (accessed July 8, 2004).

Piantadosi S, Byar DP, Green SB. The ecological fallacy. *Am J Epidemiol* 1988;127:893–904.

Piattelli-Palmarini M. *Inevitable illusions*. New York: Wiley, 1994.

Pickett KE, Pearl M. Multilevel analyses of neighborhood socioeconomic context and health outcomes: a critical review. *J Epidemiol Comm Health* 2001;55:111–122.

Pickle LW, Hartman AM. Indicator foods for vitamin A assessment. *Nutr Cancer* 1985;7:3–23.

Pickle LW, Mungiole M, Jones GK, White AA. Atlas of United States mortality. Hyattsville, Maryland: National Center for Health Statistics. 1996. DHHS Publication No. (PHS) 97–1015, page 67.

Piegorsch WW, Weinberg CR, Taylor JA. Non-hierarchical logistic models and case-only designs for assessing susceptibility in population-based case-control studies. *Stat Med* 1994;13:153–162.

Pietinen P, Hartman AM, Haapa E, Räsänen L, Haapakoski J, Palmgren J, Albanes D, Virtamo J, Huttunen JK. Reproducibility and validity of dietary assessment instruments, II: a qualitative food frequency questionnaire. *Am J Epidemiol* 1988;128:667–676.
Pietinen P, Aro A, Tuomilehto J, Uusitalo U, Korhonen H. Consumption of boiled coffee is correlated with serum cholesterol in Finland. *Int J Epidemiol* 1990;19:586–590.
Pike MC, Andersen J, Day NE. Some insights into Miettinen's multivariate confounder score approach to case-control study analysis. *J Epidemiol Comm Health* 1979;33:104–106.
Pike MC, Hill AP, Smith PG. Bias and efficiency in logistic analyses of stratified case-control studies. *Int J Epidemiol* 1980;9:89–95.
Pilcher CD, Tien HC, Eron JJ Jr, Vernazza PL, Leu SY, Stewart PW, Goh LE, Cohen MS; Quest Study; Duke-UNC-Emory Acute HIV Consortium. Brief but efficient: acute HIV infection and the sexual transmission of HIV. *J Infect Dis* 2004;189:1785–1792.
Pinner RW, Rebmann CA, Schuchat A, Hughes JM. Disease surveillance and the academic, clinical, and public health communities. *Emerging Infect Dis J* 2003;9:781–787.
Pinsky L, Atkins D, Ramsey S, Burke W. Developing guidelines for the clinical use of genetic tests: a U.S. perspective. In Khoury MJ, Little J, Burke W, eds. *Human genome epidemiology: a scientific foundation for using genetic information to improve health and prevent disease*. Oxford University Press, New York, 2004;264–282.
Pinto SS, Henderson VV, Enterline PE. Mortality experience of arsenic-exposed workers. *Arch Environ Health* 1978;33:325–331.
Platt JR. Strong inference. *Science* 1964;146:347–353.
Plummer M, Clayton D. Estimation of population exposure in ecological studies. *J R Stat Soc Ser B* 1996;58:113–126.
Pocock SJ, Cook DG, Beresford SAA. Regression of area mortality rates on explanatory variables: what weighting is appropriate? *Appl Stat* 1981;30:286–295.
Pocock SJ, Hughes MD, Lee RJ. Statistical problems in the reporting of clinical trials. *N Eng J Med* 1987;317:426–432.
Pocock SJ, Hughes MD. Practical problems in interim analyses, with particular regard to estimation. *Control Clin Trials* 1989;10 (Supplement): 209S–221S.
Podolsky DK. Inflammatory bowel disease. *N Engl J Med* 2002;347:417–429.
Polissar L. The effect of migration on comparison of disease rates in geographic studies in the United States. *Am J Epidemiol* 1980;111:175–182.
Pollock DA, Holmgreen P, Lui K, Kirk ML. Discrepancies in the reported frequency of cocaine-related deaths, United States, 1983 through 1988. *JAMA* 1991;266:2233–2237.
Poole C. Exposure opportunity in case-control studies. *Am J Epidemiol* 1986;123:352–358.
Poole C. Beyond the confidence interval. *Am J Public Health* 1987a;77:195–199.
Poole C. Confidence intervals exclude nothing. *Am J Public Health* 1987b;77:492–493.
Poole C. Exceptions to the rule about nondifferential misclassification (abstract). *Am J Epidemiol* 1985;122:508.
Poole C. Controls who experienced hypothetical causal intermediates should not be excluded from case-control studies. *Am J Epidemiol* 1999;150:547–551.
Poole C. Positivized epidemiology and the model of sufficient and component causes. *Int J Epidemiol* 2001a;30:707–709.
Poole C. Causal values. *Epidemiology* 2001b;12:139–141.
Poole C. Low P-values or narrow confidence intervals: Which are more durable? *Epidemiology* 2001c;12:291–294.
Poole C, Greenland S. Random-effects meta-analyses are not always conservative. *Am J Epidemiol* 1999;150:469–475.
Poole C, Greenland S, Luetters C, Kelsey JL, Mezei G. The relation of socioeconomic status to childhood leukemia: a review of the literature. *Int J Epidemiol* 2006;35:370–385.
Popper KR: Logik der Forschung. Vienna: Julius Springer, 1934.
Popper KR. *The logic of scientific discovery* (in German). New York: Basic Books, 1959.
Portes A. The two meanings of social capital. *Sociological Forum* 2000;15:1–12.
Posner BM, Borman CL, Morgan JL, Borden WS, Ohls JC. The validity of a telephone-administered 24-hour dietary recall methodology. *Am J Clin Nutr* 1982;36:546–553.
Potter J, Slattery M, Bostick R, Gapstur S. Colon cancer: a review of the epidemiology. *Epidemiol Rev* 1993;15:499–545.
Poumadere M, Mays C, Le Mer S. The 2003 heat wave in France: dangerous climate change here and now. *Risk Anal* 2005;25:1483–1494.
Pregibon D. Logistic regression diagnostics. *Ann Stat* 1981;9:705–724.
Prentice RL. A case-cohort design for epidemiologic studies and disease prevention trials. *Biometrika* 1986;73:1–11.
Prentice RL, Breslow NE. Retrospective studies and failure-time models. *Biometrika* 1978;65:153–158.
Prentice RL, Kalbfleisch JD. Author's reply. *Biometrics* 1988;44:1205.
Prentice RL, Pyke R. Logistic disease incidence models and case-control studies. *Biometrika* 1979;66:403–411.
Prentice RL, Sheppard L. Validity of international, time trend, and migrant studies of dietary factors and disease risk. *Prev Med* 1989;18:167–179.
Prentice RL, Sheppard L. Aggregate data studies of disease risk factors. *Biometrika* 1995;82:113–125.
Prentice RL, Thomas DC. Methodologic research needs in environmental epidemiology: data analysis. *Environ Health Perspect* 1993;101(suppl 4):39–48.
Prentice RL, Thomson CA, Caan B, Hubbell FA, Anderson GL, Beresford SA, Pettinger M, Lane DS, Lessin L, Yasmeen S, Singh B, Khandekar J, Shikany JM, Satterfield S, Chlebowski RT. Low-fat dietary pattern and risk of invasive breast cancer: the Women's Health Initiative Randomized Controlled Dietary Modification Trial. *JAMA* 2006;295:629–642.

Prentice RL, Kakar F, Hursting S, Sheppard L, Klein R, Kushi LH. Aspects of the rationale for the Women's Health Trial. *J Natl Cancer Inst* 1988;80:802–814.

Prentice RL, Langer R, Stefanick ML, Howard BV, Pettinger M, Anderson G, Barad D, Curb JD, Kotchen J, Kuller L, Limacher M, Wactawski-Wende J, for the Women's Health Initiative Investigators. Combined postmenopausal hormone therapy and cardiovascular disease: toward resolving the discrepancy between observational studies and the Women's Health Initiative clinical trial (with discussion). *Am J Epidemiol.* 2005;162:404–420.

Preston SH. Relations among standard epidemiologic measures in a population. *Am J Epidemiol* 1987;126:336–345.

Prevots R, Sutter RW, Strebel PM, Cochi SL, Hadler S. Tetanus surveillance-United States, 1989–1990. *MMWR Morb Mortal Wkly Rep* 1992;41(no SS-8):1–10.

Prostate Cancer Trialists' Collaborative Group: Maximum androgen blockade in advanced prostate cancer: an overview of 22 randomised trials with 3283 deaths in 5710 patients. *Lancet* 1995;346:265–269.

Public Health Leadership Society. *Principles of ethical practice of public health, version 2.2*, 2002. Accessed June 2002. Available at URL: http://www.phls.org.

Public Population Project in Genomics. Website accessed May, 2004 at http://www.p3gconsortium.org/index.cfm.

Quine WVO. Two dogmas of empiricism. *The philosophical review* 1951;60:20–43. Reprinted with edits in Quine WVO, *From a logical point of view* (Harvard University Press, 1953; second, revised, edition 1961).

Radloff L. The CES-D scale: a self-report depression scale for research in the general population. *Journal of Applied Psychological Measurement* 1977;1:385–401.

Raftery AE. Bayesian model selection in social research (with discussion). *Sociological Methodology* 1995;25:111–196.

Rahman P, Bartlett S, Siannis F, Pellett FJ, Farewell VT, Peddle L, Schentag CT, Alderdice CA, Hamilton S, Khraishi M, Tobin Y, Hefferton D, Gladman DD. CARD15: a pleiotropic autoimmune gene that confers susceptibility to psoriatic arthritis. *Am J Hum Genet* 2003;73:677–681.

Ramsey FR Truth and probability. In Kyburg HE, Smokler HE, eds. *Studies in subjective probability.* New York, Wiley, 1964. (Original publication, 1931.)

Rappaport SM, Symanski E, Yager JW, Kupper LL. The relationship between environmental monitoring and biological markers in exposure assessment. *Environ Health Perspect* 1995;103(suppl 3):49–54.

Raudenbush SW, Bryk AS. Empirical Bayes meta-analysis. *J Educ Stat* 1985;10:75–98.

Raudenbush SW, Sampson R. Ecometrics: Toward a science of assessing ecological settings, with application to the systematic social observations of neighborhoods. *Sociological Methodology* 1999;29:1–41.

Ray WA. Population-based studies of adverse drug effects. *N Engl J Med* 2003;349:592–594.

Reeder AL, Foley GL, Nichols DK, Hansen LG, Wikoff B, Faeh S, Eisold J,Wheeler MB, Warner R, Murphy JE, Beasley VR. Forms and prevalence of intersexuality and effects of environmental contaminants on sexuality in cricket frogs (Acris crepitans). *Environ Health Perspect* 1998;106:261–266.

Reingold A. If syndromic surveillance is the answer, what is the question? *Biosecur Bioterror* 2003;1:77–81.

Reissman DB, Staley F, Curtis BG, Kaufmann RB. Use of geographic information system technology to aid health department decision making about childhood lead poisoning prevention activities. *Environ Health Persp* 2001;109:89–94.

Reynolds P, VonBehren J, Gunier RB, Goldberg DE, Hertz A, Smith DF. Childhood cancer incidence rates and hazardous air pollutants in California: An exploratory analysis. *Environ Health Perspect* 2003;111:663–668.

Rhoads GG, Kagan A. The relation of coronary disease, stroke, and mortality to weight in youth and middle age. *Lancet* 1983;2:492–495.

Richardson S, Hemon D. Ecological bias and confounding (letter). *Int J Epidemiol* 1990;19:764–766.

Richardson S, Stucker I, Hemon D. Comparison of relative risks obtained in ecological and individual studies: some methodological considerations. *Int J Epidemiol* 1987;16:111–120.

Richardson S, Thomson A, Best N, Elliott P. Interpreting posterior relative risk estimates in disease-mapping studies. *Environ Health Perspect* 2004;112:1016–1025.

Rifat SL. Graphic representations of effect estimates: an example from a meta-analytic review. *J Clin Epidemiol* 1990;43:1267–1271.

Riley LW, Remis RS, Helgerson SD, McGee HB, Wells JG, Davis BR, Hebert RJ, Olcott ES, Johnson LM, Hargrett NT, Blake PA, Cohen ML. Hemorrhagic colitis associated with a rare *Escherichia coli* serotype. *N Engl J Med* 1983;308:681–685.

Rimm EB, Giovannucci EL, Stampfer MJ, Colditz GA, Litin LB, Willett WC. Reproducibility and validity of an expanded self-administered semi-quantitative food frequency questionnaire among male health professionals. *Am J Epidemiol* 1992a;135:1114–1126.

Rimm EB, Giovannucci EL, Stampfer MJ, Colditz GA, Litin LB, Willett WC. Authors' response to "Invited commentary: some limitations of semi-quantitative food frequency questionnaires." *Am J Epidemiol* 1992b;135:1133–1136.

Rioux JD, Daly MJ, Silverberg MS, Lindblad K, Steinhart H, Cohen Z, Delmonte T, Kocher K, Miller K, Guschwan S, Kulbokas EJ, O'Leary S, Winchester E, Dewar K, Green T, Stone V, Chow C, Cohen A, Langelier D, Lapointe G, Gaudet D, Faith J, Branco N, Bull SB, McLeod RS, Griffiths AM, Bitton A, Greenberg GR, Lander ES, Siminovitch KA, Hudson TJ. Genetic variation in the 5q31 cytokine gene cluster confers susceptibility to Crohn disease. *Nat Genet* 2001;29:223–228.

Robert SA, House JS. SES differentials in health by age and alternative indicators of SES. *J Aging Health* 1996;8:359–388.

Robbins JM, Vaccarino V, Zhang HP, Kasl SV. Socioeconomic status and diagnosed diabetes incidence. *Diabetes Res Clin Pract* 2005:68:230–236.

Robins JM. A new approach to causal inference in mortality studies with a sustained exposure period-application to control of the healthy worker survivor effect. *Math Model* 1986;7:1393–1512.

Robins JM. A graphical approach to the identification and estimation of causal parameters in mortality studies with sustained exposure periods. *J Chronic Dis* 1987;40(suppl 2):139S–161S.

Robins JM. The control of confounding by intermediate variables. *Stat Med* 1989;8:679–701.

Robins JM. Estimation of the time-dependent accelerated failure time model in the presence of confounding factors. *Biometrika* 1992;79:321–334.

Robins JM. Analytic methods for HIV treatment and cofactor effects. In: Ostrow SG, Kessler R, eds. *Methodologic issues in AIDS behavioral research.* New York: Plenum, 1993:213–287.

Robins JM. Causal inference from complex longitudinal data. In: Berkane M, ed. *Latent variable modeling with applications to causality.* New York: Springer-Verlag, 1997, 69–117.

Robins JM. Structural nested failure time models. In: Armitage P, Colton T, eds. *The encyclopedia of biostatistics.* New York: Wiley, 1998a:4372–4389.

Robins JM. Marginal structural models. In: 1997 Proceedings of the Section on Bayesian Statistical Science, Alexandria, VA: American Statistical Association; 1998b:pp. 1–10.

Robins JM. Marginal Structural Models versus Structural Nested Models as Tools for Causal Inference. Statistical Models in Epidemiology: The Environment and Clinical Trials. Halloran ME, Berry D, Eds, IMA Volume 116, NY: Springer-Verlag, 1999:pp. 95–134.

Robins JM. Data, design, and background knowledge in etiologic inference. *Epidemiology* 2001;12:313–320.

Robins JM, Greenland S. The role of model selection in causal inference from nonexperimental data. *Am J Epidemiol* 1986;123:392–402.

Robins JM, Greenland S. Estimability and estimation of excess and etiologic fractions. *Stat Med* 1989a;8:845–859.

Robins JM, Greenland S. The probability of causation under a stochastic model for individual risks. *Biometrics* 1989b;45:1125–1138.

Robins JM, Greenland S. Estimability and estimation of expected years of life lost due to a hazardous exposure. *Stat Med* 1991;10:79–93.

Robins JM, Greenland S. Identifiability and exchangeability for direct and indirect effects. *Epidemiology* 1992;3:143–155.

Robins JM, Greenland S. Adjusting for differential rates of prophylaxis therapy for PCP in high versus low dose AZT treatment arms in an AIDS randomized trial. *J Am Stat Assoc* 1994;89:737–749.

Robins JM, Morgenstern H. The foundations of confounding in epidemiology. *Comp Math Appl* 1987;14:869–916.

Robins JM, Pike M. The validity of case-control studies with non-random selection of controls. *Epidemiology* 1990;1:273–284.

Robins JM, Tsiatis AA. Correcting for non-compliance in randomized trials using rank-preserving structural failure-time models. *Commun Stat* 1991;20:2609–2631.

Robins J, Wasserman L. On the impossibility of inferring causation from association without background knowledge. In: Glymour C, Cooper G, eds. *Computation, causation, and discovery.* Menlo Park, CA and Cambridge, MA, AAAI Press/ The MIT Press, 1999:305–321.

Robins JM, Gail MH, Lubin JH. More on biased selection of controls for case-control analyses of cohort studies. *Biometrics* 1986a;42:293–299.

Robins JM, Greenland S, Breslow NE. A general estimator for the variance of the Mantel-Haenszel odds ratio. *Am J Epidemiol* 1986b;124:719–723.

Robins JM, Breslow NE, Greenland S. Estimators of the Mantel-Haenszel variance consistent in both sparse-data and large-strata limiting models. *Biometrics* 1986c;42:311–323.

Robins JM, Blevins D, Ritter G, Wulfsohn M. G-estimation of the effect of prophylaxis therapy for *Pneumocystis carinii* pneumonia on the survival of AIDS patients. *Epidemiology* 1992a;3:319–336. Errata: *Epidemiology* 1993;4:189.

Robins JM, Mark SD, Newey WK. Estimating exposure effects by modeling the expectation of exposure conditional on confounders. *Biometrics* 1992b;48:479–495.

Robins JM, Rotnitzky A, Zhao LP. Estimation of regression coefficients when some regressors are not always observed. *J Am Stat Assoc* 1994;89:846–866.

Robins JM, Rotnitzky A, Scharfstein DO. Sensitivity analysis for selection bias and unmeasured confounding in missing data and causal inference models. In: Halloran ME, Berry DA, eds. *Statistical models in epidemiology.* New York: Springer-Verlag, 1999a:1–92.

Robins JM, Greenland S, Hu F. Estimation of the causal effect of a time-varying exposure on the marginal mean of a repeated binary outcome (with discussion). *J Am Stat Assoc* 1999b;94:687–712.

Robins JM, Hernán MA, Brumback B. Marginal structural models and causal inference in epidemiology. *Epidemiology* 2000;11:550–560.

Robins JM, Hernán MA, Brumback B. Marginal structural models and causal inference in epidemiology. *Epidemiology* 2000;11:561–570.

Robins JM, Scheines R, Spirtes P, Wasserman L. Uniform consistency in causal inference. *Biometrika* 2003:90:491–515.

Robinson GK. That BLUP is a good thing: the estimation of random effects. *Stat Sci* 1991;6:15–51.

Robinson WS. Ecological correlations and the behavior of individuals. *Am Sociol Rev* 1950;15:351–357.

Rockhill B. Proteomic patterns in serum and identification of ovarian cancer [letter]. *Lancet* 2002;360:169.

Rodgers A, MacMahon S. Systematic underestimation of treatment effects as a result of diagnostic test inaccuracy: implications for the interpretation and design of thromboprophylaxis trials. *Thromb Haemost* 1995;73:167–171.

Rodriguez EM, Staffa JA, Graham DJ. The role of databases in drug postmarketing surveillance. *Pharmacoepidemiol Drug Saf* 2001;10:407–410.

Rogerson PA. Statistical methods for the detection of spatial clustering in case-control data. *Stat Med* 2006;25:811–823.

Rogot E, Sorlie PD, Johnson NJ, Schmitt C. *A mortality study of 1.3 million persons by demographic, social, and economic factors: 1979–1985*. Bethesda, MD.:NIH, 1992.
Rohan TE, Potter JD. Retrospective assessment of dietary intake. *Am J Epidemiol* 1984;120:876–887.
Rooth G. Low birthweight revised. *Lancet* 1980;1:639–641.
Rose G. Sick individuals and sick populations. *Int J Epidemiol* 1985;14:32–38.
Rosner B, Willett WC, Spiegelman D. Correction of logistic regression relative risk estimates and confidence intervals for systematic within-person measurement error. *Stat Med* 1989;8:1051–1069; discussion 1071–1073.
Rosenbaum PR. Model-based direct adjustment. *J Am Stat Assoc* 1987;82:387–394.
Rosenbaum PR. *Observational studies*, 2nd ed. New York: Springer, 2002.
Rosenbaum PR, Rubin DB. The central role of the propensity score in observational studies for causal effects. *Biometrika* 1983;70:41–55.
Rosenbaum PR, Rubin DB. Difficulties with regression analyses of age-adjusted rates. *Biometrics* 1984;40:437–443.
Rosenberg L, Slone D, Shapiro S, Kaufman DW, Stolley PD, Miettinen OS. Coffee drinking and myocardial infarction in young women. *Am J Epidemiol* 1980;111:675–681.
Rosenberg L, Slone D, Shapiro S, Kaufman DW, Miettinen OS. Case-control studies on the acute effects of coffee upon the risk of myocardial infarction: problems in the selection of a hospital control series. *Am J Epidemiol* 1981;113:646–652.
Rosenberg L, Werler MM, Kaufman DW, Shapiro S. Coffee drinking and myocardial infarction in young women: an update. *Am J Epidemiol* 1987;126:147–149.
Rosenberg L, Palmer JR, Kelly JP, Kaufman DW, Shapiro S. Coffee drinking and nonfatal myocardial infarction in men under 55 years of age. *Am J Epidemiol* 1988;128:570–578.
Rosengren A, Wilhelmsen L. Coffee, coronary heart disease and mortality in middle-aged Swedish men: findings from the Primary Prevention Study. *J Intern Med* 1991;230:67–71.
Rosenthal RB, Rubin DR. A note on percent variance explained as a measure of importance of effects. *J Appl Soc Psychol* 1979;9:395–396.
Rosner B, Hennekens CH, Kass EH, Miall WE. Age-specific correlation analysis of longitudinal blood pressure data. *Am J Epidemiol* 1977;106:306–313.
Rosner B, Willett WC, Spiegelman D. Correction of logistic regression relative risk estimates and confidence intervals for systematic within-person measurement error. *Stat Med* 1989;8:1051–1069.
Rosner B, Spiegelman D, Willett WC. Correction of logistic regression relative risk estimates and confidence intervals for measurement error: the case of multiple covariates measured with error. *Am J Epidemiol* 1990:132: 734–745.
Rothman KJ. Causes. *Am J Epidemiol* 1976;104:587–592.
Rothman KJ. Synergy and antagonism in cause-effect relationships. *Am J Epidemiol* 1974;99:385–388.
Rothman KJ. Causes. *Am J Epidemiol* 1976a;104:587–592.
Rothman KJ. The estimation of synergy or antagonism. *Am J Epidemiol* 1976b;103:506–511.
Rothman KJ. Epidemiologic methods in clinical trials. *Cancer* 1977;39:1771–1775.
Rothman KJ. A show of confidence. *N Engl J Med* 1978a;299:1362–1363.
Rothman KJ. Estimation of confidence limits for the cumulative probability of survival in life-table analysis. *J Chron Dis* 1978b;31:557–560.
Rothman KJ. Induction and latent periods. *Am J Epidemiol* 1981;114:253–259.
Rothman KJ. Sleuthing in hospitals. *N Engl J Med* 1985;313:258–260.
Rothman KJ. *Modern epidemiology.* Boston: Little, Brown, 1986.
Rothman KJ, ed. *Causal inference.* Boston: Epidemiology Resources, 1988.
Rothman KJ. No adjustments are needed for multiple comparisons. *Epidemiology* 1990a;1:43–46.
Rothman KJ. A sobering start for the cluster buster's conference. *Am J Epidemiol* 1990b;132(suppl):6–13.
Rothman KJ, Boice JD. *Epidemiologic analysis with a programmable calculator,* 2nd ed. Newton, MA: Epidemiology Resources, 1982.
Rothman KJ, Keller AZ. The effect of joint exposure to alcohol and tobacco on risk of cancer of the mouth and pharynx. *J Chronic Dis* 1972;25:711–716.
Rothman KJ, Michels KB. The continuing unethical use of placebo controls. *N Engl J Med* 1994;331:394–398.
Rothman KJ, Michels KB. "When is it appropriate to use a placebo arm in a trial?", In: Guess HA, Kleinman A, Kusek JW, Engel LW, eds. *The science of the placebo: toward an interdisciplinary research agenda*. BMJ Books: London, 2002.
Rothman KJ, Poole C. A strengthening programme for weak associations. *Int J Epidemiol* 1988;17(suppl):955–959.
Rothman KJ, Fyler DC, Goldblatt A, Kreidberg MB. Exogenous hormones and other drug exposures of children with congenital heart disease. *Am J Epidemiol* 1979;109:433–439.
Rothman KJ, Greenland S, Walker AM. Concepts of interaction. *Am J Epidemiol* 1980;112:467–470.
Rothman KJ, Johnson ES, Sugano DS. Is flutamide effective in patients with bilateral orchiectomy? *Lancet* 1999;353:1184.
Rothman KJ, Funch DP, Alfredson T, Brady J, Dreyer NA. Randomized field trial of vaginal douching, pelvic inflammatory disease, and pregnancy. *Epidemiology* 2003;14;340–348.
Rothman KJ, Lanes S, Sacks ST. The reporting odds ratio and its advantages over the proportional reporting ratio. *Pharmacoepidemiol Drug Saf* 2004;13:519–523.
Royall RM. Model robust confidence intervals using maximum likelihood estimators. *Int Stat Rev* 1986;54:221–226.
Royall R. *Statistical inference: a likelihood paradigm*. New York: Chapman and Hall, 1997.
Royston P, Altman DG. Regression using fractional polynomials of continuous covariates: parsimonious parametric modeling (with discussion). *Appl Stat* 1994;43:425–467.
Rozeboom WM. The fallacy of null-hypothesis significance test. *Psych Bull* 1960;57:416–428.

Rubin DB. Estimating causal effects of treatments in randomized and nonrandomized studies. *J Educ Psychol* 1974:66:688–701.

Rubin DB. Bayesian inference for causal effects: the role of randomization. *Ann Stat* 1978;6:34–58.

Rubin DB. Bayesianly justifiable and relevant frequency calculations. *Ann Stat* 1984;12:1151–1172.

Rubin DB. Comment: Neyman (1923) and causal inference in experiments and observational studies. *Stat Sci* 1990a;5:472–480.

Rubin DB. A new perspective. In: Wachter KW, Straf ML, eds. *The future of meta-analysis.* New York: Russell Sage Foundation, 1990b:155–165.

Rubin DB. Practical implications of modes of statistical inference for causal effects, and the critical role of the assignment mechanism. *Biometrics* 1991;47:1213–1234.

Rubin DB. Meta-analysis: literature synthesis or effect-size estimation? *J Educ Stat* 1992;17:363–374.

Rubin DB. Multiple imputation after 18+ years. *J Am Stat Assoc* 1996;91:473–489.

Rubin DB. Estimating effects from large data sets using propensity scores. *Ann Intern Med* 1997;127:757–763.

Rubin DB. *Matched sampling for causal effects.* New York: Cambridge University Press, 2006.

Rubin DB, Thomas N. Combining propensity score matching with additional adjustments for prognostic covariates. *J Am Stat Assoc* 2000;95:573–585.

Rundle A, Tang D, Mooney L, Grumet S, Perera F. The interaction between alcohol consumption and GSTM1 genotype on Polycyclic Aromatic Hydrocarbon-DNA adduct levels in breast tissue. *Cancer Epidemiol Biomarkers Prev* 2003;12:911–914.

Russell B. *A history of western philosophy.* New York: Simon and Schuster, 1945.

Russell-Briefel R, Bates MW, Kuller LH. The relationship of plasma carotenoids to health and biochemical factors in middle-aged men. *Am J Epidemiol* 1985;122:741–749.

Rutstein DD, Mullan RJ, Frazier TM, Halperin WE, Melius JM, Sestito JP. Sentinel health events (occupational): a basis for physician recognition and public health surveillance. *Am J Public Health* 1983;73:1054–1062.

Sackett DL, Haynes RB, Guyatt GH, Tugwell P. *Clinical epidemiology: a basic science for clinical medicine.* Boston: Little, Brown, 1991.

Sacks FM, Handysides GH, Marais GE, Rosner B, Kass EH. Effects of a low-fat diet on plasma lipoprotein levels. *Arch Intern Med* 1986;146:1573–1577.

Sacks HS, Berrier J, Reitman D, Ancona-Berk VA, Chalmers TC. Meta-analysis of randomized controlled trials. *N Engl J Med* 1987;316:450–455.

Salsburg DS. The religion of statistics as practiced in medical journals. *Am Statist* 1985;39:220–223.

Saltelli A, Chan K, Scott EM (eds.). *Sensitivity Analysis.* New York: Wiley, 2000.

Salvaggio A, Periti M, Miano L, Quaglia G, Marzorati D. Coffee and cholesterol, an Italian study. *Am J Epidemiol* 1991;134;149–156.

Salvan A, Stayner L, Steenland K, Smith R. Selecting an exposure lag period. *Epidemiology* 1995;6:387–390.

Salvini S, Hunter DJ, Sampson L, Stampfer MJ, Colditz GA, Rosner B, Willett WC. Food based validation of a dietary questionnaire: the effects of week-to-week variation in food consumption. *Int J Epidemiol* 1989;18:858–867.

Samet JM, Humble CG, Skipper BE. Alternatives in the collection and analysis of food frequency interview data. *Am J Epidemiol* 1984;120:572–581.

Sampson L. Food frequency questionnaires as a research instrument. *Clin Nutr* 1985;9:171–173.

Saracci R. Interaction and synergism. *Am J Epidemiol* 1980;112:465–466.

Sartwell P. On the methodology of investigations of etiologic factors in chronic diseases further comments. *J Chronic Dis* 1960;11:61–63.

Sato T. On the variance estimator for the Mantel-Haenszel risk difference (letter). *Biometrics* 1989;45:1323–1324.

Sato T. Maximum likelihood estimation of the risk ratio in case-cohort studies. *Biometrics* 1992a;48:1215–1221.

Sato T. Estimation of a common risk ratio in stratified case-cohort studies. *Stat Med* 1992b;11:1599–1605.

Sato T, Matsuyama Y. Marginal structural models as a tool for standardization. *Epidemiology* 2003;14:680–686.

Savage LJ. *The foundations of statistics.* New York: Dover, 1972.

Savitz DA. *Interpreting epidemiologic evidence: strategies for study design and analysis.* New York, Oxford University Press, 2001.

Savitz DA, Baron AE. Estimating and correcting for confounder misclassification. *Am J Epidemiol* 1989;129:1062–1071.

Savitz DA, Olshan AF. Multiple comparisons and related issues in epidemiologic research. *Am J Epidemiol* 1995;142:904–908.

Savitz DA, Olshan AF. Describing data requires no adjustment for multiple comparisons: a reply from Savitz and Olshan. *Am J Epidemiol* 1998;147:813–814.

Savitz DA, Wachtel H, Barnes FA, John EM, Tvrdik JG. Case-control study of childhood cancer and exposure to 60-Hz magnetic fields. *Am J Epidemiol* 1988;128:21–38.

Sayrs LW. *Pooled time series analysis.* Newbury Park, CA: Sage Foundation, 1989.

Schaid DJ, Sommer SS. Genotype relative risks: methods for design and analysis of candidate gene association studies. *Am J Hum Genet* 1993;53:1114–1126.

Scharfstein DO, Rotnitsky A, Robins JM. Adjusting for nonignorable drop-out using semiparametric nonresponse models. *J Am Stat Assoc* 1999;94,1096–1120.

Schatzkin A, Lanza E, Freedman LS, Tangrea J, Cooper MR, Marshall JR, Murphy PA, Selby JV, Shike M, Schade RR, Burt RW, Kikendall JW, Cahill J. The Polyp Prevention Trial I: rationale, design, recruitment, and baseline participant characteristics. *Cancer Epidemiol Biomarkers Prev* 1996;5:375–383.

Schlesselman JJ. Sample size requirements in cohort and case-control studies of disease. *Am J Epidemiol* 1974;99:381–384.

Schlesselman JJ. Assessing effects of confounding variables. *Am J Epidemiol* 1978;108:3–8.

Schouten EG, Dekker JM, Kok FJ, Le Cessie S, Van Houwelingen HC, Pool J, Vanderbroucke JP. Risk ratio and rate ratio estimation in case-cohort designs. *Stat Med* 1993;12:1733–1745.

Schrag SJ, Brooks JT, Van Beneden C, Parashar UD, Griffin PM, Anderson LJ, Bellini WJ, Benson RF, Erdman DD, Klimov A, Ksiazek TG, Peret TC, Talkington DF, Thacker WL, Tondella ML, Sampson JS, Hightower AW, Nordenberg DF, Plikaytis BD, Khan AS, Rosenstein NE, Treadwell TA, Whitney CG, Fiore AE, Durant TM, Perz JF, Wasley A, Feikin D, Herndon JL, Bower WA, Klibourn BW, Levy DA, Coronado VG, Buffington J, Dykewicz CA, Khabbaz RF, Chamberland ME. SARS surveillance during emergency public health response, United States, March-July 2003. *Emerging Infect Dis J* 2004;10:185–194.

Schrenk HH, Heimann H, Clayton GD, Gafafer, W.M.; Wexler, H. *Air pollution in Donora, Pa., epidemiology of the unusual smog episode of October 1948.* Washington, DC: Federal Security Agency, Public Health Service, Bureau of State Services, Division of Industrial Hygiene, 1949. Public Health Bulletin No 306.

Schulman KA, Berlin JA, Harless W, Kerner JF, Sistrunk S, Gersh BJ, Dubé R, Taleghani CK, Burke JE, Williams S, Eisenberg JM, Escarce JJ. The effect of race and sex on physicians' recommendations for cardiac catheterization. *N Engl J Med* 1999;340:618–626.

Schulte PA. Some implications of genetic biomarkers in occupational epidemiology and practice. *Scand J Work Environ Health* 2004;30:71–79.

Schulte PA, Perera FP, eds. *Molecular epidemiology: principles and practice.* New York: Academic Press, 1993.

Schulte PA, Perera FP. Transitional studies. In: Toniolo P, Boffeta P, Shuker DEG, Rothman N, Hulka B, Pearce N, eds. *Application of biomarkers in cancer epidemiology*. IARC Scientific Publications: Lyon, France, 1997;19–29.

Schulte PA, Lomax GP, Ward EM, Colligan MJ. Ethical issues in the use of genetic markers in occupational epidemiologic research. *J Occup Environ Med* 1999;41:639–646.

Schulze MB, Hu FB. Primary prevention of diabetes: what can be done and how much can be prevented? *Annu Rev Public Health* 2005;26:445–467.

Schwartz S, Carpenter KM. The right answer for the wrong question: consequences of type III error for public health research. *Am J Public Health* 1999;89:1175–1180.

Schwingl P. *Prenatal smoking exposure in relation to female adult fecundability.* Chapel Hill, NC: Department of Epidemiology, the University of North Carolina at Chapel Hill, 1992. Doctor of philosophy thesis.

Sclove SL, Morris C, Radhakrishna R. Non-optimality of preliminary-test estimators for the mean of a multivariate normal distribution. *Ann Math Stat* 1972;43:1481–1490.

Scott A, Wild C. On the robustness of weighted methods for fitting models to case-control data. *J R Stat Soc Ser B* 2002;64:207–219.

Secretary's Advisory Committee on Genetic Testing: Enhancing the oversight of genetic tests: Recommendations of the SACGT, 2000 http://www4.od.nih.gov/oba/sacgt/gtdocuments.html.

Seifert B. Validity criteria for exposure assessment methods. *Sci Total Environ* 1995;168:101–107.

Selby JV, Peng T, Karter AJ, Alexander M, Sidney S, Lian J, Arnold A, Pettitt D. High rates of co-occurrence of hypertension, elevated low-density lipoprotein cholesterol, and diabetes mellitus in a large managed care population. *Am J Manag Care* 2004;10:163–170.

Selén J. Adjusting for errors in classification and measurement in the analysis of partly and purely categorical data. *J Am Stat Assoc* 1986;81:75–81.

Selevan S, Lemasters G. The dose-response fallacy in human reproductive studies of toxic exposures. *J Occup Med* 1987;29:451–454.

Self SG, Liang K-Y. Asymptotic properties of maximum likelihood estimators and likelihood ratio tests under non-standard conditions. *J Am Stat Assoc* 1987;82:605–610.

Self SG, Longton G, Kopecky KJ, Liang KY. On estimating HLA/disease association with application to a study of aplastic anemia. *Biometrics* 1991;47:53–61.

Selhub J, Jacques PF, Wilson PW, Rush D, Rosenberg IH. Vitamin status and intake as primary determinants of homocysteinemia in an elderly population. *JAMA* 1993;270:2693–2698.

Seligman PJ, Halperin WE, Mullan RJ, Frazier TM. Occupational lead poisoning in Ohio: surveillance using workers' compensation data. *Am J Public Health* 1986;76:1299–1302.

Sellers TA, Yates JR. Review of proteomics with applications to genetic epidemiology. *Genet Epidemiol* 2003;24:83–98.

Selvin HC. Durkheim's "Suicide" and problems of empirical research. *Am J Sociol* 1958;63:607–619.

Semenza JC, Tolbert PE, Rubin CH, Guillette LJ Jr, Jackson RJ. Reproductive toxins and alligator abnormalities at Lake Apopka, Florida. *Environ Health Perspect* 1997;105:1030–1032.

Senn S. The many modes of meta. *Drug Inf J* 2002;34:535–549.

Shapiro S. Meta-analysis/shmeta-analysis. *Am J Epidemiol* 1994;140:771–778.

Sheehe PR. Dynamic risk analysis in retrospective matched-pair studies of disease. *Biometrics* 1962;18:323–341.

Shekelle RB, Shryock AM, Paul O, Lepper M, Stamler J, Liu S, Raynor WJ Jr. Diet, serum cholesterol, and death from coronary heart disease: the Western Electric study. *N Engl J Med* 1981;304:64–70.

Shen X, Huang H, Ye J. Inference after model selection. *J Am Stat Assoc* 2004;99:751–762.

Sheppard L, Prentice RL. On the reliability and precision of within- and between-population estimates of relative rate parameters. *Biometrics* 1995;51:853–863.

Sheppard L, Slaughter JC, Schildcrout J, Liu LJ, Lumley T. Exposure and measurement contributions to estimates of acute air pollution effects. *J Expo Anal Environ Epidemiol* 2005;15:366–376.

Sheps M. Shall we count the living or the dead? *N Engl J Med* 1958;259:12210–12214.

Sheps MC, Mencken JA. *Mathematical models of conception and birth.* Chicago: University of Chicago Press, 1973.

Sherman DI, Ward RJ, Yoshida A, Peters TJ. Alcohol and aldehyde dehydrogenase gene polymorphism and alcoholism. *EXS* 1994;71:291–300.

Shi JQ, Copas JB. Publication bias and meta-analysis for 2×2 tables. *J R Stat Soc Ser B* 2002;64:221–236.

Shimizu H, Ross RK, Bernstein L, Yatani R, Henderson BE, Mack TM. Cancers of the prostate and breast among Japanese and white immigrants in Los Angeles County. *Br J Cancer* 1991;63:963–966.

Shore RE, Pasternack BS, Curnen MG. Relating influenza epidemics to childhood leukemia in tumor registries without a defined population base. *Am J Epidemiol* 1976;103:527–535.

Shriver MD, Smith MW, Jin L, Marcini A, Akey JM, Deka R, Ferrell RE. Ethnic-affiliation estimation by use of population-specific DNA markers. *Am J Hum Genet* 1997;60:957–964.

Siemiatycki J, Friendly control bias. *J Clin Epidemiol* 1989;42:687–688.

Siemiatycki J, Thomas DC. Biological models and statistical interactions: an example from multistage carcinogenesis. *Int J Epidemiol* 1981;10:383–387.

Sieswerda LE, Soskolne CL, Newman SC, Schopflocher D, Smoyer KE. Toward measuring the impact of ecological disintegrity on human health. *Epidemiology* 2001;12:28–32.

Silverman DI, Reis GJ, Sacks FM, Boucher TM, Pasternak RC. Usefulness of plasma phospholipid n-3 fatty acid levels in predicting dietary fish intake in patients with coronary artery disease. *Am J Cardiol* 1990;66:860–862.

Silverman DT, Hoover RN, Swanson GM, Hartge P. The prevalence of coffee drinking among hospitalized and population-based control groups. *JAMA* 1983;249:1877–1880.

Simon JL, Burstein P. *Basic research methods in social science,* 3rd ed. New York: Random House, 1985.

Simon R. Length-biased sampling in etiologic research. *Am J Epidemiol* 1980a;111:444–452.

Simon R. Re: "Assessing effect of confounding variables." *Am J Epidemiol* 1980b;111:127–128.

Simon R, Wittes RE. Methodologic guidelines for reports of clinical trials. *Cancer Treat Rep* 1985;69:1–3.

Simonoff JS. *Smoothing methods in statistics*. New York: Springer, 1996.

Singer E. The use of incentives to reduce nonresponse in household surveys. In: Groves R, Dillman D, Eltinge J, Little R, eds. *Survey nonresponse.* New York: John Wiley & Sons, 2002.

Sinha R, Rothman N, Salmon CP, Knize MG, Brown ED, Swanson CA, Rhodes D, Rossi S, Felton JS, Levander OA. Heterocyclic amine content in beef cooked by different methods to varying degrees of doneness and gravy made from meat drippings. *Food Chem Toxicol* 1998;36:279–287.

Sinha R, Chow WH, Kulldorff M, Denobile J, Butler J, Garcia-Closas M, Weil R, Hoover RN, Rothman N. Well-done grilled red meat increases the risk of colorectal adenomas. *Cancer Res* 1999;59:4320–4324.

Skjaerven R, Wilcox A, Russell D. Birthweight and perinatal mortality of second births conditional on weight of the first. *Int J Epidemiol* 1988;17:830–838.

Skrondal A, Rabe-Hesketh S. *Generalized latent variable modeling: multilevel, longitudinal, and structural equation models*. Boca Raton, FL: Chapman and Hall/CRC, 2004.

Smans M, Esteve J. Practical approaches to disease mapping. In: Elliott P, Cuzick J, English D, Stern R eds. *Geographical and environmental epidemiology: methods for small-area studies*. New York: Oxford University Press, 1992:141–150.

Smith AH, Bates M. Confidence limit analyses should replace power calculations in the interpretation of epidemiologic studies. *Epidemiology* 1992;3:449–452.

Smith AH, Lingas EO, Rahman M. Contamination of drinking-water by arsenic in Bangladesh: a public health emergency. *Bull World Health Org* 2000;78:1093–1103.

Smith DC, Prentice R, Thompson DJ, Herrmann WL. Association of exogenous estrogen and endometrial carcinoma. *N Engl J Med* 1975;293:1164–1167.

Smith HV, Spalding JMR. Outbreak of paralysis in Morocco due to ortho-cresyl phosphate poisoning. *Lancet* 1959;2:1019–1021.

Smith J. Healthy bodies and thick wallets: The dual relationship between health and socioeconomic status. *J Econ Perspect* 1999;13:145–167.

Smith PG, Day NE. Matching and confounding in the design and analysis of epidemiological case-control studies. In: Blithell JF, Coppi R, eds. *Perspectives in medical statistics*. New York: Academic Press, 1981.

Smith PG, Day NE. The design of case-control studies: the influence of confounding and interaction effects. *Int J Epidemiol* 1984;13:356–365.

Smith-Warner SA, Ritz J, Hunter DJ, Albanes D, Beeson WL, van den Brandt PA, Colditz G, Folsom AR, Fraser GE, Freudenheim JL, Giovannucci E, Goldbohm RA, Graham S, Kushi LH, Miller AB, Rohan TE, Speizer FE, Virtamo J, Willett WC. Dietary fat and risk of lung cancer in a pooled analysis of prospective studies. *Cancer Epidemiol Biomarkers Prev* 2002;11:987–992.

Smith-Warner SA, Spiegelman D, Yaun SS, Albanes D, Beeson WL, van den Brandt PA, Feskanich D, Folsom AR, Fraser GE, Freudenheim JL, Giovannucci E, Goldbohm RA, Graham S, Kushi LH, Miller AB, Pietinen P, Rohan TE, Speizer FE, Willett WC, Hunter DJ. Fruits, vegetables and lung cancer: a pooled analysis of cohort studies. *Int J Cancer* 2003;107:1001–1011.

Smithells RW, Shepard S. Teratogenicity testing in humans: a method demonstrating the safety of Bendectin. *Teratology* 1978;17:31–36.

Snijder MB, Zimmet PZ, Visser M, Dekker JM, Seidell JC, Shaw JE. Independent and opposite associations of waist and hip circumferences with diabetes, hypertension and dyslipidemia: the AusDiab Study. *Int J Obes Relat Metab Disord* 2004;28:402–409.

Snow J. On the Mode of Communication of Cholera. London. John Churchill, New Burlington Street 1855.

Sobel ME. Spatial concentration and social stratification: does the clustering of disadvantage "beget" bad outcomes? In: Bowles S, Durlauf SN, Hoff K, eds. *Poverty traps*. Princeton University Press: Princeton, NJ, 2006:204–230.

Somes GW. The generalized Mantel-Haenszel statistic. *Am Statist* 1986;40:106–108.

Sommer AS, Zeger S. On estimating efficacy from clinical trials. *Stat Med* 1991;10:45–52.

Speizer H, Buckley P. Automated coding of survey data. In: Couper M, Baker R, Bethlehem J, Clark CZF, Martin J, Nicholls, WL II, O'Reilly WL, eds. *Computer-assisted survey information collection.* New York: John Wiley & Sons, 1998.

Spielgelhalter DJ, Freedman LS, Parmar MKB. Bayesian approaches to randomized trials (with discussion). *J R Stat Soc Ser A* 1994;156:357–416.

Spiegelhalter DJ. Bayesian methods for cluster randomized trials with continuous responses. *Stat Med* 2001;20:435–452.

Spiegelhalter David J, Abrams KR, Myles JP. *Bayesian approaches to clinical trials and health-care evaluation.* New York: Wiley, 2004.

Spiegelman D. Commentary: Correlated errors and energy adjustment—where are the data? *Int J Epidemiol* 2004; 33:1387–1388.

Spiegelman D, Israel RG, Bouchard C, Willett WC. Absolute fat mass, percent body, and body fat distribution: which is the real determinant of blood pressure and serum glucose? *Am J Clin Nutr* 1992;55:1033–1044.

Spiegelman D, Schneeweiss S, McDermott A. Measurement error correction for logistic regression models with an "alloyed gold standard." *Am J Epidemiol* 1997a;145:184–196.

Spiegelman D, McDermott A, Rosner B. Regression calibration method for correcting measurement-error bias in nutritional epidemiology. *Am J Clin Nutr* 1997b;65(suppl):1179S–1186S.

Spiegelman D, Rosner B, Logan R. Estimation and inference for logistic regression with covariate misclassification and measurement error in main study/validation study designs. *J Am Stat Assoc* 2000;95:51–61.

Spiegelman D, Carroll RJ, Kipnis V. Efficient regression calibration for logistic regression in main study/internal validation study designs with an imperfect reference instrument. *Stat Med* 2001;20:139–160.

Spiegelman D, Zhao B, Kim J. Correlated errors in biased surrogates: study designs and methods for measurement error correction. *Stat Med* 2005;24:1657–1682.

Spielman RS, McGinnis RE, Ewens WJ. Transmission test for linkage disequilibrium: the insulin gene region and insulin dependent diabetes mellitus. *Am J Hum Genet* 1993;52:506–516.

Spirtes P. *Directed cyclic graphical representation of feedback.* 11th Conference on Uncertainty in Artificial Intelligence, San Mateo, CA, Morgan Kaufman, 1995.

Spirtes P, Glymour C, Scheines R. *Causation, prediction, and search.* Cambridge, MA, MIT Press, 2001.

Staffa JA, Chang J, Green N. Cerivastatin and reports of fatal rhabdomyolysis. *N Engl J Med* 2002;346:539–540.

Stallones RA. The rise and fall of ischemic heart disease. *Sci Am* 1980;243:53–59.

Stampfer MJ, Colditz GA. Estrogen replacement therapy and coronary heart disease: a quantitative assessment of the epidemiologic evidence. *Prev Med* 1991;20:47–63.

Stampfer MJ, Willett WC, Speizer FE, Dysert DC, Lipnick R, Rosner B, Hennekens CH. Test of the National Death Index. *Am J Epidemiol* 1984;119:837–839.

Stampfer MJ, Kang JH, Chen J, Cherry R, Grodstein F. Effects of moderate alcohol consumption on cognitive function in women. *N Engl J Med* 2005;352:245–253.

Stansfeld SA, Marmot MG. *Stress and the heart: psychosocial pathways to coronary heart disease.* London: BMJ Books, 2002.

Staszewski J, Haenszel W. Cancer mortality among the Polish-born in the United States. *J Natl Cancer Inst* 1965;35:291–297.

Stavraky KM. The role of ecologic analysis in studies of the etiology of disease: a discussion with reference to large bowel cancer. *J Chronic Dis* 1976;29:435–444.

Steenland K, Greenland S. Monte-Carlo sensitivity analysis and Bayesian analysis of smoking as an unmeasured confounder in a study of silica and lung cancer. *Am J Epidemiol* 2004;160:384–392.

Steenland K, Bray I, Greenland S, Boffetta, P. Empirical-Bayes adjustments for occupational surveillance analysis. *Cancer Epidemiol Biomarkers Prev* 2000;9:895–903.

Steinberg KK, Cogswell ME, Chang JC, Caudill SP, McQuillan GM, Bowman BA, Grummer-Strawn LM, Sampson EJ, Khoury MJ, Gallagher ML. Prevalence of C282Y and H63D mutations in the hemochromatosis (HFE) gene in the United States. *JAMA* 2001;285:2216–2222.

Stelfox HT, Chua G, O'Rourke K, Detsky AS. Conflict of interest in the calcium channel antagonist debate. *N Engl J Med* 1998;338:101–106.

Stensvold I, Tverdal A, Foss OR. The effect of coffee on blood lipids and blood pressure: results from a Norwegian cross-sectional study, men and women, 40–42 years. *J Clin Epidemiol* 1989;42:877–884.

Stensvold I, Tverdal A, Jacobsen BK. Cohort study of coffee intake and death from coronary heart disease. *Br Med J* 1996;312:544–545.

Stephanik PA, Trulson ME. Determining the frequency of foods in large group studies. *Am J Clin Nutr* 1962;2:335–343.

Stewart AW, Kuulasmaa K, Beaglehole R. Ecological analysis of the association between mortality and major risk factors of cardiovascular disease. *Int J Epidemiol* 1994;23:505–516.

Stewart PA, Lemanski D, White D, Zey J, Herrick RF, Masters M, Rayner J, Dosemeci M, Gomez M, Pottern L. Exposure assessment for a study of workers exposed to acrylonitrile, I: job exposures profiles: a computerized data management system. *Appl Occup Environ Hyg* 1992;7:820–825.

Stidley C, Samet JM. Assessment of ecologic regression in the study of lung cancer and indoor radon. *Am J Epidemiol* 1994;139:312–322.

Stijnen T, van Houwelingen HC. Empirical Bayes methods in clinical trials meta-analysis. *Biometr J* 1990;32:335–346.

Stijnen T, van Houwelingen HC. Relative risk, risk difference and rate difference models for sparse stratified data: a pseudolikelihood approach. *Stat Med* 1993;12:2285–2303.

Stiratelli R, Laird NM, Ware JH. Random-effects models for serial observations with binary response. *Biometrics* 1984;40:961–971.

Stram DO. Meta-analysis of published data using a linear mixed-effects model. *Biometrics* 1996;52:936–944.

Strom BL. *Pharmacoepidemiology*, 3rd edition. John Wiley, West Sussex, 2000.

Stromberg U. Collapsing ordered outcome categories: a note of concern. *Am J Epidemiol* 1996;144:421–424.

Struewing JP, Hartge P, Wacholder S, Baker SM, Berlin M, McAdams M, Timmerman MM, Brody LC, Tucker MA. The risk of cancer associated with specific mutations of *BRCA1* and *BRCA2* among Ashkenazi Jews. *N Engl J Med* 1997;336:1401–1408.

Stryker WS, Kaplan LA, Stein EA, Stampfer MJ, Sober A, Willett WC. The relation of diet, cigarette smoking, and alcohol consumption to plasma beta-carotene and alpha-tocopherol levels. *Am J Epidemiol* 1988;127:283–296.

Stukel TA, Glynn RJ, Fisher ES, Sharp SM, Lu-Yao G, Wennberg JE. Standardized rates of recurrent outcomes. *Stat Med* 1994;13:1781–1791.

Stunkard AJ, Albaum JM. The accuracy of self-reported weights. *Am J Clin Nutr* 1981;34:1593–1599.

Stürmer T, Brenner H. Degree of matching and gain in power and efficiency in case-control studies. *Epidemiology* 2001;12:101–108.

Stürmer T, Brenner H. Flexible matching strategies to increase power and efficiency to detect and estimate gene-environment interactions in case-control studies. *Am J Epidemiol* 2002;155:593–602.

Stürmer T, Thürigen D, Spiegelman D, Blettner M, Brenner H. The performance of methods for correcting measurement error in case-control studies. *Epidemiology* 2002;13:507–516.

Stürmer T, Schneeweiss S, Brookhart MA, Rothman KJ, Avorn J, Glynn RJ. Analytic strategies to adjust confounding using exposure propensity scores and disease risk scores: nonsteroidal anti-inflammatory drugs and short-term mortality in the elderly. *Am J Epidemiol* 2005;161:891–898.

Stürmer T, Rothman KJ, Glynn R. Insights into different results from different causal contrasts in the presence of effect-measure modification. *Pharmacoepidemiol Drug Saf* 2006;698–709.

Subar AF, Kipnis V, Troiano RP, Midthune D, Schoeller DA, Bingham S, Sharbaugh CO, Trabulsi J, Runswick S, Ballard-Barbash R, Sunshine J, Schatzkin A. Using intake biomarkers to evaluate the extent of dietary misreporting in a large sample of adults: the OPEN study. *Am J Epidemiol* 2003;158:1–13.

Subramanian SV, Kawachi I. Income inequality and health: What have we learned so far? *Epidemiologic Reviews* 2004;26:78–91.

Suissa S. The case-time-control design. *Epidemiology* 1995;6:248–253.

Sullivan KM, Foster DA. Use of the confidence interval function. *Epidemiology* 1990;1:39–42.

Sun F, Flanders WS, Yang Q, Khoury MJ. A new method for estimating the risk ratio in studies using case-parental control design. *Am J Epidemiol* 1998;148:902–909.

Sundararajan V, Mitra N, Jacobson JS, Grann VR, Heitjan DF, Neugut AI. Survival associated with 5-Fluorouracil-based adjuvant chemotherapy among elderly patients with node-positive colon cancer. *Ann Intern Med* 2002;136:349–357.

Susser M. *Causal thinking in the health sciences*. New York: Oxford, 1973.

Susser M. Judgment and causal inference. *Am J Epidemiol* 1977;105:1–15.

Susser M. What is a cause and how do we know one? A grammar for pragmatic epidemiology. *Am J Epidemiol* 1991;133:635–648.

Susser M. The logic in ecological: II. The logic of design. *Am J Public Health* 1994;84:830–835.

Susser M, Susser E. Choosing a future for epidemiology, II: from black box to Chinese boxes and eco-epidemiology. *Am J Public Health* 1996;86:674–677. Erratum in: *Am J Public Health* 1996;86:1093.

Sussman MP, Jones SE, Wilson TW, Kann L. The youth risk behavior surveillance system: updating policy and program applications. *J School Health* 2002:72:13–17.

Sutton AJ, Abrams KR, Jones DR. *Methods for meta-analysis in medical research*. Chichester: Wiley, 2000.

Swan S, Shaw G, Shulman J. Reporting and selection bias in case-control studies of congenital malformations. *Epidemiology* 1992;3:356–363.

Sweeney BP. Watson and Crick 50 years on. From double helix to pharmacogenomics. *Anaesthesia* 2004;59:150–165.

Sytkowski PA, Kannel WB, D'Agostino RB. Changes in risk factors and the decline in mortality from cardiovascular disease: the Framingham Heart Study. *N Engl J Med* 1990;322:1635–1641.

Szklo M, Nieto FJ. *Epidemiology: beyond the basics*. Aspen Publishers: Gaithersburg, MD; 2000.

Szmuness W. Hepatitis B vaccine: demonstration of efficacy in a controlled clinical trial in a high-risk population in the United States. *N Engl J Med* 1980;303:833–841.

Tang MC, Weiss NS, Malone KE. Induced abortion in relation to breast cancer among parous women: A birth certificate registry study. *Epidemiology* 2000;11:177–180.

Tanur JM, ed. *Questions about questions: inquiries into the cognitive bases of surveys*. New York: Sage Foundation, 1992.

Tarone RE. On summary estimators of relative risk. *J Chronic Dis* 1981;34:463–468.

Tarone RE, Chu KC. Implications of birth cohort patterns in interpreting trends in breast cancer rates. *J Natl Cancer Inst* 1992;84:1402–1410.

Task force on genetic testing: Promoting safe and effective genetic testing in the United States. Final report 1997 http://www.genome.gov/10001733.

Tate RB, Manfreda J, Cuddy TE. The effect of age on risk factors for ischemic heart disease: The Manitoba Follow Up Study, 1948–1993. *Ann Epidemiol* 1998;8:415–421.

Taubes G. *Bad science: the short life and weird times of cold fusion*. New York: Random House, 1993.

Taubes G. Fields of fear. *The Atlantic* 1994;274:94–100.

Taubes G. Epidemiology faces its limits. *Science* 1995;269:164–169.

Taubes G. Do we really know what makes us healthy? *The New York Times Magazine*, Sept. 16, 2007, 52–59.
Taussig HB. A study of the German outbreak of phocomelia, the thalidomide syndrome. *JAMA* 1962;180:80:80–88.
Taylor DM, Wright SC, Moghaddam FM, Lalonde RN. The personal group discrimination discrepancy - perceiving my group, but not myself, to be a target for discrimination. *Pers Soc Psychol B* 1990;16:254–262.
Tennenbein A. A double sampling scheme for estimating from binomial data with misclassification. *J Am Stat Assoc* 1970;65:1350–1361.
Terry MB, Neugut AL. Cigarette smoking and the colorectal adenoma-carcinoma sequence: a hypothesis to explain the paradox. *Am J Epidemiol* 1998;147:903–910.
Thacker SB, Berkelman RL. Public health surveillance in the United States. *Epidemiol Rev* 1988;10:164–190.
Thacker SB, Berkelman RL. History of public health surveillance. In: Halperin W, Baker EL, Monson RR, eds. *Public health surveillance.* New York: Van Nostrand Reinhold, 1992:1–15.
The Esprit Team. Estrogen therapy for the prevention of reinfarction in postmenopausal women: a randomized placebo controlled trial. *Lancet* 2002;360:2001–2008.
Thomas DB. Relationship of oral contraceptives to cervical carcinogenesis. *Obstet Gynecol* 1972;40:508–518.
Thomas DC. Are dose-response, synergy, and latency confounded? In: *Abstracts of the joint statistical meetings.* Alexandria, VA: American Statistical Association, 1981a.
Thomas DC. General relative risk models for survival time and matched case-control analysis. *Biometrics* 198lb;37:673–686.
Thomas DC. Statistical methods for analyzing effects of temporal patterns of exposure on cancer risks. *Scand J Work Environ Health* 1983;9:353–366.
Thomas DC. Models for exposure-time-response relationships with applications to cancer epidemiology. *Annu Rev Public Health* 1988;9:451–482.
Thomas DC. Re: "When will nondifferential misclassification of an exposure preserve the direction of a trend?" *Am J Epidemiol* 1995;142:782–783.
Thomas DC. *Statistical methods in genetic epidemiology*. Oxford University Press: New York, 2004a.
Thomas DC. Statistical issues in the design and analysis of gene-disease association studies. In: Khoury MJ, Little J, Burke W, eds. *Human genome epidemiology: a scientific foundation for using genetic information to improve health and prevent disease*. New York: Oxford University Press, 2004b:92–110.
Thomas DC, Greenland S. The relative efficiencies of matched and independent sample designs for case-control studies. *J Chronic Dis* 1983;36:685–697.
Thomas DC, Greenland S. The efficiency of matching case-control studies of risk factor interactions. *J Chronic Dis* 1985;38:569–574.
Thomas DC, Semiatycki J, Dewar R, Robins J, Goldberg M, Armstrong BG. The problem of multiple inference in studies designed to generate hypotheses. *Am J Epidemiol* 1985;122:1080–1095.
Thomas DC, Witte JS. Point: population stratification: a problem for case-control studies of candidate-gene associations? *Cancer Epidemiol Biomarkers Prev* 2002;11:505–512.
Thomas JC, Thomas KK. Things ain't what they ought to be: social forces underlying racial disparities in rates of sexually transmitted diseases in a rural North Carolina county. *Soc Sci Med* 1999;49:1075–1084.
Thompson JR. Re: "Multiple comparisons and related issues in the interpretation of epidemiologic data." *Am J Epidemiol* 1998a;147:801–806.
Thompson JR. A response to "Describing data requires no adjustment for multiple comparisons." *Am J Epidemiol* 1998b;147:815.
Thompson SG. Why sources of heterogeneity in meta-analysis should be investigated. *Br Med J* 1994;309:1351–1355.
Thompson SG, Pocock SL. Can meta-analyses be trusted? *Lancet* 1991;338:1127–1130.
Thompson WD. Statistical criteria in the interpretation of epidemiologic data. *Am J Public Health* 1987;77:191–194.
Thompson WD. Effect modification and the limits of biological inference from epidemiologic data. *J Clin Epidemiol* 1991;44:221–232.
Thompson WD, Kelsey JL, Walter SD. Cost and efficiency in the choice of matched and unmatched case-control studies. *Am J Epidemiol* 1982;116:840–851.
Thornton R. The Navajo-US population mortality crossover since the mid-20th century. *Popul Res Policy Rev* 2004;23:291–308.
Thurigen D, Spiegelman D, Blettner M, Heuer C, Brenner H. Measurement error correction using validation data: a review of methods and their applicability in case-control studies. *Stat Methods Med Res* 2000;9:447–474.
Tilling K, Sterne JA, Szklo M. Estimating the effect of cardiovascular risk factors on all-cause mortality and incidence of coronary heart disease using g-estimation: the ARIC study. *Am J Epidemiol* 2002;155:710–718.
Timmer A. Environmental influences on inflammatory bowel disease manifestations. Lessons from epidemiology. *Dig Dis* 2003;21:91–104.
Titterington DM. Common structure of smoothing techniques in statistics. *Int Stat Rev* 1985;53:141–170.
Titus-Ernstoff L, Egan KM, Newcomb PA, Ding J, Trentham-Dietz A, Greenberg ER, Baron JA, Trichopoulos D, Willett WC. Early life factors in relation to breast cancer risk in postmenopausal women. *Cancer Epidemiol Biomarkers Prev* 2002;11:207–210.
Tobi M, Luo FC, Ronai Z. Detection of K-ras mutation in colonic effluent samples from patients without evidence of colorectal carcinoma. *J Natl Cancer Inst* 1994;86:1007–1010.
Traverso G, Shuber A, Levin B, Johnson C, Olsson L, Schoetz DJ Jr, Hamilton SR, Boynton K, Kinzler KW, Vogelstein B. Detection of APC mutations in fecal DNA from patients with colorectal tumors. *New Eng J Med* 2002;346:311–320.
Treloar AE, Boynton RE, Behn BG, Brown BW. Variation of the human menstrual cycle through reproductive life. *Int J Fertil* 1967;12:77–126.

Trichopoulou A, Costacou T, Bamia C, Trichopoulos D. Adherence to a Mediterranean diet and survival in a Greek population. *N Engl J Med* 2003;348:2599–2608.

Trichopoulos D, Lipman RD. Mammary gland mass and breast cancer risk. *Epidemiology* 1992;3:523–526.

Truett J, Cornfield J, Kannel W. A multivariate analysis of the risk of coronary heart disease in Framingham. *J Chronic Dis* 1967;20:511–524.

Tsiatis AA. *Semiparametric theory and missing data.* New York: Springer, 2006.

Tugwood JD, Hollins LE, Cockerill MJ. Genomics and the search for novel biomarkers in toxicology. *Biomarkers* 2003;8:79–92.

Tukey JW. *EDA: exploratory data analysis.* Reading, MA: Addison-Wesley, 1977.

Turner RM, Omar RZ, Thompson SG. Bayesian methods of analysis for cluster randomized trials with binary outcome data. *Stat Med* 2001;20:453–472.

Tverdal A, Stensvold I, Solvoll K, Foss OP, Lund-Larsen P, Bjartveit K. Coffee consumption and death from coronary heart disease in middle-aged Norwegian men and women. *Br Med J* 1990;300:566–569.

Uemura K, Pisa Z. Trends in cardiovascular disease mortality in industrialized countries since 1950. *World Health Stat Q* 1988;41:155–178.

Umbach D, Wilcox A. A technique for measuring epidemiologically useful features of birthweight distributions. *Stat Med* 1996;15:1333–1348.

Umbach DM, Weinberg CR. The use of case-parent triads to study joint effects of genotype and exposure. *Am J Hum Genet* 2000;66:251–261.

United Church of Christ Commission for Racial Justice. *Toxic wastes and race in the United States: a national report on the racial and socio-economic characteristics of communities with hazardous waste sites.* 1987.

UKCCS (United Kingdom Childhood Cancer Study). Exposure to power-frequency magnetic fields and the risk of childhood cancer. *Lancet*, 1999;354:1925–1931.

United States Congress, Office of Technology Assessment. *Infertility: medical and social choices.* Washington, DC: U.S. Government Printing Office, 1988. OTA-BA-358.

United States Congress, Office of Technology Assessment. *The CDC's case definition of AIDS: implications of the proposed revisions-background paper.* Washington, DC: U.S. Government Printing Office, 1992. OTA-BP-H-89.

United States Department of Health, Education and Welfare. *Smoking and health: report of the Advisory Committee to the Surgeon General of the Public Health Service.* Washington, DC: Government Printing Office, 1964. PHS Publ No 1103.

United States Environmental Protection Agency. Guidelines for cancer risk assessment. *Fed Reg* 1986;51:33992.

United States Environmental Protection Agency. *Toxics in the community: national and local perspectives: the 1989 toxics release inventory national report.* Washington, DC: U.S. EPA, Office of Toxic Substances, Economics and Technology Division, 1991.

United States Environmental Protection Agency. *Environmental equity: reducing risk for all communities.* Washington, DC: U.S. EPA, 1992.

United States General Accounting Office. *Siting of hazardous waste landfills and their correlation with racial and economic status of surrounding communities.* Washington, DC: U.S. GAO, 1983.

University Group Diabetes Program. A study of the effects of hypoglycemic agents on vascular complications in patients with adult onset diabetes. *Diabetes* 1970;19(suppl 2):747–830.

Vach W, Blettner M. Biased estimation of the odds ratio in case-control studies due to the use of *ad hoc* methods of correcting for missing values of confounding variables. *Am J Epidemiol* 1991;134:895–907. Erratum: *Am J Epidemiol* 1994;140:79.

Valdiserri RO, Ogden LL, McCray E. Accomplishments in HIV prevention science: implications for stemming the epidemic. *Nature Medicine* 2003;9:881–886.

Valkonen T. Individual and structural effects in ecological research. In: Dogan M, Rokkan S, eds. *Social ecology.* Cambridge, MA: MIT Press, 1969:53–68.

Valleron AJ, Bouvet E, Garnerin P, Ménarès J, Heard I, Letrait S, Lefaucheux J. A computer network for the surveillance of communicable diseases: the French experiment. *Am J Public Health* 1986;76:1289–1292.

Vandenbroucke JP, Koster T, Briët E, Reitsma PH, Bertina RM, Rosendaal FR. Increased risk of venous thrombosis in oral-contraceptive users who are carriers of factor V Leiden mutation. *Lancet* 1994;344:1453–1457.

Vandentorren S, Suzan F, Medina S, Pascal M, Maulpoix A, Cohen JC, Ledrans M. Mortality in 13 French cities during the August 2003 heat wave. *Am J Public Health* 2004;94:1518–1520.

Van der Laan M, Robins JM. *Unified methods for censored longitudinal data and causality.* New York: Springer, 2003.

van der Leun JC, de Gruijl FR. Climate change and skin cancer. *Photochem Photobiol Sci* 2002;1:324–326.

VanderWeele TJ, Hernán MA. From counterfactuals to sufficient component causes and vice versa. *Eur J Epidemiol* 2006;21:855–858.

VanderWeele TJ, Robins JM. The identification of synergism in the sufficient-component cause framework. *Epidemiology* 2007a;18:329–339.

VanderWeele TJ, Robins JM. Directed acyclic graphs, sufficient causes and the properties of conditioning on a common effect. *Am J Epidemiol* 2007b;166:1096–1104.

VanderWeele TJ, Robins JM. Empirical and counterfactual conditions for sufficient-cause interactions. *Biometrika* 2008a;in press.

VanderWeele TJ, Robins JM. Signed directed acyclic graphs for causal inference. *J R Stat Soc Ser B* 2008b;in press.

van den Brandt PA, Spiegelman D, Yaun SS, Adami HO, Beeson L, Folsom AR, Fraser G, Goldbohm RA, Graham S, Kushi L, Marshall JR, Miller AB, Rohan T, Smith-Warner SA, Speizer FE, Willett WC, Wolk A, Hunter DJ. Pooled analysis of prospective cohort studies on height, weight, and breast cancer risk. *Am J Epidemiol* 2000;152:514–527.

van Ommen B, Stierum R. Nutrigenomics: exploiting systems biology in the nutrition and health arena. *Curr Opin Biotechnol* 2002;13:517–521.

Vaupel JW, Yashin AI. Heterogeneity ruses - some surprising effects of selection on population-dynamics. *Am Stat* 1985;39:176–185.

Vermeire S, Louis E, Rutgeerts P, De Vos M, Van Gossum A, Belaiche J, Pescatore P, Fiasse R, Pelckmans P, Vlietinck R, Merlin F, Zouali H, Thomas G, Colombel JF, Hugot JP; Belgian Group of Infliximab Expanded Access Program and Fondation Jean Dausset CEPH, Paris, France. NOD2/CARD15 does not influence response to infliximab in Crohn's disease. *Gastroenterology* 2002;123:106–111.

Viallefont V, Raftery AE, Richardson S. Variable selection and Bayesian model averaging in epidemiological case-control studies. *Stat Med* 2001;20:3215–3230.

Vineis P, Malats N, Lang M, d'Errico A, Caporaso N, Cuzick J, Boffetta P. Metabolic polymorphisms and susceptibility to cancer. IARC Scientific Publications, No. 148. International Agency for Research on Cancer. Lyon, France, 1999.

Vines SK, Farrington CP. Within-subject exposure dependency in case-crossover studies. *Stat Med* 2001;20:3039–3049.

Virtamo J, Pietinen P, Huttunen JK, Korhonen P, Malila N, Virtanen MJ, Albanes D, Taylor PR, Albert P; ATBC Study Group. Incidence of cancer and mortality following alpha-tocopherol and beta-carotene supplementation: a postintervention follow-up. *JAMA* 2003;290:476–485.

von Ehrenstein OS, Mazumder DN, Yuan Y, Samanta S, Balmes J, Sil A, Ghosh N, Hira-Smith M, Haque R, Purushothamam R, Lahiri S, Das S, Smith AH. Decrements in lung function related to arsenic in drinking water in West Bengal, India. *Am J Epidemiol* 2005;162:533–541.

Von Korff M, Koepsell T, Curry S, Diehr P. Multi-level analysis in epidemiologic research on health behaviors and outcomes. *Am J Epidemiol* 1992;135:1077–1082.

Von Reyn CF, Levy BS, Arbeit RD, Friedland G, Crumpacker CS. Infective endocarditis: an analysis based on strict case definitions. *Ann Intern Med* 1981;94:505–518.

Vose D. *Risk analysis*. New York: John Wiley and Sons 2000.

Wacholder S. Practical considerations in choosing between the case-cohort and nested case-control design. *Epidemiology* 1991;2:155–158.

Wacholder S. The case-control study as data missing by design: estimating risk differences. *Epidemiology* 1996;7:144–150.

Wacholder S, Dosemeci M, Lubin JH. Blind assignment of exposure does not prevent differential misclassification. *Am J Epidemiol* 1991;134:433–437.

Wacholder S, McLaughlin JK, Silverman DT, Mandel JS. Selection of controls in case-control studies, I: principles. *Am J Epidemiol* 1992a;135:1019–1028.

Wacholder S, Silverman DT, McLaughlin JK, Mandel JS. Selection of controls in case-control studies, II: types of controls. *Am J Epidemiol* 1992b;135:1029–1041.

Wacholder S, Silverman DT, McLaughlin JK, Mandel JS. Selection of controls in case-control studies, III: design options. *Am J Epidemiol* 1992c;135:1042–1050.

Wacholder S, Armstrong B, Hartge P. Validation studies using an alloyed gold standard. *Am J Epidemiol* 1993;137:1251–1258.

Wacholder S, Hartge P, Streuwing JP, Pee D, McAdams M, Brody L, Tucker M. The kin-cohort study for estimating penetrance. *Am J Epidemiol* 1998:148:623–630.

Wacholder S, Rothman N, Caporaso N. Counterpoint: bias from population stratification is not a major threat to the validity of conclusions from epidemiological studies of common polymorphisms and cancer. *Cancer Epidemiol Biomarkers Prev* 2002;11:513–520.

Wacholder S, Chanock S, Garcia-Closas M, El Ghormli L, Rothman N. Assessing the probability that a positive report is false: an approach for molecular epidemiology studies. *J Natl Cancer Inst* 2004;96:434–442.

Wahba G. *Spline models for observational data*. Boston: Cambridge University Press, 1990.

Wahba G, Gu C, Wang Y, Chappel R. Soft classification, a.k.a. risk estimation, via penalized log likelihood and smoothing spline analysis of variance. In: Wolper D, ed. *The mathematics of generalization*. Reading, MA: Addison-Wesley, 1995.

Waksberg J. Sampling methods for random digit dialing. *J Am Stat Assoc* 1978;73:40–46.

Wakefield AJ, Murch SH, Anthony A, Linnell J, Casson DM, Malik M, Berelowitz M, Dhillon AP, Thomson MA, Harvey P, Valentine A, Davies SE, Walker-Smith JA. Ileal-lymphoid-nodular hyperplasia, non-specific colitis, and pervasive developmental disorder in children. *Lancet* 1998;351:637–641.

Wakefield J. Ecological inference for 2 × 2 tables. *J R Stat Soc Ser A* 2004;167(Part 2):385–445.

Wakefield J, Salway R. A statistical framework for ecological and aggregate studies. *J R Stat Soc Ser A* 2001;164 (Part 1):119–137.

Wald NA. Smoking. In: Vessey MP, Gray M, eds. *Cancer risks and prevention*. New York: Oxford University Press, 1985. Chapter 3.

Wald N, Boreham J, Bailey A. Serum retinol and subsequent risk of cancer. *Br J Cancer* 1986;54:957–961.

Walker AM. Proportion of disease attributable to the combined effect of two factors. *Int J Epidemiol* 1981;10:81–85.

Walker AM. Anamorphic analysis: sampling and estimation for covariate effects when both exposure and disease are known. *Biometrics* 1982a;38:1025–1032.

Walker AM. Efficient assessment of confounder effects in matched cohort studies. *Appl Stat* 1982b;31:293–297.

Walker AM. Small sample properties of some estimators of a common hazard ratio. *Appl Stat* 1985;34:42–48.

Walker AM. Reporting the results of epidemiologic studies. *Am J Public Health* 1986;76:556–558.

Walker AM, Blettner M. Comparing imperfect measures of exposure. *Am J Epidemiol* 1985;121:783–790.

Walker AM, Rothman KJ. Models of varying parametric form in case-referent studies. *Am J Epidemiol* 1982;115:129–137.

Walker AM, Martin-Moreno JM, Artalejo FR. Odd man out: a graphical approach to meta-analysis. *Am J Public Health* 1988;78:961–966.

Walker LJ, Aldhous MC, Drummond HE, Smith BR, Nimmo ER, Arnott ID, Satsangi J. Anti-Saccharomyces cerevisiae antibodies (ASCA) in Crohn's disease are associated with disease severity but not NOD2/CARD15 mutations. *Clin Exp Immunol* 2004;135:490–496.

Wallenstein S, Bodian C. Inferences on odds ratios, relative risks, and risk differences based on standard regression programs. *Am J Epidemiol* 1987;126:346–355.

Waller L. Detecting disease clustering in time or space. In: Brookmeyer R, Stroup DF, Eds. *Monitoring the health of populations: statistical principles and methods for public health surveillance.* Oxford: Oxford University Press, 2004:167–201.

Weinstein RA. Planning for epidemics—the lessons of SARS. *N Eng J Med* 2004;350:2332–2334.

Walter SD. The estimation and interpretation of attributable risk in health research. *Biometrics* 1976;32:829–849.

Walter SD. Determination of significant relative risks and optimal sampling procedures in prospective and retrospective comparative studies of various sizes. *Am J Epidemiol* 1977;105:387–397.

Walter SD. The ecologic method in the study of environmental health, I: overview of the method. *Environ Health Perspect* 1991a;94:61–65.

Walter SD. The ecologic method in the study of environmental health, II: methodologic issues and feasibility. *Environ Health Perspect* 1991b;94:67–73.

Walter SD. The analysis of regional patterns in health data, I: distributional considerations. *Am J Epidemiol* 1992a;136:730–741.

Walter SD. The analysis of regional patterns in health data, II: the power to detect environmental effects. *Am J Epidemiol* 1992b;136:742–759.

Walter SD, Holford TR. Additive, multiplicative, and other models for disease risks. *Am J Epidemiol* 1978;108:341–346.

Wang J, Miettinen OS. Occupational mortality studies: principles of validity. *Scand J Work Environ Health* 1982;8:153–158.

Warburton D, Stein Z, Kline J. *In utero* selection against fetuses with trisomy. *Am J Hum Genet* 1983;35:1059–1064.

Ware JH, Mosteller F, Ingelfinger JA. P values. In: *Medical uses of statistics.* Waltham, MA: NEJM Books, 1986.

Warkany J. Terathanasia. *Teratology* 1978;17:187–192.

Wasserman L. *All of nonparametrics*. New York: Springer, 2006.

Wasserman GA, Liu X, Parvez F, Ahsan H, Factor-Litvak P, van Geen A, Slavkovich V, LoIacono NJ, Cheng Z, Hussain I, Momotaj H, Graziano JH. Water arsenic exposure and children's intellectual function in Araihazar, Bangladesh. *Environ Health Perspect* 2004;112:1329–1333.

Wasserman S, Faust K. *Social Network Analysis*. Cambridge: Cambridge University Press, 1994.

Wasserman SL, Berg JW, Finch JL, Kreiss K. Investigation of an occupational cancer cluster using a population-based tumor registry and the national death index. *J Occup Med* 1992;34:1008–1012.

Wattenberg LW, Loub WD. Inhibition of polycyclic aromatic hydrocarbon-induced neoplasia by naturally occurring indoles. *Cancer Res* 1978;38:1410–1413.

Waxweiler R, Stringer W, Wagoner JK, Jones J. Neoplastic risk among workers exposed to vinyl chloride. *Ann N Y Acad Sci* 1976;271:40–48.

Webster PJ, Holland GJ, Curry JA, Chang H-R. Changes in tropical cyclone number, duration, and intensity in a warming environment. *Science* 2005;309:1844–1846.

Weed DL. On the logic of causal inference. *Am J Epidemiol* 1986;123:965–979.

Weed DL, Gorelic LS. The practice of causal inference in cancer epidemiology. *Cancer Epidemiol Biomarkers Prev* 1996;5:303–311.

Weed DL, Selmon M, Sinks T. Links between categories of interaction. *Am J Epidemiol* 1988;127:117–127.

Weinberg CR. On pooling across strata when frequency matching has been followed in a cohort study. *Biometrics* 1985;41:103–116.

Weinberg CR. Applicability of the simple independent-action model to epidemiologic studies involving two factors and a dichotomous outcome. *Am J Epidemiol* 1986;123:162–173.

Weinberg CR. Infertility and the use of illicit drugs. *Epidemiology* 1990;1:189–192.

Weinberg CR. Toward a clearer definition of confounding. *Am J Epidemiol* 1993;137:1–8.

Weinberg CR. Methods for detection of parent-of-origin effects in genetic studies of case-parents triads. *Am J Hum Genet* 1999;65:229–235.

Weinberg CR, Gladen BC. The beta-geometric distribution applied to comparative fecundability studies. *Biometrics* 1986:42:547–560.

Weinberg CR, Sandler DR. Randomized recruitment in case-control studies. *Am J Epidemiol* 1991;134:421–432.

Weinberg CR, Baird DD, Wilcox AJ. Sources of bias in studies of time to pregnancy. *Stat Med* 1994;13:671–681.

Weinberg CR, Wacholder S. The design and analysis of case-control studies with biased sampling. *Biometrics* 1990;46:963–975.

Weinberg CR, Wacholder S. Prospective analysis of case-control data under general multiplicative-intercept risk models. *Biometrika* 1993;80:461–465.

Weinberg CR, Wilcox AJ. A model for estimating the potency and survival of human gametes *in vivo. Biometrics* 1995;51:405–412.

Weinberg CR, Hertz-Picciotto I, Baird DD, Wilcox AJ. Efficiency and bias in studies of early pregnancy loss. *Epidemiology* 1992;3:17–22.

Weinberg CR, Baird DD, Rowland A. Pitfalls inherent in retrospective time-to-event data: the example of time to pregnancy. *Stat Med* 1993;12:867–879.

Weinberg CR, Baird DD, Wilcox AJ. Bias in retrospective studies of spontaneous abortion based on the outcome of the most recent pregnancy. In: Campbell KL, Wood JW, eds. *Human reproductive ecology: interactions of environment, fertility, and behavior.* New York: The New York Academy of Sciences, 1994a:280–286.

Weinberg CR, Gladen BC, Wilcox AJ. Models relating the timing of intercourse to the probability of conception and the sex of the baby. *Biometrics* 1994b;50:358–367.

Weinberg CR, Baird DD, Wilcox AJ. Sources of bias in studies of time to pregnancy. *Stat Med* 1994c;13:671–681.

Weinberg CR, Umbach DM, Greenland S. When will nondifferential misclassification preserve the direction of a trend? *Am J Epidemiol* 1994d;140:565–571.

Weinberg CR, Wilcox AJ, Lie RT. A log-linear approach to case-parent-triad data: assessing effects of disease genes that act either directly or through maternal effects and that may be subject to parental imprinting. *Am J Hum Genet* 1998;62:969–978.

Weinstein RA. Planning for epidemics—the lessons of SARS. *N Eng J Med* 2004;350:2332–2334.

Weiss NS. Can the specificity of an association be rehabilitated as a basis for supporting a causal hypothesis? *Epidemiology* 2002;13:6–8.

Weiss NS. *Clinical epidemiology: the study of the outcome of illness*, 3rd ed. New York: Oxford University Press, 2006.

Weiss RE. The influence of variable selection. *J Am Stat Assoc* 1995;90:619–625.

Welsh SO, Marston RM. Review of trends in food use in the United States, 1909 to 1980. *J Am Diet Assoc* 1982;81:120–128.

Wen SW, Kramer MS. Uses of ecologic studies in the assessment of intended treatment effects. *J Clin Epidemiol* 1999;52:7–12.

Weninger BJ, Limpakarnjanarat K, Ungchusak K, Thanprasertsuk S, Choopanya K, Vanichseni S, Uneklabh T, Thongcharoen P, Wasi C. The epidemiology of HIV infection and AIDS in Thailand. *AIDS* 1991;5(suppl 2):S71–S85.

Werler M, Pober B, Nelson K, Holmes L. Reporting accuracy among mothers of malformed and nonmalformed infants. *Am J Epidemiol* 1989;129:415–421.

Wheatley K, Clayton D. Be skeptical about unexpected large apparent treatment effects: the case of an MRC AML12 randomization. *Control Clin Trials* 2003;24:66–70.

White H. Maximum likelihood estimation in misspecified models. *Econometrica* 1982a;50:1–9.

White H. *Estimation, inference, and specification analysis.* New York: Cambridge University Press, 1993.

White IR, Walker S, Babiker A. strbee: Randomization-based efficacy estimator. *The Stata Journal* 2002;2:140–150.

White JE. A two-stage design for the study of the relationship between a rare exposure and a rare disease. *Am J Epidemiol* 1982b;115:119–128.

White ME, McDonnell SM. Public health surveillance in low- and middle-income countries. In: Teutsch SM, Churchill RE, eds. *Principles and practice of public health surveillance*, 2nd ed. New York: Oxford University Press, 2000:287–315.

Whitehead A. *Meta-analysis of controlled clinical trials.* Oxford: John Wiley and Sons, 2002.

Wiehl DG, Reed R. Development of new or improved dietary methods for epidemiological investigation. *Am J Public Health* 1960;50:824–828.

Wilcox A. Birthweight and perinatal mortality: the effect of maternal smoking. *Am J Epidemiol* 1993;137:1098–1104.

Wilcox A, Russell I. Why small black infants have lower mortality than small white infants: the case for population-specific standards for birth weight. *J Pediatr* 1990;116:7–10.

Wilcox A, Skjaerven R. Birthweight and perinatal mortality: the effect of gestational age. *Am J Public Health* 1992;82:378–382.

Wilcox AJ, Weinberg CR, O'Connor JF, Baird DD, Schlatterer JP, Canfield RE, Armstrong EG, Nisula BC. Incidence of early loss of pregnancy. *N Engl J Med* 1988;319:189–194.

Wilcox AJ, Gladen BC. Spontaneous abortion: the role of heterogeneous risk and selective fertility. *Early Hum Dev* 1982;7:165–178.

Wilhelmsen L. Role of the data and safety monitoring committee. *Stat Med* 2002;21:2823–2829.

Wilhelmsen L, Tibblin G, Elmfeldt D, Wedel H, Werkö L. Coffee consumption and coronary heart disease in middle-aged Swedish men. *Acta Med Scand* 1977;201:547–552.

Wilkinson RG. Class mortality differentials, income distribution, and trends in poverty 1921–1981. *J Soc Policy* 1989; 18:307–335.

Willett WC. Nutritional epidemiology: issues and challenges. *Int J Epidemiol* 1987;16:312–317.

Willett WC. *Nutritional epidemiology*, 2nd ed. New York: Oxford University Press, 1998.

Willett WC. Isocaloric diets are of primary interest in experimental and epidemiological studies. *Int J Epidemiol* 2002;31:694–695.

Willett WC. Invited Commentary: OPEN Questions. *Am J Epidemiol* 2003;158:22–24.

Willett WC, Stampfer MJ. Total energy intake: implications for epidemiologic analyses. *Am J Epidemiol* 1986;124:17–27.

Willett WC, Stampfer MJ, Underwood BA, Speizer FE, Rosner B, Hennekens CH. Validation of a dietary questionnaire with plasma carotenoid and a-tocopherol levels. *Am J Clin Nutr* 1983;38:631–639.

Willett WC, Sampson L, Stampfer MJ, Rosner B, Bain C, Witschi J, Hennekens CH, Speizer FE. Reproducibility and validity of a semiquantitative food frequency questionnaire. *Am J Epidemiol* 1985;122:51–65

Willett WC, Reynolds RD, Cottrell-Hoehner S, Sampson L, Browne ML. Validation of a semi-quantitative food frequency questionnaire: comparison with a one-year diet record. *J Am Diet Assoc* 1987;87:43–47.
Willett WC, Hunter DJ, Stampfer MJ, Colditz G, Manson JE, Spiegelman D, Rosner B, Hennekens CH, Speizer FE. Dietary fat and fiber in relation to risk of breast cancer: an eight-year follow-up. *JAMA* 1992;268:2037–2044.
Willett WC, Stampfer MJ, Manson JE, Colditz GA, Rosner BA, Speizer FE, Hennekens CH. Coffee consumption and heart disease in women: a ten-year follow-up. *JAMA* 1996;275:458–462.
Willett WC, Stampfer M, Chu N, Spiegelman D, Holmes M, Rimm E. Assessment of questionnaire validity for measuring total fat intake using plasma lipid levels as criteria. *Am J Epidemiol* 2001;154:1107–1112.
Williams DR. Race and health: basic questions, emerging directions. *Ann Epidemiol* 1997;7:322–333.
Wingo PA, Ory HW, Layde PM, Lee NC. Cancer and steroid hormone study group. *Am J Epidemiol* 1988;128:206–217.
Winn DM, Blot WJ, Shy CM, Pickle LW, Toledo A, Fraumeni JF Jr. Snuff dipping and oral cancer among women in the southern United States. *N Engl J Med* 1981;304:745–749.
Witte JS, Greenland S. Simulation study of hierarchical regression. *Stat Med* 1996;15:1161–1170.
Witte JS, Greenland S, Haile RW, Bird CL. Hierarchical regression analysis applied to a study of multiple dietary exposures and breast cancer. *Epidemiology* 1994;5:612–621.
Witte JS, Longnecker MP, Bird CL, Frankl HD, Lee ER, Haile RW. Relation of vegetable, fruit, and grain consumption to colorectal adenomatous polyps. *Am J Epidemiol* 1996;144:1015–1025.
Witte JS, Greenland S, Kim LL, Arab LK. Multilevel modeling in epidemiology with GLIMMIX. *Epidemiology* 2000;11:684–688.
Witteman JCM, D Agostino RB, Stijnen T, Kannel WB, Cobb JC, de Ridder MAJ, Hofman A, Robins JM. G-estimation of causal effects: isolated systolic hypertension and cardiovascular death in the Framingham Study. *Am J Epidemiol* 1998;148:390-401.
Women's Health Initiative. Study findings: Women's Health Initiative Participant Website, http://www.whi.org/findings/index.php (accessed July 14, 2004).
Wong GY, Mason WM. The hierarchical logistic regression model for multilevel analysis. *J Am Stat Assoc* 1985; 80:513–524.
Wong GY, Mason WM. Contextually specific effects and other generalizations for the hierarchical linear model for comparative analysis. *J Am Stat Assoc* 1991;86:487–503.
Woolf B. On estimating the relation between blood group and disease. *Ann Hum Genet* 1955;19:251–253.
World Cancer Research Fund, American Institute for Cancer Research. Food, Nutrition and the Prevention of Cancer: a Global Perspective. Washington, DC: American Institute for Cancer Research, 1997.
World Health Organization and UNAIDS. *Reconciling antenatal clinic-based surveillance and population-based survey estimates of HIV prevalence in Sub-Saharan Africa.* Issued August 2003. Accessed June 2004. Available at URL: http://www.unaids.org.
Wright AF, Carothers AD, Campbell H. Gene environment interactions–the BioBank UK study. *Pharmacogenomics J* 2002;2:75–82.
Wright EO. *Class counts: comparative studies in class analysis*. New York: Cambridge University Press, 1996.
Writing group for the woman's health initiative investigators. Risks and benefits of estrogen plus progestin in healthy postmenopausal women. Principal results from the Women's Health Initiative randomized controlled trial. *JAMA* 2002;288:321–333.
Wulff HR. Confidence limits in evaluating controlled therapeutic trials. *Lancet* 1973;2:969–970.
Wynder EL, Graham EA. Tobacco smoking as a possible etiologic factor in bronchogenic carcinoma: a study of six hundred and eighty-four proved cases. *JAMA* 1950;143:329–336.
Yamazaki K, Takazoe M, Tanaka T, Kazumori T, Nakamura Y. Absence of mutation in the NOD2/CARD15 gene among 483 Japanese patients with Crohn's disease. *J Hum Genet* 2002;47:469–472.
Yanagawa T. Case-control studies: assessing the effect of a confounding factor. *Biometrika* 1984;71:191–194.
Yanagawa T, Fujii Y. Generalized Mantel-Haenszel procedures for 2 × J tables. *Environ Health Perspect* 1994;102 (suppl 8):57–60.
Yanagimoto T, Kashiwagi N. Empirical Bayes methods for smoothing data and for simultaneous estimation of many parameters. *Environ Health Perspect* 1990;87:109–114.
Yanez ND, Kronmal RA, Shemanski LR. The effects of measurement error in response variables and tests of association of explanatory variables in change models. *Stat Med* 1998;17:2597–2606.
Yano K, Rhoads GG, Kagan A. Coffee, alcohol and risk of coronary heart disease among Japanese men living in Hawaii. *N Engl J Med* 1977;297:405–409.
Yano K, Reed DM, MacLean CJ. Letter to editor. *N Engl J Med* 1987;316:946.
Yasnoff WA, O'Carroll PW, Koo D, Linkins RW, Kilbourne EM. Public health informatics: improving and transforming public health in the information age. *J Public Health Management Practice* 2000;6:67–75.
Yates F. Contingency tables involving small numbers and the chi-square test. *JR Stat Soc Suppl* 1934;1:217–235.
Yates F, Cochran WG. The analysis of groups of experiments. *Journal of Agricultural Science* 1938;28:556–580.
Ye J. On measuring and correcting the effects of data mining and model selection. *J Am Stat Assoc* 1998;93:120–131.
Yinger J. Measuring racial discrimination with fair housing audits: caught in the act. *Am Econ Rev* 1986;26:881–893.
Youkeles LH. Loss of power through ineffective pairing of observations in small two-treatment all-or-none experiments. *Biometrics* 1963;19:175–180.
Young GA. Bootstrap: more than just a stab in the dark? (with discussion). *Stat Sci* 1994;9:382–415.
Youroukos S, Lyberatos C, Philippidou A, Gardikas C, Tsomi A. Increased blood lead levels in mentally retarded children in Greece. *Arch Environ Health* 1978;33:297–300.
Yule GU. On some points related to vital statistics, more especially statistics of occupational mortality. *J R Stat Soc* 1934;97:1–84.

Yudkin J, Roddy J. Levels of dietary sucrose in patients with occlusive atherosclerotic disease. *Lancet* 1964;2:6–8.

Yusuf S, Simon R, Ellenberg S, eds. Proceedings of the workshop on methodologic issues in overviews of randomized clinical trials, May 1986. *Stat Med* 1987;6.

Zaffanella LE, Savitz DA, Greenland S, Ebi KL. The residential case-specular method to study wire codes, magnetic fields, and disease. *Epidemiology* 1998;9:16–20.

Zeger SL. Statistical reasoning in epidemiology. *Am J Epidemiol* 1991;134:1062–1066.

Zeger SL, Irizarry R, Peng RD. On time series analysis of public health and biomedical data. *Ann Rev Public Health* 2006;27:57–79.

Zeger SL, Liang KY. An overview of methods for the analysis of longitudinal data. *Stat Med* 1992;11:1825–1839.

Zhang H, Yu CY, Singer B, Xiong M. Recursive partitioning for tumor classification with gene expression microarray data. *Proc Natl Acad Sci USA* 2001;98:6730–6735.

Zhao LP, Kolonel L. Efficiency loss from categorizing quantitative exposures into qualitative exposures in case-control studies. *Am J Epidemiol* 1992;136:464–474.

Zhou H, Weinberg CR. Modeling conception as an aggregated Bernoulli outcome with latent variables, via the EM algorithm. *Biometrics* 1996;52:945–954.

Ziel HK, Finkle WD. Increased risk of endometrial carcinoma among users of conjugated estrogens. *N Engl J Med* 1975;293:1167–1170.

Ziliak ST, McCloskey DN. Size matters: the standard error of regressions in the *American Economic Review*. *Journal of Socio-Economics* 2004;33:527–546.

Zimmerman HJ, Lewis JH, Ishak KG, Maddrey WC. Ticrynafen-associated hepatic injury: Analysis of 340 cases. *Hepatology* 1984;4:315–323.

Zock PL, Katan MB, Merkus MP, van Dusseldorp M, Harryvan JL. Effect of a lipid-rich fraction from boiled coffee on serum cholesterol. *Lancet* 1990;335:1235–1237.

Zohoori N, Savitz DA. Econometric approaches to epidemiologic data: Relating endogeneity and unobserved heterogeneity to confounding. *Ann Epidemiol* 1997;7:251–257.

Zou G, Donner A. A simple alternative confidence interval for the difference between two proportions. *Control Clin Trials* 2004;25:3–12.

Index

Note: Page numbers followed by *f* indicate figures; page numbers followed by *t* indicate tables.

Absence of effect, evidence of, 159–162
Absolute effect, 52
Absolute measures, 52, 53
Absolute rate, 40
Absolute statistics, *P*-value, 220. *See also P*-value
Abstracts
  data capture and, 499
  form, 500
ACASI. *See* Audio computer-assisted self-interviewing
Accelerated failure-time model, 295, 396. *See also* Structural nested models
Accelerated-life model, 295, 396
Acceptability of surveillance systems, 479
Accuracy. *See also* Bias; Measurement error; Misclassification; Precision; Validity
  of data, 213
  of diagnostic test, 642–646
  of estimation, 128, 213, 231, 314, 331, 419, 436
  generalizability and, 146–147
  matching and, 171–181
  of measurement or classification, 143–146
  of models, 389–390, 419, 449–450
  of prediction, 389–390, 436
  random error and, 149
  of recall, 138
  smoothing and, 314
  of statistical approximations, 220, 225, 227–229, 243, 245, 247, 249, 250, 324, 334, 340, 342
  study design and, 168–182
Acquired immunodeficiency syndrome. *See* AIDS
Active surveillance, 476
  passive surveillance v., 472
Acute respiratory syndrome (SARS). *See* Severe acute respiratory syndrome
Acyclic graphs, 187. *See also* Causal diagrams
Adaptive randomization, clinical trials and, 90
Additive log-risk equation, 73, 74,
Additive risk model, 73, 77, 404
Additivity conditions
  and biologic interaction, 77–78, 298–299
  public-health implications, 83
  response-type distributions v., 77–79
Adherence, in clinical trials, 90, 202–204, 647–648
Adjacent-category logistic models, 414–415
Adjacent-category logit models, 414
Adjusted attributable fraction estimates, 295–297
Adjusted odds ratios, unadjusted odds ratios v., 351–352
Adjustment. *See* Confounding; Confounders; External adjustment; Mantel-Haenszel methods; Regression analysis; Standardization; Stratified analysis
Adverse Event Reporting System (AERS), 98
Adverse events, studying, 646–647, 649
AERS. *See* Adverse Event Reporting System
Age at event. *See* Average age at event
Age groups, 39
Agent-related factors, infection occurrence, 556
Age-period-cohort analysis, exploratory mixed design study, 517
Aggregate measures, ecologic studies, 512
Aggregation bias. *See* ecologic bias
  in meta-analysis, 678
AIC. *See* Akaike information criterion
AIDS (Acquired immunodeficiency syndrome). *See also* HIV (Human immunodeficiency virus)
  confidentiality, 470
  record linkages, 475
  surveillance, 463
  criteria, 468
Air pollution, 615–616
Akaike information criterion (AIC), 426
Alpha level, 151, 153, 154, 155
Alternative hypothesis, 155–156
Analogy, causal inference and, 30
Analysis. *See also specific entries, e.g.,* sensitivity analysis
  of change, baseline adjustment and, 206, 207, 207*f*, 208*f*
  ecologic, 514
  methods, classification of, 240
  prior literature, 330
  surveillance data, 476–478
Analytic studies, hypothesis generation v., 99
Analytic validity, of biomarker, 566, 567*t*
Anomalies, 21
Antagonism, 76–82. *See also* Biologic interaction
Anthropometry, measures of body composition, 594–595
Antibiotic, in animals, surveillance, 463
Apportionment ratios, study efficiency and, 169–171
Approximate statistics
  accuracy of, 220, 225, 227–229, 243, 245, 247, 249, 250, 324, 334, 340, 342
  Bayesian, 333–341
  likelihood-ratio method, 229–230
  score method, 225–226
  Wald method, 226–227
Area-based sampling, case-control studies, 496

ARIMA models. *See* Autoregressive integrated moving-average models
Assessing risk, infection, 555–560
Association, 57, 184–185. *See also* Measures of association; Regression
  biased, 191
  in causal diagrams and, 187–190
  causal structures and, 186
  causation v., 59–60, 59*t*, 185, 383, 385–388
  confounding and, 56–60, 192–194
  standardized, 67
  unbiased, 191
  validity of, 128–129
Associational ratio, confounding and, 60
Asymptotic methods. *See* Large-sample methods
Atkinson index, segregation, 539
Attack rate, 40
  as risk measure, 553
Attributable fractions, 54, 62–67, 295–297, 385, 387, 440. *See also* Preventable fractions
  estimation, 295–297, 430, 440, 443, 445
  etiologic fraction v., 63–64, 297–298
  exposure pattern and, 67
  model-based, 440
  probability of causation v., 64–65, 297–298
  population, 67, 295–297
  terminology and, 65–66
Attributable proportion, 13–15, 67. *See also* Attributable fractions
  population disease impact, 65–67
Attributable risk, 63. *See also* Attributable fractions
Attributable risk percent, 63. *See also* Attributable fractions
  Levin and, 65
Attrition-related bias, fertility and, 621
Audio computer-assisted self-interviewing (ACASI), 500
"Audit studies,"538
Autism, vaccines and, secondary data, 485–486
Auto-regression, time-series analyses, 610–611
Autoregressive integrated moving-average (ARIMA) models, 515, 516
Auxiliary hypotheses, 23
Average age
  at death, 34
  at event, 48–49
Average exposure assignment schema, 106
Average exposure measures, 103
Average incidence time, survival proportion v., 45
Average intensity, and alternatives, 106
Average risk, 40, 73, 101
  case-cohort studies, 123
  effects on incidence rates v., 67
  response-type distributions v., 77–78
Average survival time, estimation of, 293–294

Back-door paths, 192
Backward deletion, Backward elimination, 262, 438 *See also* Contracting model search
Bacon, Francis, philosophy of, 18
Bacterial pathogens, laboratory-based surveillance, 472–473
Baker, George, 619
Balancing scores, 446–447. *See also* Confounder scores
Barker's hypothesis, 546
Base priors, sensitivity analyses, 380
Baseline adjustment, bias and, 206, 207, 207*f*, 208*f*
Baseline incidence proportion, 13
Baseline values, bias and, 206, 207*f*
Basic reproductive number, state of infectiousness, 550*f*, 560
Bayes empirical-Bayes modeling, 437
Bayesian analysis, 165–167, 230–231, 328–344, 388–389. *See also* Bayesianism; Hierarchical regression; Semi-Bayes analysis; Subjective probability
  bias analysis, 378–380
  criticism summary, 333
  frequentist methods v., 166–167, 331–333, 388–389
  in genetics, 571–572
  intervals, 165–167, 330–335
  likelihoods in, 230–231
  regression, 329, 344, 388
  reverse, 338–339
  semi-Bayes v., 337
  sensitivity analyses, 342
Bayesian information criterion (BIC), 426
Bayesian intervals, Bayesian limits 165–167, 330–335 *See also* Prior intervals; Posterior intervals
  calibrated, 166
Bayesian regression, 329, 344, 388
  frequentist regression v., 388–389
Bayesian statistics. *See* Bayesian analysis
Bayesianism, 22–24, 165–167, 329–333. *See also* Bayesian analysis; Subjective probability
  objective, 343
  subjective, 165–166, 328–333
Bayes' theorem, 166, 330, 331, 333
Behavioral Risk Factor Surveillance System (BRFSS), 473–474
Berksonian bias, 135–136, 185, 197. *See also* Collider bias; Selection bias
Bernoulli distribution, model fitting and, 421
Beta error. *See* Type II error
Between-community studies, air pollution, 616
Bias, 128. *See also specific entries, e.g., ecologic bias*
  baseline values, 206–207
  complete populations, 483
  confounder-selection strategies, 263
  control groups and, 122
  control of, graphical representation of, 191–209
  equal accuracy principle, 121
  exposure misclassification, 301
  exposures assessment, 603
  friend controls and, 120
  intentional selection, 196–198
  misclassification and, quantification of, 488–490
  missing-data categories, 199–200
  missing-data indicators, 199–200
  outcome definition and, 144
  overmatching and, 180–181
  parameters, distributions of results, as output, 345
  quantification, residual confounding and, 198–199
  recognized fetal loss, 629
  time-to-pregnancy studies, 627–628
Bias analysis, 345–380. *See also specific topics, e.g.,* Confounding; Misclassification; Selection bias
  Bayesian, 378–380
  caveats, 347–348
  need for, 346–347

Biasing path, 191
BIC. *See* Bayesian information criterion
Binary exposure variables, 131
  notification for risks, 73*t*
  potential outcomes and, 75, 76*t*
Binary regression, 383–384. *See also* Binomial regression; Logistic models
Binomial coefficient, 223
Binomial distribution (model), 225, 245, 246, 421
Binomial likelihood, 246
Binomial regression, 421–422. *See also* Logistic models
  extravariation, 422
Binomial test, the null and, 680
Biochemical indicators, nutrient intake,592, 594
Biologic effect, ecologic effect v., 513
Biologic gradient, causal inference and, 28
Biologic inferences, individual risks and, 513
Biologic interaction, 13, 17, 74–83. *See also* Additive risk model; Additivity conditions; Statistical interaction; Synergism
  additivity conditions and, 298–299
  analysis of, 298–299
  qualitative statistical interactions v., 299
  regression models and, 406–407
  statistical interaction v., 82–83
  in sufficient cause model, 13,17,80–81
Biomarker epidemiology, 565–568, 565*t*, 619
Biomarkers
  evaluation of, 566–568, 566*t*
  exposure assessment, 601–602
  validation, 565–566
Biospecimen collection, epidemiologic studies, 505, 506*f*
Bioterrorism-related epidemics, syndromic surveillance systems and, 464
Birth cohort, 38
Birth cohort analysis, mapping, 608
Birth control definitions, 627
Birth defects, 636–637
Birth weight, 632–633
  distribution shifts, 634
  mortality and, 636
  summaries, 633, 635
Blinding, clinical trials and, 90–91
Blocked randomization, 174
Blood collection, protocol, 505, 506*f*
Bonferroni method, 236. *See also* Multiple comparisons
Bootstrapping, 369, 427, 428–429, 440, 443. *See also* Resampling
BRFSS. *See* Behavioral Risk Factor Surveillance System

Calibrated confidence levels, 231
Caliper matching, 120, 284
Callbacks, refusal conversion, 499
Cancer
  causes, 14–15
  migrant studies, nutritional exposures, 581–582
  screening, "Omic" tools, 577
Candida infection, colonization of, 556
CAPI. *See* Computer-assisted personal interviewing; Computer-assisted telephone interviewing
Carcinogenesis, cause, 16
Case definition, surveillance systems, 467–469
Case fatality rate, 41
Case fatality ratio, 41
Case selection, source population and, 115
Case surveillance data, estimation from, 286
Case-cohort studies, 114, 123–124
  analysis of, 252–253, 280–281, 432
  for pregnancy complications, 632
Case-control data, 250–252, 269
Case-control ratios. *See* Pseudo-rates
  graphing, 308–309
Case-control studies, 88, 95, 111–127, 136, 137. *See also* Case-cohort studies; Case-crossover studies; Case-only studies; Case-specular studies; Odds ratio; Two-stage studies
  birth defects, 637
  common elements of, 113–122
  cost reduction and, 109
  disease registers, epidemiologic studies, 483
  ecologic studies, nutritional exposures, 582–583, 584*f*, 585
  gene-environment interaction analysis, methodologic issues in, 571, 572*t*
  genetic variants, conventional epidemiologic studies, 568
  GWA analysis, 564
  illness, natural history of, 642
  matching in, 175–176
    analysis, 283–288, 434–435
    benefits, 178–179
    cost of, 178
    efficiency in, 176
    selection bias and, 205, 205*f*
  models for, 431–432
  nested, 114, 122–123, 432
  prevalent, 97, 127
  reproductive epidemiology, 624–625
  scoring methods, 451
  standardization in, 445
  subject identification, 496–497
  variants of, 122–127
  with prevalent cases, 127
Case-crossover studies, 125–126, 605
  analysis, 288–289
Case fatality rate, 41
Case-load reduction, 83, 296. *See also* Excess caseload
Case-only studies, 125–126, 573–575. *See also* Case-crossover studies; Case-specular studies
  analysis, 288–289
Case-parent studies, 575, 638
Case-specular studies, 125–126
  analysis, 288–289
Categorical models, power models v., 410
Categorical regressors, 407–408
Categorical statistics, 238–257
Categorical trends, multiple regression, 409–410
Categorization of variables, 303–305. *See also* Category
Category
  boundaries, variable, 217–218
  choice of, 217–218
  codes, in trend models, 409
  contingency table, 217
  external information and, 304
  horizontal scaling and, 312, 313*f*
  indicator variables, 407
  means, horizontal scaling and, 312
  medians, horizontal scaling and, 312

Category (*Contd.*)
midpoints, 410
scores
horizontal scaling and, 312–313, 313*f*
regression with, 410
Category matching, 120, 284
Category-specific relative-risk estimates, dose-response, 308
meta analysis and, 674
Causal criteria, 26–31
Causal diagrams, 183–209
applications, 194
bias and, 191–209
confounding path, 193*f*
instrumental variables, 202, 202*f*
no confounding, 186*f*
preliminaries for, 183–186
residual confounding and, 198
unconfounded direct effect, 201, 201*f*
Causal effects, 6–10, 59. *See also* Cause; Effect; Preventive effects; Potential outcomes
definition of, 52
bias analyses and, 347
conditioning sets identifying, 192
social epidemiology, 532–533
Causal exposure, 65
Causal graphs. *See* Causal diagrams
Causal inference, 25–31. *See also* Bias analysis; Causal diagrams; Causation; Confounding
Hill's considerations for, 26–31
post hoc ergo propter hoc fallacy, 19
Causal Markov assumption (CMA), 190
Causal mechanisms, 15
Causal models. *See specific models, e.g.,* Causal diagrams; Marginal-structural models; Potential outcomes; Structural nested models; Sufficient-cause model
Causal monotonicity, 208
Causal odds ratios, 53, 62
Causal path, 186
Causal rate difference, 52, 53
Causal rate ratio, 53
Causal ratio of disease-free time, 53
Causal relationships, association v., 59–60, 185
Causal risk difference, 52, 53
Causal risk ratio, 53
Causal structure. *See* Causal diagrams; Structural equations
Causation, 5–18, 59–60, 185, 385–388. *See also* Causal effects; Causal inference; Effects; Potential outcomes; Sufficient-cause model
association v., 59–60, 185, 383, 385–386, 533–534
regression v., 383, 385–386
in social epidemiology, 533–534
Cause, 6, 9–10. *See also* Causal effects; Causation; Effect; Biologic interaction
component, 6
interaction among, 13
sufficient, 6
CDC (Centers for Disease Control and Prevention)
confidentiality, surveillance systems, 469, 470
consent form template, on-line, 568
notifiable disease reporting, 472
rates of events, 477*f*
Censoring, 34–35, 45, 289–293. *See also* Competing risks; Loss to follow-up; Survival analysis
g-estimation and, 454
risk-estimation and, 289–293
Centering of variables, 392
Centers for Disease Control and Prevention. *See* CDC
Centers for Epidemiologic Studies Depression scale (CESD), 206
Centralization, segregation, 539
Certainties, 165, 338*t*, 343. *See also* Bayesian analysis; Bayesianism; Uncertainty
CES-D. See Centers for Epidemiologic Studies Depression scale
Chance variation, 17, 88. *See also* Random error; Random sampling; Randomization
Change-in-estimate criteria. *See also* Collapsibility
selecting confounders for control, 261–263, 419
Chi-square, 216
Chlamydia trachomatis, incubation periods, infection occurrence, 558
Cholera, Snow's study of, 94, 608, 615
Chronic exposure, 103–104
Chronic infection. *See* Persistent infection
Cigarette smoking, surveillance systems, 469
Classification error, 138. *See also* Misclassification; Bias analysis
Climatologists, global climate change, 617, 618*f*
Clinical disease, subclinical infection v., 551, 641–651
Clinical fertility, 624
Clinical trials, 87, 89–92, 240
cohort studies, 100
field trials v., 92
Clinical validity, of biomarker, 566, 567*t*
Clinic-based controls, 118–119
Closed cohort, 101
Closed populations, 36–37, 37*t*, 41, 101
event times and intervals, 42*f*, 42*t*
open populations v., 38
Closed-cohort studies, 240
Cluster randomized trials, community intervention trials and, 92–93
Clustered binary outcomes, recognized loss, 630
Clustering segregation, 540
Clusters, analysis of, 611–613
Cluster-specific models, 544
CMA. *See* Causal Markov assumption
CMLE. *See* Conditional maximum-likelihood estimate
Coaction, causal, 80. *See also* Biologic Interaction; Synergism
Coding, 508
incremental, in trend models, 409
schemes, choosing, 408
Coefficient(s). *See also* Regression modeling
adjustment, external, 661
standardized measures v., 443–444
Coherence, causal inference and, 29
Coherence of probability assessments, 166. *See also* Bayesianism
Cohorts, 38, 100–103
assembly of, 495–496
defining for study, 100–107
populations v., 38
response types and, 77
Cohort studies, 88, 94–95, 100–110
case-control study designs v., 111–127
cost reduction, 108–109
disease, nondifferential misclassification, 142–143

ecologic studies, nutritional exposures, 582–583, 585
expense, 108
genetic variants, conventional epidemiologic studies, 568–569, 569*t*
hypothetical data from, *P*-value and, 158*t*
illness, natural history of, 642
mapping, 609
matched risk factors, stratification in, 284
matching in, 174–175
odds ratios, 352
selection bias, 136–137
tracing subjects, 109
Collapsibility, 261–263. *See also* Noncollapsibility
Collider, 187
unconditional d-separation, 187–188
Collider bias, 137, 185–186, 193, 193*f*. *See also* Berksonian bias; Selection bias
Collinearity, ecologic studies, 527–528
Colorectal cancer, "Omic" tools, 575–577
Combinatorial argument, 222
Combinatorial coefficient, 223
Common exposures, cohort studies and, 110
Community diagnosis, surveillance, 462
Community intervention trials, 87
fluoride supplementation and, 1
Community trials, subject identification, 494
Comparative analysis, Monte-Carlo analyses and, 376, 377*t*, 378
Compatibility, in causal graphs, 189–191
Competing causes, 322
Competing risks, 39, 44–45, 55–56, 68, 289–290. *See also* Censoring; Competing causes; Survival analysis
attributable fractions, problems with, 296
effects mediated by, 55–56
removal, problems with, 45, 55–56, 296
Competitive interaction, 76
Complementary component cause, 7
Complementary log-log model, 417
Complete populations, secondary data analysis, 482–483
Complete-subject analysis, 219
Complex disease, epidemiology and, examples, 579
Compliance, in clinical trials, 90, 202–204, 647–648
Component causes, 6, 9, 16
defining, 7
Computer-assisted interviewing, 500, 501, 502*f*
Concentration, segregation, 539
Conception, 620
Concordant pairs, 288
Conditional analysis, unconditional analysis v., 272–273
Conditional association, 184, 261. *See also* Association; Conditional probability
Conditional d-separation, 188–189
Conditional likelihood, 257, 272–273, 422, 433
Conditional logistic regression, 433
Conditional maximum likelihood(CML), 257, 272–273, 422, 433
Conditional probability, 184–185. *See also* Probability
Conditional risk, 44
independent-censoring assumption, 289
Conditioning bias, on descendant of outcome, 204–205, 205*f*
Conditioning sets, causal effects and, 192
Confidence band, 310
surveillance systems, 472
Confidence intervals and limits, 157–158, 221, 238, 239, 267–269. *See also specific estimates, e.g.,* Risk ratio, *and specific methods, e.g.,* Wald limits
hypothesis tests v., 157–158
in meta-analysis, 671–673
model-based, 440
P-value function, 158–159
plotting, 309–310
problems with, 163
significance tests v., 157–158
statistical estimation and, 156–157
Confidence levels, 157, 234–235
Confidence region, 324
Confidentiality, surveillance systems, 470, 478
Confounded trial, diagram for, 203*f*
Confounders, 58–59, 129, 193–196. *See also* Confounding, Control of Confounding
as extraneous risk factors, 131
identifying, 194–196
intercommunity comparisons, 611–612
misclassification of, 359–360
in ecologic analysis, 518–519, 522–523, 527
properties of, 139
scores, 446
selecting for control, 261–263
study variables, meta-analysis, 656
surrogate confounders, 130–131
in propensity scores, 448
in trend models, 409
unmeasured, 348–352
Confounder categories, 218, 305. *See also* Measured confounders
selecting, 263–264
Confounder-disease associations, 352
Confounder scores, 446–451. *See also* Doubly robust estimation; Exposure scores; Outcome scores; Prognostic scores; Propensity scores
Confounding, 28, 57–60, 129–134, 137, 193–196, 570. *See also* Confounders, Control of Confounding
adjustment for, 202–204, 265–278, 336, 348–352, 365–370, 442–455
assessment of, 260–264
association and, 56–60
associational ratio, 60
bounds for, 352, 662
causal diagrams and, 186*f*, 641
collapsibility and, 261–263
contingency table, 217
conventional rules, unreliability of, 194–196
design options for control, 168–169
external estimates of, adjustments using, meta-analysis, 660–662
factor, criteria for, 132–134
genetic susceptibility, 570
by group, ecologic bias, 520
heterogeneity v., 259
by indication, 650
matching and, 171–176
as mixing of effects, 129
noncollapsibility v., 62
path, 193
causal diagrams, 193*f*

Confounding (*Contd.*)
population causal relations and, multiple bias analyses and, 363
randomized controlled trials, 647
selection bias v., 136–137, 192–194
time-series analyses, 610–611
variable, misclassification of, 144–145
Congenital malformations, 127. *See also* Birth defects, reproductive epidemiology
incidence of, 47
prevalence and, 47
Conjecture and refutation model
hypothesis and, 20–21
science and, 20
Connectors in graphs, 187
Consensus, naturalism and, 21–22
Consent form template, on-line, CDC, 568
Consistency, causal inference, 27
Constant across strata, 61. *See also* Homogeneity; Homogeneity assumptions
Constant models, 391
Contextual analysis, 529
Contextual association, 513
Contextual effect, 513
Contingency tables, data analysis and, 216
Continuation-ratio model, 415
Continuity corrections, 232–233
Contracting model search, 420–421, 438
Control of confounding, 58–59. *See also* Confounding, adjustment; External adjustment; Mantel-Haenszel; Standardization
design options for, 168–169, 171
matching and, 171–175
scoring methods, 446–451
Control groups,
number of, 121
sources, 117–120
Control sampling fractions, 123
Controlled direct effect, 200
Control selection, 112, 115–120
fallacies, 117
Controlled trials. *See* Clinical trials
Conventional statistical analysis, 213
flaws of, 343
random error and, 364
randomized controlled trials, 648
Correlated error, 138, 378. *See also* Dependent error
Correlation coefficients, 70, 424–425
meta-analysis and, 681
Correlated-outcome logistic regression, 452
Corynebacterium diphtheriae, infectivity and, 558
Cost efficiency
case-control studies and, 109
complete populations, 482–483
ecologic studies, 513
overmatching and, 181
Count data
incidence and survival proportions, 40–41
classification of subjects, 218–219
large sample methods, 245–252
small sample statistics for, 255–257
standardization of, 265–270
Mantel-Haenszel estimation, 274–276
model fitting, 423
Count regression, 423, 444. *See also* Log-linear models
Counterfactual outcomes, 54–55, 129. *See also* Potential outcomes
in confounding, 57–58
Counterfactual models of causation, 18, 54–55. *See also* Potential outcomes
Countermatching, 177
Couple-specific fecundability, 626
Covariate, 383. *See also* Confounder; Regressor
categorical, 407–410
time-dependent, 397–398, 452
Cox (proportional-hazards) model, Cox regression 397–398, 422, 429, 451–453, 626
accelerated failure-time models v., 397
in meta-analysis, 658
structural nested models v., 453–454
time-dependent, 397–398, 451–453
Credible model form, 420. *See also* Model specification
Crohn's disease, 578–579
Cross-level bias, 520, 521*t*, 523, 524*t*. *See also* Ecologic bias; Ecologic studies
Cross-level inferences, 513. *See also* Ecologic studies
Crossover studies, 648–649
Cross-product ratio, 114. *See* Odds ratio
Cross-sectional studies, 88, 97, 497, 569–570
Cross-validation sum of squares, 442
Crude analysis, 239–257
Cubic spline, 411–412
Cumulative case-control studies, 125
Cumulative exposure assignment schema, 106
Cumulative exposures, exposures assessment, 602–604
Cumulative incidence, 44
Cumulative odds model, 415
Cyclic patterns, 606, 607–608

DAG. *See* Directed acyclic graph
Data. *See also* Computerized databases; Data collection; Exposure assessment; Sparse data
description and summarization of, 216–219
discussion of, 341
editing, 213, 214–215
fitted model v., 423
interpretation, 214
lack of, ecologic studies, 527
pooling, 509, 652
quality
complete populations, 483
secondary data, 487–488
surveillance systems, 479
sparse, bias from, 263, 386, 422, 433
sparse, methods for, 272–278, 280–281, 283–288, 294, 296, 314, 316, 381, 386, 425, 433–435, 446–451
summarization, 214
tabulation, 216
Data analysis, 213–215. *See also specific topics, e.g.,* categorization, stratified analysis, regression analysis
Data and Safety Monitoring Board (DSMB), 91
Data capture, 499–509
Data coding questionnaires, 214
Data collection, 499–510
errors in, 214–216

epidemiologic investigation, 460
methods of, epidemiologic studies, 492
Data editing, 214–216
Data entry, questionnaires, 214
Data grouping, model fitting and, 423
Data priors, 337–342. *See also* Priors
as diagnostic device, 338–339, 341–342
frequentist interpretation, 337–338
methods, extensions, 340
and reverse-Bayes analysis, 338–339
Data probability. *See* Probability
Databases, study populations, 482–483, 493
Dead controls, 120
Dead subjects, proportional mortality studies and, 97–99
Death. *See also* Occurrence of death
sufficient-component cause model and, 9
Death certificates, surveillance, 474–475
Declaration of Helsinki, 89
Decomposition of effects, 200–202, 545–546
Deforestation, weather patterns and, 618
Delta-beta analysis, 428
Denominators. *See* Count data; Incidence proportion; Incidence rate; Person time
case-control studies and, 113
exposure affected, 68, 296–297
reproductive epidemiology, 621
Density sampling, 116. *See also* Risk-set sampling
Density studies
case-control studies, 124–125
multiplicative-intercept models, 430–431
Dental caries, community intervention trials; 1, 92
Dependent error, 138, 143, 145, 360. *See also* Correlated error
Dependent happenings, transmission, 561
Dependent variables. *See also* Outcome variables; Regressand simulation generation, 371–372
Depression score, 32, 206
Deprivation, 538
DES. *See* Diethystilbestrol
Descriptive statistics, 216–219
meta-analysis and, 668–670
Descriptive studies, birth defects, 637
Design strategies, 85–99, 168–182
ecologic studies, 514–517
genetic studies, 568–570, 573–575
study accuracy and, 168–182
Detection bias, 25–26
Deviance statistics, 229, 425–427. *See also* Likelihood functions; Likelihood ratios
model checking, 425–426
Diabetes, global trends, 466–467
Diagnostic laboratories, laboratory-based surveillance, 472–473
Diagnostic tests, accuracy of, 642–646
"Diary" menstrual cycle data, 623
Dichotomous-outcome analysis, multiple outcomes analysis, 322
Diet. *See also* Food intake assessment; Nutritional epidemiology
biochemical indicators, 592, 594
pattern measurement, 586–588
records, 589
Dietary-assessment methods, 588–592
Diethylstilbestrol, 16
Difference measures, 52–53, 53. *See also specific measures, e.g.,* Rate difference; Risk difference
Differential misclassification, 138, 373–374
Direct effect, 187
controlled, 200
estimating, complications in, 200–202
intermediate adjustment, 200–202
natural, 200–201
pure, 200–201
Directed acyclic graph (DAG), 187. *See also* Causal diagrams
assumptions, statistical implications of, 189*t*
Directed-graph separation rules. *See* d-Separation rules
Directed path, 186
Directional statistics, 156
Discordant pairs, 286–288
Discrete variables, 138
Discrete-time model, 640
Discrimination, social, 537–538
Disease. *See also* CDC; Confounder-disease associations; Genetic epidemiology; Infectious disease; Mapping; Multiple diseases; Notifiable disease; Public health; *specific diseases, e.g.,* Crohn's disease
causal mechanisms and, 80
chronic, surveillance systems, 468
cohort studies and, 111, 112
confounding factor and, 132
control selection and, 119
exposure on, 325
effects of, 51
field trials and, 92
frequency of, 33
induction period, 15
infection v., infectious agents and, 551
intensity, 34
measures of frequency, 45, 553–555
misclassification, 358–359
monitoring, 488–490, 490*f*
nondifferential misclassification, 142–143
occurrence, 41
potential confounder v., 131
presence, binary regression, 384
prevalence, cross-sectional studies, 97
proportion, sufficient-cause mechanisms, 13–15
rare, mapping, 609
rates, population estimates v., 466
registers, 483–484
self-reported, 473
sufficient-causes of, 6, 6*f*, 63, 63*f*
surveillance and, 459
Disease-confounder associations, 352
Disjoint category coding, 407
in trend models, 409
Dissimilarity index, segregation, 539
Distributions. *See also* Probability distributions and densities
of disease and health events, 32–34, 41, 46, 66–67
standard, 49–50, 68–69, 265–266
Dose-response. *See also* Trend
analysis, 314–317
causal criterion, 28
graphing, 308–314

Dose-response (*Contd.*)
modeling, 404–405
in meta-analysis, 674
zero exposure handling, 317
Dosimetric model, 601
"Double loss" of subjects, 284
Double-blind studies, 91
Doubly robust estimation, 450–451
d-Separation rules, 187–191
statistical independence and, 189–190
DSMB. *See* Data and Safety Monitoring Board
Duhem-Quine thesis, 21
Duration of contact, 601
Duration of disease, and prevalence 47–48
Dynamic population. *See* Open population

Ecologic analysis. *See* Ecologic studies
Ecologic bias, ecologic fallacy, 519–522. *See also* Cross-level bias
Ecologic inference, 513
Ecologic studies, 88, 99, 511–531, 606
analysis, 517–530
biases, 519–528
concepts and rationale, 511–514
designs, 514–517
interpretation problems, 528, 530–531
methodologic problems, 519–528
nutritional exposures, 581–586
rationale for, 513–514
Edges in graphs, 187
Education, 467, 535
E-estimation, 449
Effects, 5–8. *See also* Causal effects; Causality; Causation; Effect measures; Effect-measure modification; Interaction
direct,187, 200
generalized definitions of, 66–67
indirect, 13, 200
preventive, 8, 9, 17, 54, 59, 65
public health, 14,
strength of, 10–13
Effect decomposition, direct-indirect, 200–202, 545–546
Effect estimation. *See specific topics, e.g.,* Bias; Bias analysis; Confounding; Maximum likelihood; Precision; Selection bias; Study design; Validity
Effect measures, 51–56, 59–70. *See also* Causal effects; Effects; Effect-measure modification
defining exposure in, 55
generalized, 66–67
measures of association v., 59–60, 59*t*, 185, 385–388
null state and, 54–56
regression, 385–386
relations among, 60–62
standardized, 67–69, 386–388
theoretical nature of, 54–55
Effective reproductive number, infectious disease, 563
Effect-measure modification, 61–62, 72–74, 76. *See also* Heterogeneity; Statistical interaction
confounding v., 259
by group, ecologic bias, 520
Effect modification. *See* Effect-measure modification
Effect size, divided by standard deviation, 681
Effect-size modeling, 673–677
Efficiency. *See also* Cost efficiency
cohort study v. case-control study, 93, 112
definition of, 168
matching and, in cohort studies, 174–175
matching and, in case-control studies, 176–181
statistical, 169–171
study 150
Efficient score statistic, maximum-likelihood estimate (MLE), 226
Eligibility criteria, meta-analysis, 653
ELSI (Ethical, legal, and social issues), biomarkers, epidemiologic research, 567–568
Empirical-Bayes modeling, 331, 337, 436, 439. *See also* Hierarchical regression
Empirical priors, 331–332
Endocarditis, culture technique and, 553
Endogeneity, 622
Endogenous variables, 186, 453
Endometrial cancer and estrogens, 2
Berksonian bias and, 135–136, 137
Energy adjustment, 596
Entamoeba histolytica, infection occurrence, 556
Environment, 598
causation and, 15
exposure assessment, 619
measures, ecologic studies, 512
surveillance, 460
Environmental epidemiology, 598–619
domain of, 598–600
study designs for, 604–610
Environmental hazards
health surveillance, 613–614
risk assessment, 614–615
Environmental reservoir, human host and, 555
Environmental samples, 505
Environmental trials, 93
Epidemic case-control studies, 125
Epidemic curves, 39–40
Epidemic outbreaks, 552
Epidemiologic data analysis. *See* Data; Data analysis
Epidemiologic investigation, 460. *See also* Investigator
Epidemiologic studies. *See also specific e.g.,* case-crossover studies
case-control studies, 95, 111–127
clinical trials, 88
cohort studies, 94, 100–110
existing registers, 483–484
genetics, methodologic issues, 570–573
measurement of diet, 586–594
physical examinations and, 504–505
precision and statistics, 148–167
target population, 146
types, 87–99
validity in, 128–147
Epidemiology
criticism of, 2
defined, 32
field methods, 492–510
Equal accuracy principle, 121
Equally spaced boundaries, percentiles v., 304
Equipoise, 89–90
Equivalence testing, 156
Equivalent models, 390
Error
alpha, 153
beta, 153

classification, 137, 352–353. *See also* Misclassification
In disease onset, 359
measurement, 137–138, 346, 352–353, 361
random, 148–149, 213, 332–333, 346, 364, 366–369, 376, 379
type I, 153
type II, 153
Estimating equations, 422. *See also* Generalized estimating equations
Estimability, graphical, 192
Estimation, 128
accuracy of, 128, 213, 231, 314, 331, 419, 436
analysis and, 214
effect of errors and, 346
methods of, 219–234
Estrogens, 2, 565*t*, 616, 623, 631. *See also* Endometrial cancer and estrogens
Ethics
nonexperimental studies, 93
secondary data access, 490–491
validity v., human subjects, 89
Etiologic fractions, 63–66, 297–298
Etiologic mixed design, 517
Etiologic multiple-group study, 515
Etiologic time-trend study, 516
Event time, 33. *See also* Incidence time
Evidence of absence of an effect, 159–162
Exact 2X2 programs, application
person-time data and, 257
single-group data and, 257
Exact confidence levels, mid-*P* v., 231
Exact logistic regression, 422
Exact statistics, 220–225, 231, 256. *See also* Small-sample methods
Examination forms, 504–505
Excess caseload, 63, 83
Excess causal rate ratio, 53–54
Excess fractions, 63, 65. *See also* Attributable fractions; Rate fractions
etiologic fractions v., 64, 297–298
probability of causation v., 64–65, 297–298
Excess relative risks, 53
Excess risk, 52, 54
Exogenous variables, 186, 453
Expanding model search, 419, 438
Expected years-of-life-lost, 53, 70
Expense, cohort studies and, 108
Experimental epidemiology, 87
Experimental evidence, causal inference and, 29
Experimental studies, 87–93, 168–169
ecologic studies, nutritional exposures, 585–586
human subjects, validity v. ethical considerations, 89
social epidemiology, 547
Exploratory study designs, 514–515
Exploratory time-trend study, ecologic studies, 515–516
Exponential curve, exponential risk model, 404
Exponential decay, 37
Exponential formula, 43–44
Exponential function, natural log function v., 416
Exponential models. *See also* Log-linear models; Multiplicative models
for counts, 423, 444
for incidence times, 396
for odds, 394
for rates, 396–398
for risks, 393–394
exponential curve and, 404
for risks, 393–394, 398
Exposed subjects, unexposed time in, 104
Exposure(s), 92. *See also* Exposure assessment
average risk and, 61
case-crossover studies, 126
categories of, 105–106, 105*f*, 142, 305
chronic, 103–104
classification, predictive values, 357, 641
data, types of, 600–602
differential misclassification, 138
dose v., 601
effect measures, 55
analyses of, 300
matching factor and, 175, 176*t*
occurrence of disease and, 51
environmental, 598–600
etiologic fractions, 63*f*, 64
frequencies, 11*t*
groups
defining, 100–107
person time and, 101
special, nutritional exposures, 582
herd immunity and, 561, 562*t*
history, 119
infection occurrence, factors influencing, 556–557
intensity, 106
measurement error, 137–138
in meta-analysis, 656
misclassification, 137–146
nondifferential misclassification, 139–145
nonexperimental studies, 93
patterns, 66–67
person-time, 102–103, 218–219
PMR study and, 97
scaling, 313, 392–393
segregation, 539
social, 534–542
standardization, 265
standardized measures, 259
susceptibility, 64–65
summaries, 101–102
weighting distribution and, 266
zero level, 316–317
Exposure assessment, 598–604. *See also* Data collection; Exposure; Measurement
"Omic" tools, 575–57
Exposure lagging, 301
Exposure level
definition of, 103
trend graphing, 308
Exposure measure, induction periods, 300–302
Exposure misclassification, 137–142, 353–355. *See also* Misclassification
bias from, 301
epidemiologic studies and, genetics, 570
Exposure models
adjustment via, 450
IPW, standardization using, 444–445
outcome models v., 449–450
standardization using, 444–445

Exposure occurrence, infectious agents, factors influencing, 555–556
Exposure odds ratio, 114
Exposure opportunity, 117
Exposure patterns. *See* Patterns of exposure
Exposure prevalence, equations, 354
Exposure scores. *See also* Confounder scores; Propensity scores
for confounder control, 447–449
for exposure categories, 314
Exposure status, 104
Exposure values, percentile boundaries v., 304
Exposure variable
data and, 217
polytomous exposure, 305, 306–307, 306*t*
Exposure-balancing score, 447
Exposure-disease association, 56–57, 281, 323
cross-sectional studies and, 97
P-value, 340
Exposure-probability modeling, confounder-selection strategies, 263
External adjustment for confounding, 348–352, 363, 660–662
External reference population, SMR and, 664–665
External validity, 128. *See* Generalizability
Extra-binomial variation, 422
Extraneous risk factors, confounders, 131. *See also* Confounders
Extra-Poisson variation, 422

Failure time, 33. *See also* Incidence time
Failure-time analysis, 41
Failure-time model, 33, 396
Faithfulness assumption in causal diagrams, 191
Fallacy of affirming the consequent, 19
False-negative probability, 138
False-positive associations, gene-disease association, 572
False-positive probability, 138
Falsificationism, 20
Family based analysis, genetic factors, 638
Fatal Accident Reporting System (FARS), 286
Fatality ratio, 41
Fecundability ratio, 640
Fecundability, 626
Fertility
attrition-related bias, 621
reproductive epidemiology, 624–625
Fetal growth retardation, monitoring, 489
Field methods, in epidemiology, 492–510
Field trials, 87
clinical trials v., 92
cluster randomized trials, 92–93
First-stage model, 436. *See also* Hierarchical regression
Fisher *P*-value, 223. *See also* Exact statistics
Fisher's exact test, 256
Fitted model, 389
data v., 423
Fitted scores, 448
Fitted second-stage frequentist model, 332
Fixed cohorts, 38, 101
Floating absolute risk, 310
Follow-up, 103–108. *See also* Censoring; Losses to follow-up
data, person-time analysis, 287
disease prevalence, estimation of, 554
losses, basic survival analysis, 289
studies needing, 240
techniques, 507–508
Food intake assessment methods, 589
Food-frequency questionnaires, 589–591
dietary-assessment methods v., 593*t*
Foods, measurement of, 586–588
Force of morbidity, force of mortality, 34. *See also* Hazard rate; Incidence rate
Forward selection, 438. *See also* Expanding model search
Fractional polynomial models, 410. *See also* Smoothers and Smoothing; Spline models
Framingham Heart Study, 1
Frequency matching, 171
Frequency of outcome, 170
Frequency-based priors, 332
Frequentist methods. *See also specific methods, e.g.,* Confidence intervals, *P*-values, Significance tests
Bayesian interpretation v., 335–336
Bayesian regression v., 388–389
interpretations, 163
regression, 382–383
subjective Bayesianism v., 329–333
Friend controls, 119–120, 496

G-computation algorithm, 208. *See* G-estimation
GEE. *See* Generalized estimating equations
Gene discovery, inflammatory bowel disease study, 577–578
Gene-environment interaction, 15, 639
epidemiologic studies and, methodologic issues in, 570–571, 571*t*, 572*t*
Gene-disease associations, epidemiologic study designs, 565
Gene-gene-environment interactions, epidemiologic study designs, 565
Generalizability, 128, 129, 146–147. *See also* accuracy and, 146–147
of randomized trials, 90
Generalized additive models, 442
Generalized estimating equations (GEE) logistic regression, 452, 628
structural-nested modeling v. 453
Generalized linear models, 416–417, 640
outcome transformation v., 400
General population
cohorts, 109–110
information, cost reduction and, 109
Genetic epidemiology, 564–579
Genetic population stratification, 638–639
Genetic susceptibility
colorectal cancer, "Omic" tools, 575–576
inflammatory bowel disease study, 577–578
privacy issues, 509
Genetic variants
case-control studies, conventional epidemiologic studies, 568
cohort studies, conventional epidemiologic studies, 568–569, 569*t*
cross-sectional studies, conventional epidemiologic studies, 569–570
Type I and II errors, 571

Genetics
causal mechanisms and, 15
exposure assessment, 603
factors, 637–639
studies, 125–126
Genome-wide association analysis (GWA analysis), case-control studies, 564
Genomics, 564
infection occurrence, 556
Genotype misclassification, epidemiologic studies and, 570
Genotype-phenotype correlations, 574
Genotyping tools, genetic factors, 639
Geographic clustering, 464
Geographic information systems (GIS)
epidemiologic studies, 507
exposures assessment, 603
surveillance data, 477
Gestation, recognized loss, 629
Gestational-age-specific mortality, 636
G-estimation, 208, 302, 396, 449, 453–455. *See also* Structural nested models
Gini coefficient, 539, 540
GIS. *See* Geographic information systems; Global positioning systems
Global climate change, climatologists, 617, 618*f*
Global measures, ecologic studies, 512
Global positioning systems (GIS), epidemiologic studies, 507
Global Tests of fit, model checking and, 427
Global warming, 617, 618*f*
Graphical analyses. *See also* Causal diagrams; Smoothers and Smoothing
meta-analysis and, 668–670
of confounding, 192–194
of selection bias, 192–194, 196
surveillance data, 478–479
of trends, 308–314
Graphical models. *See* Causal diagrams
Greenwood's formula, 290
Group-specific models, 442
Growth retardation, 633
GWA analysis. *See* Genome-wide association analysis

Haack, Susan, philosophy of, 24
Hair biomarker measurements, 594
Hazard of outcome at time, 397. *See also* Cox model
Hazard rate, 34, 397
Health
epidemiologic studies and, 1
problems, descriptive epidemiology of, 462–467
services, planning and projections, 466–467
surveillance, 110, 457
Health-related behavior, 468
Health-related exposure, 468
Healthy worker effect, 109, 135, 622
Herd immunity
exposure and, 561, 562*t*
transmission, 561
Heritability indices, limitations of, 15
Heterogeneity, 61–62, 258–259. *See also* Effect-measure modification; Statistical Interaction
of association, 259
confounding v., 259
of effect, 61–62, 72–74, 259
in meta-analysis, 671–673
tests for, 270, 279–280
Hierarchical regression, 337, 435–439, 529, 630. *See also* Bayesian analysis
confounder control and, 263
model selection and, 437–438
multiple comparisons and, 237
smoothing with, 438–439
Hierarchy principle, in modeling, 405, 406
Hill's considerations for causal inference, 26–31
Historical ascertainment, 96
Historical cohorts, 109
HIV (Human immunodeficiency virus)
confidentiality, 470
incubation periods, 557*f*
infection occurrence, 557
factors influencing, 556
infectivity and, 558
surveillance, 463
data, 466
record linkages, 475
Homogeneity. *See also* Heterogeneity
assumptions, 239–240, 258, 259, 270
of effect, 61–62, 72, 259
estimation assuming, 270–276
in meta-analysis, 657, 671
tests assuming, 277–278
tests, of, 270, 279–280
Horizontal scaling of graphs, 312–313, 313*f*
Hormonal events, subclinical pregnancy loss, 630, 631*f*
Horvitz-Thompson estimation, 445
Hospital-based case-control studies, 23, 118–119, 496
Hospitalization records, follow up techniques, 508
Host immunity, infectivity and, 558
Host-related factors, infection occurrence, 556
Household wealth, 536–537
Human chorionic gonadotropin (hCG), subclinical pregnancy loss, 630, 631*f*
Human genome epidemiology, 565
Human hosts, infectious agents and, 555
Human subjects, validity v. ethical considerations, 88–89
Hume, David, philosophy of, 19
Hybrid (multilevel) design, and ecologic analyses, 530
Hypergeometric distribution, 256, 272, 422
Hypothesis, 88. *See also* Alternative hypothesis; Joint hypothesis; Null hypothesis; Test hypothesis
competing, 25–26
conjecture and refutation, 20–21
Hypothesis generation, 99
Hypothesis testing, 150–158, 213–214, 236. *See also* Neyman-Pearson hypothesis tests; Null hypothesis; *P*-values; Significance testing
confidence intervals v., 157–158
Hypothesis-screening studies, 99

IC. *See* Interaction contrast
ICD codes, cocaine, surveillance, 474
Identifiability, graphical 192
instrumental variables and, 202
Identifiers, entry of, 509
Illness. *See* Disease
Illness, natural history of, studies of, 642
Illness outcomes, 641
Immortal person-time, 106–107

Impact fractions, 67. *See also* Attributable fractions;
Imprinting, 639
Incentives, 498, 498*t*
Incidence, 47–48
  model-based estimates, 439–440
Incidence density. *See* Incidence rate
Incidence measures, 33–36, 40–45
  prevalence v., 46
  relations among, 41–45
Incidence odds, 41
  case-control studies, 113
  risk-based measures and, 58
  models, 394–395
Incidence proportion, 33, 40–41. *See also* Risk
  case-control studies, 113–122
  causes and, 11, 11*t*
  component causes and, 12, 12*t*
  case-cohort study of, 123–124
  models. *See* Risk models
Incidence rate, 33, 34–35, 40, 41, 42
  absolute, 40
  case-control studies, 113
  incidence times v., in special populations, 37*f*, 39
  models, 395–398
  person time and, 34, 101
  of population, 34
  proper interpretation of, 35–36
  of recurrent events, 36
Incidence rate difference. *See* Rate difference
Incidence rate ratio. *See* Rate ratio
Incidence studies. *See* Cohort studies
Incidence time, 33–34
  models, 396–398
  ratios, 53, 397
Incident case-control studies, 94. *See* Case-control studies
Income, 535
Incomplete matching, 177. *See also* Marginal matching; Partial matching
Incremental plots (Slope plots), 311–312, 312*f*
Incubation periods, 551
  agents with, infection occurrence, 557, 557*f*
  persistent infection v., progression-related states, 551
Independence. *See also* Association; D-Separation
  conditional, 190
  marginal, 184,188
  statistical, 184–185
Independent censoring, 34–35, 45, 289–290
Independent competing risks, 44–45, 289–290
Independent error, 138
Independent outcome, 239
Independent variables. *See also* Covariate; Regressor
  in regression, 383
  statistically, 184–185
Index condition, counterfactual measures and, 55
Index level, regressors and, 407
Indicator variables, 407–408
Indirect adjustment. *See* Standardized morbidity ratio
Indirect effects, 200
  direct effect v., 545, 545*f*
  sufficient cause model and, 13
Indirectly adjusted rate, 665
Individual matching, 170–171, 178
Individual risks, 40
Individual studies, statistical reanalysis of, meta-analysis, 659–668
Individual-level analysis, 512
Induction period, 15–17, 603
  analysis of, 300–302
Induction, 18–19
Inductivism, 18–19
  Refutationism v., 20
Inequality, 540–541
Infection, 549. *See also* Preinfectiousness; Subclinical infection
  cure, factors influencing, 559–560
  death from, factors influencing, 559–560
  disease v., infectious agents and, 551
  factors influencing, 557–559
  measures of frequency, 553–555
  occurrence of, factors influencing, 557–559
  occurrence of exposure, 556–557
  persistent, factors influencing, 559–560
  subclinical, 551
  transmission, factors influencing, 561–562
  transmission-related states, 551, 552
Infectious agents
  exposure occurrence, factors influencing, 555–556
  persistent infection, 559
Infectious disease
  emerging, outbreak investigations, 553
  epidemiology, 549–563
  process, states of, 551
  progression axis, 549, 550*f*
  public health, 617
  surveillance and, 460
  transmission models, 562–563
Infectivity factors, infection occurrence, 556
Inferential statistics, 221. *See also* Confidence limits; *P*-values
  data descriptors v., 216
Infertile worker effect, 622
Infertility, 624–628
Inflammatory bowel disease, genetic susceptibility, 577–578
Influence analysis, 221
  meta-analysis and, 675
  sensitivity, 221–222
Information
  accuracy, comparability of, 121
  needs, epidemiologic investigation, 460
  systems, surveillance, 474
  weighting, 334–337
Information bias, 137–146. *See also* Misclassification
Information-weighted averaging, 334–337. *See also* Inverse-variance weighting
Informative cluster size, recognized loss, 630
Informed consent, 90
Initiator, in carcinogensis, 16
In-person interviews, questionnaires and, 503
Instrumental variables, 91, 202–204
Instrument-outcome association, 203
Intensity of disease, 34. *See also* hazard, incidence rate
Intensity scoring, 449
Intentional selection, bias from, 196–198
Intent-to-treat analysis (ITT), 203, 647

Interaction, 10, 13, 71–83. *See also* Biologic Interaction; Public health interaction; Statistical interaction; Synergism
analysis of, 298–300
Interaction contrast (IC), 75–79, 298–299
Interaction response types, 79–80, 80*t*
Interaction terms, 406. *See also* Product terms
Interactive voice response (IVR), 500
Intercept. *See* Zero level, special handling in trend evaluation
Intercommunity comparisons, social class, 611–612
Intermediate variables, 131–134, 186–188, 545–546
adjusting for, problems of, 131–134, 200–202, 260, 545–546
in meta-analysis, 656
Internal reference group, ratios derived, meta-analysis, 665–666
Internal validity, 128–129
International ecologic studies, limitations, 581
Internet. *See also* Software
sites, follow-up techniques, 508
surveillance data, 478
surveillance systems, 471
Interval estimation, 157–158, 163–167. *See also* Bayesian intervals; Confidence intervals; Likelihood intervals
Intervening variables. *See* Intermediate variables
Intervention measure, 648–649
Intervention studies, recruitment to, 494
Interview response rates, epidemiologic research, 497–498
Interviews. *See also* Recall bias
longitudinal studies, 503–504
response rates and, 509
techniques and training, 504
Inverse-probability weighting (IPW), 266, 444–445, 449. *See also* Doubly robust estimation; Marginal models; Model-based standardization
exposure models, standardization using, 444–445
and propensity scores, 445
stabilized, 446
Inverse-variance weighting, 334–337, 670–671. *See also* Information-weighted averaging
IP. *See* Incidence proportion
IPW. *See* Inverse-probability weighting
Item non-response. *See* Missing values, handling
ITT association. *See* Intent-to-treat association
IVR. *See* Interactive voice response

Join points, of spline, 411
Joint action, 82. *See also* Interaction, concepts of
Joint analysis, of multiple exposure levels, 323
Joint confidence regions, 235–236, 324, 324*f*
Joint effects, model searching, 419
Joint hypothesis, 237, 307, 322–327
Joint null hypothesis, Pearson χ^2 statistic, 307
Joint *P*-value, 235
Joint trend statistic, 326

Kaplan-Meier formula, 42–43, 290–292
censoring and, 45, 290
Kernels, 314, 318–320, 440, 441
Knots, of spline, 411
Kuhn, Thomas, philosophy of, 21

Laboratory-based surveillance, 472–473
Lagged analysis, 301
Large-sample methods, 216, 220, 225–230, 240–253, 263, 267–282, 307, 314–316, 422
and model fitting, 422–423
person-time data, 240–245
pure count data, 245–253
sparse data and, 263
trend statistics, 314–316
Latency
of effects, 16, 603
preinfectiousness v., transmission-related states, 551
reactivation disease, 559
Latency periods, exposure assessment, 603
Latent effects model, 546
Latent period, 16, 603. *See also* Induction period
Levels of analysis, ecologic studies, 512–513
Levels of inference, ecologic studies, 513
Levels of measurement, ecologic studies, 512
Life-course model, 546
Life expectancy, 34
"Life trajectory" effect, 547
Life-table analysis, 37, 290. *See also* Log-rank test; Product-limit estimator
Likelihood function, 164, 165*f*, 227–228
conditional, 257, 272–273, 422, 433
partial, 422
statistical theory and, 227–229
Likelihood inference, pure, 164–165, 227–229
Likelihood intervals, pure, 164–165, 229
Likelihood ratio, 228–231, 425–426
in Bayesian analysis, 230–231
confidence limits, 229–230
statistics, 229–230
tests, 229–230, 425–426
Linear hypothesis, 314
Linear models, 392, 395, 396, 398. *See also* Generalized linear models
in ecologic analysis, 517, 520
in hierarchical regression, 436
for odds, 395
for rates, 396
for risks, 392
for trends, 398, 402–403
Linear predictor, 416
Linear risk models, 392, 395, 398, 402–403
Linear spline, 411
trend, 411
Link function
generalized linear models, 416
secondary data, 486
Linkage analysis, 565
List-based sampling, 496
Locally linear regression, 441
LOESS procedures, 442
Log additive model. *See* Log-linear model, Multiplicative model
Logarithmic curve, 398
Logarithmic plot scales, 310–313, 313*f*
Logic checks, 215, 509
Logistic distributions, 370

Logistic models, 394–395, 399, 414–415, 442
adjacent-category, 414–415
conditional, 433
continuation ratio, 415
cumulative-odds, 415
group-specific, 442
exact, 422
hierarchical, 435–439
marginal, 446
for matched data, 434
ordinal, 414–415
polytomous, 413–414
proportional-odds, 415
stratified, 433
Logistic transform, 246, 391
Logit-logistic distribution, 371
Logit-normal distribution, 371
Logit, 231, 246, 391
Logit models, 395, 414–415. *See also* Logistic models
Log-likelihood function, 165
Log-linear hypothesis, 314
Log-linear models, 395, 416, 420. *See also* Multiplicative models
for counts, 423, 444
ecologic studies and, 517
genetic factors, 638
for incidence times, 396
for odds, 394, 416
for rates, 396, 416
for risks, 393, 416
Log-log risk model, 417
Log-rank test, 295
Log-risk scale, 74
Longitudinal causal modeling, 46, 453–455
Longitudinal cohort studies, 569. *See also* Cohort studies
Longitudinal data, 46
modeling, 451–455
Longitudinal monitoring, 489
Longitudinal sampling, 116. *See also* Density sampling
Longitudinal studies. *See also* Cohort studies
follow-up techniques, 507–508
interviews, 503–504
Longitudinal trends, 606, 608
Log-likelihoods. *See* Deviance statistics; Likelihood functions; Likelihood ratios
Log-rank test, 295
Lorenz curve, 540, 541*f*, 542
Loss to follow-up, 100–101, 108–109, 289. *See also* Censoring
Low birth-weight paradox, 633
Lower *P*-value, 220
Lower-tailed *P*-value, 152, 220
LOWESS procedures, 442
Lung cancer, 18, 103, 263, 604, 607*f*, 609
Lyme disease, culture technique and, 553

"M" diagram, 188*f*
Malformations, prevalence and, 47
Mantel trend statistic, 314–316
Mantel-Haenszel methods, 271
case-cohort, 281
homogeneity assumption, 271
model fitting, 433
odds ratio, 276, 276*t*
rate difference, 273
rate ratio, 273
risk difference, 274–275
risk ratio 274–275, 281, 285
sparse-data, 272, 275, 281
statistic for person-time data, 277
statistic for pure-count data, 278
statistic for polytomous exposures, 307
study size, 679
survival analysis, 294–295
two-stage data, 282
Mapping, disease rates, 608–609
Marginal averages, 387
Marginal independence, 184
Marginal matching, 182
Marginal models, 442, 446, 447, 450, 451, 544–545. *See also* Inverse probability weighting; Marginal structural models; Model based standardization
Marginal structural models (MSM), 208, 446, 454–455
Marginally unbiased, 191
Marginal outcome modeling, 446
Markov-chain Monte Carlo (MCMC), 342
Matched data. *See also* Matched pair; Matching
analysis of, 283–288
modeling, 434–435
Matched designs, 171–182. *See also* Matching
Matched pair
analysis, 284–288
case-control data, 287–288
cohort data, 284–287
odds ratio, 287–288
risk ratio, 285
test, 286
Matched randomization, 175
Matching, 171–179. *See also* Matched data; Matched pairs; Overmatching
in case-control studies, 175–179
cost of, 178
selection bias and, 174–176, 205, 205*f*
in cohort studies, 174–175
effect of, 171–174, 205
information accuracy, indicators of, 181
marginal, 182
partial, 177, 182
purpose of, 171–174
stratification variables, 150
Matrix adjustment methods for misclassification, 360–361
Maximum likelihood estimate (MLE), 164, 221, 228, 271–272. *See also* Likelihood function; Likelihood ratio
homogeneity assumption, 271
of homogenous measure, 271
model fitting and, 421, 425
overdispersion and, 422
priors, 342
score statistic and, 226
Maximum likelihood test statistic, 230. *See* Wald statistic
Maximal models, 421
MCMC. *See* Markov-chain Monte Carlo program
McNemar test statistic, 286, 288

MCSA. *See* Monte-Carlo sensitivity analysis of biases
MDR method. *See* Multifactor dimensionality-reduction method
Measles vaccine
  prevention programs and, 462, 463*f*
  register, secondary data, 485–486
Measurement error, 137–138, 346, 352–353, 361. *See also* Misclassification
  in dietary and nutritional assessment, 591–592, 595, 596–597
Measures of association, 51–70, 57. *See also* Association
  Measures of effect v., 59–60, 59*t*, 185, 385–388
  standardized measures of, 67–69
Measures of body composition, anthropometry, 594–595
Measures of occurrence, 33–35, 40, 46
Measures of effect, 51–56, 59–70; *See also* Causal effects; Effects; Effect-measure modification
  defining exposure in, 55
  generalized, 66–67
  measures of association v., 59–60, 59*t*, 185, 385–388
  null state and, 54–56
  regression, 385–386
  relations among, 60–62
  standardized, 67–69, 386–388
  theoretical nature of, 54–55
Measures of frequency, infection and disease, 553–555
Median-unbiased estimates, 221, 224, 253, 255, 257
Mediating variables. *See* Intermediate variables
Medical testing, 643, 644*t*
Medical-record abstracts, 499
Mendelian transmission, 565
Menopause, 622–623
Menstrual cycle, 623
Meta-analysis, 652–682. *See also* Publication bias
  goals of, 654–655
  nature of, 652–653
  protocol for, 655
  quality scores, 679, 681
  quantification of effects, 657–658
  role and limitations, 681
  statistical methods, 668–677
  study identification, 656–657
  summary statistics for, 670*t*
  vote counting, 680–681
Meta-regression methods, 673–677
Methods, classes of, 220
Mid-*P*-values, 232–233, 255–257
  v. continuity corrections, 232–233
Migrant studies, nutritional exposures, 582
Migration across groups, ecologic studies, 527
Mill, John Stuart, philosophy of, 19
Minimally sufficient conditioning sets, 192
Minimal models, 420–421
Miscarriage studies, 629
Misclassification, 138–144
  analysis of, 352–361, 372
  bias related to, quantification of, 352–361, 488
  of confounders, 144–145
  dependent, 138, 143, 145, 360
  of multiple variables, 360
  in meta-analysis, 662–663
  multiple-bias analyses and, 363
Misspecification. *See* Model specification; Specification bias; Specification error
Missing at random (MAR), 219
Missing completely at random (MCAR), 219
Missing data, 215, 219
  bias, 199–200, 200*f*, 346
  methods, 219
Missing-data indicators, bias from, 199–200, 219
Mixed effects model, 130, 529. *See also* Hierarchical regression
  in meta regression, 677
MLE. *See* Maximum-likelihood estimate
Mobility. *See* Social mobility
Model accuracy, 389–390, 419, 449–450
Model averaging, 427
Model-based estimates, 424, 439–440
Model-based standardization, 442–446; *See also* Inverse probability weighting; Marginal modeling; Regression standardization
Model checking, 423–429, 425*t*
Model combination, doubly robust estimation, 450–451
Model diagnostics, model checking and, 423, 427–428
Model fitting, 389–390, 421–423
  background example, 390
Model parameter, 389
Model selection, 419–421
  hierarchical regression and, 437–438
  confounder scoring and, 449–450
Model sensitivity analysis, 346, 429
Model specification, 382, 389–390, 420–421, 449–450. *See also* Model selection
Modifiers. *See* Effect measure modification
Modular questionnaire, multipurpose studies and, 503
Molecular epidemiology, 561 579
Monitoring of disease, 488–490, 490*f*
Monotone trend, 308
Monte-Carlo sensitivity analysis (MCSA), 364–378
Bayesian analysis v., 378–380
  combined, 376–378
  intervals, 365
  probabilistic bias analysis and, 364
  simulation histograms, 368*f*
Mortality rates
  follow-up, 109–110
  monitoring disease, 488–490, 489*f*
  patterns of, 33, 33*t*
  time-series analyses, 611
Mosquito, environmental reservoir, 555
Moving To Opportunity study (MTO study), 547
Moving averages, 317–321. *See also* Smoothers and Smoothing categorical estimates as, 321
MRFIT. *See* Multiple Risk Factor Intervention Trial
MSM. *See* Marginal structural model
MTO study. *See* Moving To Opportunity study
Multidimensional outcome, 56
Multifactor dimensionality-reduction (MDR) method, gene-disease association, 572
Multifactorial causation and etiology, 5, 14
Multigeneration registers, secondary data, 484
Multilevel analyses, 513
  and designs, ecologic studies, 528–530
Multilevel modeling, 337, 435–439, 529, 530, 542–544. *See also* Hierarchical regression
Multi-linear regression, 674*t*
Multiple bias analyses, 363–364, 376–378

Multiple comparisons, 234–237, 322–327
hierarchical regression and, 237
single-comparisons v., 326–327
in trend analyses, 307, 326
Multiple control groups, case-control studies, 122, 322
Multiple correlation, 424–425
Multiple diseases, analysis of. *See* Multiple outcomes analysis
Multiple group designs, ecologic studies, 514
Multiple group ecologic analysis, confounders, 518–519
Multiple group ecologic studies, within-group misclassification, 526
Multiple imputation, 219
Multiple inference procedures. *See* Multiple comparisons
Multiple logistic model, 401. *See also* Logistic models
extensions of, 413–416
single-logistic model v., 401
Multiple outcomes analysis, 321–323, 322*t*, 325–326. *See also* Longitudinal data; Recurrent events
simultaneous analysis of, 325, 325*t*
Multiple probabilistic bias analysis, Monte-Carlo analyses and, 376, 377*t*, 378
Multiple regression, 384
models, 400–408. *See also specific models, e.g.,* Logistic models
trend models, 408–413
Multiple Risk Factor Intervention Trial (MRFIT), 92
Multiple testing. *See* Multiple comparisons
Multiplicative models, 404–405. *See also* Exponential models; Log-linear models
Multiplicative-intercept models
conditional fitting, 433
cumulative studies, 431
density studies, 430–431
prevalence studies, 431
Multipurpose studies, modular questionnaire, 503
Multistage model, 82
Multivariable modeling. *See* Multiple regression; Multivariate regression
Multivariate outcome, with competing risks, 56
Multivariate regression, 388
Mycobacterium avium, infectivity and, 558
Mycobacterium leprae, culture technique and, 553
Mycobacterium tuberculosis
infection occurrence, 556
surveillance, 464

Nails, biochemical measurements, 594
Naive direct-effect analysis, 201
Narrative historical approach, 548
National Death Index (NDI), tracing, epidemiologic studies, 507
National genetic testing committees, terminology by, 566, 566*t*
National Health and Nutrition Examination Survey. *See* NHANES survey
Natural direct effect, 200–201
Natural log function, exponential function v., 416
Naturalism, consensus and, 21–22
NDI. *See* National Death Index
Nearest-neighbor windows, 321
Necessary cause, 7, 9
Negative adjustments, treatment of, in bias analysis, 373
Neighborhood controls, 117, 121
Neisseria meningitidis, colonization of, 556
Nelson-Aalen estimator, 292. *See also* Exponential formula; Kaplan-Meier formula
Neonatal mortality, 633–635, 634*f*
Nested case-control studies, 114, 122–123
and missing data models, 432
Nested confidence intervals, 157*f*
Nested indicator coding, 407
Next-step investigations, surveillance data, 478
Neyman-Pearson hypothesis testing, 150, 153–155. *See also* Hypothesis test; *P*-values; Statistical significance
statistical estimation and, 157–158
NHANES survey (National Health and Nutrition Examination Survey), 569, 611
surveillance, 474
Nodes. *See* Vertices
Nominal-scale variables, 214
Nonadherence. *See* adherence
Noncausal associations, 26
Noncollapsibility, 58, 62. *See also* Collapsibility
confounding v., 62
Noncompliance. *See* compliance
g-estimation and, 454
Nondependent error, 138. *See* Independent error
Nondifferential misclassification, 139, 372–373
of disease, 142–143
of exposure, 139–142
incidence-rate difference and, incidence-rate ratio and, 139*t*
pervasiveness of misinterpretation, 143
requirements for, 355–356
with three exposure categories, 141*t*
with two exposure categories, 140*t*
Nonexperimental studies, 93–99
types of, 87–88
Noninformative priors, 167, 335–337, 343, 348, 379–380
Nonnested models, 426
Non-normal priors, 340, 370–372
Nonparametric bootstrapping, model checking and, 429
Nonparametric regression, 421, 440–442. *See also* Smoothers and Smoothing
Nonrandomized clinical studies, 641, 650
Nonsignificance of a statistical test, proper interpretation of, 151–152
In meta-analysis, 657, 680
Notifiable disease
reporting, 472
surveillance and, 460
Novum Organum, scientific method and, 18
Null hypergeometric distribution, 256, 257
Null hypothesis, 60, 88, 151, 156, 314
bias and, 144
P-value, 153, 315, 454
test for, 158
true, cross-level bias, 523, 525*t*
Null state, effect measure and, 54–56
Null studies, publication bias and, meta-analysis and, 678–679
Nutrient content, measurement of, epidemiologic studies, 586–588
Nutrient, definition complexity, 580

Nutritional epidemiology, 580–597
  methodological issues, 595–597
Nutritional exposures, 581–586

Observational studies, 19, 87–88, 332–333
  confounding and, 129
Occam's razor, 389
Occupation, as social variable, 537
Occupational cohort study, 495
Occupational epidemiology, 599
Occurrence measures, 33–50
Occurrence time, 33. *See also* Incidence time
Odds models, 394–395
Odds ratio, 61, 62, 74
  case-control studies, 127
  pseudo-frequencies and, 113–114
Oil disease, 603
"Omic" tools, 564–566
One step study, 646
One-sided *P*-value, 156
One-sided tests, 156
One-tailed *P*-value, 152
Open populations, 38, 101. *See also* Dynamic population
  closed populations v., 38
  steady state, 38–39
Open-ended categories, confounder stratification, 218, 304–305, 410
"Optimal" control distribution, case-control studies, 176, 177
Ordered variables, categorization of, 303–305
Ordering of classification, multiple-bias analyses and, 363
Ordinal logistic models, 414–415
Ordinal category scores, 312–313, 410
Outbreak bias, 553
Outbreak investigations, emerging infectious diseases, 553
Outcome events. *See also* Causal effects; Effects; Outcome variables
  sufficient-component cause model and, 9
  timing of, exposure category and, 107–108
Outcome measures. *See specific measures, e.g.,* Incidence times; Rates
Outcome models
  exposure models v., 449–450
  standardization using, 443
Outcome scores, 447–448. *See also* Confounder scores
Outcome transformations, 400
Outcome variables, 382–383. *See also* Causal effects; Effects; Outcome events; Regressand
  in meta-analysis, 655–656
  in regression v. causation, 383
  transformed, 400
Outliers, 410
Overadjustment, 181, 260
Overconclusiveness, meta-analysis and, 677
Overdispersion, 422
Overmatching, 179–181, 260
  bias and, 180–181
  cost efficiency, 181
  statistical efficiency and, 179–180
Ovulation, 623

Pair matching, 283–289
Pairwise blocking, 174
Parallel linear trends, 404
Partial likelihood, 422
Partial-Bayes analysis. *See* Semi-Bayes analysis
Partial matching, 177, 182
Partially ecologic analysis, 512, 512*f*
Passive surveillance, 476
  active surveillance v., 472
Pathway model, 546
Patterns of exposure, 66
  attributable fractions, 67
  distinguishing, 67
Pearson global test statistics, 427
Pearson χ^2 statistic, 307
Penalized splines, 440–441
Penalized estimation, 271, 331, 341, 421, 423, 436, 437–439. *See also* Hierarchical regression; Shrinkage estimation
  maximum likelihood v., 271
Per protocol analysis, randomized controlled trials, 648
Percentile boundaries, problems with, 217–218, 264, 303–305
Perfect compatibility, in causal graphs, 191
Perinatal mortality, 635–636
Period effect, 606, 608
Persistent infection (Chronic infection), 552
  incubation period v., progression-related states, 551
  infectious agents and, 559
Persistent organic pollutants, 616–617
Personal identifiers, secondary data access, ethics of, 491
Person-count cohort data, 240
Person-time, 294. *See also* Follow-up
  analysis, follow-up data, 287
  classifying, 102–103
  data
    large-sample methods, 240–245
    small-sample methods, 253–255
    unstratified data with, 243, 243*t*
  distribution, 49–50, 68
  exposure, 106
  follow-up data, disease misclassification, 358–359
  immortal, 106–107
  rate, 34
  at risk, 34, 39
  units, classification of, 218–219
  weights, Mantel-Haenszel estimation, 275
Physical examinations, epidemiologic studies, 504–505
Placebo, 91
  equipoise and, 89
  response, 91
Plausibility, causal inference and, 28–29
PMR. *See* Proportional mortality ratio
Point estimate, 156
Point prevalence, 46
Point sources, clustering analysis, 613
Point-source outbreaks, epidemic outbreaks, 552
Poisson distribution (model), 241–243
  clusters, 612
Poisson regression, 421–422. *See also* Exponential models for rates
  case-parent studies, genotype distribution and, 575
  extravariation, 422
  genetic factors, 638
Policy, and bias analysis, 347, 380
Policy, surveillance data, 467

Polynomial regression, 410
Polytomous exposures, and outcomes, analysis of, 303–327
Polytomous logistic models, 413–414
Pooled estimate, 271
Popper, Karl, philosophy of, 20
Population. *See also* Case selection; Complete populations; Confounding; General-population; Impact fractions; Incidence rate; Population-based case-control studies; Source population; Superpopulation; Target population
  closed, 36–37
  cohorts v., 38
  concepts of, 383
  individual rates and, 34–35
  open, 38, 101
  regression, 383
  at risk, 34
    of recurrent events, 36
  steady state, 38–39
  source, 114–115, 128–129, 383
  target, 60, 90, 146–147, 383, 471
  under surveillance, 460
  types of, 36–39
Population-attributable fractions, 67, 295–297
Population-attributable risk percent, 67
Population-average models, 544–545
Population-averaged regression, 387
Population-based case-control studies, 114, 123 *See also* Nested case-control studies
Population-based prevalence study, 569
Population-based surveillance systems, 469–470
Population effects, 52
Population incidence rate, 34, 35
Population time at risk, 34
Post hoc ergo propter hoc fallacy, 19
Posterior probability, 23, 166–167, 330–331, 337, 345, 364, 379–380
Postexposure events, person-time allocation, 107
Potential biases. *See* Systematic errors
Potential outcomes, 54, 385–386. *See also* Counterfactual outcomes
  binary exposure variables and, 75, 76*t*
  causal models and, 60
  causation, 18
  model, 59–60, 59*t*
  in regression, 385–388
  in standardization, 387–388
  sufficient-cause models v., 81–82, 81*f*
Poverty, 536
Power models, 410
Power of statistical test, 153–154
Pr. *See* Probability
Precision
  data stratification and, 150
  definition of, 1498–149
  statistical significance and, 162, 162*f*
  weighting, 271, 334–337, 670–671. *See also* Information-weighted averaging
Prediction, 421
Prediction accuracy, 389–390, 436
Predictive values
  diagnostic tests, 643–644,644t
  exposure misclassification, 138, 353–354
  negative, 138, 353, 643–644,644t
  positive, 138, 353, 643–644, 644t
  screening tests, 643–644, 644*t*
  sensitivity and specificity v., 357–358, 643–644, 644*t*
  surveillance systems, 479
Pregnancy. *See also* Subclinical pregnancy loss
  complications, 632
  hormone, 621
  loss, 628–631
  reproductive epidemiology, 620, 621
Preinfectiousness, latency v., 551. *See also* Infection
Pretesting, nonresponse and, 499
Prevalence, 46–48
  case-control studies, 97, 127
  duration of disease, 47–48
  etiologic research and, 46–47
  model-based estimates, 439–440
  multiplicative-intercept models, 431
  odds, 48
  pool, 46, 47
  proportion, 46, 47
  rate, 46
  ratios, 69
  studies, 88, 97
Preventable fractions, 54, 67. *See also* Attributable fractions
Prevention programs, measles vaccine and, 462, 463*f*
Preventive effects, 8, 9, 17, 54, 59, 65. *See also* Causal effects; Potential outcomes
Primary base study, 114–115
Primary data, secondary data v., 481
Prior data, 337–342. *See also* Data priors; Priors
Prior information, in model searching, 419–420. *See also* Bayesian analysis; Priors
Prior limits, 330. *See also* Priors
Prior model, in hierarchical regression, 436
Prior probability. *See* Priors
Prior parameters, Bayesian analysis and, 330
Prior standard deviation, hierarchical regression, 436–437
Prior data, 337–342
  as diagnostic device, 338–339, 341–342
  frequentist interpretation, 337–338
  methods, extensions, 340
  and reverse Bayes analysis, 338–339
Priors, 23, 166–167, 330–332, 337–343, 366–373, 378–380. *See also* Prior data; Probability; Probability distributions
  cautions, 342–343
  correlated, 371–372
  noninformative, 167, 335–337, 343, 348, 379–380
  reference, 343
  realistic, 335–336, 337, 365, 369–370, 371, 373
Privacy rights, surveillance, 462
Probabilistic bias analysis, 364–380
Probabilistic sensitivity analysis (PSA), 364–365. *See also* Monte-Carlo sensitivity analysis
  Bayesian analysis v., 378–380
Probability, 9–10. *See also* Likelihood; Probability distributions and densities; Risk
  conditional, 184–185
  data, 331
  frequency, 10, 331–332

in graphs, 187–190
marginal, 184
mass functions, 378
models for counts, 240–247
population, 184–185, 387
posterior, 23, 166–167, 330–331, 337, 345, 364, 379–380
prior, 23, 166–167, 330–332, 337–343, 366–373, 378–380
propensity, 10
standardized, 442–445
subjective, 10, 23–24, 165–167, 330–331
unconditional, 184
Probability distributions and densities, 184–185, 222–225, 370–372, 378–380
binomial, 223–225, 245–247, 254
graphical models for, 186–195
exact statistics and, 222–225
log F, 370
logistic, 367*f*, 370
logit logistic, 371
log normal, 371
logit normal, 371
normal, 367*f*
parameter, 223
Poisson, 241–245
population, 184–185, 387
posterior, 23, 166–167, 330–331, 337, 345, 364, 379–380
prior, 23, 166–167, 330–332, 337–343, 366–373, 378–380
trapezoidal, 367*f*, 371
uniform, 365, 369
Probability of causation (of a case), 64–65, 297–298
Probit model, 395
Product terms, 402–407. *See also* Statistical interaction
biologic interactions v., 407
interpreting, 405–406
trends and, 404–405
Product-limit estimator, 290–292
Nelson-Aalen estimator v., 292
Product-limit formula, 42–43, 42*f*, 42*t*, 43, 290–292
censoring and, 45, 290
Prognostic scores, 447. *See also* Confounder scores; Outcome scores
Progression axis, infectious disease and, 549, 550*f*
Progression-related studies, 553–560
Promoter, in carcinogenesis, 16
Propagated outbreaks, epidemic outbreaks, 552
Propensity scores, 445, 448–450. *See also* Confounder scores; Doubly robust estimation; Exposure scores
inverse-weighting by, 445, 448
Proportional hazards model. *See* Cox model
Proportional mortality ratio (PMR), 97–98
Proportional mortality studies, 97–99, 127
Proportional odds model, 415
Prospective ascertainment, 96
Prospective studies, retrospective studies v., 95–97
Prostate cancer, surveillance, 464, 465*f*
PSA. *See* Probabilistic sensitivity analysis
Pseudo-denominators, in case-cohort studies, 252–253
Pseudo-frequencies, 113–114, 125
Pseudo-likelihood, 422
Pseudo-rates, 113–114
Pseudo-risks, 123–124
Puberty, 622–623
Public health
bias analysis and, 347, 380
effects, 14
functions of, 462
interaction, 83
interventions, evaluation, 465–466, 466*f*
laws, notifiable disease reporting, 472
services, planning and projections, 466–467
surveillance, history of, 460–462, 461*t*
Public resources, secondary data access, ethics of, 491
Publication bias
In meta-analysis, 656–657, 678–679
from study exclusion, 679
Pure count data. *See* Count Data
Pure direct effect, 200–201
Pure likelihood equation, 230
Pure likelihood inference, 228
Pure likelihood limits, 229
P-values, 151–153, 156–163, 364. *See also* Confidence intervals and limits; Evidence of absence of an effect; Hypothesis tests; Joint *P*-value; Lower-*P*-value; Mantel trend *P*-value; Mid-*P*-values; Nonsignificance; One-sided *P*-value; Significance tests; Two-sided *P*-value
Bayesian theory and, 166
confidence intervals and, 158–159
continuity corrected, 232
data and, 216
deviance, 229–230
exact, 220
function, 158–159, 160, 160*f*, 161*f*, 239
hypothetical data, 158*t*
interpretation, 151–152, 159–163
likelihood ratio, 229–230
linear hypothesis, 314–316
lower-tailed, 152
Mantel trend, 314–316
mid, 232–233
misinterpretations, 151–152
multiple testing, 234–237, 322–327
null hypothesis and, 153, 315, 454
one-sided, 156
from Pearson χ^2 statistic, 307
practice guidelines, 162–163
random error and, 156
score, 225–226
test statistics, 220–221
trend, 314–316
two-sided, 156, 221, 234
two-tailed, 152
types, 152–153
upper-tailed, 152
Wald, 220, 226–227

Quadratic model, 398
Quadratic spline, 411–412
Qualitative statistical interaction, 79–80
biologic interaction v., 299
Qualitative tally (vote counting), in meta-analysis, 680
Quality scoring, 681

Quantification of effects, 51–52. *See also* Effect measures
in meta-analysis, 657–658
Quantiles, 217–218, 304
Quantitative criterion, variables and, 261
Quasi-experiments, 88–89, 547
Quasi-likelihood, 422
Questionnaires. *See also* Data coding questionnaires; Data entry questionnaires; Food-frequency questionnaires; Modular questionnaire; Self-administered questionnaires; Semiquantitative food-frequency questionnaires
administration method, 500–501
data and, 214
modular, multipurpose studies, 503
respondent burden, 503–504

R. *See* Effective reproductive number (*R*)
R^2, 424–425
Race/ethnicity, as social variable, 534–535
Racism, 537–538
Random allocation. *See* Randomization
Random coefficient models, 331, 423, 426, 427, 439. *See also* Hierarchical regression
Random digit dialing (RDD), 117–118, 496
Random effects models, 452, 542–544, 628. *See also* Hierarchical regression
in meta-analysis, 675–677
Random error, 24, 128, 148–167, 332–333; *See also* Confidence Limits; Probability distributions; *P*-values; Random sampling
adjustment for, in bias analysis, 346, 366–369, 376, 379
conventional statistical analysis, 364
distributions, 222–225, 241–247, 421
P-values, 151–153, 156
P-value functions, 158–159
statistical precision and, 148–149
study size and, 149–150
systematic errors v., 346
Random sampling, 10, 213, 220, 222, 224, 346. *See also* Sampling error; Selection bias
of cases, case-control studies, 115
of controls, case-control studies, 114, 122–123
for validation data, 361
Random variation, components, 148–149. *See also* Random error
Randomization (Random allocation), 88–89
clinical studies, 641
d-separated unconditionally v., 187
experiments and, 168–169
of exposure assignment, 346
intervention studies, recruitment to, 494
Randomized experiments. *See* Experimental studies
Randomized recruitment, 604
Randomized trials, 18, 203*f*. *See also* Experimental studies
dietary hypothesis, 585–586
subject selection, 647–648
therapeutic interventions and, 646–649
Rare disease assumption in case-control studies, 114, 125
Rate fractions, 54, 63. *See also* Attributable fractions
etiologic fractions v., 63–64, 297–298
probability of causation v., 64–65, 297–298
Rate, 34–36, 39–40. *See also specific types, e.g.,* Case fatality rate; Incidence rate; Prevalence; Mortality rates
standardized, 49–50
Rate difference, 52–53, 277
crude data, 243, 244, 245
Mantel-Haenszel, 273–274
standardized, 67–69, 266–267
Rate models, 395–398
in meta-analysis, 663
Rate ratio (RR), 61, 62, 116, 241
crude data, 243, 244, 245, 251, 254–255
ecologic studies and, 517, 518f
Mantel-Haenszel, 273–274
relation to other ratio measures, 250
standardized, 67–69, 267–269
unconditional v. conditional, 272
Ratio measures, 53. *See also* Rate ratio; Relative risk; Risk ratio
relations among, 250
Rationally coherent probability assessments, 166. *See also* Bayesianism
RDD. *See* Random-digit dialing
Reactivation disease, latency and, 559
Reanalysis, for meta-analysis and, 659–668, 669*t*
Recall, in interviews, 96
Recall bias, 111, 112, 138, 356–357
birth defects, 637
Recentering variables, 392
Recognized loss, 628–630
Record abstraction, 499
Record linkage, 486
in surveillance, 475, 476
Record-level adjustment, in bias analysis, 373
Recurrent events, recurrent outcomes, 36, 452–453. *See also* Longitudinal data
Red blood cells, biochemical measurements, 594
Reference level, regressors and, 407
Reference model, in checking model fit, 425
Reference priors, 343. *See also* Noninformative priors
Referent, for causes, 7
Refutationism, 20–21, 24, 30
Registries, use of in epidemiologic research, 481–491
surveillance, 473
of vaccinations, 488
Regressand, 383–384. *See also* Outcome variables
in multivariate regression, 388
Regression, 382
Bayesian, 388
binary, 383–384
causal, 385–386
frequentist, 382–383, 388–389
hierarchical, 237, 263, 435–439, 529, 630
meta-analytic, 673–677
multiple, 384
multivariate, 388
ridge, 331, 423, 436, 437, 439. *See also* Shrinkage estimation
standardization, 386–388, 442–445
Regression analysis, 381–382, 418–456
Regression measures of effect, 385–388
Regression functions, 382–389

Regression models, 381–417. *See also specific entries, e.g.,* Generalized linear models; Linear models; Logistic models; Log-linear models
biologic interactions and, 406–407
contingency table data and, 216
in meta-analysis, 658–659, 673–677
smoothed curves and, 321
transformed, 400
Regression splines, 410–412. *See also* Nonparametric regression; Power models; Smoothers and Smoothing
Regressor, 383–384
transformed, 398–400
Regressor-specific predictions, fitted model v., 423
Relative birth weight, 635
Relative difference, 54, 65
Relative effect measures, 52
Relative excess measures, 53–54
Relative risk scale, meta-analysis and, 670
Relative risk (RR), 53, 67. *See also* Rate ratio; Risk ratio
adjustment of, in Bayesian-analysis, 336
factorization of, meta-analysis, 660–661
relations among ratio effect measures, 60–61
single two-way table, 334–335, 334*t*
Relative tests of regression models, 425
Repeated-measures, 451
Representativeness
generalizability and, 146–147
in case-control studies, 120–121
surveillance systems, 479
Reproductive endpoints, 621–622
Reproductive epidemiology, 620–641
Reproductive systems, 620
Reproductively unhealthy worker effect, 622
Resampling, 368–369, 376
model checking and, 428–429
Rescaling variables, 392–393
Research
biomarkers, ELSI and, 567–568
conduct, 21
links to, surveillance, 464–465
objective, 32–33
questions, meta-analysis, 655
resources, secondary data access, 491
secondary data access, ethics of, 490–491
sponsors, suppression bias and, 678
staff, occupational cohort study, 495
Research synthesis. *See* Bias analysis; Meta-analysis
Reservoirs, infectious agents and, 555
Residual confounding, 69, 198–199, 199*f,* 259
bias quantification and, 198–199
Residual degrees of freedom
global tests of fit, 427
meta-regression methods, 673
Residual distributions, model fitting and, 421–422
Residual effects, 435
Residual sum of squares, 427
meta-regression, 673
Register-based search, secondary data, 488
Respondent burden of questionnaires, 503–504
Response rates
epidemiologic research, 497–499
interviews and, 509
Response types, causal and preventive, 59–60
and additivity, 78–79
cohorts and, equivalent interaction contrast and, 80*t*
sufficient cause models and, 82
Restriction in study design, 169
Retention time of toxic exposures, 602–603
Retrospective ascertainment, 96, 112. *See also* Recall bias
Retrospective cohort selection, 109
Retrospective studies, prospective studies v., 95–97, 112
Reference event, in incidence times, 33
Reverse causation, 28, 30, 622
Reverse-Bayes analysis, 338–339
Reverse-continuation-ratio model, 415
Ridge regression, 331, 423, 436, 437, 439. *See also* Hierarchical regression; Shrinkage estimation
Risk, 9–10
analysis, 347
assessment, 347
difference, 52–53
environmental hazards, 614
estimation, 290–293
fraction, 54, 65
history, 41, 42*f*
models, 395
ratio, 61, 73, 116
score, 447
standardized, 49–50
Risk difference, 52–53, 260–261
crude data, 247, 249, 250
Mantel-Haenszel, 274–276
standardized, 68, 266–267
Risk-difference additivity, biologic interactions and, 78–79, 298–299, 406
Risk factors
coronary heart disease, 14
lung cancer, 18
non-causal, 28
Risk fraction, 54. *See also* Excess fraction
Risk models, 393–395, 417
Risk period, 33, 34
Risk ratio, 61, 73, 116
case-cohort data, 252–253, 280–281
crude data, 246, 247, 250
Mantel-Haenszel, 274–276
standardized, 68, 267–269
Risk scores, 447. *See also* Confounder scores, Outcome scores
Risk-set sampling, 124, 125
RR. *See* Rate ratio; Relative risk; Risk ratio
Run-in phase, subject selection, randomized controlled trials, 647
Running mean, 317
Running-weighted regression curve, 321. *See also* Nonparametric regression; Smoothers and Smoothing
Russell, Bertrand, philosophy of, 19

Salk vaccine field trial, 1
Salmonella, infection occurrence, factors influencing, 556
Salmonella newport, surveillance, 463
Sample-size, considerations, 239. *See also* Study size
model fitting and, 422–423

Sampling
error, 149, 346. *See also* Random error; Random sampling; Selection bias
fractions, case-control studies, 115, 123–125, 430–432
rates, case-control studies, 113, 430
variation, 149
SARS. *See* Severe acute respiratory syndrome
Saturated regression model, 427
Scale dependence
of effect-measure modification, 72–74
of regression coefficients, 392–393
Scaling,
of graphs, 310–311, 312–313,
of regressors, 392–393
Scanned forms, 500
Scatterplot smoothers, 321. *See also* Nonparametric regression; Smoothers and Smoothing
Scatterplots, 216, 321
of test statistics, 681
Schwarz information criterion. *See* Bayesian information criterion
Scientific inference, philosophy of, 18–25
Scientific proof, impossibility of, 24–25
Score limits, 226
Score statistics, 225–226. *See also* Mantel-Haenszel statistics
for case-cohort data, 252
for case-control data, 251
for person-time data, 242–245
for pure count data, 245–250
Score test, 225–226
Scoring methods for confounder control. *See* Confounder scoring
Scoring of categories, 312–313, 410
Screening tests, studies, 642–646
SD. *See* Standard deviation
SE. *See* Standard error
Seasonal variation, 605, 608, 609, 611. *See also* Cyclic patterns
Second stage model, hierarchical regression and, 438
Second stage standard deviations, hierarchical regression, 436
Secondary attack rate, 560–561
Secondary data, 481–491
access, ethics of, 490–491
analysis, complete populations, 482–483
use of, examples, 484
validity and, 483
Second-stage model, 435–437. *See also* Hierarchical regression
Secular trends, migrant studies and, nutritional exposures, 582
Segregation analysis, genetic, 565
Segregation, racial/social, 539
Selection bias, 2, 134–137, 186, 193, 193*f*, 194, 362–363. *See also* Berksonian bias; Collider bias; Publication bias; Sampling error; Source population; Target population
analysis of, 362–363, 375–376, 662–663
case-control studies, matching, 205, 205*f*
complete populations, 482–483
confounding v., 136–137
graphical representation and analysis, 192–198
and publication bias, 654–655
quantitatively v. qualitatively, 136
substudies and, 488
Selection time, study design and, 122
Self-administered questionnaires, 500
Self-reported disease, surveillance, 473
Self-selection bias, 134
Semen quality, 623–624
Semi-Bayes analysis, 337, 345, 378–380, 437, 439. *See also* Bayesian analysis; Hierarchical regression; Shrinkage estimation
biases and, 378–380
Semilogarithmic plotting, 310, 311*f*
Semiquantitative food-frequency questionnaires, 591
Sensitivity
in bias analysis, 354–360
of diagnostic or screening test, 643–644
of exposure measurement method, 138
influence analysis and, 221–222
in probabilistic bias analysis, 372–375
relation of predictive values to, 357–358
surveillance systems, 479
Sensitivity analysis, 208, 355, 488. *See also* Bias analysis
base priors and, 380
Bayesian analysis, 342, 378–380
external adjustment process and, 351, 351*t*
meta-analysis, 661–662, 675
multiple bias analyses and, 363
unmeasured confounders, 349
Sentinel events, surveillance, 475
Sequelae prevention, clinical trials and, 90
Serial interval, state of infectiousness, 550*f*, 560
Serotyping, 553
Seroconversion, HIV, 557
Seventh Day Adventists studies, 582
Severe acute respiratory syndrome (SARS), infection occurrence, factors influencing, 556
Sex/gender, as social variable, 535
Sharp null hypothesis, 60
Shep's relative difference, 65
Short-term recall, food intake, 589
Shrinkage estimation, 331, 337, 423, 436, 437, 439. *See also* Bayesian analysis; Hierarchical regression
confounder control and, 263
Siblings records, secondary data, 484
Side effects of treatments. *See* Adverse events
Sign test, 680
Significance tests, 150, 151–153
confidence intervals v., 157–158
model searching and, 419
Simplifying search, model searching, 419
Simulation intervals, 365
Simultaneous analysis, 323–327. *See also* Multiple comparisons
of exposure levels, 323–324
of multiple outcomes, 325–327
single-comparison v., 326–327
of trends, 326
Simultaneous misclassification, 145–146
Sine curve, cyclic patterns, 608
Single study group
large-sample methods, 245–247, 247*t*
person-time data, large-sample methods, 240–243
small-sample statistics, person time data and, 253–254

Single-regression models, 401
multiple-regression models v., 401–402
SIRs. *See* Standardized incidence ratios
Small-sample methods, 220, 239, 253–257, 276. *See also* Exact statistics; Sparse data
person-time data, 253–255
count data, 255–257
Smoking 1, 2, 8–10, 13–14, 24, 26–30, 52, 55–56, 64–66, 117, 118, 119, 121, 122, 251, 263, 264, 266–267, 274, 280, 424, 483, 488, 608, 616
in pregnancy, 602, 624, 632, 634, 635
Smoothed curves, 319–321, 410–412
Smoothers and Smoothing, 313–14, 317–321, 410–412, 421, 438–442. *See also* Moving averages; Nonparametric regression; Power models; Spline models
fractional polynomial, 410
graphical, 313–314
with hierarchical regression, 438–439
kernels, 314, 318–320, 440, 441
locally linear, 441
power model, 410
regression splines, 410–412
for surveillance data, 478
variable span, 321, 442
windows, 317–321
Smoothing parameter, 441–442
Smoothing splines, 440–441. *See also* Nonparametric regression; Spline models
SMR. *See* Standardized morbidity ratio
SNFT. *See* Structural nested failure-time models
SNM models. *See* Structural nested mean models
Snow's natural experiment, 94, 95. *See also* Cholera, Snow's study of
Social capital, 541–542
Social class, 537, 548
intercommunity comparisons, 611–612
Social epidemiology, 532–548
analytic approaches, 542–548
covariate assessment, 534–542
exposure, 534–542
Social factors, 534–542
aggregate level, 538–542
individual level, 534–542
Social mobility, 539, 547
Software
for Bayesian analysis, 338
for hierarchical modeling, 436
problems in distinguishing models, 402
Source population, 114–115, 128–129, 383. *See also* Sampling error; Selection bias; Superpopulation; Target population
confounding and, 129–133
subject identification, 496
target population v., 129, 383
Sparse data. *See also* Small-sample methods
bias from, 263, 386, 422, 433
methods for, 272–278, 280–281, 283–288, 294, 296, 314, 316, 381, 386, 425, 433–435, 446–451
Spatial-data analysis, time-trend designs v., 609–610
Special-exposure cohorts, 109–110
Specification accuracy, 449–450
Specification biases, 346
Specification error, 346
Specificity, as causal criterion, 27–28
Specificity
in bias analysis, 354–360
of diagnostic or screening test, 643–644
of exposure measurement method, 138
in probabilistic bias analysis, 372–375
relation to predictive values, 357–358
Spline models, 410–412, 440–441. *See also* Nonparametric regression; Power models; Smoothers and Smoothing
Spontaneous abortion, 621, 628
Square-root model, 398
Stability assumption in causal diagrams, 191
Standard, choice of, 266
Standard deviation (SD). *See also* Variance
flaws in conventional estimates, 239, 346–347
flaws in rescaling by, 393, 681
Standard distribution, 49–50, 68–69, 265–266, 386–388. *See also* Standardization
Standard error (SE). *See also specific estimates, e.g.,* Risk ratio
of externally adjusted estimates, meta-analysis, 661–662
impact of model searching on, 419
Standardization, 49–50, 67–69, 265–269, 386–388, 442–445. *See also* Inverse-probability weighting; Standard distribution; Standardized measures; Standardized morbidity ratio
in case-control studies, 269, 445
by exposure models, 444–445
by full-data models, 444
by outcome models, 443
of regression, 386–388
Standardized coefficients, 681. *See also* Standard deviation, flaws in rescaling by
Standardized incidence ratio (SIR), 68. *See* Standardized morbidity ratio
Standardized measures, 33, 386–388. *See also* Standardization
of association, 67–69
of effect, 67–69, 386–388
of outcome, 33, 387
probability, 442–445
rate, 49, 67, 265, 442
rate difference, 68, 266
rate ratio, 68, 267, 269
regression, 386–388, 442–445
risk, 50, 265
risk difference, 68, 266
risk ratio, 68, 267
regression coefficients v., 443–444
Standardized morbidity ratio (SMR), 68–69, 241–242, 267, 269, 664–665
Standardized mortality ratio, 68. *See* Standardized morbidity ratio
State of infectiousness, 550*f,* 560
assessing risk of, 561–563
progression-related infectious process and, 550*f,* 560
Stationary population, 38–39, 47
Statistical approximations, accuracy of, 220, 225, 227–229, 243, 245, 247, 249, 250, 324, 334, 340, 342
Statistical biases, variable selection, 263, 419
Statistical efficiency, overmatching and, 176*t,* 179–180
Statistical estimation, 156–167

Statistical independence, 184–185
absence of open paths and, rules linking, 187–190
and d-separation rules, 189–190
Statistical inference, philosophies of. *See* Bayesianism; Frequentist methods; Pure likelihood inference
Statistical interaction, 72–74, 402–404. *See also* Effect-measure modification; Heterogeneity; Product terms
and biologic interactions, 82–83, 298–300, 407
effect-measure modification v., 72
qualitative, 79–80
Statistical precision, 149
Statistical significance, 151. *See also* Hypothesis tests; *P*-values; Significance tests;
inference and, 160*f*, 161
Statistical tests. *See* Hypothesis tests; *P*-values; Significance tests
Statistics, epidemiology and, 167
Steady state population, 38–39
Stein estimation, 331, 423, 439. *See also* Bayesian analysis; Hierarchical regression; Shrinkage estimation
Stepwise model searching, 419, 420
Stereotype model, 415
Stillbirth mortality, 635–636
Stratification of data, and precision, 150
Stratified analysis, 258–302
problems with, 179
Stratified count data, polytomous exposure, 305, 306*t*
Stratified logistic model, 433
Stratified models, 432–433
Stratified null hypothesis, *P*-values, 277–278
Stratified person-count data. *See* Stratified count data, polytomous exposure
Stratified person-time data, polytomous exposure, 305, 305*t*
Stratified pure count data, *P*-values, 278
Stratum-specific
estimates, 258, 264–265
measures, overall measures v., 62
models, 433
Strength associations, causal inference, 26–27
Strength of effects, 6*f*, 10–13, 14*t*
Streptococcus pneumoniae, laboratory-based surveillance, 472–473
Stress, during pregnancy, 485
Structural equations, 60, 208, 453
Structural nested models, 453–455. *See also* G-estimation
Structural nested failure-time (SNFT) models, 453–454
Structural nested mean (SNM) models, 453
Study. *See also* Epidemiologic studies
base, in case-control studies, 112
efficiency, 150
apportionment ratios and, 169–171
endpoints, 648–649
exposure, levels of, 440
hypothesis, person-time and, 102
populations, variations, 493–494
primary base, secondary base v., 114–115
size
binomial likelihood, 247
formulas, 149–150
meta-analysis and, 679
random error and, 149–150
small, publication bias and, 679
variables, in meta-analysis, 655–656
Subclinical infection, clinical disease v., 551
Subclinical pregnancy loss, 630–631, 631*f*
Subcutaneous fat, biochemical measurements, 594
Subinterval-specific incidence rates, survival proportion and, 45
Subject selection
case-control studies, 120–121, 496–497
community trials, 494
and recruitment, epidemiologic studies, 493–499
run-in phase, randomized controlled trials, 647
Subject tracing, 109, 157
Subjective Bayesianism, 165–166, 328–333. *See also* Bayesianism; Subjective probability
frequentism v., 166–167, 329–333
Subjective probability, 10, 23–24, 165–167, 330–331
Subjects, classification of, 218–219
Subject-selection bias, meta-analysis, 656–657
Subject-specific models, 544. *See also* Group-specific models
Substudies, selection bias and, 488
Sufficient cause, 13
disease and, 6, 6*f*
mechanisms, disease proportion and, 13–15
Sufficient component cause model, 6–18
biologic interactions under, 80–81
epidemiology and, 8–9, 8*f*
indirect effects and, 13
potential-outcome v., 81–82, 81*f*
scope of, 17–18
Sufficient conditioning sets, 192
Superpopulation, 151, 152, 383
for regression, 383
"Superspreaders," infection occurrence, 556
Suppression bias, 678
Surgeon General's *Smoking and Health,* 29
Surrogate confounders, 130
Surveillance, 459–480
approaches to, 472–476
history of, 460–462, 461*t*
objectives, 462–467
Surveillance data
analysis and interpretation, 476–478
assessing completeness, 478
education and policy, 467
presentation of, 478–479
Surveillance methods, combinations of, 475–476
Surveillance reports, surveillance data, 478
Surveillance systems, 459
attributes of, 479
cycles of, 470
elements of, 467–472
participation incentives, 470–471
SARS, 480
Surveys, 473. *See also* Cross-sectional studies; Prevalence studies
Survival analysis, 41, 290–294, 291*t*. *See also* Accelerated failure-time model; Cox model
average incidence time v., 45
subinterval-specific incidence rates and, 45
Survival proportion, 40

Survival time. *See* Incidence time
Survivor bias, 198
Susceptibility measures, 64–65
Susceptibility factors, infection occurrence, 556
Syndromic surveillance systems, bioterrorism-related epidemics and, 464
Synergism, 76–82. *See also* Biologic interaction
Synthetic meta-analysis, problem with, 654
Systematic errors (biases), 128–146, 345–380
  random errors v., 346

Tabular analysis. *See* stratified analysis
Tabular checks, regression model checking and, 423–424
Tabular data, simultaneous statistics for, 323
Tabular presentation, surveillance data, 478–479
Target population, 60, 90, 146–147, 383. *See also* Source population; Sampling error; Selection bias
  confounding and, 60
  generalizability of trial results, 90
  matching, 172
  source population v., 129, 383
  surveillance systems, 471
TDT. *See* Transmission disequilibrium test
Temporal ambiguity, ecologic studies, 527
Temporality, causal inference and, 28
Test hypothesis, 152–154, 156, 165, 220. *See also* Null hypothesis
Test of fit, 425–427
Test statistics, 152, 219–237
Test validity, screening tests, 642, 643, 643*t*. *See also* Misclassification
Test-based method for extraction of estimates, meta-analysis, 660
Tetanus, surveillance, 464
Therapy, studies of, 646–650
Time at risk, 102
  time of exposure v., 102
Time clustering, 606–607, 607*f*
Time unit, incidence rates and, 36
Time windows, induction analysis, 300–302
Time-dependent exposures, 300–302, 397–398, 452. *See also* Longitudinal data
Time-dependent covariates, 397–398, 452
Time-related disease patterns, 606–608
Time-series analyses, 517, 610–611
Time-stratified referent periods, case-crossover studies, 605, 605*f*
Time-to-pregnancy studies, 625–628
Time-trend designs
  ecologic studies, 515–517
  spatial-data analysis v., 609–610
Time-varying covariates, 397–398, 452. *See also* Longitudinal data
Tissue analysis, biochemical measurements, 594
Tobacco. *See* Smoking
Total energy intake, dietary intake and, 596–597
Townsend and Carstairs deprivation indices, 538
Toxic shock syndrome, surveillance, 465, 466*f*
Tracing, epidemiologic studies, 109, 507
Transformed regressors, 398–400
Transformed-outcome models, 400
  generalized linear models v., 416
Transmission axis, 549, 550*f*
Transmission disequilibrium test (TDT), 638
Transmission, factors influencing, 561
Transmission-related states, infection and, 551, 552
Transmission-related studies, epidemiologic issues in, 560–563
Trapezoidal distribution, 371
Treatment assignment, clinical trials and, 90
Trend. *See also* Dose response
  analysis, 314–317
  dose-response and, 308–314, 308*t*
  graphing, 308–14
  modeling, product terms and, 404–405
  P-value, 314–316
  in surveillance data, 477–478, 477*f*
Trend models, 398–399, 408–413
  category codes in, 409
  hierarchical, 438
  trend variation models, 412–413
Trend statistics, 314–316
Triple-blind studies, 91
Tumor heterogeneity, 577
Tumor promoter, 16
Twin studies, 15, 568–569
Two-binomial model
  large-sample methods, 247–250
  Wald confidence limits, 250
Two-by-two tables, 247, 247t, 345. *See also* Contingency tables, data analysis and
Two-phase studies. *See* Two-stage studies
Two-Poisson model, 245
Two-sided confidence interval, 158, 221
Two-sided *P*-value, 156, 221
Two-stage studies, 127, 496, 604
  analysis of, 281–282, 432
Two-tailed *P*-value, 152
Type I error (alpha error), 153, 154
  DSMB and, 91
  gene-disease association, 571–572
Type II error (beta error), 153, 154, 155*f*
Typhoid fever, evolution of, 553, 554*f*

Uncertainty, 329, 331, 346–347, 364–365, 370, 376, 378, 379, 380
Uncertainty analysis, 346–347. *See also* Bayesian analysis; Bias analysis; Uncertainty
Unconditional analysis, conditional analysis v., 272–273
Unconditional d-separation, 187–188. *See also* d-Separation
Unconditionally unbiased, in causal diagrams, 191
Unconditional probability, 184. *See also* Probability
Uncontrolled confounders, analysis of, 348–352, 365–371
Unconfounded dependence, in causal diagrams, 193
Unconfounded direct effect, diagram, 201*f*
Unemployment, 537
Unexposed group, bias and, in trend evaluation, 317
Unexposed time in exposed subjects, cohort studies, 104
Unhealthy worker effect, 622. *See also* Healthy worker effect
Uniformity of effect measures, 61, 259. *See also* Homogeneity
Uniform prior distributions, 365, 369
Univariate analysis. *See* Descriptive statistics
Univariate exposure transforms, 398–399
Unmatched case-control studies, modeling in, 429–432

Upper *P*-value, 220
Upper-tailed *P*-value, 152, 220
U.S. Surgeon General's *Smoking and Health,* 29
UV-B radiation, cancer and, 617

Vaccines
  and autism, secondary data, 485–486
Vacuous models, 390–391
Validation data, 361
  dietary assessment methods, 591–592
  secondary data, 487
Validity. *See also* Bias; Generalizability; Precision; *specific validity topics, e.g.*, Confounding; Selection bias; Sparse-data bias
  of biomarkers, 566
  external, 128
  in epidemiologic studies, 128–147
  of estimation, 128–129
  ethical considerations v., 89
  internal, 128
  secondary data and, 483
Variables. *See also specific types, e.g.,* Regressors
  in causal graphs, 186–187
  in regression and causation, 383
Variable selection, 261–263, 419–421
Variable-span smoothers, 321, 442. *See also* Nonparametric regression; Smoothers and Smoothing
Variance. *See also specific estimates, e.g.,* Standardized estimates
  bootstrap estimation, 429, 443
  and confounder scores, 447
  estimates, 149, 225, 226, 231, 243, 246, 248, 253, 254, 256, 422, 440, 443
  model, 436
  residual, 422, 425
Variance component models. *See* Hierarchical regression
Vectors, 384–385
Vertical scaling of graphs, 310–311
Vertices, in causal diagrams, 187
Virulence factors, 558
Volunteer providers, surveillance networks, 473
Vote counting, in meta-analysis, 680–681

Waiting time, 39. *See also* Incidence time
Wald limits, 227
  for binomial data, 246
  for case-cohort data, 252–253
  for case-control data, 250–252
  for person-time data, 240–245
  for pure count data, 245–250
Wald statistic, 220, 226–227, 279
Wald test, 227
Weighted averaging
  for Bayesian analysis, 334–337
  by information, 334–337
  for pooling across strata, 271
  for smoothing, 318–319, 441
  for meta-analysis, 670–671
  by inverse probability of selection. *See* inverse-probability weighting
  by inverse variance, 271, 334–337, 670–671
  by precision, 271, 334–337, 670–671
  by quality scores, 681
  in standardization, 49–50, 67–69, 265–269, 386–388
Weighted regression, 441. *See also* Inverse-probability weighting in meta-analysis, 663, 668
Weights
  in meta-analysis, 670–671, 681
  in standardization, 49–50, 67–69, 265–267, 386–388
Weight-specific mortality, 633–635, 634*f*
WHO. *See* World Health Organization
Windows, *See also* Smoothers and Smoothing
  in smoothing, 317–321
Within-community time-series analysis, air pollution, 616
Within-group bias, ecologic studies, 520
Within-group misclassification, ecologic studies, 526–527, 526*f*
Withdrawals. *See* Loss to follow-up; Censoring
Woolf method for pooling, 271. *See also* Information-weighted averaging
World Health Organization (WHO) surveillance, 466, 474

Zero level, in trend evaluation, 316–317
Z-ratio, 220. *See* Wald statistic
Z-score. *See* Wald statistic; Z-ratio